Lippincott's Illustrated Reviews: Pharmacology

3rd edition

Lippincott's Illustrated Reviews: Pharmacology

Richard D. Howland, Ph.D.
Department of Pharmacology and Toxicology
University of Medicine and Dentistry of New Jersey–
New Jersey Medical School
Newark, New Jersey

Mary J. Mycek, Ph.D.
Department of Pharmacology and Toxicology
University of Medicine and Dentistry of New Jersey–
New Jersey Medical School
Newark, New Jersey

Editors

Richard A. Harvey, Ph.D.
Department of Biochemistry
University of Medicine and Dentistry of New Jersey–
Robert Wood Johnson Medical School
Piscataway, New Jersey

Pamela C. Champe, Ph.D.
Department of Biochemistry
University of Medicine and Dentistry of New Jersey–
Robert Wood Johnson Medical School
Piscataway, New Jersey

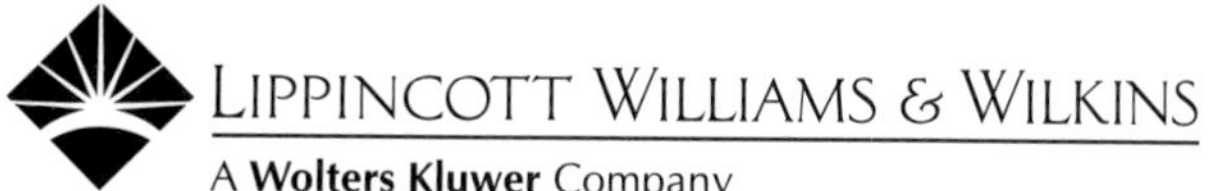

LIPPINCOTT WILLIAMS & WILKINS
A **Wolters Kluwer** Company
Philadelphia • Baltimore • New York • London
Buenos Aires • Hong Kong • Sydney • Tokyo

Acquisitions Editor: Betty Sun
Development Editor: Kathleen Scogna
Marketing Manager: Emilie Linkins
Production Editor: Jennifer Glazer
Designer: Holly McLaughlin
Printer: R.R. Donnelley—Willard

351 West Camden Street
Baltimore, MD 21201

530 Walnut Street
Philadelphia, PA 19106

Printed in the United States of America

Library of Congress Cataloging-in-Publication Data

Howland, Richard D.
Pharmacology / authors, Richard D. Howland, Mary J. Mycek; editors, Richard A.
Harvey, Pamela C. Champe.—3rd ed.
p. ; cm. — (Lippincott's illustrated reviews)
Rev. ed. of: Pharmacology / Mary J. Mycek, Richard A. Harvey, Pamela C. Champe.
2nd ed. c1997.
Includes bibliographical references and index.
ISBN 0-7817-4118-1
1. Pharmacology—Outlines, syllabi, etc. 2. Pharmacology
Examinations, questions, etc. I. Mycek, Mary Julia. II. Harvey, Richard A., Ph.D. III. Champe, Pamela C.
IV. Pharmacology. V. Title. VI. Series.
[DNLM: 1. Pharmacology—Examination Questions. 2. Pharmacology—Outlines. QV
18.2 H864p 2006]
RM301.14.P47 2006
615'.1'076—dc22
2005044251

05 06 07 08 09
1 2 3 4 5 6 7 8 9 10

Acknowledgments

We are grateful to the many friends and colleagues who generously contributed their time and effort to help us make this book as accurate and as useful as possible. We would like to acknowledge the contributions of Drs. Guojie Huang, Edward J. Flynn, and Lester G. Sultatos who provided many helpful comments. We would particularly like to express our thanks to Drs. Richard Finkel, Kathy Fuller, Kathy Graham, Michelle A. Clark, and David Gazze, whose clinical insights and suggestions were invaluable. We highly value the additional support of our other colleagues at the University of Medicine and Dentistry–Robert Wood Johnson Medical School and –New Jersey Medical School. We (RAH and PCC) owe a special thanks to our Chairman, Dr. Masayori Inouye, who has encouraged us in this and other teaching projects.

The editors and production staff of Lippincott William & Wilkins were a constant source of encouragement and discipline. We particularly want to acknowledge the tremendously helpful, supportive, creative contributions of our editor, Betty Sun, whose imagination and positive attitude helped us out of the valleys. Final editing and assembly of the book has been greatly enhanced through the efforts of Kathleen Scogna and Jennifer Glazer.

Contents

UNIT I:
Introduction to Pharmacology

Pharmacokinetics 1

I. OVERVIEW

The aim of drug therapy is to prevent, cure, or control various disease states. To achieve this goal, adequate drug doses must be delivered to the target tissues so that therapeutic yet nontoxic levels are obtained. Pharmacokinetics examines the movement of a drug over time through the body. The clinician must recognize that the speed of onset of drug action, the intensity of the drug's effect, and the duration of drug action are controlled by four fundamental pathways of drug movement and modification in the body (Figure 1.1). First, drug absorption from the site of administration (input) permits entry of the therapeutic agent (either directly or indirectly) into plasma. Second, the drug may then reversibly leave the bloodstream and distribute into the interstitial and intracellular fluids (distribution). Third, the drug may be metabolized by the liver, kidney, or other tissues. Finally, the drug and its metabolites are eliminated from the body (output) in urine, bile, or feces. This chapter describes how knowledge of these processes influences the clinician's decision as to the route of administration for a specific drug, the amount and frequency of each dose, and the dosing intervals.

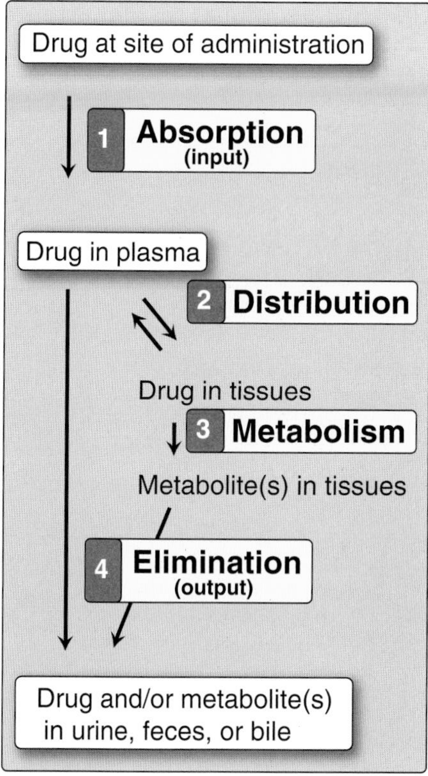

Figure 1.1
Schematic representation of drug absorption, distribution, metabolism, and elimination.

II. ROUTES OF DRUG ADMINISTRATION

The route of administration is determined primarily by the properties of the drug (for example, water or lipid solubility, ionization, etc.), and by the therapeutic objectives (for example, the desirability of a rapid onset of action or the need for long-term administration or restriction to a local site). There are two major routes of drug administration, enteral and parenteral. (Figure 1.2 illustrates the subcategories of these routes as well as other methods of drug administration.)

Lippincott's Illustrated Reviews: Pharmacology, Third Edition,
by Richard D. Howland and Mary J. Mycek.
Lippincott Williams & Wilkins, Baltimore, MD © 2006.

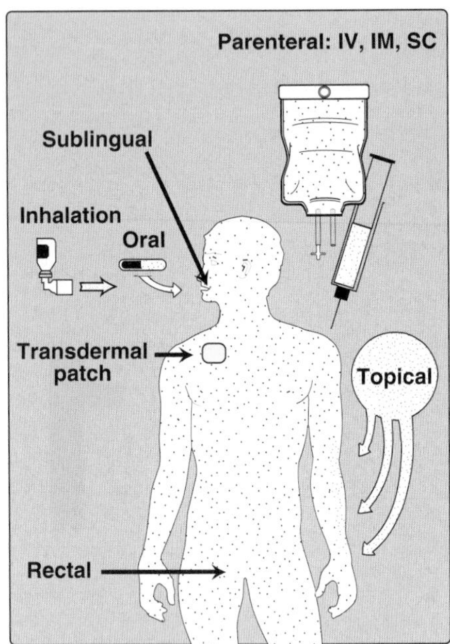

Figure 1.2
Commonly used routes of drug administration. IV = intravenous; IM = intramuscular; SC = subcutaneous.

A. Enteral

1. **Oral:** Giving a drug by mouth is the most common route of administration, but it is also the most variable, and involves the most complicated pathway to the tissues. Some drugs are absorbed from the stomach; however, the duodenum is the major site of entry to the systemic circulation because of its larger absorptive surface. [Note: Most drugs absorbed from the gastrointestinal (GI) tract enter the portal circulation and encounter the liver before they are distributed into the general circulation (Figure 1.3). First-pass metabolism by the intestine or liver limits the efficacy of many drugs when taken orally. For example, more than ninety percent of *nitroglycerin* is cleared during a single passage through the liver.] Ingestion of drugs with food can influence absorption. The presence of food in the stomach delays gastric emptying, so drugs that are destroyed by acid (for example, *penicillin*) become unavailable for absorption (see p. 356). [Note: Enteric coating of a drug protects it from the acidic environment and may prevent gastric irritation. Depending on the formulation, the release of the drug may be prolonged, producing a sustained-release effect.]

2. **Sublingual:** Placement under the tongue allows a drug to diffuse into the capillary network and, therefore, to enter the systemic circulation directly. Administration of an agent by this route has the advantage that the drug bypasses the intestine and liver and thus avoids first pass metabolism.

3. **Rectal:** Fifty percent of the drainage of the rectal region bypasses the portal circulation; thus, the biotransformation of drugs by the liver is minimized. Both the sublingual and the rectal routes of administration have the additional advantage that they prevent the destruction of the drug by intestinal enzymes or by low pH in the stomach. The rectal route is also useful if the drug induces vomiting when given orally or if the patient is already vomiting. [Note: The rectal route is commonly used to administer antiemetic agents.]

B. Parenteral

Parenteral administration is used for drugs that are poorly absorbed from the GI tract, and for agents, such as *insulin*, that are unstable in the GI tract. Parenteral administration is also used for treatment of unconscious patients, and under circumstances that require a rapid onset of action. Parenteral administration provides the most control over the actual dose of drug delivered to the body. The three major parenteral routes are intravascular (intravenous or intra-arterial), intramuscular, and subcutaneous (see Figure 1.2). Each route has advantages and drawbacks.

1. **Intravascular:** Intravenous (IV) injection is the most common parenteral route. For drugs that are not absorbed orally, there is often no other choice. With IV administration, the drug avoids the GI tract and, therefore, first-pass metabolism by the liver. This route permits a rapid effect and a maximal degree of control over the circulating levels of the drug. However, unlike drugs in the GI

tract, those that are injected cannot be recalled by strategies such as emesis or binding to activated charcoal. Intravenous injection may inadvertently introduce bacteria through contamination, at the site of injection. IV injection may also induce hemolysis, or cause other adverse reactions by the too-rapid delivery of high concentrations of drug to the plasma and tissues. Therefore, the rate of infusion must be carefully controlled. Similar concerns apply to intra-arterially injected drugs.

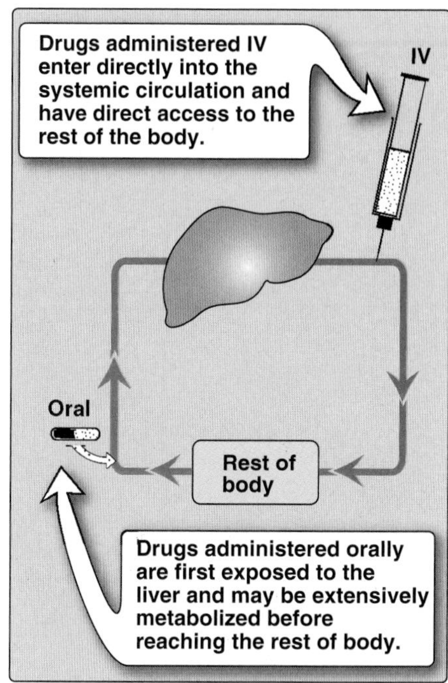

Figure 1.3
First-pass metabolism can occur with orally administered drugs. IV = intravenous.

2. **Intramuscular (IM):** Drugs administered IM can be aqueous solutions or specialized depot preparations—often a suspension of drug in a nonaqueous vehicle, such as polyethylene glycol. Absorption of drugs in aqueous solution is fast, whereas that from depot preparations is slow. As the vehicle diffuses out of the muscle, the drug precipitates at the site of injection. The drug then dissolves slowly, providing a sustained dose over an extended period of time. An example is sustained-release *haloperidol decanoate* (see p. 153), the slow diffusion of which from the muscle produces an extended neuroleptic effect.

3. **Subcutaneous (SC):** This route of administration, like that of IM injection, requires absorption and is somewhat slower than the IV route. Subcutaneous injection minimizes the risks associated with intravascular injection. [Note: Minute amounts of *epinephrine* are sometimes combined with a drug to restrict its area of action. *Epinephrine* acts as a local vasoconstrictor and decreases removal of a drug, such as *lidocaine*, from the site of administration.] Other examples of drugs utilizing SC administration include solids, such as silastic capsules containing the contraceptive *levonorgestrel* that are implanted for long-term activity (see p. 301), and also programmable mechanical pumps that can be implanted to deliver *insulin* in some diabetics.

C. Other

1. **Inhalation:** Inhalation provides the rapid delivery of a drug across the large surface area of the mucous membranes of the respiratory tract and pulmonary epithelium, producing an effect almost as rapidly as with IV injection. This route of administration is used for drugs that are gases (for example, some anesthetics), or those that can be dispersed in an aerosol. The route is particularly effective and convenient for patients with respiratory complaints (for example, asthma or chronic obstructive pulmonary disease), because the drug is delivered directly to the site of action, and systemic side effects are minimized.

2. **Intranasal:** *Desmopressin* is administered intranasally in the treatment of diabetes insipidus; salmon *calcitonin*, a peptide hormone used in the treatment of osteoporosis, is also available as a nasal spray. The abused drug, *cocaine*, is generally taken by sniffing.

3. **Intrathecal/intraventricular:** It is sometimes necessary to introduce drugs directly into the cerebrospinal fluid. For example, *amphotericin B* is used in treating cryptococcal meningitis (see p. 404).

4. **Topical:** Topical application is used when a local effect of the drug is desired. For example, *clotrimazole* is applied as a cream directly to the skin in the treatment of dermatophytosis, and *atropine* is instilled directly into the eye to dilate the pupil and permit measurement of refractive errors.

5. **Transdermal:** This route of administration achieves systemic effects by application of drugs to the skin, usually via a transdermal patch. The rate of absorption can vary markedly, depending on the physical characteristics of the skin at the site of application. This route is most often used for the sustained delivery of drugs, such as the antianginal drug *nitroglycerin* (see p. 209).

III. ABSORPTION OF DRUGS

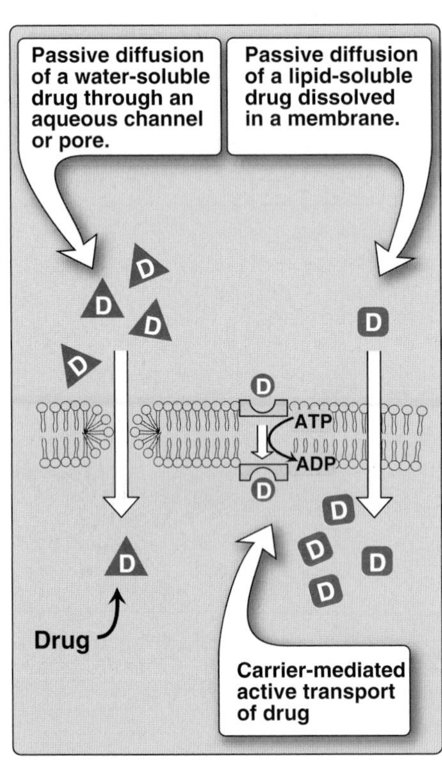

Figure 1.4
Schematic representation of drugs crossing a cell membrane of an epithelial cell of the gastrointestinal tract.

Absorption is the transfer of a drug from its site of administration to the bloodstream. The rate and efficiency of absorption depend on the route of administration. For IV delivery, absorption is complete; that is, the total dose of drug reaches the systemic circulation. Drug delivery by other routes may result in only partial absorption and, thus, lower bioavailability. For example, the oral route requires that a drug dissolve in the GI fluid and then penetrate the epithelial cells of the intestinal mucosa; disease states or the presence of food may affect this process.

A. Transport of a drug from the GI tract

Depending on their chemical properties, drugs may be absorbed from the GI tract by either passive diffusion or active transport.

1. **Passive diffusion:** The driving force for passive absorption of a drug is the concentration gradient across a membrane separating two body compartments; that is, the drug moves from a region of high concentration to one of lower concentration. Passive diffusion does not involve a carrier, the process is not saturable, and shows a low structural specificity. The vast majority of drugs gain access to the body by this mechanism. Lipid-soluble drugs readily move across most biological membranes, whereas water-soluble drugs penetrate the cell membrane through aqueous channels (Figure 1.4).

2. **Active transport:** This mode of drug entry involves specific carrier proteins that span the membrane. A few drugs that closely resemble the structure of naturally occurring metabolites are actively transported across cell membranes using these specific carrier proteins. Active transport is energy-dependent and is driven by the hydrolysis of adenosine triphosphate (see Figure 1.4). It is capable of moving drugs against a concentration gradient—that is, from a region of low drug concentration to one of higher drug concentration. The process shows saturation kinetics for the carrier, much in the same way that an enzyme-catalyzed reaction shows a maximal velocity at high substrate levels when binding to the enzyme is maximal.[1]

[1]See p. 57 in ***Lippincott's Illustrated Reviews: Biochemistry*** (3rd ed.) for a discussion of enzyme kinetics.

B. Effect of pH on drug absorption

Most drugs are either weak acids or weak bases. Acidic drugs (HA) release a H^+ causing a charged anion (A^-) to form[2]:

$$HA \rightleftarrows H^+ + A^-$$

Weak bases (BH^+) can also release a H^+. However, the protonated form of basic drugs is usually charged, and loss of a proton produces the uncharged base (B):

$$BH^+ \rightleftarrows B + H^+$$

1. **Passage of an uncharged drug through a membrane:** A drug passes through membranes more readily if it is uncharged (Figure 1.5). Thus, for a weak acid, the uncharged HA can permeate through membranes, and A^- cannot. For a weak base, the uncharged form, B, penetrates through the cell membrane, but BH^+ does not. Therefore, the effective concentration of the permeable form of each drug at its absorption site is determined by the relative concentrations of the charged and uncharged forms. The ratio between the two forms is, in turn, determined by the pH at the site of absorption, and by the strength of the weak acid or base, which is represented by the pK_a (Figure 1.6). [Note: The pK_a is a measure of the strength of the interaction of a compound with a proton. The lower the pK_a of a drug, the stronger the acid. Conversely, the higher the pK_a, the stronger the base.] Distribution equilibrium is achieved when the permeable form of a drug achieves an equal concentration in all body water spaces. [Note: Highly lipid-soluble drugs rapidly cross membranes and often enter tissues at a rate determined by blood flow.]

2. **Determination of how much drug will be found on either side of a membrane:** The relationship of pK_a and the ratio of acid-base concentrations to pH is expressed by the Henderson-Hasselbalch equation[3]:

$$pH = pK_a + \log \frac{[\text{nonprotonated species}]}{[\text{protonated species}]}$$

$$\text{For acids: } pH = pK_a + \log \frac{[A^-]}{[HA]}$$

$$\text{For bases: } pH = pK_a + \log \frac{[B]}{[BH^+]}$$

This equation is useful in determining how much drug will be found on either side of a membrane that separates two compartments that differ in pH—for example, stomach (pH 1.0–1.5) and blood plasma (pH 7.4). [Note: The lipid solubility of the non-ionized drug directly determines its rate of equilibration.]

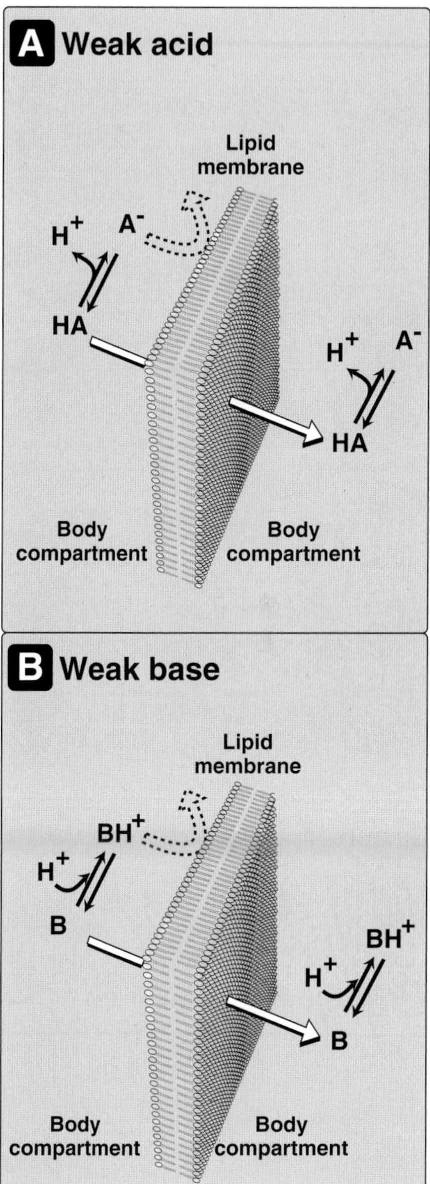

Figure 1.5
A. Diffusion of the non-ionized form of a weak acid through a lipid membrane. B. Diffusion of the non-ionized form of a weak base through a lipid membrane.

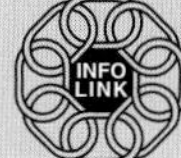

[2]See p. 8 in ***Lippincott's Illustrated Reviews: Biochemistry*** (3rd ed.) for a discussion of acid-base chemistry.
[3]See p. 6 in ***Lippincott's Illustrated Reviews: Biochemistry*** (3rd ed.) for a discussion of the Henderson-Hasselbalch equation.

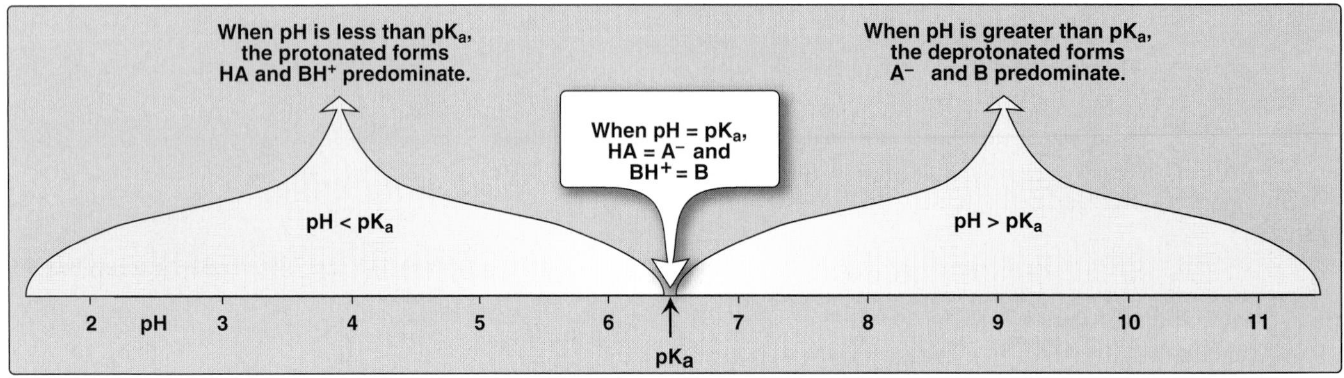

Figure 1.6
The distribution of a drug between its ionized and nonionized forms depends on the ambient pH and pK_a of the drug. For illustrative purposes, the drug has been assigned a pK_a of 6.5.

C. Physical factors influencing absorption

1. **Blood flow to the absorption site:** Blood flow to the intestine is much greater than the flow to the stomach; thus, absorption from the intestine is favored over that from the stomach. [Note: Shock severely reduces blood flow to cutaneous tissues, thus minimizing the absorption from subcutaneous administration.]

2. **Total surface area available for absorption:** Because the intestine has a surface rich in microvilli, it has a surface area about 1,000-fold that of the stomach; thus, absorption of the drug across the intestine is more efficient.

3. **Contact time at the absorption surface:** If a drug moves through the GI tract very quickly, as in severe diarrhea, it is not well absorbed. Conversely, anything that delays the transport of the drug from the stomach to the intestine delays the rate of absorption of the drug. [Note: Parasympathetic input increases the rate of gastric emptying, whereas sympathetic input (prompted, for example, by exercise or stressful emotions) prolongs gastric emptying. Also, the presence of food in the stomach both dilutes the drug and slows gastric emptying. Therefore, a drug taken with a meal is generally absorbed more slowly.]

IV. BIOAVAILABILITY

Bioavailability is the fraction of administered drug that reaches the systemic circulation. Bioavailability is expressed as the fraction of administered drug that gains access to the systemic circulation in a chemically unchanged form. For example, if 100 mg of a drug are administered orally and 70 mg of this drug are absorbed unchanged, the bioavailability is seventy percent.

A. Determination of bioavailability

Bioavailability is determined by comparing plasma levels of a drug after a particular route of administration (for example, oral administration), with plasma drug levels achieved by IV injection, in which all of the agent enters the circulation. When the drug is given orally, only part of the administered dose appears in the plasma. By plotting plasma concentrations of the drug versus time, one can measure the area under the curve (AUC). This curve reflects the extent of absorption of the drug. [Note: By definition, this is 100 percent for drugs delivered IV.] Bioavailability of a drug administered orally is the ratio of the area calculated for oral administration compared with the area calculated for IV injection (Figure 1.7).

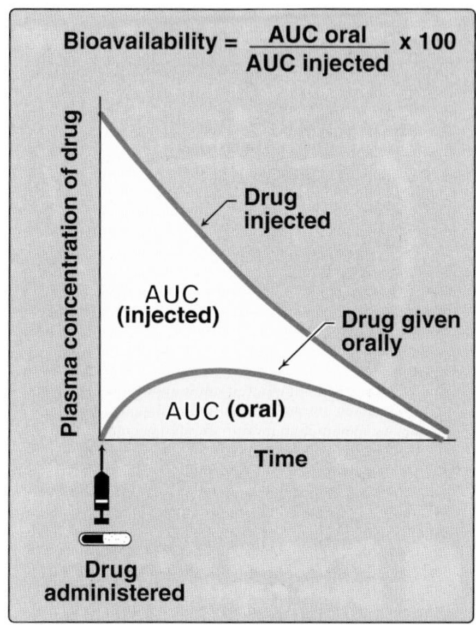

Figure 1.7
Determination of the bioavailability of a drug. (AUC = area under curve.)

B. Factors that influence bioavailability

1. **First-pass hepatic metabolism:** When a drug is absorbed across the GI tract, it enters the portal circulation before entering the systemic circulation (see Figure 1.3). If the drug is rapidly metabolized by the liver, the amount of unchanged drug that gains access to the systemic circulation is decreased. Many drugs, such as *propranolol* or *lidocaine*, undergo significant biotransformation during a single passage through the liver.

2. **Solubility of the drug:** Very hydrophilic drugs are poorly absorbed because of their inability to cross the lipid-rich cell membranes. Paradoxically, drugs that are extremely hydrophobic are also poorly absorbed, because they are totally insoluble in the aqueous body fluids and, therefore, cannot gain access to the surface of cells. For a drug to be readily absorbed, it must be largely hydrophobic yet have some solubility in aqueous solutions.

3. **Chemical instability:** Some drugs, such as *penicillin G*, are unstable in the pH of the gastric contents. Others, such as *insulin*, are destroyed in the GI tract by degradative enzymes.

4. **Nature of the drug formulation:** Drug absorption may be altered by factors unrelated to the chemistry of the drug. For example, particle size, salt form, crystal polymorphism, and the presence of excipients (such as binders and dispersing agents) can influence the ease of dissolution and, therefore, alter the rate of absorption.

C. Bioequivalence

Two related drugs are bioequivalent if they show comparable bioavailability and similar times to achieve peak blood concentrations. Two related drugs with a significant difference in bioavailability are said to be bioinequivalent.

D. Therapeutic equivalence

Two similar drugs are therapeutically equivalent if they have comparable efficacy and safety. [Note: Clinical effectiveness often depends both on maximum serum drug concentrations and on the time after administration required to reach peak concentration. Therefore, two drugs that are bioequivalent may not be therapeutically equivalent.]

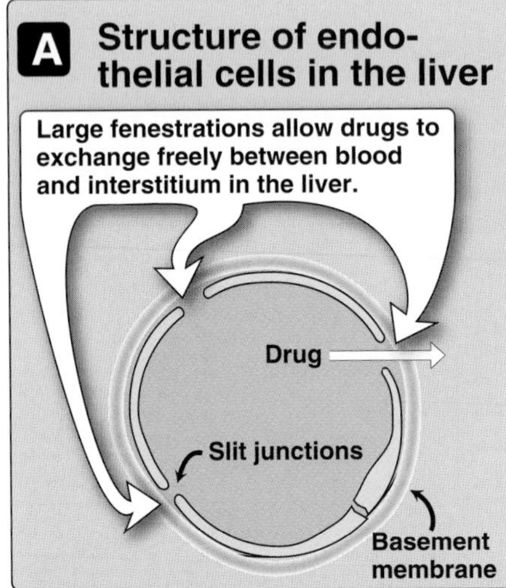
A
Structure of endothelial cells in the liver
Large fenestrations allow drugs to exchange freely between blood and interstitium in the liver.
Drug
Slit junctions
Basement membrane

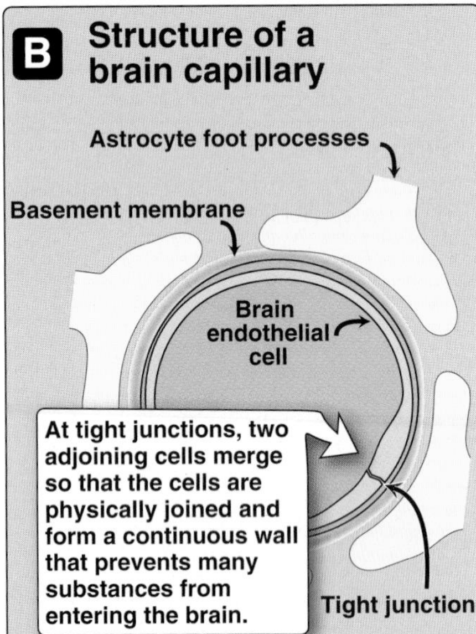
B
Structure of a brain capillary
Astrocyte foot processes
Basement membrane
Brain endothelial cell
At tight junctions, two adjoining cells merge so that the cells are physically joined and form a continuous wall that prevents many substances from entering the brain.
Tight junction

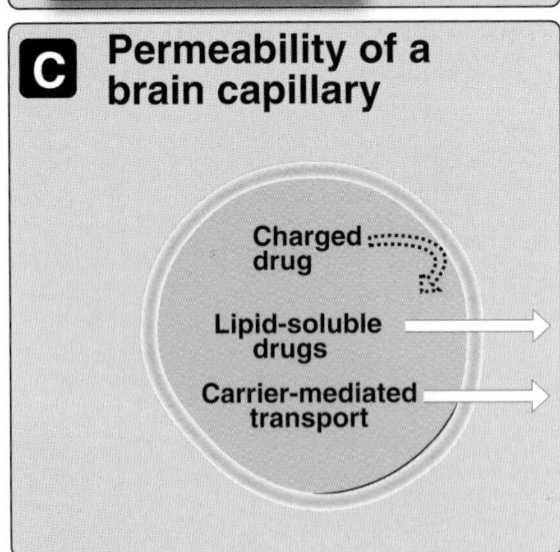
C
Permeability of a brain capillary
Charged drug
Lipid-soluble drugs
Carrier-mediated transport

Figure 1.8
Cross-section of liver and brain capillaries.

V. DRUG DISTRIBUTION

Drug distribution is the process by which a drug reversibly leaves the bloodstream and enters the interstitium (extracellular fluid) and/or the cells of the tissues. The delivery of a drug from the plasma to the interstitium primarily depends on blood flow, capillary permeability, the degree of binding of the drug to plasma and tissue proteins, and the relative hydrophobicity of the drug.

A. Blood flow

The rate of blood flow to the tissue capillaries varies widely as a result of the unequal distribution of cardiac output to the various organs. Blood flow to the brain, liver, and kidney is greater than that to the skeletal muscles, and adipose tissue has a still lower rate of blood flow. This differential blood flow partly explains the short duration of hypnosis produced by a bolus intravenous injection of *thiopental*. The high blood flow together with the superior lipid solubility of *thiopental* permit it to rapidly move into the central nervous system (CNS) and produce anesthesia. Slower distribution to skeletal muscle and adipose tissue lowers the plasma concentration sufficiently so that the higher concentrations within the CNS decrease and consciousness is regained. Although this phenomenon occurs with all drugs to some extent, redistribution accounts for the extremely short duration of action of *thiopental* and compounds of similar chemical and pharmacologic properties.

B. Capillary permeability

Capillary permeability is determined by capillary structure and by the chemical nature of the drug.

1. **Capillary structure:** Capillary structure varies widely in terms of the fraction of the basement membrane that is exposed by slit junctions between endothelial cells. In the brain, the capillary structure is continuous, and there are no slit junctions (Figure 1.8). This contrasts with the liver and spleen, where a large part of the basement membrane is exposed due to large, discontinuous capillaries through which large plasma proteins can pass.

    a. **Blood-brain barrier:** To enter the brain, drugs must pass through the endothelial cells of the capillaries of the CNS or be actively transported. For example, the large, neutral amino acid carrier transports *levodopa* into the brain. Lipid-soluble drugs readily penetrate into the CNS, because they can dissolve in the membrane of the endothelial cells. Ionized or polar drugs generally fail to enter the CNS, because they are unable to pass through the endothelial cells of the CNS, which have no slit junctions. These tightly juxtaposed cells form tight junctions that constitute the so-called blood-brain barrier.

2. **Drug structure:** The chemical nature of the drug strongly influences its ability to cross cell membranes. Hydrophobic drugs, which have a uniform distribution of electrons and no net charge, readily move across most biological membranes. These drugs can

dissolve in the lipid membranes and, therefore, permeate the entire cell's surface. The major factor influencing the hydrophobic drug's distribution is the blood flow to the area. By contrast, hydrophilic drugs, which have either a nonuniform distribution of electrons or a positive or negative charge, do not readily penetrate cell membranes and must go through the slit junctions .

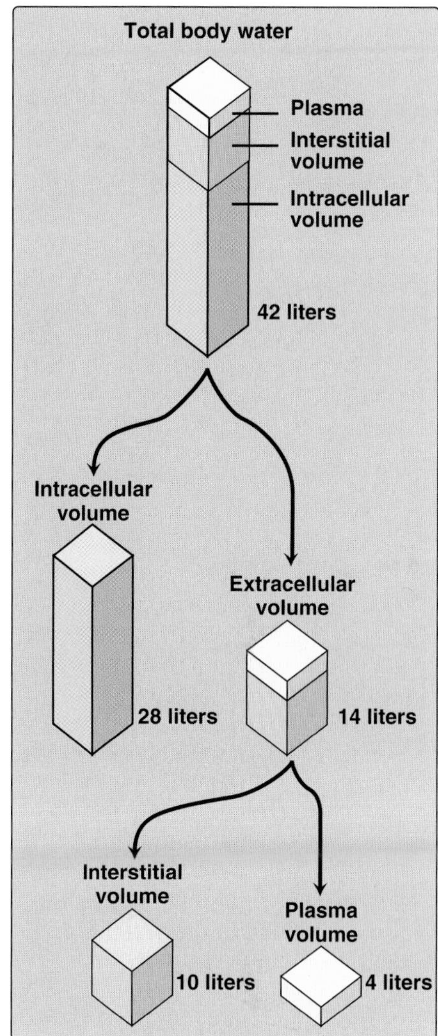

Figure 1.9
Relative size of various distribution volumes within a 70-kg individual.

C. Binding of drugs to proteins

Reversible binding to plasma proteins sequesters drugs in a nondiffusible form, and slows their transfer out of the vascular compartment. Binding is relatively nonselective as to chemical structure, and takes place at sites on the protein to which endogenous compounds, such as bilirubin, normally attach. Plasma albumin is the major drug-binding protein, and may act as a drug reservoir; that is, as the concentration of the free drug decreases due to elimination by metabolism or excretion, the bound drug dissociates from the protein. This maintains the free-drug concentration as a constant fraction of the total drug in the plasma.

VI. VOLUME OF DISTRIBUTION

The volume of distribution is a hypothetical volume of fluid into which a drug is disseminated. Although the volume of distribution has no physiologic or physical basis, it is sometimes useful to compare the distribution of a drug with the volumes of the water compartments in the body (Figure 1.9).

A. Water compartments in the body

Once a drug enters the body, from whatever route of administration, it has the potential to distribute into any one of three functionally distinct compartments of body water, or to become sequestered in some cellular site.

1. **Plasma compartment:** If a drug has a very large molecular weight or binds extensively to plasma proteins, it is too large to move out through the endothelial slit junctions of the capillaries and, thus, is effectively trapped within the plasma (vascular) compartment. As a consequence, the drug distributes in a volume (the plasma) that is about six percent of the body weight or, in a 70 kg individual, about 4 L of body fluid. Heparin (see p. 235) shows this type of distribution.

2. **Extracellular fluid:** If a drug has a low molecular weight but is hydrophilic, it can move through the endothelial slit junctions of the capillaries into the interstitial fluid. However, hydrophilic drugs cannot move across the membranes of cells to enter the water phase inside the cell. Therefore, these drugs distribute into a volume that is the sum of the plasma water and the interstitial fluid, which together constitute the extracellular fluid. This is about twenty percent of the body weight, or about 14 L in a 70 kg individual. Aminoglycoside antibiotics (see p. 371) show this type of distribution.

3. **Total body water:** If a drug has a low molecular weight and is hydrophobic, it not only can move into the interstitium through the slit junctions, but can also move through the cell membranes into the intracellular fluid. The drug therefore distributes into a volume of about sixty percent of body weight, or about 42 L in a 70 kg individual. *Ethanol* exhibits this apparent volume of distribution (see below).

4. **Other sites:** In pregnancy, the fetus may take up drugs and thus increase the volume of distribution. Drugs which are extremely lipid soluble, such as *thiopental* (see p. 134), may also have unusually high volumes of distribution.

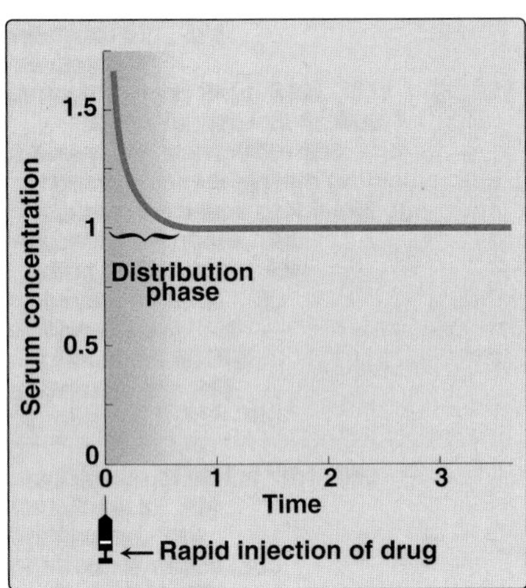

Figure 1.10
Drug concentrations in serum after a single injection of drug at time = 0. Assume that the drug distributes but is not eliminated.

B. Apparent volume of distribution

A drug rarely associates exclusively with only one of the water compartments of the body. Instead, the vast majority of drugs distribute into several compartments, often avidly binding cellular components—for example, lipids (abundant in adipocytes and cell membranes), proteins (abundant in plasma and within cells), or nucleic acids (abundant in the nuclei of cells). Therefore, the volume into which drugs distribute is called the apparent volume of distribution, or V_d. Another useful way to think of this constant is as the partition coefficient of a drug between the plasma and the rest of the body.

1. Determination of V_d

a. **Distribution of drug in the absence of elimination:** The apparent volume into which a drug distributes, V_d, is determined by injection of a standard dose of drug, which is initially contained entirely in the vascular system. The agent may then move from the plasma into the interstitium and into cells, causing the plasma concentration to decrease with time. Assume for simplicity that the drug is not eliminated from the body; the drug then achieves a uniform concentration that is sustained with time (Figure 1.10). The concentration within the vascular compartment is the total amount of drug administered divided by the volume into which it distributes, V_d

$$C = D/V_d \text{ or } V_d = D/C$$

where C = the plasma concentration of the drug, and D = the total amount of drug in the body. For example, if 25 mg of a drug (D = 25 mg) are administered, and the plasma concentration is 1 mg/L, then V_d = 25 mg/1 mg/L = 25 L.

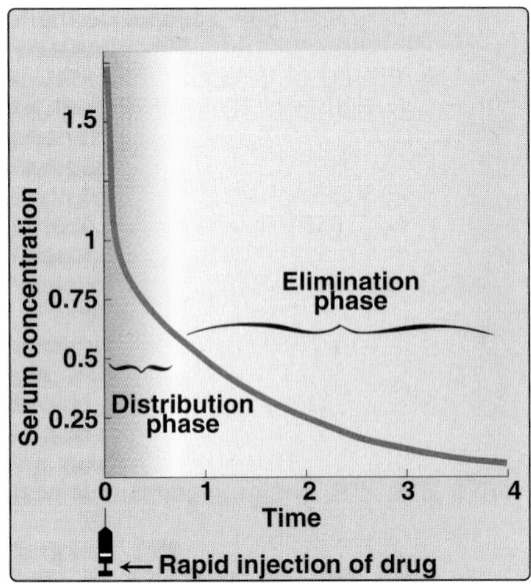

Figure 1.11
Drug concentrations in serum after a single injection of drug at time = 0. Assume that the drug distributes and is subsequently eliminated.

b. **Distribution of drug when elimination is present:** In reality, drugs are eliminated from the body, and a plot of plasma concentration versus time shows two phases. The initial decrease in plasma concentration is due to a rapid distribution phase in which the drug is transferred from the plasma into the interstitium and the intracellular water. This is followed by a slower elimination phase during which the drug leaves the plasma compartment and is lost from the body—for example, by renal or biliary excretion or by hepatic biotransformation (Figure 1.11). The rate at which the drug is eliminated is usually proportional to the concentration of drug (C); that is, the rate for most drugs is first order and shows a linear relationship with time if ln C (rather than C) is plotted versus time (Figure 1.12). This is because the elimination processes are not saturated.

c. **Calculation of drug concentration if distribution were instantaneous:** Assume that the elimination process began at the time of injection and continued throughout the distribution phase. Then, the concentration of drug in the plasma, C, can be extrapolated back to time-zero (the time of injection) to determine C_0, which is the concentration of drug that would have been achieved if the distribution phase had occurred instantly. For example, if 10 mg of drug are injected into a patient and the plasma concentration is extrapolated to time-zero, the concentration is C_0 = 1 mg/L (from the graph shown in Figure 1.12), then V_d = 10 mg/1 mg/L = 10 L.

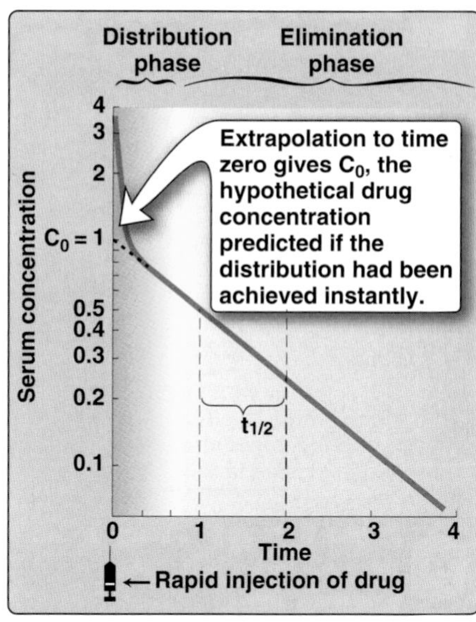

Figure 1.12
Drug concentrations in serum after a single injection of drug at time = 0. Data are plotted on a log scale.

d. **Uneven drug distribution between compartments:** The apparent volume of distribution assumes that the drug distributes uniformly in a single compartment. However, most drugs distribute unevenly in several compartments, and the volume of distribution does not describe a real, physical volume but, rather, reflects the ratio of drug in the extraplasmic spaces relative to the plasma space. Nonetheless, V_d is useful, because it can be used to calculate the amount of drug needed to achieve a desired plasma concentration. For example, assume the arrhythmia of a cardiac patient is not well controlled due to inadequate plasma levels of *digitalis*. Suppose the concentration of the drug in the plasma is C_1 and the desired level of *digitalis* (known from clinical studies) is a higher concentration, C_2. The clinician needs to know how much additional drug should be administered to bring the circulating level of the drug from C_1 to C_2.

$(V_d)(C_1)$ = amount of drug initially in the body

$(V_d)(C_2)$ = amount of drug in the body needed to achieve the desired plasma concentration

The difference between the two values is the additional dosage needed, which equals $V_d(C_2 - C_1)$.

2. **Effect of a large V_d on the half-life of a drug:** A large V_d has an important influence on the half-life of a drug, because drug elimination depends on the amount of drug delivered to the liver or kidney (or other organs where metabolism occurs) per unit of time. Delivery of drug to the organs of elimination depends not only on blood flow but also on the fraction of the drug in the plasma. If the V_d for a drug is large, most of the drug is in the extraplasmic space and is unavailable to the excretory organs. Therefore, any factor that increases the volume of distribution can lead to an increase in the half-life and extend the duration of action of the drug. [Note: An exceptionally large V_d indicates considerable sequestration of the drug in some organ or compartment.]

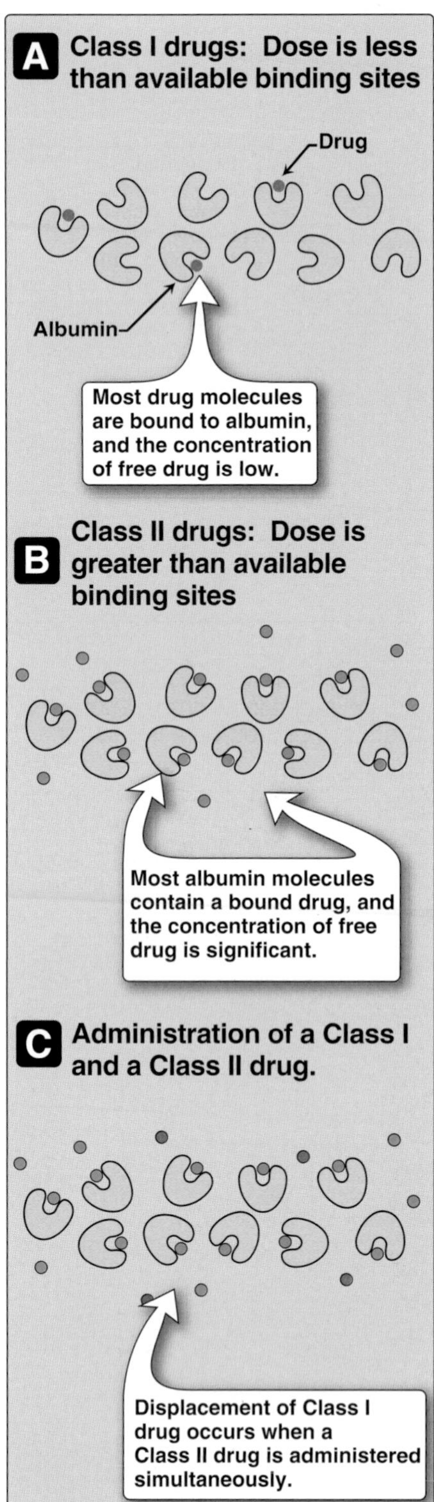
A Class I drugs: Dose is less than available binding sites
Drug
Albumin
Most drug molecules are bound to albumin, and the concentration of free drug is low.
B Class II drugs: Dose is greater than available binding sites
Most albumin molecules contain a bound drug, and the concentration of free drug is significant.
C Administration of a Class I and a Class II drug.
Displacement of Class I drug occurs when a Class II drug is administered simultaneously.

Figure 1.13
Binding of Class I and Class II drugs to albumin when drugs are administered alone (A, B), or together (C).

VII. BINDING OF DRUGS TO PLASMA PROTEINS

Drug molecules may bind to plasma proteins (usually albumin). Bound drugs are pharmacologically inactive; only the free, unbound drug can act on target sites in the tissues, elicit a biologic response, and be available to the processes of elimination. [Note: Hypoalbuminemia may alter the level of free drug.]

A. Binding capacity of albumin

The binding of drugs to albumin is reversible, and may show low capacity (one drug molecule per albumin molecule) or high capacity (a number of drug molecules binding to a single albumin molecule). Drugs can also bind with varying affinities. Albumin has the strongest affinity for anionic drugs (weak acids) and hydrophobic drugs. Most hydrophilic drugs and neutral drugs do not bind to albumin. [Note: Many drugs are hydrophobic by design, because this property permits absorption after oral administration.]

B. Competition for binding between drugs

When two drugs are given, each with high affinity for albumin, they compete for the available binding sites. The drugs with high affinity for albumin can be divided into two classes, depending on whether the dose of drug (the amount of drug found in the body under conditions used clinically) is greater than or less than the binding capacity of albumin (quantified as the number of millimoles of albumin multiplied by the number of binding sites; Figure 1.13).

1. **Class I drugs:** If the dose of drug is less than the binding capacity of albumin, then the dose/capacity ratio is low. The binding sites are in excess of the available drug, and the bound-drug fraction is high. This is the case for Class I drugs, which includes the majority of clinically useful agents.

2. **Class II drugs:** These drugs are given in doses that greatly exceed the number of albumin binding sites. The dose/capacity ratio is high, and a relatively high proportion of the drug exists in the free state, not bound to albumin.

3. **Clinical importance of drug displacement:** This assignment of drug classification assumes importance when a patient who is taking a Class I drug, such as *tolbutamide*, is given a Class II drug, such as a sulfonamide antibiotic. *Tolbutamide* is normally 95 percent bound, and only five percent is free. This means that most of the drug is sequestered on albumin, and is inert in terms of exerting pharmacologic actions. If a sulfonamide is administered, it displaces *tolbutamide* from albumin, leading to a rapid increase in the concentration of free *tolbutamide* in plasma, because almost 100 percent is now free compared with the initial five percent. [Note: The *tolbutamide* concentration does not remain elevated, because the drug moves out of the plasma into the interstitial fluid and achieves a new equilibrium.]

C. Relationship of drug displacement to V_d

The impact of drug displacement from albumin depends on both the V_d and the therapeutic index (see p. 32) of the drug. If the V_d is large, the drug displaced from the albumin distributes to the periphery, and the change in free-drug concentration in the plasma is not significant. If the V_d is small, the newly displaced drug does not move into the tissues as much, and the increase in free drug in the plasma is more profound. If the therapeutic index of the drug is small, this increase in drug concentration may have significant clinical consequences. [Note: Clinically, drug displacement from albumin is one of the most significant sources of drug interactions.]

VIII. DRUG METABOLISM

Drugs are most often eliminated by biotransformation and/or excretion into the urine or bile. The liver is the major site for drug metabolism, but specific drugs may undergo biotransformation in other tissues. [Note: Some agents are initially administered as inactive compounds (prodrugs) and must be metabolized to their active forms.]

A. Kinetics of metabolism

1. **First-order kinetics:** The metabolic transformation of drugs is catalyzed by enzymes, and most of the reactions obey Michaelis-Menten kinetics:[4]

$$v = \text{rate of drug metabolism} = \frac{V_{max}[C]}{K_m + [C]}$$

In most clinical situations, the concentration of the drug, [C], is much less than the Michaelis constant, K_m, and the Michaelis-Menten equation reduces to

$$v = \text{rate of drug metabolism} = \frac{V_{max}[C]}{K_m}$$

That is, the rate of drug metabolism is directly proportional to the concentration of free drug, and first-order kinetics are observed (Figure 1.14). This means that a constant fraction of drug is metabolized per unit of time.

2. **Zero-order kinetics:** With a few drugs, such as *aspirin*, *ethanol* and *phenytoin*, the doses are very large. Therefore the [C] is much greater than K_m, and the velocity equation becomes:

$$v = \text{rate of drug metabolism} = \frac{V_{max}[C]}{[C]} = V_{max}$$

The enzyme is saturated by a high free-drug concentration, and the rate of metabolism remains constant over time. This is called zero-order kinetics (or sometimes is referred to clinically as nonlinear kinetics). A constant amount of drug is metabolized per unit of time.

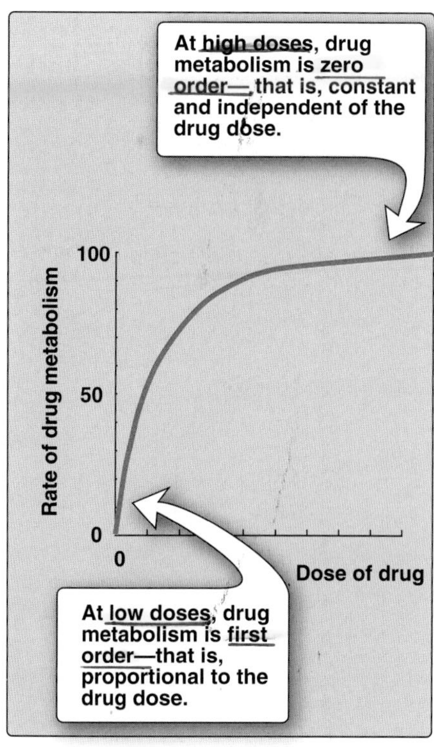
At high doses, drug metabolism is zero order—that is, constant and independent of the drug dose.
Rate of drug metabolism
100
50
0
0
Dose of drug
At low doses, drug metabolism is first order—that is, proportional to the drug dose.

Figure 1.14
Effect of drug dose on the rate of metabolism.

INFO LINK

[4]See p. 58 in ***Lippincott's Illustrated Reviews: Biochemistry*** (3rd ed.) for a discussion of Michaelis-Menten kinetics.

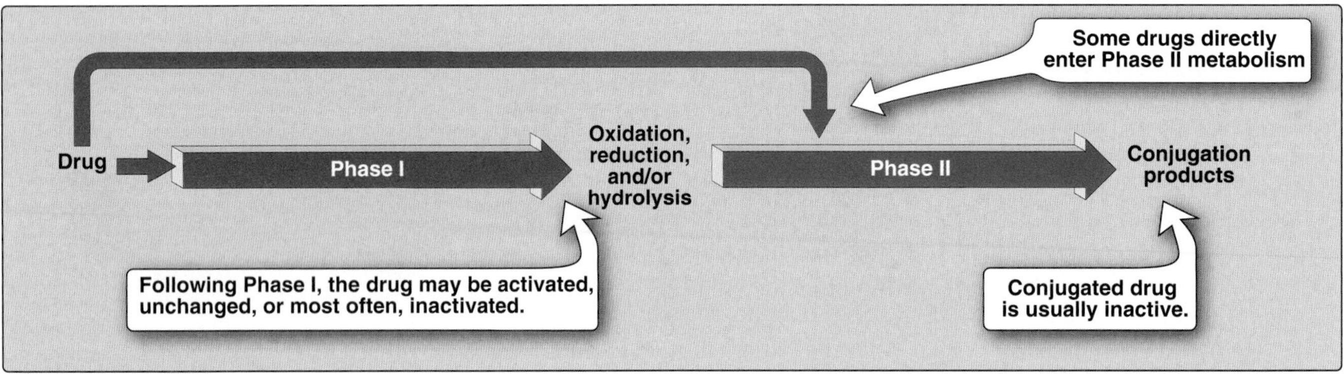

Figure 1.15
The biotransformation of drugs.

B. Reactions of drug metabolism

The kidney cannot efficiently eliminate lipophilic drugs that readily cross cell membranes and are reabsorbed in the distal tubules. Therefore, lipid-soluble agents must first be metabolized in the liver using two general sets of reactions, called Phase I and Phase II (Figure 1.15).

1. **Phase I:** Phase I reactions function to convert lipophilic molecules into more polar molecules by introducing or unmasking a polar functional group, such as –OH or $-NH_2$. Phase I metabolism may increase, decrease, or leave unaltered the drug's pharmacologic activity.

   a. **Phase I reactions utilizing the P450 system:** The Phase I reactions most frequently involved in drug metabolism are catalyzed by the cytochrome P450 system (also called microsomal mixed function oxidase):

   $$\text{Drug} + O_2 + \text{NADPH} + H^+ \rightarrow \text{Drug}_{\text{modified}} + H_2O + \text{NADP}^+$$

   The oxidation proceeds by the drug binding to the oxidized form of cytochrome P450, and then oxygen is introduced through a reductive step coupled to NADPH:cytochrome P450 oxidoreductase.

   b. **Summary of the P450 system:** The P450 system is important for the metabolism of many endogenous compounds (steroids, lipids, etc.) and for the biotransformation of exogenous substances. Cytochrome P450, designated as CYP, is composed of many families of heme-containing isozymes that are located in most cells, but mainly those in the liver and GI tract. The family name is indicated by a number followed by a capital letter for the subfamily (for example, CYP3A). Another number is added to indicate the specific isozyme (CYP3A4). Six isozymes are responsible for the vast majority of P450 catalyzed reactions: CYP3A4, CYP2D6, CYP2C9/10, CYP2C19, CYP2E1, and CYP1A2. The percentages of currently available drugs that are substrates for these isozymes is 60, 25, 15, 15, 2, and 2 percent, respectively. [Note: An individual drug may be a substrate for more than one isozyme.] Considerable amounts of CYP3A4 are found in intestinal mucosa, accounting for first-pass metabolism of drugs such as *chlorpromazine* and *clonazepam.* As might be expected, these enzymes exhibit considerable genetic variability, which has implications for individual dosing regimens, and, even more importantly, as determinants of therapeutic responsiveness and the risk of adverse events. CYP2D6, in particular, has been shown to exhibit genetic polymorphism.[5] Mutations result in very low capacities to metabolize substrates. Some individuals, for example, obtain no benefit from the opioid analgesic *codeine*, because it must be O-demethylated for activation. This reaction is CYP2D6-dependent. The frequency of this polymorphism is racially determined, with a prevalence of five to ten percent in European Caucasians as compared to less than two percent of Southeast Asians. Similar polymorphisms have been characterized for the CYP2C subfamily of isozymes. Although CYP3A4 exhibits a greater than ten-fold interindividual variability, no polymorphisms have been identified for this P450 isozyme.

c. **Inducers:** The cytochrome P450-dependent enzymes are an important target for pharmacokinetic drug interactions. One such interaction is the induction of selected CYP isozymes. Certain drugs, most notably *phenobarbital*, *rifampin*, and *carbamazepine*, are capable of increasing the synthesis of one or more CYP isozymes. The increased biotransformation rates can lead to significant decreases in plasma concentrations of drugs as measured by AUC, with concurrent loss of pharmacologic effect. For example, *rifampin*, an antituberculosis drug (see p. 449), significantly decreases the plasma concentrations of HIV protease inhibitors,[6] diminishing their ability to suppress HIV viron maturation. Figure 1.16 lists some of the more important inducers for representative CYP isozymes.

d. **Inhibitors:** Inhibition of CYP isozyme activity is an important source of drug interactions that leads to serious adverse events. The most common form of inhibition is through competition for the same isozyme. Some drugs, however, are capable of inhibiting reactions for which they are not substrates (for example, *ketoconazole*). Numerous drugs have been shown to inhibit one or more of the CYP-dependent biotransformation pathways of *warfarin*. For example, *omeprazole* is a potent inhibitor of three of the CYP isozymes responsible for *warfarin* metabolism. If the two drugs are taken together, plasma concentrations of *warfarin* increase, which leads to greater inhibition of coagulation and risk of hemorrhage and serious bleeding reactions. [Note: The more important CYP inhibitors are *erythromycin*, *ketoconazole*, and *ritonavir*, because they each inhibit several CYP isozymes.]

e. **Phase I reactions not involving the P450 system:** These include amine oxidation (for example, oxidation of catecholamines or histamine), alcohol dehydrogenation (for example, ethanol oxidation), and hydrolysis (for example, of *procaine*).

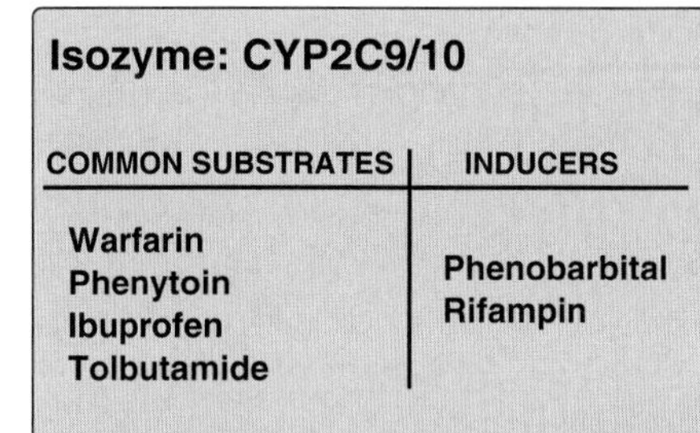

Isozyme: CYP2C9/10

COMMON SUBSTRATES	INDUCERS
Warfarin Phenytoin Ibuprofen Tolbutamide	Phenobarbital Rifampin

Isozyme: CYP2D6

COMMON SUBSTRATES	INDUCERS
Desipramine Imipramine Haloperidol Propanolol	

Isozyme: CYP3A4/5

COMMON SUBSTRATES	INDUCERS
Carbamazepine	Carbamazepine
Cyclosporine	Dexamethasone
Erythromycin	Phenobarbital
Nifedipine	Phenytoin
Verapamil	Rifampin

Figure 1.16
Some representative P450 isozymes.

INFO LINK

[5]See p. 454 in ***Lippincott's Illustrated Reviews: Biochemistry*** (3rd ed.) for a discussion of genetic polymorphism.
[6]See p. 374 in ***Lippincott's Illustrated Reviews: Microbiology*** for a discussion of HIV protease inhibitors.

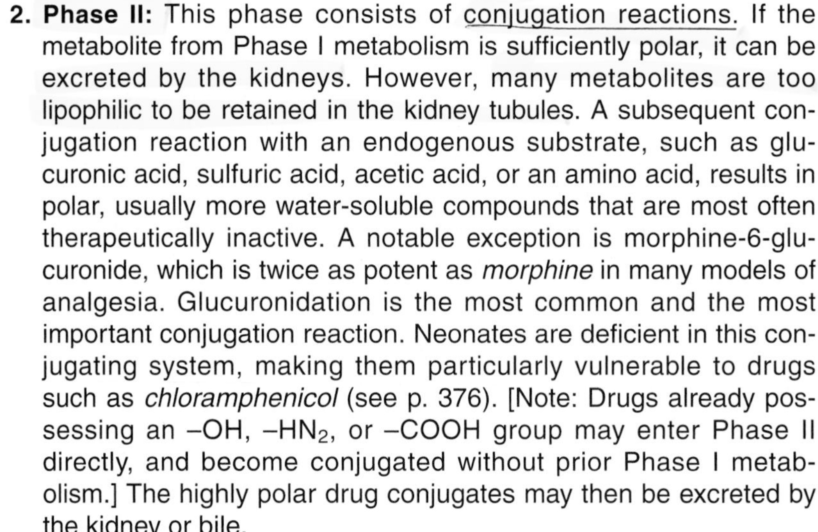

2. **Phase II:** This phase consists of conjugation reactions. If the metabolite from Phase I metabolism is sufficiently polar, it can be excreted by the kidneys. However, many metabolites are too lipophilic to be retained in the kidney tubules. A subsequent conjugation reaction with an endogenous substrate, such as glucuronic acid, sulfuric acid, acetic acid, or an amino acid, results in polar, usually more water-soluble compounds that are most often therapeutically inactive. A notable exception is morphine-6-glucuronide, which is twice as potent as *morphine* in many models of analgesia. Glucuronidation is the most common and the most important conjugation reaction. Neonates are deficient in this conjugating system, making them particularly vulnerable to drugs such as *chloramphenicol* (see p. 376). [Note: Drugs already possessing an –OH, $-HN_2$, or –COOH group may enter Phase II directly, and become conjugated without prior Phase I metabolism.] The highly polar drug conjugates may then be excreted by the kidney or bile.

3. **Reversal of order of the phases:** Not all drugs undergo Phase I and II reactions in that order. For example, *isoniazid* is first acetylated (a Phase II reaction) and then hydrolyzed to isonicotinic acid (a Phase I reaction).

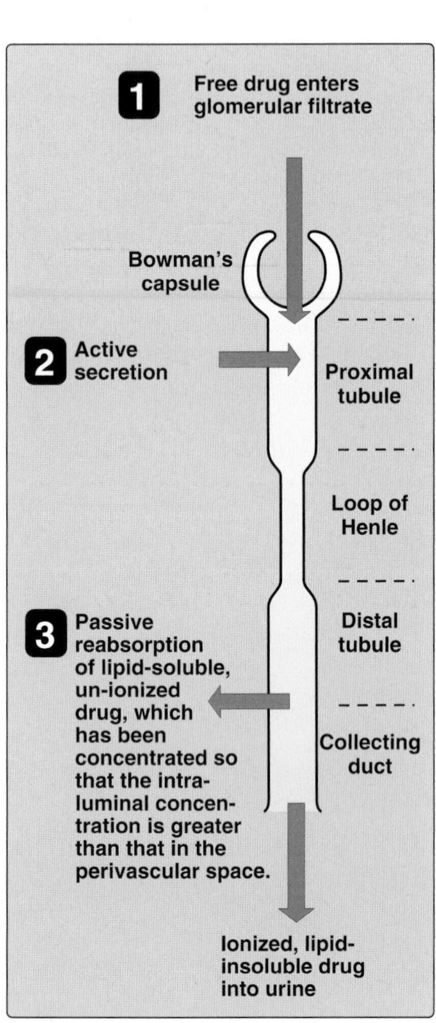
1 Free drug enters glomerular filtrate
Bowman's capsule
2 Active secretion
Proximal tubule
Loop of Henle
Distal tubule
3 Passive reabsorption of lipid-soluble, un-ionized drug, which has been concentrated so that the intra-luminal concentration is greater than that in the perivascular space.
Collecting duct
Ionized, lipid-insoluble drug into urine

Figure 1.17
Drug elimination by the kidney.

IX. DRUG ELIMINATION

Removal of a drug from the body may occur via a number of routes, the most important being through the kidney into the urine. Other routes include the bile, intestine, lung, or milk in nursing mothers. A patient in renal failure may undergo extracorporeal dialysis, which will remove small molecules, such as drugs.

A. Renal elimination of a drug

1. **Glomerular filtration:** Drugs enter the kidney through renal arteries, which divide to form a glomerular capillary plexus. Free drug (not bound to albumin) flows through the capillary slits into Bowman's space as part of the glomerular filtrate (Figure 1.17). The glomerular filtration rate (125 ml/min) is normally about twenty percent of the renal plasma flow (600 ml/min). [Note: Lipid solubility and pH do not influence the passage of drugs into the glomerular filtrate.]

2. **Proximal tubular secretion:** Drug that was not transferred into the glomerular filtrate leaves the glomeruli through efferent arterioles, which divide to form a capillary plexus surrounding the nephric lumen in the proximal tubule. Secretion primarily occurs in the proximal tubules by two energy-requiring active transport (carrier-requiring) systems, one for anions (for example, deprotonated forms of weak acids) and one for cations (protonated forms of weak bases). Each of these transport systems shows a low specificity and can transport many compounds; thus, competition between drugs for the carriers can occur within each transport system (for example, see *probenecid*, p. 513). [Note: Premature

infants and neonates have an incompletely developed tubular secretory mechanism and, thus, may retain certain drugs.]

3. **Distal tubular reabsorption:** As a drug moves toward the distal convoluted tubule, its concentration increases and exceeds that of the perivascular space. The drug, if uncharged, may diffuse out of the nephric lumen back into the systemic circulation. Manipulating the pH of the urine to increase the ionized form of the drug in the lumen may be used to minimize the amount of back-diffusion and, hence, increase the clearance of an undesirable drug. For example, a patient presenting with a *phenobarbital* overdose can be given *bicarbonate*, which alkalinizes the urine and keeps the drug ionized, thereby decreasing its reabsorption. If the drug is a weak base, acidification of the urine with NH_4Cl leads to protonation of the drug and an increase in its clearance. This process is called "ion trapping."

4. **Role of drug metabolism:** Most drugs are lipid soluble and diffuse out of the kidney's tubular lumen when the drug concentration in the filtrate becomes greater than that in the perivascular space. To minimize this reabsorption, drugs are modified by the body to be more polar using two types of reactions: Phase I reactions (see p. 14) that involve either the addition of hydroxyl groups or the removal of blocking groups from hydroxyl, carboxyl, or amino groups, and Phase II reactions (see p. 16) that use conjugation with sulfate, glycine, or glucuronic acid to increase drug polarity. The conjugates are ionized, and the charged molecules cannot back-diffuse out of the kidney lumen (Figure 1.18).

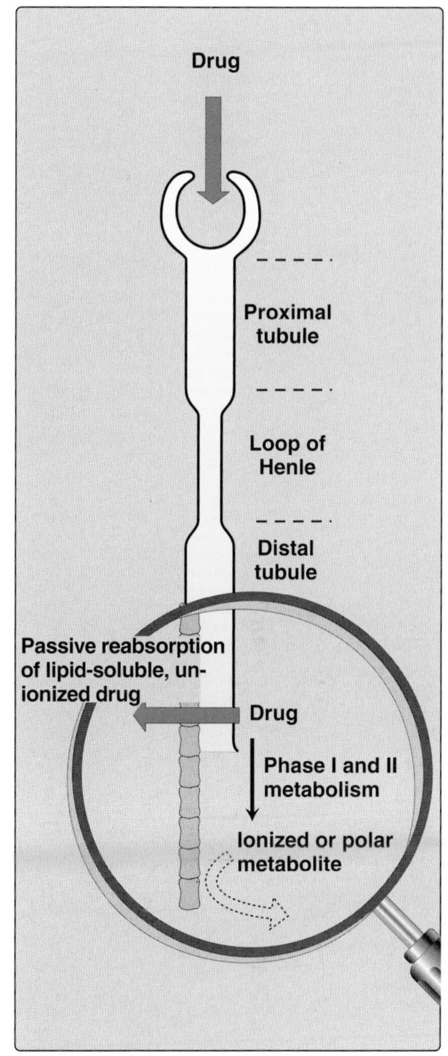

Figure 1.18
Effect of drug metabolism on reabsorption in the distal tubule.

B. Quantitative aspects of renal drug elimination

Plasma clearance is expressed as the volume of plasma from which all drug appears to be removed in a given time—for example, as ml/min. Clearance equals the amount of renal plasma flow multiplied by the extraction ratio, and because these are normally invariant over time, clearance is constant.

1. **Extraction ratio:** This ratio is the decline of drug concentration in the plasma from the arterial to the venous side of the kidney. The drugs enter the kidneys at concentration C_1 and exit the kidneys at concentration C_2. The extraction ratio = C_2/C_1

2. **Excretion rate:**

$$\underset{\text{mg/min}}{\text{Excretion rate}} = \underset{\text{ml/min}}{(\text{clearance})}\underset{\text{mg/ml}}{(\text{plasma concentration})}$$

The elimination of a drug usually follows first-order kinetics, and the concentration of drug in plasma drops exponentially with time. This can be used to determine the half-life of the drug (the time during which the concentration of the drug decreases from C to $\frac{1}{2}$C):

$$t_{1/2} = \ln 0.5/k_e = 0.693\ V_d/CL$$

where k_e = the first-order rate constant for drug elimination from the total body and CL = clearance.

C. Total body clearance

The total body (systemic) clearance (CL_{total} or CL_t) is the sum of the clearances from the various drug metabolizing and drug-eliminating organs. The kidney is often the major organ of excretion; however, the liver also contributes to drug loss through metabolism and/or excretion into the bile. A patient in renal failure may sometimes benefit from a drug that is excreted by this pathway into the intestine and feces rather than through the kidney. Some drugs may also be reabsorbed through the enterohepatic circulation, thus prolonging their half-life. Total clearance can be calculated by using the following equation:

$$CL_{total} = CL_{hepatic} + CL_{renal} + CL_{pulmonary} + CL_{other}$$

It is not possible to measure and sum these individual clearances. However, total clearance can be derived from the steady-state equation:

$$CL_{total} = k_e V_d$$

D. Clinical situations resulting in increased drug half-life

When a patient has an abnormality that alters the half-life of a drug, adjustment in dosage is required. It is important to be able to predict in which patients a drug is likely to have a longer half-life. The half-life of a drug is increased by: 1) diminished renal plasma flow or hepatic blood flow—for example, in cardiogenic shock, heart failure, or hemorrhage; 2) decreased extraction ratio—for example, as seen in renal disease; and 3) decreased metabolism—for example, when another drug inhibits its biotransformation or in hepatic insufficiency, as with cirrhosis.

X. KINETICS OF CONTINUOUS ADMINISTRATION

The preceding discussion describes the pharmacokinetic processes that determine the rates of absorption, distribution, and elimination of a drug. Pharmacokinetics also describes the quantitative, time-dependent changes of both the plasma drug concentration and the total amount of drug in the body, following the drug's administration by various routes, with the two most common being IV infusion and oral fixed-dose/fixed-time interval regimens (for example, "one tablet every four hours"). The interactions of the processes previously described determine the pharmacokinetic profile of a drug. The significance of identifying the pharmacokinetics of a drug lies not only in defining the factors that influence its levels and persistence in the body, but also in tailoring the therapeutic use of drugs that have a high toxic potential. [Note: The following discussion assumes that the administered drug distributes into a single body compartment. In actuality, most drugs equilibrate between two or three compartments and, thus, display complex kinetic behavior. However, the simpler model suffices to demonstrate the concepts.]

A. Kinetics of IV infusion

With continuous IV infusion, the rate of drug entry into the body is constant. In the majority of cases, the elimination of a drug is first-order; that is, a constant fraction of the agent is cleared per unit of time. Therefore, the rate of drug exit from the body increases proportionately as the plasma concentration increases, and at every point in time, it is proportional to the plasma concentration of the drug.

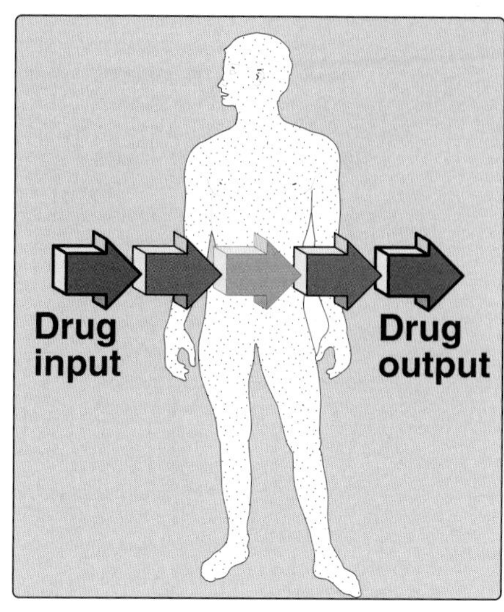

Figure 1.19
At steady state, input (rate of infusion) equals output (rate of elimination).

1. **Steady-state drug levels in blood:** Following the initiation of an intravenous infusion, the plasma concentration of drug rises until the rate of drug eliminated from the body precisely balances the input rate. Thus a steady-state is achieved in which the plasma concentration of drug remains constant. [Note: The rate of drug elimination from the body = $(CL_t)(C)$, where CL_t is total body clearance (see p 18) and C is the plasma concentration of drug.] Two questions can be asked about achieving the steady-state. First, what is the relationship between the rate of drug infusion and the plasma concentration of drug achieved at the plateau, or steady-state? Second, what length of time is required to reach the steady-state drug concentration?

2. **Influence of the rate of drug infusion on the steady-state:** A steady-state plasma concentration of a drug occurs when the rate of drug elimination is equal to the rate of administration (Figure 1.19), as described by the following equation

$$C_{ss} = R_o/k_eV_d = R_o/CL_t$$

where C_{ss} = the steady-state concentration of the drug, R_o = the infusion rate (for example, mg/min), K_e is the first-order elimination rate constant, and V_d = the volume of distribution. Because k_e, CL_t, and V_d are constant for most drugs showing first-order kinetics, C_{ss} is directly proportional to R_o; that is, the steady-state plasma concentration is directly proportional to the infusion rate. For example, if the infusion rate is doubled, the plasma concentration ultimately achieved at the steady-state is doubled (Figure 1.20). Furthermore, the steady-state concentration is inversely proportional to the clearance of the drug, CL_t. Thus, any factor that decreases clearance, such as liver or kidney disease, increases the steady-state concentration of an infused drug (assuming V_d remains constant).

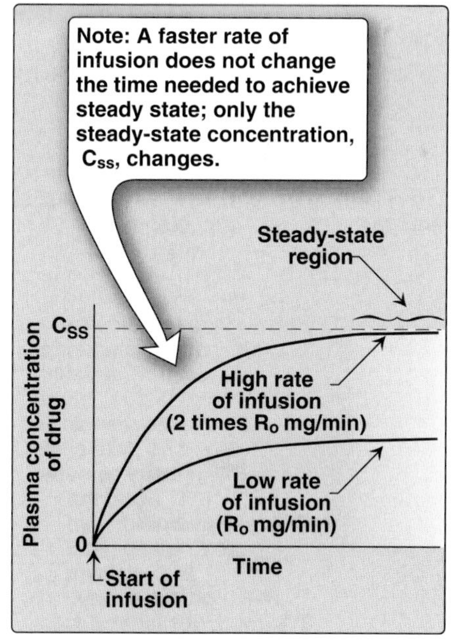

Figure 1.20
Effect of infusion rate on the steady-state concentration of drug in the plasma. (R_o = rate of infusion of a drug.)

3. **Time required to reach the steady-state drug concentration:** The concentration of drug rises from zero at the start of the infusion to its ultimate steady-state level, C_{ss} (Figure 1.21). The fractional rate of approach to a steady-state is achieved by a first-order process.

   a. **Exponential approach to steady-state:** The rate constant for attainment of steady-state is the rate constant for total body elimination of the drug, k_e. Thus, fifty percent of the final steady-state concentration of drug is observed after the time

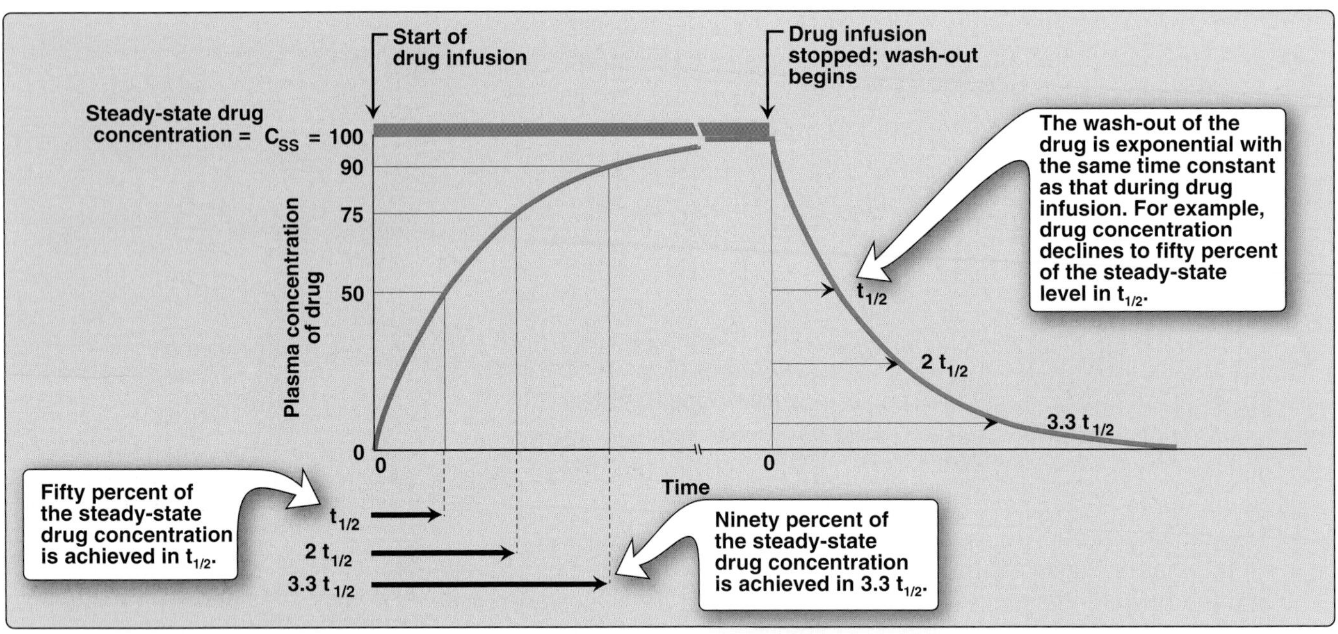

Figure 1.21
Rate of attainment of steady-state concentration of a drug in the plasma.

elapsed since the infusion, t, is equal to $t_{1/2}$, where $t_{1/2}$ (or half-life) is the time required for the drug concentration to change by fifty percent. Waiting another half-life allows the drug concentration to approach 75 percent of C_{SS} (see Figure 1.21). The drug concentration is ninety percent of the final steady-state concentration in 3.3 times $t_{1/2}$. For convenience, therefore, one can assume that a drug will reach steady-state in about four half-lives. The time required to reach a specific fraction of the steady-state is described by:

$$f = 1 - e^{-k_e t}$$

where f is the fractional shift (for example, 0.9 if the time to reach ninety percent of the steady-state concentration was being calculated) and t is the time elaspsed since the start of the infusion.

b. **Effect of the rate of drug infusion:** The sole determinant of the rate that a drug approaches steady-state is the $t_{1/2}$ or k_e, and this rate is influenced only by the factors that affect the half-life. The rate of approach to steady-state is not affected by the rate of drug infusion. Although increasing the rate of infusion of a drug increases the rate at which any given concentration of drug in the plasma is achieved, it does not influence the time required to reach the ultimate steady-state concentration. This is because the steady-state concentration of drug rises directly with the infusion rate (see Figure 1.20).

c. **Rate of drug decline when the infusion is stopped:** When the infusion is stopped, the plasma concentration of a drug declines (washes out) to zero with the same time course observed in approaching the steady-state (see Figure 1.21). This relationship is expressed as

$$C_t = C_0 – e^{-k_e t}$$

where C_t is the plasma concentration at any time, C_0 is the starting plasma concentration, k_e is the first-order elimination rate constant, and t is the time elapsed.

d. **Loading dose:** A delay in achieving the desired plasma levels of drug may be clinically unacceptable. Therefore, a "loading dose" of drug can be injected as a single dose to achieve the desired plasma level rapidly, followed by an infusion to maintain the steady-state (maintenance dose). In general, the loading dose can be calculated as

Loading dose = (V_d)(desired steady-state plasma concentration)

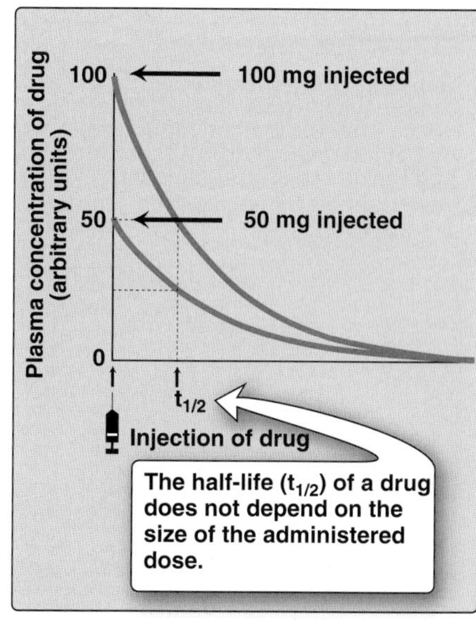

Figure 1.22
Effect of the dose of a single intravenous injection of drug on plasma levels.

B. Kinetics of fixed-dose/fixed-time-interval regimens

Administration of a drug by fixed doses rather than by continuous infusion is often more convenient. However, fixed doses, given at fixed-time intervals, result in time-dependent fluctuations in the circulating level of drug.

1. **Single IV injection:** For simplicity, assume the injected drug rapidly distributes into a single compartment. Because the rate of elimination is usually first order in regard to drug concentration, the circulating level of drug decreases exponentially with time (Figure 1.22). [Note: The $t_{1/2}$ does not depend on the dose of drug administered.]

2. **Multiple intravenous injections:** When a drug is given repeatedly at regular intervals, the plasma concentration increases until a steady-state is reached (Figure 1.23). Because most drugs are given at intervals shorter than five half-lives and are eliminated exponentially with time, some drug from the first dose remains in the body at the time that the second dose is administered, and some from the second dose remains at the time that the third dose is given, and so forth. Therefore, the drug accumulates until, within the dosing interval, the rate of drug loss (driven by an elevated plasma concentration) exactly balances the rate of drug administration—that is, until a steady-state is achieved.

   a. **Effect of dosing frequency:** The plasma concentration of a drug oscillates about a mean. Using smaller doses at shorter intervals reduces the amplitude of the swings in drug concentration. However, the steady-state concentration of the drug and the rate at which the steady-state is approached are not affected by the frequency of dosing.

   b. **Example of achievement of steady-state using different dosage regimens:** Curve B of Figure 1.23 shows the amount of drug in the body when 1g of drug is administered IV to a

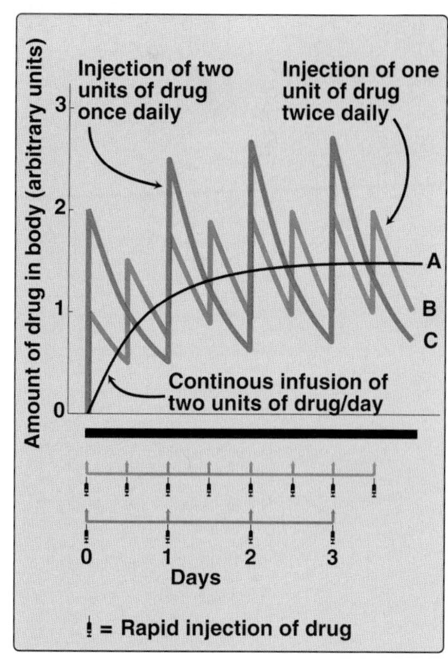

Figure 1.23
Predicted plasma concentrations of a drug given by infusion (A), twice daily injection (B), or once daily injection (C). Model assumes rapid mixing in a single body compartment and a $t_{1/2}$ of twelve hours.

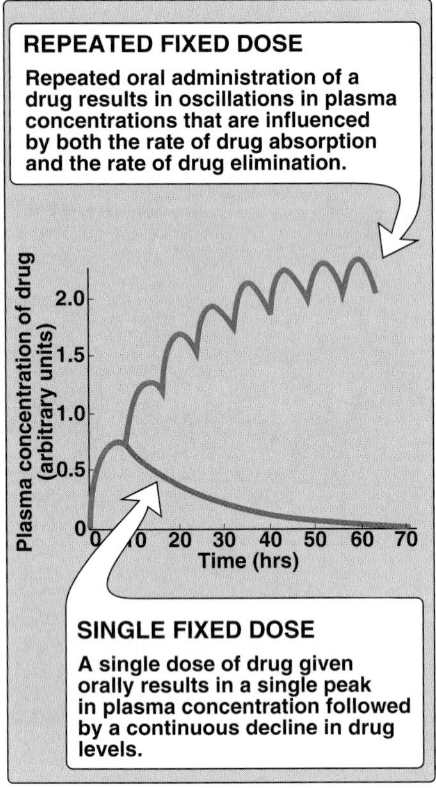

REPEATED FIXED DOSE
Repeated oral administration of a drug results in oscillations in plasma concentrations that are influenced by both the rate of drug absorption and the rate of drug elimination.
Plasma concentration of drug (arbitrary units)
2.0
1.5
1.0
0.5
0
0 10 20 30 40 50 60 70
Time (hrs)
SINGLE FIXED DOSE
A single dose of drug given orally results in a single peak in plasma concentration followed by a continuous decline in drug levels.

Figure 1.24
Predicted plasma concentrations of a drug given by repeated oral administrations.

patient, and the dose is repeated at a time interval that corresponds to the half-life of the drug. At the end of the first dosing interval, 0.50 units of drug remain from the first dose when the second dose is administered. At the end of the second dosing interval, 0.75 units are present when the third dose is taken. The minimal amount of drug during the dosing interval progressively increases and approaches a value of 1.00 unit, whereas the maximal value immediately following drug administration progressively approaches 2.00 units. Therefore, at the steady-state, 1.00 unit of drug is lost during the dosing interval, which is exactly matched by the rate at which the drug is administered; that is, the "rate in" equals the "rate out." As in the case for IV infusion, ninety percent of the steady-state value is achieved in 3.3 times $t_{1/2}$.

3. **Orally administered drugs:** Most drugs that are administered on an outpatient basis are taken orally on a fixed-dose/fixed-time-interval regimen—for example, a specific dose taken one, two or three times daily. In contrast to iv injection, orally administered drugs may be absorbed slowly, and the plasma concentration of the drug is influenced by both the rate of absorption and the rate of drug elimination (Figure 1.24). This relationship can be expressed as

$$C_{ss} = \frac{1}{(k_e)(V_d)} \frac{(D)(F)}{T}$$

where D = the dose, F = the fraction absorbed (bioavailability), T = dosage interval, C_{ss} = the steady-state concentration of the drug, k_e = the first-order rate constant for drug elimination from the total body, and V_d = the volume of distribution.

Study Questions

Choose the ONE best answer.

1.1 Which one of the following statements is CORRECT?

A. Weak bases are absorbed efficiently across the epithelial cells of the stomach.

B. Coadministration of atropine speeds the absorption of a second drug.

C. Drugs showing a large V_d can be efficiently removed by dialysis of the plasma.

D. Stressful emotions can lead to a slowing of drug absorption.

E. If the V_d for a drug is small, most of the drug is in the extraplasmic space.

Correct answer = D. Both exercise and strong emotions prompt sympathetic output, which slows gastric emptying. In the stomach, a weak base is primarily in the protonated, charged form, which does not readily cross the epithelial cells of the stomach. Atropine is a parasympathetic blocker and slows gastric emptying. This delays the rate of drug absorption. A large V_d indicates that most of the drug is outside the plasma space, and dialysis would not be effective. A small V_d indicates extensive binding to plasma proteins.

1.2 Which one of the following is TRUE for a drug whose elimination from plasma shows first-order kinetics?

A. The half-life of the drug is proportional to the drug concentration in plasma.

B. The amount eliminated per unit of time is constant.

C. The rate of elimination is proportional to the plasma concentration.

D. Elimination involves a rate-limiting enzymic reaction operating at its maximal velocity (V_m).

E. A plot of drug concentration versus time is a straight line.

Correct answer = C. The direct proportionality between concentration and rate is the definition of first-order. The half-life of a drug is a constant. For first-order reactions, the fraction of the drug eliminated not the amount of drug is constant. A rate limiting reaction operating at V_m would show zero-order kinetics. First-order kinetics show a linear plot of log [drug concentration] versus time.

1.3 A patient is treated with drug A, which has a high affinity for albumin and is administered in amounts that do not exceed the binding capacity of albumin. A second drug, B, is added to the treatment regimen. Drug B also has a high affinity for albumin, but is administered in amounts that are 100 times the binding capacity of albumin. Which of the following occurs after administration of drug B?

A. An increase in the tissue concentrations of drug A.

B. A decrease in the tissue concentrations of drug A.

C. A decrease in the volume of distribution of drug A.

D. A decrease in the half-life of drug A.

E. Addition of more drug A significantly alters the serum concentration of unbound drug B.

Correct answer = A. Drug A is largely bound to albumin, and only a small fraction is free. Most of drug A is sequestered on albumin and is inert in terms of exerting pharmacologic actions. If drug B is administered, it displaces drug A from albumin, leading to a rapid increase in the concentration of free drug A in plasma, because almost 100 percent is now free. Drug A moves out of the plasma into the interstitial water and the tissues. The V_d of drug A increases, providing less drug to the organ of excretion and prolonging the overall lifetime of the drug. Because drug B is already in 100-fold excess of its albumin-binding capacity, dislodging some of drug B from albumin does not significantly affect its serum concentration.

1.4 The addition of glucuronic acid to a drug:

A. decreases its water solubility.
B. usually leads to inactivation of the drug.
C. is an example of a Phase I reaction.
D. occurs at the same rate in adults and newborns.
E. involves cytochrome P450.

Correct answer = B. The addition of glucuronic acid prevents recognition of the drug by its receptor. Glucuronic acid is charged, and the drug conjugate has increased water solubility. Conjugation is a Phase II reaction. Neonates are deficient in the conjugating enzymes. Cytochrome P450 is involved in Phase I reactions.

1.5 Drugs showing zero-order kinetics of elimination:

A. are more common than those showing first-order kinetics.
B. decrease in concentration exponentially with time.
C. have a half-life independent of dose.
D. show a plot of drug concentration versus time that is linear.
E. show a constant fraction of the drug eliminated per unit time.

Correct answer = D. Drugs with zero-order kinetics of elimination show a linear relationship between drug concentration and time. In most clinical situations, the concentration of a drug is much less than the Michaelis-Menten constant (K_m). A decrease in drug concentration is linear with time. The half-life of the drug increases with dose. A constant amount of drug is eliminated per unit of time.

1.6 A drug, given as a 100 mg single dose, results in a peak plasma concentration of 20 μg/ml. The apparent volume of distribution is (assume a rapid distribution and negligible elimination prior to measuring the peak plasma level):

A. 0.5 L.
B. 1 L.
C. 2 L.
D. 5 L.
E. 10 L.

Correct answer = D. V_d = D/C, where D = the total amount of drug in the body and C = the plasma concentration of drug. Thus, V_d = 100mg/20 mg/ml = 100 mg/20 mg/L = 5 L.

1.7 A drug with a half-life of twelve hours is administered by continuous IV infusion. How long will it take for the drug to reach ninety percent of its final steady-state level?

A. 18 hours.
B. 24 hours.
C. 30 hours.
D. 40 hours.
E. 90 hours.

Correct answer = D. One approaches ninety percent of the final steady-state in (3.3)($t_{1/2)}$ = (3.3)(12) = ~40 hours.

1.8 Which of the following results in a doubling of the steady-state concentration of a drug?

A. Doubling the rate of infusion.
B. Maintaining the rate of infusion, but doubling the loading dose.
C. Doubling the rate of infusion and doubling the concentration of the infused drug.
D. Tripling the rate of infusion.
E. Quadrupling the rate of infusion.

Correct answer = A. The steady-state concentration of a drug is directly proportional to the infusion rate. Increasing the loading dose provides a transient increase in drug level, but the steady-state level remains unchanged. Doubling both the rate of infusion and the concentration of infused drug leads to a four-fold increase in the steady-state drug concentration. Tripling or quadrupling the rate of infusion leads to either a three- or four-fold increase in the steady-state drug concentration.

Drug-Receptor Interactions and Pharmacodynamics

2

I. OVERVIEW

Most drugs exert their effects, both beneficial and harmful, by interacting with receptors—that is, specialized target macromolecules—present on the cell surface or intracellularly. Receptors bind drugs and mediate their pharmacologic actions (Figure 2.1). Drugs may interact with enzymes (for example, inhibition of dihydrofolate reductase by *trimethoprim,* see p. 387), nucleic acids (for example, blockade of transcription by *dactinomycin,* see p. 465), or membrane receptors (for example, alteration of membrane permeability by *pilocarpine,* see p. 49). In each case, the formation of the drug-receptor complex leads to a biologic response, and the magnitude of the response is proportional to the number of drug-receptor complexes:

$$\text{Drug} + \text{Receptor} \rightleftarrows \text{Drug–receptor complex} \rightarrow \text{Biologic effect}$$

This concept is closely related to the formation of complexes between enzyme and substrate[1], or antigen and antibody[2]; these interactions have many common features, perhaps the most noteworthy being specificity of the receptor for a specific ligand. However, the receptor not only has the ability to recognize a ligand (drug), but can also couple or transduce this binding into a response by causing a conformational change or a biochemical effect. Although much of this chapter will be centered on the interaction of drugs with specific receptors, it is important to be aware that not all drugs exert their effects by interacting with a receptor; for example, antacids chemically neutralize excess gastric acid, reducing the symptoms of "heartburn". This chapter introduces the study of pharmacodynamics—the influence of drug concentrations on the magnitude of the response. It deals with the interaction of drugs with receptors, the molecular consequences of these interactions, and their effects in the living organism. A fundamental principle of pharmacodynamics is that drugs only modify underlying biochemical and physiological processes; they do not create effects de novo.

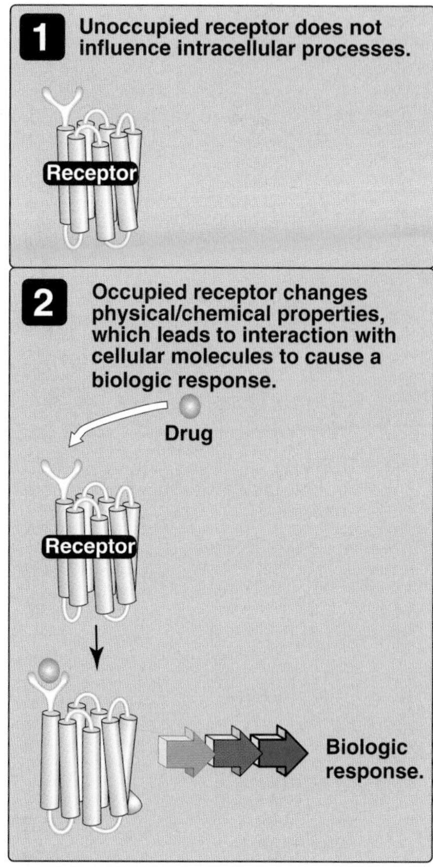

1 Unoccupied receptor does not influence intracellular processes.
Receptor
2 Occupied receptor changes physical/chemical properties, which leads to interaction with cellular molecules to cause a biologic response.
Drug
Receptor
Biologic response.

Figure 2.1
The recognition of a drug by a receptor triggers a biologic response.

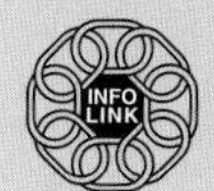

[1]See p. 58 in ***Lippincott's Illustrated Reviews: Biochemistry*** (3rd ed.) for a discussion of the interaction of enzyme and substrate.
[2]See p. 80 in ***Lippincott's Illustrated Reviews: Microbiology*** for a discussion of the interaction between antigens and antibodies.

II. CHEMISTRY OF RECEPTORS AND LIGANDS

Interaction of receptors with ligands involves the formation of chemical bonds, most commonly electrostatic and hydrogen bonds, as well as weak interactions involving van der Waals forces. These bonds are important in determining the selectivity of receptors, because the strength of these noncovalent bonds is related inversely to the distance between the interacting atoms. Therefore, the successful binding of a drug requires an exact fit of the ligand atoms with the complementary receptor atoms. The bonds are usually reversible, except for a handful of drugs that covalently bond to their targets. The size, shape, and charge distribution of the drug molecule determines which of the myriad binding sites in the cells and tissues of the patient can interact with the ligand. The metaphor of the "lock and key" is a useful concept for understanding the interaction of receptors with their ligands. The precise fit required of the ligand echoes the characteristics of the "key," whereas the opening of the "lock" reflects the activation of the receptor. The interaction of the ligand with its receptor thus exhibits a high degree of specificity.

III. MAJOR RECEPTOR FAMILIES

Pharmacology defines a receptor as any biologic molecule to which a drug binds and produces a measurable response. Thus, enzymes and structural proteins can be considered to be pharmacologic receptors. However, the richest sources of therapeutically exploitable pharmacologic receptors are proteins that are responsible for transducing extracellular signals into intracellular responses. These receptors may be divided into four families: 1) ligand-gated ion channels, 2) G protein-coupled receptors, 3) enzyme-linked receptors, and 4) intracellular receptors.

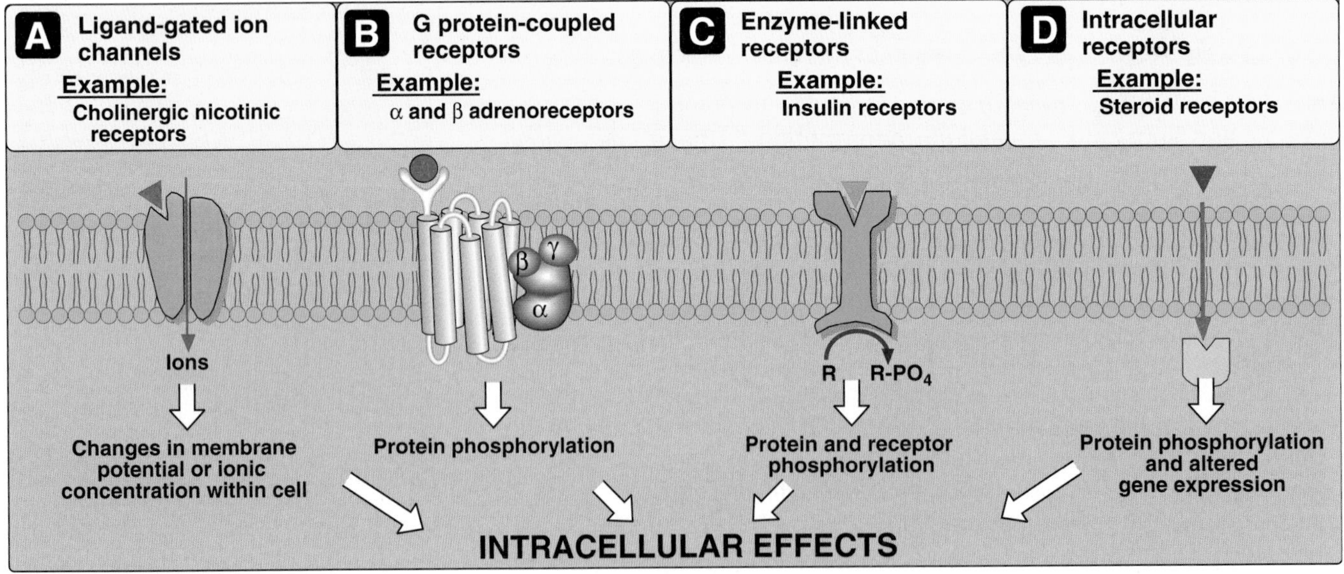

Figure 2.2
Transmembrane signaling mechanisms. A. Ligand binds to the extracellular domain of a ligand-gated channel. B. Ligand binds to a domain of the serpentine receptor, which is coupled to a G protein. C. Ligand binds to the extracellular domain of a receptor that activates a kinase enzyme. D. Lipid-soluble ligand diffuses across the membrane to interact with its intracellular receptor. GABA = γ-aminobutyric acid.

A. Ligand-gated ion channels

The first receptor family comprises ligand-gated ion channels that are responsible for regulation of the flow of ions across cell membranes (see Figure 2.2A). The activity of these channels is regulated by the binding of a ligand to the channel. Response to these receptors is very rapid, having durations of a few milliseconds. The nicotinic receptor and the γ-aminobutyric acid (GABA) receptor are important examples of ligand-gated receptors, the functions of which are modified by numerous drugs. Stimulation of the nicotinic receptor by acetylcholine results in sodium influx and the activation of contraction in skeletal muscle. Benzodiazepines, on the other hand, enhance the stimulation of the GABA-receptor by GABA, resulting in increased chloride influx and hyperpolarization of the respective cell. Although not ligand-gated, ion channels, such as the voltage-gated sodium channel, are important drug receptors for several drug classes, including the local anesthetics.

B. G protein-coupled receptors

A second family of receptors consists of G protein-coupled receptors. Comprised of a single peptide that has seven membrane-spanning regions, these receptors are linked to a G protein (G_s) having three subunits, an α subunit that binds guanosine triphosphate (GTP), and a βγ subunit (Figure 2.3). Binding of the appropriate ligand to the extracellular region of the receptor activates the G protein so that GTP replaces guanosine diphosphate (GDP) on the α-subunit. Dissociation of the G protein occurs, and both the α-GTP subunit and the βγ subunit subsequently interact with other cellular effectors. These effectors are known as second messengers, because they are responsible for further actions within the cell. Stimulation of these receptors results in responses that last several seconds to minutes.

1. **Second messengers:** A common pathway turned on by G_s is the activation of adenylyl cyclase by α-GTP subunits, which results in the production of cyclic-adenosine monophosphate (cAMP), a second messenger that regulates protein phosphorylation. G proteins also activate phospholipase C, which is responsible for the generation of two other second messengers, namely inositol-1,4,5-triphosphate (IP_3) and diacylglycerol. These effectors are responsible for the regulation of free calcium concentrations within the cell. This family of receptors transduces signals derived from odors, light, and numerous neurotransmitters, including norepinephrine, dopamine, serotonin, and acetylcholine.

C. Enzyme-linked receptors

A third major family of receptors consists of those that have a cytosolic enzyme activity as an integral component of their structure or function (see Figure 2.2C). Binding of a ligand to an extracellular domain activates or inhibits this cytosolic enzyme activity. Duration of responses to stimulation of these receptors is on the order of minutes to hours. The most common are those that have a tyrosine kinase activity as part of their structure. Binding of a ligand to two such receptors activates the kinase, resulting in the phosphorylation

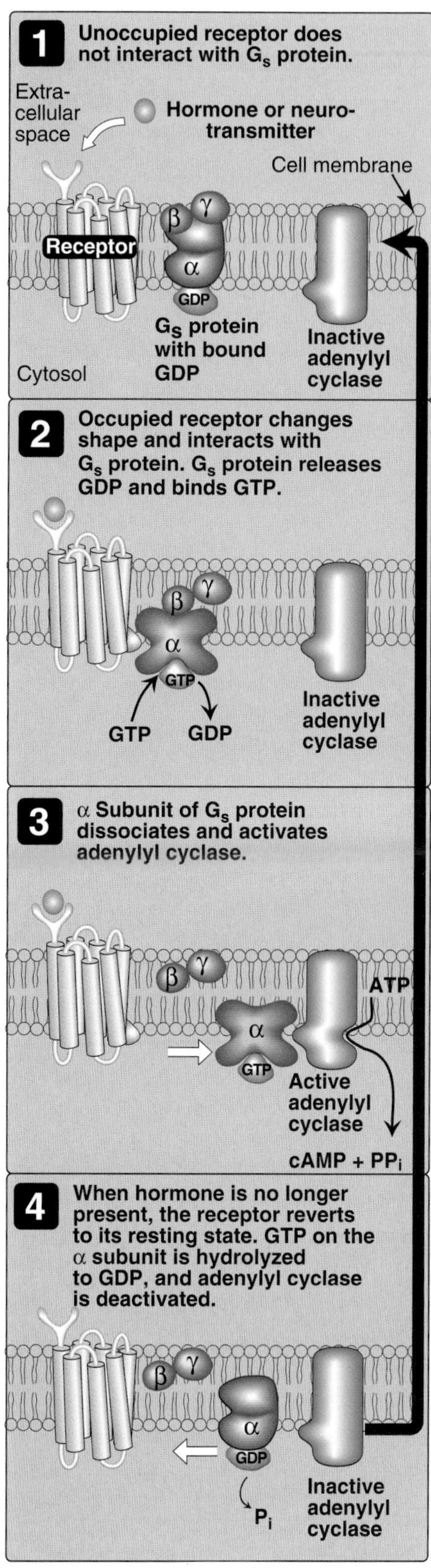

Figure 2.3
The recognition of chemical signals by G-protein coupled membrane receptors triggers an increase (or, less often, a decrease) in the activity of adenylyl cyclase.

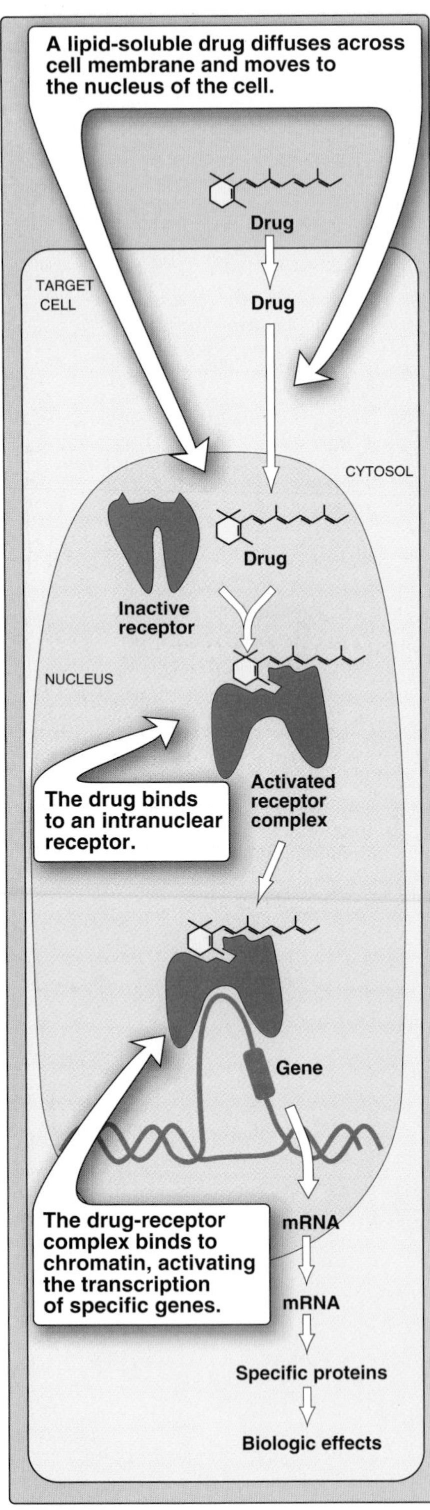

Figure 2.4
Mechanism of intracellular receptors.

of tyrosine residues of specific proteins. The addition of a phosphate group can substantially modify the three-dimensional structure of the target protein, thereby acting as a molecular switch. For example, when the peptide hormone insulin binds two receptor molecules, their intrinsic tyrosine kinase activity causes autophosphorylation of the receptor itself. In turn, the phosphorylated receptor phosphorylates target molecules—insulin-receptor substrate peptides—that subsequently activate other important cellular signals such as IP3, and the mitogen-activated protein kinase system. This cascade of activations results in a multiplication of the initial signal, much like that which occurs with G protein-coupled receptors.

D. Intracellular receptors

The fourth family of receptors differs considerably from the other three in that the receptor is entirely intracellular and, therefore, the ligand must diffuse into the cell to interact with the receptor (Figure 2.4). This places constraints on the physical-chemical properties of the ligand in that it must have sufficient lipid solubility to be able to move across the target cell membrane. For example, steroid hormones exert their action on target cells via this receptor mechanism. Binding of the ligand with its receptor follows a general pattern in which the receptor becomes activated because of the dissociation of a small repressor peptide. The activated ligand-receptor complex migrates to the nucleus, where it binds to specific DNA sequences, resulting in the regulation of gene expression. The time course of activation and response of these receptors is much longer than the other mechanisms described above. Because gene expression—and, therefore, protein synthesis—is modified, cellular responses are not observed until considerable time has elapsed (thirty minutes or more), and the duration of the response (hours to days) is much greater than that of other receptor families.

E. Spare receptors

A characteristic of many receptors, particularly those that respond to hormones, neurotransmitters, and peptides, is their ability to amplify signal duration and intensity. The family of G protein-linked receptors exemplifies many of the possible responses initiated by ligand binding to a receptor. Specifically, two phenomena account for the amplification of the ligand-receptor signal. First, a single ligand/receptor complex can interact with many G proteins, thereby multiplying the original signal many-fold. Second, the activated G proteins persist for a longer duration than the original ligand-receptor complex. The binding of *albuterol*, for example, may only exist for a few milliseconds, but the subsequent activated G proteins may last for hundreds of milliseconds. Further prolongation and amplification of the initial signal is mediated by the interaction between G proteins and their respective intracellular targets. Because of this amplification, only a fraction of the total receptors for a specific ligand may need to be occupied to elicit a maximal response from a cell. Systems that exhibit this behavior are said to have spare receptors. Spare receptors are exhibited by insulin receptors, where it has been estimated that 99 percent of the receptors are "spare." This constitutes an immense functional reserve that ensures adequate amounts of glucose enter the cell. On the other end of the scale is the human heart, in which about five to ten percent of the total β adrenoceptors are spare. An important implication of this observation is that little functional reserve exists in the failing heart; most receptors must be occupied to obtain maximum contractility.

F. Desensitization of receptors

Repeated or continuous administration of an agonist (or an antagonist) may lead to changes in the responsiveness of the receptor. To prevent potential damage to the cell (for example, high concentrations of calcium initiating cell death), several mechanisms have evolved to protect a cell from excessive stimulation. When repeated administration of a drug results in a diminished effect, the phenomenon is called tachyphylaxis. The receptor becomes desensitized to the action of the drug (Figure 2.5). Other types of desensitization occur when receptors are down-regulated. Binding of the agonist results in molecular changes in the membrane-bound receptors such that the receptor undergoes endocytosis and is sequestered from further agonist interaction. These receptors may be recycled to the cell surface, restoring sensitivity, or, alternatively, may be further processed and degraded, decreasing the total number of receptors available. Some receptors, particularly voltage-gated channels, require a finite time (rest period) following stimulation before they can be activated again. During this recovery phase they are said to be "refractory" or "unresponsive."

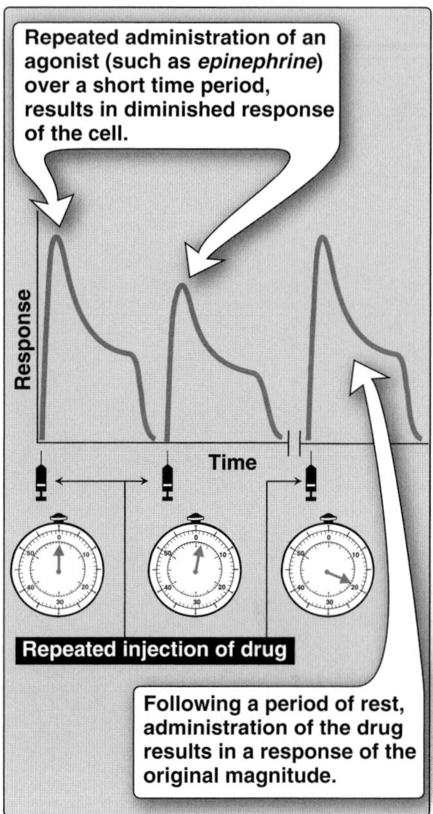

Figure 2.5
Desensitization of receptors.

IV. DOSE-RESPONSE RELATIONSHIPS

An agonist is defined as an agent that can bind to a receptor and elicit a response. The magnitude of the drug effect depends on its concentration at the receptor site, which in turn is determined by the dose of drug administered and by factors characteristic of the drug, such as rate of absorption, distribution, and metabolism.

A. Graded dose-response relations

As the concentration of a drug increases, the magnitude of its pharmacologic effect also increases. The relationship between dose and response is a continuous one, and can be mathematically described for many systems by application of the law of mass action, assuming the most simple model of drug binding:

$$[\text{Drug}] + [\text{Receptor}] \rightleftarrows [\text{Drug-receptor complex}]$$

The response is a graded effect, meaning that the response is continuous and gradual. This contrasts with a quantal, which describes an all-or-nothing response. A graph of the relationship is known as a graded dose-response curve. Plotting the magnitude of the response against increasing doses of a drug produces a graph that has the general shape depicted in Figure 2.6A. The curve can be described as a rectangular hyperbola—a very familiar curve in biology, because it can be applied to diverse biological events, such as ligand binding, enzymatic activity, and responses to pharmacologic agents.

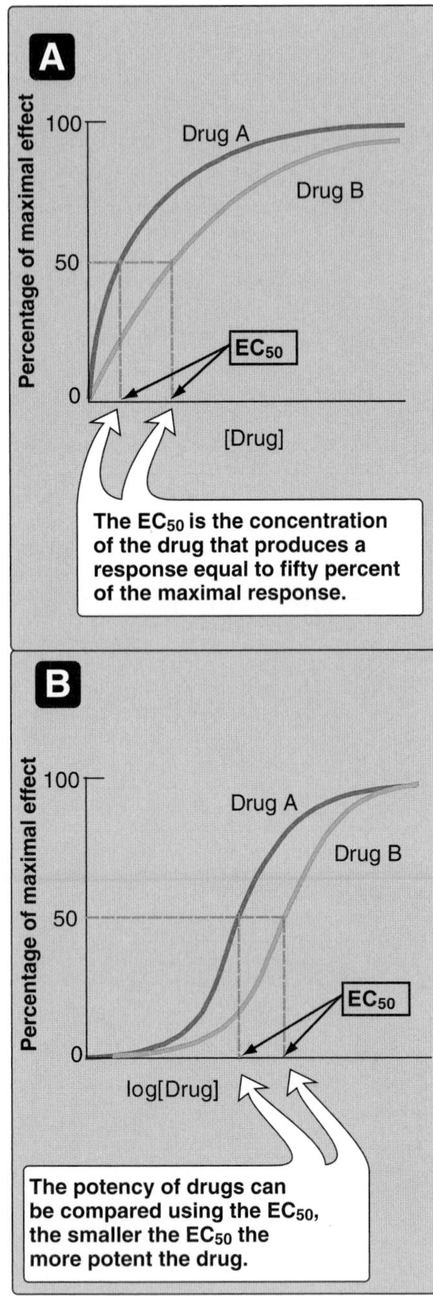

Figure 2.6
The effect of dose on the magnitude of pharmacologic response. Panel A is a linear graph. Panel B is a semi-logarithmic plot of the same data.

1. **Potency:** Two important properties of drugs can be determined by graded dose-response curves. The first is potency, a measure of the amount of drug necessary to produce an effect of a given magnitude. For a number of reasons, the concentration producing an effect that is fifty percent of the maximum is used to determine potency; it commonly designated as the EC_{50}. In Figure 2.6 the EC_{50} for Drugs A and B are indicated. Drug A is more potent than Drug B. An important contributing factor to the dimension of the EC_{50} is the affinity of the drug for the receptor. Semilogarithmic plots are often employed, because the range of doses (or concentrations) may span several orders of magnitude. By plotting the log of the concentration, the complete range of doses can be graphed. As shown in Figure 2.6B, the curves become sigmoidal in shape. It is also easier to visually estimate the EC_{50}.

2. **Efficacy:** The second drug property that can be determined from graded dose-response plots is the efficacy of the drug. Efficacy is dependent on the number of drug-receptor complexes formed, and the efficiency of coupling of receptor activation to cellular responses. Analogous to the maximal velocity for enzyme catalyzed reactions, the maximal response (E_{max}) or efficacy is more important than drug potency. A drug with greater efficacy is more therapeutically beneficial than one that is more potent. Figure 2.7 shows the response to drugs of differing potency and efficacy.

3. **Drug-receptor binding:** The quantitative relationship between drug concentration and receptor occupancy applies the law of mass action to the kinetics of the binding of drug and receptor molecules. By making the assumption that the binding of one drug molecule does not alter the binding of subsequent molecules, we can mathematically express the relationship between the percentage or fraction of bound receptors and the drug concentration

$$\frac{[D-R]}{[R_t]} = \frac{[D]}{K_d + [D]} \qquad (1)$$

where [D] = the concentration of free drug; [D – R] = the concentration of bound drug; $[R_t]$ = the total concentration of receptors, and is equal to the sum of the concentrations of unbound (free) receptors and bound receptors; and K_d = [D][R]/[DR], and is the dissociation constant for the drug from the receptor. Equation (1) defines a curve that has the shape of a rectangular hyperbola (Figure 2.8). As the concentration of free drug increases, the ratio of the concentrations of bound receptor to total receptor approaches unity. Doses are often plotted on a logarithmic scale, because the range from lowest to highest concentrations or doses often spans several orders of magnitude. It is important to note the similarity between these curves and those representing the relationship between dose and effect.

4. Relationship of binding to effect: The binding of the drug to its receptor initiates events that ultimately lead to a measurable biologic response. The mathematical model that describes drug concentration and receptor binding can be applied to dose (drug concentration) and response (or effect), providing the following assumptions are met: 1) the magnitude of the response is proportional to the amount of receptors bound or occupied, 2) the E_{max} occurs when all receptors are bound, and 3) binding of the drug to the receptor exhibits no cooperativity. In this case,

$$\frac{[E]}{[E_{max}]} = \frac{[D]}{K_d + [D]} \quad (2)$$

where [E] = the effect of the drug at concentration [D], and $[E_{max}]$ = the maximal efffect of the drug.

5. Agonists: If a drug binds to a receptor and produces a biologic response that mimics the response to the endogenous ligand, it is known as an agonist. For example, *phenylephrine* is an agonist at α_1 adrenoceptors, because it produces effects that resemble the action of the endogenous ligand, *norepinephrine*. Upon binding to α_1 adrenoceptors on the membranes of vascular smooth muscle, *phenylephrine* mobilizes intracellular Ca^{2+}, causing contraction of the actin and myosin filaments. The shortening of the muscle cells decreases the diameter of the arteriole, causing an increase in resistance to flow of blood through the vessel. Blood pressure therefore rises to maintain the blood flow. As this brief description illustrates, an agonist may have many effects that can be measured, including actions on intracellular molecules, cells, tissues, and intact organisms. All of these actions are attributable to interaction of the drug molecule with the receptor molecule.

6. Antagonists: Antagonists are drugs that decrease the actions of another drug or endogenous ligand. Antagonism may occur in several ways. Many antagonists act on the identical receptor macromolecule as the agonist. Antagonists, however, have no intrinsic activity and, therefore, produce no effect by themselves. If both the antagonist and the agonist bind to the same site on the receptor, they are said to be "competitive." For example, the antihypertensive drug *prazosin* competes with the endogenous ligand, norepinephrine, at α_1 adrenoceptors, decreasing vascular smooth muscle tone and reducing blood pressure. Plotting the effect of the competitive antagonist characteristically causes a shift of the agonist dose-response curve to the right. Competitive antagonists have no intrinsic activity. If the antagonist binds to a site other then where the agonist binds, the interaction is "noncompetitive" or "allosteric" (Figure 2.9). [Note: A drug may also act as a chemical antagonist by combining with another drug and rendering it inactive. For example, *protamine* ionically binds to *heparin*, rendering it inactive and antagonizing *heparin's* anticoagulant effect.]

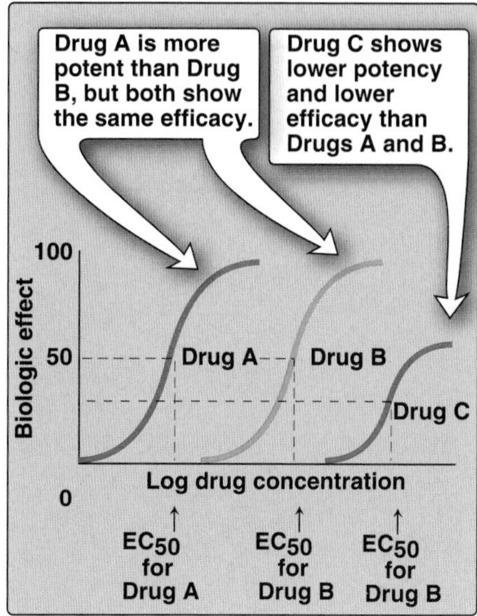

Figure 2.7
Typical dose-response curve for drugs showing differences in potency and efficacy. (EC_{50} = drug dose that shows fifty percent of maximal response.)

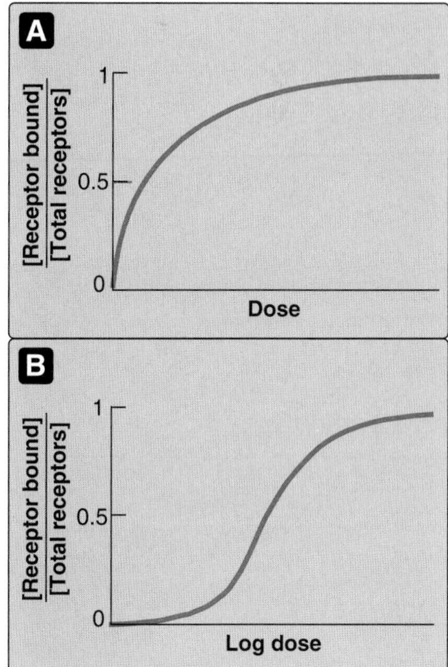

Figure 2.8
The effect of dose on the magnitude of drug binding.

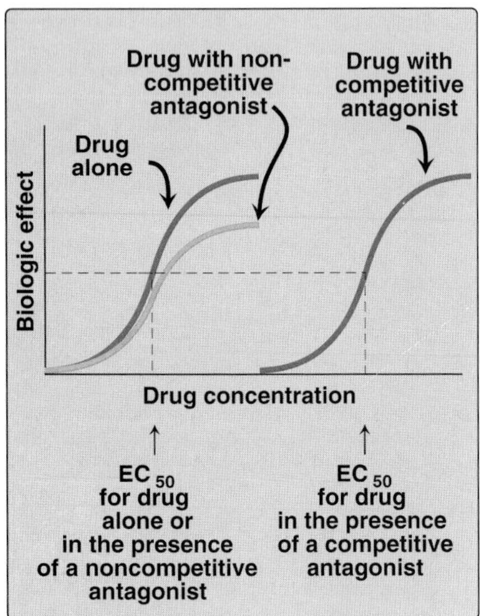

Figure 2.9
Effects of drug antagonists.

7. **Functional antagonism:** An antagonist may act at a completely separate receptor, initiating effects that are functionally the opposite of the agonist. A classic example is the antagonism by *epinephrine* to histamine-induced bronchoconstriction. Histamine binds to H_1 histamine receptors on bronchial smooth muscle, causing contraction and narrowing of the bronchial tree. Epinephrine is an agonist at β_2 adrenoceptors on bronchial smooth muscle, which causes the muscles to actively relax. This functional antagonism is also known as "physiologic antagonism."

8. **Partial agonists:** Partial agonists have efficacies (intrinsic activities) greater than zero but less than that of a full agonist. Even if all the receptors are occupied, partial agonists cannot produce an E_{max} of as great a magnitude as that of a full agonist. However, a partial agonist may have an affinity that is greater than, less than, or equivalent to that of a full agonist. A unique feature of these drugs is that under appropriate conditions, a partial agonist may act as an antagonist of a full agonist. Consider what would happen to the E_{max} of an agonist in the presence of increasing concentrations of a partial agonist (Figure 2.10). As the number of receptors occupied by the partial agonist increases, the E_{max} would decrease until it reached the E_{max} of the partial agonist. This potential of partial agonists to act both agonistically and antagonistically may be therapeutically exploited. For example, *aripiperazole*, an atypical neuroleptic agent, is a partial agonist at selected dopamine receptors. Dopaminergic pathways that were overactive would tend to be inhibited by the partial agonist, whereas pathways that were underactive may be stimulated. This might explain the ability of *aripiperazole* to improve many of the symptoms of schizophrenia, with a small risk of causing extrapyramidal adverse effects.

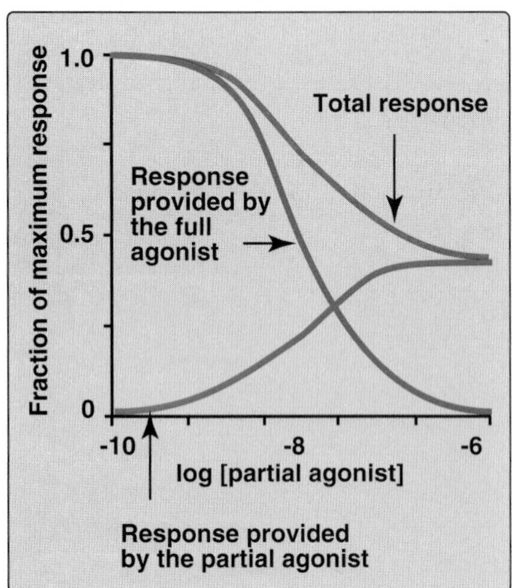

Figure 2.10
Effects of partial agonists.

V. QUANTAL DOSE-RESPONSE RELATIONSHIPS

Another important dose-response relationship is that of the influence of the magnitude of the dose on the proportion of a population that responds. These responses are known as quantal responses, because, for any individual, the effect either occurs or it does not. Even graded responses can be considered to be quantal if a predetermined level of the graded response is designated as the point at which a response occurs or not. For example, a quantal dose-response relationship can be determined in a population for the antihypertensive drug *atenolol*. A positive response is defined as at least a 5 mm Hg fall in diastolic blood pressure. Quantal dose-response curves are useful for determining doses to which most of the population responds.

A. Therapeutic index

The therapeutic index of a drug is the ratio of the dose that produces toxicity to the dose that produces a clinically desired or effective response in a population of individuals:

$$\text{Therapeutic index} = TD_{50}/ED_{50}$$

where TD_{50} = the drug dose that produces a toxic effect in half the population, and ED_{50} = the drug dose that produces a therapeutic or desired response in half the population. The therapeutic index is thus a measure of a drug's safety, because a large value indicates that there is a wide margin between doses that are effective and doses that are toxic.

B. Determination of therapeutic index

The therapeutic index is determined by measuring the frequency of desired response and toxic response at various doses of drug. By convention, the doses that produce the therapeutic effect and the toxic effect in fifty percent of the population are employed; these are known as the ED_{50} and TD_{50}, respectively. For example, Figure 2.11 shows the responses to *warfarin*, an oral anticoagulant with a narrow therapeutic index, and *penicillin*, an antimicrobial drug with a large therapeutic index.

1. **Warfarin (example of a drug with a small therapeutic index):** As the dose of warfarin is increased, a greater fraction of the patients respond (for this drug, the desired response is a two-fold increase in prothrombin time) until eventually all patients respond (see Figure 2.11A). However, at higher doses of *warfarin*, a toxic response occurs, namely a high degree of anticoagulation that results in hemorrhage. Note that when the therapeutic index is low, it is possible to have a range of concentrations where the effective and toxic responses overlap. That is, some patients hemorrhage, whereas others achieve the desired two-fold prolongation of prothrombin time. Variation in patient response is therefore most likely to occur with a drug showing a narrow therapeutic index, because the effective and toxic concentrations are similar. Agents with a low therapeutic index—that is, drugs in which dose is critically important—are those drugs in which bioavailability critically alters the therapeutic effects (see p. 7).

2. **Penicillin (example of a drug with a large therapeutic index):** For drugs with a large therapeutic index, such as *penicillin* (see Figure 2.11B), it is safe and common to give doses in excess (often about ten-fold excess) of that which is minimally required to achieve a desired response. In this case, bioavailability does not critically alter the therapeutic effects.

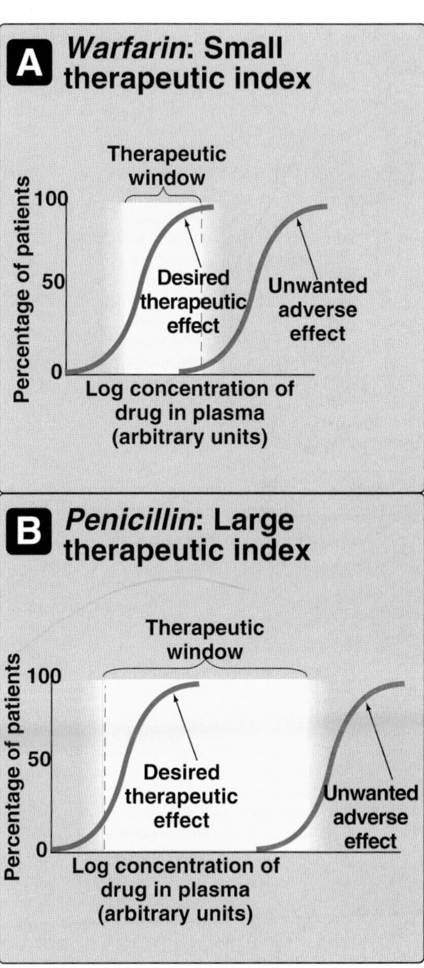

Figure 2.11
Cumulative percentage of patients responding to plasma levels of a drug.

Study Questions

Choose the ONE best answer.

2.1 Which of the following statements is correct?

A. If 10 mg of Drug A produces the same response as 100 mg of Drug B, Drug A is more efficacious than Drug B.
B. The greater the efficacy, the greater the potency of a drug.
C. In selecting a drug, potency is usually more important than efficacy.
D. A competitive antagonist increases the ED_{50}.
E. Variation in response to a drug among different individuals is most likely to occur with a drug showing a large therapeutic index.

Correct answer = D. In the presence of a competitive antagonist, a higher concentration of drug is required to elicit a given response. Efficacy and potency can vary independently, and the maximal response obtained is often more important than the amount of drug needed to achieve it. For example, in Choice A, no information is provided about the efficacy of Drug A, so all one can say is that Drug A is more potent than Drug B. Variability between patients in the pharmacokinetics of a drug is most important clinically when the effective and toxic doses are not very different, as is the case with a drug that shows a small therapeutic index.

2.2 Variation in the sensitivity of a population of individuals to increasing doses of a drug is best determined by which of the following?

A. Efficacy
B. Potency
C. Therapeutic Index
D. Graded dose-response curve
E. Quantal dose-response curve

Correct answer = E. Only a quantal dose-response curve gives information about differences in the sensitivity of individuals to increasing doses of a drug.

2.3 Which of the following statements most accurately describes a system having spare receptors?

A. The number of spare receptors determines the maximum effect.
B. Spare receptors are sequestered in the cytosol.
C. A single drug-receptor interaction results in many cellular response elements being activated.
D. Spare receptors are active even in the absence of agonist.
E. Agonist affinity for spare receptors is less than their affinity for non-spare receptors.

Correct answer = C. One explanation for the existence of spare receptors is that any one agonist-receptor binding event can lead to the activation of many more cellular response elements. Thus, only a small fraction of the total receptors need to be bound in order to elicit a maximum cellular response.

UNIT II: Drugs Affecting the Autonomic Nervous System

The Autonomic Nervous System

3

I. OVERVIEW

The autonomic nervous system, along with the endocrine system, coordinates the regulation and integration of bodily functions. The endocrine system sends signals to target tissues by varying the levels of blood-borne hormones. In contrast, the nervous system exerts its influence by the rapid transmission of electrical impulses over nerve fibers that terminate at effector cells, which specifically respond to the release of neuromediator substances. Drugs that produce their primary therapeutic effect by mimicking or altering the functions of the autonomic nervous system are called autonomic drugs and are discussed in the following four chapters. These autonomic agents act either by stimulating portions of the autonomic nervous system or by blocking the action of the autonomic nerves. This chapter outlines the fundamental physiology of the autonomic nervous system, and it describes the role of neurotransmitters in the communication between extracellular events and chemical changes within the cell.

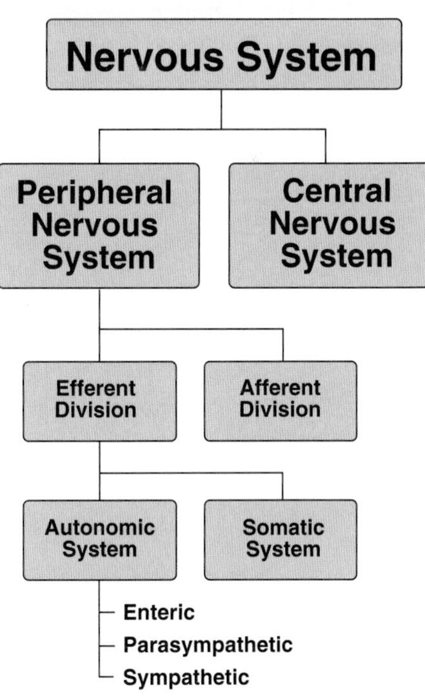

Figure 3.1
Organization of the nervous system.

II. INTRODUCTION TO THE NERVOUS SYSTEM

The nervous system is divided into two anatomical divisions: the central nervous system (CNS), which is composed of the brain and spinal cord, and the peripheral nervous system, which includes neurons located outside the brain and spinal cord—that is, any nerves that enter or leave the CNS (Figure 3.1). The peripheral nervous system is subdivided into the efferent division, the neurons of which carry signals away from the brain and spinal cord to the peripheral tissues, and the afferent division, the neurons of which bring information from the periphery to the CNS. Afferent neurons provide sensory input to modulate the function of the efferent division through reflex arcs.

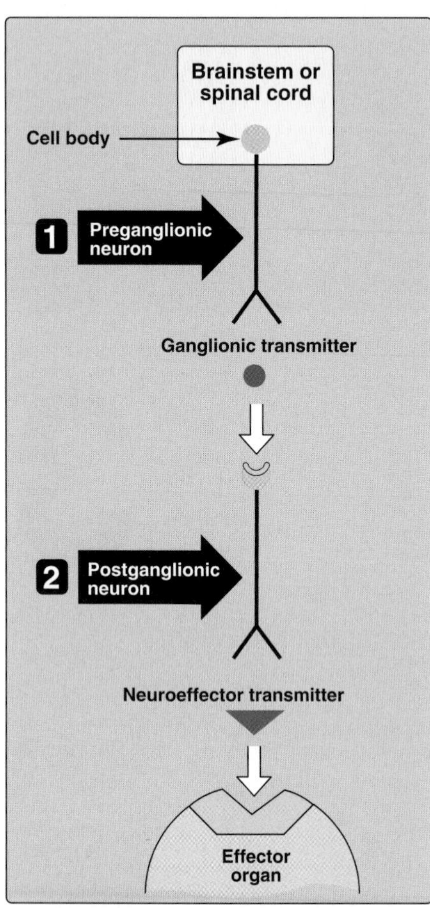

Figure 3.2
Efferent neurons of the autonomic nervous system.

A. Functional divisions within the nervous system

The efferent portion of the peripheral nervous system is further divided into two major functional subdivisions, the somatic and the autonomic systems (see Figure 3.1). The somatic efferent neurons are involved in the voluntary control of functions such as contraction of the skeletal muscles essential for locomotion. On the other hand, the autonomic system involuntarily regulates the everyday needs and requirements of the vital bodily functions without the conscious participation of the mind. It is composed of efferent neurons that innervate smooth muscle of the viscera, cardiac muscle, vasculature, and the exocrine glands, thereby controlling digestion, cardiac output, blood flow, and glandular secretions.

B. Anatomy of the autonomic nervous system

1. **Efferent neurons:** The autonomic nervous system carries nerve impulses from the CNS to the effector organs by way of two types of efferent neurons (Figure 3.2). The first nerve cell is called a preganglionic neuron, and its cell body is located within the CNS. Preganglionic neurons emerge from the brainstem or spinal cord and make a synaptic connection in ganglia (an aggregation of nerve cell bodies located in the peripheral nervous system). These ganglia function as relay stations between the preganglionic neuron and a second nerve cell, the postganglionic neuron. The latter neuron has a cell body originating in the ganglion. It is generally nonmyelinated and terminates on effector organs, such as smooth muscles of the viscera, cardiac muscle, and the exocrine glands.

2. **Afferent neurons:** The afferent neurons (fibers) of the autonomic nervous system are important in the reflex regulation of this system (for example, by sensing pressure in the carotid sinus and aortic arch), and signaling the CNS to influence the efferent branch of the system to respond (see below).

3. **Sympathetic neurons:** The efferent autonomic nervous system is divided into the sympathetic and the parasympathetic nervous systems (see Figure 3.1). Anatomically, they originate in the CNS and emerge from two different spinal cord regions. The preganglionic neurons of the sympathetic system come from thoracic and lumbar regions of the spinal cord, and they synapse in two cord-like chains of ganglia that run in parallel on each side of the spinal cord. The preganglionic neurons are short in comparison to the postganglionic ones. Axons of the postganglionic neuron extend from these ganglia to the tissues that they innervate and regulate (see Chapter 6). [Note: The adrenal medulla, like the sympathetic ganglia, receives preganglionic fibers from the sympathetic system. Lacking axons, the adrenal medulla, in response to stimulation by the ganglionic neurotransmitter acetylcholine, influences other organs by secreting the hormone epinephrine, also known as adrenaline, and lesser amounts of norepinephrine into the blood.]

4. **Parasympathetic neurons:** The parasympathetic preganglionic fibers arise from the cranium and from the sacral areas of the spinal cord and synapse in ganglia near or on the effector organs.

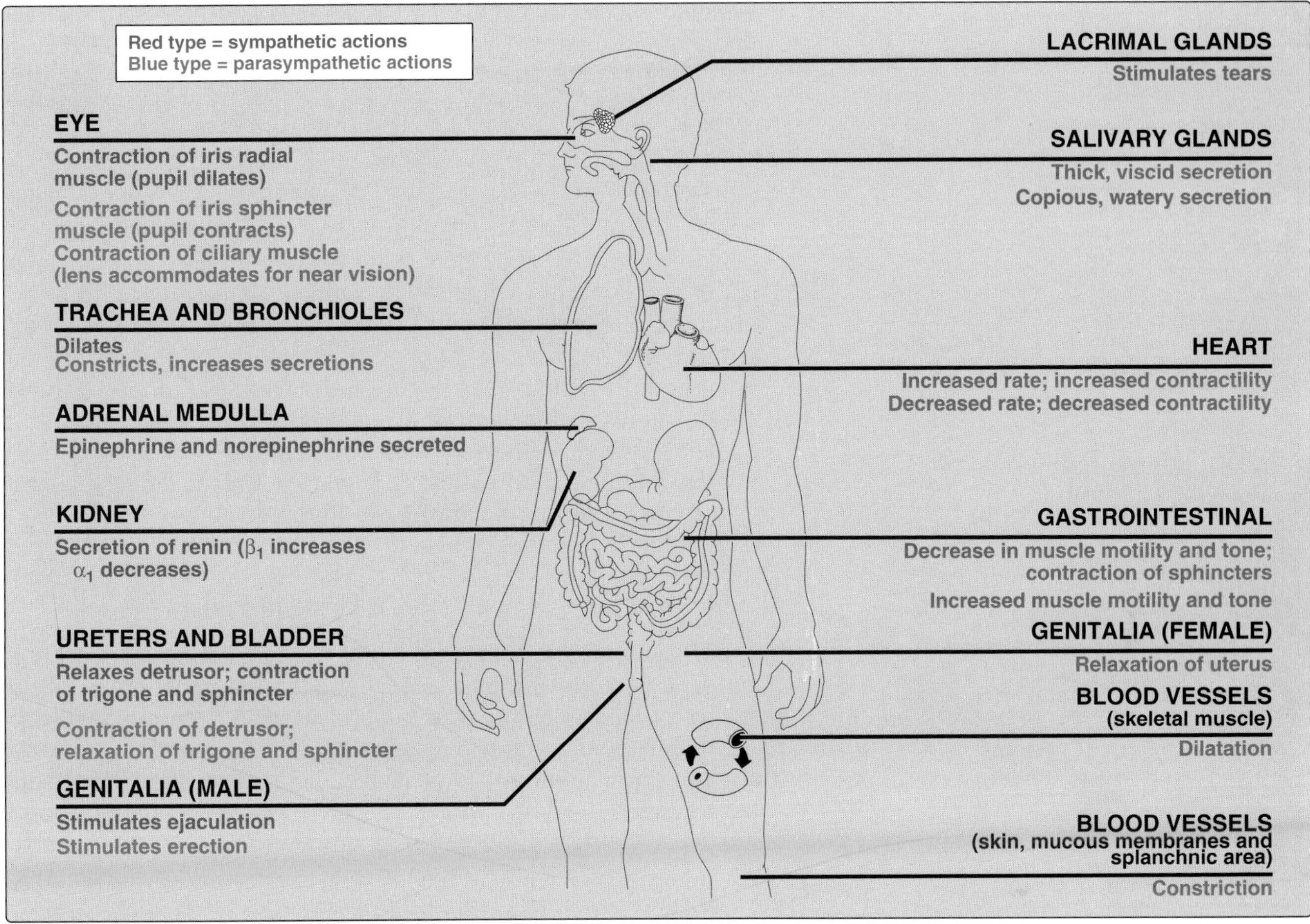

Figure 3.3
Action of sympathetic and parasympathetic nervous systems on effector organs.

Thus, in contrast to the sympathetic system, the preganglionic fibers are long, and the postganglionic ones are short.

5. **Enteric neurons:** The enteric nervous system is the third division of the autonomic nervous system. It is a collection of nerve fibers that innervate the gastrointestinal tract, pancreas, and gallbladder, and it constitutes the "brain of the gut." This system functions independently of the CNS and controls the motility, exocrine and endocrine secretions, and microcirculation of the gastrointestinal tract. It is modulated by both the sympathetic and parasympathetic nervous systems.

C. Functions of the sympathetic nervous system

Although continually active to some degree (for example, in maintaining the tone of vascular beds), the sympathetic division has the property of adjusting in response to stressful situations, such as trauma, fear, hypoglycemia, cold, or exercise.

1. **Effects of stimulation of the sympathetic division:** The effect of sympathetic output is to increase heart rate and blood pressure, to mobilize energy stores of the body, and to increase blood flow to

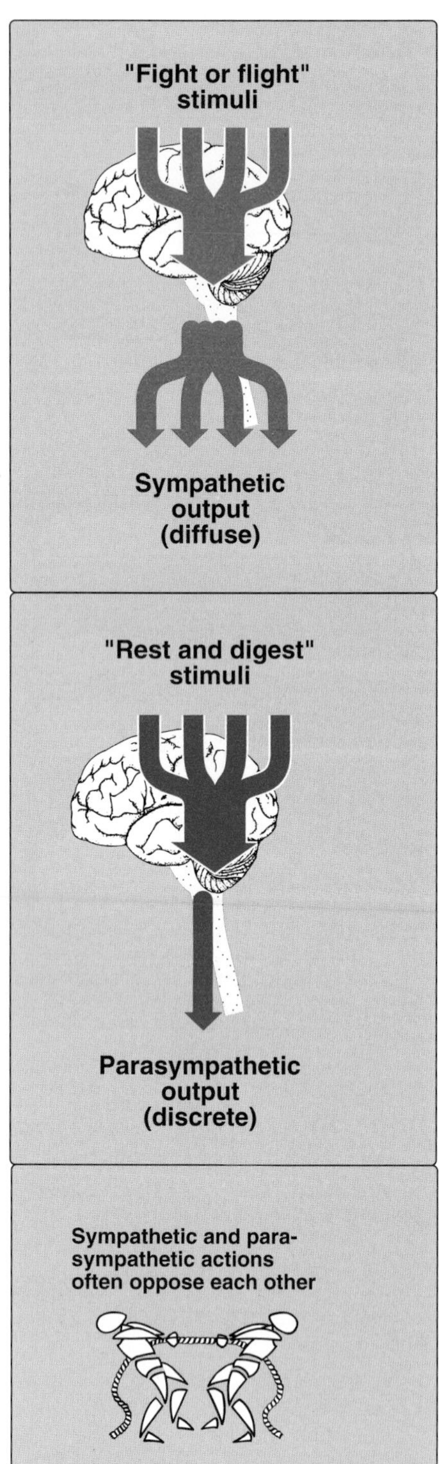

Figure 3.4
Sympathetic and parasympathetic actions are elicited by different stimuli.

skeletal muscles and the heart while diverting flow from the skin and internal organs. Sympathetic stimulation results in dilation of the pupils and the bronchioles (Figure 3.3). It also affects gastrointestinal motility, and the function of the bladder and sexual organs.

2. **Fight or flight response:** The changes experienced by the body during emergencies have been referred to as the "fight or flight" response (Figure 3.4). These reactions are triggered both by direct sympathetic activation of the effector organs, and by stimulation of the adrenal medulla to release epinephrine and lesser amounts of norepinephrine. These hormones enter the bloodstream and promote responses in effector organs that contain adrenergic receptors (see Figure 6.6). The sympathetic nervous system tends to function as a unit, and it often discharges as a complete system—for example, during severe exercise or in reactions to fear (see Figure 3.4). This system, with its diffuse distribution of postganglionic fibers, is involved in a wide array of physiologic activities, but it is not essential for life.

D. Functions of the parasympathetic nervous system

The parasympathetic division maintains essential bodily functions, such as digestive processes and elimination of wastes, and is required for life. It usually acts to oppose or balance the actions of the sympathetic division and is generally dominant over the sympathetic system in "rest and digest" situations. The parasympathetic system is not a functional entity as such, and never discharges as a complete system. If it did, it would produce massive, undesirable, and unpleasant symptoms. Instead, discrete parasympathetic fibers are activated separately, and the system functions to affect specific organs, such as the stomach or eye.

E. Role of the CNS in autonomic control functions

Although the autonomic nervous system is a motor system, it does require sensory input from peripheral structures to provide information on the state of affairs in the body. This feedback is provided by streams of afferent impulses, originating in the viscera and other autonomically innervated structures, that travel to integrating centers in the CNS—that is, the hypothalamus, medulla oblongata, and spinal cord. These centers respond to the stimuli by sending out efferent reflex impulses via the autonomic nervous system (Figure 3.5).

1. **Reflex arcs:** Most of the afferent impulses are translated into reflex responses without involving consciousness. For example, a fall in blood pressure causes pressure-sensitive neurons (baroreceptors in the heart, vena cava, aortic arch, and carotid sinuses) to send fewer impulses to cardiovascular centers in the brain. This prompts a reflex response of increased sympathetic output to the heart and vasculature and decreased parasympathetic output to the heart, which results in a compensatory rise in blood pressure and tachycardia (see Figure 3.5)

2. **Emotions and the autonomic nervous system:** Stimuli that evoke feelings of strong emotion, such as rage, fear, or pleasure, can modify the activity of the autonomic nervous system.

F. Innervation by the autonomic nervous system

1. **Dual innervation:** Most organs in the body are innervated by both divisions of the autonomic nervous system. Thus, vagal parasympathetic innervation slows the heart rate, and sympathetic innervation increases the heart rate. Despite this dual innervation, one system usually predominates in controlling the activity of a given organ. For example, in the heart, the vagus nerve is the predominant factor for controlling rate.

2. **Organs receiving only sympathetic innervation:** Although most tissues receive dual innervation, some effector organs, such as the adrenal medulla, kidney, pilomotor muscles, and sweat glands, receive innervation only from the sympathetic system. The control of blood pressure is also mainly a sympathetic activity, with essentially no participation by the parasympathetic system.

G. Somatic nervous system

The efferent somatic nervous system differs from the autonomic system in that a single myelinated motor neuron, originating in the CNS, travels directly to skeletal muscle without the mediation of ganglia. As noted earlier, the somatic nervous system is under voluntary control, whereas the autonomic is an involuntary system.

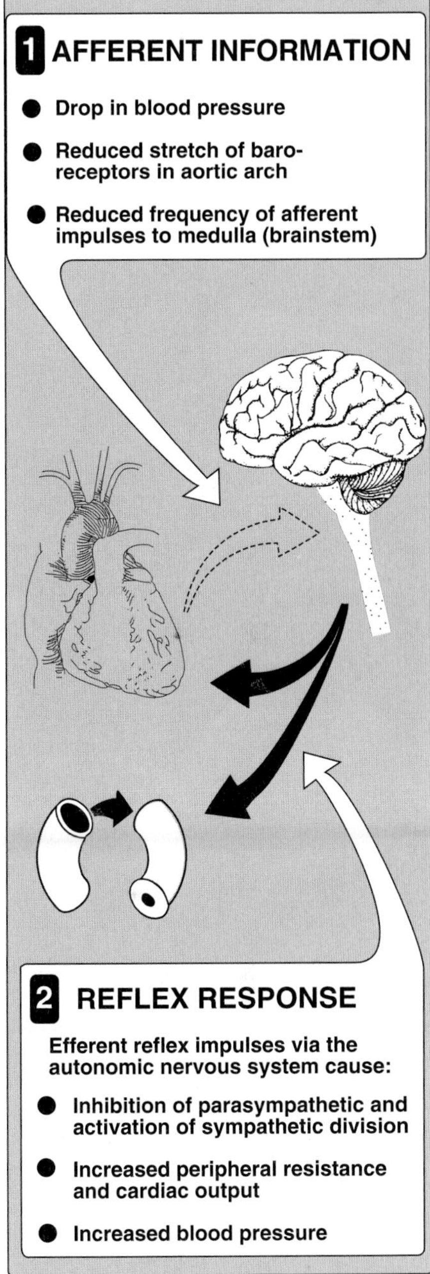

1 AFFERENT INFORMATION
Drop in blood pressure
Reduced stretch of baroreceptors in aortic arch
Reduced frequency of afferent impulses to medulla (brainstem)
2 REFLEX RESPONSE
Efferent reflex impulses via the autonomic nervous system cause:
Inhibition of parasympathetic and activation of sympathetic division
Increased peripheral resistance and cardiac output
Increased blood pressure

Figure 3.5
Baroreceptor reflex arc responds to a decrease in blood pressure.

III. CHEMICAL SIGNALING BETWEEN CELLS

Neurotransmission in the autonomic nervous system is an example of the more general process of chemical signaling between cells. In addition to neurotransmission, other types of chemical signaling are the release of local mediators and the secretion of hormones.

A. Local mediators

Most cells in the body secrete chemicals that act locally—that is, on cells in their immediate environment. These chemical signals are rapidly destroyed or removed; therefore they do not enter the blood and are not distributed throughout the body. Histamine (see p. 516) and the prostaglandins (see p.515) are examples of local mediators.

B. Hormones

Specialized endocrine cells secrete hormones into the bloodstream, where they travel throughout the body exerting effects on broadly distributed target cells in the body. (Hormones are described in Chapters 23 through 26.)

C. Neurotransmitters

All neurons are distinct anatomic units, and no structural continuity exists between most neurons. Communication between nerve cells—and between nerve cells and effector organs—occurs through the release of specific chemical signals, called neurotransmitters, from the nerve terminals. This release is triggered by the arrival of the action potential at the nerve ending, leading to depolarization. Uptake of Ca^{2+} ensues to initiate docking of the synaptic vesicles and release of their contents.The neurotransmitters rapidly

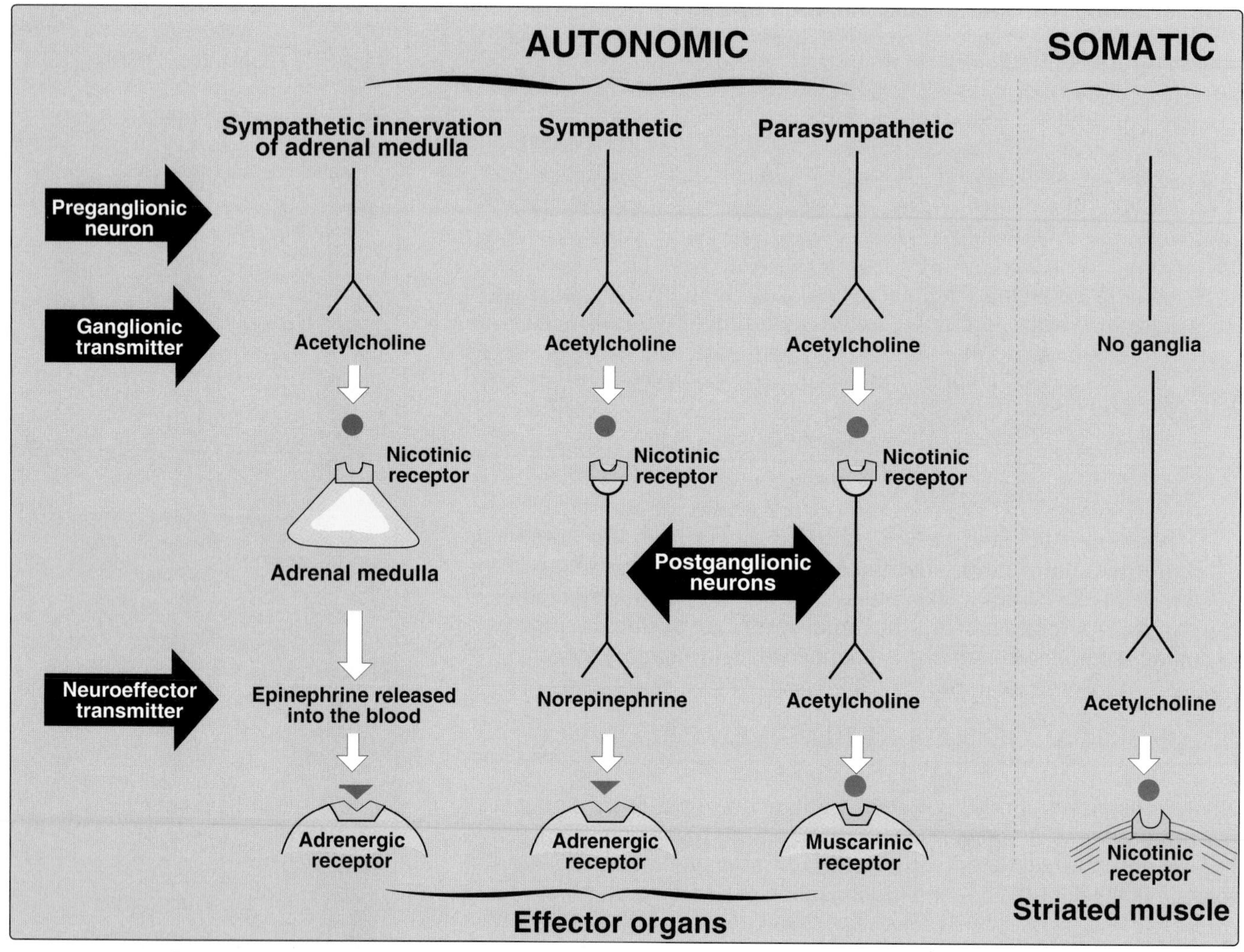

Figure 3.6
Summary of the neurotransmitters released and the types of receptors found within the autonomic and somatic nervous systems. [Note: This schematic diagram does not show that the parasympathetic ganglia are close to or on the surface of the effector organs and that the postganglionic fibers are usually shorter than the preganglionic fibers. By contrast, the ganglia of the sympathetic nervous system are close to the spinal cord. The postganglionic fibers are long, allowing extensive branching to innervate more than one organ system. This allows the sympathetic nervous system to discharge as a unit.]

diffuse across the synaptic cleft or gap (synapse) and combine with specific receptors on the postsynaptic (target) cell (Figure 3.6 and see Chapter 2).

1. **Membrane receptors:** All neurotransmitters and most hormones and local mediators are too hydrophilic to penetrate the lipid bilayer of target-cell plasma membranes. Instead, their signal is mediated by binding to specific receptors on the cell surface of target organs. [Note: A receptor is defined as a recognition site for a substance. It has a binding specificity, and it is coupled to processes that eventually evoke a response. Most receptors are proteins. They need not be located in the membrane.]

2. **Types of neurotransmitters:** Although over fifty signal molecules in the nervous system have tentatively been identified, six signal compounds—norepinephrine (and the closely related epinephrine), acetylcholine, dopamine, serotonin, histamine, and γ-aminobutyric acid—are most commonly involved in the actions of therapeutically useful drugs. Each of these chemical signals binds to a specific family of receptors. Acetylcholine and norepinephrine are the primary chemical signals in the autonomic nervous system, whereas a wide variety of neurotransmitters function in the CNS. Not only are these neurotransmitters released on nerve stimulation, cotransmitters, such as adenosine, often accompany them, and modulate the transmission process.

   a. **Acetylcholine:** The autonomic nerve fibers can be divided into two groups based on the chemical nature of the neurotransmitter released. If transmission is mediated by acetylcholine, the neuron is termed cholinergic (see Chapters 4 and 5). Acetylcholine mediates the transmission of nerve impulses across autonomic ganglia in both the sympathetic and parasympathetic nervous systems. It is the neurotransmitter at the adrenal medulla. Transmission from the autonomic postganglionic nerves to the effector organs in the parasympathetic system also involves the release of acetylcholine. In the somatic nervous system, transmission at the neuromuscular junction (that is, between nerve fibers and voluntary muscles) is also cholinergic (see Figure 3.6).

   b. **Norepinephrine and epinephrine:** When norepinephrine or epinephrine is the transmitter, the fiber is termed adrenergic (adrenaline being another name for epinephrine). In the sympathetic system, norepinephrine mediates the transmission of nerve impulses from autonomic postganglionic nerves to effector organs. Norepinephrine and adrenergic receptors are discussed in Chapters 6 and 7. A summary of the neuromediators released and the type of receptors within the peripheral nervous system is shown in Figure 3.6. [Note: A few sympathetic fibers, such as those involved in sweating, are cholinergic; for simplicity, they are not shown in the figure.]

IV. SECOND MESSENGER SYSTEMS IN INTRACELLULAR RESPONSE

The binding of chemical signals to receptors activates enzymatic processes within the cell membrane that ultimately result in a cellular response, such as the phosphorylation of intracellular proteins or changes in the conductivity of ion channels. A neurotransmitter can be thought of as a signal and a receptor as a signal detector and transducer. "Second messenger" molecules, produced in response to neurotransmitter binding to a receptor, translate the extracellular signal into a response that may be further propagated or amplified within the cell. Each component serves as a link in the communication between extracellular events and chemical changes within the cell (see Chapter 2).

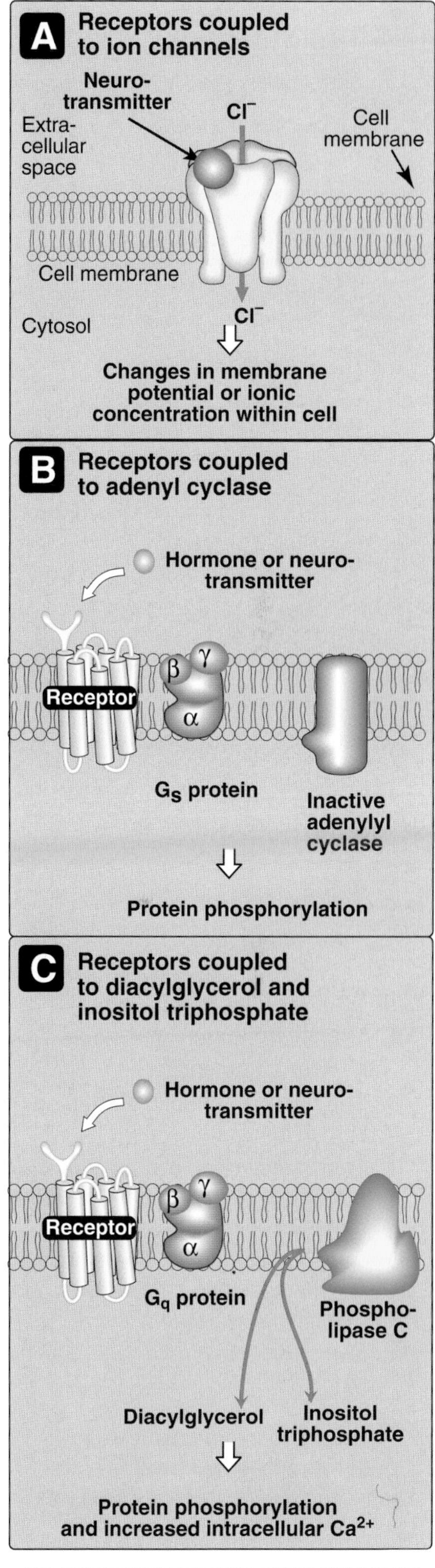

Figure 3.7
Three mechanisms whereby binding of a neurotransmitter leads to a cellular effect.

A. Membrane receptors affecting ion permeability

Neurotransmitter receptors are membrane proteins that provide a binding site that recognizes and responds to neurotransmitter molecules. Some receptors, such as the postsynaptic receptors of nerve or muscle, are directly linked to membrane ion channels; thus, binding of the neurotransmitter occurs rapidly (within fractions of a millisecond) and directly affects ion permeability (Figure 3.7A). [Note: The effect of acetylcholine on these chemically gated ion channels is discussed on p. 27.]

B. Regulation involving second messenger molecules

Many receptors are not directly coupled to ion gates. Rather, the receptor signals its recognition of a bound neurotransmitter by initiating a series of reactions, which ultimately results in a specific intracellular response. "Second messenger" molecules—so named because they intervene between the original message (the neurotransmitter or hormone) and the ultimate effect on the cell—are part of the cascade of events that translates neurotransmitter binding into a cellular response, usually through the intervention of a G protein. The two most widely recognized second messengers are the adenylyl cyclase system and the calcium/phosphatidylinositol system (Figure 3.7B and C). [Note: G_s is the protein involved in the activation of adenylyl cyclase, and G_q is the subunit that activates phospholipase C to release diacylglycerol and inositol triphosphate (see p. 27).]

Study Questions

Choose the ONE best answer.

3.1 Which one of the following statements concerning the parasympathetic nervous system is correct?

A. The parasympathetic system uses norepinephrine as a neurotransmitter.
B. The parasympathetic system often discharges as a single, functional system.
C. The parasympathetic division is involved in accommodation of near vision, movement of food, and urination.
D. The postganglionic fibers of the parasympathetic division are long compared to those of the sympathetic nervous system.
E. The parasympathetic system controls the secretion of the adrenal medulla.

Correct answer = C. The parasympathetic system maintains essential bodily functions, such as vision, movement of food, and urination. It uses acetylcholine, not norepinephrine, as a neurotransmitter, and it discharges as discrete fibers that are activated separately. The postganglionic fibers of the parasympathetic system are short compared to those of the sympathetic division. The adrenal medulla is under control of the sympathetic system.

3.2 Which one of the following is characteristic of parasympathetic stimulation?

A. Decrease in intestinal motility.
B. Inhibition of bronchial secretion.
C. Contraction of sphincter muscle in the iris of the eye (miosis).
D. Contraction of sphincter of urinary bladder.
E. Increase in heart rate.

Correct answer = C.

Cholinergic Agonists

4

I. OVERVIEW

Drugs affecting the autonomic nervous system are divided into two groups according to the type of neuron involved in their mechanism of action. The cholinergic drugs, which are described in this and the following chapter, act on receptors that are activated by acetylcholine. The second group—the adrenergic drugs (discussed in Chapters 6 and 7)—act on receptors that are stimulated by norepinephrine or epinephrine. The cholinergic and adrenergic drugs both act by either stimulating or blocking receptors of the autonomic nervous system. Figure 4.1 summarizes the cholinergic agonists discussed in this chapter.

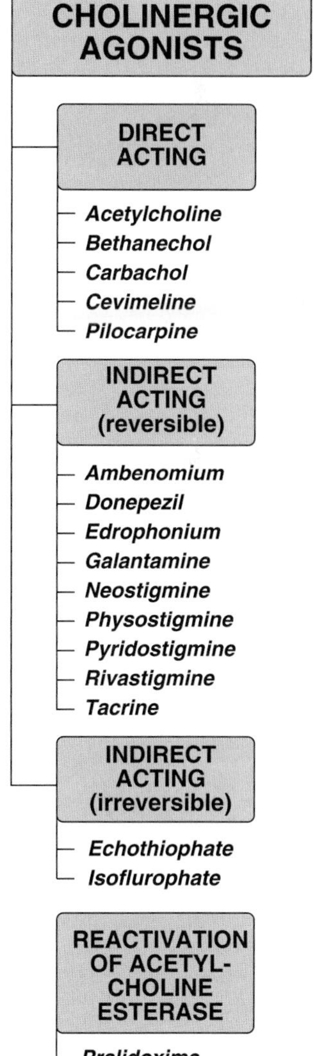

Figure 4.1
Summary of cholinergic agonists.

II. THE CHOLINERGIC NEURON

The preganglionic fibers terminating in the adrenal medulla, the autonomic ganglia (both parasympathetic and sympathetic), and the postganglionic fibers of the parasympathetic division use acetylcholine as a neurotransmitter (Figure 4.2). In addition, cholinergic neurons innervate the muscles of the somatic system, and also play an important role in the central nervous system (CNS). [Note: Patients with Alzheimer disease have a significant loss of cholinergic neurons in the temporal lobe and entorhinal cortex. Most of the drugs available to treat the disease at this time are acetylcholinesterase inhibitors (see p. 52).]

A. Neurotransmission at cholinergic neurons

Neurotransmission in cholinergic neurons involves six steps. The first four—synthesis, storage, release, and binding of the acetylcholine—to a receptor, are followed by the fifth step, degradation of the neurotransmitter in the synaptic gap (that is, the space between the nerve endings and adjacent receptors located on nerves or effector organs), and the sixth step, the recycling of choline (Figure 4.3).

1. **Synthesis of acetylcholine:** Choline is transported from the extracellular fluid into the cytoplasm of the cholinergic neuron by a carrier system that cotransports sodium, and can be inhibited by the drug *hemicholinium*. [Note: Choline has a quarternary nitrogen and carries a permanent positive charge and, thus, cannot dif-

fuse through the membrane.] The uptake of choline is the rate-limiting step in acetylcholine synthesis. Choline acetyltransferase catalyzes the reaction of choline with acetyl CoA to form acetylcholine—an ester—in the cytosol.

2. **Storage of acetylcholine in vesicles:** The acetylcholine is packaged into vesicles by an active transport process coupled to the efflux of protons. The mature vesicle contains not only acetylcholine but also adenosine triphosphate (ATP) and proteoglycan. The function of the latter substances in the nerve terminal is not completely understood. [Note: ATP has been suggested to act at prejunctional purinergic receptors to inhibit the release of acetylcholine or norepinephrine.]

3. **Release of acetylcholine:** When an action potential propagated by the action of voltage-sensitive sodium channels arrives at a nerve ending, voltage-sensitive calcium channels in the presynaptic membrane open, causing an increase in the concentration of intracellular calcium. Elevated calcium levels promote the fusion

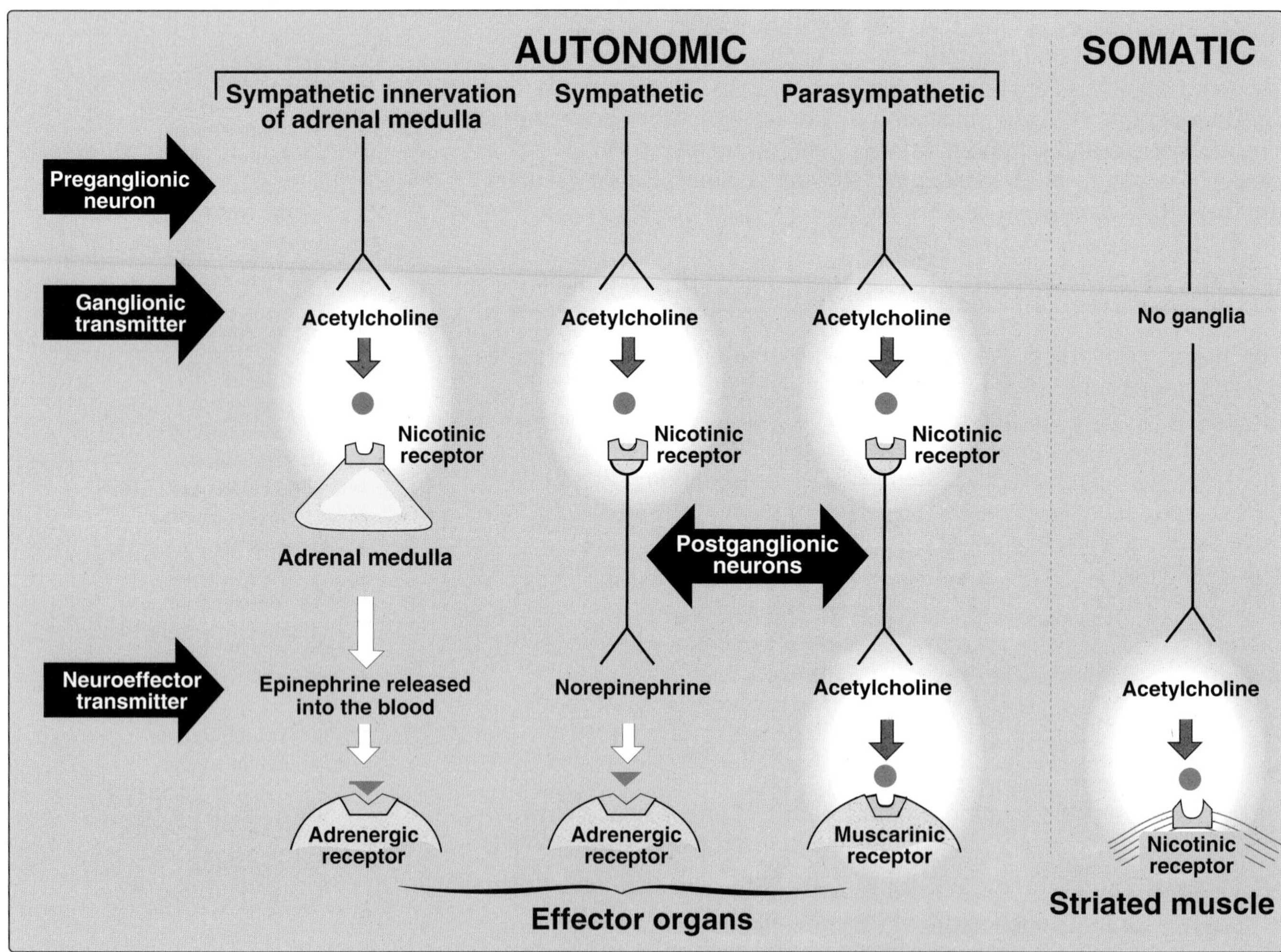

Figure 4.2
Sites of actions of cholinergic agonists in the autonomic and somatic nervous systems.

of synaptic vesicles with the cell membrane and release of their contents into the synaptic cleft. This release can be blocked by botulinum toxin. In contrast, the toxin in black widow spider venom causes all the acetylcholine stored in synaptic vesicles to empty into the synaptic gap.

4. **Binding to the receptor:** Acetylcholine released from the synaptic vesicles diffuses across the synaptic space, and binds to either of two postsynaptic receptors on the target cell or to presynaptic receptors in the membrane of the neuron that released the acetylcholine. [Note: The two different classes of postsynaptic cholinergic receptors on the membrane surface of the effector cell are called muscarinic and nicotinic. (See Figure 4.2 and below.)] Binding to a receptor leads to a biological response within the cell,

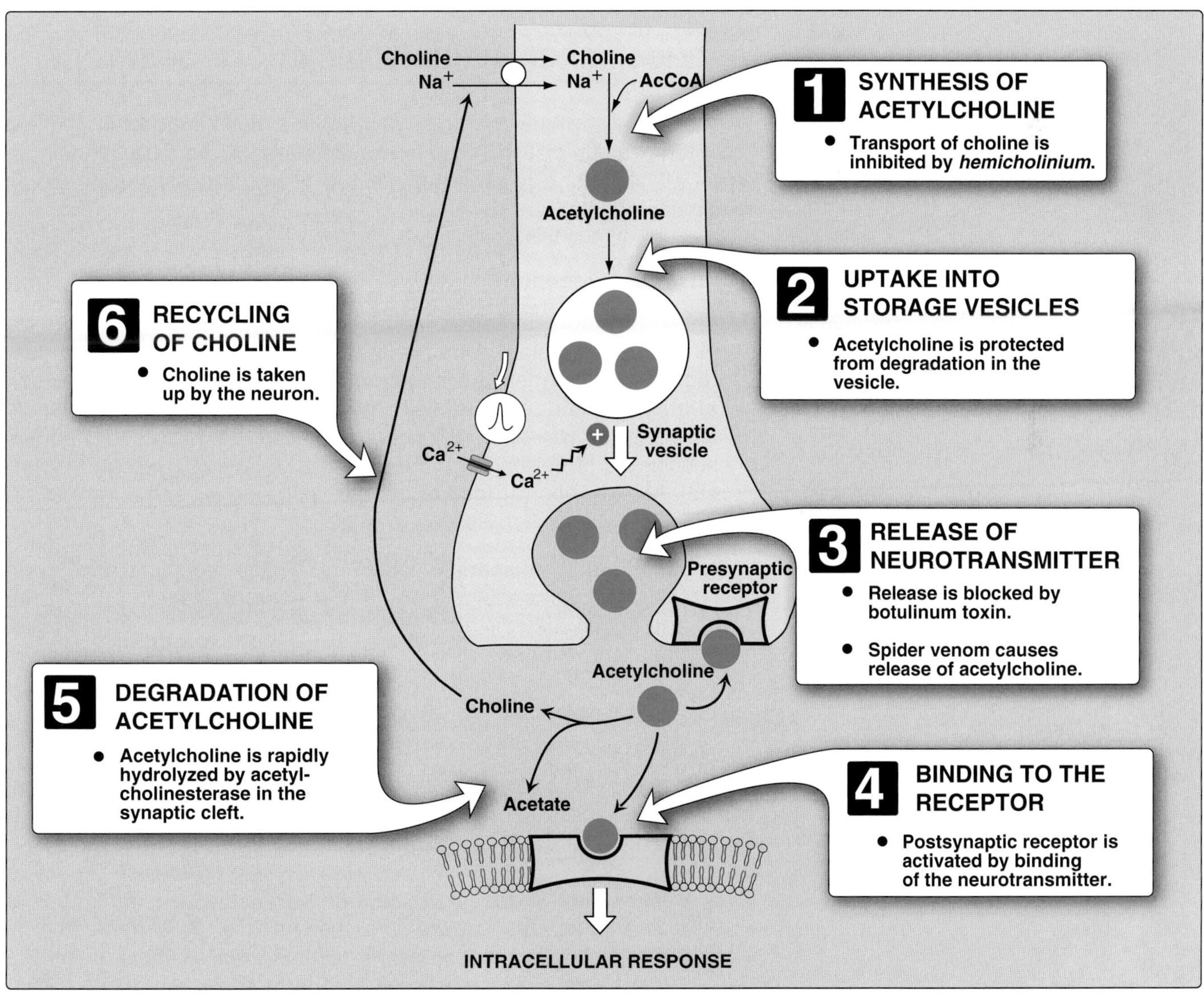

Figure 4.3
Synthesis and release of acetylcholine from the cholinergic neuron. AcCoA = acetyl CoA.

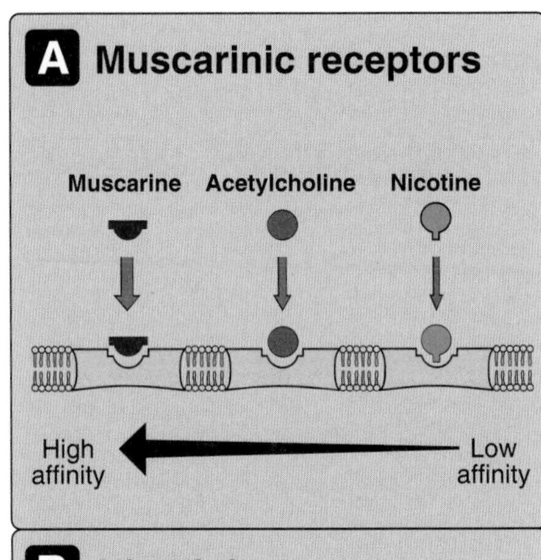

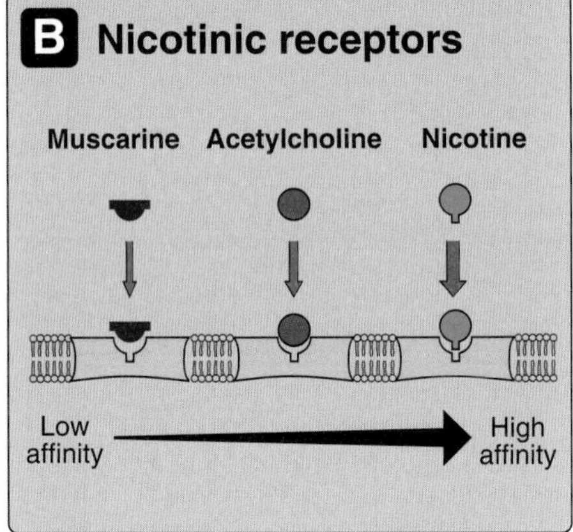

Figure 4.4
Types of cholinergic receptors.

such as the initiation of a nerve impulse in a postganglionic fiber or activation of specific enzymes in effector cells as mediated by second messenger molecules (see p. 27 and below).

5. **Degradation of acetylcholine:** The signal at the postjunctional effector site is rapidly terminated, because acetylcholinesterase cleaves acetylcholine to choline and acetate in the synaptic cleft (see Figure 4.3). [Note: Butyrylcholinesterase, sometimes called pseudocholinesterase, is found in the plasma, but it does not play a significant role in termination of the acetylcholine's effect in the synapse.]

6. **Recycling of choline:** Choline may be recaptured by a sodium-coupled, high-affinity uptake system that transports the molecule back into the neuron, where it is acetylated and stored until released by a subsequent action potential.

III. CHOLINERGIC RECEPTORS (CHOLINOCEPTORS)

Two families of cholinoceptors, designated muscarinic and nicotinic receptors, can be distinguished from each other on the basis of their different affinities for agents that mimic the action of acetylcholine (cholinomimetic agents).

A. Muscarinic receptors

These receptors, in addition to binding acetylcholine, also recognize muscarine, an alkaloid that is present in certain poisonous mushrooms. By contrast, the muscarinic receptors show only a weak affinity for nicotine (Figure 4.4A). Binding studies and specific inhibitors, as well as cDNA characterization, have distinguished five subclasses of muscarinic receptors: M_1, M_2, M_3, M_4, and M_5. In general, M_1, M_3, and M_5 lead to cellular excitation, whereas M_2 and M_4 inhibit cellular excitability.

1. **Locations of muscarinic receptors:** These receptors have been found on ganglia of the peripheral nervous system and on the autonomic effector organs, such as the heart, smooth muscle, brain and exocrine glands (see Figure 3.3, p. 37). Specifically, although all five subtypes have been found on neurons, M_1 receptors are also found on gastric parietal cells, M_2 receptors on cardiac cells and smooth muscle, and M_3 receptors on the bladder, exocrine glands, and smooth muscle. [Note: Drugs with muscarinic actions preferentially stimulate muscarinic receptors on these tissues, but at high concentration they may show some activity at nicotinic receptors.]

2. **Mechanisms of acetylcholine signal transduction:** A number of different molecular mechanisms transmit the signal generated by acetylcholine occupation of the receptor. For example, when the M_1 or M_3 receptors are activated, the receptor undergoes a conformational change and interacts with a G protein, designated G_q, which in turn activates phospholipase C.[1] This leads to the

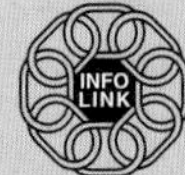

[1]See p. 203 in ***Lippincott's Illustrated Reviews: Biochemistry*** (3rd ed.) for a discussion of of inositol trisphosphate and intracellular signaling.

hydrolysis of phoshatidylinositol-(4,5)-bisphosphate (PIP_2) to yield diacylglycerol (DAG) and inositol (1,4,5)-trisphosphate (IP_3), which cause an increase in intracellular Ca^{2+} (see Figure 3.7C, p. 41). This cation can then interact to stimulate or inhibit enzymes, or cause hyperpolarization, secretion, or contraction. In contrast, activation of the M_2 subtype on the cardiac muscle stimulates a G protein, designated G_i, that inhibits adenylyl cyclase[2], and increases K^+ conductance (see Figure 3.7B, p. 41), to which the heart responds with a decrease in rate and force of contraction.

3. **Muscarinic agonists and antagonists:** Attempts are currently underway to develop muscarinic agonists and antagonists that are directed against specific receptor subtypes. For example, *pirenzepine*, a tricyclic anticholinergic drug, has a greater selectivity for inhibiting M_1 muscarinic receptors, such as in the gastric mucosa. At therapeutic doses, *pirenzepine* does not cause many of the side effects seen with the non-subtype-specific drugs; however, it does produce a reflex tachycardia on rapid infusion due to blockade of M_2 receptors in the heart. Therefore, the usefulness of *pirenzepine* as an alternative to proton pump inhibitors in the treatment of gastric and duodenal ulcers is questionable. *Darifenacin* is a competitive muscarinic receptor antagonist with a greater affinity for the M_3 receptor than for the other muscarinic receptors. The drug is used in the treatment of overactive bladder. [Note: At present, there are no clinically important agents that interact solely with the M_4 and M_5 receptors.]

4. **Nicotinic receptors:** These receptors, in addition to binding acetylcholine, also recognize nicotine but show only a weak affinity for muscarine (see Figure 4.4B). The nicotinic receptor is composed of five subunits, and functions as a ligand-gated channel (see Figure 3.7A). Binding of two acetylcholine molecules elicits a conformational change that allows the entry of sodium ions, resulting in the depolarization of the effector cell. Nicotine (or acetylcholine) initially stimulates and then blocks the receptor. Nicotinic receptors are located in the CNS, adrenal medulla, autonomic ganglia, and the neuromuscular junction. Those at the neuromuscular junction are sometimes designated N_M and the others N_N. The nicotinic receptors of autonomic ganglia differ from those of the neuromuscular junction. For example, ganglionic receptors are selectively blocked by *hexamethonium*, whereas neuromuscular junction receptors are specifically blocked by *tubocurarine*.

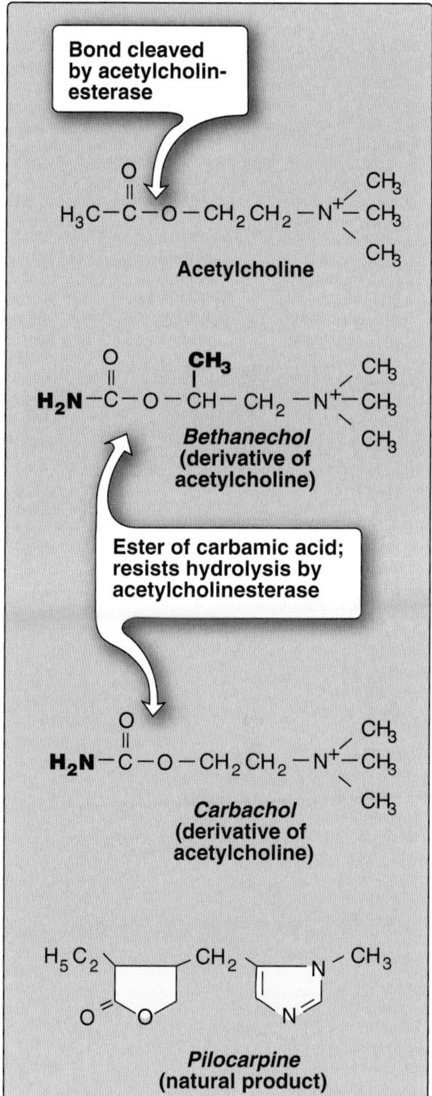

Figure 4.5
Comparison of the structures of some cholinergic agonists.

IV. DIRECT-ACTING CHOLINERGIC AGONISTS

Cholinergic agonists mimic the effects of acetylcholine by binding directly to cholinoceptors. These agents are synthetic esters of choline, such as *carbachol* and *bethanechol*, or naturally occurring alkaloids, such as *pilocarpine* (Figure 4.5). All the direct-acting cholinergic drugs have longer durations of action than acetylcholine. Some of the more therapeutically useful drugs (*pilocarpine* and *bethanechol*) preferentially bind to muscarinic receptors, and are sometimes referred to as mus-

INFO LINK [2]See p. 92 in ***Lippincott's Illustrated Reviews: Biochemistry*** (3rd ed.) for a discussion of adenylyl cyclase and intracellular signaling.

carinic agents. [Note: Muscarinic receptors are located primarily, but not exclusively, at the neuroeffector junction of the parasympathetic nervous system.] However, as a group, the direct-acting agonists show little specificity in their actions, which limits their clinical usefulness.

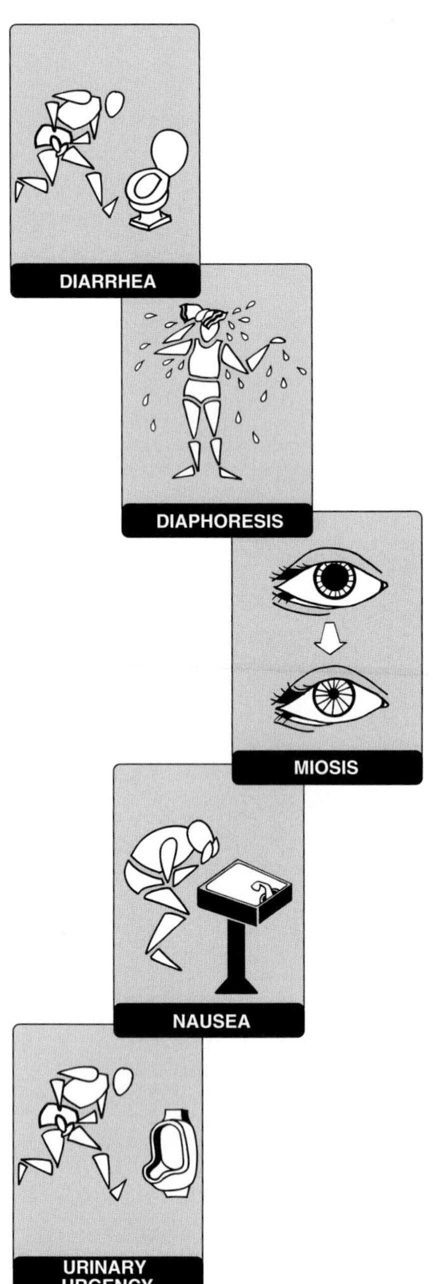

Figure 4.6
Some adverse effects observed with cholinergic drugs.

A. Acetylcholine

Acetylcholine [a se teel KOE leen] is a quarternary ammonium compound that cannot penetrate membranes. Although it is the neurotransmitter of parasympathetic and somatic nerves as well as ganglia, it is therapeutically of no importance because of its multiplicity of actions, and its rapid inactivation by the cholinesterases. Acetylcholine has both muscarinic and nicotinic activity. Its actions include:

1. **Decrease in heart rate and cardiac output:** The actions of acetylcholine on the heart mimic the effects of vagal stimulation. For example, acetylcholine, if injected intravenously, produces a brief decrease in cardiac rate and stroke volume as a result of a reduction in the rate of firing at the sinoatrial (SA) node. [Note: It should be remembered that normal vagal activity regulates the heart by the release of acetylcholine at the SA node.]

2. **Decrease in blood pressure:** Injection of acetylcholine causes vasodilation and lowering of blood pressure. Although no innervation of the vasculature by the parasympathetic system exists, there are cholinergic receptors on the blood vessels that respond by causing vasodilation. The vasodilation is due to an acetylcholine-induced rise in intracellular Ca^{2+}, caused by the phosphatidylinositol system, that results in the formation of nitric oxide (NO) from arginine in endothelial cells.[3] [Note: NO is also known as endothelium-derived relaxing factor (EDRF).] (See p. 208 for more detail on nitric oxide.) In the absence of administered cholinergic agents, the vascular receptors have no known function, because acetylcholine is never released into the blood in any significant quantities. *Atropine* blocks these muscarinic receptors and prevents acetylcholine from producing vasodilation.

3. **Other actions:** In the gastrointestinal tract, acetylcholine increases salivary secretion and stimulates intestinal secretions and motility. Bronchiolar secretions are also enhanced. In the genitourinary tract, the tone of the detrusor urinae muscle is increased. In the eye, acetylcholine is involved in stimulating ciliary muscle contraction for near vision, and in the constriction of the pupillae sphincter muscle, causing miosis (marked constriction of the pupil).

B. Bethanechol

Bethanechol [be THAN e kole] is structurally related to acetylcholine, in which the acetate is replaced by carbamate and the choline methylated (see Figure 4.5). Hence, it is not hydrolyzed by acetylcholinesterase, although it is inactivated through hydrolysis by other esterases. It lacks nicotinic actions but does have strong muscarinic activity. Its major actions are on the smooth musculature of

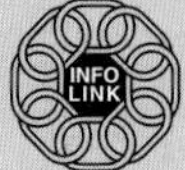

[3]See p. 383 in ***Lippincott's Illustrated Reviews: Biochemistry*** (3rd ed.) for a discussion of the roles of nitric oxide.

the bladder and gastrointestinal tract. It has a duration of action of about one hour.

1. **Actions:** *Bethanechol* directly stimulates muscarinic receptors, causing increased intestinal motility and tone. It also stimulates the detrusor muscles of the bladder while the trigone and sphincter are relaxed, causing expulsion of urine.

2. **Therapeutic applications:** In urologic treatment, *bethanechol* is used to stimulate the atonic bladder, particularly in postpartum or postoperative, nonobstructive urinary retention.

3. **Adverse effects:** *Bethanechol* causes the effects of generalized cholinergic stimulation (Figure 4.6). These include sweating, salivation, flushing, decreased blood pressure, nausea, abdominal pain, diarrhea, and bronchospasm.

C. Carbachol (carbamylcholine)

Carbachol [KAR ba kole] has both muscarinic as well as nicotinic actions. Like *bethanechol*, *carbachol* is an ester of carbamic acid and a poor substrate for acetylcholinesterase (see Figure 4.5). It is biotransformed by other esterases, but at a much slower rate. A single administration can last as long as one hour.

1. **Actions:** *Carbachol* has profound effects on both the cardiovascular system and the gastrointestinal system because of its ganglion-stimulating activity, and it may first stimulate and then depress these systems. It can cause release of epinephrine from the adrenal medulla by its nicotinic action. Locally instilled into the eye, it mimics the effects of acetylcholine, causing miosis and a spasm of accomodation.

2. **Therapeutic uses:** Because of its high potency and relatively long duration of action, *carbachol* is rarely used therapeutically except in the eye as a miotic agent to treat glaucoma by causing pupillary contraction and a decrease in intraocular pressure.

3. **Adverse effects:** At doses used ophthalmologically, little to no side effects occur.

D. Pilocarpine

The alkaloid *pilocarpine* [pye loe KAR peen] is a tertiary amine, and is stable to hydrolysis by acetylcholinesterase (see Figure 4.5). Compared with acetylcholine and its derivatives, it is far less potent. *Pilocarpine* exhibits muscarinic activity and is used primarily in ophthalmology.

1. **Actions:** Applied topically to the cornea, *pilocarpine* produces a rapid miosis and contraction of the ciliary muscle. The eye undergoes miosis and a spasm of accommodation; the vision is fixed at some particular distance, making it impossible to focus (Figure 4.7). [Note the opposing effects of *atropine*, a muscarinic blocker, on the eye (see p. 57).] *Pilocarpine* is one of the most potent stimulators of secretions such as sweat, tears, and saliva, but its use for producing these effects has been limited due to its lack of selectivity. Recent studies have shown that mouth sprays of the

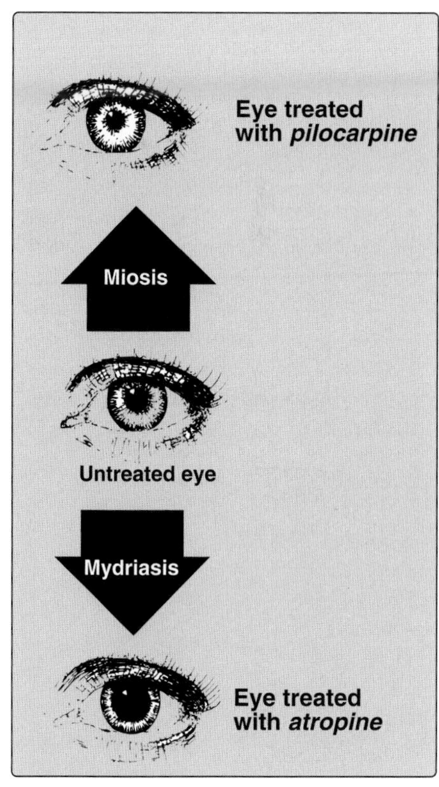

Figure 4.7
Actions of *pilocarpine* and *atropine* on the iris and ciliary muscle of the eye.

drug are beneficial in promoting salivation in patients with xerostomia resulting from irradiation of the head and neck. Sjögren syndrome, which is characterized by dry mouth and lack of tears is usually treated with *cevimeline*, a cholinergic drug that also has the drawback of being non-specific.

2. **Therapeutic use in glaucoma:** *Pilocarpine* is the drug of choice in the emergency lowering of intraocular pressure of both narrow-angle (also called closed-angle) and wide-angle (also called open-angle) glaucoma. *Pilocarpine* is extremely effective in opening the trabecular meshwork around Schlemm canal, causing an immediate drop in intraocular pressure as a result of the increased drainage of aqueous humor. This action lasts up to one day and can be repeated. The organophosphate *echothiophate* inhibits acetylcholinesterase, and exerts the same effect for a longer duration. [Note: Carbonic anhydrase inhibitors, such as *acetazolamide*, *epinephrine*, and the β-adrenergic blocker *timolol*, are effective in treating glaucoma chronically, but are not used for emergency lowering of intraocular pressure.]

3. **Adverse effects:** *Pilocarpine* can enter the brain and cause CNS disturbances. It stimulates profuse sweating and salivation.

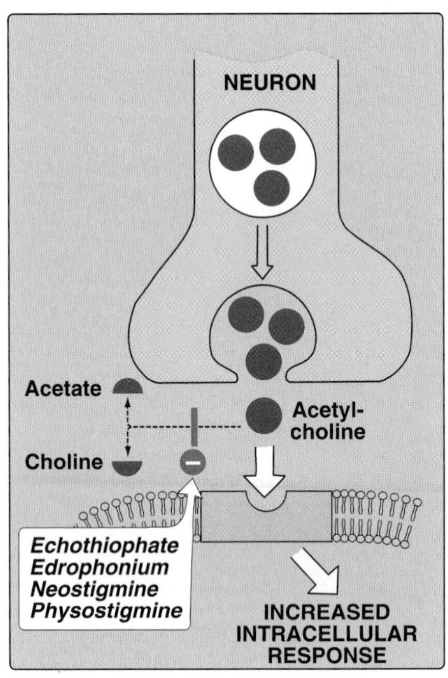

Figure 4.8
Mechanisms of action of indirect (reversible) cholinergic agonists.

V. ANTICHOLINESTERASES (REVERSIBLE)

Acetylcholinesterase is an enzyme that specifically cleaves acetylcholine to acetate and choline and, thus, terminates its actions. It is located both pre- and postsynaptically in the nerve terminal, where it is membrane bound. Inhibitors of acetylcholinesterase indirectly provide a cholinergic action by prolonging the lifetime of acetylcholine produced endogenously at the cholinergic nerve endings. This results in the accumulation of acetylcholine in the synaptic space (Figure 4.8). These drugs can thus provoke a response at all cholinoceptors in the body, including both muscarinic and nicotinic receptors of the autonomic nervous system, as well as at neuromuscular junctions and in the brain.

A. Physostigmine

Physostigmine [fi zoe STIG meen] is an alkaloid (a nitrogenous compound found in plants) and a tertiary amine. It is a carbamic acid ester and a substrate for acetylcholinesterase, and it forms a relatively stable carbamoylated intermediate with the enzyme, which then becomes reversibly inactivated. The result is potentiation of cholinergic activity throughout the body.

1. **Actions:** *Physostigmine* has a wide range of effects as a result of its action, and not only the muscarinic and nicotinic sites of the autonomic nervous system but also the nicotinic receptors of the neuromuscular junction are stimulated. Its duration of action is about two to four hours. *Physostigmine* can enter and stimulate the cholinergic sites in the CNS.

2. **Therapeutic uses**: The drug increases intestinal and bladder motility, which serve as its therapeutic action in atony of either organ (Figure 4.9). Placed topically in the eye, it produces miosis and spasm of accommodation, as well as a lowering of intraocular pressure. It is used to treat glaucoma, but *pilocarpine* is more effective. *Physostigmine* is also used in the treatment of overdoses of drugs with anticholinergic actions, such as *atropine*, *phenothiazines*, and tricyclic antidepressants.

3. **Adverse effects:** The effects of *physostigmine* on the CNS may lead to convulsions when high doses are used. Bradycardia and a fall in cardiac output may also occur. Inhibition of acetylcholinesterase at the skeletal neuromuscular junction causes the accumulation of acetylcholine and, ultimately, results in paralysis of skeletal muscle. However, these effects are rarely seen with therapeutic doses.

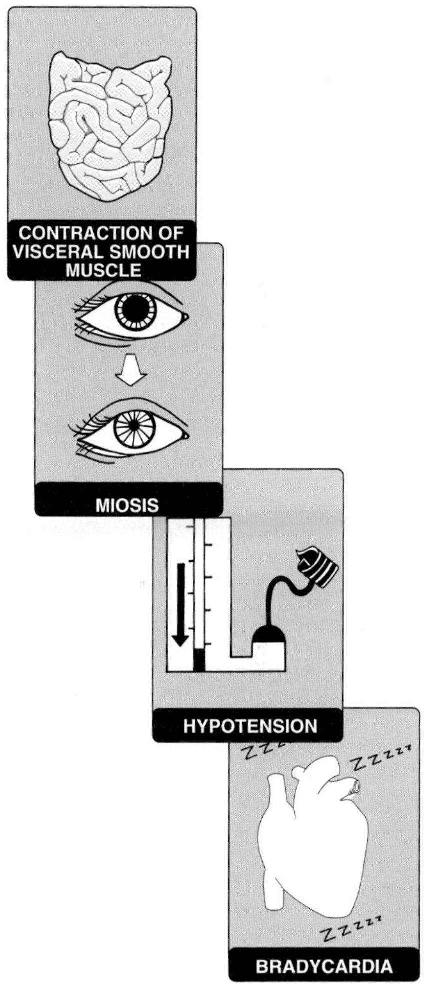

Figure 4.9
Some actions of *physostigmine*.

B. Neostigmine

Neostigmine [nee oh STIG meen] is a synthetic compound that is also a carbamic acid ester, and reversibly inhibits acetylcholinesterase in a manner similar to that of *physostigmine*. Unlike *physostigmine*, *neostigmine* has a quarternary nitrogen; hence, it is more polar and does not enter the CNS. Its effect on skeletal muscle is greater than that of *physostigmine*, and it can stimulate contractility before it paralyzes. *Neostigmine* has a moderate duration of action, usually thirty minutes to two hours. It is used to stimulate the bladder and GI tract, and it is also used as an antidote for *tubocurarine* and other competitive neuromuscular blocking agents (see p. 60). *Neostigmine* has found use in symptomatic treatment of myasthenia gravis, an autoimmune disease caused by antibodies to the nicotinic receptor at neuromuscular junctions. This causes their degradation and, thus, makes fewer receptors available for interaction with the neurotransmitter. Adverse effects of *neostigmine* include those of generalized cholinergic stimulation, such as salivation, flushing, decreased blood pressure, nausea, abdominal pain, diarrhea, and bronchospasm.

C. Pyridostigmine and ambenomium

Pyridostigmine [peer id oh STIG meen] and *ambenomium* [am be NOE mee um] are other cholinesterase inhibitors that are used in the chronic management of myasthenia gravis. Their durations of action (three to six hours and four to eight hours, respectively) are longer than that of *neostigmine*, but their adverse effects are similar.

D. Edrophonium

The actions of *edrophonium* [ed roe FOE nee um] are similar to those of *neostigmine*, except that it is more rapidly absorbed and has a short duration of action (ten to twenty minutes). *Edrophonium* is a quarternary amine and is used in the diagnosis of myasthenia gravis. Intravenous injection of *edrophonium* leads to a rapid increase in muscle strength. Care must be taken, because excess drug may provoke a cholinergic crisis. *Atropine* is the antidote.

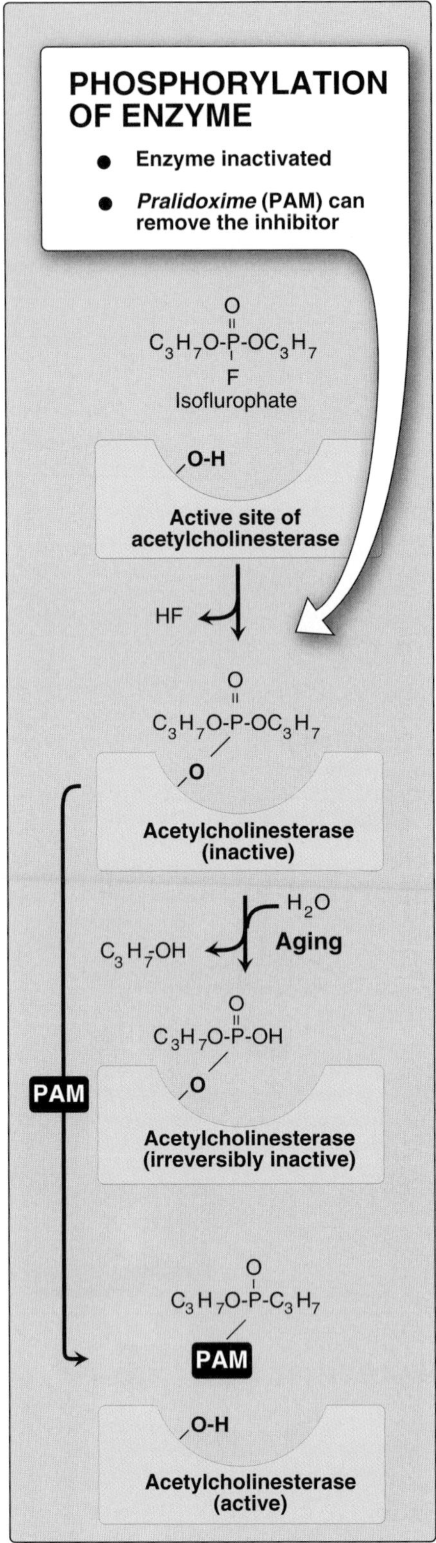

Figure 4.10
Covalent modification of acetylcholinesterase by isoflurophate; also shown is the reactivation of the enzyme with *pralidoxime*.

E. Tacrine, donezepil, rivastigmine, and galantamine

As mentioned above, patients with Alzheimer disease have a deficiency of cholinergic neurons in the CNS. This observation led to the development of anticholinesterases as possible remedies for the loss of cognitive function. *Tacrine* [TAK reen] was the first to become available, but it has been replaced by the others because of its hepatotoxicity. Despite the ability of *donezepil* [doe NEP e zil], *rivastigmine* [ri va STIG meen], and *galantamine* [gaa LAN ta meen] to delay the progression of the disease, none can stay its progression. Gastrointestinal distress is their primary adverse effect.

VI. ANTICHOLINESTERASES (IRREVERSIBLE)

A number of synthetic organophosphate compounds have the capacity to bind covalently to acetylcholinesterase. The result is a long-lasting increase in acetylcholine at all sites where it is released. Many of these drugs are extremely toxic and were developed by the military as nerve agents. Related compounds, such as *parathion*, are employed as insecticides. The prototype agent, *isoflurophate*, is described, because it has been the best studied.

A. Isoflurophate

1. **Mechanism of action:** *Isoflurophate* [eye soe FLURE oh fate] (diisopropylfluorophosphate, DFP) is an organophosphate that covalently binds to a serine-OH at the active site of acetylcholinesterase (Figure 4.10). Once this occurs, the enzyme is permanently inactivated, and restoration of acetylcholinesterase activity requires the synthesis of new enzyme molecules. Following covalent modification of acetylcholinesterase, the phosphorylated enzyme slowly releases one of its isopropyl groups (see Figure 4.10). The loss of an alkyl group, which is called aging, makes it impossible for chemical reactivators, such as *pralidoxime* (see below), to break the bond between the remaining drug and the enzyme. DFP ages in six to eight hours, whereas newer nerve agents, available to the military, age in minutes or seconds.

2. **Actions:** Actions include generalized cholinergic stimulation, paralysis of motor function (causing breathing difficulties), and convulsions. *Isoflurophate* produces intense miosis and, thus, has found therapeutic use. *Atropine* in high dosage can reverse many of the muscarinic and central effects of *isoflurophate*.

3. **Therapeutic uses:** An ophthalmic ointment of the drug is used topically in the eye for the chronic treatment of open-angle glaucoma. The effects may last for up to one week after a single administration. [Note: *Echothiophate* [ek oe THI oh fate] covalently bonds to acetylcholinesterase, and has largely replaced *isoflurophate* as a therapy for this condition.]

4. **Reactivation of acetylcholinesterase:** *Pralidoxime* (PAM) can reactivate inhibited acetylcholinesterase. However, it is unable to penetrate into the CNS. The presence of a charged group allows

it to approach an anionic site on the enzyme, where it essentially displaces the organophosphate and regenerates the enzyme. If given before aging of the alkylated enzyme occurs, it can reverse the effects of *isoflurophate*, except for those in the CNS. With the newer nerve agents, which produce aging of the enzyme complex within seconds, *pralidoxime* is less effective.

A summary of the actions of some of the cholinergic agonists is presented in Figure 4.11.

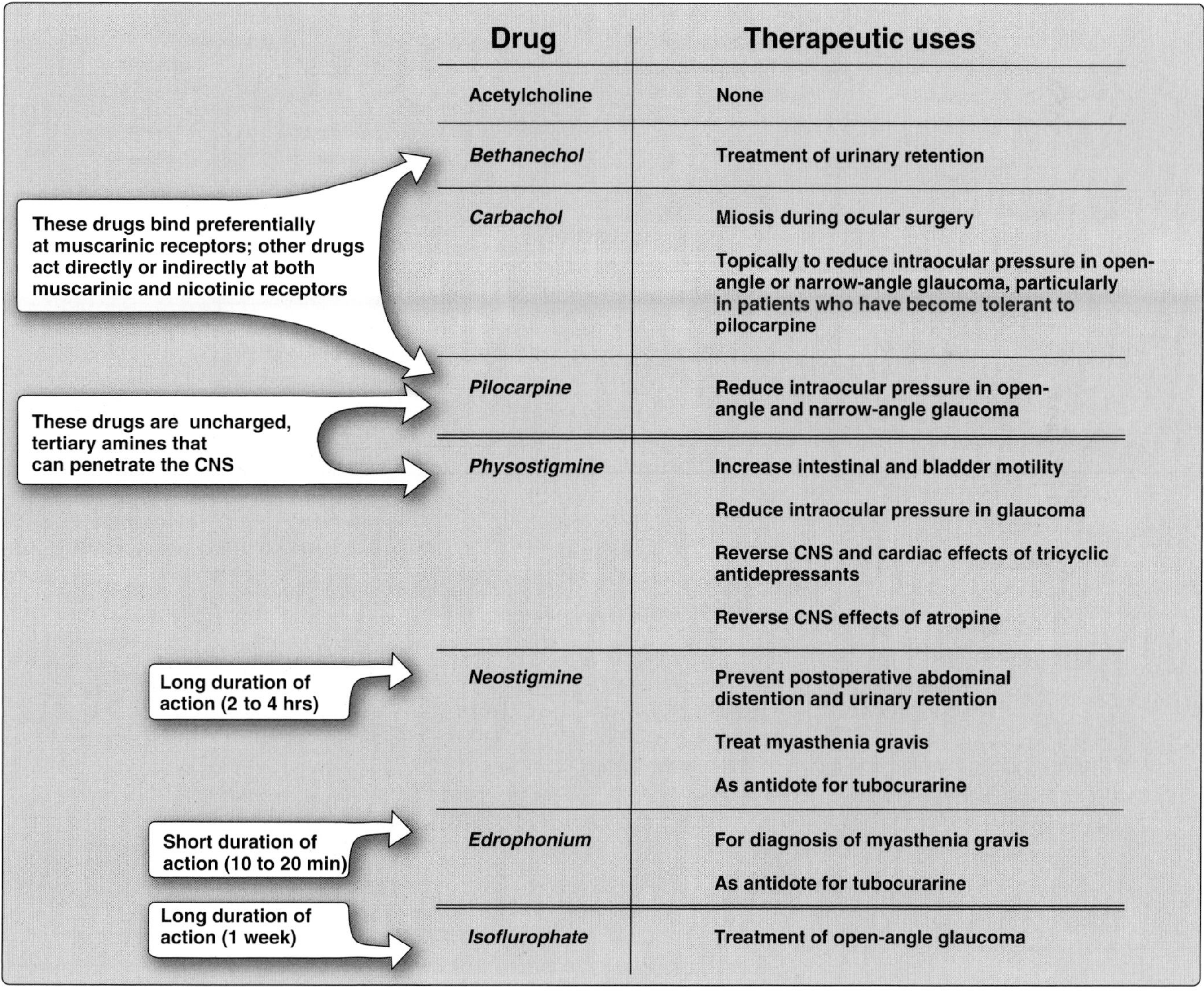

Drug	Therapeutic uses
Acetylcholine	None
Bethanechol	Treatment of urinary retention
Carbachol	Miosis during ocular surgery Topically to reduce intraocular pressure in open-angle or narrow-angle glaucoma, particularly in patients who have become tolerant to pilocarpine
Pilocarpine	Reduce intraocular pressure in open-angle and narrow-angle glaucoma
Physostigmine	Increase intestinal and bladder motility Reduce intraocular pressure in glaucoma Reverse CNS and cardiac effects of tricyclic antidepressants Reverse CNS effects of atropine
Neostigmine	Prevent postoperative abdominal distention and urinary retention Treat myasthenia gravis As antidote for tubocurarine
Edrophonium	For diagnosis of myasthenia gravis As antidote for tubocurarine
Isoflurophate	Treatment of open-angle glaucoma

Figure 4.11
Summary of actions of some cholinergic agonists.

Study Questions

Choose the ONE best answer.

4.1 A patient with an acute attack of glaucoma is treated with pilocarpine. The primary reason for its effectiveness in this condition is its:

A. action to terminate acetylcholinesterase.
B. selectivity for nicotinic receptors.
C. ability to inhibit secretions, such as tears, saliva, and sweat.
D. ability to lower intraocular pressure.
E. inability to enter the brain.

Correct answer = D. Pilocarpine can abort an acute attack of glaucoma, because it causes pupillary constriction to lower intraocular pressure. It binds mainly to muscarinic receptors, and can enter the brain. It is effective in inhibiting secretions.

4.2 A soldier's unit has come under attack with a nerve agent. The symptoms exhibited are skeletal muscle paralysis, profuse bronchial secretions, miosis, bradycardia, and convulsions. The alarm indicates exposure to an organophosphate. What is the correct treatment?

A. Do nothing until you can confirm the nature of the nerve agent.
B. Administer atropine, and attempt to confirm the nature of the nerve agent.
C. Administer atropine and 2-PAM (pralidoxime).
D. Administer 2-PAM.

Correct answer = C. Organophosphates exert their effect by irreversibly binding to acetylcholinesterase and, thus, can cause a cholinergic crisis. Administration of atropine will block the muscarinic sites, However, it will not reactivate the enzyme, which will remain blocked for a long period of time. Therefore, it is essential to also administer 2-PAM as soon as possible to reactivate the enzyme before aging occurs. Administering 2-PAM alone will not protect the patient against the effects of acetylcholine resulting from acetylcholinesterase inhibition.

4.3 A patient being diagnosed for myasthenia gravis would be expected to have improved neuromuscular function after being treated with:

A. donezepil.
B. edrophonium.
C. atropine.
D. isoflurophate.
E. neostigmine.

Correct answer = B. Edrophonium is a short-acting inhibitor of acetylcholinesterase that is used to diagnose myasthenia gravis. It is a quartenary compound and does not enter the CNS. Donezepil, isoflurophate, and neostigmine are also anticholinesterases but with longer actions. Donezepil is used in the the treatment of Alzheimer disease. Isoflurophate has some activity in treating open-angle glaucoma. Neostigmine is used in the treatment of myasthenia gravis, but is not employed in its diagnosis. Atropine is a cholinergic antagonist and, thus, would have the opposite effects.

4.4 The drug of choice for treating decreased salivation accompanying head and neck irradiation is:

A. physostigmine.
B. scopolamine.
C. carbachol.
D. acetylcholine.
E. pilocarpine.

Correct answer = E. Pilocarpine has proven beneficial in this situation. All the others except scopolamine are cholinergic agonists. However, their ability to stimulate salivation is less than that of pilocarpine, and their other effects are more troublesome.

Cholinergic Antagonists

5

I. OVERVIEW

The cholinergic antagonists (also called cholinergic blockers or anticholinergic drugs) bind to cholinoceptors, but they do not trigger the usual receptor-mediated intracellular effects. The most useful of these agents selectively block at the muscarinic synapses of the parasympathetic nerves. The effects of parasympathetic innervation are thus interrupted, and the actions of sympathetic stimulation are left unopposed. A second group of drugs, the ganglionic blockers, show a preference for the nicotinic receptors of the sympathetic and parasympathetic ganglia. Clinically, they are the least important of these drugs. A third family of compounds, the neuromuscular blocking agents, interfere with transmission of efferent impulses to skeletal muscles. Figure 5.1 summarizes the cholinergic antagonists discussed in this chapter.

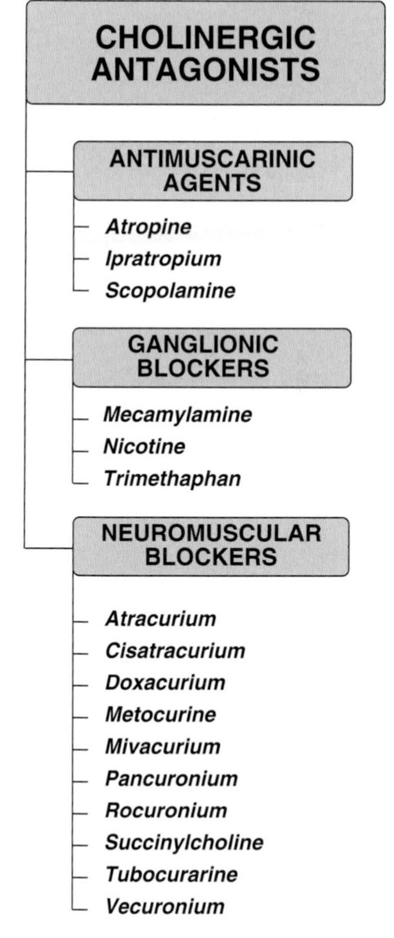

Figure 5.1
Summary of cholinergic antagonists.

II. ANTIMUSCARINIC AGENTS

These agents (for example, *atropine* and *scopolamine*) block muscarinic receptors (Figure 5.2), causing inhibition of all muscarinic functions. In addition, these drugs block the few exceptional sympathetic neurons that are cholinergic, such as those innervating salivary and sweat glands. In contrast to the cholinergic agonists, which have limited usefulness therapeutically, the cholinergic blockers are beneficial in a variety of clinical situations. Because they do not block nicotinic receptors, the antimuscarinic drugs have little or no action at skeletal neuromuscular junctions or autonomic ganglia. [Note: A number of antihistaminic and antidepressant drugs also have antimuscarinic activity.]

A. Atropine

Atropine [A troe peen], a belladonna alkaloid, has a high affinity for muscarinic receptors, where it binds competitively, preventing acetylcholine from binding to those sites (Figure 5.3). *Atropine* acts both centrally and peripherally. Its general actions last about four hours except when placed topically in the eye, where the action may last for days.

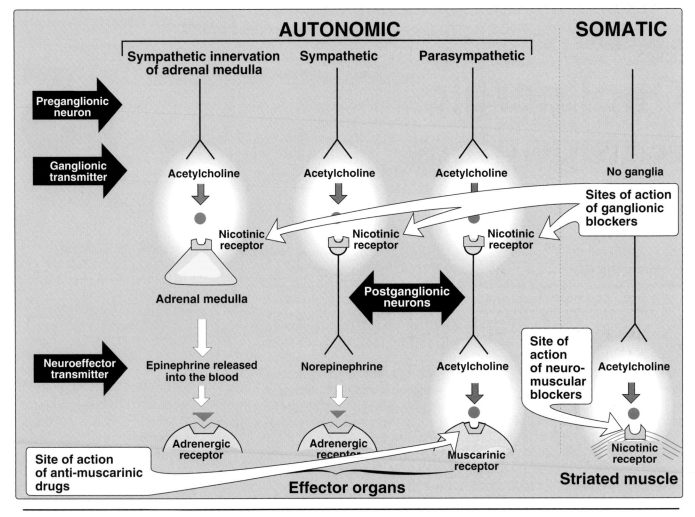

Figure 5.2
Sites of actions of cholinergic antagonists.

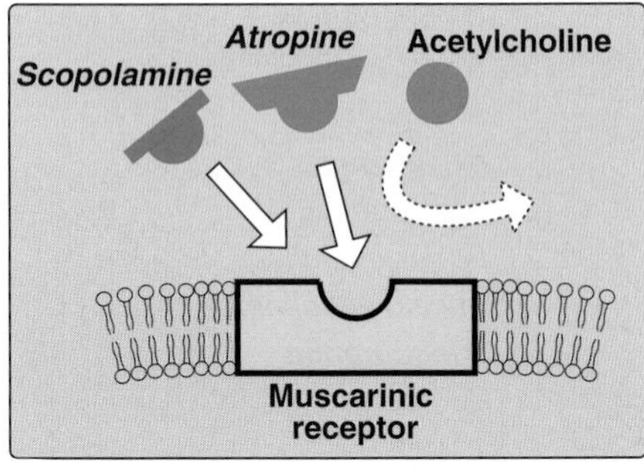

Figure 5.3
Competition of *atropine* and *scopolamine* with acetylcholine for the muscarinic receptor.

1. Actions:

a. Eye: *Atropine* blocks all cholinergic activity on the eye, resulting in persistent mydriasis (dilation of the pupil, see Figure 4.6, p. 46), unresponsiveness to light, and cycloplegia (inability to focus for near vision). In patients with narrow-angle glaucoma, intraocular pressure may rise dangerously. Shorter-acting agents, such as the antimuscarinic *tropicamide*, or an α-adrenergic drug, like *phenylephrine*, are generally favored for producing mydriasis in ophthalmic examinations.

b. Gastrointestinal (GI): *Atropine* can be used as an antispasmodic to reduce activity of the GI tract. *Atropine* and *scopolamine* (which is discussed below) are probably the most potent drugs available that produce this effect. Although gastric motility is reduced, hydrochloric acid production is not significantly affected. Thus, the drug is not effective in promoting healing of peptic ulcer. [Note: *Pirenzepine* (see p. 47), an M_1-muscarinic antagonist, does reduce gastric acid secretion at doses that do not antagonize other systems.]

c. **Urinary system:** *Atropine* is also employed to reduce hypermotility states of the urinary bladder. It is still occasionally used in enuresis (involuntary voiding of urine) among children, but α-adrenergic agonists with fewer side effects may be more effective.

d. **Cardiovascular:** *Atropine* produces divergent effects on the cardiovascular system, depending on the dose (Figure 5.4). At low doses, the predominant effect is a decreased cardiac rate (bradycardia). Originally thought to be due to central activation of vagal efferent outflow, newer data indicate that the effect results from blockade of the M_1 receptors on the inhibitory prejunctional neurons, thus permitting increased acetylcholine release. With higher doses of *atropine*, the M_2 receptors on the sinoatrial node are blocked, and the cardiac rate increases modestly. This generally requires at least 1 mg of *atropine*, which is a higher dose than ordinarily given. Arterial blood pressure is unaffected, but at toxic levels, *atropine* will dilate the cutaneous vasculature.

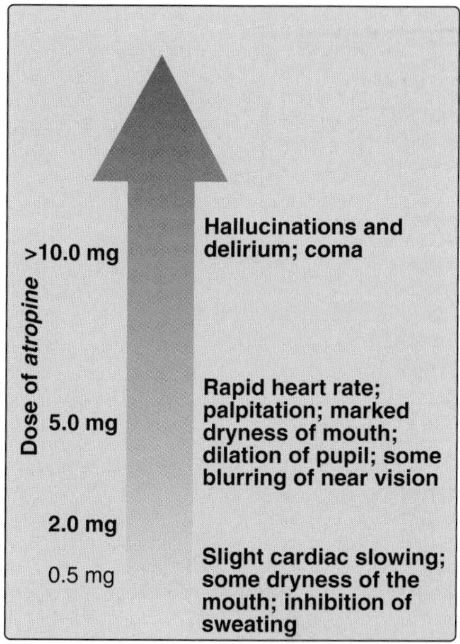

Figure 5.4
Dose-dependent effects of *atropine*.

e. **Secretions:** *Atropine* blocks the salivary glands, producing a drying effect on the oral mucus membranes (xerostomia). The salivary glands are exquisitely sensitive to *atropine*. Sweat and lacrimal glands are also affected. [Note: Inhibition of secretions by sweat glands can cause elevated body temperature.]

2. Therapeutic uses:

a. **Ophthalmic:** In the eye, topical *atropine* exerts both mydriatic and cycloplegic effects, and it permits the measurement of refractive errors without interference by the accommodative capacity of the eye. [Note: *Phenylephrine* or similar α-adrenergic drugs are preferred for pupillary dilation if cycloplegia is not required. Also, individuals forty years of age and older have decreased ability to accommodate, and drugs are not necessary for an accurate refraction.] *Atropine* may induce an attack in individuals with narrow-angle glaucoma.

b. **Antispasmodic agent:** *Atropine* is used as an antispasmodic agent to relax the GI tract and bladder.

c. **Antidote for cholinergic agonists:** *Atropine* is used for the treatment of overdoses of cholinesterase inhibitor insecticides and some types of mushroom poisoning (certain mushrooms contain cholinergic substances that block cholinesterases). Massive doses of the antagonist may be required over a long period of time to counteract the poisons. The ability of *atropine* to enter the central nervous system (CNS) is of particular importance. The drug also blocks the effects of excess acetylcholine resulting from acetylcholinesterase inhibitors, such as *physostigmine*.

d. **Antisecretory agent:** The drug is sometimes used as an antisecretory agent to block secretions in the upper and lower respiratory tracts prior to surgery.

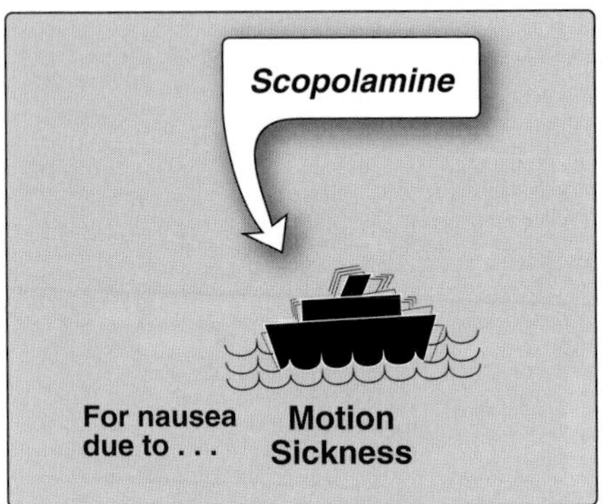

Figure 5.5
Scopolamine is an effective anti-motion sickness agent.

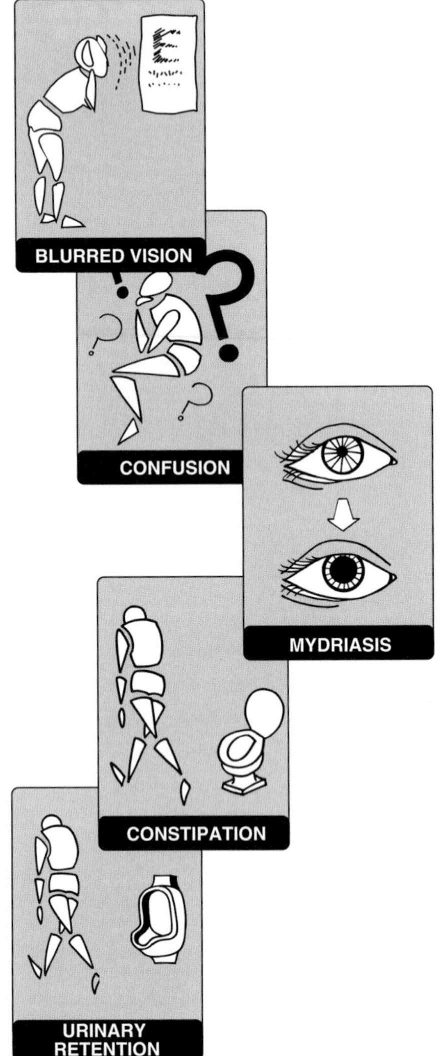

Figure 5.6
Adverse effects commonly observed with cholinergic antagonists.

3. **Pharmacokinetics:** *Atropine* is readily absorbed, partially metabolized by the liver, and eliminated primarily in the urine. It has a half-life of about four hours.

4. **Adverse effects:** Depending on the dose, *atropine* may cause dry mouth, blurred vision, "sandy eyes," tachycardia, and constipation. Effects on the CNS include restlessness, confusion, hallucinations, and delirium, which may progress to depression, collapse of the circulatory and respiratory systems, and death. In older individuals, the use of *atropine* to induce mydriasis and cycloplegia is considered to be too risky, because it may exacerbate an attack of glaucoma in someone with a latent condition.

B. Scopolamine

Scopolamine [skoe POL a meen], another belladonna alkaloid, produces peripheral effects similar to those of *atropine*. However, *scopolamine* has greater action on the CNS and a longer duration of action in comparison to those of *atropine*. It has some special actions as indicated below.

1. **Actions:** *Scopolamine* is one of the most effective anti-motion sickness drugs available (Figure 5.5). *Scopolamine* also has the unusual effect of blocking short-term memory. In contrast to *atropine*, *scopolamine* produces sedation, but at higher doses it can produce excitement instead.

2. **Therapeutic uses:** Although similar to *atropine*, therapeutic use of *scopolamine* is limited to prevention of motion sickness (for which is particularly effective), and to block short-term memory. [Note: As with all such drugs used for motion sickness, it is much more effective prophylactically than for treating motion sickness once it occurs. The amnesic action of *scopolamine* makes it an important adjunct drug in anesthetic procedures.]

3. **Pharmacokinetics and adverse effects:** These aspects are similar to those of *atropine*.

C. Ipratropium

Inhaled *ipratropium* [i pra TROE pee um], a quaternary derivative of *atropine*, is useful in treating asthma in patients who are unable to take adrenergic agonists. *Ipratropium* is also beneficial in the management of chronic obstructive pulmonary disease. It is inhaled for these conditions. Because of its positive charge, it does not enter the systemic circulation nor the CNS. Important characteristics of the muscarinic antagonists are summarized in Figure 5.6 and 5.7.

III. GANGLIONIC BLOCKERS

Ganglionic blockers specifically act on the nicotinic receptors of both parasympathetic and sympathetic autonomic ganglia. Some also block the ion channels of the autonomic ganglia. These drugs show no selectivity toward the parasympathetic or sympathetic ganglia, and are not effective as neuromuscular antagonists. Thus, these drugs block the entire output of the autonomic nervous system at the nicotinic receptor. Except for *nicotine*, the other drugs mentioned in this category are nondepolarizing, competitive antagonists. The responses observed are complex and unpredictable, making it impossible to achieve selective actions. Therefore, ganglionic blockade is rarely used therapeutically. However, they often serve as tools in experimental pharmacology.

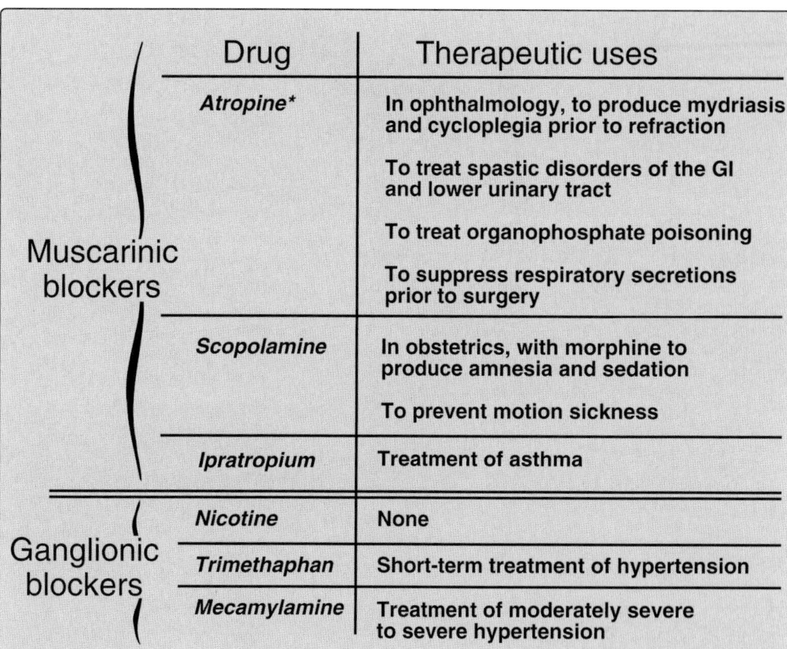

	Drug	Therapeutic uses
Muscarinic blockers	*Atropine**	In ophthalmology, to produce mydriasis and cycloplegia prior to refraction To treat spastic disorders of the GI and lower urinary tract To treat organophosphate poisoning To suppress respiratory secretions prior to surgery
	Scopolamine	In obstetrics, with morphine to produce amnesia and sedation To prevent motion sickness
	Ipratropium	Treatment of asthma
Ganglionic blockers	*Nicotine*	None
	Trimethaphan	Short-term treatment of hypertension
	Mecamylamine	Treatment of moderately severe to severe hypertension

Figure 5.7
Summary of cholinergic antagonists. *Contraindicated in narrow-angle glaucoma.

A. Nicotine

A component of cigarette smoke, *nicotine* [NIC oh teen] has many undesirable actions. It is without therapeutic benefit and is deleterious to health. [Note: *Nicotine* patches are available for application to the skin. The drug is absorbed and is effective in reducing the craving for *nicotine* in people who wish to stop smoking.] Depending on the dose, *nicotine* depolarizes ganglia, resulting first in stimulation and then paralysis of all ganglia. The stimulatory effects are complex, including increased blood pressure and cardiac rate (due to release of transmitter from adrenergic terminals and from the adrenal medulla), and increased peristalsis and secretions. At higher doses, the blood pressure falls because of ganglionic blockade, and activity both in the GI tract and bladder musculature ceases. (See p. 116 for a full discussion of *nicotine*.)

B. Trimethaphan

Trimethaphan [trye METH a fan] is a short-acting, competitive nicotinic ganglionic blocker that must be given by intravenous infusion. Today, the drug is used for the emergency lowering of blood pressure—for example, in hypertension caused by pulmonary edema or dissecting aortic aneurysm when other agents cannot be used.

C. Mecamylamine

Mecamylamine [mek a MILL a meen] produces a competitive nicotinic blockade of the ganglia. The duration of action is about ten hours after a single administration. The uptake of the drug via oral absorption is good in contrast to that of *trimethaphan*.

IV. NEUROMUSCULAR BLOCKING DRUGS

These drugs block cholinergic transmission between motor nerve endings and the nicotinic receptors on the neuromuscular end plate of skeletal muscle (see Figure 5.2). These neuromuscular blockers are structural analogs of acetylcholine, and act either as antagonists (nondepolarizing type) or agonists (depolarizing type) at the receptors on the end plate of the neuromuscular junction. Neuromuscular blockers are clinically useful during surgery for producing complete muscle relaxation, without having to employ higher anesthetic doses to achieve comparable muscular relaxation. A second group of muscle relaxants, the central muscle relaxants, are used to control spastic muscle tone. These drugs include *diazepam*, which binds at γ-aminobutyric acid (GABA) receptors, *dantrolene*, which acts directly on muscles by interfering with the release of calcium from the sarcoplasmic reticulum, and *baclofen*, which probably acts at GABA receptors in the central nervous system.

A. Nondepolarizing (competitive) blockers

The first drug that was found to be capable of blocking the skeletal neuromuscular junction was *curare*, which the native hunters of the Amazon in South America used to paralyze game. The drug *tubocurarine* [too boe kyoo AR een] was ultimately purified and introduced into clinical practice in the early 1940s. The neuromuscular blocking agents have significantly increased the safety of anesthesia, because less anesthetic is required to produce muscle relaxation.

1. Mechanism of action:

a. At low doses: Nondepolarizing neuromuscular blocking drugs combine with the nicotinic receptor and prevent the binding of acetylcholine (Figure 5.8). These drugs thus prevent depolarization of the muscle cell membrane and inhibit muscular contraction. Because these agents compete with acetylcholine at the receptor, they are called competitive blockers. Their action can be overcome by increasing the concentration of acetylcholine in the synaptic gap—for example, by administration of cholinesterase inhibitors, such as *neostigmine*, *pyridostigmine*, or *edrophonium*. Anesthesiologists often employ this strategy to shorten the duration of the neuromuscular blockade.

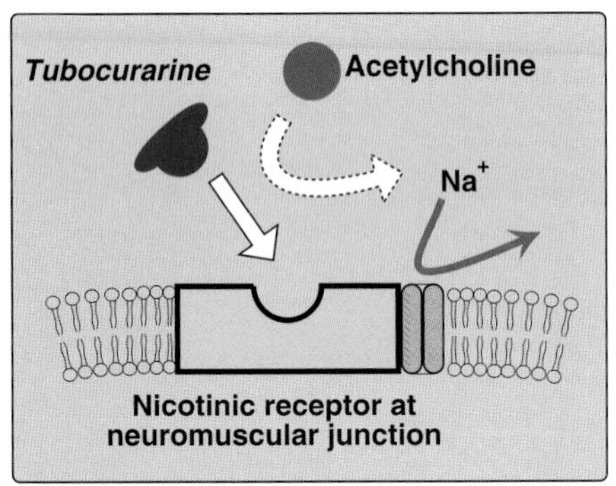

Figure 5.8
Mechanism of action of competitive neuromuscular blocking drugs.

b. At high doses: Nondepolarizing blockers can block the ion channels of the end plate. This leads to further weakening of neuromuscular transmission, and it reduces the ability of acetylcholinesterase inhibitors to reverse the actions of nondepolarizing muscle relaxants.

2. Actions: Not all muscles are equally sensitive to blockade by competitive blockers. Small, rapidly contracting muscles of the face and eye are most susceptible and are paralyzed first, followed by the fingers. Thereafter, the limbs, neck, and trunk muscles are paralyzed, then the intercostal muscles are affected, and lastly, the diaphragm muscles are paralyzed. Those agents (for example, *tubocurarine*, *mivacurium*, and *atracurium*), which release histamine, can produce a fall in blood pressure, flushing, and bronchoconstriction.

3. Therapeutic uses: These blockers are used therapeutically as adjuvant drugs in anesthesia during surgery to relax skeletal muscle.

4. **Pharmacokinetics:** All neuromuscular blocking agents are injected intravenously because their uptake via oral absorption is minimal. They penetrate membranes very poorly and do not enter cells or cross the blood-brain barrier. Many of the drugs are not metabolized; their actions are terminated by redistribution (Figure 5.9). For example, *tubocurarine*, *pancuronium*, *mivacurium*, *metocurine*, and *doxacurium* are excreted in the urine unchanged. *Atracurium* is degraded spontaneously in the plasma and by ester hydrolysis. [Note: *Atracurium* has been replaced by its isomer, *cisatracurium*. *Atracurium* releases histamine and is metabolized to laudanosine, which can provoke seizures. *Cisatracurium*, which has the same pharmacokinetic properties as *atracurium*, is less likely to have these effects.] The aminosteroid drugs (*vecuronium* and *rocuronium*) are deacetylated in the liver, and their clearance may be prolonged in patients with hepatic disease. These drugs are also excreted unchanged in the bile. The onset and duration of action as well as other characteristics of the neuromuscular blocking drugs are shown in Figure 5.10.

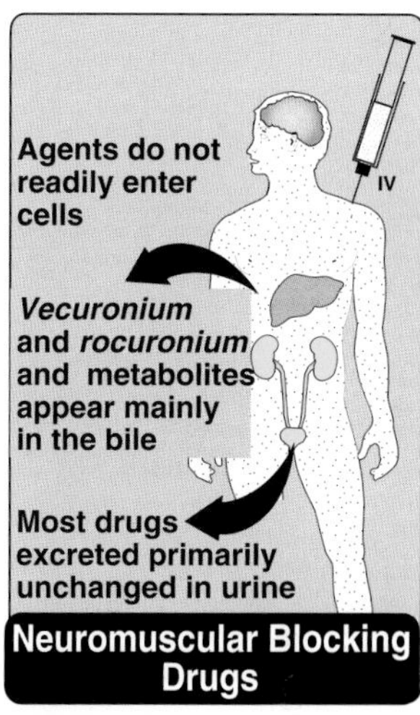

Figure 5.9
Pharmacokinetics of the neuromuscular blocking drugs.

5. **Adverse effects:** The adverse effects of the neuromuscular blocking drugs are shown in Figure 5.10.

6. **Drug interactions:**

   a. **Cholinesterase inhibitors:** Drugs such as *neostigmine*, *physostigmine*, *pyridostigmine*, and *edrophonium* can overcome the action of nondepolarizing neuromuscular blockers, but with increased dosage, cholinesterase inhibitors can cause a depolarizing block as a result of elevated acetylcholine concentrations at the end-plate membrane.

   b. **Halogenated hydrocarbon anesthetics:** Drugs such as *halothane* act to enhance neuromuscular blockade by exerting a stabilizing action at the neuromuscular junction.

   c. **Aminoglycoside antibiotics:** Drugs such as *gentamicin* or *tobramycin* inhibit acetylcholine release from cholinergic nerves by competing with calcium ions. They synergize with *tubocurarine* and other competitive blockers, enhancing the blockade.

   d. **Calcium-channel blockers:** These agents may increase the neuromuscular block of *tubocurarine* and other competitive blockers as well as depolarizing blockers.

B. Depolarizing agents

1. **Mechanism of action:** The depolarizing neuromuscular blocking drug *succinylcholine* [suk sin ill KOE leen] attaches to the nicotinic receptor and acts like acetylcholine to depolarize the junction (Figure 5.11). Unlike acetylcholine, which is instantly destroyed by acetylcholinesterase, the depolarizing agent persists at high concentrations in the synaptic cleft, remaining attached to the receptor for a relatively longer time and providing a constant stimulation

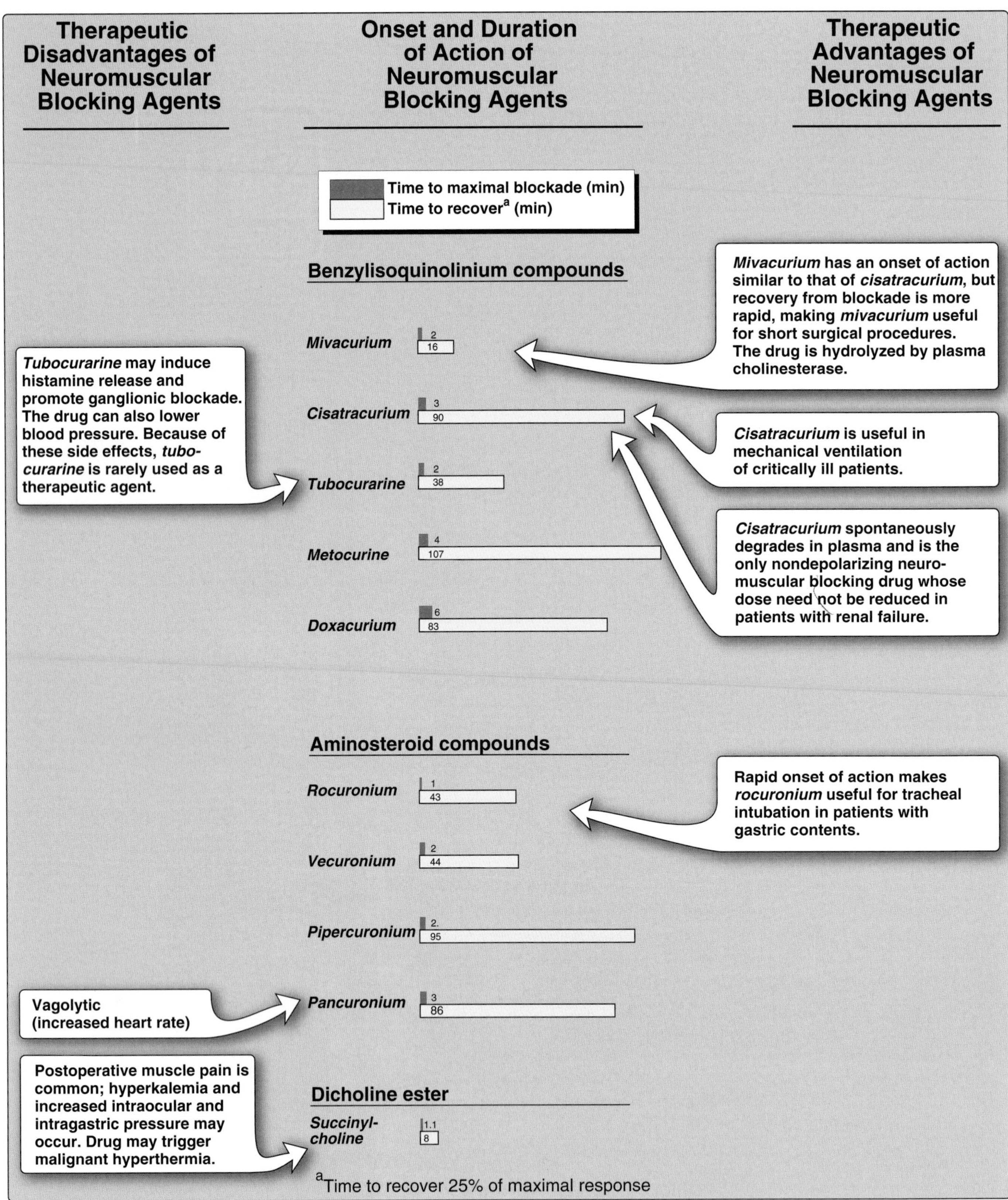

Figure 5.10
Onset and duration of action of neuromuscular blocking drugs (center column), with a summary of therapeutic considerations.

of the receptor. [Note: The duration of action of *succinylcholine* is dependent on diffusion from the motor end plate and hydrolysis by plasma cholinesterase.] The depolarizing agent first causes the opening of the sodium channel associated with the nicotinic receptors, which results in depolarization of the receptor (Phase I). This leads to a transient twitching of the muscle (fasciculations). The continued binding of the depolarizing agent renders the receptor incapable of transmitting further impulses. With time, the continuous depolarization gives way to gradual repolarization as the sodium channel closes or is blocked. This causes a resistance to depolarization (Phase II) and a flaccid paralysis.

2. **Actions:** The sequence of paralysis may be slightly different, but as with the competitive blockers, the respiratory muscles are paralyzed last. *Succinylcholine* initially produces short-lasting muscle fasciculations, followed within a few minutes by paralysis. The drug does not produce a ganglionic block except in high doses, but it does have weak histamine-releasing action. Normally, the duration of action of *succinylcholine* is extremely short, because this drug is rapidly broken down by plasma cholinesterase. [Note: Genetic variants in which plasma cholinesterase levels are low or absent leads to prolonged neuromuscular paralysis.]

3. **Therapeutic uses:** Because of its rapid onset and short duration of action, *succinylcholine* is useful when rapid endotracheal intubation is required during the induction of anesthesia (a rapid action is essential if aspiration of gastric contents is to be avoided during intubation). It is also employed during electroconvulsive shock treatment.

4. **Pharmacokinetics:** *Succinylcholine* is injected intravenously. Its brief duration of action (several minutes) results from redistribution and rapid hydrolysis by plasma cholinesterase. It therefore is usually given by continuous infusion.

5. **Adverse effects:**

   a. **Hyperthermia:** When *halothane* (see p. 132) is used as an anesthetic, administration of *succinylcholine* has occasionally caused malignant hyperthermia (with muscular rigidity and hyperpyrexia) in genetically susceptible people (see Figure 5.10). This is treated by rapidly cooling the patient, and by administration of *dantrolene*, which blocks release of Ca^{2+} from the sarcoplasmic reticulum of muscle cells, thus reducing heat production and relaxing muscle tone.

   b. **Apnea:** Administration of *succinylcholine* to a patient who is genetically deficient in plasma cholinesterase or has an atypical form of the enzyme can lead to prolonged apnea due to paralysis of the diaphragm.

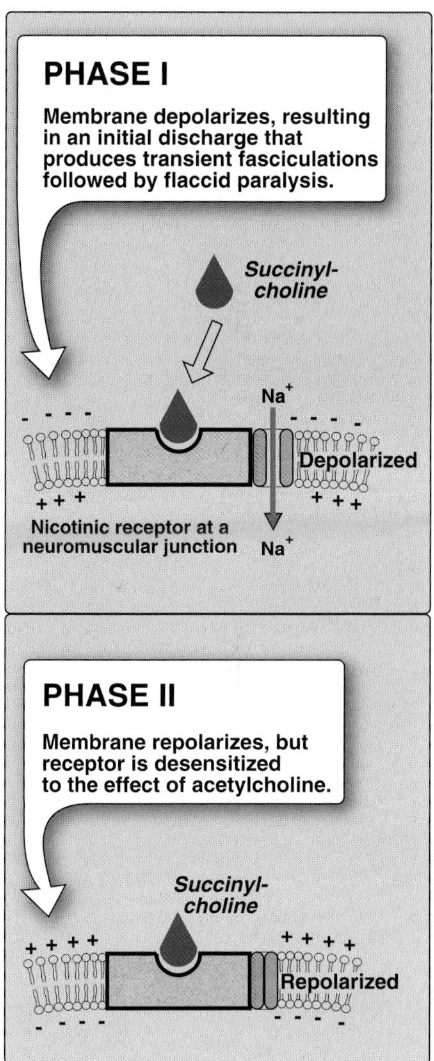

Figure 5.11
Mechanism of action of depolarizing neuromuscular blocking drugs.

Study Questions

Choose the ONE best answer.

5.1 A 75-year-old man who was a smoker is diagnosed with chronic obstructive pulmonary disease and suffers from occasional bronchospasm. Which of the following would be effective in treating him?

A. Ipratoprium aerosol
B. Scopolamine patches
C. Mecamylamine
D. Oxygen

Correct answer = A. This is a drug of choice especially in a patient who cannot tolerate an adrenergic agonist, which would dilate the bronchioles. Scopolamine's main effect is atropinic and is the most effective anti-motion sickness drug. Mecamylamine is a ganglionic blocker and completely inappropriate in this situation. Oxygen would improve aeration but would not dilate the bronchial musculature.

5.2 Which of the following may precipitate an attack of open-angle glaucoma if instilled into the eye?

A. Physostigmine
B. Atropine
C. Pilocarpine
D. Echothiophate

Correct answer = B. The mydriatic effect of atropine can result in the narrowing of the canal of Schlemm leading to an increase in intracocular pressure. The other agents would cause miosis.

5.3 The prolonged apnea sometimes seen in patients who had undergone an operation in which succinylcholine was employed as a muscle relaxant has been shown to be due to:

A. urinary atony.
B. depressed levels of plasma cholinesterase.
C. a mutation in acetylcholinesterase.
D. a mutation in the nicotinic receptor at the neuromuscular junction.

Answer: B. These patients have a genetic deficiency of the non-specific plasma cholinesterase which is required for the termination of succinylcholine's action.

5.4 A 50-year-old male farm worker is brought to the emergency room. He was found confused in the orchard and since then has lost consciousness. His heart rate is 45 and his blood pressure is 80/40 mm Hg. He is sweating and salivating profusely. Which of the following treatments is indicated?

A. Physostigmine
B. Norepinephrine
C. Trimethaphan
D. Atropine
E. Edrophonium

Correct answer = D. The patient is exhibiting signs of cholinergic stimulation. Since he is a farmer, insecticide poisoning is a likely diagnosis. Thus either intravenous or intramuscular doses of atropine are indicated to antagonize the muscarinic symptoms. Physostigmine and edrophonium are cholinesterase inhibitors and would exacerbate the problem. Norepinephrine would not be effective in combatting the cholinergic stimulation. Trimethaphan being a ganglionic blocker would also worsen the condition.

Adrenergic Agonists

6

I. OVERVIEW

The adrenergic drugs affect receptors that are stimulated by *norepinephrine* or *epinephrine*. Some adrenergic drugs act directly on the adrenergic receptor (adrenoceptor) by activating it, and are said to be sympathomimetic. Others, which will be dealt with in Chapter 7, block the action of the neurotransmitters at the receptors, whereas still other drugs affect adrenergic function by interrupting the release of *norepinephrine* from adrenergic neurons. This chapter describes agents that either directly or indirectly stimulate the adrenoceptor (Figure 6.1).

ADRENERGIC AGONISTS

DIRECT-ACTING

- ***Albuterol***
- ***Clonidine***
- ***Dobutamine****
- ***Dopamine****
- ***Epinephrine****
- ***Formoterol***
- ***Isoproterenol****
- ***Metaproterenol***
- ***Methoxamine***
- ***Norepinephrine****
- ***Phenylephrine***
- ***Piruterol***
- ***Salmeterol***
- ***Tamsulosine***
- ***Terbutaline***

INDIRECT-ACTING

- ***Amphetamine***
- ***Tyramine***

DIRECT and INDIRECT ACTING (mixed action)

- ***Ephedrine***

Figure 6.1
Summary of adrenergic agonists. Agents marked with an asterisk (*) are catecholamines.

II. THE ADRENERGIC NEURON

Adrenergic neurons release *norepinephrine* as the neurotransmitter. These neurons are found in the central nervous system (CNS) and also in the sympathetic nervous system, where they serve as links between ganglia and the effector organs. The adrenergic neurons and receptors, located either presynaptically on the neuron or postsynaptically on the effector organ, are the sites of action of the adrenergic drugs (Figure 6.2).

A. Neurotransmission at adrenergic neurons

Neurotransmission in adrenergic neurons closely resembles that already described for the cholinergic neurons (see p. 43), except that *norepinephrine* is the neurotransmitter instead of acetylcholine. Neurotransmission takes place at numerous bead-like enlargements called varicosities. The process involves five steps: the synthesis, storage, release, and receptor binding of the *norepinephrine*, followed by removal of the neurotransmitter from the synaptic gap (Figure 6.3).

1. **Synthesis of norepinephrine:** Tyrosine is transported by a Na^+-linked carrier into the axoplasm of the adrenergic neuron, where it is hydroxylated to dihydroxyphenylalanine (DOPA) by tyrosine hydroxylase.[1] This is the rate-limiting step in the formation of *norepinephrine*. DOPA is then decarboxylated to form *dopamine*.

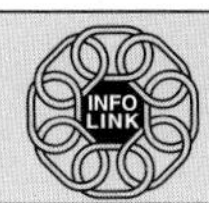

[1]See p. 284 in ***Lippincott's Illustrated Reviews: Biochemistry*** (3rd ed.) for a discussion of the synthesis of DOPA.

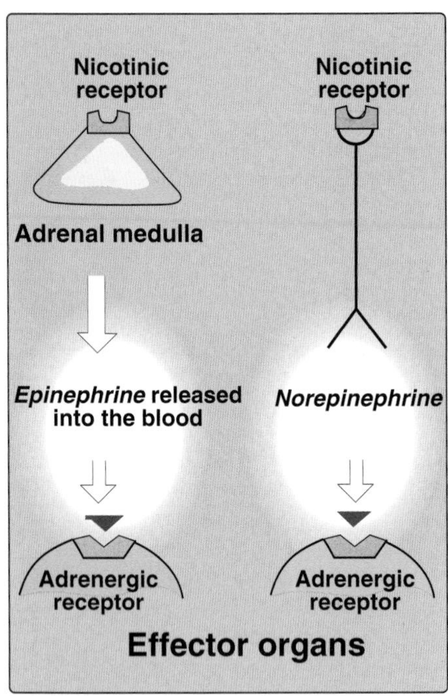

Figure 6.2
Sites of actions of adrenergic agonists.

2. **Storage of norepinephrine in vesicles:** *Dopamine* is transported into synaptic vesicles by an amine transporter system that is also involved in the re-uptake of preformed *norepinephrine*. This carrier system is blocked by *reserpine* (see p. 89). *Dopamine* is hydroxylated to form *norepinephrine* by the enzyme, *dopamine* β-hydroxylase. [Note: Synaptic vesicles contain *dopamine* or *norepinephrine* plus adenosine triphosphate (ATP) and the β-hydroxylase.] In the adrenal medulla, *norepinephrine* is methylated to yield *epinephrine*, both of which are stored in chromaffin cells. On stimulation, the adrenal medulla releases about 85 percent *epinephrine* and fifteen percent *norepinephrine*.

3. **Release of norepinephrine:** An action potential arriving at the nerve junction triggers an influx of calcium ions from the extracellular fluid into the cytoplasm of the neuron. The increase in calcium causes vesicles inside the neuron to fuse with the cell membrane and expel their contents into the synapse. This release is blocked by drugs such as *guanethidine* (see p. 89).

4. **Binding to a receptor:** *Norepinephrine* released from the synaptic vesicles diffuses across the synaptic space and binds to either postsynaptic receptors on the effector organ or to presynaptic receptors on the nerve ending. The recognition of *norepinephrine* by the membrane receptors triggers a cascade of events within the cell, resulting in the formation of intracellular second messengers that act as links (transducers) in the communication between the neurotransmitter and the action generated within the effector cell. Adrenergic receptors use both the cyclic adenosine monophosphate (cAMP) second messenger system,[2] and the phosphatidylinositol cycle,[3] to transduce the signal into an effect.

5. **Removal of norepinephrine:** *Norepinephrine* may 1) diffuse out of the synaptic space and enter the general circulation, 2) be metabolized to O-methylated derivatives by postsynaptic cell membrane-associated catechol O-methyltransferase (COMT) in the synaptic space, or 3) be recaptured by an uptake system that pumps the *norepinephrine* back into the neuron. The uptake by the neuronal membrane involves a sodium/potassium-activated ATPase that can be inhibited by tricyclic antidepressants, such as *imipramine*, or by *cocaine* (see Figure 6.3).

6. **Potential fates of recaptured norepinephrine:** Once *norepinephrine* reenters the cytoplasm of the adrenergic neuron, it may be taken up into adrenergic vesicles via the amine transporter system and be sequestered for release by another action potential, or it may persist in a protected pool. Alternatively, *norepinephrine* can be oxidized by monoamine oxidase (MAO), present in neuronal mitochondria. The inactive products of *norepinephrine* metabolism are excreted in the urine as vanillylmandelic acid, metanephrine, and normetanephrine.

INFO LINK
[2]See p. 93 in ***Lippincott's Illustrated Reviews: Biochemistry*** (2nd ed.) for a discussion of the cyclic AMP second messenger system.
[3]See p. 203 in ***Lippincott's Illustrated Reviews: Biochemistry*** (2nd ed.) for a discussion of the phosphatidylinositol cycle.

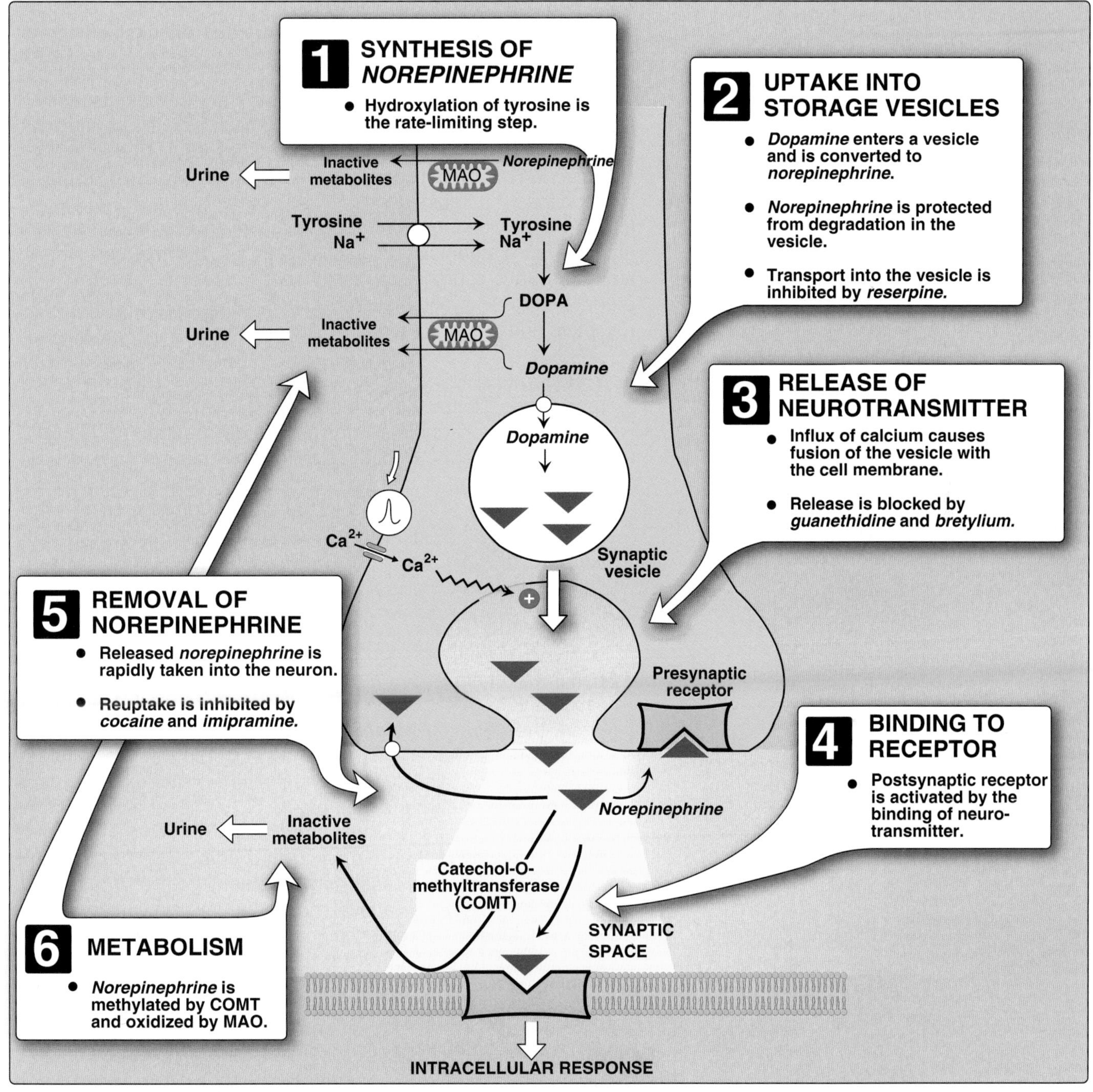

Figure 6.3
Synthesis and release of *norepinephrine* from the adrenergic neuron. (MAO = monoamine oxidase.)

B. Adrenergic receptors (adrenoceptors)

In the sympathetic nervous system, several classes of adrenoceptors can be distinguished pharmacologically. Two families of receptors, designated α and β, were initially identified on the basis of their responses to the adrenergic agonists *epinephrine*, *norepinephrine*, and *isoproterenol*. The use of specific blocking drugs and the cloning of genes have revealed the molecular identities of a number

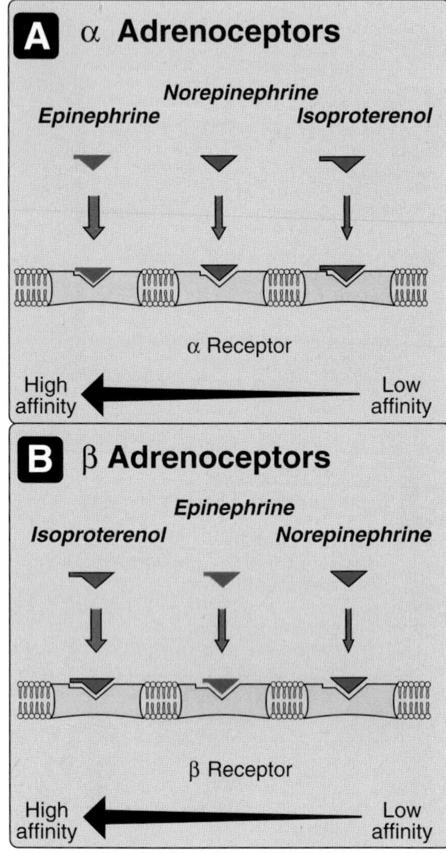

Figure 6.4
Types of adrenergic receptors.

of subtypes. These proteins belong to a multigene family. Alterations in the primary structure of the receptors influence their affinity for various agents.

1. **α_1 And α_2 receptors:** The α adrenoceptors show a weak response to the synthetic agonist *isoproterenol*, but are responsive to the naturally occurring catecholamines *epinephrine* and *norepinephrine* (Figure 6.4). For α receptors, the rank order of potency is *epinephrine* ≥ *norepinephrine* >> *isoproterenol.* The α adrenoceptors are subdivided into two subgroups, α_1 and α_2, based on their affinities for α agonists and blocking drugs. For example, the α_1 receptors have a higher affinity for *phenylephrine* than do the α_2 receptors. Conversely, the drug *clonidine* selectively binds to α_2 receptors and has less effect on α_1 receptors.

   a. **α_1 Receptors:** These receptors are present on the postsynaptic membrane of the effector organs and mediate many of the classic effects—originally designated as α-adrenergic—involving constriction of smooth muscle. Activation of α_1 receptors initiates a series of reactions through a G protein activation of phospholipase C, resulting in the generation of inositol-1,4,5-trisphosphate (IP_3) from phosphatidylinositol, causing the release of Ca^{2+} from the endoplasmic reticulum into the cytosol (Figure 6.5).

   b. **α_2 Receptors:** These receptors, located primarily on presynaptic nerve endings and on other cells, such as the β cell of the pancreas, control adrenergic neuromediator and insulin output, respectively. When a sympathetic adrenergic nerve is stimulated, the released *norepinephrine* traverses the synaptic cleft and interacts with the α_1 receptor. A portion of the released *norepinephrine* "circles back" and reacts with the α_2 receptor on the neuronal membrane (see Figure 6.5). The stimulation of the α_2 receptor causes feedback inhibition of the ongoing release of *norepinephrine* from the stimulated adrenergic neuron. This inhibitory action decreases further output from the adrenergic neuron and serves as a local modulating mechanism for reducing sympathetic neuromediator output when there is high sympathetic activity. In contrast to α_1 receptors, the effects of binding at α_2 receptors are mediated by inhibition of adenylyl cyclase and a fall in the levels of intracellular cAMP.

   c. **Further subdivisions:** The α_1 and α_2 receptors are further divided into α_1A, α_1B, α_1C, and α_1D, and α_2A, α_2B, α_2C, and α_2D. This extended classification is necessary for understanding the selectivity of some drugs. For example, *tamsulosine* is a selective α_1A antagonist that is used to treat benign prostate hypertrophy. The drug is clinically useful because it targets α_1A receptors found primarily in the urinary tract.

2. **β Receptors:** β Receptors exhibit a set of responses different from those of the α receptors. These are characterized by a strong response to *isoproterenol*, with less sensitivity to *epinephrine* and *norepinephrine* (see Figure 6.4). For β receptors, the rank order of potency is *isoproterenol* > *epinephrine* > *norepinephrine*. The

β adrenoceptors can be subdivided into two major subgroups, β_1 and β_2, based on their affinities for adrenergic agonists and antagonists, although several others have been identified by gene cloning. β_1 Receptors have approximately equal affinities for *epinephrine* and *norepinephrine*, whereas β_2 receptors have a higher affinity for *epinephrine* than for *norepinephrine*. Thus, tissues with a predominance of β_2 receptors (such as the vasculature of skeletal muscle) are particularly responsive to the hormonal effects of circulating *epinephrine* released by the adrenal medulla. Binding of a neurotransmitter at the β_1 or β_2 receptor results in activation of adenylyl cyclase and, therefore, increased concentrations of cAMP within the cell.

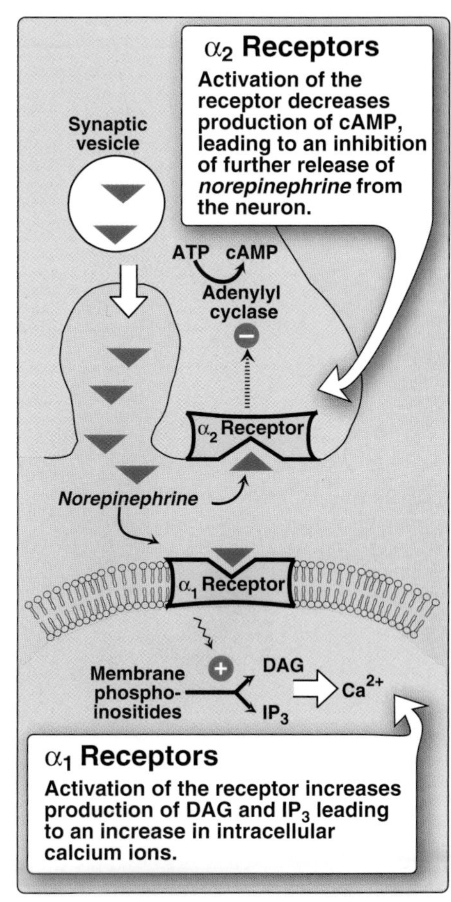

Figure 6.5
Second messengers mediate the effects of α receptors. DAG = diacylglycerol; IP_3 = inositol trisphosphate.

3. **Distribution of receptors:** Adrenergically innervated organs and tissues tend to have a predominance of one type of receptor. For example, tissues such as the vasculature to skeletal muscle have both α_1 and β_2 receptors, but the β_2 receptors predominate. Other tissues may have one type of receptor exclusively, with practically no significant numbers of other types of adrenergic receptors. For example, the heart contains predominantly β_1 receptors.

4. **Characteristic responses mediated by adrenoceptors:** It is useful to organize the physiologic responses to adrenergic stimulation according to receptor type, because many drugs preferentially stimulate or block one type of receptor. Figure 6.6 summarizes the most prominent effects mediated by the adrenoceptors. As a generalization, stimulation of α_1 receptors characteristically produces vasoconstriction (particularly in skin and abdominal viscera) and an increase in total peripheral resistance and blood pressure. Conversely, stimulation of β_1 receptors characteristically causes cardiac stimulation, whereas β_2 produces vasodilation (in skeletal vascular beds) and bronchiolar relaxation.

5. **Desensitization of receptors:** Prolonged exposure to the catecholamines reduces the responsiveness of these receptors, a phenomenon known as desensitization. Three mechanisms have

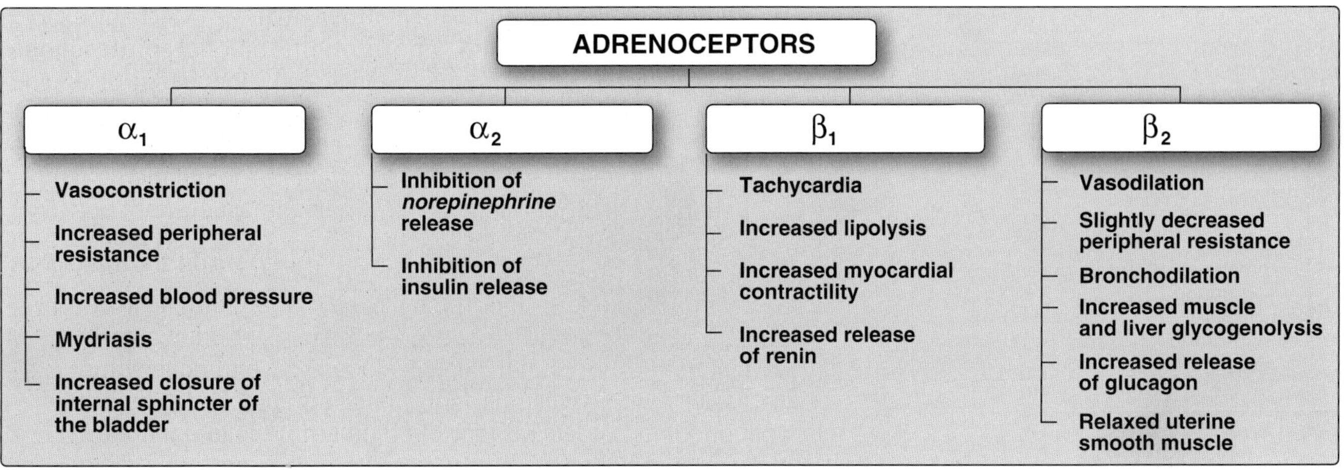

ADRENOCEPTORS
α1
Vasoconstriction
Increased peripheral resistance
Increased blood pressure
Mydriasis
Increased closure of internal sphincter of the bladder
α2
Inhibition of *norepinephrine* release
Inhibition of insulin release
β1
Tachycardia
Increased lipolysis
Increased myocardial contractility
Increased release of renin
β2
Vasodilation
Slightly decreased peripheral resistance
Bronchodilation
Increased muscle and liver glycogenolysis
Increased release of glucagon
Relaxed uterine smooth muscle

Figure 6.6
Major effects mediated by α and β adrenoceptors.

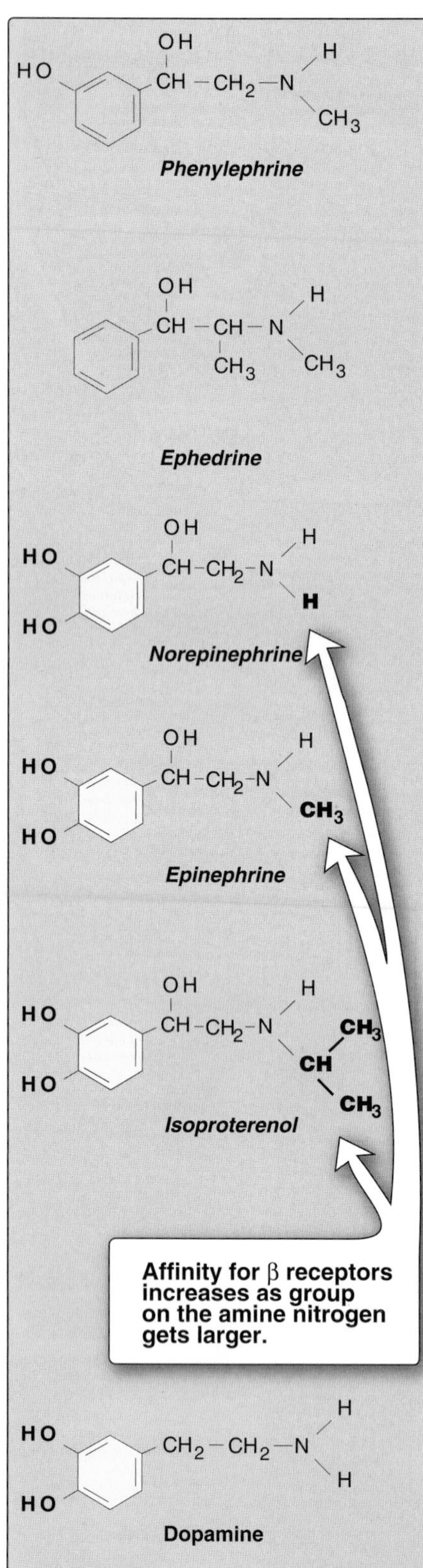

Figure 6.7
Structures of several important adrenergic agonists. Drugs containing the catechol ring are shown in yellow.

been suggested to explain this phenomenon: 1) sequestration of the receptors so that they are unavailable for interaction with the ligand; 2) down-regulation, that is, a disappearance of the receptors either by destruction or decreased synthesis; and 3) an inability to couple to G protein, because the receptor has been phosphorylated on the cytoplasmic side by either protein kinase A or β-adrenergic receptor kinase.

III. CHARACTERISTICS OF ADRENERGIC AGONISTS

Most of the adrenergic drugs are derivatives of β-phenylethylamine (Figure 6.7). Substitutions on the benzene ring or on the ethylamine side chains produce a great variety of compounds with varying abilities to differentiate between α and β receptors and to penetrate the CNS. Two important structural features of these drugs are the number and location of OH substitutions on the benzene ring, and the nature of the substituent on the amino nitrogen.

A. Catecholamines

Sympathomimetic amines that contain the 3,4-dihydroxybenzene group (such as *epinephrine*, *norepinephrine*, *isoproterenol*, and *dopamine*) are called catecholamines. These compounds share the following properties:

1. **High potency:** Drugs that are catechol derivatives (with –OH groups in the 3 and 4 positions on the benzene ring) show the highest potency in activating α or β receptors.

2. **Rapid inactivation:** Not only are the catecholamines metabolized by COMT postsynaptically and by MAO intraneuronally, they are also metabolized in other tissues. For example, COMT is in the gut wall, and MAO is in the liver and gut wall. Thus, catecholamines have only a brief period of action when given parenterally, and are ineffective when administered orally because of inactivation.

3. **Poor penetration into the CNS:** Catecholamines are polar and, therefore, do not readily penetrate into the CNS. Nevertheless, most of these drugs have some clinical effects (anxiety, tremor, and headaches) that are attributable to action on the CNS.

B. Noncatecholamines

Compounds lacking the catechol hydroxyl groups have longer half-lives, because they are not inactivated by COMT. These include *phenylephrine*, *ephedrine*, and *amphetamine*. *Phenylephrine*, an analog of *epinephrine*, has only a single –OH at position 3 on the benzene ring, whereas *ephedrine* lacks hydroxyls on the ring but has a methyl substitution at the α-carbon. These are poor substrates for MAO and, thus, show a prolonged duration of action, because MAO is an important route of detoxification. Increased lipid solubility of many of the noncatecholamines permits greater access to the CNS. [Note: *Ephedrine* and *amphetamine* may act indirectly by causing the release of stored catecholamines.]

C. Substitutions on the amine nitrogen

The nature and bulk of the substituent on the amine nitrogen is important in determining the β selectivity of the adrenergic agonist. For example, *epinephrine*, with a $-CH_3$ substituent on the amine nitrogen, is more potent at β receptors than *norepinephrine*, which has an unsubstituted amine. Similarly, *isoproterenol*, with an isopropyl substituent $-CH(CH_3)_2$ on the amine nitrogen (see Figure 6.7), is a strong β agonist with little α activity (see Figure 6.4).

D. Mechanism of action of the adrenergic agonists

1. **Direct-acting agonists:** These drugs act directly on α or β receptors, producing effects similar to those that occur following stimulation of sympathetic nerves or release of the hormone *epinephrine* from the adrenal medulla (Figure 6.8). Examples of direct-acting agonists include *epinephrine*, *norepinephrine*, *isoproterenol*, and *phenylephrine*.

2. **Indirect-acting agonists:** These agents, which include *amphetamine* and *tyramine*, are taken up into the presynaptic neuron and cause the release of *norepinephrine* from the cytoplasmic pools or vesicles of the adrenergic neuron (see Figure 6.8). As with neuronal stimulation, the *norepinephrine* then traverses the synapse and binds to the α or β receptors.

3. **Mixed-action agonists:** Some agonists, such as *ephedrine* and *metaraminol*, have the capacity both to stimulate adrenoceptors directly and to release *norepinephrine* from the adrenergic neuron (see Figure 6.8).

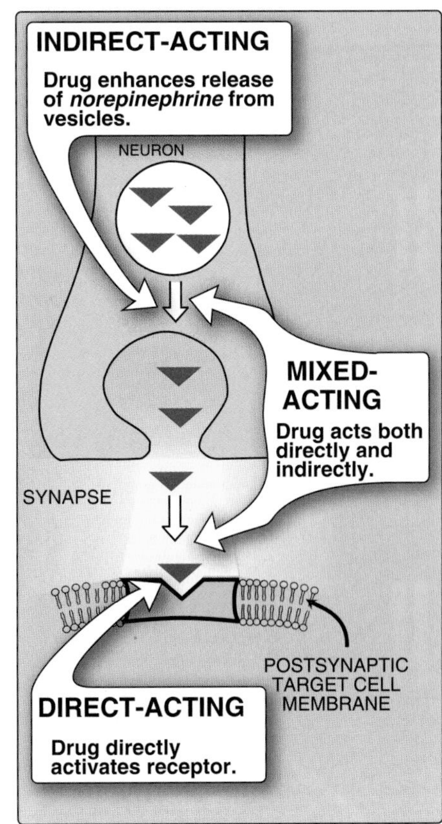

Figure 6.8
Sites of action of direct-, indirect-, and mixed-acting adrenergic agonists.

IV. DIRECT-ACTING ADRENERGIC AGONISTS

Direct-acting agonists bind to adrenergic receptors without interacting with the presynaptic neuron. The activated receptor initiates synthesis of second messengers and subsequent intracellular signals. As a group, these agents are widely used clinically.

A. Epinephrine

Epinephrine [ep i NEF rin] is one of four catecholamines—*epinephrine*, *norepinephrine*, *dopamine*, and *dobutamine*—commonly used in therapy. The first three catecholamines occur naturally, the latter is a synthetic compound. *Epinephrine* is synthesized from tyrosine in the adrenal medulla and released, along with small quantities of *norepinephrine*, into the bloodstream. *Epinephrine* interacts with both α and β receptors. At low doses, β effects (vasodilation) on the vascular system predominate, whereas at high doses, α effects (vasoconstriction) are strongest.

1. **Actions:**

   a. **Cardiovascular:** The major actions of *epinephrine* are on the cardiovascular system. *Epinephrine* strengthens the contractility of the myocardium (positive inotropic: β_1 action) and

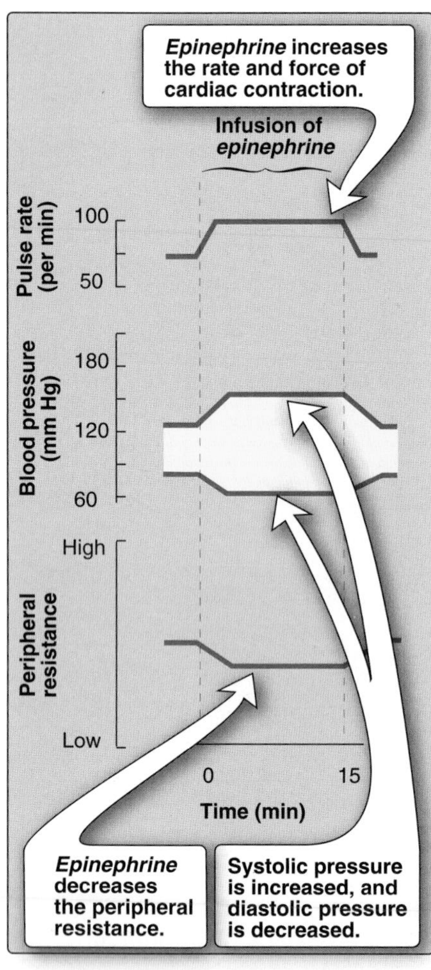

Figure 6.9
Cardiovascular effects of intravenous infusion of low doses of *epinephrine*.

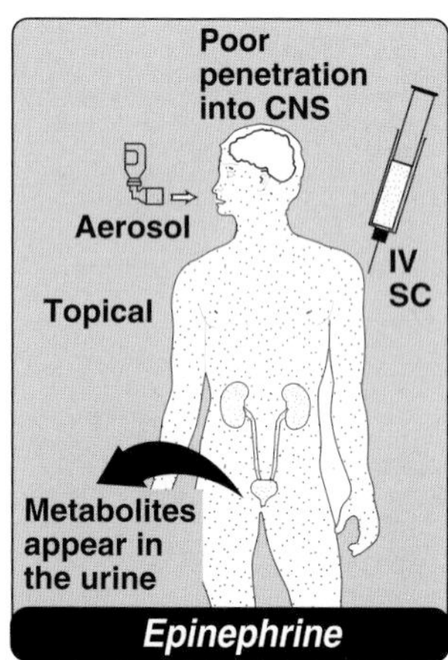

Figure 6.10
Pharmacokinetics of *epinephrine*.

increases its rate of contraction (positive chronotropic: β_1 action). Cardiac output therefore increases. With these effects comes increased oxygen demands on the myocardium. *Epinephrine* constricts arterioles in the skin, mucous membranes, and viscera (α effects), and dilates vessels going to the liver and skeletal muscle (β_2 effects). Renal blood flow is decreased. Therefore, the cumulative effect is an increase in systolic blood pressure, coupled with a slight decrease in diastolic pressure (Figure 6.9).

b. **Respiratory:** *Epinephrine* causes powerful bronchodilation by acting directly on bronchial smooth muscle (β_2 action). This action relieves all known allergic- or histamine-induced bronchoconstriction. In the case of anaphylactic shock, this can be lifesaving. In individuals suffering from an acute asthmatic attack, *epinephrine* rapidly relieves the dyspnea (labored breathing) and increases the tidal volume (volume of gases inspired and expired).

c. **Hyperglycemia:** *Epinephrine* has a significant hyperglycemic effect because of increased glycogenolysis in the liver (β_2 effect), increased release of glucagon (β_2 effect), and a decreased release of insulin (α_2 effect). These effects are mediated via the cyclic AMP mechanism.

d. **Lipolysis:** *Epinephrine* initiates lipolysis through its agonist activity on the β receptors of adipose tissue, which upon stimulation activate adenylyl cyclase to increase cyclic AMP levels. Cyclic AMP stimulates a hormone-sensitive lipase, which hydrolyzes triacylglycerols to free fatty acids and glycerol.[4]

2. **Biotransformations:** *Epinephrine*, like the other catecholamines, is metabolized by two enzymatic pathways: MAO, and COMT, which has S-adenosylmethionine as a cofactor (see Figure 6.3). The final metabolites found in the urine are metanephrine and vanillylmandelic acid. [Note: Urine also contains normetanephrine, a product of *norepinephrine* metabolism.]

3. **Therapeutic uses**

a. **Bronchospasm:** *Epinephrine* is the primary drug used in the emergency treatment of any condition of the respiratory tract when bronchoconstriction has resulted in diminished respiratory exchange. Thus, in treatment of acute asthma and anaphylactic shock, *epinephrine* is the drug of choice; within a few minutes after subcutaneous administration, greatly improved respiratory exchange is observed. Administration may be repeated after a few hours. However, selective β_2 agonists, such as *albuterol*, are presently favored in the chronic treatment of asthma because of a longer duration of action and minimal cardiac stimulatory effect.

b. **Glaucoma:** In ophthalmology, a two-percent *epinephrine* solution may be used topically to reduce intraocular pressure in

[4]See p. 187 in ***Lippincott's Illustrated Reviews: Biochemistry*** (3rd ed.) for a discussion of hormone-sensitive lipase activity.

open-angle glaucoma. It reduces the production of aqueous humor by vasoconstriction of the ciliary body blood vessels.

c. **Anaphylactic shock:** *Epinephrine* is the drug of choice for the treatment of Type I hypersensitivity reactions in response to allergens.

d. **In anesthetics:** Local anesthetic solutions usually contain 1:100,000 parts *epinephrine*. The effect of the drug is to greatly increase the duration of the local anesthesia. It does this by producing vasoconstriction at the site of injection, thereby allowing the local anesthetic to persist at the site before being absorbed into the circulation and metabolized. Very weak solutions of *epinephrine* (1:100,000) can also be used topically to vasoconstrict mucous membranes to control oozing of capillary blood.

4. **Pharmacokinetics:** *Epinephrine* has a rapid onset but a brief duration of action. In emergency situations, *epinephrine* is given intravenously for the most rapid onset of action. It may also be given subcutaneously, by endotracheal tube, by inhalation, or topically to the eye (Figure 6.10). Oral administration is ineffective, because *epinephrine* and the other catecholamines are inactivated by intestinal enzymes. Only metabolites are excreted in the urine.

5. **Adverse effects:**

a. **CNS disturbances:** *Epinephrine* can produce adverse CNS effects that include anxiety, fear, tension, headache, and tremor.

b. **Hemorrhage:** The drug may induce cerebral hemorrhage as a result of a marked elevation of blood pressure.

c. **Cardiac arrhythmias:** *Epinephrine* can trigger cardiac arrhythmias, particularly if the patient is receiving *digitalis*.

d. **Pulmonary edema:** *Epinephrine* can induce pulmonary edema.

6. **Interactions:**

a. **Hyperthyroidism:** *Epinephrine* may have enhanced cardiovascular actions in patients with hyperthyroidism. If *epinephrine* is required in such an individual, the dose must be reduced. The mechanism appears to involve increased production of adrenergic receptors on the vasculature of the hyperthyroid individual leading to a hypersensitive response.

b. **Cocaine:** In the presence of *cocaine*, *epinephrine* produces exaggerated cardiovascular actions. This is due to the ability of *cocaine* to prevent re-uptake of catecholamines into the adrenergic neuron; thus, like *norepinephrine*, *epinephrine* remains at the receptor site for longer periods of time (see Figure 6.3).

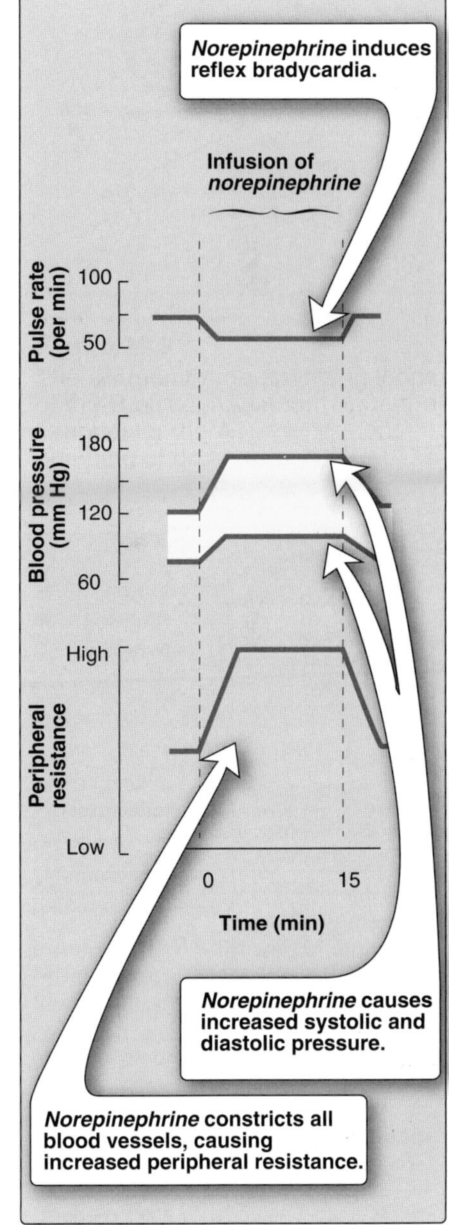

Figure 6.11
Cardiovascular effects of intravenous infusion of *norepinephrine*.

B. Norepinephrine

Because *norepinephrine* [nor ep i NEF rin] is the neuromediator of adrenergic nerves, it should theoretically stimulate all types of

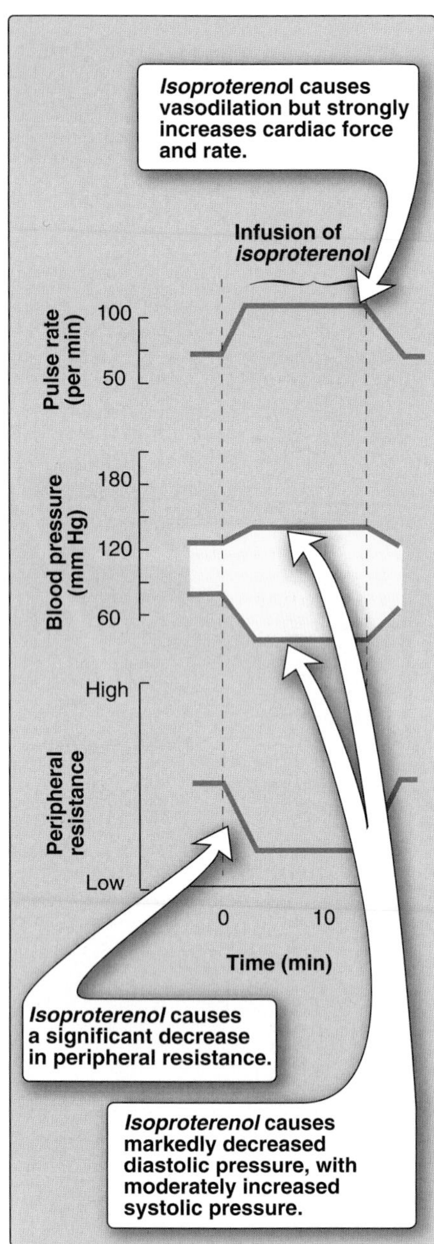

Figure 6.12
Cardiovascular effects of intravenous infusion of *isoproterenol.*

adrenergic receptors. In practice, when the drug is given in therapeutic doses to humans, the α-adrenergic receptor is most affected.

1. **Cardiovascular actions:**

   a. **Vasoconstriction:** *Norepinephrine* causes a rise in peripheral resistance due to intense vasoconstriction of most vascular beds, including the kidney (α_1 effect). Both systolic and diastolic blood pressures increase (Figure 6.11). [Note: *Norepinephrine* causes greater vasoconstriction than does *epinephrine* because it does not induce compensatory vasodilation via β_2 receptors of blood vessels supplying skeletal muscles, etc. The weak β_2 activity of *norepinephrine* also explains why it is not useful in the treatment of asthma.]

   b. **Baroreceptor reflex:** In isolated cardiac tissue, *norepinephrine* stimulates cardiac contractility; however, in vivo, little if any cardiac stimulation is noted. This is due to the increased blood pressure that induces a reflex rise in vagal activity by stimulating the baroreceptors. This bradycardia is sufficient to counteract the local actions of *norepinephrine* on the heart, although the reflex compensation does not affect the positive inotropic effects of the drug (see Figure 6.11).

   c. **Effect of atropine pretreatment:** If *atropine*, which blocks the transmission of vagal effects, is given before *norepinephrine*, then *norepinephrine* stimulation of the heart is evident as tachycardia.

2. **Therapeutic uses:** *Norepinephrine* is used to treat shock, because it increases vascular resistance and, therefore, increases blood pressure. However, *metaraminol* is favored, because it does not reduce blood flow to the kidney, as does *norepinephrine*. Other actions of *norepinephrine* are not considered to be clinically significant. It is never used for asthma. [Note: When *norepinephrine* is used as a drug, it is sometimes called *levarterenol* [leev are TER a nole].]

C. Isoproterenol

Isoproterenol [eye soe proe TER e nole] is a direct-acting synthetic catecholamine that predominantly stimulates both β_1 and β_2 adrenergic receptors. Its non-selectivity is one of its drawbacks. Its action on α receptors is insignificant.

1. **Actions:**

   a. **Cardiovascular:** *Isoproterenol* produces intense stimulation of the heart to increase its rate and force of contraction, causing increased cardiac output (Figure 6.12). It is as active as *epinephrine* in this action and, therefore, is useful in the treatment of atrioventricular block or cardiac arrest. *Isoproterenol* also dilates the arterioles of skeletal muscle (β_2 effect), resulting in a decreased peripheral resistance. Because of its cardiac stimulatory action, it may increase systolic blood pressure slightly, but it greatly reduces mean arterial and diastolic blood pressure (see Figure 6.12).

b. **Pulmonary:** A profound and rapid bronchodilation is produced by the drug (β_2 action, Figure 6.13). *Isoproterenol* is as active as *epinephrine* and rapidly alleviates an acute attack of asthma when taken by inhalation (which is the recommended route). This action lasts about one hour and may be repeated by subsequent doses.

c. **Other effects:** Other actions on β receptors, such as increased blood sugar and increased lipolysis, can be demonstrated but are not clinically significant.

2. **Therapeutic uses:** *Isoproterenol* is now rarely used as a bronchodilator in asthma. It can be employed to stimulate the heart in emergency situations.

3. **Pharmacokinetics:** *Isoproterenol* can be absorbed systemically by the sublingual mucosa but is more reliably absorbed when given parenterally or as an inhaled aerosol. It is a marginal substrate for COMT and is stable to MAO action.

4. **Adverse effects:** The adverse effects of *isoproterenol* are similar to those of *epinephrine*.

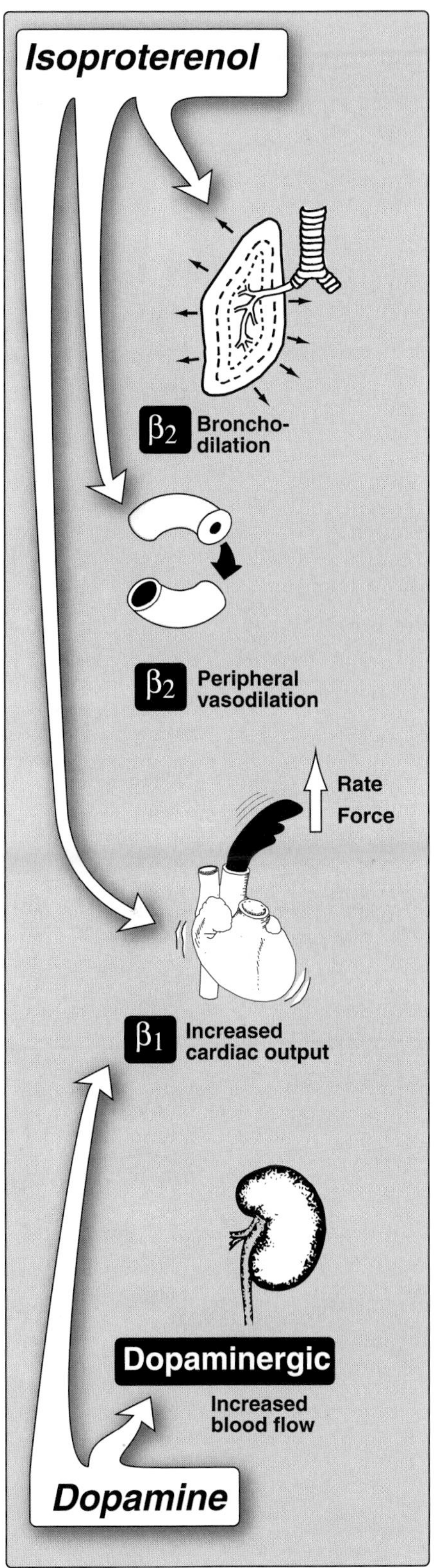

Figure 6.13
Clinically important actions of *isoproterenol* and *dopamine*.

D. Dopamine

Dopamine [DOE pa meen], the immediate metabolic precursor of *norepinephrine*, occurs naturally in the CNS in the basal ganglia, where it functions as a neurotransmitter, as well as in the adrenal medulla. *Dopamine* can activate α- and β-adrenergic receptors. For example, at higher doses, it can cause vasoconstriction by activating α receptors, whereas at lower doses, it stimulates β_1 cardiac receptors. In addition, D_1 and D_2 dopaminergic receptors, distinct from the α- and β-adrenergic receptors, occur in the peripheral mesenteric and renal vascular beds, where binding of *dopamine* produces vasodilatation. D_2 receptors are also found on presynaptic adrenergic neurons, where their activation interferes with *norepinephrine* release.

1. **Actions:**

a. **Cardiovascular:** *Dopamine* exerts a stimulatory effect on the β_1 receptors of the heart, having both inotropic and chronotropic effects (see Figure 6.13). At very high doses, *dopamine* activates α receptors on the vasculature, resulting in vasoconstriction.

b. **Renal and visceral:** *Dopamine* dilates renal and splanchnic arterioles by activating dopaminergic receptors, thus increasing blood flow to the kidneys and other viscera (see Figure 6.13). These receptors are not affected by α- or β-blocking drugs. Therefore, *dopamine* is clinically useful in the treatment of shock, in which significant increases in sympathetic activity might compromise renal function. [Note: Similar *dopamine* receptors are found in the autonomic ganglia and in the CNS.]

2. **Therapeutic uses:**

a. **Shock:** *Dopamine* is the drug of choice for shock, and is given by continuous infusion. It raises the blood pressure by stimulating the heart (α_1 action). In addition, it enhances perfusion to the kidney and splanchnic areas, as described above. An increased blood flow to the kidney enhances the glomerular filtration rate and causes sodium diuresis. In this regard, *dopamine* is far superior to *norepinephrine*, which diminishes the blood supply to the kidney and may cause renal shutdown.

3. **Adverse effects:** An overdose of *dopamine* produces the same effects as sympathetic stimulation. *Dopamine* is rapidly metabolized to homovanillic acid, and its adverse effects (nausea, hypertension, arrhythmias) are therefore short-lived.

E. Dobutamine

1. **Actions:** *Dobutamine* [doe BYOO ta meen] is a synthetic, direct-acting catecholamine that is a β_1-receptor agonist. It is available as a racemic mixture. One of the stereoisomers has a stimulatory activity. It increases cardiac rate and output with few vascular effects.

2. **Therapeutic uses:** *Dobutamine* is used to increase cardiac output in congestive heart failure (see p. 192). The drug increases cardiac output with little change in heart rate, and does not significantly elevate oxygen demands of the myocardium—a major advantage over other sympathomimetic drugs.

3. **Adverse effects:** *Dobutamine* should be used with caution in atrial fibrillation, because the drug increases atrioventricular conduction. Other adverse effects are the same as those for *epinephrine*. Tolerance may develop on prolonged use.

F. Phenylephrine

Phenylephrine [fen ill EF rin] is a direct-acting, synthetic adrenergic drug that binds primarily to α receptors and favors α_1 receptors over α_2 receptors. It is not a catechol derivative and, therefore, not a substrate for COMT. *Phenylephrine* is a vasoconstrictor that raises both systolic and diastolic blood pressures. It has no effect on the heart itself but rather induces reflex bradycardia when given parenterally. It is often used topically on the nasal mucous membranes and in ophthalmic solutions for mydriasis. *Phenylephrine* acts as a nasal decongestant, and produces prolonged vasoconstriction. The drug is used to raise blood pressure and to terminate episodes of supraventricular tachycardia (rapid heart action arising both from the atrioventricular junction and atria). Large doses can cause hypertensive headache and cardiac irregularities.

G. Methoxamine

Methoxamine [meth OX a meen] is a direct-acting, synthetic adrenergic drug that binds primarily to α receptors, with α_1 receptors favored over α_2 receptors. *Methoxamine* raises blood pressure by stimulating α_1 receptors in the arterioles, causing vasoconstriction. This causes an increase in total peripheral resistance. Because of its effects on the vagus nerve, *methoxamine* is used clinically to relieve attacks of paroxysmal supraventricular tachycardia. It is also used to overcome hypotension during surgery involving *halothane* anesthetics. In contrast to most other adrenergic drugs, *methoxamine* does not tend to trigger cardiac arrhythmias in the heart, which is sensitized by these general anesthetics. Adverse effects include hypertensive headache and vomiting.

H. Clonidine

Clonidine [KLOE ni deen] is an α_2 agonist that is used in essential hypertension to lower blood pressure because of its action in the CNS (see p. 223). It can be used to minimize the symptoms that accompany withdrawal from opiates or benzodiazepines. *Clonidine* acts centrally to produce inhibition of sympathetic vasomotor centers.

I. Metaproterenol

Metaproterenol [met a proe TER a nole], although chemically similar to *isoproterenol*, is not a catecholamine, and is resistant to methylation by COMT. It can be administered orally or by inhalation. The drug acts primarily at β_2 receptors, producing little effect on the heart. *Metaproterenol* produces dilation of the bronchioles and improves airway function. The drug is useful as a bronchodilator in the treatment of asthma and to reverse bronchospasm (Figure 6.14).

J. Albuterol, pirbuterol, and terbutaline

Albuterol [al BYOO ter ole], *pirbuterol* [peer BYOO ter ole], and *terbutaline* [ter BYOO te leen] are short-acting β_2 agonists used primarily as broncodilators, and administered by a metered-dose inhaler (see Figure 6.14). Compared with the nonselective β-adrenergic agonists, such as *metaproterenol*, these drugs produce equivalent bronchodilation with less cardiac stimulation.

K. Salmeterol and formoterol

Salmeterol [sal ME ter ole] and *formoterol* [for MOH ter ole] are β_2-adrenergic selective, long-acting bronchodilators. A single dose by a metered-dose inhaler provides sustained bronchodilation over twelve hours compared with less than three hours for *albuterol.* Unlike *formoterol*, however, *salmeterol* has a somewhat delayed onset of action (see Figure 6.14).

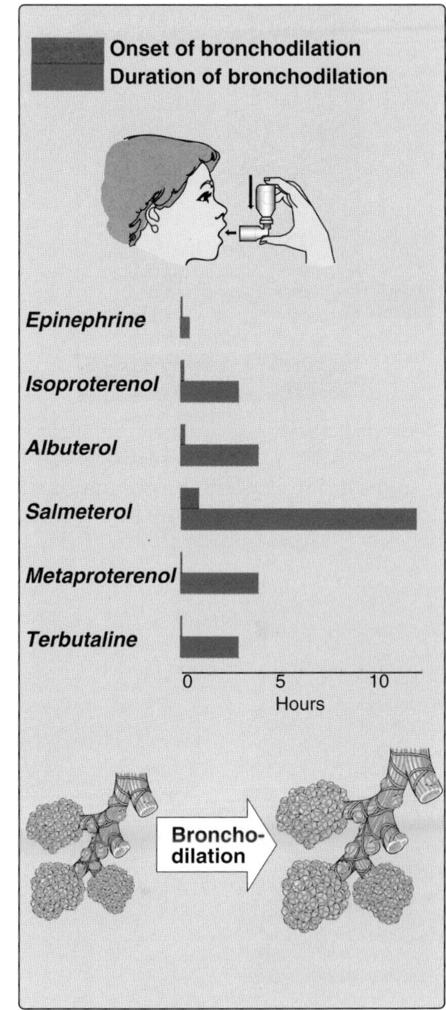

Figure 6.14
Onset and duration of bronchodilation effects of inhaled adrenergic agonists.

V. INDIRECT-ACTING ADRENERGIC AGONISTS

Indirect-acting adrenergic agonists cause *norepinephrine* release from presynaptic terminals (see Figure 6.8). They potentiate the effects of *norepinephrine* produced endogenously, but these agents do not directly affect postsynaptic receptors.

A. Amphetamine

The marked central stimulatory action of *amphetamine* [am FET a meen] is often mistaken by drug abusers as its only action. However, the drug can increase blood pressure significantly by α-agonist action on the vasculature as well as β-stimulatory effects on the heart. Its peripheral actions are mediated primarily through the cellular release of stored catecholamines; thus, *amphetamine* is an indirect-acting adrenergic drug. The actions and uses of *amphetamines* are discussed under stimulants of the CNS (see p. 119). The CNS stimulant effects of *amphetamine* and its derivatives have led to their use for treating hyperactivity in children, narcolepsy, and appetite control. Its use in pregnancy should be avoided because of adverse effects on development of the fetus.

B. Tyramine

Tyramine [TIE ra meen] is not a clinically useful drug, but it is found in fermented foods, such as ripe cheese and Chianti wine (see MAO inhibitors, p. 145). It is a normal byproduct of tyrosine metabolism. Normally, it is oxidized by MAO, but if the patient is taking MAO inhibitors, it can precipitate serious vasopressor episodes. Like *amphetamine*, *tyramine* can enter the nerve terminal and displace stored *norepinephrine*. The released catecholamine then acts on adrenoceptors.

VI. MIXED-ACTION ADRENERGIC AGONISTS

Mixed-action drugs induce the release of *norepinephrine* from presynaptic terminals, and activate adrenergic receptors on the postsynaptic membrane (see Figure 6.8).

A. Ephedrine

Ephedrine [e FED rin], a plant alkaloid, is now made synthetically. The drug is a mixed-action adrenergic agent. It not only releases stored *norepinephrine* from nerve endings (see Figure 6.8), but also directly stimulates both α and β receptors. Thus, a wide variety of adrenergic actions ensue that are similar to those of *epinephrine*, although less potent. *Ephedrine* is not a catechol and is a poor substrate for COMT and MAO; thus, the drug has a long duration of action. *Ephedrine* has excellent absorption orally, and penetrates into the CNS. It is eliminated unchanged in the urine. *Ephedrine* raises systolic and diastolic blood pressures by vasoconstriction and cardiac stimulation. *Ephedrine* produces bronchodilation, but it is less potent than *epinephrine* or *isoproterenol* in this regard and produces its action more slowly. It is therefore sometimes used prophylactically in chronic treatment of asthma to prevent attacks rather than to treat the acute attack. *Ephedrine* enhances contractility and improves motor function in myasthenia gravis, particularly when used in conjunction with anticholineesterases (see p. 50). *Ephedrine* produces a mild stimulation of the CNS. This increases alertness, decreases fatigue, and prevents sleep. It also improves athletic performance. *Ephedrine* has been used to treat asthma, as a nasal decongestant (due to its local vasoconstrictor action), and to raise blood pressure. [Note: The clinical use of *ephedrine* is declining due to the availability of better, more potent agents that cause fewer adverse effects. *Ephedrine*-containing herbal supplements (mainly Ephedra-containing products) were banned by the FDA in April 2004 because of life-threatening cardiovascular reactions.]

Important characteristics of the adrenergic agonists are summarized in Figures 6.15 and 6.16.

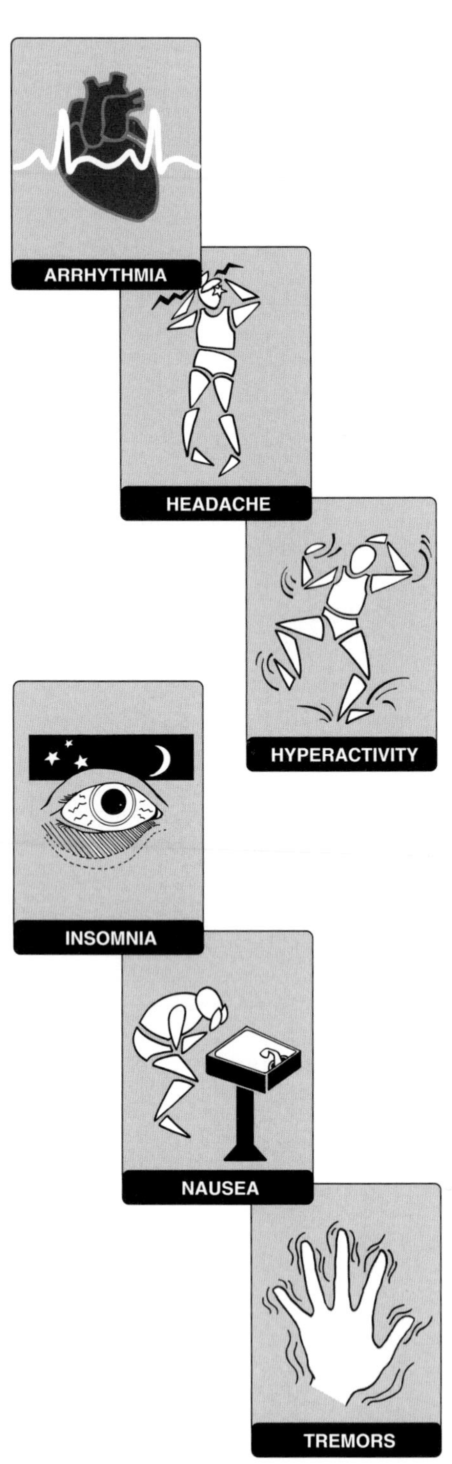

Figure 6.15
Some adverse effects observed with adrenergic agonists.

CATECHOLAMINES

- Rapid onset of action
- Brief duration of action
- Not administered orally
- Do not penetrate the blood-brain barrier

NONCATECHOLAMINES

Compared to catecholamines:

- Longer duration of action
- All can be administered orally

Drug	Receptor specificity	Therapeutic uses
Epinephrine	α_1, α_2 β_1, β_2	Acute asthma Treatment of open-angle glaucoma Anaphylactic shock In local anesthetics to increase duration of action
Norepinephrine	α_1, α_2 β_1	Treatment of shock
Isoproterenol	β_1, β_2	As a cardiac stimulant
Dopamine	Dopaminergic α_1, β_1	Treatment of shock Treatment of congestive heart failure Raise blood pressure
Dobutamine	β_1	Treatment of congestive heart failure
Phenylephrine	α_1	As a nasal decongestant Raise blood pressure Treatment of paroxysmal supraventricular tachycardia
Methoxamine	α_1	Treatment of supraventricular tachycardia
Clonidine	α_2	Treatment of hypertension
Metaproterenol	$\beta_2 > \beta_1$	Treatment of bronchospasm and asthma
Terbutaline *Albuterol*	β_2	Treatment of bronchospasm (short acting)
Salmeterol *Formoterol*	β_2	Treatment of bronchospasm (long acting)
Amphetamine	α, β, CNS	As a CNS stimulant in treatment of children with attention deficit syndrome, narcolepsy, and appetite control
Ephedrine	α, β, CNS	Treatment of asthma As a nasal decongestant Raise blood pressure

Figure 6.16
Summary of the adrenergic agonists.

Study Questions

Choose the ONE best answer.

6.1 A 68-year-old man presents to the emergency department with acute heart failure. You decide that this patient requires immediate drug therapy to improve his cardiac function. Which one of the following drugs would be most beneficial?

A. Albuterol
B. Dobutamine
C. Epinephrine
D. Norepinephrine
E. Phenylephrine

Correct answer = B. Dobutamine increases cardiac output without significantly increasing heart rate—a complicating condition in heart failure. Because epinephrine can significantly increase heart rate, it is not usually employed for acute heart failure. Both norepinephrine and phenylephrine have significant α_1-receptor–stimulating properties. The subsequent increase in blood pressure would worsen the heart failure. Albuterol, a β_2-selective–receptor agonist, would not improve contractility of the heart significantly.

6.2 Remedies for nasal stuffiness often contain which one of the following drugs?

A. Albuterol
B. Atropine
C. Epinephrine
D. Norepinephrine
E. Phenylephrine

Correct answer = E. Phenylephrine is an α agonist that constricts the nasal mucosa, thereby decreasing airway resistance. Norepinephrine and epinephrine also constrict the mucosa but have much too short a duration of action. Albuterol is a β_2 agonist and has no effect on mucosal volume. Atropine, a muscarinic antagonist, only dries the mucosa—it does not decrease its volume.

6.3 Which one of the following drugs, when administered intravenously, can decrease blood flow to the skin, increase blood flow to skeletal muscle, and increase the force and rate of cardiac contraction?

A. Epinephrine
B. Isoproterenol
C. Norepinephrine
D. Phenylephrine
E. Terbutaline

Correct answer = A. Exogenous epinephrine stimulates α and β receptors equally well, leading to the constriction of blood vessels in tissues such as skin and dilation of other blood vessels in tissues such as skeletal muscle. Epinephrine also has positive chronotropic and inotropic effects in the heart. Exogenous norepinephrine constricts blood vessels only and causes a reflex bradycardia because of its strong α-adrenergic stimulating properties. Phenylephrine has similar effects. Isoproterenol stimulates β receptors and would not cause vasoconstriction of cutaneous vessels.

6.4 The following circles represent pupillary diameter in one eye prior to and following the topical application of Drug X.

Control

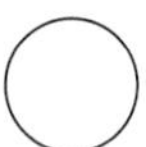

Drug X

Which of the following is most likely to be Drug X?

A. Physostimine
B. Acetylcholine
C. Terbutaline
D. Phenylephrine
E. Isoproterenol

Correct answer = D. Phenylephrine is the only drug on the list that causes mydriasis, because it stimulates α receptors. Both physostigmine and acetylcholine cause pupillary constriction. The β-blockers, terbutaline and isoproterenol, do not influence pupillary diameter.

Adrenergic Antagonists

7

I. OVERVIEW

The adrenergic antagonists (also called blockers or sympatholytic agents) bind to adrenoceptors but do not trigger the usual receptor-mediated intracellular effects. These drugs act by either reversibly or irreversibly attaching to the receptor, thus preventing its activation by endogenous catecholamines. Like the agonists, the adrenergic antagonists are classified according to their relative affinities for α or β receptors in the peripheral nervous system. [Note: Antagonists that block dopamine receptors are most important in the central nervous system and are therefore considered in that section (see p. 150).] The receptor-blocking drugs discussed in this chapter are summarized in Figure 7.1.

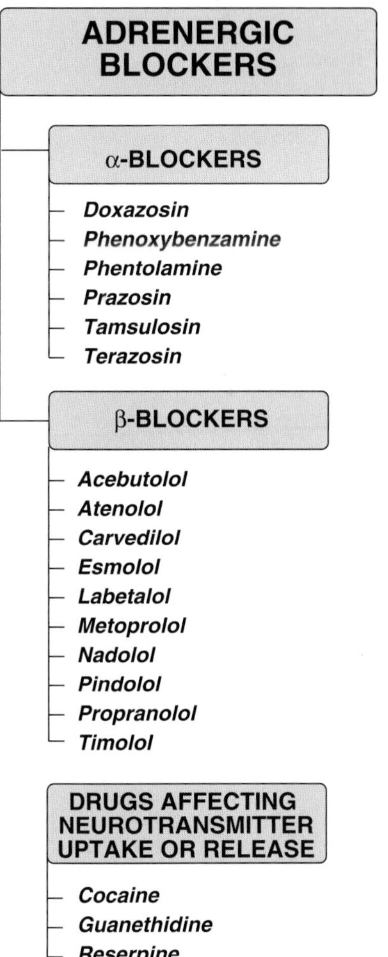

ADRENERGIC BLOCKERS
α-BLOCKERS
Doxazosin
Phenoxybenzamine
Phentolamine
Prazosin
Tamsulosin
Terazosin
β-BLOCKERS
Acebutolol
Atenolol
Carvedilol
Esmolol
Labetalol
Metoprolol
Nadolol
Pindolol
Propranolol
Timolol
DRUGS AFFECTING NEUROTRANSMITTER UPTAKE OR RELEASE
Cocaine
Guanethidine
Reserpine

Figure 7.1
Summary of blocking agents and drugs affecting neurotransmitter uptake or release.

II. α-ADRENERGIC BLOCKING AGENTS

Drugs that block α adrenoceptors profoundly affect blood pressure. Because normal sympathetic control of the vasculature occurs in large part through agonist actions on α-adrenergic receptors, blockade of these receptors reduces the sympathetic tone of the blood vessels, resulting in decreased peripheral vascular resistance. This induces a reflex tachycardia resulting from the lowered blood pressure. [Note: β receptors, including β_1 adrenoceptors on the heart, are not affected by α blockade.] The α-adrenergic blocking agents, *phenoxybenzamine* and *phentolamine*, have limited clinical applications.

A. Phenoxybenzamine

Phenoxybenzamine [fen ox ee BEN za meen], a drug related to the nitrogen mustards, is nonselective, linking covalently to both α_1-postsynaptic and α_2-presynaptic receptors (Figure 7.2). The block is irreversible and noncompetitive, and the only mechanism the body has for overcoming the block is to synthesize new adrenoceptors, which requires a day or more. Therefore, the actions of *phenoxybenzamine* last about 24 hours after a single administration. After

Lippincott's Illustrated Reviews: Pharmacology, Third Edition, by Richard D. Howland and Mary J. Mycek.

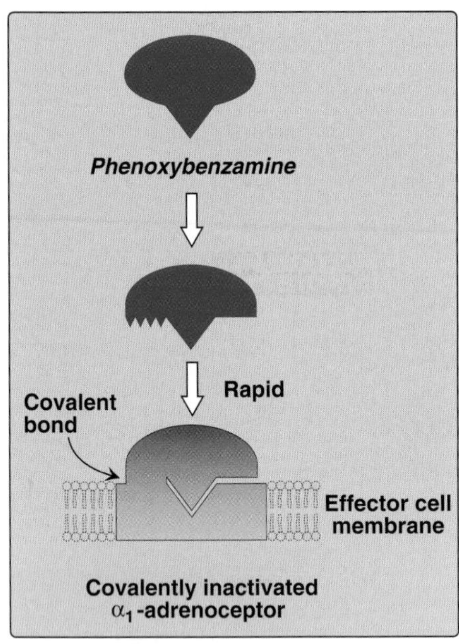

Figure 7.2
Covalent inactivation of α_1 adrenoceptor by *phenoxybenzamine*.

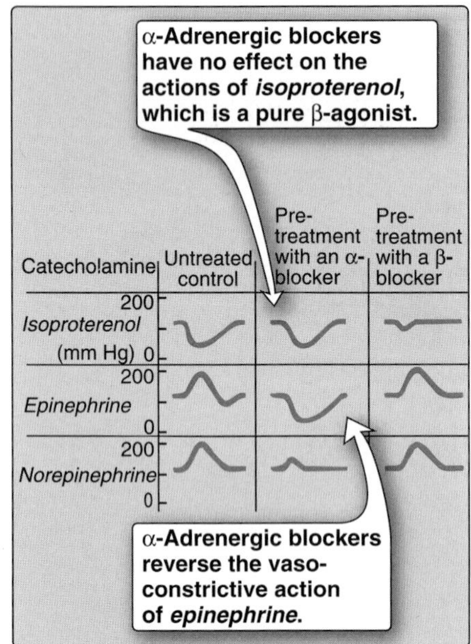

Figure 7.3
Summary of effects of adrenergic blockers on the changes in blood pressure induced by *isoproterenol*, *epinephrine*, and *norepinephrine*.

the drug is injected, a delay of a few hours occurs before a blockade develops, because the molecule must undergo biotransformation to the active form.

1. **Actions:**

   a. **Cardiovascular effects:** By blocking α receptors, *phenoxybenzamine* prevents vasoconstriction of peripheral blood vessels by endogenous catecholamines. The decreased peripheral resistance provokes a reflex tachycardia. Furthermore, the ability to block presynaptic α_2 receptors in the heart can contribute to an increased cardiac output. Thus, the drug has been unsuccessful in maintaining lowered blood pressure in hypertension and has been discontinued for this purpose.

   b. **Epinephrine reversal:** All α-adrenergic blockers reverse the α-agonist actions of *epinephrine*. For example, the vasoconstrictive action of *epinephrine* is interrupted, but vasodilation of other vascular beds caused by stimulation of β receptors is not blocked. Therefore, the systemic blood pressure decreases in response to *epinephrine* given in the presence of *phenoxybenzamine* (Figure 7.3). [Note: The actions of *norepinephrine* are not reversed but are diminished, because *norepinephrine* lacks significant β-agonist action on the vasculature.] *Phenoxybenzamine* has no effect on the actions of *isoproterenol*, which is a pure β agonist (see Figure 7.3).

2. **Therapeutic uses:** *Phenoxybenzamine* is used in the treatment of pheochromocytoma, a catecholamine-secreting tumor of cells derived from the adrenal medulla. Prior to surgical removal of the tumor, patients are treated with *phenoxybenzamine* to preclude the hypertensive crisis that can result from manipulation of the tissue. This drug also finds use in the chronic management of these tumors, particularly when the catecholamine-secreting cells are diffuse and, therefore, inoperable. *Phenoxybenzamine* or *phentolamine* are sometimes effective in treating Raynaud disease. Autonomic hyperreflexia, which predisposes paraplegics to strokes, can be managed with *phenoxybenzamine*.

3. **Adverse effects:** *Phenoxybenzamine* can cause postural hypotension, nasal stuffiness, nausea, and vomiting. It can inhibit ejaculation. The drug also may induce tachycardia, mediated by the baroreceptor reflex, and is contraindicated in patients with decreased coronary perfusion.

B. Phentolamine

In contrast to *phenoxybenzamine*, *phentolamine* [fen TOLE a meen] produces a competitive block of α_1 and α_2 receptors. The drug's action lasts for approximately four hours after a single administration. Like *phenoxybenzamine*, it produces postural hypotension and causes *epinephrine* reversal. *Phentolamine*-induced reflex cardiac stimulation and tachycardia are mediated by the baroreceptor reflex and by blocking the α_2 receptors of the cardiac sympathetic nerves.

The drug can also trigger arrhythmias and anginal pain, and is contraindicated in patients with decreased coronary perfusion.

C. Prazosin, terazosin, doxazosin, and tamsulosin

Prazosin [PRAY zoe sin], *terazosin* [ter AY zoe sin], *doxazosin* [dox AY zoe sin], and *tamsulosin* [tam SUE loh sin] are selective competitive blockers of the α_1 receptor. In contrast to *phenoxybenzamine* and *phentolamine*, the first three drugs are useful in the treatment of hypertension. *Tamsulosin* is indicated for the treatment of benign prostatic hypertrophy. Metabolism leads to inactive products that are excreted in the urine except for those of *doxazosin*, which appear in the feces. *Doxazosin* is the longest acting of these drugs.

1. **Cardiovascular effects:** All of these agents decrease peripheral vascular resistance and lower arterial blood pressure by causing the relaxation of both arterial and venous smooth muscle. *Tamsulosin* has the least effect on blood pressure. These drugs, unlike *phenoxybenzamine* and *phentolamine*, cause minimal changes in cardiac output, renal blood flow, and the glomerular filtration rate.

2. **Therapeutic uses:** Individuals with elevated blood pressure who have been treated with one of these drugs do not become tolerant to its action. However, the first dose of these drugs produces an exaggerated hypotensive response that can result in syncope (fainting). This action, termed a "first-dose" effect, may be minimized by adjusting the first dose to one-third or one-fourth of the normal dose, and by giving the drug at bedtime. An increase in the risk of congestive heart failure has been reported when α_1-blockers have been used as monotherapy in hypertension. The α_1 antagonists have been used as an alternative to surgery in patients with symptomatic benign prostatic hypertrophy. Blockade of the α receptors decreases tone in the smooth muscle of the bladder neck and prostate and improves urine flow. *Tamsulosin* is a more potent inhibitor of the α_{1A} receptors found on the smooth muscle of the prostate. This selectivity accounts for *tamsulosin's* minimal effect on blood pressure. [Note: *Finasteride*, which inhibits dihydrotestosterone synthesis, has been approved for treatment of benign prostatic hypertrophy, but its effects are not evident for several weeks.]

3. **Adverse effects:** α_1-Blockers may cause dizziness, a lack of energy, nasal congestion, headache, drowsiness, and orthostatic hypotension (although to a lesser degree than that observed with *phenoxybenzamine* and *phentolamine*). An additive antihypertensive effect occurs when *prazosin* is given with either a diuretic or a β-blocker, thereby necessitating a reduction in its dose. Due to a tendency to retain sodium and fluid, *prazosin* is frequently used along with a diuretic. Male sexual function is not as severely affected by these drugs as it is by *phenoxybenzamine* and *phentolamine*. Figure 7.4 summarizes some adverse effects observed with α-blockers.

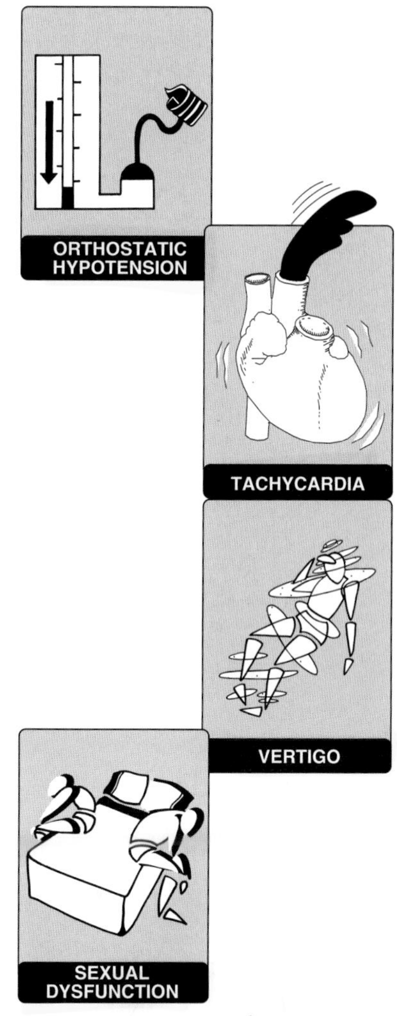

Figure 7.4
Some adverse effects commonly observed with nonselective α-adrenergic blocking agents.

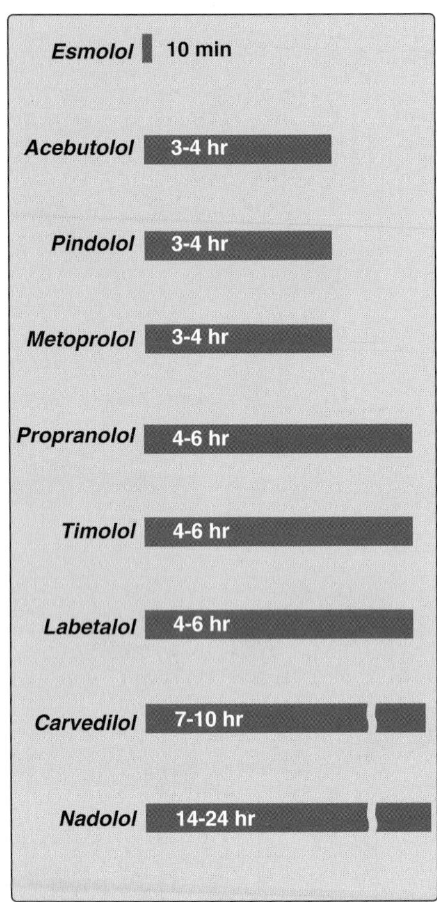

Figure 7.5
Elimination half-lives for some β-blockers.

III. β-ADRENERGIC BLOCKING AGENTS

All the clinically available β-blockers are competitive antagonists. Nonselective β-blockers act at both β_1 and β_2 receptors, whereas cardioselective β antagonists primarily block β_1 receptors. These drugs also differ in intrinsic sympathomimetic activity, in central nervous system (CNS) effects, and in pharmacokinetics (Figure 7.5). Although all β-blockers lower blood pressure in hypertension, they do not induce postural hypotension, because the α adrenoceptors remain functional. Therefore, normal sympathetic control of the vasculature is maintained. β-Blockers are also effective in treating angina, cardiac arrhythmias, myocardial infarction, and glaucoma, as well as serving in the prophylaxis of migraine headaches. [Note: The names of all β-blockers end in "-olol" except for *labetalol* and *carvedilol*.]

A. Propranolol: A nonselective β antagonist

Propranolol [proe PRAN oh lole] is the prototype β-adrenergic antagonist and blocks both β_1 and β_2 receptors. Sustained release preparations for once-a-day dosing are available.

1. Actions:

a. Cardiovascular: *Propranolol* diminishes cardiac output, having both negative inotropic and chronotropic effects (Figure 7.6). It directly depresses sinoauricular and atrioventricular activity. The resulting bradycardia usually limits the dose of the drug. Cardiac output, work, and oxygen consumption are decreased by blockade of β_1 receptors; these effects are useful in the treatment of angina (see p. 209). The β-blockers are effective in attenuating supraventricular cardiac arrhythmias but generally are not effective against ventricular arrhythmias (except those induced by exercise).

b. Peripheral vasoconstriction: Blockade of β receptors prevents β_2-mediated vasodilation (see Figure 7.6). The reduction in cardiac output leads to decreased blood pressure. This hypotension triggers a reflex peripheral vasoconstriction that is reflected in reduced blood flow to the periphery. On balance, there is a gradual reduction of both systolic and diastolic blood pressures in hypertensive patients. No postural hypotension occurs, because the α_1-adrenergic receptors that control vascular resistance are unaffected.

c. Bronchoconstriction: Blocking β_2 receptors in the lungs of susceptible patients causes contraction of the bronchiolar smooth muscle (see Figure 7.6). This can precipitate a respiratory crisis in patients with chronic obstructive pulmonary disease or asthma. β-Blockers are thus contraindicated in patients with asthma.

d. Increased Na^+ retention: Reduced blood pressure causes a decrease in renal perfusion, resulting in an increase in Na^+ retention and plasma volume (see Figure 7.6). In some cases, this compensatory response tends to elevate the blood pressure. For these patients, β-blockers are often combined with a diuretic to prevent Na^+ retention.

e. Disturbances in glucose metabolism: β-blockade leads to decreased glycogenolysis and decreased glucagon secretion. Therefore, if an insulin-dependent diabetic is to be given *propranolol*, very careful monitoring of blood glucose is essential, because pronounced hypoglycemia may occur after insulin injection. β-Blockers also attenuate the normal physiologic response to hypoglycemia.

f. Blocked action of isoproterenol: All β-blockers, including *propranolol*, have the ability to block the actions of *isoproterenol* on the cardiovascular system. Thus, in the presence of a β-blocker, *isoproterenol* does not produce either the typical reductions in mean arterial pressure and diastolic pressure, or cardiac stimulation (see Figure 7.3). [Note: In the presence of a β-blocker, *epinephrine* no longer lowers diastolic blood pressure or stimulates the heart, but its vasoconstrictive action (mediated by α receptors) remains unimpaired. The actions of *norepinephrine* on the cardiovascular system are mediated primarily by α receptors and are, therefore, unaffected.]

2. Therapeutic effects:

a. Hypertension: *Propranolol* lowers blood pressure in hypertension by decreasing cardiac output.

b. Glaucoma: *Propranolol* and other β-blockers, particularly *timolol*, are effective in diminishing intraocular pressure in glaucoma. This occurs by decreasing the secretion of aqueous humor by the ciliary body. Many patients with glaucoma have been maintained with these drugs for years. They neither affect the ability of the eye to focus for near vision nor change pupil size, as do the cholinergic drugs. However, in an acute attack of glaucoma, *pilocarpine* is still the drug of choice. The β-blockers are only used to treat this disease chronically.

c. Migraine: *Propranolol* is also effective in reducing migraine episodes (see p. 523). The value of the β-blockers is in the treatment of chronic migraine, in which the drug decreases the incidence and severity of the attacks. The mechanism may depend on the blockade of catecholamine-induced vasodilation in the brain vasculature. [Note: During an attack, the usual therapy with *sumatripan* or other drugs is used.]

d. Hyperthyroidism: *Propranolol* and other β-blockers are effective in blunting the widespread sympathetic stimulation that occurs in hyperthyroidism. In acute hyperthyroidism (thyroid storm), β-blockers may be lifesaving in protecting against serious cardiac arrhythmias.

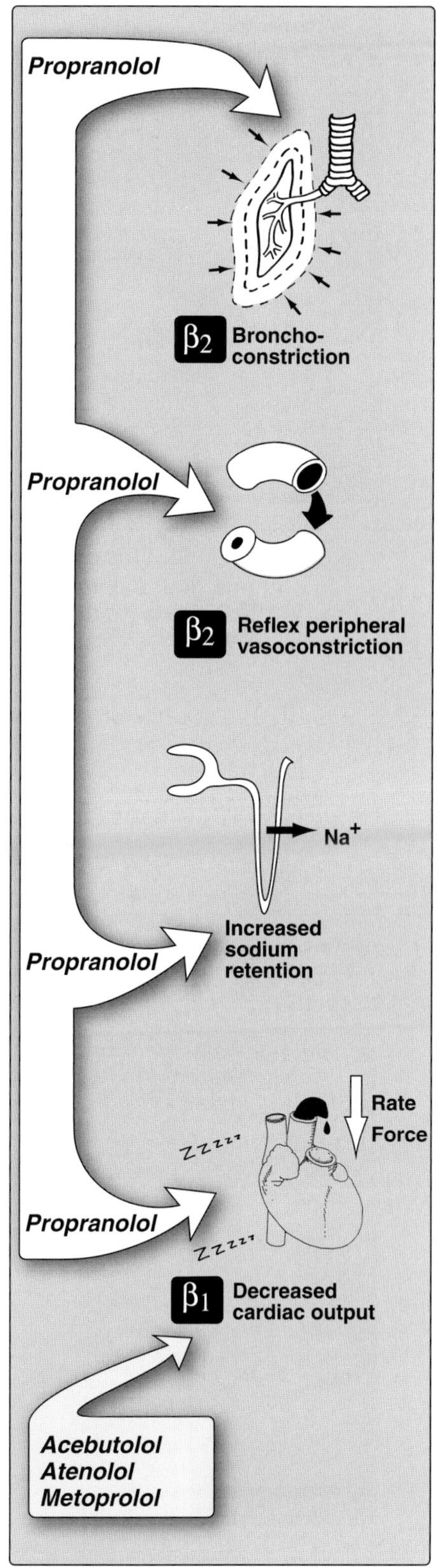

Figure 7.6
Actions of *propranolol* and other β-blockers.

e. **Angina pectoris:** *Propranolol* decreases the oxygen requirement of heart muscle and, therefore, is effective in reducing the chest pain on exertion that is common in angina. *Propranolol* is therefore useful in the chronic management of stable angina, but not for acute treatment. Tolerance to moderate exercise is increased, and this is measurable by improvement in the electrocardiogram. However, treatment with *propranolol* does not allow strenuous physical exercise, such as tennis.

f. **Myocardial infarction:** *Propranolol* and other β-blockers have a protective effect on the myocardium. Thus, patients who have had one myocardial infarction appear to be protected against a second heart attack by prophylactic use of β-blockers. In addition, administration of a β-blocker immediately following a myocardial infarction reduces infarct size and hastens recovery. The mechanism for these effects may be a blocking of the actions of circulating catecholamines, which would increase the oxygen demand in an already ischemic heart muscle. *Propranolol* also reduces the incidence of sudden arrhythmic death after myocardial infarction.

3. **Adverse effects:**

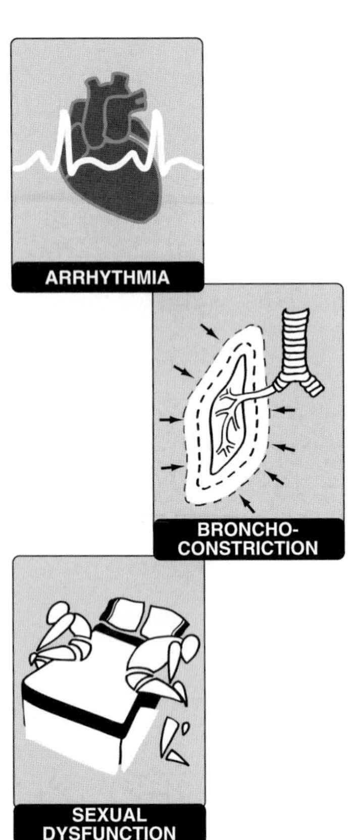

Figure 7.7
Adverse effects commonly observed in individuals treated with *propranolol*.

a. **Bronchoconstriction:** *Propranolol* has a serious and potentially lethal side effect when administered to an asthmatic (Figure 7.7). An immediate contraction of the bronchiolar smooth muscle prevents air from entering the lungs. Deaths by asphyxiation have been reported for asthmatics who were inadvertently administered the drug. Therefore, *propranolol* must never be used in treating any individual with chronic obstructive pulmonary disease.

b. **Arrhythmias:** Treatment with β-blockers must never be stopped quickly because of the risk of precipitating cardiac arrhythmias, which may be severe. The β-blockers must be tapered off gradually for one week. Long-term treatment with a β antagonist leads to up-regulation of the β-receptor. On suspension of therapy, the increased receptors can worsen angina or hypertension.

c. **Sexual impairment:** Because sexual function in the male occurs through α-adrenergic activation, β-blockers do not affect normal ejaculation or the internal bladder sphincter function. On the other hand, some men do complain of impaired sexual activity. The reasons for this are not clear, and they may be independent of β-receptor blockade.

d. **Disturbances in metabolism:** β-Blockade leads to decreased glycogenolysis and decreased glucagon secretion. Fasting hypoglycemia may occur. [Note: Cardioselective β-blockers are preferred in treating insulin-dependent asthmatics (see below).]

e. **Drug interactions:** Drugs that interfere with the metabolism of *propranolol*, such as *cimetidine*, *furosemide*, and *chlorpromazine*, may potentiate its antihypertensive effects. Conversely, those that stimulate its metabolism, such as barbiturates, *phenytoin* and *rifampin*, can mitigate its effects.

B. Timolol and nadolol: Nonselective β antagonists

Timolol [TIM o lole] and *nadolol* [NAH doh lole] also block β_1 and β_2 adrenoceptors, and are more potent than *propranolol*. *Nadolol* has a very long duration of action (see Figure 7.5). *Timolol* reduces the production of aqueous humor in the eye. It is used topically in the treatment of chronic open-angle glaucoma and, occasionally, for systemic treatment of hypertension.

C. Acebutolol, atenolol, metoprolol, and esmolol: Selective β_1 antagonists

Drugs that preferentially block the β_1 receptors have been developed to eliminate the unwanted bronchoconstrictor effect (β_2 effect) of *propranolol* seen among asthmatic patients. Cardioselective β-blockers, such as *acebutolol* [a se BYOO toe lole], *atenolol* [a TEN oh lole], and *metoprolol* [me TOE proe lole], antagonize β_1 receptors at doses 50- to 100-fold less than those required to block β_2 receptors. This cardioselectivity is thus most pronounced at low doses and is lost at high doses. [Note: *Acebutolol* has some intrinsic agonist activity.]

1. **Actions:** These drugs lower blood pressure in hypertension and increase exercise tolerance in angina (see Figure 7.6). *Esmolol* [EZ moe lole] has a very short lifetime (see Figure 7.5) due to metabolism of an ester linkage. It is only given intravenously if required during surgery or diagnostic procedures (for example, cystoscopy). In contrast to *propranolol*, the cardiospecific blockers have relatively little effect on pulmonary function, peripheral resistance, and carbohydrate metabolism. Nevertheless, asthmatics treated with these agents must be carefully monitored to make certain that respiratory activity is not compromised.

2. **Therapeutic use in hypertension:** The cardioselective β-blockers are useful in hypertensive patients with impaired pulmonary function. Because these drugs have less effect on peripheral vascular β_2 receptors, coldness of extremities, a common side effect of β-blocker therapy, is less frequent. Cardioselective β-blockers are useful in diabetic hypertensive patients who are receiving insulin or oral hypoglycemic agents.

D. Pindolol and acebutolol: Antagonists with partial agonist activity

1. **Actions:**

a. **Cardiovascular:** *Acebutolol* and *pindolol* [PIN doe lole] are not pure antagonists; instead, they have the ability to weakly stimulate both β_1 and β_2 receptors (Figure 7.8), and are said to have intrinsic sympathomimetic activity (ISA). These partial agonists

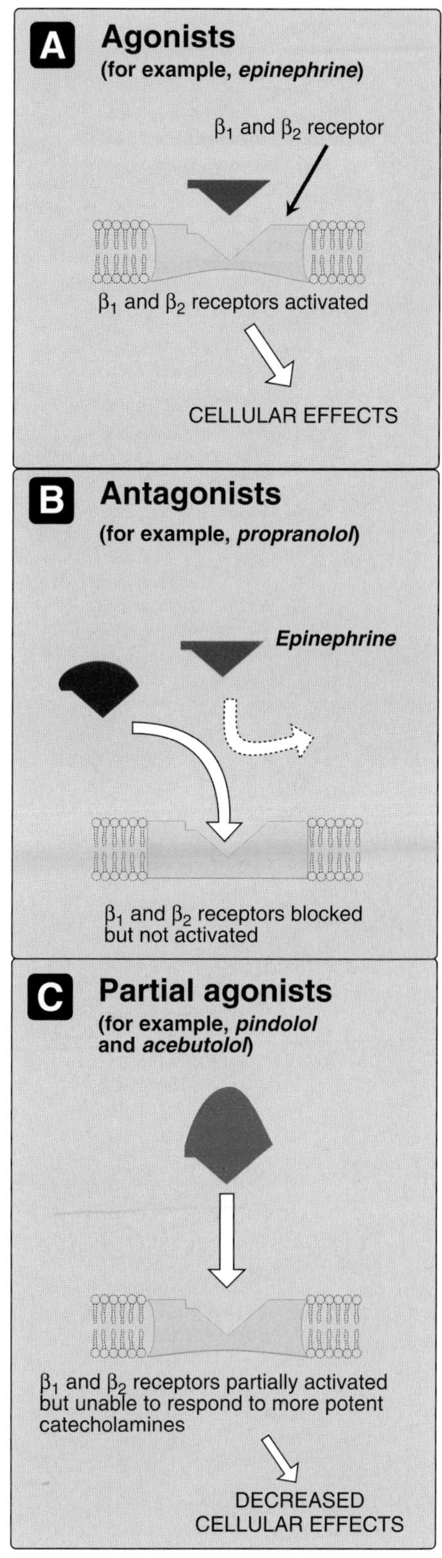

Figure 7.8
Comparison of agonists, antagonists, and partial agonists of β adrenoceptors.

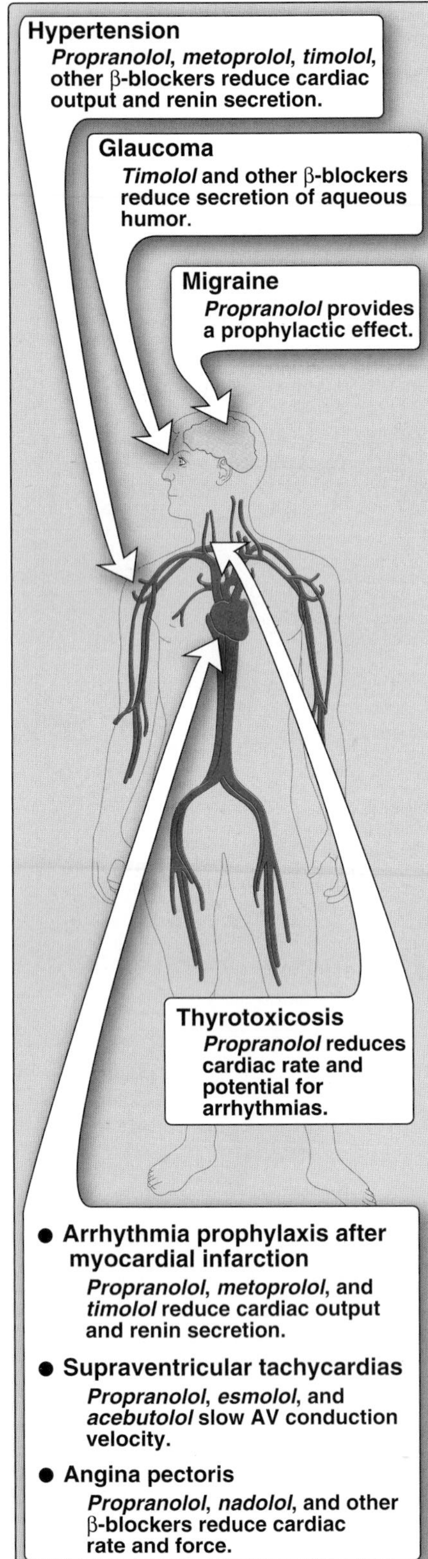

Hypertension
Propranolol, metoprolol, timolol, other β-blockers reduce cardiac output and renin secretion.
Glaucoma
Timolol and other β-blockers reduce secretion of aqueous humor.
Migraine
Propranolol provides a prophylactic effect.
Thyrotoxicosis
Propranolol reduces cardiac rate and potential for arrhythmias.
Arrhythmia prophylaxis after myocardial infarction
Propranolol, metoprolol, and timolol reduce cardiac output and renin secretion.
Supraventricular tachycardias
Propranolol, esmolol, and acebutolol slow AV conduction velocity.
Angina pectoris
Propranolol, nadolol, and other β-blockers reduce cardiac rate and force.

Figure 7.9
Some clinical applications of β-blockers. AV = atrioventricular.

stimulate the β-receptor to which they are bound, yet they inhibit stimulation by the more potent endogenous catecholamines, *epinephrine* and *norepinephrine*. The result of these opposing actions is a much diminished effect on cardiac rate and cardiac output compared to that of β-blockers without ISA.

b. **Decreased metabolic effects:** Blockers with ISA minimize the disturbances of lipid and carbohydrate metabolism that are seen with other β-blockers.

2. **Therapeutic use in hypertension:** β-Blockers with ISA are effective in hypertensive patients with moderate bradycardia, because a further decrease in heart rate is less pronounced with these drugs. Carbohydrate metabolism is less affected with *acebutolol* and *pindolol* than it is with *propranolol*, making them valuable in the treatment of diabetics. Figure 7.9 summarizes some of the indications for β-blockers.

E. Labetalol and carvedilol: Antagonists of both α and β adrenoceptors

1. **Actions:** *Labetalol* [lah BET a lole] and *carvedilol* [CAR ve dil ol] are reversible β-blockers with concurrent α_1-blocking actions that produce peripheral vasodilation, thereby reducing blood pressure. They contrast with the other β-blockers that produce peripheral vasoconstriction, and are therefore useful in treating hypertensive patients for whom increased peripheral vascular resistance is undesirable. They do not alter serum lipid or blood glucose levels. *Carvedilol* also decreases lipid peroxidation and vascular wall thickening, effects that have benefit in heart failure.

2. **Therapeutic use in hypertension:** *Labetalol* is useful for treating the elderly or black hypertensive patient in whom increased peripheral vascular resistance is undesirable. [Note: In general, black hypertensive patients are not well controlled with β-blockers.] *Labetalol* may be employed as an alternative to *hydralazine* in the treatment of pregnancy-induced hypertension. *Labetalol* is also used to treat hypertensive emergencies because it can rapidly lower blood pressure.

3. **Adverse affects:** Orthostatic hypotension and dizziness are associated with α_1 blockade. Figure 7.10 summarizes the receptor specificities and uses of the β-adrenergic antagonists.

IV. DRUGS AFFECTING NEUROTRANSMITTER RELEASE OR UPTAKE

As was noted on p. 119, some agonists, such as *amphetamine* and *tyramine*, do not act directly on the adrenoceptor. Instead, they exert their effects indirectly on the adrenergic neuron by causing the release of neurotransmitter from storage vesicles. Similarly, some agents act on the adrenergic neuron, either to interfere in neurotransmitter release or to alter the uptake of the neurotransmitter into the adrenergic nerve.

A. Reserpine

Reserpine [re SER peen], a plant alkaloid, blocks the Mg^{2+}/adenosine triphosphate (ATP)-dependent transport of biogenic amines, *norepinephrine*, *dopamine*, and *serotonin* from the cytoplasm into storage vesicles in the adrenergic nerves of all body tissues. This causes an ultimate depletion of *norepinephrine* levels in the adrenergic neuron, because monoamine oxidase can degrade the *norepinephrine* in the cytoplasm. Sympathetic function, in general, is impaired because of decreased release of *norepinephrine*. Hypertensive patients taking the drug show a gradual decline in blood pressure, with a concomitant slowing of the cardiac rate. The drug has a slow onset and a long duration of action. When the drug is discontinued, the actions persist for many days. *Reserpine* is only used to treat hypertension that fails to repond to other treatments.

B. Guanethidine

Guanethidine [gwahn ETH i deen] inhibits the response of the adrenergic nerve to stimulation or to indirectly acting sympathomimetic amines. *Guanethidine* acts by blocking the release of stored *norepinephrine*. This results in a gradual lowering of blood pressure in hypertensive patients, and a decrease in cardiac rate. [Note: There is also an accentuation of parasympathetic tone of the gastrointestinal tract.] *Guanethidine* also displaces *norepinephrine* from storage vesicles (thus producing a transient increase in blood pressure). This leads to gradual depletion of *norepinephrine* in nerve endings except for those in the CNS. *Guanethidine* is now rarely used in the treatment of hypertension. *Guanethidine* commonly causes orthostatic hypotension and interferes with male sexual function. Supersensitivity to *norepinephrine* due to depletion of the amine can result in hypertensive crises in patients with pheochromocytoma.

C. Cocaine

Cocaine [koe KANE] is unique among local anesthetics in having the ability to block the Na^+/K^+-activated ATPase (required for cellular uptake of *norepinephrine*) across the cell membrane of the adrenergic neuron. Consequently, *norepinephrine* accumulates in the synaptic space, resulting in enhancement of sympathetic activity and potentiation of the actions of *epinephrine* and *norepinephrine*. Therefore, small doses of the catecholamines produce greatly magnified effects in an individual taking cocaine as compared to those in one who is not. In addition, the duration of action of *epinephrine* and *norepinephrine* is increased. [Note: Cocaine as a CNS stimulant and drug of abuse is discussed on p. 118.]

DRUG	RECEPTOR SPECIFICITY	USES
Propranolol	β_1, β_2	Hypertension Glaucoma Migraine Hyperthyroidism Angina pectoris Myocardial infarction
Nadolol *Timolol*	β_1, β_2	Glaucoma Hypertension
Acebutolol[1] *Atenolol* *Esmolol* *Metoprolol*	β_1	Hypertension
Pindolol[1]	β_1, β_2	Hypertension
Carvedilol *Labetalol*	$\alpha_1, \beta_1, \beta_2$	Hypertension Congestive heart failure

Figure 7.10
Summary of β-adrenergic antagonists. [1]*Acebutolol* and *pindolol* are partial agonists.

Study Questions

Choose the ONE best answer.

7.1 The graphs below depict the changes in blood pressure caused by the intravenous administration of epinephrine before and after an unknown Drug X.

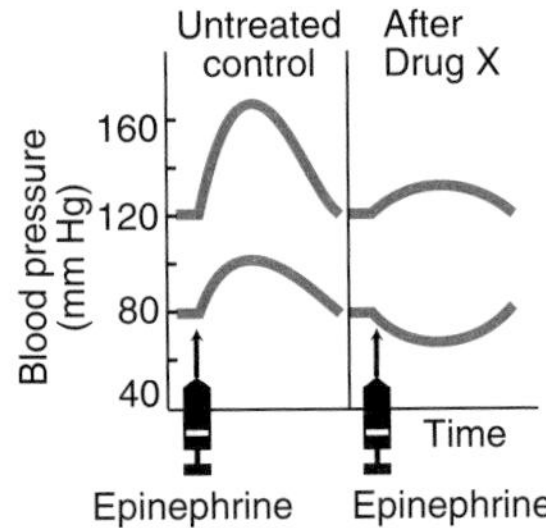

Which of the following drugs is most likely Drug X?

A. Atropine
B. Phenylephrine
C. Physostigmine
D. Prazosin
E. Propranolol

Correct answer = D. The dose of epinephrine increased both systolic and diastolic pressures, but because epinephrine dilates some and constricts other vessel beds, the rise in diastolic pressure is not as much. There is a marked increase in the pulse pressure. An α-blocker, such as prazosin, prevents the peripheral vasoconstrictor effects of epinephrine, leaving the vasodilator (β_2-stimulation) unopposed. This results in a marked decrease in the diastolic pressure coupled with a slight increase in systolic pressure due to increased cardiac output. This phenomenon is known as "epinephrine reversal", and is characteristic of the effect of α-blockers on the cardiovascular effects of epinephrine. None of the other drugs have α–blocking activity and, therefore, cannot produce this interaction.

7.2 A 38-year-old male has recently started monotherapy for mild hypertension. At his most recent office visit, he complains of tiredness and not being able to complete three sets of tennis. Which one of the following drugs is he most likely to be taking for hypertension?

A. Albuterol
B. Atenolol
C. Ephedrine
D. Phentolamine
E. Prazosin

Correct answer = B. Atenolol is a β_1 antagonist, and is effective in lowering blood pressure in patients with hypertension. Side effects of β-blockers include fatigue and exercise intolerance. Albuterol and ephedrine are not antihypertensive medications. Phentolamine and prazosin are antihypertensive drugs, but the side effects of α antagonists are not characterized by these symptoms.

7.3 A 60-year-old asthmatic man comes in for a checkup and complains that he is having some difficulty in "starting to urinate." Physical examination indicates that the man has a blood pressure of 160/100 mm Hg and a slightly enlarged prostate. Which of the following medications would be useful in treating both of these conditions?

A. Doxazosin
B. Labetalol
C. Phentolamine
D. Propranolol
E. Isoproterenol

Correct answer = A. Doxazosin is an competitive blocker at the α_1 receptor and lowers blood pressure. In addition, it blocks the α receptors in the smooth muscle of the bladder neck and prostate to improve urine flow. Labetalol and propranolol, although effective for treating the hypertension, are contraindicated in an asthmatic. They would not improve urine flow. Phentolamine has too many adverse effects to be used as an hypertensive agent. Isoproterenol is a β agonist and is not employed as a hypertensive, nor would it affect urinary function.

UNIT III:
Drugs Affecting the
Central Nervous System

Treatment of Neurodegenerative Diseases

8

I. OVERVIEW

Most drugs that affect the central nervous system (CNS) act by altering some step in the neurotransmission process. Drugs affecting the CNS may act presynaptically by influencing the production, storage, release, or termination of action of neurotransmitters. Other agents may activate or block postsynaptic receptors. This chapter provides an overview of the CNS, with a focus on those neurotransmitters that are involved in the actions of the clinically useful CNS drugs. These concepts are useful in understanding the etiology and treatment strategies of Parkinson and Alzheimer diseases—the two neurodegenerative disorders that respond to drug therapy (Figure 8.1).

ANTI-PARKINSON DRUGS

- *Amantadine*
- *Benzotropine*
- *Biperiden*
- *Bromocriptine*
- *Carbidopa*
- *Entacapone*
- *Levodopa*
- *Pergolide*
- *Pramipexole*
- *Ropinirole*
- *Selegiline* (*Deprenyl*)
- *Tolcapone*
- *Trihexphenidyl*

ANTI-ALZEHEIMER DRUGS

- *Donepezil*
- *Galantamine*
- *Memantine*
- *Rivastigmine*
- *Tacrine*

Figure 8.1
Summary of agents used in the treatment of Parkinson and Alzheimer diseases.

II. NEUROTRANSMISSION IN THE CNS

In many ways, the basic functioning of neurons in the CNS is similar to that of the autonomic nervous system described in Chapter 3. For example, transmission of information in the CNS and in the periphery both involve the release of neurotransmitters that diffuse across the synaptic space to bind to specific receptors on the postsynaptic neuron. In both systems, the recognition of the neurotransmitter by the membrane receptor of the postsynaptic neuron triggers intracellular changes. However, several major differences exist between neurons in the peripheral autonomic nervous system and those in the CNS. The circuitry of the CNS is much more complex than that of the autonomic nervous system, and the number of synapses in the CNS is far greater. The CNS, unlike the peripheral autonomic nervous system, contains powerful networks of inhibitory neurons that are constantly active in modulating the rate of neuronal transmission. In addition, the CNS communicates

Lippincott's Illustrated Reviews: Pharmacology, Third Edition,
by Richard D. Howland and Mary J. Mycek.
Lippincott Williams & Wilkins, Baltimore, MD © 2006.

NEUROTRANSMMITER		POSTSYNAPTIC EFFECTS
	Acetylcholine	Excitatory: Involved in arousal, short-term memory, and learning.
BIOGENIC AMINES	Norepinephrine	Excitatory: Involved in arousal, wakefulness, mood, and cardiovascular regulation.
	Dopamine	Excitatory: Involved in emotion and reward systems.
	Serotonin	Excitatory: Feeding behavior, control of body temperature, modulation of sensory pathways including nociception (pain), regulation of mood and emotion, and in sleep/wakefulness.
AMINO ACIDS	GABA	Inhibitory: Mediates the majority of inhibitory postsynaptic potentials.
	Glycine	Inhibitory: Increases Cl^- flux into the postsynaptic neuron, resulting in hyperpolarization.
	Gutamate	Excitatory: Mediates excitatory Na^+ influx into the postsynaptic neuron.
NEURO-PEPTIDES	Substance P	Excitatory: Mediates nociception (pain) within the spinal cord.
	Met-enkephalin	Generally inhibitory: Mediates analgesia as well as other central nervous system effects.

Figure 8.2
Summary of some neurotransmitters of the central nervous system (CNS). GABA = γ-aminobutyric acid.

through the use of more than ten (and perhaps as many as fifty) different neurotransmitters. In contrast, the autonomic system uses only two primary neurotransmitters, acetylcholine and norepinephrine. Figure 8.2 describes some of the more important neurotransmitters in the CNS.

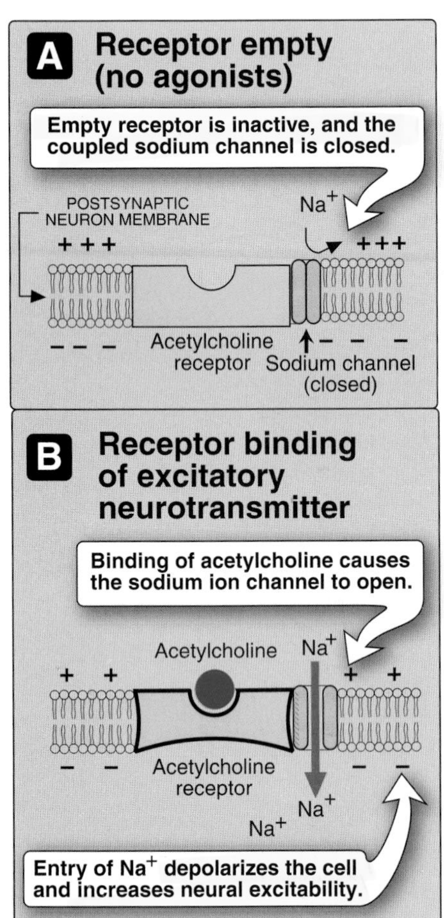

Figure 8.3
Binding of the excitatory neurotransmitter, acetylcholine, causes depolarization of the neuron.

III. SYNAPTIC POTENTIALS

In the CNS, receptors at most synapses are coupled to ion channels; that is, binding of the neurotransmitter to the postsynaptic membrane receptors results in a rapid but transient opening of ion channels. Open channels allow specific ions inside and outside the cell membrane to flow down their concentration gradients. The resulting change in the ionic composition across the membrane of the neuron alters the postsynaptic potential, producing either depolarization or hyperpolarization of the postsynaptic membrane, depending on the specific ions that move and the direction of their movement.

A. Excitatory pathways

Neurotransmitters can be classified as excitatory or inhibitory, depending on the nature of the action they elicit. Stimulation of excitatory neurons causes a movement of ions that results in a depolarization of the postsynaptic membrane. These excitatory postsynaptic potentials (EPSP) are generated by the following: 1) Stimulation of an excitatory neuron causes the release of neurotransmitter molecules, such as norepinephrine or acetylcholine, which bind to receptors on the postsynaptic cell membrane. This causes a transient increase in the permeability of sodium (Na^+) ions. 2) The influx of Na^+ causes a weak depolarization or EPSP. 3) If the number of excitatory fibers stimulated increases, more excitatory neurotransmitter is released. This ultimately causes the EPSP depolarization of the postsynaptic cell to pass a threshold, thereby generating an all-or-none action potential. [Note: The generation of a nerve impulse typically reflects the activation of synaptic receptors by thousands of excitatory neurotransmitter molecules released from many nerve fibers.] (See Figure 8.3 for an example of an excitatory pathway.)

B. Inhibitory pathways

Stimulation of inhibitory neurons causes movement of ions that results in a hyperpolarization of the postsynaptic membrane. These inhibitory postsynaptic potentials (IPSP) are generated by the following: 1) Stimulation of inhibitory neurons releases neurotransmitter molecules, such as γ-aminobutyric acid (GABA) or glycine, which bind to receptors on the postsynaptic cell membrane. This causes a transient increase in the permeability of specific ions, such as potassium (K^+) and chloride (Cl^-) ions. 2) The influx of Cl^- and efflux of K^+ cause a weak hyperpolarization or IPSP that moves the postsynaptic potential away from its firing threshold. This diminishes the generation of action potentials. (See Figure 8.4 for an example of an inhibitory pathway.)

C. Combined effects of the EPSP and IPSP

Most neurons in the CNS receive both EPSP and IPSP input. Thus, several different types of neurotransmitters may act on the same neuron, but each binds to its own specific receptor. The overall resultant action is due to the summation of the individual actions of the various neurotransmitters on the neuron. The neurotransmitters are not uniformly distributed in the CNS but are localized in specific clusters of neurons, the axons of which may synapse with specific regions of the brain. Many neuronal tracts thus seem to be chemically coded, and this may offer greater opportunity for selective modulation of certain neuronal pathways.

IV. NEURODEGENERATIVE DISEASES

Neurodegenerative diseases of the CNS include Alzheimer disease, Parkinson disease, Huntington disease, and amyotrophic lateral sclerosis. These devastating illnesses are characterized by the progressive loss of selected neurons in discrete brain areas, resulting in characteristic disorders of movement, cognition, or both. For example, Alzheimer disease is characterized by the loss of cholinergic neurons in the nucleus basalis of Maynert, whereas Parkinson disease is associated with a loss of dopaminergic neurons in the substantia niagra. The most prevalent of these disorders is Alzheimer, affecting some four million people. The number of cases is expected to increase as the proportion of elderly in the population increases. Parkinson disease is the second most frequent, affecting approximately 1.5 million Americans. Discussion of pharmacologic agents to treat these neurodegenerative diseases will be confined to those agents effective in Parkinson disease and Alzheimer disease, because specific agents for the other disorders listed above do not exist.

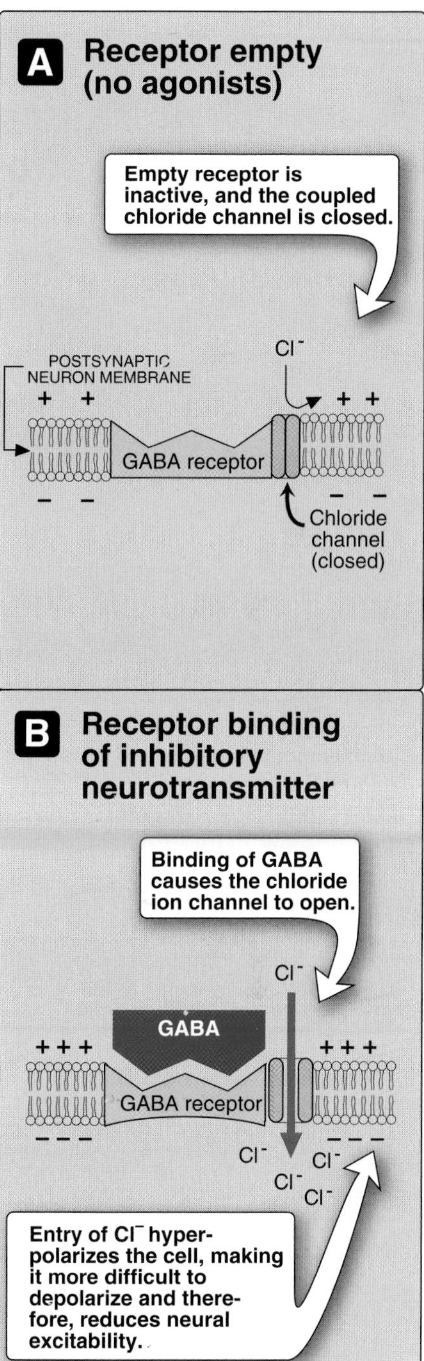

Figure 8.4
Binding of the inhibitory neurotransmitter, γ-aminobutyric acid (GABA), causes hyperpolarization of the neuron.

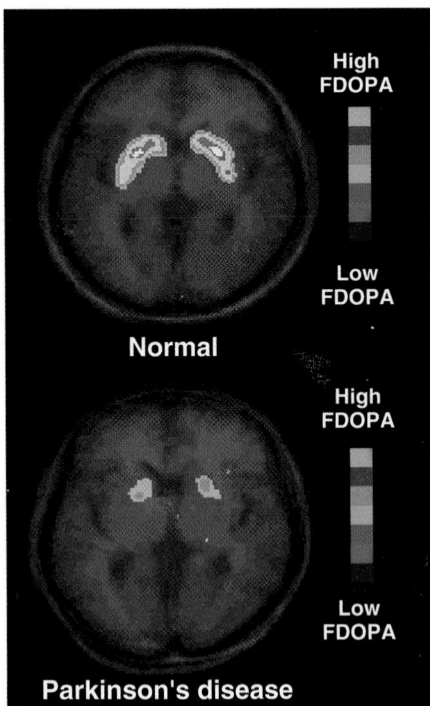

Figure 8.5
Positron-emission tomography scan of the brain showing the difference in fluorodopa (F-DOPA) levels between those with and without Parkinson disease.

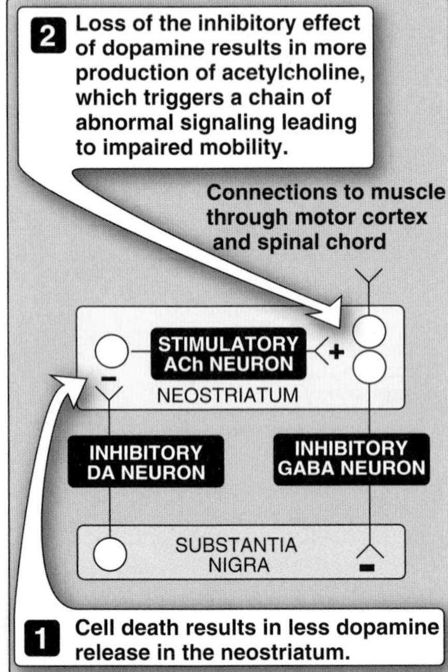

Figure 8.6
Role of substantia nigra in Parkinson's disease. DA = dopamine; GABA = γ-aminobutyric acid.

V. OVERVIEW OF PARKINSON DISEASE

Parkinsonism is a progressive neurologic disorder of muscle movement, characterized by tremors, muscular rigidity, bradykinesia (slowness in initiating and carrying out voluntary movements), and postural and gait abnormalities. Most cases involve people over the age of 65, among whom the incidence is about 1 in 100 individuals.

A. Etiology

The cause of Parkinson disease is unknown for most patients. The disease is correlated with a reduction in the activity of inhibitory dopaminergic neurons in the substantia nigra and corpus striatum—parts of the brain's basal ganglia system that are involved in motor control. This results in a decrease in dopamine in these nerve tracts, which can be visualized using positron-emission tomography and the dopamine analog *fluorodopa* (Figure 8.5). Genetic factors do not play a dominant role in the etiology of Parkinson disease, although they may exert some influence on an individual's susceptibility to the disease. It appears increasingly likely that an as-yet-unidentified environmental factor may play a role in the loss of dopaminergic neurons.

1. **Substantia nigra:** The substantia nigra, part of the extrapyramidal system, is the source of dopaminergic neurons that terminate in the striatum (Figure 8.6). Each dopaminergic neuron makes thousands of synaptic contacts within the neostriatum and, therefore, modulates the activity of a large number of cells. These dopaminergic projections from the substantia nigra fire tonically, rather than in response to specific muscular movements or sensory input. Thus, the dopaminergic system appears to serve as a tonic, sustaining influence on motor activity, rather than participating in specific movements.

2. **Neostriatum:** Normally, the neostriatum is connected to the substantia nigra by neurons that secrete the inhibitory transmitter GABA at their termini in the substantia nigra. In turn, cells of the substantia nigra send neurons back to the neostriatum, secreting the inhibitory transmitter dopamine at their termini. This mutual inhibitory pathway normally maintains a degree of inhibition of the two separate areas. In Parkinson disease, destruction of cells in the substantia nigra results in the degeneration of neurons responsible for secreting dopamine in the neostriatum. Thus, the normal modulating inhibitory influence of dopamine on cholinergic neurons in the neostriatum is significantly diminished, resulting in overproduction of acetylcholine. This triggers a chain of abnormal signaling, resulting in loss of the control of muscle movements (see Figure 8.6).

3. **Secondary parkinsonism:** Parkinsonian symptoms infrequently follow viral encephalitis or multiple small vascular lesions. Drugs such as the phenothiazines and *haloperidol*, whose major pharmacologic action is blockade of dopamine receptors in the brain, may also produce parkinsonian symptoms. These drugs should not be used in parkinsonian patients.

B. Strategy of treatment

In addition to an abundance of inhibitory dopaminergic neurons, the neostriatum is also rich in excitatory cholinergic neurons that oppose the action of dopamine (see Figure 8.6). Many of the symptoms of parkinsonism reflect an imbalance between the excitatory cholinergic neurons and the greatly diminished number of inhibitory dopaminergic neurons. Therapy is aimed at restoring dopamine in the basal ganglia and antagonizing the excitatory effect of cholinergic neurons, thus reestablishing the correct dopamine/acetylcholine balance. Because long-term treatment with *levodopa* is limited by fluctuations in therapeutic responses, strategies to maintain CNS dopamine levels as constant as possible have been devised.

VI. DRUGS USED IN PARKINSON DISEASE

Currently available drugs offer temporary relief from the symptoms of the disorder, but do not arrest or reverse the neuronal degeneration caused by the disease.

A. Levodopa and carbidopa

Levodopa [lee voe DOE pa] is a metabolic precursor of dopamine (Figure 8.7). It restores dopamine levels in the extrapyramidal centers (substantia nigra) that atrophy in parkinsonism. In patients with early disease, the number of residual dopaminergic neurons in the substantia nigra (typically about twenty percent of normal) is adequate for conversion of *levodopa* to dopamine. Thus, in new patients, the therapeutic response to *levodopa* is consistent, and the patient rarely complains that the drug effects "wear off." Unfortunately, with

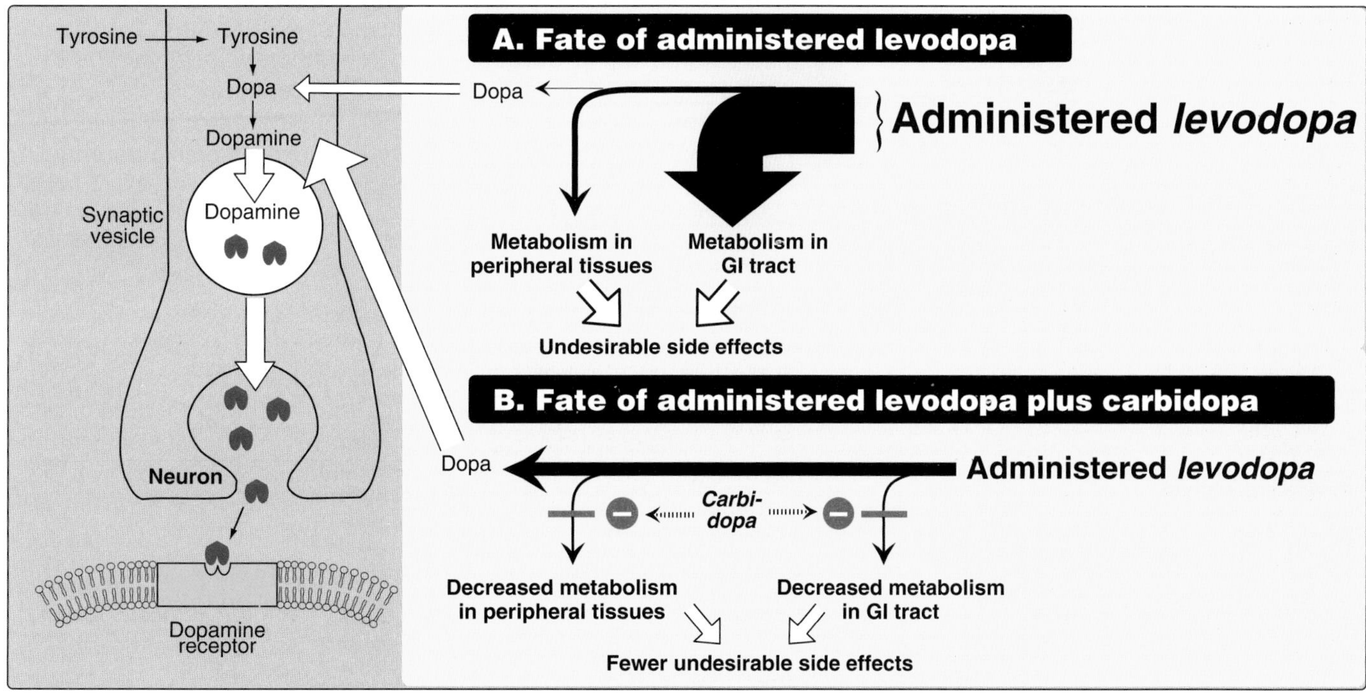

Figure 8.7
Synthesis of dopamine from *levodopa* in the absence and presence of *carbidopa*, an inhibitor of dopamine decarboxylase in the peripheral tissues. GI = gastrointestinal.

time, the number of neurons decreases, and fewer cells are capable of taking up exogenously administered *levodopa* and converting it to dopamine for subsequent storage and release. Consequently, motor control fluctuation develops. Relief provided by *levodopa* is only symptomatic, and it lasts only while the drug is present in the body.

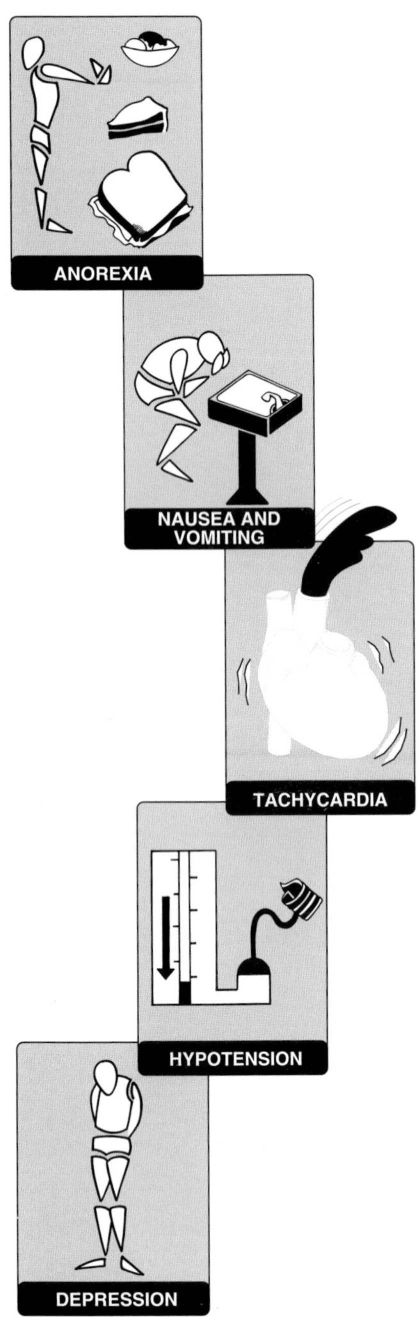

Figure 8.8
Adverse effects of *levodopa*.

1. Mechanism of action

a. Levodopa: Because parkinsonism results from insufficient dopamine in specific regions of the brain, attempts have been made to replenish the dopamine deficiency. Dopamine itself does not cross the blood-brain barrier, but its immediate precursor, *levodopa*, is readily transported into the CNS and is converted to dopamine in the brain (see Figure 8.7). Large doses of *levodopa* are required, because much of the drug is decarboxylated to dopamine in the periphery, resulting in side effects that include nausea, vomiting, cardiac arrhythmias, and hypotension.

b. Carbidopa: The effects of *levodopa* on the CNS can be greatly enhanced by coadministering *carbidopa* [kar bi DOE pa], a dopa decarboxylase inhibitor that does not cross the blood-brain barrier. *Carbidopa* diminishes the metabolism of *levodopa* in the gastrointestinal (GI) tract and peripheral tissues; thus, it increases the availability of *levodopa* to the CNS. The addition of *carbidopa* lowers the dose of *levodopa* needed by four- to five-fold and, consequently, decreases the severity of the side effects of peripherally formed dopamine.

2. Actions: *Levodopa* decreases the rigidity, tremors, and other symptoms of parkinsonism.

3. Therapeutic uses: *Levodopa* in combination with *carbidopa* is a potent and efficacious drug regimen currently available to treat Parkinson disease. In approximately two-thirds of patients with Parkinson disease, *levodopa-carbidopa* treatment substantially reduces the severity of the disease for the first few years of treatment. Patients then typically experience a decline in response during the third to fifth year of therapy.

4. Absorption and metabolism: The drug is absorbed rapidly from the small intestine (when empty of food). *Levodopa* has an extremely short half-life (one to two hours), which causes fluctuations in plasma concentration. This may produce fluctuations in motor response ("on-off" phenomenon), which may cause the patient to suddenly lose normal mobility and experience tremors, cramps, and immobility. Ingestion of meals, particularly if high in protein content, interferes with the transport of *levodopa* into the CNS. Large, neutral amino acids (for example, leucine and isoleucine) compete with *levodopa* for absorption from the gut and for transport across the blood-brain barrier. Thus, *levodopa* should be taken on an empty stomach, typically 45 minutes before a meal. Withdrawal from the drug must be gradual.

5. Adverse effects:

a. Peripheral effects: Anorexia, nausea, and vomiting occur because of stimulation of the emetic center (Figure 8.8). Tachycardia and ventricular extrasystoles result from dopaminergic action on the heart. Hypotension may also develop. Adrenergic action on the iris causes mydriasis, and in some individuals, blood dyscrasias and a positive reaction to the Coombs test are seen. Saliva and urine are a brownish color because of the melanin pigment produced from catecholamine oxidation.

b. CNS effects: Visual and auditory hallucinations and abnormal involuntary movements (dyskinesia) may occur. These CNS effects are the opposite of parkinsonian symptoms and reflect the overactivity of dopamine at receptors in the basal ganglia. *Levodopa* can also cause mood changes, depression, and anxiety.

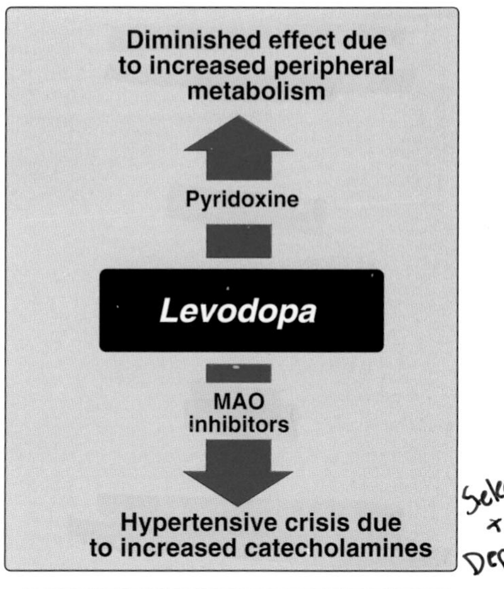

Figure 8.9
Some drug interactions observed with *levodopa*.

6. Interactions: The vitamin pyridoxine (B_6) increases the peripheral breakdown of *levodopa* and diminishes its effectiveness (Figure 8.9). Concomitant administration of *levodopa* and monoamine oxidase (MAO) inhibitors, such as *phenelzine*, can produce a hypertensive crisis caused by enhanced catecholamine production; therefore, caution is required when they are used simultaneously. In many psychotic patients, *levodopa* exacerbates symptoms, possibly through the buildup of central amines. In patients with glaucoma, the drug can cause an increase in intraocular pressure. Cardiac patients should be carefully monitored because of the possible development of cardiac arrhythmias. Antipsychotic drugs are contraindicated in parkinsonian patients, because these block dopamine receptors and produce a parkinsonian syndrome themselves.

B. Selegiline

Selegiline [seh LEDGE ah leen], also called *deprenyl* [DE pren ill], selectively inhibits MAO B (which metabolizes dopamine), but does not inhibit MAO A (which metabolizes norepinephrine and serotonin). By thus decreasing the metabolism of dopamine, *selegiline* has been found to increase dopamine levels in the brain (Figure 8.10). Therefore, it enhances the actions of *levodopa*, and when these drugs are administered together, *selegiline* substantially reduces the required dose of *levodopa*. Unlike nonselective MAO inhibitors, *selegiline* at recommended doses has little potential for causing hypertensive crises. However, if *selegiline* is administered at high doses, the selectivity of the drug is lost, and the patient is at risk for severe hypertension. [Note: Early reports of possible neuroprotective effects of *selegiline* have not been supported by long-term studies.]

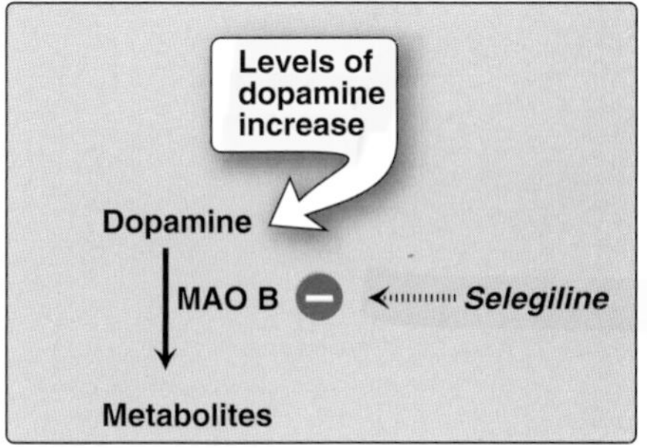

Figure 8.10
Action of *selegiline* (*deprenyl*) in dopamine metabolism. MAO = monoamine oxidase.

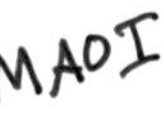

C. Catechol-O-methyltransferase inhibitors

Normally, the methylation of *levodopa* by catechol-O-methyltransferase (COMT) to 3-O-methyldopa is a minor pathway for *levodopa*

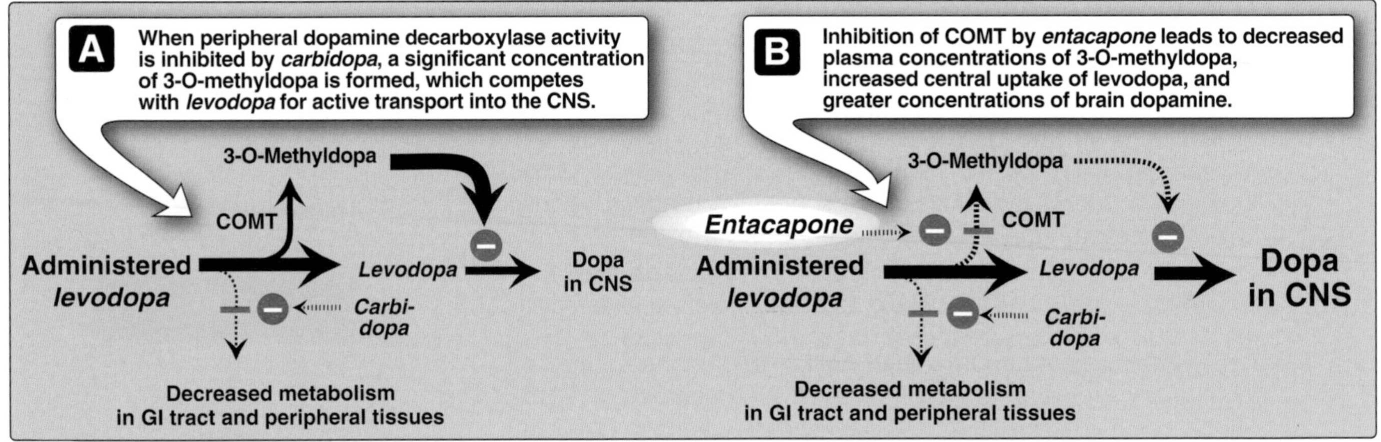

Figure 8.11
Effect of *entacapone* on dopa concentration in the central nervous system (CNS).
COMT = catechol-O-methyltransferase.

metabolism. However, when peripheral dopamine decarboxylase activity is inhibited by *carbidopa*, a significant concentration of 3-O-methyldopa is formed that competes with *levodopa* for active transport into the CNS (Figure 8.11). Inhibition of COMT by *entacapone* [en TA ka pone] or *tolcapone* [TOLE ka pone] leads to decreased plasma concentrations of 3-O-methyldopa, increased central uptake of *levodopa*, and greater concentrations of brain dopamine. Both of these agents have been demonstrated to reduce the symptoms of "wearing-off" phenomena seen in patients on *levodopa-carbidopa*. *Entacapone* and *tolcapone* are nitrocatechol derivatives that selectively and reversibly inhibit COMT. The two drugs differ primarily in their pharmacokinetics and in some adverse effects.

1. **Pharmacokinetics:** Oral absorption of both drugs occurs readily and is not influenced by food. They are extensively bound to plasma albumin (>98 percent), with limited volumes of distribution. *Tolcapone* differs from *entacapone* in that the former penetrates the blood-brain barrier and inhibits COMT in the CNS. However, the inhibition of COMT in the periphery appears to be the primary therapeutic action. *Tolcapone* has a relatively long duration of action (probably due to its affinity for the enzyme) compared to *entacapone*, which requires more frequent dosing. Both drugs are extensively metabolized and eliminated in the feces and urine. Dosage may need to be adjusted in patients with moderate or severe cirrhosis.

2. **Adverse effects:** Both drugs exhibit adverse effects that are observed in patients taking *levodopa-carbidopa,* including diarrhea, postural hypotension, nausea, anorexia, dyskinesias, hallucinations, and sleep disorders. Most seriously, fulminating hepatic necrosis is associated with *tolcapone* use. Therefore, it should be used—along with appropriate hepatic function monitoring—only in patients in whom other modalities have failed. *Entacapone* does not exhibit this toxicity and has largely replaced *tolcapone*.

D. Dopamine receptor agonists

This group of anti-Parkinson compounds includes two older agents that are ergot derivatives, *bromocriptine* and *pergolide*, and two newer, non-ergot drugs, *ropinirole* and *pramipexole*. These agents have durations of action longer than that of *levodopa* and, thus, have been effective in patients exhibiting fluctuations in their response to *levodopa*. Initial therapy with the newer drugs is associated particularly with less risk of developing dyskinesias and motor fluctuations when compared to patients started with *levodopa* therapy. *Bromocriptine*, *pergolide*, *pramipexole*, and *ropinirole* are all effective in patients with advanced Parkinson disease complicated by motor fluctuations and dyskinesias. However, these drugs are ineffective in patients who have shown no therapeutic response to *levodopa*.

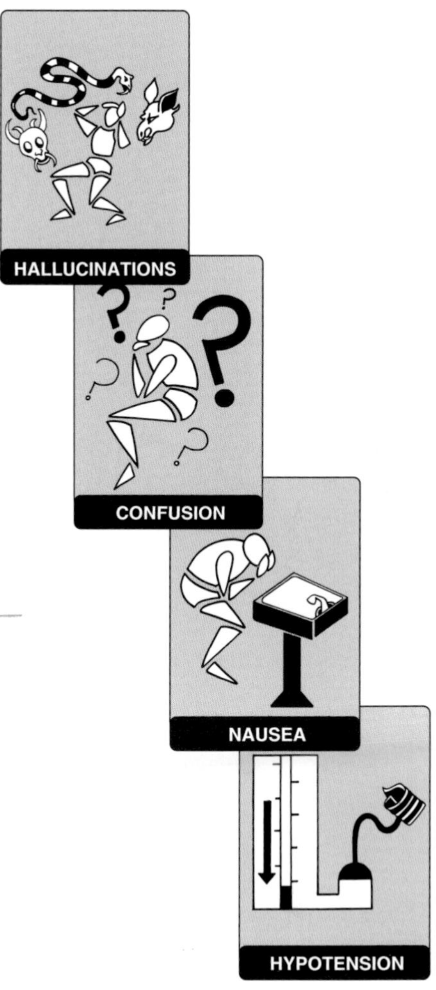

Figure 8.12
Some adverse effects of *bromocriptine*.

1. **Bromocriptine and pergolide:** *Bromocriptine* [broe moe KRIP teen] and *pergolide* [PER go lide], both ergotamine (an alkaloid with vasoconstrictor action) derivatives, are dopamine receptor agonists. *Pergolide* is the more potent of the two. The dose is increased gradually during a period of two to three months. Side effects severely limit the utility of the dopamine agonists (Figure 8.12). The actions of the ergotamine derivatives are similar to those of *levodopa*, except that hallucinations, confusion, delirium, nausea, and orthostatic hypotension are more common, whereas dyskinesia is less prominent. In psychiatric illness, they may cause the mental condition to worsen. Serious cardiac problems may develop, particularly in patients with a history of myocardial infarction. In patients with peripheral vascular disease, a worsening of the vasospasm occurs, and in patients with peptic ulcer, there is a worsening of the ulcer. Because they are ergot derivatives, both have the potential to cause pulmonary and retroperitoneal fibrosis.

2. **Pramipexole and ropinirole:** These are non-ergot dopamine agonists that have been approved for the treatment of Parkinson disease. *Pramipexole* [pra mi PEX ole] and *ropinirole* [roe PIN i role] are non-ergot agonists at dopamine receptors. They alleviate the motor deficits in both *levodopa*-naïve patients (patients who have never been treated with *levodopa*) and patients with advanced Parkinson disease taking *levodopa*. These dopamine agonists may delay the need to employ *levodopa* therapy in early Parkinson, and may decrease the dose of *levodopa* in advanced Parkinson. Unlike the ergotamine derivatives, *pramipexole* and *ropinirole* do not exacerbate peripheral vasospasm, nor do they cause fibrosis. Nausea, hallucinations, insomnia, dizziness, constipation, and orthostatic hypotension are among the more distressing side-effects of these drugs; dyskinesias are less frequent than with *levodopa*. The dependence of *pramipexole* on renal function for its elimination cannot be overly stressed. For example, *cimetidine*, which inhibits renal tubular secretion of organic bases, increases the half-life of *pramipexole* by forty percent. The fluoroquinolone antibiotics (see p. 381) have been shown to inhibit the metabolism of *ropinirole*, and enhance the AUC (area under

	Pramipexole	*Ropinirole*
Bioavailability	>90%	55%
V_d	7 L/kg	7.5 L/kg
Half-life	8 hours[1]	6 hours
Metabolism	Negligible	Extensive
Elimination	Renal	Renal[2]

[1]Increases to 12 hours in patients greater than 65 years old
[2]Less than 10 percent excreted unchanged

Figure 8.13
Pharmacokinetic properties of dopamine agonists of *pramipexole* and *ropinirole*. V_d = volume of distribution.

	Pramipexole	*Ropinirole*
Somnolence	+++	++
Insomnia	++++	+
Dizziness or light-headedness	+++	++
Hallucinations or confusion	++	++
Headache		++
Orthostasis	++	+++
Nausea	++++	++
Constipation	++	
Others		
Arthralgia		++
Blurred vision	+	
Dry mouth	++	
Upper respiratory infection		++

+ = Incidence of 1 to 5 percent;
++ = incidence of 6 to 15 percent;
+++ = incidence of 16 to 25 percent;
++++ = incidence of greater than 25 percent.

Figure 8.14
Side effects of dopamine agonists *pramipexole* and *ropinirole*.

the concentration vs. time curve) by some eighty percent. Figures 8.13 and 8.14 summarize some properties of *pramipexole* and *ropinirole*.

E. Amantadine

It was accidentally discovered that the antiviral drug *amantadine* [a MAN ta deen], effective in the treatment of influenza (see p. 434), has an antiparkinsonism action. *Amantadine* has several effects on a number of neurotransmitters implicated in causing parkinsonism including increasing the release of dopamine, blockading cholinergic receptors, and inhibiting the N-methyl-D-aspartate (NMDA) type of glutamate receptors. Current evidence supports an action at NMDA receptors as the primary action at therapeutic concentrations. [Note: If dopamine release is already at a maximum, *amantadine* has no effect.] The drug may cause restlessness, agitation, confusion, and hallucinations, and at high doses, it may induce acute toxic psychosis. Orthostatic hypotension, urinary retention, peripheral edema, and dry mouth also may occur. *Amantadine* is less efficacious than *levodopa*, and tolerance develops more readily. However, *amantadine* has fewer side effects. The drug has little effect on tremor, but is more effective than the anticholinergics against rigidity and bradykinesia.

F. Antimuscarinic agents

The antimuscarinic agents are much less efficacious than *levodopa* and play only an adjuvant role in antiparkinsonism therapy. The actions of *benztropine*, *trihexyphenidyl*, and *biperiden* are similar, although individual patients may respond more favorably to one drug. All these drugs can induce mood changes and produce xerostomia (dryness of the mouth) and visual problems, as do all muscarinic blockers. They interfere with gastrointestinal peristalsis, and are contraindicated in patients with glaucoma, prostatic hypertrophy, or pyloric stenosis. Blockage of cholinergic transmission produces effects similar to augmentation of dopaminergic transmission (again, because of the creation of an imbalance in the dopamine/acetylcholine ratio). Adverse effects are similar to those caused by high doses of *atropine*—for example, pupillary dilation, confusion, hallucination, urinary retention, and dry mouth.

VII. DRUGS USED IN ALZHEIMER DISEASE

Pharmacologic intervention for Alzheimer disease is only palliative and provides modest short-term benefit. None of the current therapeutic agents alter the underlying neurodegenerative process. Alzheimer dementia has three distinguishing features: 1) accumulation of senile plaques (β-amyloid accumulations), 2) formation of numerous neurofibrillary tangles, and 3) loss of cortical neurons—particularly cholinergic neurons. Current therapies are aimed at either improving cholinergic transmission within the CNS or preventing the excitotoxicity actions of NMDA glutamate receptors in selected brain areas.

A. Acetylcholinesterase inhibitors

Numerous studies have linked the progressive loss of cholinergic neurons and, presumably, cholinergic transmission within the cortex, to the memory loss that is a hallmark symptom of Alzheimer disease. It is postulated that inhibition of acetylcholinesterase (AChE) within the CNS will improve cholinergic transmission, at least at those neurons that are still functioning. Currently, four reversible AChE inhibitors are approved for the treatment of mild to moderate Alzheimer disease. They are *donepezil* [dahn ee PEH zeel], *galantamine* [ga LAN ta meen], *rivastigmine* [ri va STIG meen] and *tacrine* [TAK reen]. Except for *galantamine*, which is competitive, all are uncompetitive inhibitors of AChE, and appear to have some selectivity for AChE in the CNS as compared to the periphery. At best, these compounds provide a modest reduction in the rate of loss of cognitive functioning in Alzheimer patients. *Rivastigmine* is hydrolyzed by AChE to a carbamylate metabolite, and has no interactions with drugs that alter the activity of P450-dependent enzymes. The other agents are substrates for P450 and have a potential for such interactions. Common adverse effects include nausea, diarrhea, vomiting, anorexia, and muscle cramps—all of which are predicted by the actions of the drugs (Figure 8.15). Unlike the others, *tacrine* is associated with hepatotoxicity.

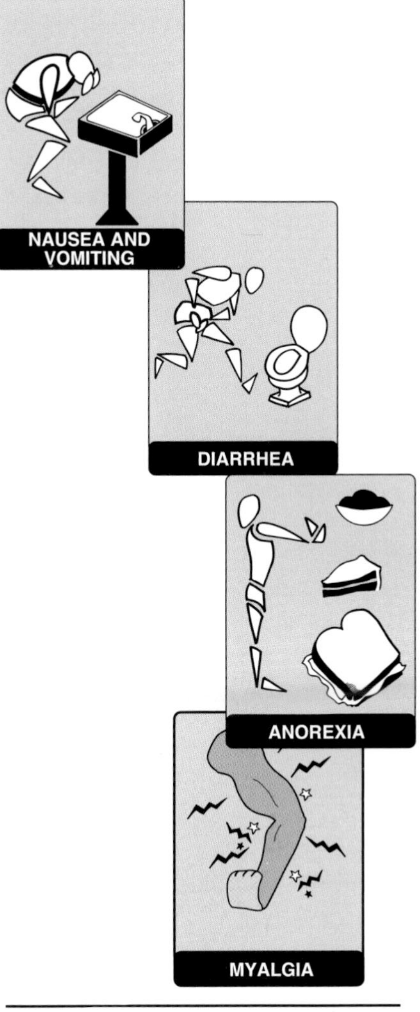

Figure 8.15
Adverse efffects of acetylcholinesterase inhibitors.

B. NMDA receptor antagonists

Overstimulation of glutamate receptors, particularly of the NMDA type, has been shown to result in excitotoxic effects on neurons, and is suggested as a mechanism for neurodegenerative processes. Antagonists of the NMDA glutamate receptor are often neuroprotective, preventing the loss of neurons following ischemic and other injuries. *Memantine* [MEM an teen] is a dimethyl adamantane derivative related to *amantadine*. It is an uncompetitive inhibitor of NMDA receptors, and has been shown to prevent or slow the rate of memory loss in both vascular-associated and Alzheimer dementia, even in patients with moderate to severe cognitive losses. However, there is no evidence that *memantine* prevents or slows the neurodegeneration in patients with Alzheimer disease. *Memantine* is well tolerated, with few dose-dependent adverse events. Expected side-effects, such as confusion, agitation, and restlessness, are indistinguishable from the symptoms of Alzheimer disease.

Study Questions

Choose the ONE best answer.

8.1 Which one of the following combinations of antiparkinson drugs is an appropriate therapy?

A. Amantadine, carbidopa, and entacapone
B. Levodopa, carbidopa, and entacapone
C. Pergolide, carbidopa, and entacapone
D. Ropinirole, selegiline, and entacapone
E. Ropinirole, carbidopa, and selegiline

Correct answer = B. To reduce the dose of levodopa and its peripheral side effects, the peripheral decarboxylase inhibitor, carbidopa, is coadministered. As a result of this combination, more levodopa is available for metabolism by COMT to 3-methyldopa, which competes with dopa for the active transport processes into the CNS. By administering entacapone (inhibitor of COMT), the competing product is not formed, and more dopa enters the brain. The other choices are not appropriate, because neither peripheral decarboxylase nor COMT nor MAO metabolize amantadine or the direct-acting dopamine agonists, ropinirole and pergolide.

8.2 Peripheral adverse effects of levodopa, including nausea, hypotension, and cardiac arrhythmias, can be diminished by including which of the following drugs in the therapy?

A. Amantadine,
B. Bromocriptine
C. Carbidopa
D. Entacapone
E. Ropinirole

Correct answer = C. Carbidopa inhibits the peripheral decarboxylation of levodopa to dopamine, thereby diminishing the gastrointestinal and cardiovascular side effects of levodopa.

8.3 Which of the following antiparkinson drugs may cause peripheral vasospasm?

A. Amantadine,
B. Bromocriptine
C. Carbidopa
D. Entacapone
E. Ropinirole

Correct answer = B. Ropinirole directly stimulate sdopamine receptors, but it does not cause vasospasm. The other drugs do not act directly on dopamine receptors.

8.4 Modest improvement in the memory of patients with Alzheimer disease may occur with drugs that increase transmission at which of the following receptors?

A. Adrenergic
B. Cholinergic
C. Dopaminergic
D. GABAergic
E. Serotonergic

Correct answer = B. Acetylcholinesterase inhibitors, such as rivastigmine, increase cholinergic transmission in the CNS, and cause a modest delay in the progression of Alzheimer disease.

Anxiolytic and Hypnotic Drugs

9

I. OVERVIEW

Anxiety is an unpleasant state of tension, apprehension, or uneasiness—a fear that seems to arise from an unknown source. Disorders involving anxiety are the most common mental disturbances. The symptoms of severe anxiety are similar to those of fear (such as tachycardia, sweating, trembling, and palpitations) and involve sympathetic activation. Episodes of mild anxiety are common life experiences and do not warrant treatment. However, the symptoms of severe, chronic, debilitating anxiety may be treated with antianxiety drugs (sometimes called anxiolytic or minor tranquilizers) and/or some form of behavioral or psychotherapy. Because all of the antianxiety drugs also cause some sedation, the same drugs often function clinically as both anxiolytic and hypnotic (sleep-inducing) agents. In addition, some have anticonvulsant activity. Figure 9.1 summarizes the anxiolytic and hypnotic agents.

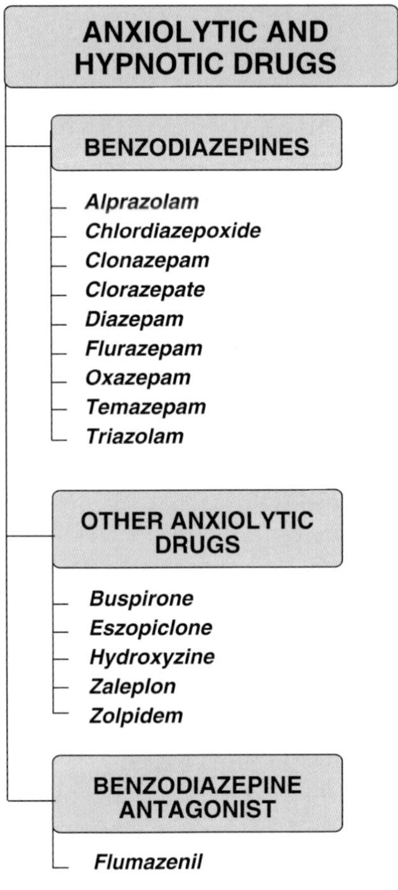

ANXIOLYTIC AND HYPNOTIC DRUGS
BENZODIAZEPINES
Alprazolam
Chlordiazepoxide
Clonazepam
Clorazepate
Diazepam
Flurazepam
Oxazepam
Temazepam
Triazolam
OTHER ANXIOLYTIC DRUGS
Buspirone
Eszopiclone
Hydroxyzine
Zaleplon
Zolpidem
BENZODIAZEPINE ANTAGONIST
Flumazenil

Figure 9.1
Summary of anxiolytic and hypnotic drugs.
(Figure continues on next page.)

II. BENZODIAZEPINES

Benzodiazepines are the most widely used anxiolytic drugs. They have largely replaced barbiturates and *meprobamate* in the treatment of anxiety, because the benzodiazepines are safer and more effective (Figure 9.2).

A. Mechanism of action

The targets for benzodiazepine actions are the γ-aminobutyric acid ($GABA_A$) receptors. [Note: GABA is the major inhibitory neurotransmitter in the central nervous system (CNS).] These receptors are composed of α, β, and γ subunit families of which a combination of five or more span the postsynaptic membrane (Figure 9.3). Depending on the types, number of subunits, and brain region localization, the activation of the receptors results in different pharmacologic effects. Benzodiazepines modulate the GABA effects by binding to a specific, high-affinity site located at the interface of the α subunit and the γ_2 subunit (see Figure 9.3). [Note: These binding sites are sometimes labeled benzodiazepine receptors, which are

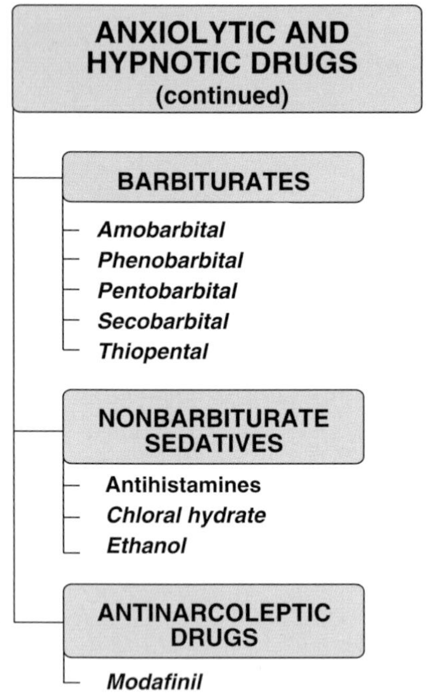

Figure 9.1 (continued)
Summary of anxiolytic and hypnotic drugs.

designated as BZ_1 or BZ_2, depending on their affinity for a particular α subunit. The benzodiazepine receptor locations in the CNS parallel those of the GABA neurons. Binding of GABA to its receptor triggers an opening of a chloride channel, which leads to an increase in chloride conductance (see Figure 9.3). Benzodiazipines increase the frequency of channel openings produced by GABA. The influx of chloride ions causes a small hyperpolarization that moves the postsynaptic potential away from its firing threshold and, thus, inhibits the formation of action potentials. [Note: Benzodiazepines and GABA mutually increase the affinity of their binding sites without actually changing the total number of sites.] The clinical effects of the various benzodiazepines correlate well with each drug's binding affinity for the GABA receptor-chloride ion channel complex.

B. Actions

The benzodiazepines have neither antipsychotic activity nor analgesic action, and they do not affect the autonomic nervous system. All benzodiazepines exhibit the following actions to a greater or lesser extent:

1. **Reduction of anxiety:** At low doses, the benzodiazepines are anxiolytic. They are thought to reduce anxiety by selectively enhancing GABAergic transmission in neurons having the α_2 subunit in their $GABA_A$ receptors, thereby inhibiting neuronal circuits in the limbic system of the brain.

2. **Sedative and hypnotic actions:** All the benzodiazepines used to treat anxiety have some sedative properties, and some can produce hypnosis (artificially-produced sleep) at higher doses. Their effects have been shown to be mediated by the α_1-$GABA_A$ receptors.

3. **Anterograde amnesia:** The temporary impairment of memory with use of the benzodiazepines is also mediated by the α_1-$GABA_A$ receptors.

4. **Anticonvulsant:** Several of the benzodiazepines have anticonvulsant activity, and are used to treat epilepsy and other seizure disorders. This effect is partially, although not completely, mediated by α_1-$GABA_A$ receptors.

5. **Muscle relaxant:** At high doses, the benzodiazepines relax the spasticity of skeletal muscle, probably by increasing presynaptic inhibition in the spinal cord, where the α_2-$GABA_A$ receptors are largely located.

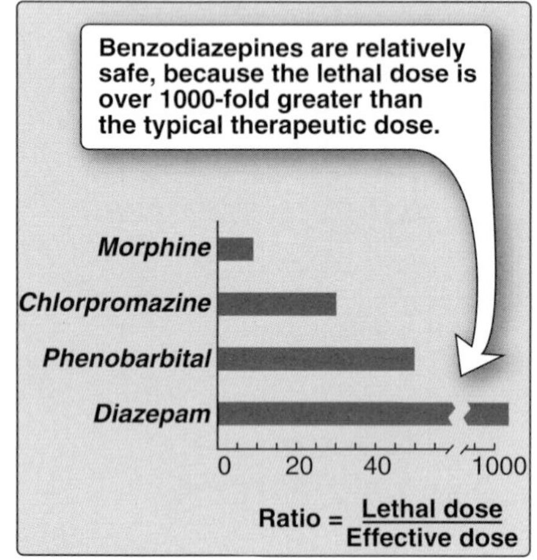

Figure 9.2
Ratio of lethal dose to effective dose for *morphine* (an opioid, see Chapter 14), *chlorpromazine* (a neuroleptic, see Chapter 13), and the anxiolytic, hypnotic drugs, *phenobarbital* and *diazepam.*

C. Therapeutic uses

The individual benzodiazepines show small differences in their relative anxiolytic, anticonvulsant, and sedative properties. However, the duration of action varies widely among this group, and pharmacokinetic considerations are often important in choosing a drug.

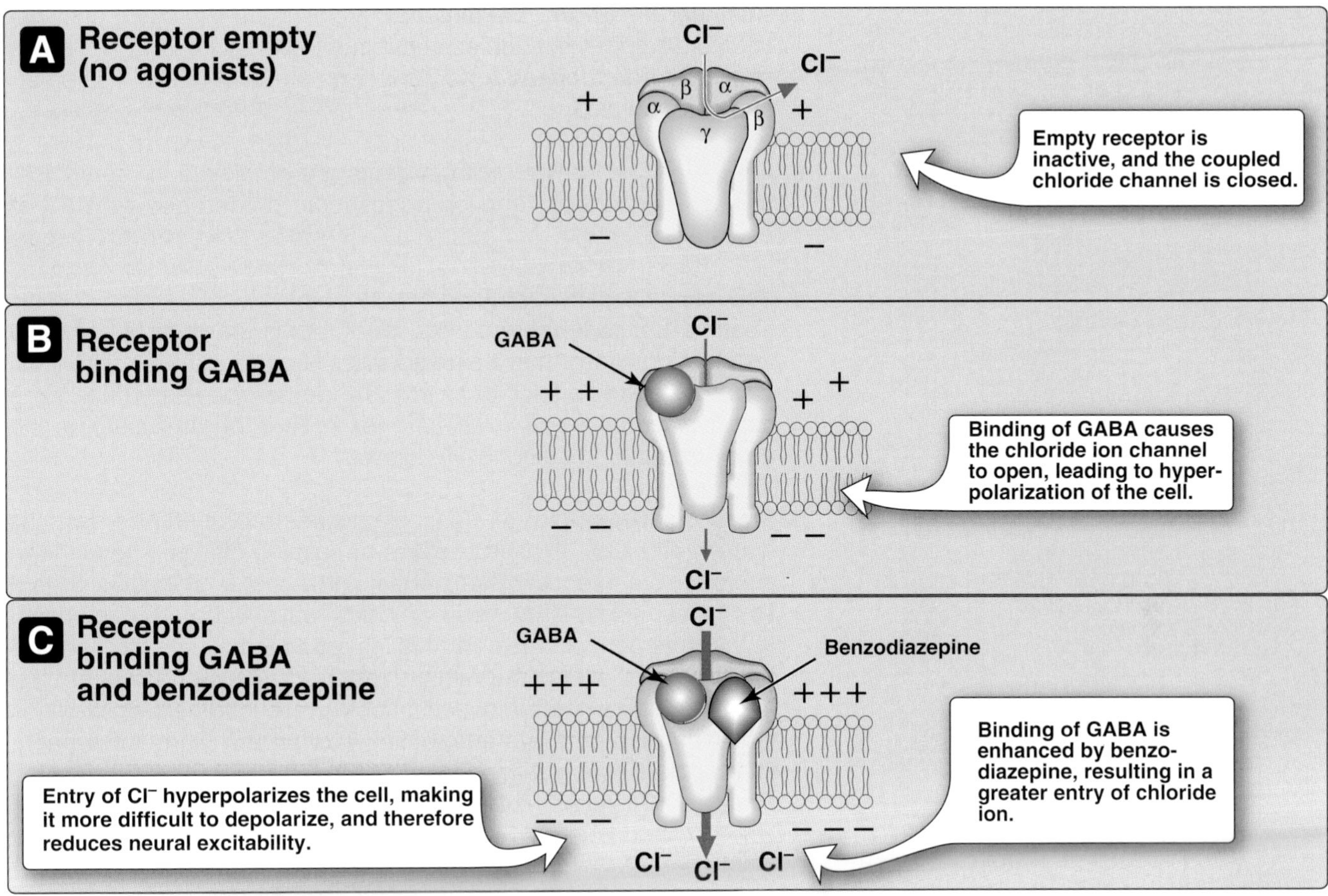
A Receptor empty (no agonists)
Cl⁻
Cl⁻
α
β
α
γ
β
Empty receptor is inactive, and the coupled chloride channel is closed.
B Receptor binding GABA
GABA
Cl⁻
Binding of GABA causes the chloride ion channel to open, leading to hyperpolarization of the cell.
Cl⁻
C Receptor binding GABA and benzodiazepine
GABA
Cl⁻
Benzodiazepine
Binding of GABA is enhanced by benzodiazepine, resulting in a greater entry of chloride ion.
Entry of Cl⁻ hyperpolarizes the cell, making it more difficult to depolarize, and therefore reduces neural excitability.
Cl⁻ Cl⁻ Cl⁻

Figure 9.3
Schematic diagram of benzodiazepine-GABA-chloride ion channel complex. GABA = γ–aminobutyric acid.

1. **Anxiety disorders:** The benzodiazepines are useful in treating the anxiety that accompanies some forms of depression and schizophrenia. These drugs should not be used to alleviate the normal stress of everyday life. They should be reserved for continued severe anxiety, and then should only be used for short periods of time because of addiction potential. The longer-acting agents, such as *diazepam* [dye AZ e pam], are often preferred in those patients with anxiety that may require treatment for prolonged periods of time. The antianxiety effects of the benzodiazepines are less subject to tolerance than the sedative and hypnotic effects. [Note: Tolerance—that is, decreased responsiveness to repeated doses of the drug—occurs when used for more than one to two weeks. Cross-tolerance exists among this group of agents as well as with ethanol. It has been shown that tolerance is associated with a decrease in GABA receptor density.] For panic disorders, *alprazolam* [al PRAY zoe lam] is effective for short- and long-term treatment, although it may cause withdrawal reactions in about thirty percent of sufferers.

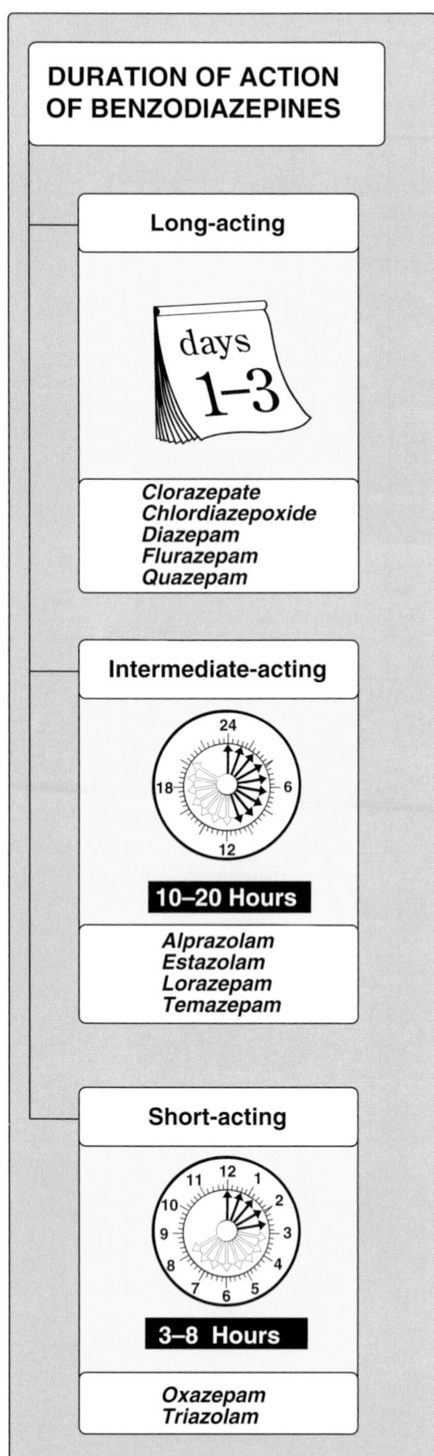

Figure 9.4
Comparison of the durations of action of the benzodiazepines.

2. **Muscular disorders:** *Diazepam* is useful in the treatment of skeletal muscle spasms, such as occur in muscle strain, and in treating spasticity from degenerative disorders, such as multiple sclerosis and cerebral palsy.

3. **Amnesia:** The shorter-acting agents are employed in premedication for endoscopic and bronchoscopic procedures as well as angioplasty.

4. **Seizures:** *Clonazepam* [kloe NA ze pam] is useful in the chronic treatment of epilepsy, whereas *diazepam* is the drug of choice in terminating grand mal epileptic seizures and status epilepticus. *Chlordiazepoxide* [klor di az e POX ide], *clorazepate* [klor AZ e pate], *diazepam*, and *oxazepam* [ox A ze pam] are useful in the acute treatment of alcohol withdrawal.

5. **Sleep disorders:** Not all benzodiazepines are useful as hypnotic agents, although all have sedative or calming effects. They tend to decrease the latency to sleep onset and increase stage two of non-REM sleep. Both REM sleep and slow-wave sleep are decreased. In the treatment of insomnia, it is important to balance the sedative effect needed at bedtime with the residual sedation ("hangover") on awakening. The three most commonly prescribed benzodiazepines for sleep disorders are long-acting *flurazepam* [flure AZ e pam], intermediate-acting *temazepam* [te MAZ e pam], and short-acting *triazolam* [trye AY zoe lam]. Two nonbenzodiazepine drugs, *zolpidem* and *zaleplon*, are also effective (see p. 108).

   a. **Flurazepam:** This long-acting benzodiazepine significantly reduces both sleep-induction time and the number of awakenings, and it increases the duration of sleep. *Flurazepam* has a long-acting effect (Figure 9.4) and causes little rebound insomnia. With continued use, the drug has been shown to maintain its effectiveness for up to four weeks. *Flurazepam* and its active metabolites have a half-life of approximately 85 hours, which may result in daytime sedation and accumulation of the drug.

   b. **Temazepam:** This drug is useful in patients who experience frequent wakening. However, the peak sedative effect occurs two to three hours after an oral dose; therefore, it may be given several hours before bedtime.

   c. **Triazolam:** This benzodiazepine has a relatively short duration of action and, therefore, is used to induce sleep in patients with recurring insomnia. Whereas *temazepam* is useful for insomnia caused by the inability to stay asleep, *triazolam* is effective in treating individuals who have difficulty in going to sleep. Tolerance frequently develops within a few days, and withdrawal of the drug often results in rebound insomnia, leading the patient to demand another prescription. Therefore, this drug is best used intermittently rather than daily. In general, hypnotics should be given for only a limited time, usually less than two to four weeks.

D. Pharmacokinetics

1. **Absorption and distribution:** The benzodiazepines are lipophilic, and they are rapidly and completely absorbed after oral administration and distribute throughout the body.

2. **Duration of actions:** The half-lives of the benzodiazepines are very important clinically, because the duration of action may determine the therapeutic usefulness. The benzodiazepines can be roughly divided into short-, intermediate-, and long-acting groups (see Figure 9.4). The longer-acting agents form active metabolites with long half-lives.

3. **Fate:** Most benzodiazepines, including *chlordiazepoxide* and *diazepam*, are metabolized by the hepatic microsomal system to compounds that are also active. For these benzodiazepines, the apparent half-life of the drug represents the combined actions of the parent drug and its metabolites. The drugs' effects are terminated not only by excretion but also by redistribution. The benzodiazepines are excreted in the urine as glucuronides or oxidized metabolites. All the benzodiazepines cross the placental barrier and may depress the newborn if given before birth. Nursing infants may also become exposed to the drugs in breast milk.

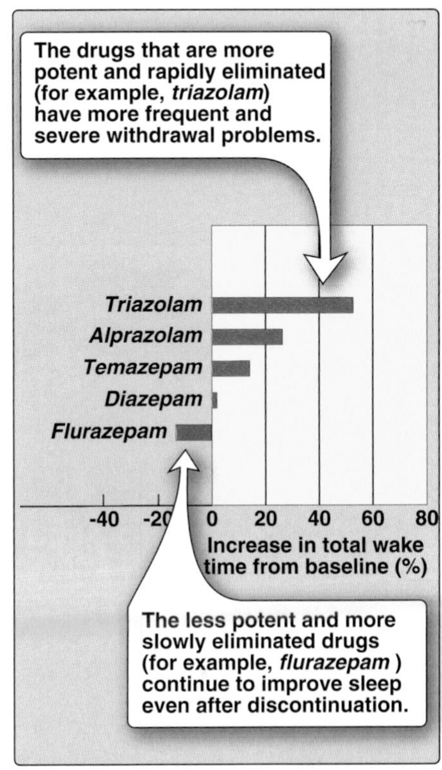

Figure 9.5
Frequency of rebound insomnia resulting from discontinuation of benzodiazepine therapy.

E. Dependence

Psychological and physical dependence on benzodiazepines can develop if high doses of the drug are given over a prolonged period. Abrupt discontinuation of the benzodiazepines results in withdrawal symptoms, including confusion, anxiety, agitation, restlessness, insomnia, and tension. Because of the long half-lives of some benzodiazepines, withdrawal symptoms may occur slowly and last a number of days after discontinuation of therapy. Benzodiazepines with a short elimination half-life, such as *triazolam*, induce more abrupt and severe withdrawal reactions than those seen with drugs that are slowly eliminated, such as *flurazepam* (Figure 9.5).

F. Adverse effects

1. **Drowsiness and confusion:** These effects are the two most common side effects of the benzodiazepines. Ataxia occurs at high doses, and precludes activities that require fine motor coordination, such as driving an automobile. Cognitive impairment (decreased long-term recall and acquisition of new knowledge) can occur with use of benzodiazepines. *Triazolam*, the benzodiazepine with the most rapid elimination, often shows a rapid development of tolerance, early morning insomnia, and daytime anxiety, along with amnesia and confusion.

2. **Precautions:** Benzodiazepines should be used cautiously in treating patients with liver disease. They should be avoided in patients with acute narrow-angle glaucoma. Alcohol and other CNS depressants enhance the sedative-hypnotic effects of the benzodiazepines. Benzodiazepines are, however, considerably less dangerous than other anxiolytic and hypnotic drugs. As a result, a

drug overdose is seldom lethal, unless other central depressants, such as alcohol, are taken concurrently.

III. OTHER ANXIOLYTIC AND HYPNOTIC AGENTS

A. Zolpidem

Although the hypnotic *zolpidem* [ZOL pie dem] is not a benzodiazepine, it acts on a subset of the benzodiazepine receptor family, BZ_1. *Zolpidem* has no anticonvulsant or muscle-relaxing properties. It shows no withdrawal effects, exhibits minimal rebound insomnia, and little or no tolerance occurs with prolonged use. *Zolpidem* is rapidly absorbed from the gastrointestinal tract, and it has a rapid onset of action and short elimination half-life (about two to three hours). [Note: An extended-release formulation is now available.] *Zolpidem* undergoes hepatic oxidation by the cytochrome P450 system to inactive products. Thus, drugs such as *rifampin*, which induce this enzyme system, shorten the half-life of *zolpidem*. Adverse effects of *zolpidem* include nightmares, agitation, headache, gastrointestinal upset, dizziness, and daytime drowsiness.

B. Zaleplon

Zaleplon (ZAL e plon) is very similar to *zolpidem* in its hypnotic actions, but it causes fewer residual effects on psychomotor and cognitive functions compared to *zolpidem* or the benzodiazepines. This may be due to its rapid elimination, with a half-life that is less than one hour. The drug is metabolized by CYP3A4 (see p. 15).

C. Buspirone

Buspirone [byoo SPYE rone] is useful in the treatment of generalized anxiety disorders, and has an efficacy comparable to the benzodiazepines. The actions of *buspirone* appear to be mediated by serotonin (5-HT_{1A}) receptors, although other receptors could be involved, because *buspirone* displays some affinity for DA_2 dopamine receptors and 5-HT_{2A} serotonin receptors. Thus, its mode of action differs from that of the benzodiazepines. [Note: "5-HT" not "S" is the accepted abbreviation for serotonin (5-hydroxytryptamine) receptors.] In addition, *buspirone* lacks anticonvulsant and muscle-relaxant properties of the benzodiazepines and causes only minimal sedation. However, it causes hypothermia and increases in prolactin and growth hormone. *Buspirone* undergoes metabolism by CYP3A4; thus, its half-life is shortened if taken with *rifampin* and lengthened if taken with *erythromycin*—an inducer and an inhibitor of the enzyme, respectively. The frequency of adverse effects is low, the most common effects being headaches, dizziness, nervousness, and light-headedness. Sedation and psychomotor and cognitive dysfunction are minimal, and dependence is unlikely. *Buspirone* has the disadvantage of a slow onset of action. Figure 9.6 compares some of the common adverse effects of *buspirone* and the benzodiazepine *alprazolam*.

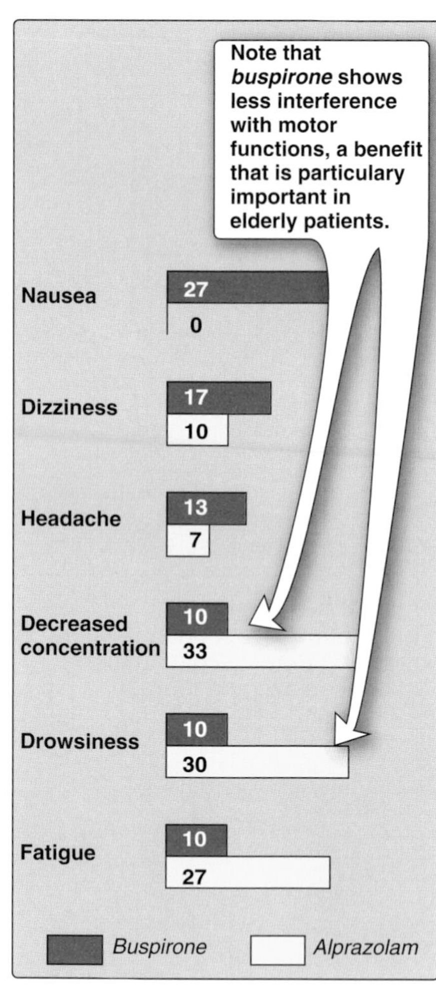

Figure 9.6
Comparison of common adverse effects of *buspirone* and *alprazolam*. Results are expressed as the percentage of patients showing each symptom.

D. Eszopiclone

Eszopiclone [es zoe PIK lone] is a nonbenzodiazepine, oral, sedative drug that is used for treating insomnia. *Eszopiclone* is unique in that it is the only drug used for insomnia that has been shown to be effective for up to six months compared to a placebo. *Eszopiclone* is rapidly absorbed (time to peak, one hour), extensively metabolized by oxidation and demethylation, and mainly excreted in the urine. Elimination half-life is approximately six hours. Adverse events reported with *eszopiclone* include anxiety, dry mouth, chest pain, headache, migraine, peripheral edema, somnolence, and unpleasant taste.

E. Hydroxyzine

Hydroxyzine [hye DROX i zeen] is an antihistamine with antiemetic activity. It has a low tendency for habituation and, thus, is useful for patients with anxiety who have a history of drug abuse. It is also often used for sedation prior to dental procedures or surgery. Drowsiness is a possible adverse effect.

IV. BENZODIAZEPINE ANTAGONIST

Flumazenil [floo MAZ eh nill] is a GABA receptor antagonist that can rapidly reverse the effects of benzodiazepines. The drug is available for intravenous (IV) administration only. Onset is rapid but duration is short, with a half-life of about one hour. Frequent administration may be necessary to maintain reversal of a long-acting benzodiazepine. Administration of *flumazenil* may precipitate withdrawal in dependent patients or cause seizures if a benzodiazepine is used to control seizure activity. Seizures may also result if the patient ingests tricyclic antidepressants. Dizziness, nausea, vomiting, and agitation are the most common side effects.

V. BARBITURATES

The barbiturates were formerly the mainstay of treatment used to sedate the patient or to induce and maintain sleep. Today, they have been largely replaced by the benzodiazepines, primarily because barbiturates induce tolerance, drug-metabolizing enzymes, physical dependence, and very severe withdrawal symptoms. Foremost is their ability to cause coma in toxic doses. Certain barbiturates, such as the very short-acting *thiopental*, are still used to induce anesthesia (see p. 134).

A. Mechanism of action

The sedative-hypnotic action of the barbiturates is due to their interaction with $GABA_A$ receptors which enhances GABAnergic transmission. The binding site is distinct from that of the benzodiazepines. Barbiturates potentiate GABA action on chloride entry into the neuron by prolonging the duration of the chloride channel openings. In addition, barbiturates can block excitatory glutamate receptors. Anesthetic concentrations of *pentobarbital* also block high frequency sodium channels. All of these molecular actions lead to decreased neuronal activity.

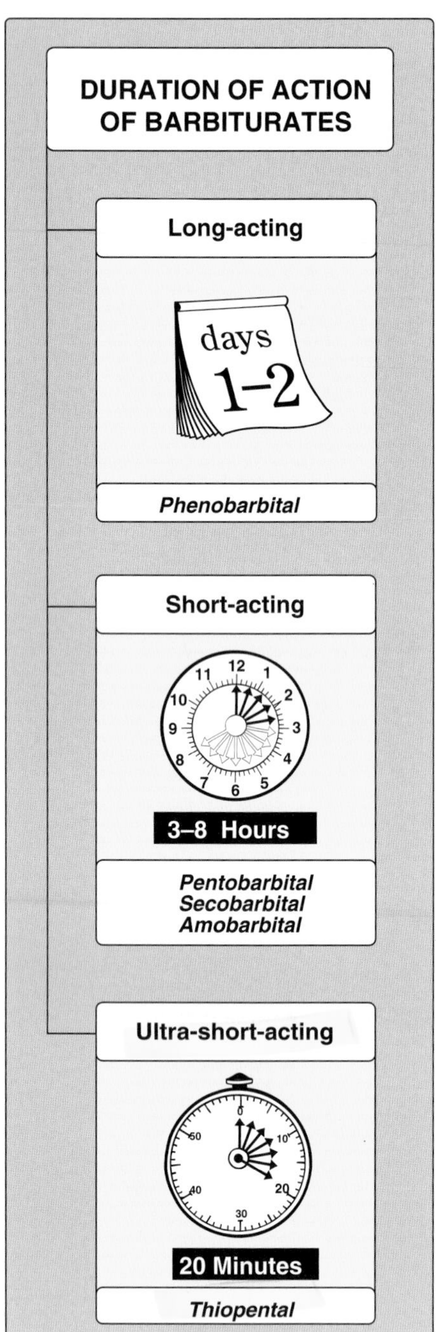

Figure 9.7
Barbiturates classified according to their durations of action.

B. Actions

Barbiturates are classified according to their duration of action (Figure 9.7). For example, *thiopental* [thye oh PEN tal], which acts within seconds and has a duration of action of about thirty minutes, is used in the intravenous induction of anesthesia. By contrast, *phenobarbital* [fee noe BAR bi tal], which has a duration of action greater than a day, is useful in the treatment of seizures (see p. 175). *Pentobarbital* [pen toe BAR bi tal], *secobarbital* [see koe BAR bi tal], and *amobarbital* [am oh BAR bi tal] are short-acting barbiturates, which are effective as sedative and hypnotic (but not antianxiety) agents.

1. **Depression of CNS:** At low doses, the barbiturates produce sedation (calming effect, reducing excitement). At higher doses, the drugs cause hypnosis, followed by anesthesia (loss of feeling or sensation), and finally, coma and death. Thus, any degree of depression of the CNS is possible, depending on the dose. Barbiturates do not raise the pain threshold and have no analgesic properties. They may even exacerbate pain. Chronic use leads to tolerance.

2. **Respiratory depression:** Barbiturates suppress the hypoxic and chemoreceptor response to CO_2, and overdosage is followed by respiratory depression and death.

3. **Enzyme induction:** Barbiturates induce P450 microsomal enzymes in the liver. Therefore, chronic barbiturate administration diminishes the action of many drugs that are dependent on P450 metabolism to reduce their concentration.

C. Therapeutic uses

1. **Anesthesia:** Selection of a barbiturate is strongly influenced by the desired duration of action. The ultra-short-acting barbiturates, such as *thiopental*, are used intravenously to induce anesthesia.

2. **Anticonvulsant:** *Phenobarbital* is used in long-term management of tonic-clonic seizures, status epilepticus, and eclampsia. *Phenobarbital* has been regarded as the drug of choice for treatment of young children with recurrent febrile seizures. However, *phenobarbital* can depress cognitive performance in children, and the drug should be used cautiously. *Phenobarbital* has specific anticonvulsant activity that is distinguished from the nonspecific CNS depression.

3. **Anxiety:** Barbiturates have been used as mild sedatives to relieve anxiety, nervous tension, and insomnia. When used as hypnotics, they suppress REM sleep more than other stages. However, most have been replaced by the benzodiazepines.

D. Pharmacokinetics

Barbiturates are absorbed orally and distributed widely throughout the body. All barbiturates redistribute in the body from the brain to the splanchnic areas, to skeletal muscle, and finally, to adipose tissue. This movement is important in causing the short duration of action of thiopental and similar short-acting derivatives. They readily cross the placenta and can depress the fetus. Barbiturates, except for *phenobarbital*, are metabolized in the liver, and inactive metabolites are excreted in the urine.

E. Adverse effects

1. **CNS:** Barbiturates cause drowsiness, impaired concentration, and mental and physical sluggishness (Figure 9.8). The CNS depressant effects of barbiturates synergize with those of *ethanol*.

2. **Drug hangover:** Hypnotic doses of barbiturates produce a feeling of tiredness well after the patient wakes. This drug hangover leads to impaired ability to function normally for many hours after waking. Occasionally, nausea and dizziness occur.

3. **Precautions:** As noted previously, barbiturates induce the P450 system and, therefore, may decrease the duration of action of drugs that are metabolized by these hepatic enzymes. Barbiturates increase porphyrin synthesis, and are contraindicated in patients with acute intermittent porphyria.

4. **Physical dependence:** Abrupt withdrawal from barbiturates may cause tremors, anxiety, weakness, restlessness, nausea and vomiting, seizures, delirium, and cardiac arrest. Withdrawal is much more severe than that associated with opiates and can result in death.

5. **Poisoning:** Barbiturate poisoning has been a leading cause of death among drug overdoses for many decades. Severe depression of respiration is coupled with central cardiovascular depression, and results in a shock-like condition with shallow, infrequent breathing. Treatment includes artificial respiration and purging the stomach of its contents if the drug has been recently taken. [Note: No specific barbiturate antagonist is available.] Hemodialysis may be necessary if large quantities have been taken. Alkalinization of the urine often aids in the elimination of *phenobarbital*.

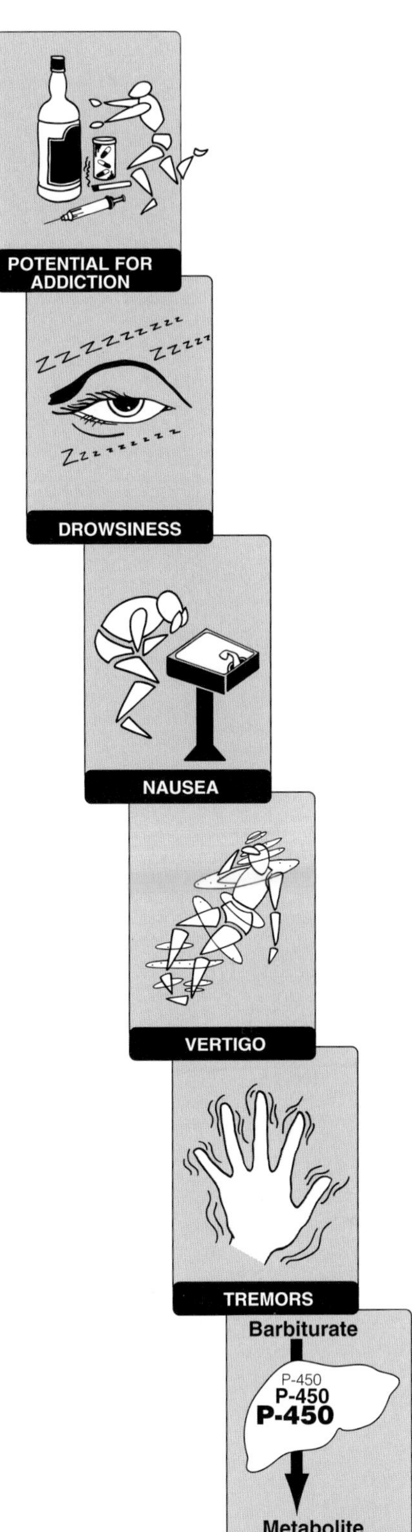

Figure 9.8
Adverse effect of barbiturates.

VI. NONBARBITURATE SEDATIVES

A. Chloral hydrate

Chloral hydrate [klor al HYE drate] is a trichlorinated derivative of acetaldehyde that is converted to the active metabolite, trichloroethanol, in the body. The drug is an effective sedative and hypnotic that induces sleep in about thirty minutes and lasts about six hours. *Chloral hydrate* is irritating to the gastrointestinal tract and causes epigastric distress. It also produces an unusual, unpleasant taste sensation. It synergizes with *ethanol*.

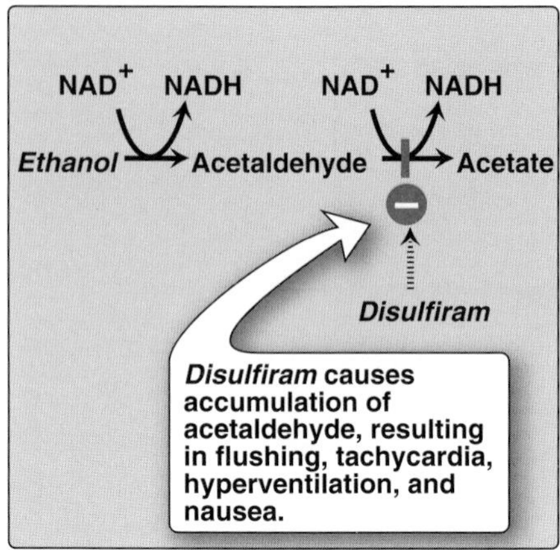

Figure 9.9
Metabolism of *ethanol*, and the effect of *disulfiram.*

B. Antihistamines

Nonprescription antihistamines with sedating properties, such as *diphenhydramine* and *doxylamine*, are effective in treating mild types of insomnia. However, these drugs are usually ineffective for all but the milder form of situational insomnia. Furthermore, they have numerous undesirable side effects that make them less useful than the benzodiazepines. These sedative antihistamines are marketed in numerous over-the-counter products.

C. Ethanol

Ethanol (*ethyl alcohol*) has antianxiety and sedative effects, but its toxic potential outweighs its benefits. Alcoholism is a serious medical and social problem. *Ethanol* [ETH an ol] is a CNS depressant, producing sedation and, ultimately, hypnosis with increasing dosage. *Ethanol* has a shallow dose-response curve; therefore, sedation occurs over a wide dosage range. It is readily absorbed orally, and has a volume of distribution close to that of total body water. *Ethanol* is metabolized primarily in the liver, first to acetaldehyde by alcohol dehydrogenase and then to acetate by aldehyde dehydrogenase (Figure 9.9). Elimination is mostly through the kidney, but a fraction is excreted through the lungs. *Ethanol* synergizes with many other sedative agents and can produce severe CNS depression with antihistamines or barbiturates. Chronic consumption can lead to severe liver disease, gastritis, and nutritional deficiencies. Cardiomyopathy is also a consequence of heavy drinking. The treatment of choice for alcohol withdrawal are the benzodizepines. *Carbamazepine* is effective in treating convulsive episodes during withdrawal.

1. **Disulfiram:** *Disulfiram* [dye SUL fi ram] blocks the oxidation of acetaldehyde to acetic acid by inhibiting aldehyde dehydrogenase (see Figure 9.9). This results in the accumulation of acetaldehyde in the blood, causing flushing, tachycardia, hyperventilation, and nausea. *Disulfiram* has found some use in the patient seriously desiring to stop alcohol ingestion. A conditioned avoidance response is induced so that the patient abstains from alcohol to prevent the unpleasant effects of *disulfiram*-induced acetaldehyde accumulation.

Figure 9.10 summarizes the therapeutic disadvantages and advantages of some of the anxiolytic and hypnotic drugs.

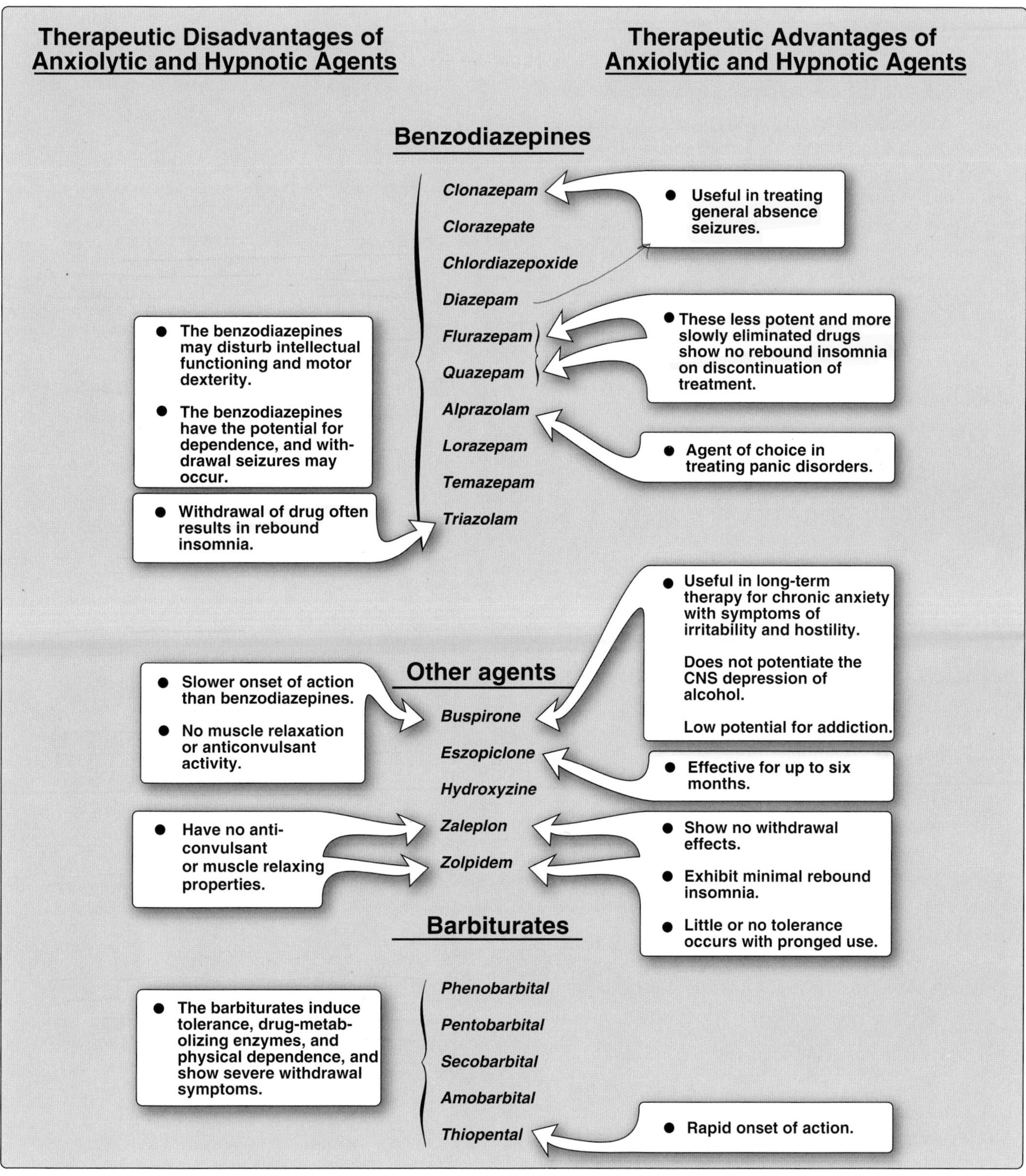

Figure 9.10
Therapeutic disadvantages and advantages of some anxiolytic and hypnotic agents. CNS = central nervous system.

Study Questions

Choose the ONE best answer

9.1 Which one of the following statements is correct?

A. Benzodiazepines directly open chloride channels.
B. Benzodiazepines show analgesic actions.
C. Clinical improvement of anxiety requires two to four weeks of treatment with benzodiazepines.
D. All benzodiazepines have some sedative effects.
E. Benzodiazepines, like other CNS depressants, readily produce general anesthesia.

Correct answer = D. Although all benzodiazepines can cause sedation, the drugs labeled "benzodiazepine hypnotics" in Figure 9.1 are promoted for the treatment of sleep disorder. Benzodiazepines enhance the binding of GABA to its receptor, which increases the permeability of chloride. The benzodiazepines do not relieve pain but may reduce the anxiety associated with pain. Unlike the tricyclic antidepressants and the monoamine oxidase (MAO) inhibitors, the benzodiazepines are effective within hours of administration. Benzodiazepines do not produce general anesthesia and are, therefore, relatively safe drugs with a high therapeutic index.

9.2 Which one of the following is a short-acting hypnotic?

A. Phenobarbital
B. Diazepam
C. Chlordiazepoxide
D. Thiopental
E. Flurazepam

Correct answer = D. Thiopental is an ultra-short-acting drug used as an adjuvant to anesthesia.

9.3 Which one of the following statements is CORRECT?

A. Phenobarbital shows analgesic properties.
B. Diazepam and phenobarbital induce the P450 enzyme system.
C. Phenobarbital is useful in the treatment of acute intermittent porphyria.
D. Phenobarbital induces respiratory depression, which is enhanced by the consumption of ethanol.
E. Buspirone has actions similar to the benzodiazepines.

Correct answer = D. Barbiturates and ethanol are a potentially lethal combination. Phenobarbital is unable to alter the pain threshold. Only phenobarbital strongly induces the synthesis of the hepatic cytochrome P450 drug metabolizing system. Phenobarbital is contraindicated in the treatment of acute intermittent porphyria. Buspirone lacks the anticonvulsant and muscle-relaxant properties of the benzodiazepines and causes only minimal sedation.

9.4 A 45-year-old man who has been injured in a car accident is brought into the emergency room. His blood alcohol level on admission is 275 mg/dL. Hospital records show a prior hospitalization for alcohol-related seizures. His wife confirms that he has been drinking heavily for three weeks. What treatment should be provided to the patient if he goes into withdrawal?

A. None
B. Lorazepam
C. Pentobarbital
D. Phenytoin

Correct answer = B. It is important to treat the seizures associated with alcohol withdrawal. Benzodiazepines, such as chlordiazepoxide, diazepam, or the shorter-acting lorazepam, are effective in controlling this problem. They are less sedating than pentobarbital or phenytoin.

Central Nervous System Stimulants

10

I. OVERVIEW

This chapter describes two groups of drugs that act primarily to stimulate the central nervous system (CNS) (Figure 10.1). The first group, the psychomotor stimulants, cause excitement and euphoria, decrease feelings of fatigue, and increase motor activity. The second group, the hallucinogens, or psychotomimetic drugs, produce profound changes in thought patterns and mood, with little effect on the brainstem and spinal cord. As a group, the CNS stimulants have few clinical uses, but they are important as drugs of abuse, as are the CNS depressants described in Chapter 9 and the narcotics described in Chapter 14 (Figure 10.2).

II. PSYCHOMOTOR STIMULANTS

A. Methylxanthines

Methylxanthines include *theophylline* [thee OFF i lin] found in tea, *theobromine* [thee o BRO min] found in cocoa, and *caffeine* [kaf EEN]. *Caffeine*, the most widely consumed stimulant in the world, is found in highest concentration in coffee, but is also present in tea, cola drinks, chocolate candy, and cocoa.

1. **Mechanism of action:** Several mechanisms have been proposed for the actions of methylxanthine, including translocation of extracellular calcium, increase in cyclic adenosine monophosphate and cyclic guanosine monophosphate caused by inhibition of phosphodiesterase, and blockade of adenosine receptors. The latter most likely accounts for the actions achieved by the usual consumption of *caffeine*-containing beverages.

2. **Actions:**

   a. **CNS:** The *caffeine* contained in one to two cups of coffee (100–200 mg) causes a decrease in fatigue and increased mental alertness as a result of stimulating the cortex and other areas of the brain. Consumption of 1.5 g of *caffeine* (twelve to fifteen cups of coffee) produces anxiety and tremors. The spinal cord is stimulated only by very high doses (2–5 g) of *caffeine*. Tolerance can rapidly develop to the stimulating properties of *caffeine*; withdrawal consists of feelings of fatigue and sedation.

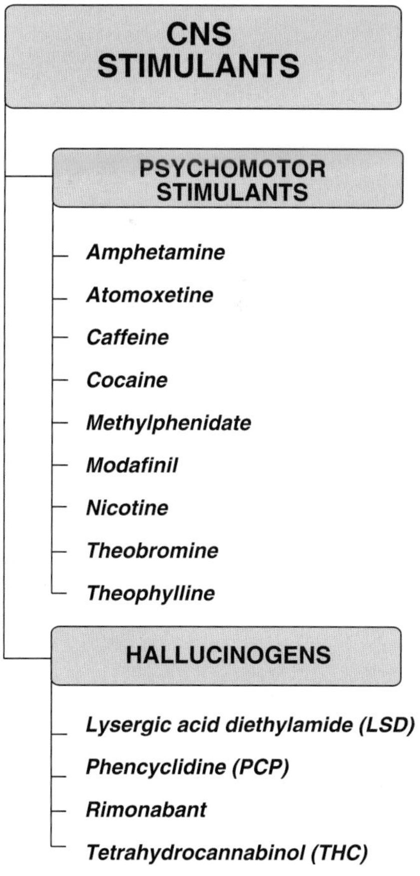
CNS STIMULANTS
PSYCHOMOTOR STIMULANTS
Amphetamine
Atomoxetine
Caffeine
Cocaine
Methylphenidate
Modafinil
Nicotine
Theobromine
Theophylline
HALLUCINOGENS
Lysergic acid diethylamide (LSD)
Phencyclidine (PCP)
Rimonabant
Tetrahydrocannabinol (THC)

Figure 10.1
Summary of central nervous system (CNS) stimulants.

Lippincott's Illustrated Reviews: Pharmacology, Third Edition,
by Richard D. Howland and Mary J. Mycek.
Lippincott Williams & Wilkins, Baltimore, MD © 2006.

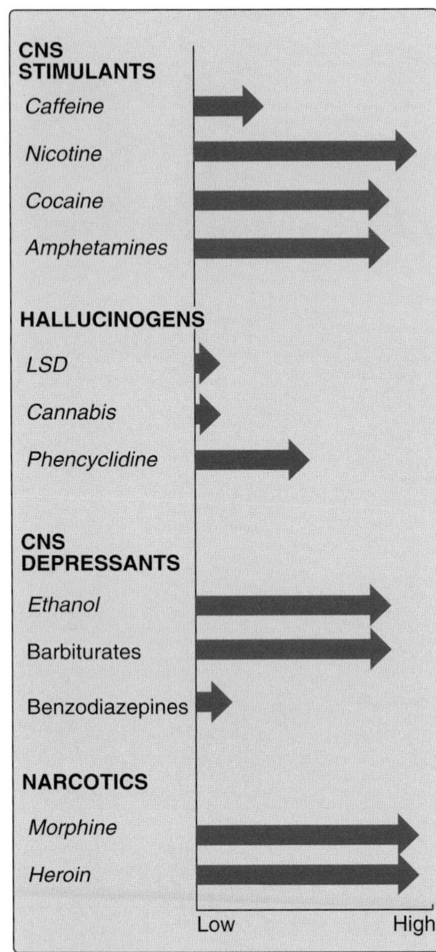

Figure 10.2
Relative potential for physical dependence on commonly abused substances.

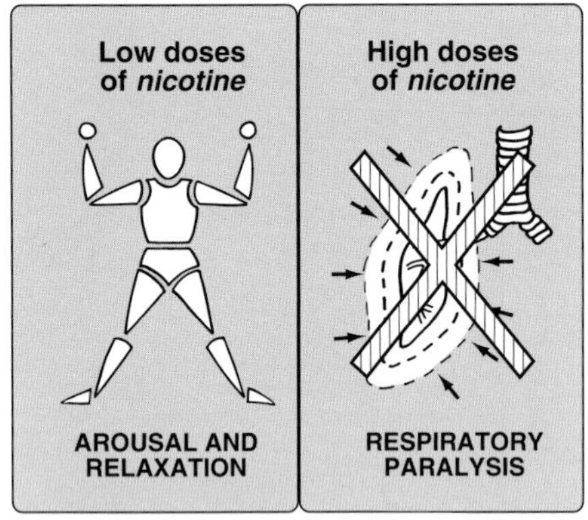

Figure 10.3
Actions of *nicotine* on the central nervous system.

b. **Cardiovascular system:** A high dose of *caffeine* has positive inotropic and chronotropic effects on the heart. [Note: Increased contractility can be harmful to patients with angina pectoris. In others, an accelerated heart rate can trigger premature ventricular contractions.]

c. **Diuretic action:** *Caffeine* has a mild diuretic action that increases urinary output of sodium, chloride, and potassium.

d. **Gastric mucosa:** Because all methylxanthines stimulate secretion of hydrochloric acid from the gastric mucosa, individuals with peptic ulcers should avoid beverages containing methylxanthines.

3. **Therapeutic uses:** *Caffeine* and its derivatives relax the smooth muscles of the bronchioles. [Note: Previously the mainstay of asthma therapy, *theophylline* has been largely replaced by other agents, such as β agonists and corticosteroids.]

4. **Pharmacokinetics:** The methylxanthines are well absorbed orally. *Caffeine* distributes throughout the body, including the brain. The drugs cross the placenta to the fetus, and are secreted into the mother's milk. All the methylxanthines are metabolized in the liver, and the metabolites are then excreted in the urine.

5. **Adverse effects:** Moderate doses of *caffeine* cause insomnia, anxiety, and agitation. A high dosage is required for toxicity, which is manifested by emesis and convulsions. The lethal dose is about 10 g of *caffeine* (about 100 cups of coffee), which induces cardiac arrhythmias; death from *caffeine* is thus highly unlikely. Lethargy, irritability, and headache occur in users who have routinely consumed more than 600 mg of *caffeine* per day (roughly six cups of coffee per day) and then suddenly stop.

B. Nicotine

Nicotine [NIC o teen] is the active ingredient in tobacco. Although this drug is not currently used therapeutically (except in smoking cessation therapy, see p. 117), *nicotine* remains important, because it is second only to *caffeine* as the most widely used CNS stimulant and second only to alcohol as the most abused drug. In combination with the tars and carbon monoxide found in cigarette smoke, *nicotine* represents a serious risk factor for lung and cardiovascular disease, various cancers, as well as other illnesses. Dependency on the drug is not easily overcome.

1. **Mechanism of action:** In low doses, *nicotine* causes ganglionic stimulation by depolarization. At high doses, *nicotine* causes ganglionic blockade. *Nicotine* receptors exist in the CNS, where similar actions occur.

2. **Actions:**

a. **CNS:** *Nicotine* is highly soluble in lipid and readily crosses the blood-brain barrier. Cigarette smoking or administration of low doses of *nicotine* produces some degree of euphoria, and arousal as well as relaxation. It improves attention, learning, problem solving, and reaction time. High doses of *nicotine* result in central respiratory paralysis and severe hypotension caused by medullary paralysis (Figure 10.3).

b. **Peripheral effects:** The peripheral effects of *nicotine* are complex. Stimulation of sympathetic ganglia as well as the adrenal medulla increases blood pressure and heart rate. Thus, use of tobacco is particularly harmful in hypertensive patients. Many patients with peripheral vascular disease experience an exacerbation of symptoms with smoking. For example, *nicotine*-induced vasoconstriction can decrease coronary blood flow, adversely affecting a patient with angina. Stimulation of parasympathetic ganglia also increases motor activity of the bowel. At higher doses, blood pressure falls, and activity ceases in both the gastrointestinal tract and bladder musculature as a result of a *nicotine*-induced block of parasympathetic ganglia.

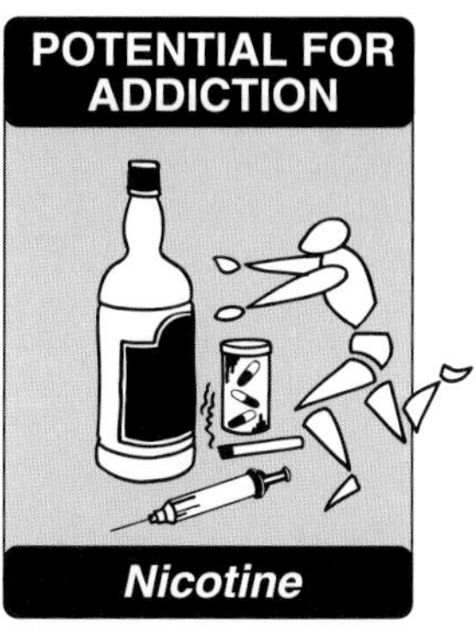

Figure 10.4
Nicotine has potential for addiction.

3. **Pharmacokinetics:** *Nicotine* is highly lipid-soluble. Thus, absorption readily occurs via the oral mucosa, lungs, gastrointestinal mucosa, and skin. *Nicotine* crosses the placental membrane and is secreted in the milk of lactating women. Most cigarettes contain 6–8 mg of *nicotine*; the acute lethal dose is 60 mg. More than ninety percent of *nicotine* inhaled in smoke is absorbed. Clearance of *nicotine* involves metabolism in the lung and the liver, and urinary excretion. Tolerance to the toxic effects of *nicotine* develops rapidly, often within days after beginning usage.

4. **Adverse effects:** The CNS effects of *nicotine* include irritability and tremors. *Nicotine* may also cause intestinal cramps, diarrhea, and increased heart rate and blood pressure. In addition, cigarette smoking increases the rate of metabolism for a number of drugs. [Note: It is not known which of the more than 3000 components of cigarette smoke are responsible for this phenomenon, although the benzopyrenes have been implicated.]

5. **Withdrawal syndrome:** As with the other drugs in this class, *nicotine* is an addictive substance, and physical dependence on *nicotine* develops rapidly and is severe (Figure 10.4). Withdrawal is characterized by irritability, anxiety, restlessness, difficulty concentrating, headaches, and insomnia. Appetite is affected, and gastrointestinal pain often occurs. [Note: Smoking cessation programs that combine pharmacologic and behavioral therapy are the most successful in helping individuals to stop smoking.] The transdermal patch and chewing gum containing *nicotine* have been shown to reduce *nicotine* withdrawal symptoms and to help smokers stop smoking. For example, the blood concentration of *nicotine* obtained from chewing gum is typically about one-half the peak level observed with smoking (Figure 10.5). *Bupropion*, an antidepressant (see p. 143), can reduce the craving for cigarettes.

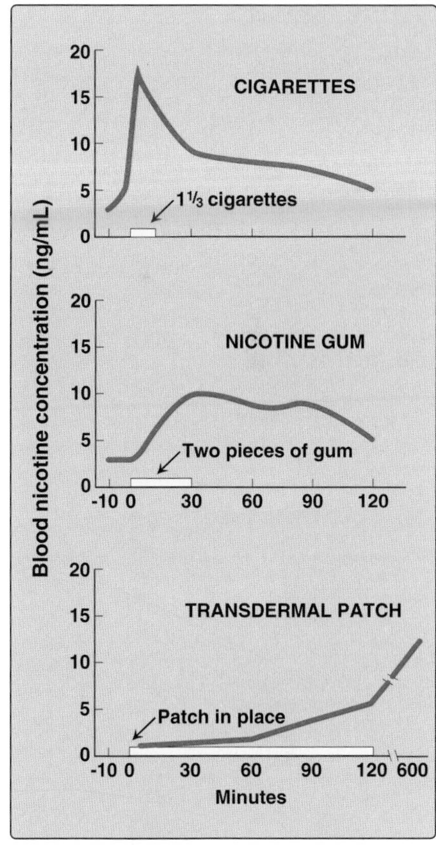

Figure 10.5
Blood concentrations of *nicotine* in individuals who smoked cigarettes, chewed nicotine gum, or received nicotine by transdermal patch.

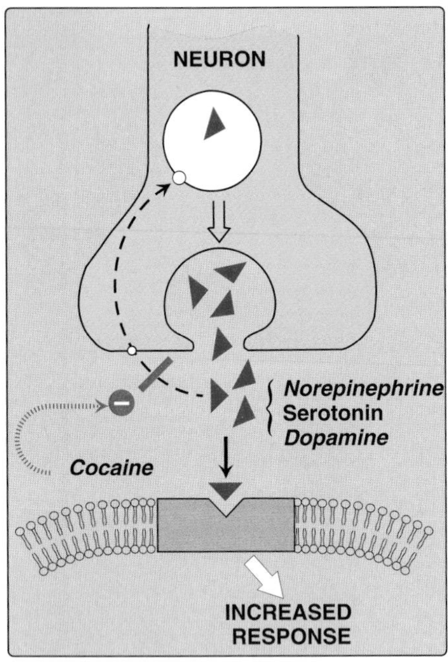

Figure 10.6
Mechanism of action of *cocaine*.

C. Cocaine

Cocaine [KOE kane] is an inexpensive, widely available, and highly addictive drug that is currently abused daily by more than three million people in the United States. Because of its abuse potential, *cocaine* is classified as a Schedule II drug by the United States Drug Enforcement Agency.

1. **Mechanism of action:** The primary mechanism of action underlying the central and peripheral effects of *cocaine* is blockade of re-uptake of the monoamines (*norepinephrine*, serotonin, and *dopamine*) into the presynaptic terminals from which these neurotransmitters are released (Figure 10.6). This blockade is effected by binding to the monoaminergic re-uptake transporters and, thus, potentiates and prolongs the CNS and peripheral actions of these monoamines. In particular, the prolongation of dopaminergic effects in the brain's pleasure system (limbic system) produces the intense euphoria that *cocaine* initially causes. Chronic intake of *cocaine* depletes *dopamine*. This depletion triggers the vicious cycle of craving for *cocaine* that temporarily relieves severe depression (Figure 10.7).

2. **Actions:**

   a. **CNS:** The behavioral effects of *cocaine* result from powerful stimulation of the cortex and brainstem. *Cocaine* acutely increases mental awareness and produces a feeling of well-being and euphoria similar to that caused by *amphetamine*. Like *amphetamine*, *cocaine* can produce hallucinations, delusions, and paranoia. *Cocaine* increases motor activity, and at high doses, it causes tremors and convulsions, followed by respiratory and vasomotor depression.

   b. **Sympathetic nervous system:** Peripherally, *cocaine* potentiates the action of *norepinephrine*, and produces the "fight or flight" syndrome characteristic of adrenergic stimulation. This is associated with tachycardia, hypertension, pupillary dilation, and peripheral vasoconstriction. Recent evidence suggests that the ability of baroreceptor reflexes to buffer the hypertensive effect may be impaired.

   c. **Hyperthermia:** *Cocaine* is unique among illicit drugs in that death can result not only as a function of dose, but also from the drug's propensity to cause hyperthermia. [Note: Mortality rates for *cocaine* overdose rise in hot weather.] Even a small dose of intranasal *cocaine* impairs sweating and cutaneous vasodilatation. Perception of thermal discomfort is also decreased.

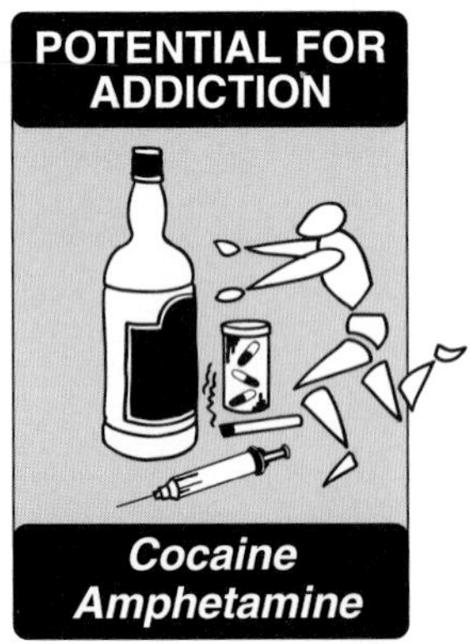

Figure 10.7
Cocaine and *amphetamine* have potential for addiction.

3. **Therapeutic uses:** *Cocaine* has a local anesthetic action that represents the only current rationale for the therapeutic use of *cocaine*. For example, *cocaine* is applied topically as a local anesthetic during eye, ear, nose, and throat surgery. Whereas the local anesthetic action of *cocaine* is due to a block of voltage-activated sodium channels, an interaction with potassium channels may contribute to the ability of *cocaine* to cause cardiac arrhythmias.

[Note: *Cocaine* is the only local anesthetic that causes vasoconstriction. This effect is responsible for the necrosis and perforation of the nasal septum seen in association with chronic inhalation of *cocaine* powder.]

4. **Pharmacokinetics:** *Cocaine* is often self-administered by chewing, intranasal snorting, smoking, or intravenous (IV) injection. The peak effect occurs at fifteen to twenty minutes after intranasal intake of *cocaine* powder, and the "high" disappears in 1 to 1.5 hours. Rapid but short-lived effects are achieved following IV injection of *cocaine* or by smoking the freebase form of the drug ("crack"). Because the onset of action is most rapid, the potential for overdosage and dependence is greatest with IV injection and crack smoking. *Cocaine* is rapidly de-esterified and demethylated to benzoylecgonine, which is excreted in the urine. Detection of this substance in the urine identifies a user.

5. **Adverse effects:**

   a. **Anxiety:** The toxic response to acute *cocaine* ingestion can precipitate an anxiety reaction that includes hypertension, tachycardia, sweating, and paranoia. Because of the irritability, many users take *cocaine* with alcohol. A product of *cocaine* metabolites and ethanol is cocaethylene, which is also psychoactive.

   b. **Depression:** Like all stimulant drugs, *cocaine* stimulation of the CNS is followed by a period of mental depression. Addicts withdrawing from *cocaine* exhibit physical and emotional depression as well as agitation. These symptoms can be treated with benzodiazepines or phenothiazines.

   c. **Heart disease:** *Cocaine* can induce seizures as well as fatal cardiac arrhythmias (Figure 10.8). IV *diazepam* and *propranolol* may be required to control *cocaine*-induced seizures and cardiac arrhythmias, respectively. The incidence of myocardial infarction in *cocaine* users is unrelated to dose, to duration of use, or to route of administration. There is no marker to identify those individuals who may have life-threatening cardiac effects after taking *cocaine*.

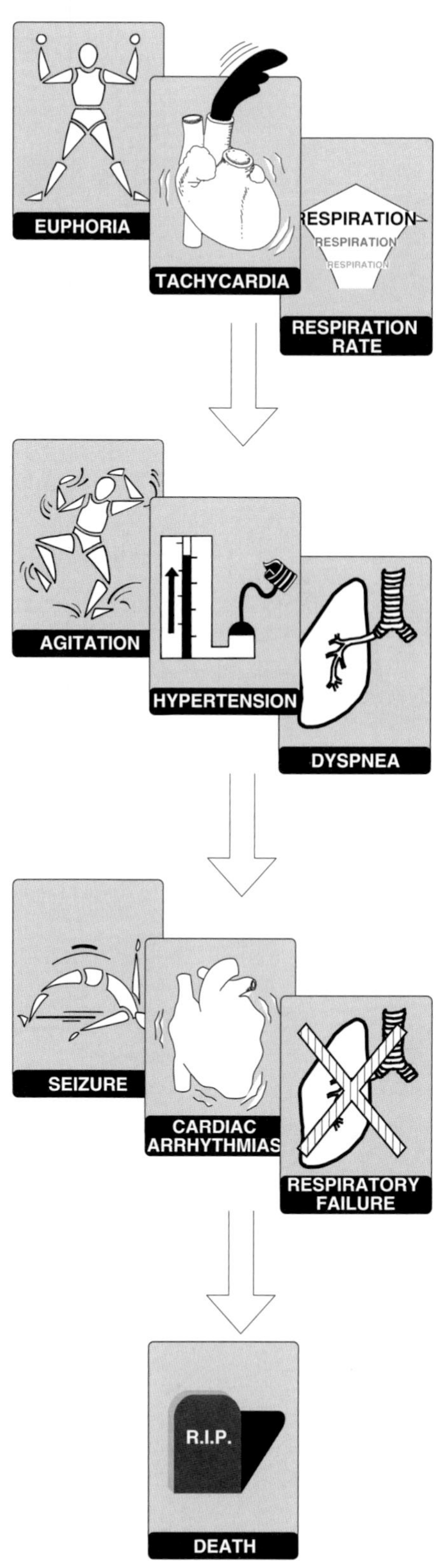

Figure 10.8
Major effects of *cocaine* use.

D. Amphetamine

Amphetamine is a noncatechoaminergic sympathetic amine that shows neurologic and clinical effects quite similar to those of *cocaine*. *Dextroamphetamine* is the major member of this class of compounds. *Methamphetamine* (also known as "speed") is a congener of *amphetamine* that can be smoked, and is preferred by many abusers.

1. **Mechanism of action:** As with *cocaine*, the effects of *amphetamine* on the CNS and peripheral nervous system are indirect; that is, both depend upon an elevation of the level of catecholamine transmitters in synaptic spaces. *Amphetamine*, however, achieves this effect by releasing intracellular stores of catecholamines (Figure 10.9). Because *amphetamine* also inhibits monoamine oxidase (MAO), high levels of catecholamines

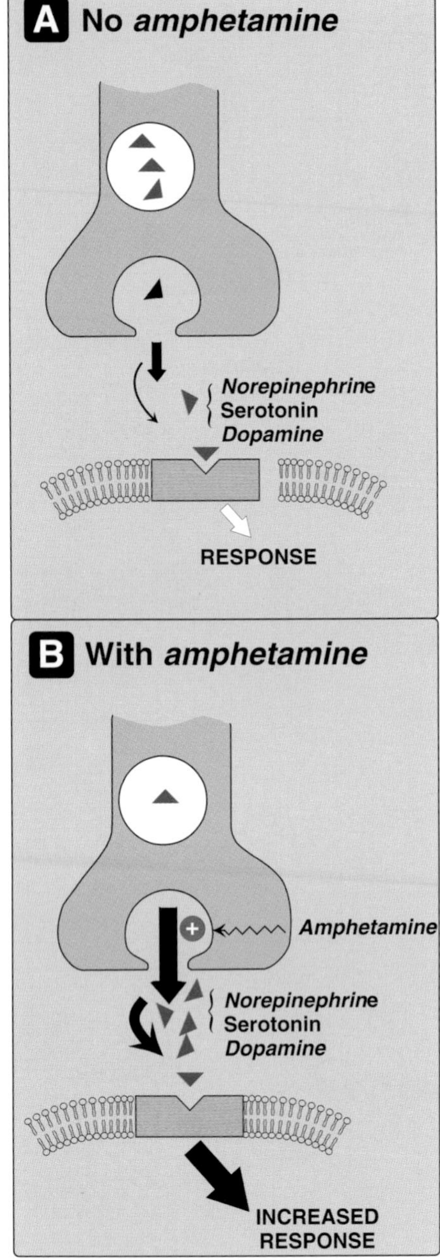

Figure 10.9
Mechanism of action of *amphetamine*.

are readily released into synaptic spaces. Despite different mechanisms of action, the behavioral effects of *amphetamine* and its congeners are similar to those of *cocaine*.

2. **Actions:**

   a. **CNS:** The major cause of the behavioral effects of *amphetamine* is probably due to release of *dopamine* rather than release of *norepinephrine*. *Amphetamine* stimulates the entire cerebrospinal axis, cortex, brainstem, and medulla. This leads to increased alertness, decreased fatigue, depressed appetite, and insomnia. At high doses, convulsions can ensue. These CNS stimulant effects of *amphetamine* and its derivatives have led to their use in therapy for hyperactivity in children, narcolepsy, and for appetite control.

   b. **Sympathetic nervous system:** In addition to its marked action on the CNS, *amphetamine* acts on the adrenergic system, indirectly stimulating the receptors through *norepinephrine* release.

3. **Therapeutic uses:** Factors that limit the therapeutic usefulness of *amphetamine* include psychologic and physiologic dependence similar to those with *cocaine*, and the development of tolerance to the euphoric and anorectic effects with chronic use. [Note: Less tolerance to the toxic CNS effects (for example, convulsions) develops.]

   a. **Attention deficit hyperactivity disorder (ADHD):** Some young children are hyperkinetic and lack the ability to be involved in any one activity for longer than a few minutes. *Dextroamphetamine* and the *amphetamine* derivative *methylphenidate* [meth ill FEN i date], paradoxically, are able to alleviate many of the behavioral problems associated with this syndrome, and to reduce the hyperkinesia that the children demonstrate. Their attention is thus prolonged, allowing them to function better in a school atmosphere. *Atomoxetine* [AT oh mox e teen] is a non-stimulant drug approved for ADHD in children and adults. [Note: It should not be taken by individuals on MAO inhibitors, and is not recommended for patients with narrow-angle glaucoma.] Unlike *methylphenidate* and *dextroamphetamine*, which block *dopamine* reuptake, *atomoxetine* is a *norepinephrine* reuptake inhibitor. It is not habit forming and is not a controlled sustance.

   b. **Narcolepsy:** Narcolepsy is a relatively rare sleep disorder that is characterized by uncontrollable bouts of sleepiness during the day. It is sometimes accompanied by catalepsy, a loss in muscle control, or even paralysis brought on by strong emotions, such as laughter. However, it is the sleepiness for which the patient is usually treated with drugs such as *amphetamine*, *methylphenidate*, or *phenelzine*. Recently, a new drug, *modafinil* (moe DAF i nil), has become available to treat narcoplepsy. *Modafinil* also produces psychoactive and euphoric effects, alterations in mood, perception, thinking, and feelings typical of other CNS stimulants. The mechanism of action remains unclear, although it has been shown to differ from that of *amphetamine*. *Modafinil* is effective orally. It is well distributed throughout the body and undergoes extensive hepatic metabolism. The metabolites are excreted in the urine. Headaches, nausea, and rhinitis are the primary adverse effects. No evidence indicates physical dependence.

4. **Pharmacokinetics:** *Amphetamine* is completely absorbed from the gastrointestinal tract, metabolized by the liver, and excreted in the urine. [Note: Administration of urinary alkalinizing agents will increase the non-ionized species of the drug and decrease its excretion.] *Amphetamine* abusers often administer the drugs by IV injection and by smoking. The euphoria caused by *amphetamine* lasts four to six hours, or four- to eight-fold longer than the effects of *cocaine*.

5. **Adverse effects:**

The *amphetamines* cause addiction, leading to dependence, tolerance, and drug-seeking behavior. In addition, they have the following undesirable effects.

a. **Central effects:** Undesirable side effects of *amphetamine* usage include insomnia, irritability, weakness, dizziness, tremor, and hyperactive reflexes (Figure 10.10). *Amphetamine* can also cause confusion, delirium, panic states, and suicidal tendencies, especially in mentally ill patients. Chronic *amphetamine* use produces a state of "*amphetamine* psychosis" that resembles an acute schizophrenic attack. Whereas *amphetamine* is associated with psychic and physical dependence, tolerance to its effects may occur within a few weeks. Overdoses of *amphetamine* are treated with *chlorpromazine* or *haloperidol*, which relieve the CNS symptoms as well as the hypertension because of their α-blocking effects. The anorectic effect of *amphetamine* is due to its action in the lateral hypothalamic feeding center.

b. **Cardiovascular effects:** In addition to its CNS effects, *amphetamine* causes palpitations, cardiac arrhythmias, hypertension, anginal pain, and circulatory collapse. Headache, chills, and excessive sweating may also occur. Because of its cardiovascular effects, *amphetamine* should not be given to patients with cardiovascular disease or those receiving MAO inhibitors.

c. **Gastrointestinal system effects:** *Amphetamine* acts on the gastrointestinal system, causing nausea, vomiting, abdominal cramps, and diarrhea. Administration of *sodium bicarbonate* will increase the absorption of *dextroamphetamine*.

d. **Contraindications:** Patients with hypertension, cardiovascular disease, hyperthyroidism, or glaucoma should not be treated with this drug nor should patients with a history of drug abuse.

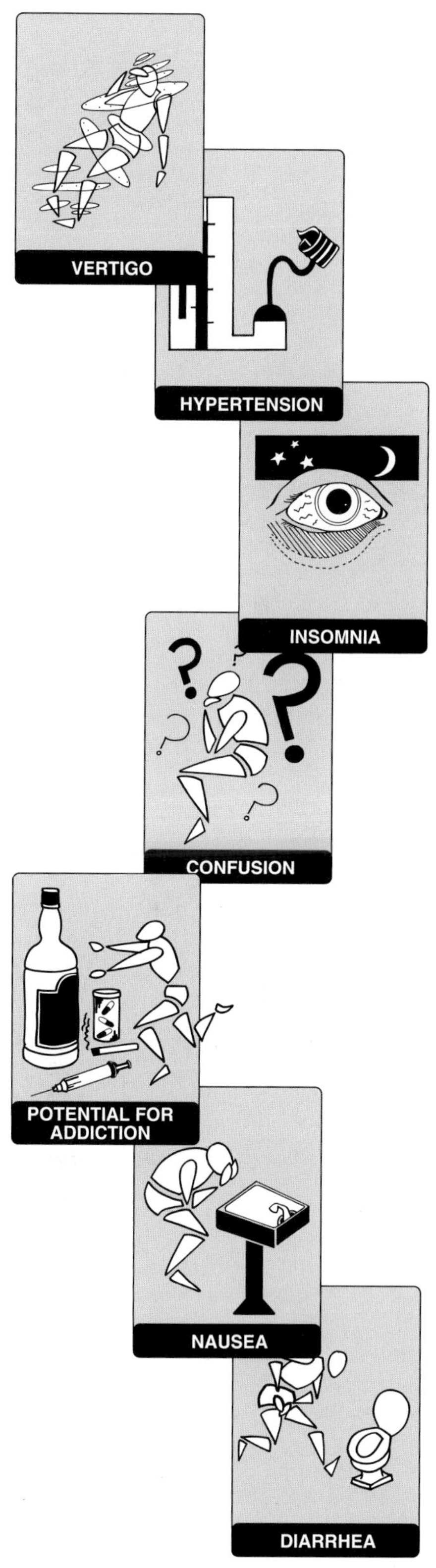

Figure 10.10
Adverse effects of amphetamines.

E. Methylphenidate

Methylphenidate has CNS stimulant properties similar to those of *amphetamine*, and may also lead to abuse, although its addictive potential is controversial. It is a Schedule II drug. It is presently one of the most prescribed medications in children. It is estimated that *methylphenidate* is taken daily by four to six million children in the United States for ADHD. The pharmacologically active isomer, *dexmethylphenidate*, has been recently approved.

1. **Mechanism of action:** Children with ADHD produce weak *dopamine* signals, which suggests that usually interesting activities provide fewer rewards to these children. At present, the basis for the stimulant effect of *methylphenidate* is not understood. However, a recent study using positron-emission tomography has opened up some interesting possibilities. It showed that *methylphenidate* is a more potent *dopamine* transport inhibitor than *cocaine*, thus making more *dopamine* available. [Note: Methylphenidate may have less potential for abuse than *cocaine*, because it enters the brain much more slowly than *cocaine* and, thus, does not increase *dopamine* levels as rapidly.]

2. **Therapeutic uses:** *Methylphenidate* has been used for several decades in the treatment of ADHD in children aged six to sixteen. It is also effective in the treatment of narcolepsy. Unlike *methylphenidate*, *dexmethylphenidate* is not indicated in the treatment of narcolepsy.

3. **Pharmacokinetics:** Both *methylphenidate* and *dexmethylphenidate* are readily absorbed on oral administration. Concentrations in the brain exceed those in the plasma. The de-esterified product, ritalinic acid, is excreted in the urine.

4. **Adverse reactions:** Gastrointestinal effects are the most common. These include abdominal pain and nausea. Other reactions include anorexia, insomnia, nervousness, and fever. In seizure patients, *methylphenidate* seems to increase the seizure frequency, especially if the patient is taking antidepressants. *Methylphenidate* is contraindicated in patients with glaucoma.

5. **Drug interactions:** Studies have shown that *methylphenidate* can interfere in the metabolism of *warfarin*, *diphenylhydantoin*, *phenobarbital*, *primidone*, and the tricyclic antidepressants.

III. HALLUCINOGENS

A few drugs have, as their primary action, the ability to induce altered perceptual states reminiscent of dreams. Many of these altered states are accompanied by bright, colorful changes in the environment and by a plasticity of constantly changing shapes and color. The individual under the influence of these drugs is incapable of normal decision making, because the drug interferes with rational thought. These compounds are known as hallucinogens or psychotomimetic drugs.

A. Lysergic acid diethylamide

Multiple sites in the CNS are affected by *lysergic acid diethylamide LSD*. The drug shows serotonin (5-HT) agonist activity at presynap-

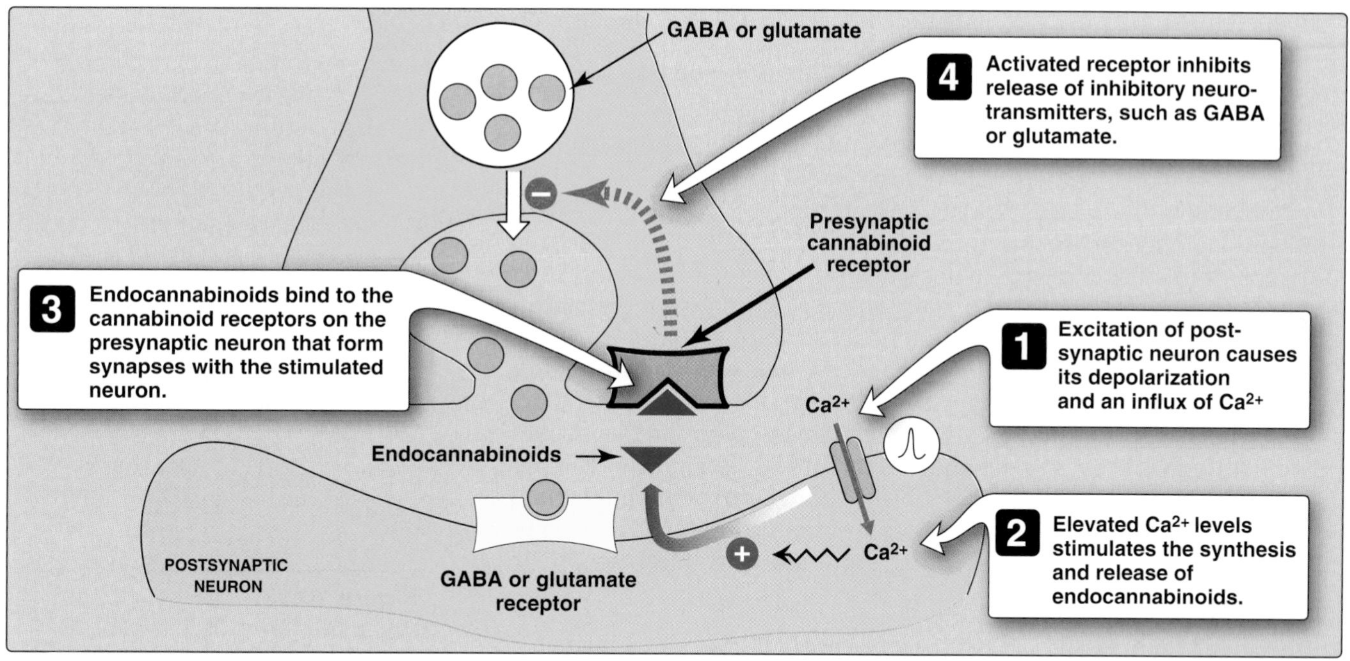

Figure 10.11
Cannabinoid receptor. GABA = γ-aminobutyric aid.

tic receptors in the midbrain, binding to both 5-HT_1 and 5-HT_2 receptors. Activation of the sympathetic nervous system occurs, which causes pupillary dilation, increased blood pressure, piloerection, and increased body temperature. Taken orally, low doses of *LSD* can induce hallucinations with brilliant colors. Mood alteration also occurs. Tolerance and physical dependence have occurred, but true dependence is rare. Adverse effects include hyperreflexia, nausea, and muscular weakness. High doses may produce long-lasting psychotic changes in susceptible individuals. *Haloperidol* and other neuroleptics can block the hallucinatory action of *LSD* and quickly abort the syndrome.

B. Tetrahydrocannabinol

The main psychoactive alkaloid contained in marijuana is Δ_9-*tetrahydrocannabinol* [tet ra hi dro can NAB i nol] (*THC*), which is available as *dronabinol* [droe NAB i nol]. Depending on the social situation, *THC* can produce euphoria, followed by drowsiness and relaxation. In addition to affecting short-term memory and mental activity, *THC* decreases muscle strength and impairs highly skilled motor activity, such as that required to drive a car. Its wide range of effects include appetite stimulation, xerostomia, visual hallucinations, delusions, and enhancement of sensory activity. *THC* receptors, designated CB1 receptors, have been found on inhibitory presynaptic nerve terminals that interact synaptically with pyramidal neurons. CB1 is coupled to a G protein. Interestingly, like the endogenous ligands of the opioid system, endocannabinoids have been identified in the CNS. These compounds, which bind to the CB1 receptors, are membrane-derived and are synthesized on demand, and they may act as local neuromodulators (Figure 10.11). The action of *THC* is believed to be mediated through the CB1 receptors, and is still under investigation. *THC* effects appear immediately after the drug is smoked, but maximal effects take about twenty minutes. By three hours, the effects largely disappear. *Dronabinol* is administered orally and has a peak effect in two to four hours. Its psychoactive effects can last up to six hours, but its appetite stimulant effects may persist for 24 hours. It is highly lipid soluble, and has a large volume of distribution. *THC* itself is extensively metabolized by the mixed-function oxidases. Elimination is largely through the biliary route. Adverse effects include increased heart rate, decreased blood pressure, and reddening of the conjunctiva. At high doses, a toxic psychosis develops (Figure 10.12). Tolerance and mild physical dependence occur with continued, frequent use of the drug. *Dronabinol* is indicated for patients with AIDS who are losing weight. It is also sometimes given for the severe emesis caused by some cancer chemotherapeutic agents (see p. 332). The CB1 receptor antagonist, *rimonabant* [rim OH nah bant] (currently in clinical trials), is effective in the treatment of obesity, and has been found to decrease appetite and body weight in humans.

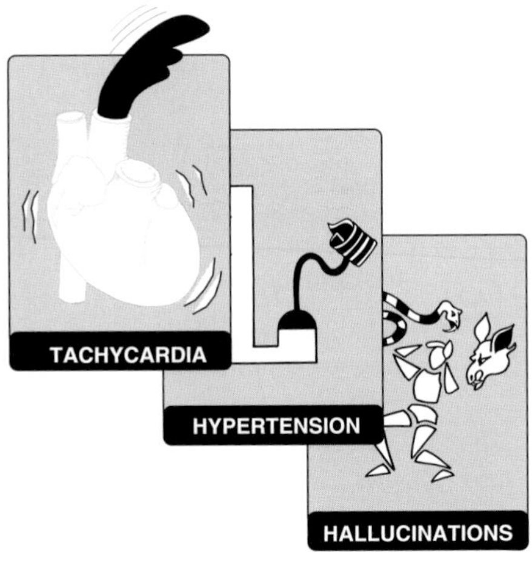

Figure 10.12
Adverse effects of *tetrahydrocannabinol.*

C. Phencyclidine (PCP)

Phencyclidine [fen SYE kli deen] (also known as PCP, or "angel dust") inhibits the re-uptake of *dopamine*, 5-HT, and *norepinephrine*. The major action of *phencyclidine* is to block the ion channel regulated by the NMDA subtype of glutamate receptor. This action prevents the passage of critical ions (particularly Ca^{2+}) through the channel. *Phencyclidine* also has anticholinergic activity but, surprisingly, produces hypersalivation. *Phencyclidine*, an analog of ketamine, causes dissociative anesthesia (insensitivity to pain, without loss of consciousness) and analgesia. In this state, it produces numbness of extremities, staggered gait, slurred speech, and muscular rigidity. Sometimes, hostile and bizarre behavior occurs. At increased dosages, anesthesia, stupor, or coma result, but strangely, the eyes may remain open. Increased sensitivity to external stimuli exists, and the CNS actions may persist for a week. Tolerance often develops with continued use.

Study Question

Choose the ONE best answer

10.1 A very agitated young male was brought to the emergency room by the police. Psychiatric examination revealed that he had snorted cocaine several times in the past few days, the last time being ten hours previously. He was given a drug that sedated him, and he fell asleep. The drug very likely used to counter this patient's apparent cocaine withdrawal was:

A. Phenobarbital
B. Lorazepam
C. Cocaine
D. Hydroxyzine
E. Fluoxetine

Correct answer = B. The anxiolytic properties of benzodiazepines, such as lorazepam, make them the drugs of choice in treating the anxiety and agitation of cocaine withdrawal. Lorazepam also has hypnotic properties. Phenobarbital has hypnotic properties, but its anxiolytic properties are inferior to those of the benzodiazepines. Cocaine itself could counteract the agitation of withdrawal, but its use would not be proper therapy. Hydroxyzine, an antihistaminic, is effective as a hypnotic, and is sometimes used to deal with anxiety, especially if emesis is a problem. Fluoxetine is an antidepressant with no immediate effects on anxiety.

Anesthetics

11

I. OVERVIEW

General anesthesia is essential to surgical practice, because it renders patients analgesic, amnesic, and unconscious, while causing muscle relaxation and suppression of undesirable reflexes. No single drug is capable of achieving these effects both rapidly and safely. Rather, several different categories of drugs are utilized to produce optimal anesthesia (Figure 11.1). Preanesthetic medication serves to calm the patient, relieve pain, and protect against undesirable effects of the subsequently administered anesthetic or the surgical procedure. Skeletal muscle relaxants facilitate intubation and suppress muscle tone to the degree required for surgery. Potent general anesthetics are delivered via inhalation or intravenous injection. With the exception of *nitrous oxide*, modern inhaled anesthetics are all volatile, halogenated hydrocarbons that derive from early research and clinical experience with *diethyl ether* and *chloroform*. On the other hand, intravenous general anesthetics consist of a number of chemically unrelated drug types that are commonly used for the rapid induction of anesthesia.

PREANESTHETIC MEDICATION
- **Anticholinergics**
- **Antiemetics**
- **Antihistamines**
- **Barbiturates**
- **Benzodiazepines**
- **Muscle relaxants**
- **Opioids**

GENERAL ANESTHETICS
- **INHALED**
  - ***Desflurane***
  - ***Enflurane***
  - ***Halothane***
  - ***Isoflurane***
  - ***Nitrous oxide***
  - ***Sevoflurane***
- **INTRAVENOUS**
  - **Barbiturates**
  - **Benzodiazepines**
  - ***Etomidate***
  - ***Ketamine***
  - **Opioids**
  - ***Propofol***

LOCAL ANESTHETICS
- ***Bupivacaine***
- ***Lidocaine***
- ***Procaine***
- ***Tetracaine***

Figure 11.1
Summary of anesthetics.

II. PATIENT FACTORS IN SELECTION OF ANESTHESIA

During the preoperative phase, the anesthesiologist selects drugs that provide a safe and efficient anesthetic regimen based on the nature of the surgical or diagnostic procedure, as well as on the patient's physiologic, pathologic, and pharmacologic state.

A. Status of organ systems

1. **Liver and kidney:** Because the liver and kidney not only influence the long-term distribution and clearance of anesthetic agents but can also be the target organs for toxic effects, the physiologic status of these organs must be considered. Of particular concern, is that the release of fluoride, bromide, and other metabolic products of the halogenated hydrocarbons can affect these organs, especially if the metabolites accumulate with repeated anesthetic administration over a short period of time.

Lippincott's Illustrated Reviews: Pharmacology, Third Edition,
by Richard D. Howland and Mary J. Mycek.
Lippincott Williams & Wilkins, Baltimore, MD © 2006.

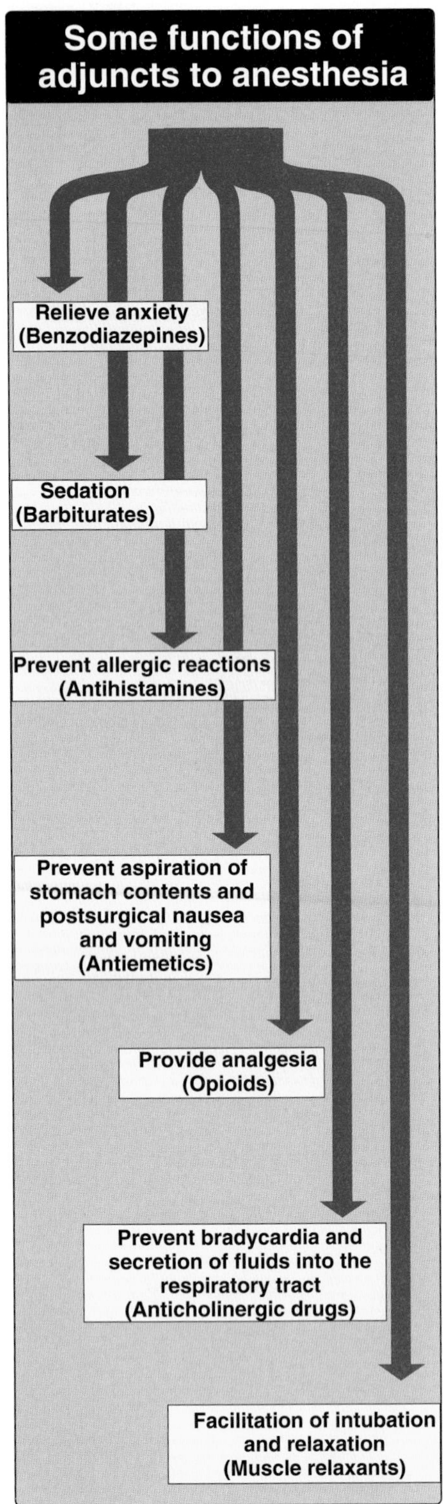

Figure 11.2
Components of balanced anesthesia.

2. **Respiratory system:** The condition of the respiratory system must be considered if inhalation anesthetics are indicated. For example, asthma or ventilation or perfusion abnormalities complicate control of an inhalation anesthetic. All inhaled anesthetics depress the respiratory system. Interestingly, they also are bronchodilators.

3. **Cardiovascular system:** Whereas the hypotensive effect of most anesthetics is sometimes desirable, ischemic injury of tissues could follow reduced perfusion pressure. If a hypotensive episode during a surgical procedure necessitates treatment, a vasoactive substance is administered. This is done after consideration of the possibility that some anesthetics, such as *halothane*, may sensitize the heart to the arrhythmogenic effects of sympathomimetic agents.

4. **Nervous system:** The existence of neurologic disorders (for example, epilepsy or myasthenia gravis) influences the selection of an anesthetic. So, too, would a patient history suggestive of a genetically determined sensitivity to halogenated hydrocarbon-induced malignant hypothermia.

5. **Pregnancy:** Some precautions should be kept in mind when anesthetics and adjunct drugs are administered to a pregnant woman. There has been at least one report that transient use of *nitrous oxide* can cause aplastic anemia in the unborn child. Oral clefts have occurred in the fetuses of women who have received benzodiazepines. *Diazepam* should not be used routinely during labor, because it results in temporary hypotonia and altered thermoregulation in the newborn.

B. Concomitant use of drugs

1. **Multiple adjunct agents:** Commonly, surgical patients receive one or more of the following preanesthetic medications: benzodiazepines, such as *midazolam* or *diazepam*, to allay anxiety and facilitate amnesia; barbiturates, such as *pentobarbital*, for sedation; antihistamines, such as *diphenhydramine*, for prevention of allergic reactions, or, *ranitidine*, to reduce gastric acidity; antiemetics, such as *ondansetron*, to prevent the possible aspiration of stomach contents; opioids, such as *fentanyl*, for analgesia; and/or anticholinergics, such as *scopolamine*, for their amnesic effect and to prevent bradycardia and secretion of fluids into the respiratory tract (Figure 11.2). These agents facilitate smooth induction of anesthesia, and when administered continuously, they also lower the dose of anesthetic required to maintain the desired level of surgical (Stage III) anesthesia. However, such coadministration can also enhance undesirable anesthetic effects (for example, hypoventilation), and may produce negative effects not observed when each drug is given individually.

2. **Concomitant use of additional nonanesthetic drugs:** Surgical patients may be chronically exposed to agents for the treatment of the underlying disease, as well as to drugs of abuse that alter the response to anesthetics. For example, alcoholics have elevated

levels of hepatic microsomal enzymes involved in the metabolism of barbiturates, and drug abusers may be overly tolerant of opioids.

III. INDUCTION, MAINTENANCE, AND RECOVERY FROM ANESTHESIA

Anesthesia can be divided into three stages: induction, maintenance, and recovery. Induction is defined as the period of time from the onset of administration of the anesthetic to the development of effective surgical anesthesia in the patient. Maintenance provides a sustained surgical anesthesia. Recovery is the time from discontinuation of administration of the anesthesia until consciousness and protective physiologic reflexes are regained. Induction of anesthesia depends on how fast effective concentrations of the anesthetic drug reach the brain; recovery is the reverse of induction, and depends on how fast the anesthetic drug diffuses from the brain.

A. Induction

During induction, it is essential to avoid the dangerous excitatory phase (Stage II delirium) that was observed with the slow onset of action of some earlier anesthetics (see below). Thus, general anesthesia is normally induced with an intravenous anesthetic like *thiopental*, which produces unconsciousness within 25 seconds after injection. At that time, additional inhalation or intravenous drugs comprising the selected anesthetic combination may be given to produce the desired depth of surgical (Stage III) anesthesia. [Note: This often includes coadministration of an intravenous skeletal muscle relaxant to facilitate intubation and relaxation. Currently used muscle relaxants include *vecuronium*, *atracurium*, and *succinylcholine*.] For children, without intravenous access, nonpungent agents, such as *halothane* or *sevoflurane*, are used to induce general anesthesia. This is termed inhalation induction.

B. Maintenance of anesthesia

Maintenance is the period during which the patient is surgically anesthetized. After administering the selected anesthetic mixture, the anesthesiologist monitors the patient's vital signs and response to various stimuli throughout the surgical procedure to carefully balance the amount of drug inhaled and/or infused with the depth of anesthesia. Anesthesia is usually maintained by the administration of volatile anesthetics, because these agents offer good minute-to-minute control over the depth of anesthesia. Opioids such as *fentanyl*, are often used for pain along with inhalation agents, because the latter are not good analgesics.

C. Recovery

Postoperatively, the anesthesiologist withdraws the anesthetic mixture and monitors the return of the patient to consciousness. For most anesthetic agents, recovery is the reverse of induction; that is, redistribution from the site of action (rather than metabolism of the anesthetic) underlies recovery. The anesthesiologist continues to monitor the patient to be sure that he or she is fully recovered with normal physiologic functions (for example, is able to breathe on his/her own). Patients are observed for delayed toxic reactions, such as hepatotoxicity caused by halogenated hydrocarbons.

D. Depth of anesthesia

The depth of anesthesia has been divided into four sequential stages. Each stage is characterized by increased CNS depression, which is caused by accumulation of the anesthetic drug in the brain (Figure 11.3). These stages were discerned and defined with *ether*, which produces a slow onset of anesthesia. However, with *halothane* and other commonly used anesthetics, the stages are difficult to characterize clearly because of the rapid onset of anesthesia.

1. **Stage I—Analgesia:** Loss of pain sensation results from interference with sensory transmission in the spinothalamic tract. The patient is conscious and conversational. Amnesia and a reduced awareness of pain occur as Stage II is approached.

2. **Stage II—Excitement:** The patient experiences delirium and violent combative behavior. There is a rise and irregularity in blood pressure. The respiratory rate may increase. To avoid this stage of anesthesia, a short-acting barbiturate, such as *thiopental*, is given intravenously before inhalation anesthesia is administered.

3. **Stage III—Surgical anesthesia:** Regular respiration and relaxation of the skeletal muscles occur in this stage. Eye reflexes decrease progressively, until the eye movements cease and the pupil is fixed. Surgery may proceed during this stage.

4. **Stage IV—Medullary paralysis:** Severe depression of the respiratory and vasomotor centers occur during this stage. Death can rapidly ensue unless measures are taken to maintain circulation and respiration.

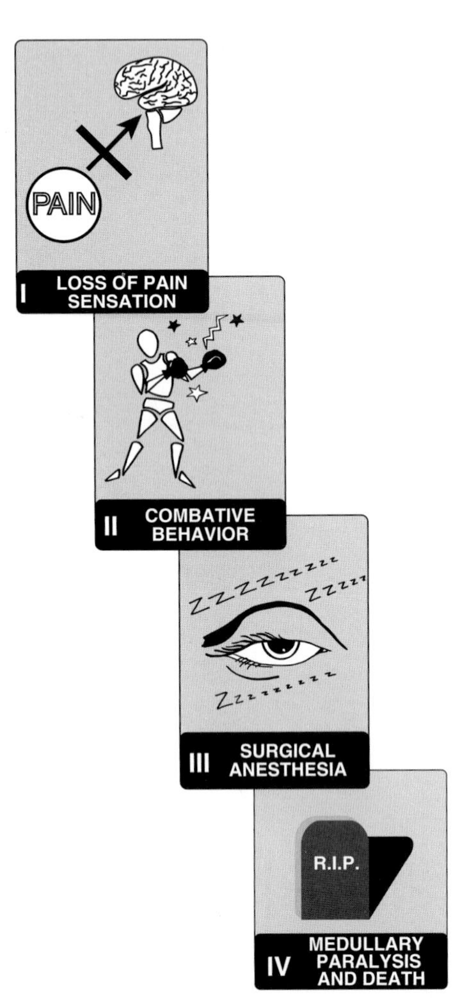

Figure 11.3
Stages of anesthesia.

IV. INHALATION ANESTHETICS

Inhaled gases are the mainstay of anesthesia, and are used primarily for the maintenance of anesthesia after administration of an intravenous agent. No one anesthetic is superior to another under all circumstances. Inhalation anesthetics have a benefit that is not available with intravenous agents, because the depth of anesthesia can be rapidly altered by changing the concentration of the drug. Inhalation anesthetics are also reversible, because most are rapidly eliminated from the body by exhalation.

A. Common features of inhaled anesthetics

Modern inhalation anesthetics are nonflammable, nonexplosive agents that include the gas *nitrous oxide*, as well as a number of volatile, halogenated hydrocarbons. As a group, these agents decrease cerebrovascular resistance, resulting in increased perfusion of the brain. They also cause bronchodilation, and decrease both minute ventilation (volume of air per unit time moved into or out of the lungs) and hypoxic pulmonary vasoconstriction (increased pulmonary vascular resistance in poorly aerated regions of the lungs, which allows redirection of pulmonary blood flow to regions that are richer in oxygen content). The movement of these agents from the lungs to the different body compartments depends upon their solubility in blood and tissues as well as on blood flow. These factors play a role not only in induction but also in recovery

B. Potency

The potency of inhaled anesthetics is defined quantitatively as the median alveolar concentration (MAC). This is the end tidal concentration of anesthetic gas needed to eliminate movement among fifty percent of patients challenged by a standardized skin incision. [Note: MAC is the median effective dose (ED_{50}) of the anesthetic.] MAC is usually expressed as the percentage of gas in a mixture required to achieve the effect. Numerically, MAC is small for potent anesthetics, such as *halothane*, and large for less potent agents, such as *nitrous oxide*. Therefore, the inverse of MAC is an index of potency of the anesthetic. The MAC values are useful in comparing pharmacologic effects of different anesthetics (Figure 11.4). The more lipid-soluble an anesthetic, the lower the concentration of anesthetic needed to produce anesthesia and, thus, the higher the potency of the anesthetic.

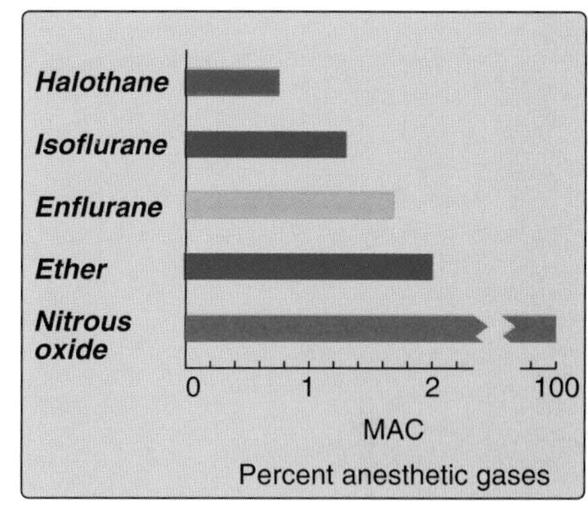

Figure 11.4
Minimal alveolar concentrations (MAC) for anesthetic gases.

C. Uptake and distribution of inhalation anesthetics

The partial pressure of an anesthetic gas at the origin of the respiratory pathway is the driving force that moves the anesthetic into the alveolar space and, thence, into the blood, which delivers the drug to the brain and various other body compartments. Because gases move from one compartment to another within the body according to partial pressure gradients, a steady state is achieved when the partial pressure in each of these compartments is equivalent to that in the inspired mixture. The time course for attaining this steady state is determined by the following factors:

1. **Alveolar wash-in:** This term refers to the replacement of the normal lung gases with the inspired anesthetic mixture. The time required for this process is directly proportional to the functional residual capacity of the lung, and inversely proportional to the ventilatory rate; it is independent of the physical properties of the gas. As the partial pressure builds within the lung, anesthetic transfer from the lung begins.

2. **Anesthetic uptake:** Anesthetic uptake is the product of gas solubility in the blood, cardiac output, and the anesthetic gradient between alveolar and venous partial pressure gradients.

   a. **Solubility in the blood:** This is determined by a physical property of the anesthetic molecule called the blood/gas partition coefficient, which is the ratio of the total amount of gas in the blood relative to the gas equilibrium phase (Figure 11.5). Drugs with low versus high solubility in blood differ in their speed of induction of anesthesia. For example, when an anesthetic gas with low blood solubility, such as *nitrous oxide*, diffuses from the alveoli into the circulation, little of the anesthetic dissolves in the

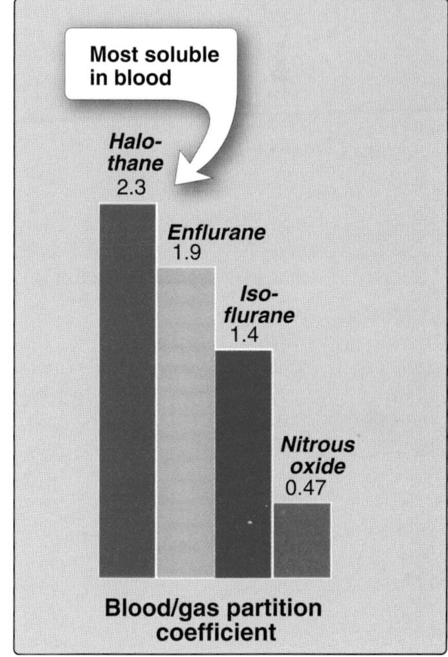

Figure 11.5
Blood/gas partition coefficients for some inhalation anesthetics.

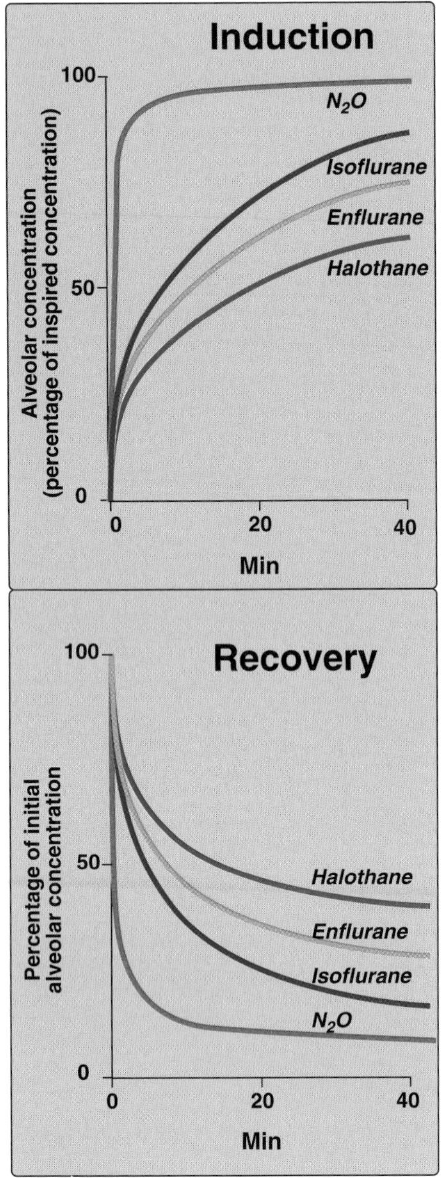

Figure 11.6
Changes in the alveolar blood concentrations of some inhalation anesthetics over time. N_20 = nitrous oxide.

blood. Therefore, the equilibrium between the inhaled anesthetic and arterial blood occurs rapidly, and relatively few additional molecules of anesthetic are required to raise arterial anesthetic partial pressure—that is, steady-state is rapidly achieved. In contrast, an anesthetic gas with high blood solubility, such as *halothane*, dissolves more completely in the blood, and greater amounts of the anesthetic and longer periods of time are required to raise arterial partial pressure. This results in increased times of induction as well as recovery, and slower changes in the depth of anesthesia in response to alterations in the concentration of the inhaled drug. Figure 11.6 illustrates the uptake curves for some inhalation anesthetics. The solubility in blood is ranked in the following order: *halothane* > *enflurane* > *isoflurane* > *sevoflurane* > *desflurane* > *nitrous oxide*.

b. **Cardiac output:** It is obvious that cardiac output affects the delivery of anesthetic to tissues. Low cardiac output will result in slow delivery of the anesthetic.

c. **Alveolar to venous partial pressure gradient of the anesthetic:** This is the driving force of anesthetic delivery. For all practical purposes, the pulmonary end-capillary anesthetic partial pressure may be considered as the anesthetic alveolar partial pressure if the patient does not have severe lung diffusion disease. The arterial circulation distributes the anesthetic to various tissues, and the pressure gradient drives free anesthetic gas into tissues. As the venous circulation returns blood depleted of anesthetic to the lung, more gas moves into the blood from the lung according to the partial pressure difference. Over time, the partial pressure in the venous blood closely approximates the partial pressure in the inspired mixture; that is, no further net anesthetic uptake from the lung occurs.

3. **Effect of different tissue types on anesthetic uptake:** The time required for a particular tissue to achieve a steady-state with the partial pressure of an anesthetic gas in the inspired mixture is inversely proportional to the blood flow to that tissue; that is, faster flow results in a more rapidly achieved steady-state. It is also directly proportional to the capacity of that tissue to store anesthetic; that is, a larger capacity results in a longer time required to achieve steady-state. Capacity, in turn, is directly proportional to the tissue's volume and the tissue/blood solubility coefficient of the anesthetic molecules. Four major tissue compartments determine the time course of anesthetic uptake.

a. **Brain, heart, liver, kidney, and endocrine glands:** These highly perfused tissues rapidly attain a steady-state with the partial pressure of anesthetic in the blood.

b. **Skeletal muscles:** These are poorly perfused during anesthesia. This, and the fact that they have a large volume, prolong the time required to achieve steady-state.

c. **Fat:** This tissue is also poorly perfused. However, potent general anesthetics are very lipid soluble. Therefore, fat has a large capacity to store anesthetic. This combination of slow delivery to a high-capacity compartment prolongs the time required to achieve steady state.

d. **Bone, ligaments, and cartilage:** These are poorly perfused and have a relatively low capacity to store anesthetic. Therefore, these tissues have only a slight impact on the time course of anesthetic distribution in the body.

4. **Wash-out:** When the administration of an inhalation anesthetic is discontinued, the body now becomes the "source" that drives the anesthetic into the alveolar space. The same factors that influence attainment of steady-state with an inspired anesthetic determine the time course of clearance of the drug from the body. Thus, *nitrous oxide* exits the body faster than *halothane* (see Figure 11.6).

D. Mechanism of action

No specific receptor has been identified as the locus of general anesthetic action. Indeed, the fact that chemically unrelated compounds produce the anesthetic state argues against the existence of such a receptor. The focus is now on interactions of the inhaled anesthetics with proteins comprising ion channels. For example, the general anesthetics increase the sensitivity of the γ-aminobutyric acid ($GABA_A$) receptors to the neurotransmitter, GABA, at clinically effective concentrations of the drug. This causes a prolongation of the inhibitory chloride ion current after a pulse of GABA release. Postsynaptic neuronal excitability is thus diminished (Figure 11.7). Other receptors are also affected by volatile anesthetics; for example, the activity of the inhibitory glycine receptors in the spinal motor neurons is increased. In addition, the inhalation anesthetics block the excitatory postsynaptic current of the nicotinic receptors. The mechanism by which the anesthetics perform these modulatory roles is not understood.

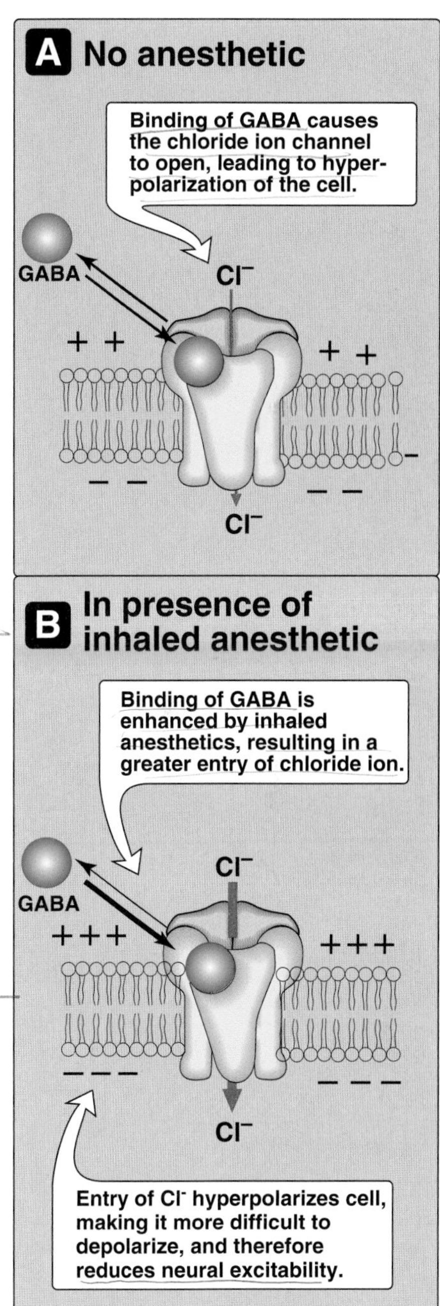

A No anesthetic
Binding of GABA causes the chloride ion channel to open, leading to hyper-polarization of the cell.
GABA
Cl⁻
+ +
+ +
– –
– –
Cl⁻
B In presence of inhaled anesthetic
Binding of GABA is enhanced by inhaled anesthetics, resulting in a greater entry of chloride ion.
GABA
Cl⁻
+++
+++
– – –
– – –
Cl⁻
Entry of Cl⁻ hyperpolarizes cell, making it more difficult to depolarize, and therefore reduces neural excitability.

Figure 11.7
An example of modulation of a ligand-gated membrane channel modulated by inhaled anthestics. GABA = γ-aminobutyric acid.

E. Halothane

This agent is the prototype to which newer inhalation anesthetics have been compared. When *halothane* (HAL oh thane) was introduced, its ability to induce the anesthetic state rapidly and to allow quick recovery—and the fact that it was nonexplosive—made it an anesthetic of choice. However, with the recognition of the adverse effects discused below, and the availabillty of other anesthetics that cause fewer complications, *halothane* is largely being replaced in the United States.

1. **Therapeutic uses:** Whereas *halothane* is a potent anesthetic, it is a relatively weak analgesic. Thus, *halothane* is usually coadministered with *nitrous oxide*, opioids, or local anesthetics. *Halothane* relaxes both skeletal and uterine muscle, and can be used in obstetrics when uterine relaxation is indicated. *Halothane* is not hepatotoxic in pediatric patients (unlike its potential effect on adults, see below), and, combined with its pleasant odor, this makes it suitable in children for inhalation induction.

2. **Pharmacokinetics:** *Halothane* is oxidatively metabolized in the body to tissue-toxic hydrocarbons (for example, trifluroethanol) and bromide ion. These substances may be responsible for the toxic reaction that some patients (especially females) develop after *halothane* anesthesia. This reaction begins as a fever, followed by anorexia, nausea, and vomiting, and patients may exhibit signs of hepatitis. [Note: Although the incidence of this reaction is low—approximately 1 in 10,000 individuals—fifty percent of such patients will die of hepatic necrosis. To avoid this condition, a *halothane* anesthesia is not repeated at intervals of less than two to three weeks.]

3. **Adverse effects:**

   a. **Cardiac effects:** Like other halogenated hydrocarbons, *halothane* is vagomimetic and causes *atropine*-sensitive bradycardia. In addition, *halothane* has the undesirable property of causing cardiac arrhythmias. [Note: These are especially serious if hypercapnia (increased arterial carbon dioxide partial pressure) develops due to reduced alveolar ventilation or to an increase in the plasma concentration of catecholamines.] *Halothane*, like the other halogenated anesthetics, produces concentration-dependent hypotension. Should it become necessary to counter excessive hypotension during *halothane* anesthesia, it is recommended that a direct-acting vasoconstrictor, such as *phenylephrine*, be given.

   b. **Malignant hyperthermia:** In a very small percentage of patients, all of the halogenated hydrocarbon anesthetics—as well as the muscle relaxant *succinylcholine*—have the potential to induce malignant hyperthermia. Whereas the etiology of this condition is poorly understood, recent investigations have identified a dramatic increase in the myoplasmic calcium ion concentration. Strong evidence indicates that malignant hyperthermia is due to an excitation-contraction coupling defect. Burn victims and individuals with Duchenne dystrophy, myotonia, osteogenesis imperfecta, and central-core disease are susceptible to malignant hyperthermia. Should a patient exhibit the characteristic symptoms of malignant hyperthermia, *dantrolene* is given as the anesthetic mixture is withdrawn. The patient must be carefully monitored and supported for respiratory, circulatory, and renal problems.

F. Enflurane

This gas is less potent than *halothane*, but produces rapid induction and recovery. About two percent of the anesthetic is metabolized to fluoride ion, which is excreted by the kidney. Therefore, *enflurane* [EN floo rane] is contraindicated in patients with kidney failure. *Enflurane* anesthesia exhibits the following differences from *halothane* anesthesia: fewer arrhythmias, less sensitization of the heart to catecholamines, and greater potentiation of muscle relaxants due to a more potent "*curare*-like" effect. A disadvantage of *enflurane* is that it causes central nervous system (CNS) excitation at twice the MAC and also at lower doses if hyperventilation reduces the pCO_2. For this reason, it is not used in patients with seizure disorders.

G. Isoflurane

This halogenated anesthetic is widely used in the United States. It is a very stable molecule that undergoes little metabolism; as a result, little fluoride is produced. *Isoflurane* [eye soe FLURE ane] is not tissue toxic. Unlike the other halogenated anesthetic gases, *isoflurane* does not induce cardiac arrhythmias and does not sensitize the heart to the action of catecholamines. However, it produces concentration-dependent hypotension due to peripheral vasodilation. It also dilates the coronary vasculature, increasing coronary blood flow and oxygen consumption by the myocardium. This property may make it beneficial in patients with ischemic heart disease. [Note: All halogenated inhalation anesthetics have been reported to cause hepatitis, but at a much lower incidence than with *halothane*. For example, *isoflurane* does so in 1 in 500,000 individuals treated with that anesthetic.]

H. Desflurane

The rapidity with which *desflurane* causes anesthesia and emergence has made this a popular anesthetic for outpatient surgery. However, *desflurane* [DES flure ane] has a low volatility and, thus, must be delivered using a special vaporizer. Like *isoflurane*, it decreases vascular resistance and perfuses all major tissues very well. Because it is irritating to the airway and can cause laryngospasm, coughing, and excessive secretions, *desflurane* is not used to induce extended anesthesia. Its degradation is minimal; thus tissue toxicity is rare.

I. Sevoflurane

Sevoflurane [see voe FLOO rane] has low pungency, allowing rapid uptake without irritating the airway during induction, thus making it suitable for induction in children. It is replacing *halothane* for this purpose. The drug has low solubility in blood, and is rapidly taken up and excreted. Recovery is faster than with other anesthetics. It is metabolized by the liver, releasing fluoride ions; thus, like *enflurane*, it may prove to be nephrotoxic.

J. Nitrous oxide

Nitrous oxide [nye truss OX ide] ("laughing gas") is a potent analgesic but a weak general anesthetic. For example, *nitrous oxide* is frequently employed at concentrations of thirty percent in combination with oxygen for analgesia, particularly in dental surgery. However, *nitrous oxide* at eighty percent (without adjunct agents) cannot produce surgical anesthesia. It is therefore frequently combined with other, more potent agents to attain pain-free anesthesia. *Nitrous oxide* is poorly soluble in blood and other tissues, allowing it to move very rapidly in and out of the body. [Note: *Nitrous oxide* can concentrate the halogenated anesthetics in the alveoli when they are concomittantly administered because of its fast uptake from the alveolar gas. This phenomenon is known as the "second gas effect."] Within closed body compartments, *nitrous oxide* can increase the volume (for example, causing a pneumothorax) or increase the pressure (for example, in the sinuses), because it replaces nitrogen in the various air spaces faster than the nitrogen leaves. Furthermore, its speed of movement allows *nitrous oxide* to retard oxygen uptake dur-

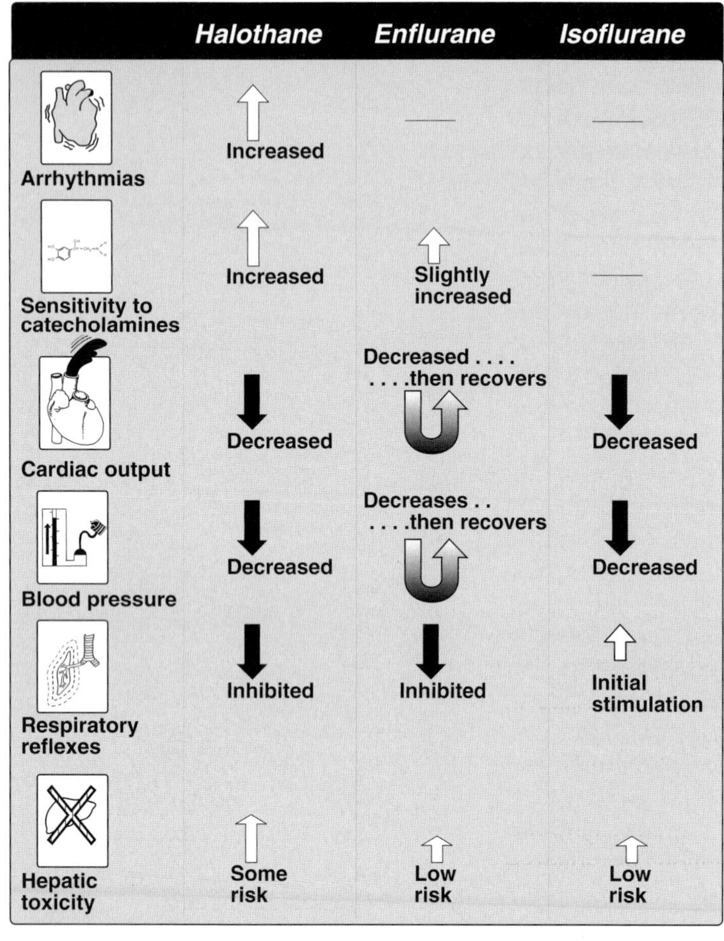

Halothane
Enflurane
Isoflurane
Arrhythmias
Increased
Sensitivity to catecholamines
Increased
Slightly increased
Cardiac output
Decreased
Decreased . . . .
. . . .then recovers
Decreased
Blood pressure
Decreased
Decreases . .
. . . .then recovers
Decreased
Respiratory reflexes
Inhibited
Inhibited
Initial stimulation
Hepatic toxicity
Some risk
Low risk
Low risk

Figure 11.8
Characteristics of some inhalation anesthetics.

ing recovery, thus causing diffusion hypoxia. This anesthetic does not depress respiration, nor does it produce muscle relaxation. Under the usual circumstances of coadministration with other anesthetics, it also has moderate to no effect on the cardiovascular system or on increasing cerebral blood flow, and it is the least hepatotoxic of the inhalation anesthetics. It is therefore probably the safest of these anesthetics, provided that at least twenty percent oxygen is always administered simultaneously.

Some characteristics of the inhaled anesthetics are summarized in Figure 11.8

V. INTRAVENOUS ANESTHETICS

Intravenous anesthetics are often used for the rapid induction of anesthesia, which is then maintained with an appropriate inhalation agent. They rapidly induce anesthesia and must therefore be injected slowly. Recovery from intravenous anesthetics is due to redistribution from sites in the CNS.

A. Barbiturates

Thiopental is a potent anesthetic but a weak analgesic. It is an ultra-short-acting barbiturate and has a high lipid solubility. When agents such as *thiopental* and *methohexital* [meth oh HEX i tal] are administered intravenously, they quickly enter the CNS and depress function, often in less than one minute. However, diffusion out of the brain can occur very rapidly as well because of redistribution of the drug to other body tissues, including skeletal muscle and ultimately adipose tissue (Figure 11.9). [Note: This latter site serves as a reservoir of drugs from which the agent slowly leaks out and is metabolized and excreted.] The short duration of anesthetic action is due to the decrease of its concentration in the brain to a level below that necessary to produce anesthesia. These drugs may remain in the body for relatively long periods of time after their administration, because only about fifteen percent of the dose of barbiturates entering the circulation is metabolized by the liver per hour. Thus, metabolism of *thiopental* is much slower than its tissue redistribution. The barbiturates are not significantly analgesic and, therefore, require some type of supplementary analgesic administration during anesthesia to avoid objectionable changes in blood pressure and autonomic function. *Thiopental* has minor effects on the cardiovascular system, but it may contribute to severe hypotension in hypovolemic or shock patients. All barbiturates can cause apnea, coughing, chest wall spasm, laryngospasm, and bronchospasm. [Note: The latter is of particular concern for asthmatic patients.] Barbiturates are contraindicated in patients with acute intermittant or variegate porphyria.

B. Benzodiazepines

The benzodiazepines are used in conjunction with anesthetics to sedate the patient. The most commonly employed is *midazolam*, which is available in many formulations, including oral. *Diazepam* and *lorazepam* are alternatives. All three facilitate amnesia while causing sedation.

C. Opioids

Because of their analgesic property, opioids are frequently used together with anesthetics; for example, the combination of *morphine* and *nitrous oxide* provides good anesthesia for cardiac surgery. The most frequently employed opioids are *fentanyl* and its congener, *sufentanil*, because they induce analgesia more rapidly than does *morphine*. They are administered either intravenously, epidurally, or intrathecally. Opioids are not good amnesics, and they can all cause hypotension, respiratory depression, and muscle rigidity as well as postanesthetic nausea and vomiting. Opioid effects can be antagonized by *naloxone* (see p. 167).

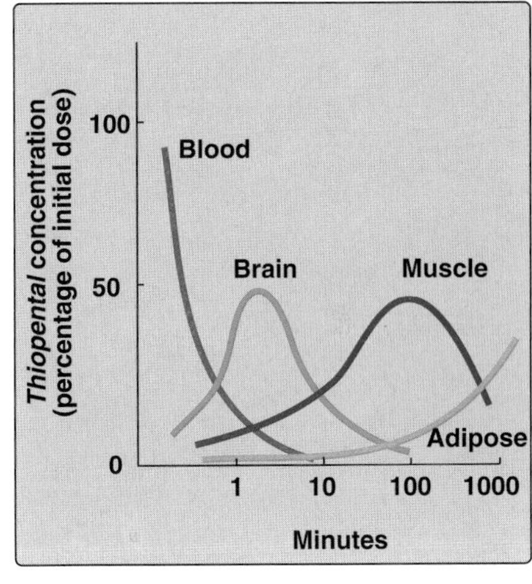

Figure 11.9
Redistribution of *thiopental* from brain to muscle and adipose tissue.

D. Etomidate

Etomidate (eh TOE mid ate) is used to induce anesthesia. It is a hypnotic agent but lacks analgesic activity. Its water solubility is poor, and *etomidate* is formulated in a propylene glycol solution. Induction is rapid, and the drug is short-acting. It is only used for patients with coronary artery disease or cardiovascular dysfunction, such as shock. *Etomidate* is hydrolyzed in the liver. Among its benefits are little to no effect on the heart and circulation. Its adverse effects include a decrease in plasma cortisol and aldosterone levels, which can persist for up to eight hours. This is apparently due to inhibition of 11-β-hydroxylase.[1] [Note: *Etomidate* should not be infused for an extended time, because prolonged suppression of these hormones can be hazardous.] Venous pain can occur, and skeletal muscle movements are not uncommon. The latter are managed by administration of benzodiazepines and opioids.

E. Ketamine

Ketamine [KET a meen], a short-acting, nonbarbiturate anesthetic, induces a dissociated state in which the patient is unconscious but appears to be awake and does not feel pain. This dissociative anesthesia provides sedation, amnesia, and immobility. *Ketamine* interacts with the N-methyl-D-aspartate receptor. It also stimulates the central sympathetic outflow, which, in turn, causes stimulation of the heart and increased blood pressure and cardiac output. This property is especially beneficial in patients with either hypovolemic or cardiogenic shock, as well as in patients with asthma. *Ketamine* is therefore used when circulatory depression is undesirable. On the other hand, these effects mitigate against the use of *ketamine* in hypertensive or stroke patients. The drug is lipophilic and enters the brain circulation very quickly, but like the barbiturates, it redistributes to other organs and tissues. It is metabolized in the liver, but small amounts can be excreted unchanged. *Ketamine* is employed mainly in children and young adults for short procedures. However, it is not

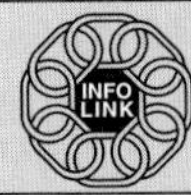

[1]See p. 236 in ***Lippincott's Illustrated Reviews: Biochemistry*** (3rd ed.) for a discussion of steroid biosynthesis.

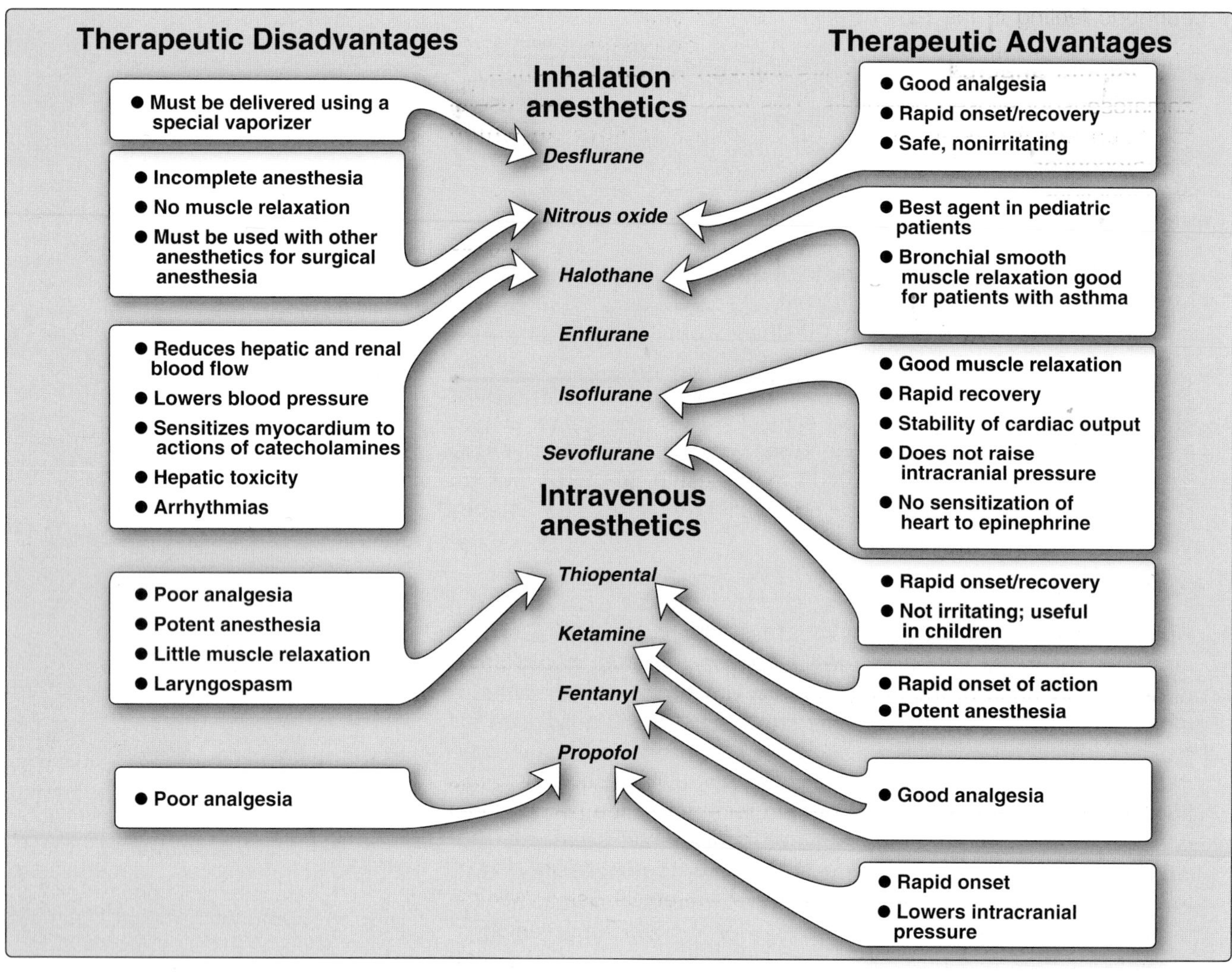

Figure 11.10
Therapeutic disadvantages and advantages of some anesthetic agents.

widely used, because it increases cerebral blood flow and induces postoperative hallucinations ("nightmares"), particularly in adults.

F. Propofol

Propofol [pro POF ol] is an intravenous sedative/hypnotic used in the induction or maintenance of anesthesia. Onset is smooth and occurs within about forty seconds of administration. Supplementation with narcotics for analgesia is required. Whereas *propofol* facilitates depression in the CNS, it is occasionally accompanied by excitatory phenomena, such as muscle twitching, spontaneous movement, or hiccups. *Propofol* decreases blood pressure without depressing the myocardium. It also reduces intracranial pressure. *Propofol* is widely used and has replaced *thiopental* as the first choice for anesthesia induction and sedation, because it produces a euphoric feeling in the patient and does not cause postanesthetic nausea and vomiting. It has much less of a depressant effect than the volatile anesthetics on CNS-evoked potentials, such as somatosensory evoked potentials. This makes *propofol* very useful for such surgeries as resection of spinal tumors, in which somatosensory evoked potentials are monitored to assess spinal cord functions.

Some therapeutic advantages and disadvantages of the anesthetic agents are summarized in Figure 11.10.

VI. LOCAL ANESTHETICS

Local anesthetics are generally applied locally, and block nerve conduction of sensory impulses from the periphery to the CNS. [Note: Some of these agents do have additional uses—for example, the antiarrthymic effect of *lidocaine*—and they are then administered by other routes.] Local anesthetics abolish sensation (and, in higher concentrations, motor activity) in a limited area of the body without producing unconsciousness (for example, during spinal anesthesia). The small, unmyelinated nerve fibers that conduct impulses for pain, temperature, and autonomic activity are most sensitive to actions of local anesthetics. The most widely used of these compounds are *bupivacaine* [byoo PIV ah kane], *lidocaine* [LYE doe kane], *procaine* [PRO kane], and *tetracaine* [TET ra kane]. Of these, *lidocaine* is the most frequently employed. At physiologic pH, these compounds are charged; it is this ionized form that interacts with the protein receptor of the Na^+ channel to inhibit its function and, thereby, achieve local anesthesia. [Note: The natural product, *cocaine*, was recognized years ago as a local anesthetic. However, its toxicity and abuse have limited its use to topical application in anesthesia of the upper respiratory tract.] The local anesthetics differ pharmacokinetically as to onset and duration of action (Figure 11.11). By adding the vasoconstrictor *epinephrine* to the local anesthetic, the rate of anesthetic absorption is decreased. This both minimizes systemic toxicity and increases the duration of action. Adverse effects result from systemic absorption of toxic amounts of the locally applied anesthetic. Seizures and cardiovascular collapse are the most significant of these systemic effects. *Bupivacaine* is noted for its cardiotoxicity. Allergic reactions may be encountered with *procaine*, which is metabolized to *p*-aminobenzoic acid.

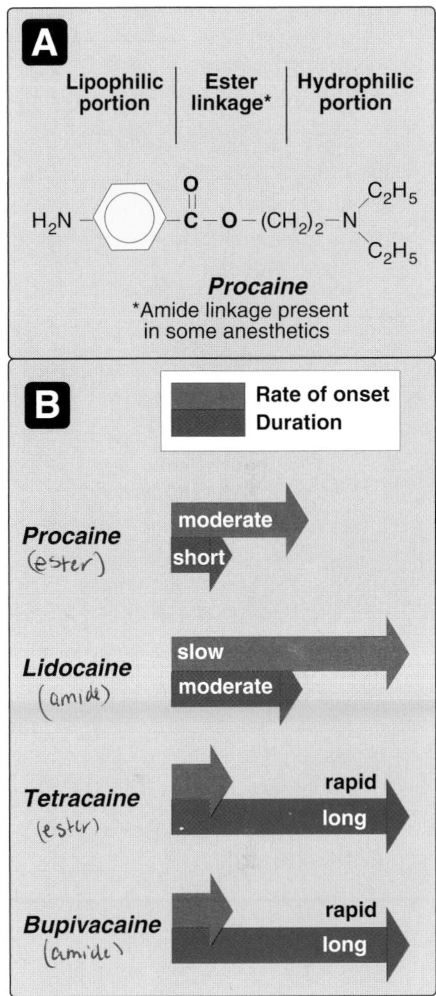

Figure 11.11
A. Structural formula of *procaine*.
B. Pharmacokinetic properties of local anesthetics.

Study Questions

Choose the ONE best answer.

11.1 Halogenated anesthetics may produce malignant hyperthermia in:

A. patients with poor renal function.
B. patients allergic to the anesthetic.
C. pregnant women.
D. alcoholics.
E. patients with a genetic defect in the muscle ryanodine receptor.

Correct answer = E. All patients undergoing anesthesia must be carefully assessed and monitored for possible adverse reactions. Malignant hyperthermia occurs in a small population who have a genetic defect and also receive succinylcholine. The other conditions are not known to dispose to this condition.

11.2 Children with asthma undergoing a surgical procedure are frequently anesthetized with sevoflurane, because it:

A. is rapidly taken up.
B. does not irritate the airway.
C. has a low nephrotoxic potential.
D. does not undergo metabolism.

Correct answer = B. Sevoflurane is an inhalational anesthetic with low pungency. It is non-irritative and, therefore, less likely to cause laryngospasm. A is true; induction and recovery are rapid. However, C and D are false.

11.3 Which one of the following is most likely to require administration of a muscle relaxant?

A. Ethyl ether
B. Halothane
C. Methoxyflurane
D. Benzodiazepines
E. Nitrous oxide

Correct answer = E. Nitrous oxide has virtually no muscle-relaxing properties. Ether, methoxyflurane, and benzodiazepine produce good muscle relaxation; halothane produces moderate muscle relaxation.

11.4 Which one of the following is a potent intravenous anesthetic but a weak analgesic?

A. Thiopental
B. Benzodiazepines
C. Ketamine
D Etomidate
E. Isoflurane

Correct answer = A. Thiopental is a potent anesthetic but a weak analgesic. It is the most widely used intravenously administered general anesthetic. It is an ultra-short-acting barbiturate and has a high lipid solubility.

11.5 Which one of the following is a potent analgesic but a weak anesthetic?

A. Methoxyflurane
B. Succinylcholine
C. Diazepam
D. Halothane
E. Nitrous oxide

Correct answer = E. Nitrous oxide is a potent analgesic but a weak general anesthetic. It is frequently employed at concentrations of thirty percent in combination with oxygen for analgesia, particularly in dental surgery.

Antidepressant Drugs

12

I. OVERVIEW

Depression is a serious disorder that afflicts approximately 14 million adults in the United States each year. The lifetime prevalence rate of depression in the United States has been estimated to include sixteen percent of adults (twenty-one percent women, thirteen percent men), or more than 32 million people. The symptoms of depression are intense feelings of sadness, hopelessness, and despair, as well as the inability to experience pleasure in usual activities, changes in sleep patterns and appetite, loss of energy, and suicidal thoughts. Mania is characterized by the opposite behavior—that is, enthusiasm, rapid thought and speech patterns, extreme self-confidence, and impaired judgment. [Note: Depression and mania are different from schizophrenia, which produces disturbances in thought.]

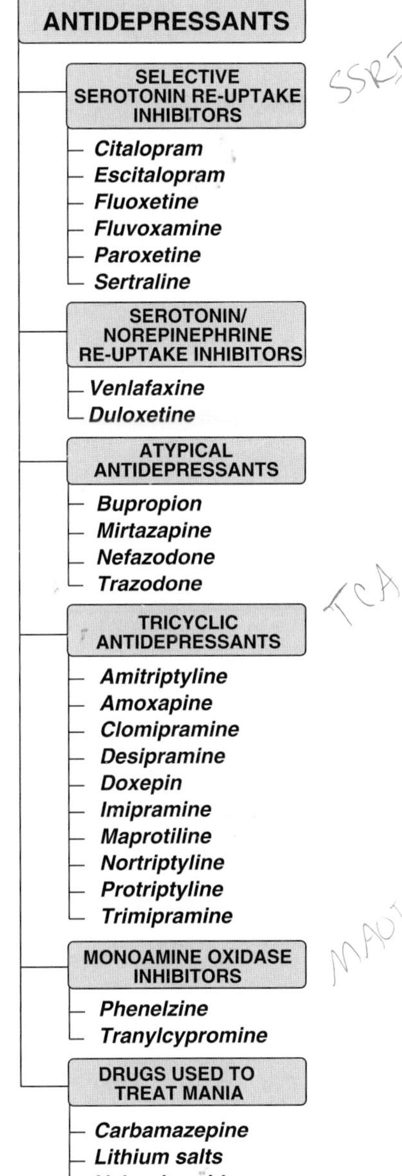

ANTIDEPRESSANTS
SELECTIVE SEROTONIN RE-UPTAKE INHIBITORS
Citalopram
Escitalopram
Fluoxetine
Fluvoxamine
Paroxetine
Sertraline
SEROTONIN/ NOREPINEPHRINE RE-UPTAKE INHIBITORS
Venlafaxine
Duloxetine
ATYPICAL ANTIDEPRESSANTS
Bupropion
Mirtazapine
Nefazodone
Trazodone
TRICYCLIC ANTIDEPRESSANTS
Amitriptyline
Amoxapine
Clomipramine
Desipramine
Doxepin
Imipramine
Maprotiline
Nortriptyline
Protriptyline
Trimipramine
MONOAMINE OXIDASE INHIBITORS
Phenelzine
Tranylcypromine
DRUGS USED TO TREAT MANIA
Carbamazepine
Lithium salts
Valproic acid

Figure 12.1
Summary of antidepressants.

II. MECHANISM OF ANTIDEPRESSANT DRUGS

Most clinically useful antidepressant drugs potentiate, either directly or indirectly, the actions of norepinephrine and/or serotonin in the brain. (See Figure 12.1 for a summary of the antidepressant agents.) This, along with other evidence, led to the biogenic amine theory, which proposes that depression is due to a deficiency of monoamines, such as norepinephrine and serotonin, at certain key sites in the brain. Conversely, the theory envisions that mania is caused by an overproduction of these neurotransmitters. However, the amine theory of depression and mania is overly simplistic. It fails to explain why the pharmacologic effects of any of the antidepressant and antimania drugs on neurotransmission occur immediately, whereas the time course for a therapeutic response occurs over several weeks. Furthermore, the potency of the antidepressant drugs in blocking neurotransmitter uptake often does not correlate with clinically observed antidepressant effects. This suggests that decreased uptake of neurotransmitter is only an initial effect of the drugs, which may not be directly responsible for the antidepressant effects. It has been proposed that presynaptic inhibitory receptor densities in the brain decrease over a two- to four-week period with antidepressant drug use. This down-regulation of inhibitory receptors permits greater synthesis and release of neurotransmitters into the synaptic cleft and enhanced signaling in the postsynaptic neurons, presumably leading to a therapeutic response (Figure 12.2)

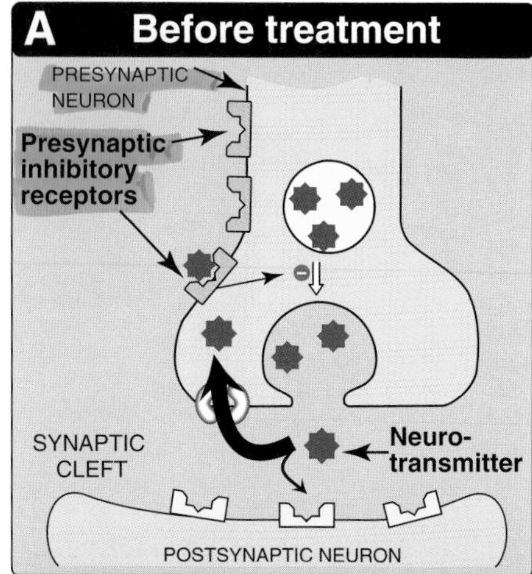

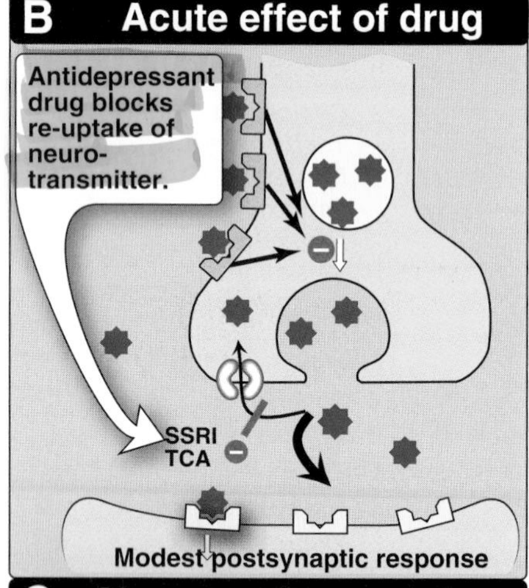

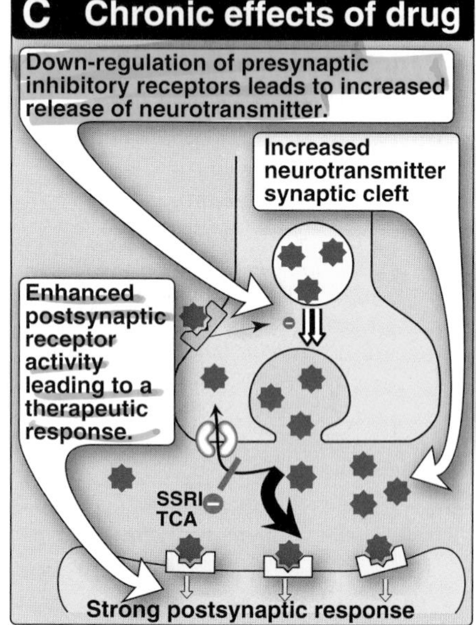

Figure 12.2
Proposed mechanism of action of selective serotonin re-uptake inhibitors (SSRI) and tricyclic anti-depressant (TCA) drugs.

III. SELECTIVE SEROTONIN RE-UPTAKE INHIBITORS

The selective serotonin re-uptake inhibitors (SSRIs) are a group of chemically unique antidepressant drugs that specifically inhibit serotonin re-uptake, having 300- to 3000-fold greater selectivity for the serotonin transporter as compared to the norepinephrine transporter. SSRIs have little ability to block the dopamine transporter. This contrasts with the tricyclic antidepressants (see p. 143) that nonselectively inhibit the uptake of norepinephrine and serotonin (Figure 12.3). Moreover, the SSRIs have little blocking activity at muscarinic, α-adrenergic, and histaminic H_1 receptors. Therefore, common side effects associated with tricyclic antidepressants, such as orthostatic hypotension, sedation, dry mouth, and blurred vision, are not seen with the SSRIs. Because they have fewer adverse effects and are relatively safe even in overdose, the SSRIs have largely replaced tricyclic antidepressants and monoamine oxidase inhibitors as the drugs of choice in treating depression. SSRIs include *fluoxetine* [floo OX e teen]—the prototypic drug, *citalopram* [sye TAL oh pram], *escitalopram* [es sye TAL oh pram], *fluvoxamine* [floo VOX e meen], *paroxetine* [pa ROX e teen], and *sertraline* [SER tra leen]. Both *citalopram* and *fluoxetine* are racemic mixtures, of which the respective S-enantiomers are the more potent inhibitors of the serotonin re-uptake pump. *Escitalopram* is the pure S-enatiomer of *citalopram.*

A. Actions

SSRIs block the re-uptake of serotonin, leading to increased concentrations of the neurotransmitter in the synaptic clefts and, ultimately, to greater postsynaptic neuronal activity. Antidepressants, including SSRIs, typically take two weeks to produce improvement in mood, and maximum benefit may require twelve weeks or more (Figure 12.4). However, none of the antidepressants is uniformly beneficial. Approximately forty percent of depressed patients treated with adequate doses of a drug for four to eight weeks do not respond to the antidepressant agent. Patients that do not respond to one antidepressant may respond to another, and approximately eighty percent or more will respond to at least one anitdepressant drug. [Note: These drugs do not produce central nervous system (CNS) stimulation or mood elevation in normal individuals.]

B. Therapeutic uses

The primary indication for SSRIs is depression, for which they are as effective as the tricyclic antidepressants. A number of other psychiatric disorders also respond favorably to SSRIs, including obsessive-compulsive disorder (the only indication for *fluvoxamine*), panic disorder, generalized anxiety, premenstrual dysphoric disorder, and bulimia nervosa.

C. Pharmacokinetics

All the SSRIs are well absorbed after oral administration. Peak levels are seen in approximately five hours on average. Food has little effect on absorption. Only *sertraline* undergoes significant first-pass metabolism. All these agents are well distributed, having volumes of distribution far in excess of body weight (15–30 L/kg). The majority

DRUG	UPTAKE INHIBITION		RECEPTOR AFFINITIES		
	Norepinephrine	Serotonin	Muscarinic	Histaminergic	Adrenergic
Selective serotonin re-uptake inhibitor *Fluoxetine*	0	++++	0	0	0
Selective serotonin/ norepinephrine re-uptake inhibitors					
Venlafaxine	++*	++++	0	0	0
Duloxetine	++++	++++	0	0	0
Tricyclic antidepressant *Imipramine*	++++	+++	++	+	+

Figure 12.3
Relative receptor specificity of some antidepressant drugs. **Venlafaxine* inhibits norepinephrine re-uptake only at high doses. ++++ = very strong affinity; +++ = strong affinity; ++ = moderate affinity; + = weak affinity; 0 = little or no affinity.

of SSRIs have plasma half-lives that range between 16 and 36 hours. Metabolism by P450-dependent enzymes and glucuronide or sulfate conjugation occur extensively. [Note: These metabolites do not contribute to the pharmacologic activity.] *Fluoxetine* differs from the other members of the class in two respects. First, it has a much longer half-life (fifty hours), and is available as a sustained release preparation allowing once-weekly dosing. Second, the metabolite of the S-enantiomer, S-norfluoxetine, is as potent as the parent compound. The half-life of the metabolite is quite long, averaging ten days. *Fluoxetine* and *paroxetine* are potent inhibitors of a hepatic cytochrome P450 isoenzyme (CYP2D6) responsible for the elimination of tricyclic antidepressant drugs, neuroleptic drugs, and some antiarrhythmic and β-adrenergic antagonist drugs. [Note: About seven percent of the white population lack this P450 enzyme and, therefore, metabolize *fluoxetine* very slowly.] Excretion of the SSRIs is primarily through the kidneys, except for *paroxetine* and *sertraline*, which also undergo fecal excretion (thirty-five and fifty percent, respectively). Dosages of all these drugs should be adjusted downward in patients with hepatic impairment.

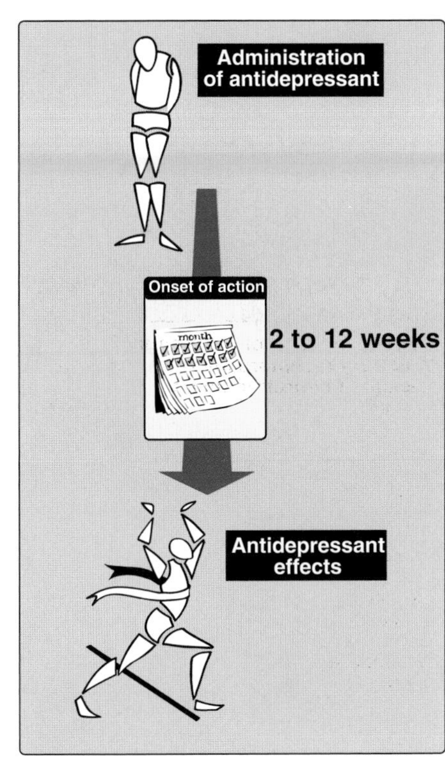

Figure 12.4
Onset of therapeutic effects of the major antidepressant drugs (tricyclic antidepressants, selective serotonin re-uptake inhibitors, and monoamine oxidase inhibitors) requires several weeks.

D. Adverse affects

Although the SSRIs have fewer and less severe adverse effects than the tricyclic antidepressants and monoamine oxidase inhibitors, the SSRIs can cause gastrointestinal effects, weakness, sexual dysfunction, sleep disturbances, and drug interactions (Figure 12.5).

1. **Sleep disturbances:** *Paroxetine* and *fluvoxamine* are sedating, and may be useful in patients who have difficulty sleeping. Conversely, patients who are fatigued may benefit from one of the more activating antidepressants, such as *fluoxetine*.

2. **Sexual dysfunction:** Loss of libido, delayed ejaculation, and anorgasmia are underreported side effects often noted by clinicians but not prominently featured in the list of standard side effects. One

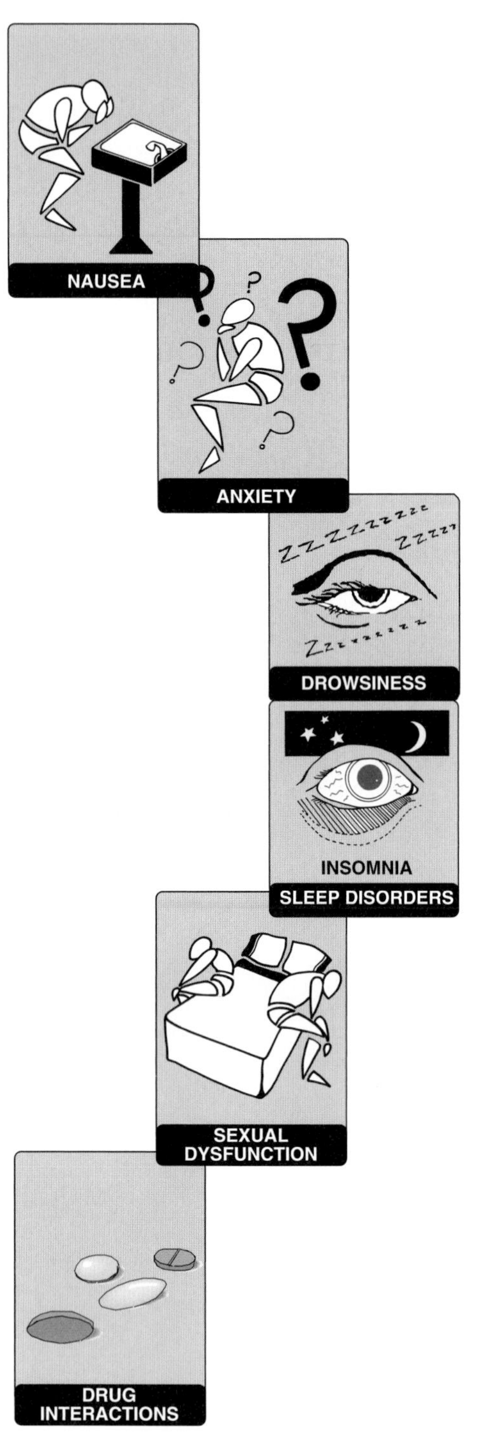

Figure 12.5
Some commonly observed adverse effects of selective serotonin re-uptake inhibitors.

option for managing SSRI-induced sexual dysfunction is to replace the offending antidepressant with a drug having fewer sexual side effects, such as *bupropion* or *mirtazapine*. Alternatively, the doses of the drug may be reduced. In men with erectile dysfunction and depression, treatment with *sildenafil*, *vardenafil*, or *tadalafil* (see p. 335) may improve sexual function.

3. **Use in children and teenagers:** Antidepressants should be used cautiously in children and teenagers, because about one out of fifty children become more suicidal as a result of SSRI treatment. Pediatric patients should be observed for worsening depression and suicidal thinking whenever one of these drugs is started or their dose is increased or decreased.

4. **Overdoses:** Large intakes of SSRIs do not cause cardiac arrhythmias, but *fluoxetine* may cause seizures. For example, in a report of patients who took an overdose of *fluoxetine* (up to 1200 mg compared with 20 mg/day as a therapeutic dose), about half the patients were adversely affected. All SSRIs have the potential to cause a serotonin syndrome characterized by hyperthermia, muscle rigidity, myoclonus (clonic muscle twitching), and changes in mental status and vital signs when used in the presence of a monoamine oxidase inhibitor. Therefore, extended periods of wash-out of each drug class must occur prior to the administration of the other class of drugs.

IV. SEROTONIN/NOREPINEPHRINE RE-UPTAKE INHIBITORS

Venlafaxine [VEN la fax een] and *duloxetine* (doo LOX e teen) selectively inhibit the re-uptake of both serotonin and norepinephrine (Figure 12.6). These agents, termed selective serotonin/norepinephrine re-uptake inhibitors (SNRIs), may be effective in treating depression in patients in which SSRIs are ineffective. Furthermore, depression is often accompanied by chronic painful symptoms (neuropathic pain), such as backache and muscle aches, against which SSRIs are also relatively ineffective. This pain is, in part, modulated by serotonin and norepinephrine pathways in the CNS. SNRIs and tricyclic antidepressants, with the dual actions of inhibiting both serotonin and norepinephrine re-uptake, are often effective in relieving physical symptoms of neuropathic pain. SNRIs, unlike the tricyclic antidepressants, have no activity at adrenergic, muscarinic, or histamine receptors and, thus, have fewer adverse effects than the tricyclic antidepressants (see Figure 12.3).

A. Venlafaxine

Venlafaxine is a potent inhibitor of serotonin re-uptake and, at higher doses, is an inhibitor of norepinephrine re-uptake. It is also a mild inhibitor of dopamine re-uptake. *Venlafaxine* has minimal inhibition of the cytochrome P450 isoenzymes. The half-life ($t_{1/2}$) of the parent compound plus its active metabolite is approximately eleven hours. The most common side effects of *venlafaxine* are nausea, dizziness, insomnia, sedation, and constipation. At high doses, there may be an increase in blood pressure.

B. Duloxetine

Duloxetine inhibits serotonin and norepinephrine re-uptake at all doses. It is extensively metabolized in the liver to numerous metabolites. *Duloxetine* should not be administered to patients with hepatic insufficiency. Metabolites are excreted in the urine, and the use of *duloxetine* is not recommended in patients with end-stage renal disease. Food delays the absorption of the drug. The $t_{1/2}$ is approximately twelve hours. Duloxetine is highly bound to plasma protein. Gastrointestinal side effects are common with *duloxetine*, including nausea, dry mouth, and constipation. Diarrhea and vomiting are seen less often. Insomnia, dizziness, somnolence, and sweating are also seen. Sexual dysfunction also occurs.

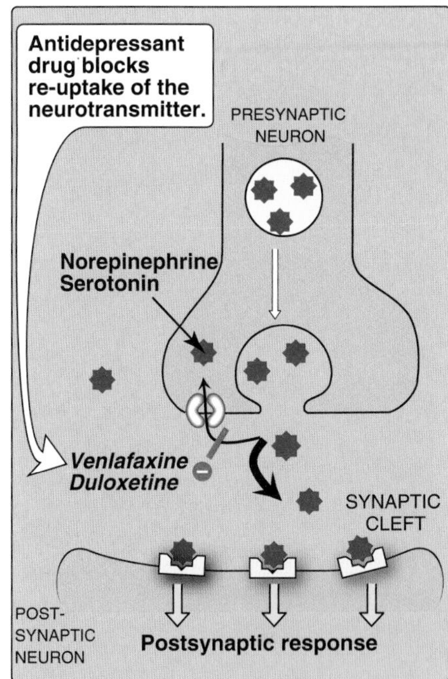

Figure 12.6
Proposed mechanism of action of selective serotonin/norepinephrine re-uptake inhibitors antidepressant drugs.

V. ATYPICAL ANTIDEPRESSANTS

The atypical antidepressants are a mixed group of agents that have actions at several different sites. This group includes *bupropion* [byoo PROE pee on], *mirtazapine* [mir TAZ a peen], *nefazodone* [nef AY zoe done], and *trazodone* [TRAZ oh done]. They are not any more efficacious than the tricyclic antidepressants (TCAs) or SSRIs, but their side effect profiles are different.

A. Bupropion

This drug acts at a still-unidentified site to alleviate the symptoms of depression. Its short half-life may require more than once-a-day dosing or the administration of an extended-release formulation. *Bupropion* is unique in that it decreases the craving for *nicotine* in tobacco abusers. Side effects include dry mouth, sweating, tremor, and seizures at high doses.

B. Mirtazapine

This drug owes at least some of its antidepressant activity to its ability to block 5-HT_2 and α_2 receptors. It is a sedative because of its potent antihistaminic activity, but it does not cause the antimuscarinic side effects of the TCAs, or interfere with sexual functioning, as do the SSRIs. Increased appetite and weight gain frequently occur. *Mirtazapine* is markedly sedating, which may be used to advantage in depressed patients having difficulty sleeping.

C. Nefazodone and trazodone

These drugs are weak inhibitors of serotonin re-uptake. Their therapeutic benefit appears to be related to their ability to block 5-HT_1 presynaptic autoreceptors and, thereby, increase serotonin release. Both agents are sedating, probably because of their potent H_1-blocking activity. *Trazodone* has been associated with causing priapism.

VI. TRICYCLIC ANTIDEPRESSANTS

The tricyclic antidepressants (TCAs) block norepinephrine and serotonin uptake into the neuron. The TCAs include the tertiary amines, *imipramine* [im IP ra meen]—the prototype drug, *amitriptyline* [a mee TRIP ti leen], *clomipramine* [kloe MIP ra meen], *doxepin* [DOX e pin] and *trimipramine* [trye MI pra meen]. The TCAs also include the secondary amines, *desipramine* ([dess IP ra meen] and *nortriptyline* [nor TRIP ti leen] (the respective N-demethylated metabolites of *imipramine* and *amitriptyline*), *amoxapine* [a MOX a peen], *maprotiline* [ma PROE ti leen], and *protriptyline* [proe TRIP ti leen]. All have similar therapeutic efficacy, and the choice of drug depends on patient tolerance of side effects and duration of action. Patients who do not respond to one TCA may benefit from a different drug in this group. These drugs are a valuable alternative for patients who do not respond to SSRIs.

A. Mechanism of action

1. **Inhibition of neurotransmitter uptake:** TCAs are potent inhibitors of the neuronal re-uptake of norepinephrine and serotonin into presynaptic nerve terminals (see Figure 12.2). However, at therapeutic concentrations, they do not block dopamine transporters. By blocking the major route of neurotransmitter removal, the TCAs lead to increased concentrations of monoamines in the synaptic cleft, ultimately resulting in antidepressant effects.

2. **Blocking of receptors:** TCAs also block serotonergic, α-adrenergic, histaminic, and muscarinic receptors (see Figure 12.3). It is not known if any of these actions accounts for the therapeutic benefit. However, actions at these receptors are probably responsible for many of the untoward effects of the TCAs.

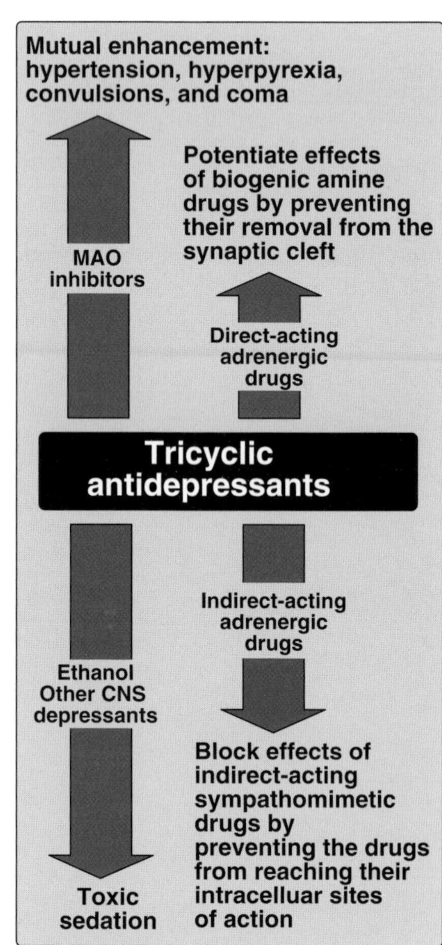

Figure 12.7
Drugs interacting with tricyclic antidepressants. CNS = central nervous system; MAO = monoamine oxidase.

B. Actions

TCAs elevate mood, improve mental alertness, increase physical activity, and reduce morbid preoccupation in fifty to seventy percent of individuals with major depression. The onset of the mood elevation is slow, requiring two weeks or longer (see Figure 12.4). These drugs do not produce CNS stimulation or mood elevation in normal individuals. Physical and psychological dependence have been reported, necessitating slow withdrawal. The drugs can be used for prolonged treatment of depression without loss of effectiveness.

C. Therapeutic uses

The TCAs are effective in treating severe major depression. Some panic disorders also respond to TCAs. *Imipramine* has been used to control bed-wetting in children (older than six years) by causing contraction of the internal sphincter of the bladder. At present, it is used cautiously because of the inducement of cardiac arrhythmias and other serious cardiovascular problems. TCAs, particularly *amitriptyline*, have been used to treat chronic pain ("neuropathic" pain) in a number of conditions in which the cause of the pain is unclear.

D. Pharmacokinetics

TCAs are well absorbed upon oral administration. Because of their lipophilic nature, they are widely distributed and readily penetrate into the CNS. This lipid solubility also causes these drugs to have long half-lives—for example, four to seventeen hours for *imipramine*. As a result of their variable first-pass metabolism in the liver, TCAs have low and inconsistent bioavailability. Therefore, the patient's response is used to adjust dosage. The initial treatment period is typically four to eight weeks. The dosage can be gradually reduced unless relapse occurs. These drugs are metabolized by the hepatic microsomal system and conjugated with glucuronic acid). Ultimately, the TCAs are excreted as inactive metabolites via the kidney.

E. Adverse effects

Blockade of acetylcholine receptors leads to blurred vision, xerostomia (dry mouth), urinary retention, constipation, and aggravation of glaucoma and epilepsy. Increased catecholamine activity results in cardiac overstimulation that can be life-threatening if an overdose of one of the drugs is taken. TCAs block α-adrenergic receptors, causing orthostatic hypotension and reflex tachycardia. In clinical practice, this is the most serious problem in the elderly. *Imipramine* is most likely and *nortriptyline* is least likely to cause orthostatic hypotension. Sedation may be prominent, especially during the first several weeks of treatment, and is related to the ability of these drugs to block histamine H_1 receptors. Weight gain is a common adverse effect of the TCAs. Sexual dysfunction, as evidenced by erectile dysfunction in men and anorgasmia in women, occurs in a significant minority of patients.

1. **Precautions:** TCAs should be used with caution in manic-depressive patients, because they may unmask manic behavior. TCAs have a narrow therapeutic index; for example, five- to six-fold the maximal daily dose of *imipramine* can be lethal. Depressed patients who are suicidal should be given only limited quantities of these drugs and be monitored closely. Drug interactions with the TCAs are shown in Figure 12.7.

VII. MONOAMINE OXIDASE INHIBITORS

Monoamine oxidase (MAO) is a mitochondrial enzyme found in nerve and other tissues, such as the gut and liver. In the neuron, MAO functions as a "safety valve" to oxidatively deaminate and inactivate any excess neurotransmitter molecules (norepinephrine, dopamine, and serotonin) that may leak out of synaptic vesicles when the neuron is at rest. The MAO inhibitors may irreversibly or reversibly inactivate the enzyme, permitting neurotransmitter molecules to escape degradation and, therefore, to both accumulate within the presynaptic neuron and leak into the synaptic space. This causes activation of norepinephrine and serotonin receptors, and it may be responsible for the antidepressant action of these drugs. Two MAO inhibitors are currently available for treatment of depression: *phenelzine* [FEN el zeen] and *tranylcypromine* [tran il SIP roe meen]. Use of MAO inhibitors is now limited due to the complicated dietary restrictions required of patients taking MAO inhibitors.

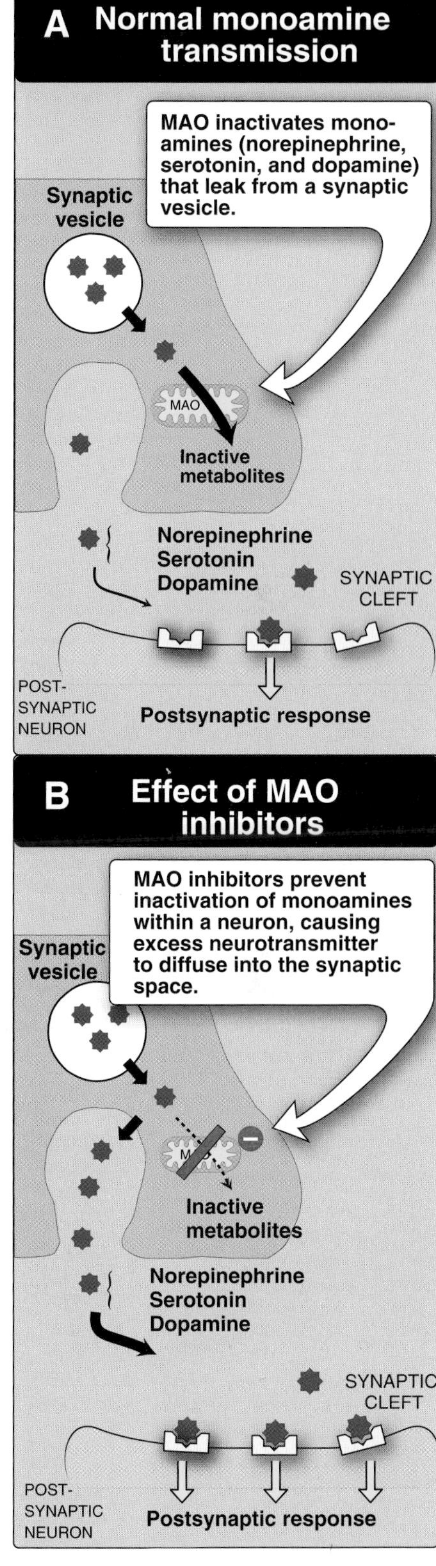

Figure 12.8
Mechanism of action of monoamine oxidase (MAO) inhibitors.

A. Mechnism of action

Most MAO inhibitors, such as *phenelzine*, form stable complexes with the enzyme, causing irreversible inactivation. This results in increased stores of norepinephrine, serotonin, and dopamine within the neuron, and subsequent diffusion of excess neurotransmitter into the synaptic space (Figure 12.8). These drugs inhibit not only MAO in the brain but also peripheral oxidases that catalyze oxidative deamination of drugs and potentially toxic substances, such as tyramine, which is found in certain foods. The MAO inhibitors therefore show a high incidence of drug-drug and drug-food interactions.

B. Actions

Although MAO is fully inhibited after several days of treatment, the antidepressant action of the MAO inhibitors, like that of the SSRIs and TCAs, is delayed several weeks. *Phenelzine* and *tranylcypromine* have a mild, amphetamine-like stimulant effect.

C. Therapeutic uses

MAO inhibitors are indicated for depressed patients who are unresponsive or allergic to TCAs, or who experience strong anxiety. Patients with low psychomotor activity may benefit from the stimulant properties of MAO inhibitors. These drugs are also useful in the treatment of phobic states. A special subcategory of depression, called atypical depression, may respond to MAO inhibitors. Atypical depression is characterized by labile mood, rejection sensitivity, and appetite disorders.

D. Pharmacokinetics

These drugs are well absorbed on oral administration, but antidepressant effects require two to four weeks of treatment. Enzyme regeneration, when irreversibly inactivated, varies, but it usually occurs several weeks after termination of the drug. Thus, when switching antidepressant agents, a minimum of two weeks of delay must be allowed after termination of MAO inhibitor therapy. MAO inhibitors are metabolized and excreted rapidly in the urine.

E. Adverse effects

Severe and often unpredictable side effects limit the widespread use of MAO inhibitors. For example, tyramine, contained in certain foods, such as aged cheeses, chicken liver, beer, and red wines, is normally inactivated by MAO in the gut. Individuals receiving an MAO inhibitor are unable to degrade tyramine obtained from the diet. Tyramine causes the release of large amounts of stored catecholamines from nerve terminals, resulting in headache, tachycardia, nausea, hypertension, cardiac arrhythmias, and stroke. Patients must therefore be educated to avoid tyramine-containing foods. *Phentolamine* or *prazosin* are helpful in the management of tyramine-induced hypertension. [Note: Treatment with MAO inhibitors may be dangerous in severely depressed patients with suicidal tendencies. Purposeful consumption of tyramine-containing foods is a possibility.] Other possible side effects of treatment with MAO inhibitors include drowsiness, orthostatic hypotension, blurred vision, dry mouth, dysuria, and constipation. MAO inhibitors and SSRIs should not be coadministered due to the risk of life-threatening "serotonin syndrome." Both types of drugs require wash-out periods of six weeks before the other type is administered. Figure 12.9 summarizes the side effects of the antidepressant drugs.

VIII. TREATMENT OF MANIA AND BIPOLAR DISORDER

Lithium salts are used prophylactically for treating manic-depressive patients and in the treatment of manic episodes. They are also effective in treating sixty to eighty percent of patients exhibiting mania and hypomania. Although many cellular processes are altered by treatment with *lithium* salts, the mode of action is unknown. [Note: Lithium is believed to attenuate signaling via receptors coupled to the phosphatidylinositol bisphosphate (PIP_2) second messenger system.[1] *Lithium* interferes with the resynthesis (recycling) of PIP_2, leading to its relative depletion in neuronal membranes of the CNS. PIP_2 levels in peripheral membranes are unaffected by lithium.] *Lithium* is given orally, and the ion is excreted by the kidney. *Lithium* salts are very toxic. Their safety factor and therapeutic index are extremely low—comparable to those of *digitalis*. Adverse effects include ataxia, tremors, confusion, and convulsions. Dry mouth, polydipsia, and polyuria are frequent complaints. [Note: The diabetes insipidus that results from taking *lithium* can be treated with *amiloride*.] Thyroid function may be decreased and should be monitored. *Lithium* causes no noticeable effect on normal individuals. It is not a sedative, euphoriant, or depressant. [Note: The antiepileptic drugs *carbamazepine* and *valproic acid* have been shown to alleviate some of the symptoms of mania.]

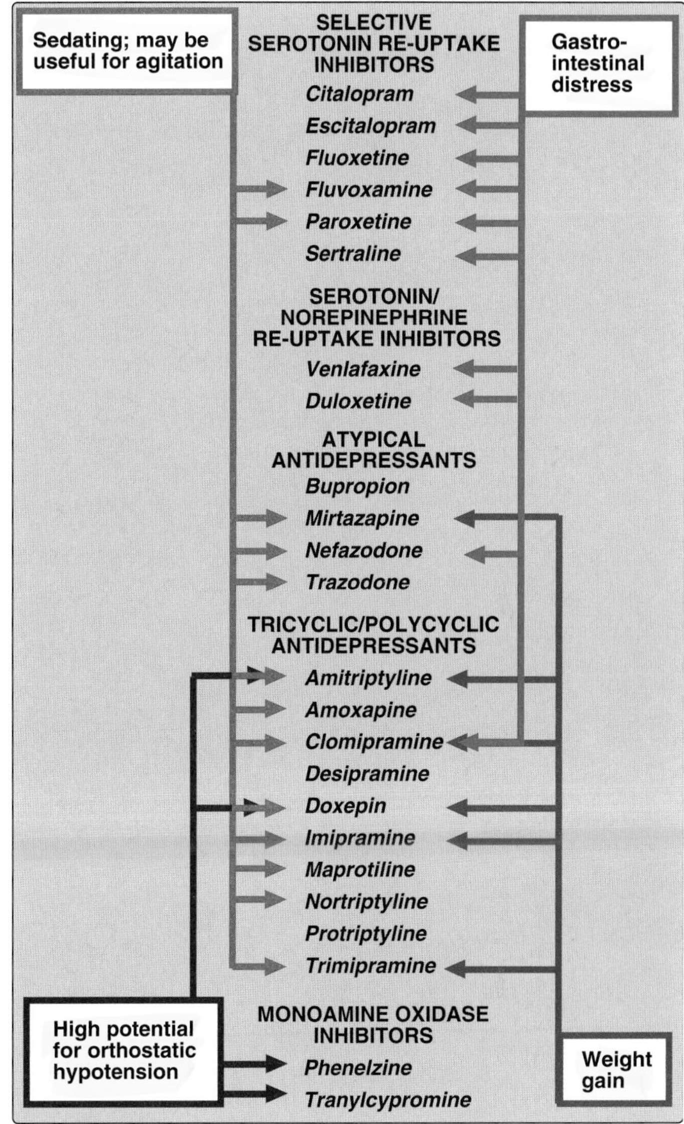

Figure 12.9
Side effects of some drugs used to treat depression.

INFO LINK [1]See p. 203 in ***Lippincott's Illustrated Reviews: Biochemistry*** (3rd ed.) for a discussion of the phosphatidylinositol bisphosphate second messenger system.

Study Questions

Choose the ONE best answer.

12.1 A 55-year-old teacher began to experience changes in mood. He was losing interest in his work and lacked the desire to play his daily tennis match. He began to have difficulty thinking and concentrating and lacked decisiveness. He was preoccupied with feelings of guilt, worthlessness, and hopelessness. In addition to the psychiatric symptoms, the patient complained of muscle aches throughout his body. Physical and laboratory tests were unremarkable. After six weeks of therapy with fluoxetine, the patient's symptoms resolved. However, the patient complains of sexual dysfunction. Which of the following drugs might be useful in this patient?

A. Fluvoxamine
B. Sertraline
C. Citalopram
D. Mirtazapine
E. Lithium

Correct answer = D. Sexual dysfunction commonly occurs with TCAs, SSRIs, and SNRIs. Mirtazapine is largely free from sexual side effects.

12.2 A 25-year-old woman had a long history of depressive symptoms accompanied by body aches. Physical and laboratory tests were unremarkable. Which of the following drugs might be useful in this patient?

A. Fluoxetine
B. Sertraline
C. Phenelzine
D. Mirtazapine
E. Duloxetine

Correct answer = E. Duoxetine is an SNRA that can be used for depression accompanied by neuropathic pain. TCAs and SSRIs have little activity against neuropathic pain.

12.3 A 51-year-old woman with symptoms of major depression also has narrow-angle glaucoma. Which of the following antidepressants should be avoided in this patient?

A. Amitriptyline
B. Sertraline
C. Bupropion
D. Mirtazepine
E. Fluvoxamine

Correct answer = A. Because of its potent antimuscarinic activity, amitriptyline should not be given to patients with glaucoma because of the risk of acute increases in ocular pressure. The other antidepressants all lack antagonist activity at the muscarinic receptor.

12.4 A 36-year-old man presents with symptoms of compulsive behavior. He must repeatedly align and realign the items on his desk throughout the day. If anything is out of order he feels that "work will not be accomplished effectively or efficiently." He realizes that his behavior is interfering with his ability to accomplish his daily tasks, but cannot seem to stop himself. Which of the following drugs would be most helpful to this patient?

A. Imipramine
B. Fluvoxamine
C. Amitriptyline
D. Tranylcypromine
E. Lithium

Correct answer = B. Serotonin selective reuptake inhibitors are particularly effective in treating obsessive/compulsive disorder; fluvoxamine is only approved for this condition. The other drugs are ineffective in the treatment of obsessive/compulsive disorder.

Neuroleptic Drugs

13

I. OVERVIEW

Neuroleptic drugs (also called antischizophrenic drugs, antipsychotic drugs, or major tranquilizers) are used primarily to treat schizophrenia, but they are also effective in other psychotic states, such as manic states and delirium. All currently available antipsychotic drugs that alleviate symptoms of schizophrenia decrease dopaminergic and/or serotonergic neurotransmission. The traditional or "typical" neuroleptic drugs are competitive inhibitors at a variety of receptors, but their antipsychotic effects reflect competitive blocking of dopamine receptors. These drugs vary in potency. For example, *chlorpromazine* is a low-potency drug, and *fluphenazine* is a high-potency agent (Figure 13.1). No one drug is clinically more effective than another. In contrast, the newer antipsychotic drugs are referred to as "atypical," because they have fewer extrapyramidal adverse effects than the traditional agents. These drugs appear to owe their unique activity to blockade of serotonin (and, perhaps, other) receptors. Current antipsychotic therapy employs the use of atypical neuroleptic drugs to minimize the risk of debilitating movement disorders associated with the typical drugs that act primarily through the D_2 dopamine receptor. All the atypical drugs exhibit an efficacy that is equivalent to or exceeds that of the typical neuroleptic agents. However, therapeutic difference among the individual atypical neuroleptic drugs have not been established, and patient response must often be used as a guide in drug selection. Neuroleptic drugs are not curative and do not eliminate the fundamental thinking disorder, but they often decrease the intensity of hallucinations and delusions and permit the psychotic patient to function in a supportive environment.

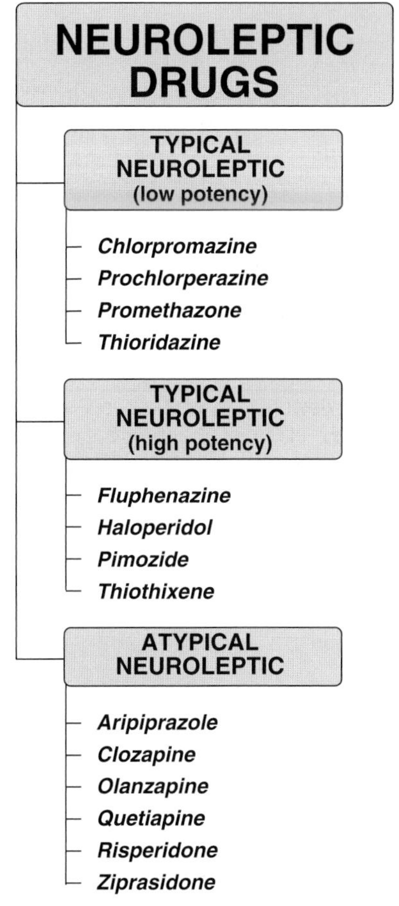

Figure 13.1
Summary of neuroleptic agents.

II. SCHIZOPHRENIA

Schizophrenia is a particular type of psychosis—that is, a mental disorder caused by some inherent dysfunction of the brain. It is characterized by delusions, hallucinations (often in the form of voices), and

Lippincott's Illustrated Reviews: Pharmacology, Third Edition,
by Richard D. Howland and Mary J. Mycek.
Lippincott Williams & Wilkins, Baltimore, MD © 2006.

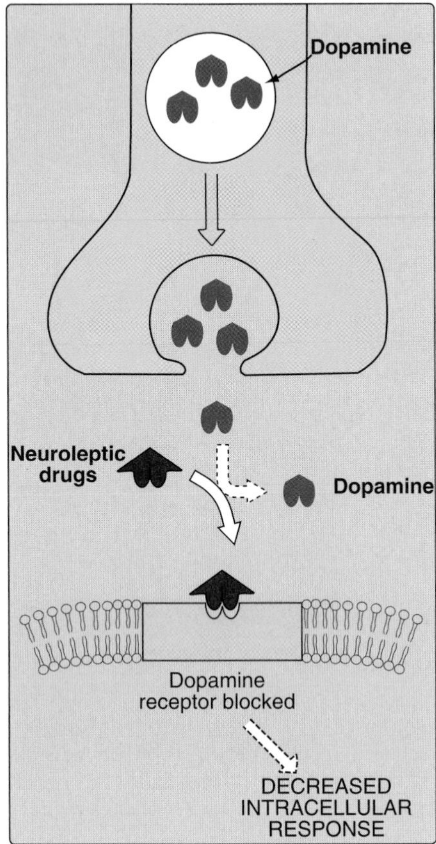

Figure 13.2
Dopamine-blocking actions of neuroleptic drugs.

thinking or speech disturbances. This mental disorder is a common affliction, occurring among about one percent of the population, or at about the same incidence as diabetes mellitus. The illness often initially affects people during adolescence and is a chronic and disabling disorder. Schizophrenia has a strong genetic component and probably reflects some fundamental biochemical abnormality, possibly an overactivity of the mesolimbic dopaminergic neurons.

III. NEUROLEPTIC DRUGS

The neuroleptic drugs represent several diverse, heterocyclic structures with markedly different potencies. The tricyclic *phenothiazine* derivative, *chlorpromazine* [klor PROE ma zeen], was the first neuroleptic drug used to treat schizophrenia. Antipsycotic drugs developed subsequently, such as *haloperidol,* are more that 100-fold as potent as *chloropromazine*, but have an increased ability to induce parkinson-like effects. Furthermore, these more potent traditional drugs are no more effective than *chlorpromazine.*

A. Mechanism of action

1. **Dopamine receptor-blocking activity in the brain:** All the neuroleptic drugs block dopamine receptors in the brain and the periphery (Figure 13.2). Five types of dopamine receptors have been identified: D_1 and D_5 receptors activate adenylyl cyclase, whereas D_2, D_3, and D_4 receptors inhibit adenylyl cyclase. The neuroleptic drugs bind to these receptors to varying degrees. However, the clinical efficacy of the typical neuroleptic drugs correlates closely with their relative ability to block D_2 receptors in the mesolimbic system of the brain. On the other hand, the atypical drug *clozapine* [KLOE za peen] has a high affinity for the D_4 receptor, which may explain its minimal ability to cause extrapyramidal side effects. (Figure 13.3 summarizes the receptor-binding properties of *clozapine*, *chlorpromazine*, and *haloperidol.*) The actions of the neuroleptic drugs are antagonized by agents that raise the dopamine concentration—for example, *levodopa* and amphetamines.

2. **Serotonin receptor-blocking activity in the brain:** The newer atypical agents appear to exert part of their unique action through inhibition of serotonin receptors (5-HT). Thus, *clozapine* has high affinity for D_1, D_2, D_4, 5-HT_2, muscarinic, and α-adrenergic receptors, but it is also a dopamine D_2 receptor antagonist. *Risperidone* [ris PEER i dohn], blocks 5-HT_2 receptors to a greater extent than it does D_2 receptors. The atypical neuroleptic *aripiprazole* [a rih PIP ra zole] is a partial agonist at D_2 and 5-HT_{1A} receptors as well as a blocker of 5-HT_{2A} receptors.

B. Actions

The antipsychotic actions of neuroleptic drugs appear to reflect a blockade at dopamine and/or serotonin receptors. However, many of these agents also block cholinergic, adrenergic, and histaminergic receptors (Figure 13.4). It is unknown what role, if any, these actions have in alleviating the symptoms of psychosis. The undesirable side effects of these agents, however, are often a result of actions at these other receptors.

1. **Antipsychotic actions:** All the neuroleptic drugs reduce the hallucinations and delusions associated with schizophrenia (the so-called "positive" symptoms) by blocking dopamine receptors in the mesolimbic system of the brain. The "negative" symptoms, such as blunted affect, anhedonia (not getting pleasure from normally pleasurable stimuli), apathy, and impaired attention, as well as cognitive impairment are not as responsive to therapy, particularly with the typical neuroleptics. Some atypical agents, such as *clozapine*, ameliorate the negative symptoms to some extent. All the drugs also have a calming effect and reduce spontaneous physical movement. In contrast to the central nervous system (CNS) depressants, such as barbiturates, the neuroleptics do not depress the intellectual function of the patient, and motor incoordination is minimal. The antipsychotic effects usually take several weeks to occur, suggesting that the therapeutic effects are related to secondary changes in the corticostriatal pathways.

2. **Extrapyramidal effects:** Dystonias, parkinson-like symptoms, akathisia (motor restlessness), and tardive dyskinesia (inappropriate postures of the neck, trunk, and limbs) occur with chronic treatment. Blocking of dopamine receptors in the nigrostriatal pathway probably causes these unwanted parkinson-like symptoms. The atypical neuroleptics exhibit a low incidence of these symptoms.

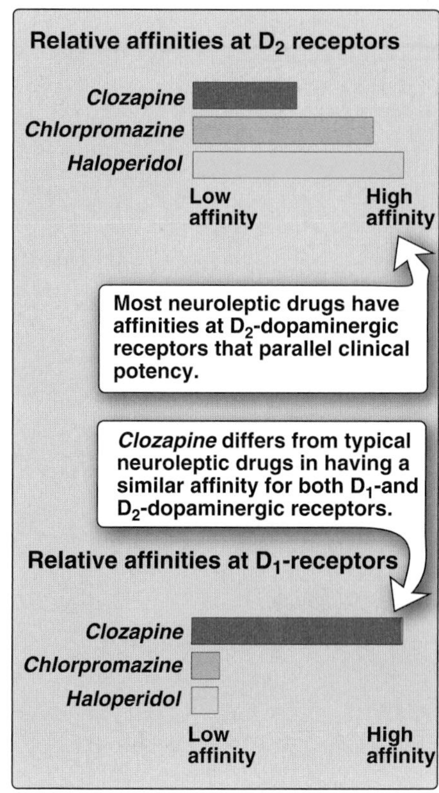

Figure 13.3
Relative affinity of *clozapine, chlorpromazine* and *haloperidol* at D_1- and D_2-dopaminergic receptors

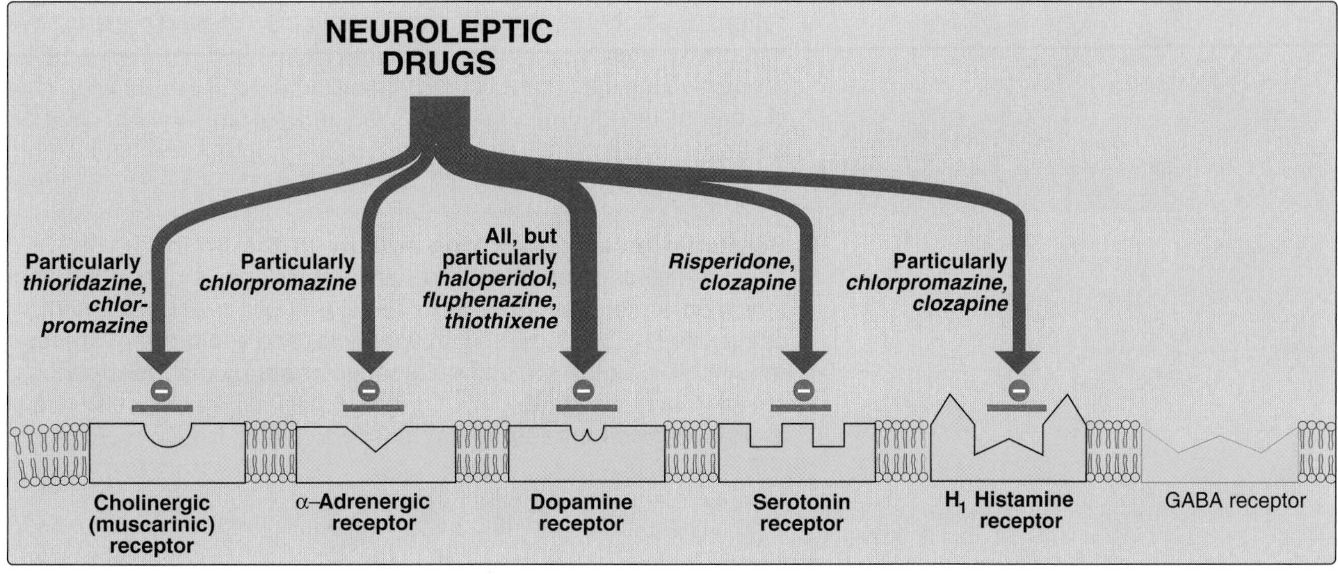

Figure 13.4
Neuroleptic drugs block at dopaminergic and serotonergic receptors as well as at adrenergic, cholinergic, and histamine-binding receptors. GABA = γ-aminobutyric acid.

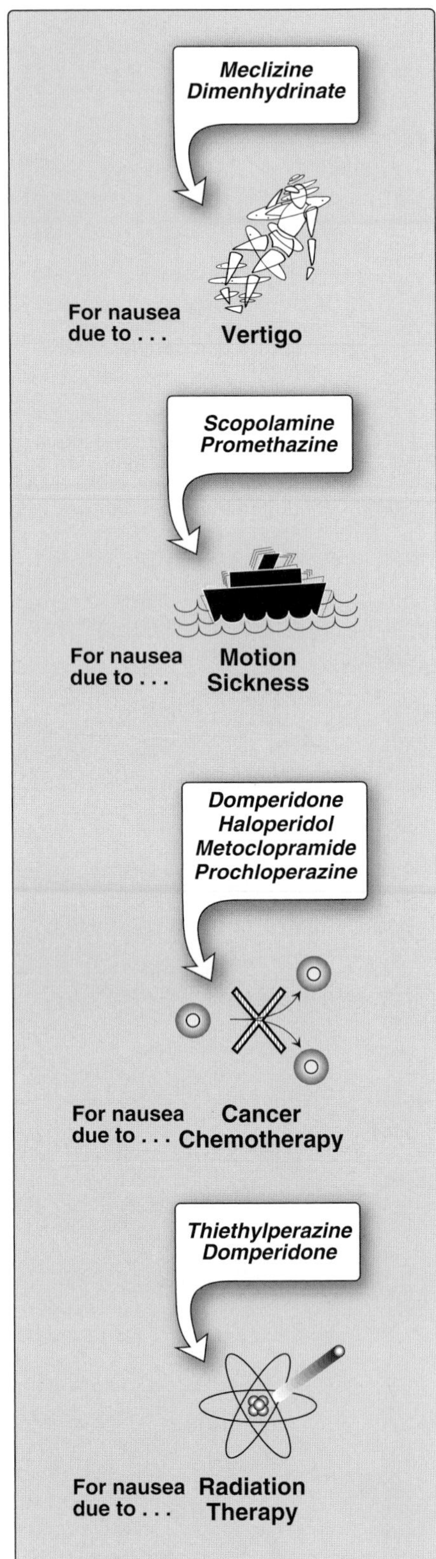

Figure 13.5
Therapeutic application of antiemetic agents.

3. **Antiemetic effects:** With the exception of *thioridazine* [thye oh RID a zeen], most of the neuroleptic drugs have antiemetic effects that are mediated by blocking D_2-dopaminergic receptors of the chemoreceptor trigger zone of the medulla. (See p. 329 for a discussion of emesis.) Figure 13.5 summarizes the antiemetic uses of neuroleptic agents, along with the therapeutic applications of other drugs that combat nausea. [Note: The atypical antipsychotic drugs are not effective antiemetics.]

4. **Antimuscarinic effects:** Some of the neuroleptics, particularly *thioridazine*, *chlorpromazine*, *clozapine*, and *olanzapine* [oh LAN za peen], cause anticholinergic effects, including blurred vision, dry mouth, sedation, confusion, and inhibition of gastrointestinal and urinary tract smooth muscle, leading to constipation and urinary retention.

5. **Other effects:** Blockade of α-adrenergic receptors causes orthostatic hypotension and light-headedness. The neuroleptics also alter temperature-regulating mechanisms and can produce poikilothermia (body temperature varies with the environment). In the pituitary, neuroleptics block D_2 receptors, leading to an increase in prolactin release. Sedation occurs in those drugs that are potent antagonists of the H_1 histamine receptor, including *chlorpromazine* and *clozapine*.

C. Therapeutic uses

1. **Treatment of schizophrenia:** The neuroleptics are the only efficacious treatment for schizophrenia. Not all patients respond, and complete normalization of behavior is seldom achieved. The traditional neuroleptics are most effective in treating positive symptoms of schizophrenia (delusions, hallucinations, and thought disorders). The newer agents with serotonin-blocking activity are effective in many patients who are resistant to the traditional agents, especially in treating negative symptoms of schizophrenia (withdrawal, blunted emotions, and reduced ability to relate to people). [Note: *Clozapine* is reserved for treatment of individuals who are unresponsive to other neurloleptics, because its use is associated with blood dyscrasias.]

2. **Prevention of severe nausea and vomiting:** The neuroleptics (most commonly *prochlorperazine*) are useful in the treatment of drug-induced nausea (see p. 329). Nausea arising from motion should be treated with sedatives and antihistamines, however, rather than with these powerful drugs. [Note: *Scopolamine* is the drug of choice for treatment of motion sickness.]

3. **Other uses:** The neuroleptic drugs can be used as tranquilizers to manage agitated and disruptive behavior. Neuroleptics are used in combination with narcotic analgesics for treatment of chronic pain with severe anxiety. *Chlorpromazine* is used to treat intractable hiccups. *Promethazine* [proe METH a zeen] is not a good antipsychotic drug; however, this agent is used in treating pruritus because of its antihistaminic properties. *Pimozide* [PI moe zide] is primarily indicated for treatment of the motor and phonic tics of Tourette disorder.

D. Absorption and metabolism

After oral administration, the neuroleptics show variable absorption that is unaffected by food. These agents readily pass into the brain, have a large volume of distribution, bind well to plasma proteins, and are metabolized to many different substances by the P450 system in the liver, particularly the CYP2D6 isozyme. Some metabolites are active. *Fluphenazine decanoate* and *haloperidol decanoate* [hal oh PER ah dole] are slow-release (up to three weeks) formulations of neuroleptics that are administered by intramuscular injection. These drugs are often used to treat outpatients and individuals who are noncompliant. However, about thirty percent of these patients develop extrapyramidal symptoms. The neuroleptic drugs produce some tolerance but little physical dependence.

E. Adverse effects

Adverse effects of the neuroleptic drugs occur in practically all patients, and are significant in about eighty percent (Figure 13.6). Although antipsychotic drugs have an array of adverse effects, their therapeutic index is high.

1. **Extrapyramidal side effects:** The inhibitory effects of dopaminergic neurons are normally balanced by the excitatory actions of cholinergic neurons. Blocking dopamine receptors alters this balance, causing a relative excess of cholinergic influence, which results in extrapyramidal motor effects. The maximal risk of appearance of the movement disorders is time dependent, with dystonias occurring within a few days of treatment, followed by akathisias (the inability to remain seated due to motor restlessness). Parkinson symptoms of bradykinesia, rigidity, and tremor occur a bit later on. Tardive dyskinesia, which is not reversible, occurs after months or years of treatment.

   a. **Effect of anticholinergic drugs:** If cholinergic activity is also blocked, a new, more nearly normal balance is restored, and extrapyramidal effects are minimized. This can be achieved by administration of an anticholinergic drug, such as *benztropine*. The therapeutic trade-off is fewer extrapyramidal effects in exchange for the side effects of parasympathetic blockade. [Note: Often, the parkinson-like actions persist, despite the anticholinergic drugs.] Those drugs that exhibit strong anticholinergic activity, such as *thioridazine*, show few extrapyramidal disturbances, because the cholinergic activity is strongly dampened. This contrasts with *haloperidol* and *fluphenazine*, which have low anticholinergic activity and produce extrapyramidal effects because of the preferential blocking of dopaminergic transmission without the blocking of cholinergic activity.

   b. **Clozapine and risperidone:** These drugs have a low potential for causing extrapyramidal symptoms and lower risk of tardive dyskinesia, which has been attributed to their block of 5-HT_{2A} autoreceptors. These drugs appear to be superior to *haloperidol* and *chlorpromazine* in treating the symptoms of schizophrenia, especially the negative symptoms. *Risperidone*

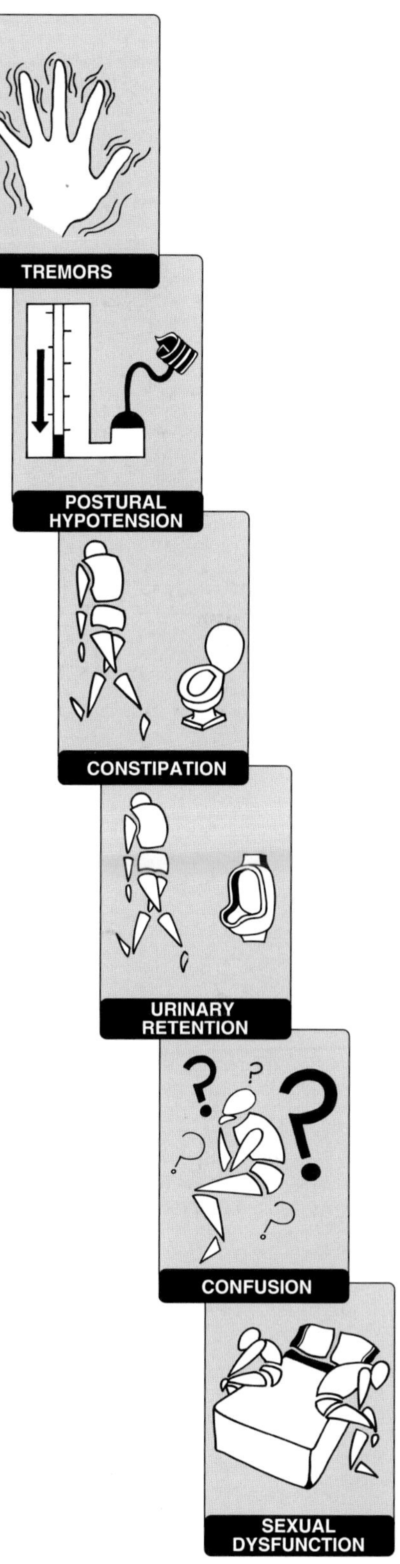

Figure 13.6
Adverse effects commonly observed in individuals treated with neuroleptic drugs.

should be included among the first-line antipsychotic drugs, whereas *clozapine* should be reserved for severely schizophrenic patients who are refractory to traditional therapy. *Clozapine* can produce bone marrow suppression and cardiovascular side effects. The risk of severe agranulocytosis necessitates frequent monitoring of white-blood-cell count.

2. **Tardive dyskinesia:** Long-term treatment with neuroleptics can cause this motor disorder. Patients display involuntary movements, including lateral jaw movements and "fly-catching" motions of the tongue. A prolonged holiday from neuroleptics may cause the symptoms to diminish or disappear within three months. However, in many individuals, dyskinesia is irreversible and persists after discontinuation of therapy. Tardive dyskinesia is postulated to result from an increased number of dopamine receptors that are synthesized in response to long-term dopamine receptor blockade. This makes the neuron supersensitive to the actions of dopamine, and it allows the dopaminergic input to this structure to overpower the cholinergic input, causing excess movement in the patient.

3. **Neuroleptic malignant syndrome:** This potentially fatal reaction to neuroleptic drugs is characterized by muscle rigidity, fever, stupor, unstable blood pressure, and myoglobinemia. Treatment necessitates discontinuation of the neuroleptic and supportive therapy. Administration of *dantrolene* or *bromocriptine* may be helpful.

4. **Other effects:** Drowsiness occurs due to CNS depression, usually during the first two weeks of treatment. Confusion is sometimes encountered. The neuroleptics often produce dry mouth, urinary retention, constipation, and loss of accommodation. They block α-adrenergic receptors, resulting in lowered blood pressure and orthostatic hypotension. The neuroleptics depress the hypothalamus, causing amenorrhea, galactorrhea, infertility, and impotence. Significant weight gain is often a reason for noncompliance.

5. **Cautions and contraindications:** Acute agitation accompanying withdrawal from alcohol or other drugs may be aggravated by the neuroleptics. Stabilization with a simple sedative, such as a benzodiazepine, is the preferred treatment. *Chlorpromazine* and *clozapine* are contraindicated in patients with seizure disorders, because these drugs can lower seizure threshold. The neuroleptics can also aggravate epilepsy. For example, the high incidence of agranulocytosis with *clozapine* may limit its use to patients who are resistant to other drugs.

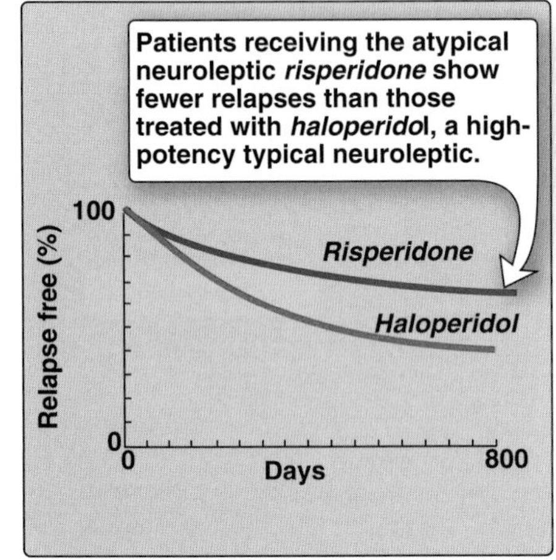

Figure 13.7
Rates of relapse among patients with schizophrenia after maintenance therapy with either *risperidone* or *haloperidol*.

F. Maintenance treatment

Patients who have had two or more schizophrenic episodes should receive maintenance therapy for at least five years, and some experts prefer indefinite therapy. Low doses of antipsychotic drugs are not as effective as higher-dose maintenance therapy in preventing relapse (Figure 13.7).

Figure 13.8 summarizes the therapeutic uses of some of the neuroleptic drugs.

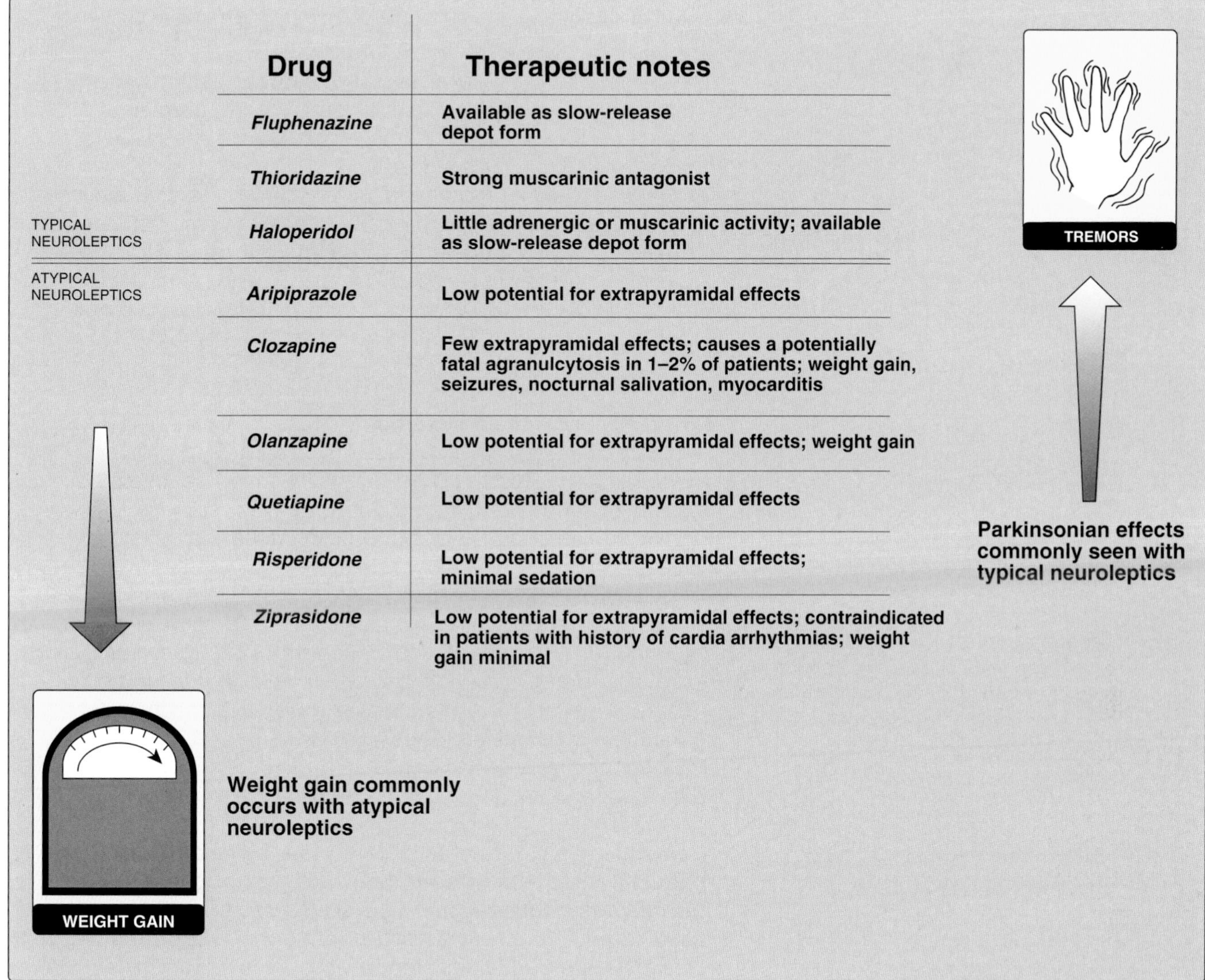

	Drug	Therapeutic notes
TYPICAL NEUROLEPTICS	*Fluphenazine*	Available as slow-release depot form
	Thioridazine	Strong muscarinic antagonist
	Haloperidol	Little adrenergic or muscarinic activity; available as slow-release depot form
ATYPICAL NEUROLEPTICS	*Aripiprazole*	Low potential for extrapyramidal effects
	Clozapine	Few extrapyramidal effects; causes a potentially fatal agranulcytosis in 1–2% of patients; weight gain, seizures, nocturnal salivation, myocarditis
	Olanzapine	Low potential for extrapyramidal effects; weight gain
	Quetiapine	Low potential for extrapyramidal effects
	Risperidone	Low potential for extrapyramidal effects; minimal sedation
	Ziprasidone	Low potential for extrapyramidal effects; contraindicated in patients with history of cardia arrhythmias; weight gain minimal

TREMORS
Parkinsonian effects commonly seen with typical neuroleptics
WEIGHT GAIN
Weight gain commonly occurs with atypical neuroleptics

Figure 13.8
Summary of neuroleptic agents.

Study Questions

Choose the ONE best answer.

13.1 An adolescent male is newly diagnosed with schizophrenia. Which of the following neuroleptic agents may improve his apathy and blunted affect?

A. Chlorpromazine
B. Fluphenazine
C. Haloperidol
D. Risperidone
E. Thioridazine

Correct answer = D. Risperidone is the only neuroleptic on the list that has some benefit in improving the negative symptoms of schizophrenia. All the agents have the potential to diminish the hallucinations and delusional thought processes.

13.2 Which one of the following neuroleptics has been shown to be a partial agonist at the D_2 receptor?

A. Aripiprazole
B. Clozapine
C. Haloperidol
D. Risperidone
E. Thioridazine

Correct answer = A. Aripiprazole is the agent that acts as a partial agonist at D_2 receptors. Theoretically, the drug would enhance action at these receptors when there is a low concentration of dopamine and would block the actions of high concentrations of dopamine. All the other drugs are only antagonistic at D_2 receptors, with haloperidol and thioridazine being particularly potent.

13.3 A 21-year-old male has recently begun pimozide therapy for Tourette disorder. He is brought to the emergency department by his parents. They describe that he has been having "different appearing tics" then before, such as prolonged contraction of the facial muscles. While being examined he experiences opisthotonus. Which of the following drugs would be beneficial in reducing these symptoms?

A. Benztropine
B. Bromocriptine
C. Lithium
D. Prochlorperazine
E. Risperidone

Correct answer = A. The patient is experiencing extrapyramidal symptoms due to pimozide, and a muscarinic antagonist such as benztropine would be effective in reducing the symptoms. The other drugs would have no effect or in the case of prochlorperazine, might increase the symptoms

13.4 A 28-year-old woman with schizoid affective disorder and difficulty sleeping would be most benefited by which of the following drugs?

A. Aripiprazole
B. Chlorpromazine
C. Haloperidol
D. Risperidone
E. Ziprasidone

Correct answer = B. Chlorpromazine has significant sedative activity as well as antipsychotic properties. Of the choices it is the drug most likely to alleviate this patient's major complaints including her insomnia.

Opioid Analgesics and Antagonists

14

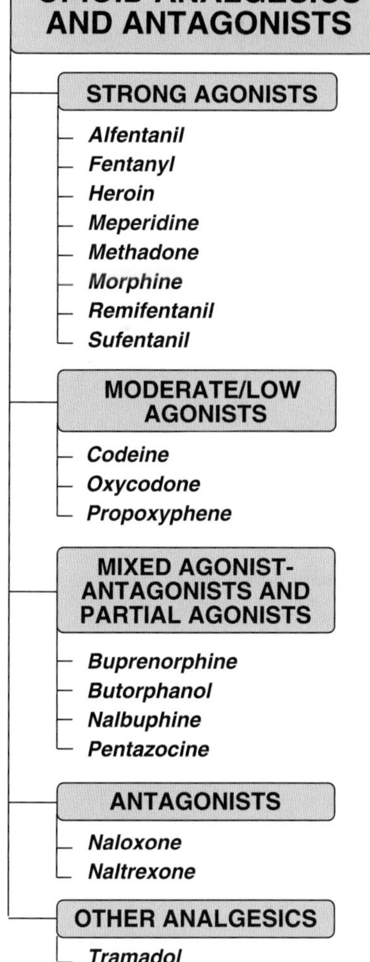

Figure 14.1
Summary of opioid analgesics and antagonists.

I. OVERVIEW

Management of pain is one of clinical medicine's greatest challenges. Pain is defined as an unpleasant sensation that can be either acute or chronic and that is a consequence of complex neurochemical processes in the peripheral and central nervous system (CNS). It is subjective, and the physician must rely on the patient's perception and description of his or her pain. Alleviation of pain depends on its type. In many cases, for example, with headache or mild to moderate arthritic pain, nonsteroidal anti-inflammatory agents (NSAIDs, see Chapter 42) are effective. Neurogenic pain responds best to tricyclic antidepressants (for example, *amitriptyline,* see p.144) or serotonin/norepinephrine reuptake inhibitors (for example, *duloxetine,* see p. 143) rather than NSAIDs or opioids. However, for severe or chronic malignant pain, opioids are usually the drugs of choice. Opioids are natural or synthetic compounds that produce *morphine*-like effects. [Note: The term opiate is reserved for drugs, such as *morphine* and *codeine*, obtained from the juice of the opium poppy.] All drugs in this category act by binding to specific opioid receptors in the CNS to produce effects that mimic the action of endogenous peptide neurotransmitters (for example, leu- and met-enkephalins). Although the opioids have a broad range of effects, their primary use is to relieve intense pain and the anxiety that accompanies it, whether that pain is from surgery or a result of injury or a disease, such as cancer. However, their widespread availability has led to abuse of those opioids with euphoric properties. [Note: Dependence is not a problem in patients being treated with these agents for severe pain.] Antagonists that can reverse the actions of opioids are also very important clinically for use in cases of overdose. Figure 14.1 lists the opioid agonists and antagonists discussed in this chapter.

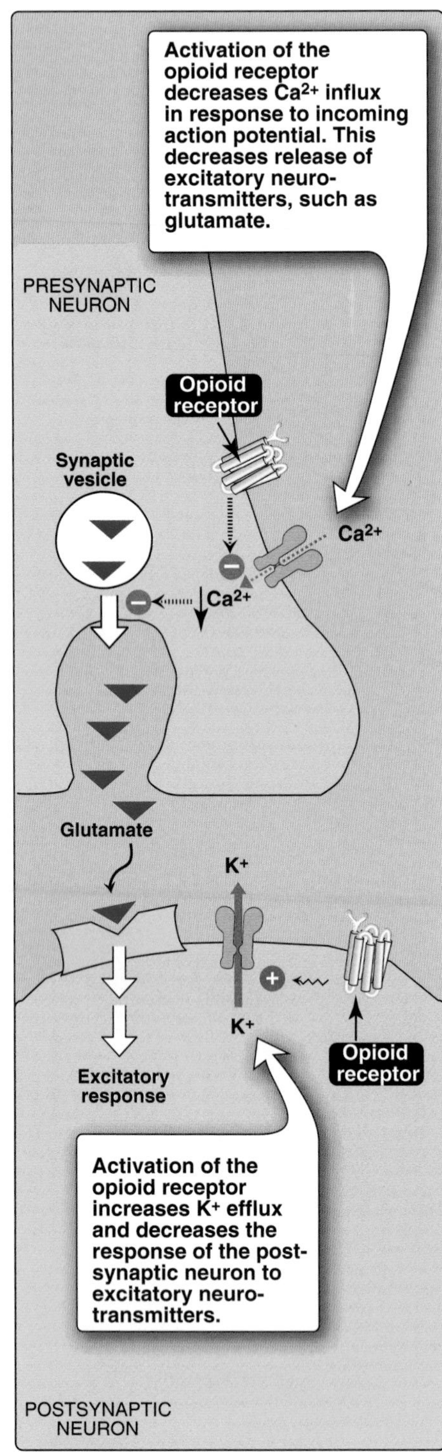

Figure 14.2
Mechanism of action of μ-opioid receptor agonists in the spinal cord.

II. OPIOID RECEPTORS

Opioids interact stereospecifically with protein receptors on the membranes of certain cells in the CNS, on nerve terminals in the periphery, and on cells of the gastrointestinal tract and other anatomic regions. The major effects of the opioids are mediated by three major receptor families. These are designated by the Greek letters μ (mu), κ (kappa), and δ (delta), each exhibiting a different specificity for the drug(s) it binds. The analgesic properties of the opioids are primarily mediated by the μ receptors; however, the κ receptors in the dorsal horn also contribute. For example, *butorphanol* and *nalbuphine* primarily owe their analgesic effect to κ-receptor activation. The enkephalins interact more selectively with the δ receptors in the periphery. All three opioid receptors are members of the G protein-coupled receptor family, and inhibit adenylyl cyclase.[1] They are also associated with ion channels, increasing postsynaptic K^+ efflux (hyperpolarization) or reducing presynaptic Ca^{2+} influx, thus impeding neuronal firing and transmitter release (Figure 14.2).

A. Distribution of receptors

High densities of opioid receptors known to be involved in integrating information about pain are present in five general areas of the CNS. They have also been identified on the peripheral sensory nerve fibers and their terminals and on immune cells. [Note: There is considerable overlap of receptor types in these various areas.]

1. **Brainstem:** Opioid receptors mediate respiration, cough, nausea and vomiting, maintenance of blood pressure, pupillary diameter, and control of stomach secretions.

2. **Medial thalamus:** This area mediates deep pain that is poorly localized and emotionally influenced.

3. **Spinal cord:** Receptors in the substantia gelatinosa are involved with the receipt and integration of incoming sensory information, leading to the attenuation of painful afferent stimuli.

4. **Hypothalamus:** Receptors here affect neuroendocrine secretion.

5. **Limbic system:** The greatest concentration of opiate receptors in the limbic system is located in the amygdala. These receptors probably do not exert analgesic action, but they may influence emotional behavior.

6. **Periphery:** Opioids also bind to peripheral sensory nerve fibers and their terminals. As in the CNS, they inhibit Ca^{2+}-dependent release of excitatory, proinflammatory substances (for example, substance P) from these nerve endings.

7. **Immune cells:** Opioid-binding sites have also been found on immune cells. The role of these receptors in nociception (response or sensitivity to painful stimuli) has not been determined.

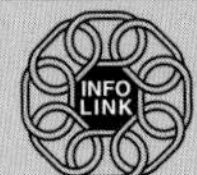

[1]See p. 92 in ***Lippincott's Illustrated Reviews: Biochemistry*** (3rd ed.) for a discussion of adenylyl cyclase.

III. STRONG AGONISTS

Morphine [MOR feen] is the major analgesic drug contained in crude opium, and is the prototype strong agonist. *Codeine* [KOE deen] is present in crude opium in lower concentrations and is inherently less potent. These drugs show a high affinity for μ receptors and varying affinities for δ and κ receptors.

A. Morphine

1. **Mechanism of action:** Opioids exert their major effects by interacting with opioid receptors in the CNS, and in other anatomic structures, such as the gastrointestinal tract and the urinary bladder. Opioids cause hyperpolarization of nerve cells, inhibition of nerve firing, and presynaptic inhibition of transmitter release. *Morphine* acts at κ receptors in lamina I and II of the substantia gelatinosa of the spinal cord, and it decreases the release of substance P, which modulates pain perception in the spinal cord. *Morphine* also appears to inhibit the release of many excitatory transmitters from nerve terminals carrying nociceptive (painful) stimuli.

2. **Actions:**

   a. **Analgesia:** *Morphine* causes analgesia (relief of pain without the loss of consciousness). Opioids relieve pain both by raising the pain threshold at the spinal cord level and, more importantly, by altering the brain's perception of pain. Patients treated with *morphine* are still aware of the presence of pain, but the sensation is not unpleasant. However, when given to an individual free of pain, its effects may be unpleasant and may cause nausea and vomiting. The maximum analgesic efficacy and the potential for addiction for representative agonists is shown in Figure 14.3.

   b. **Euphoria:** *Morphine* produces a powerful sense of contentment and well-being. Euphoria may be caused by stimulation of the ventral tegmentum.

   c. **Respiration:** *Morphine* causes respiratory depression by reduction of the sensitivity of respiratory center neurons to carbon dioxide. This occurs with ordinary doses of *morphine* and is accentuated as the dose increases until, ultimately, respiration ceases. Respiratory depression is the most common cause of death in acute opioid overdose.

   d. **Depression of cough reflex:** Both *morphine* and *codeine* have antitussive properties. In general, cough suppression does not correlate closely with analgesic and respiratory depressant properties of opioid drugs. The receptors involved in the antitussive action appear to be different from those involved in analgesia.

   e. **Miosis:** The pinpoint pupil, characteristic of *morphine* use, results from stimulation of μ and κ receptors. *Morphine* excites the Edinger-Westphal nucleus of the oculomotor nerve, which

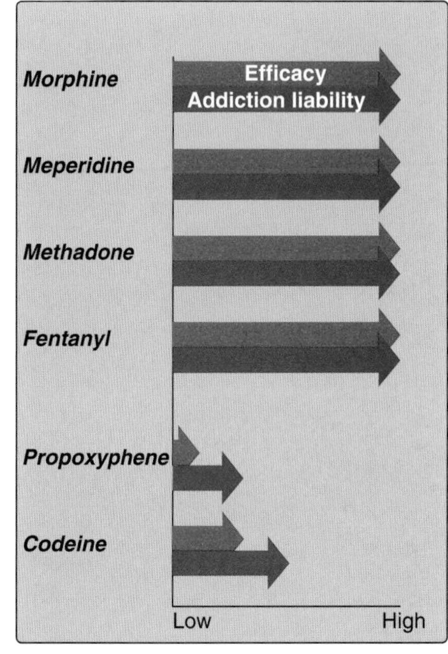

Figure 14.3
A comparison of the maximum efficacy and addiction/abuse liability of commonly used narcotic analgesics.

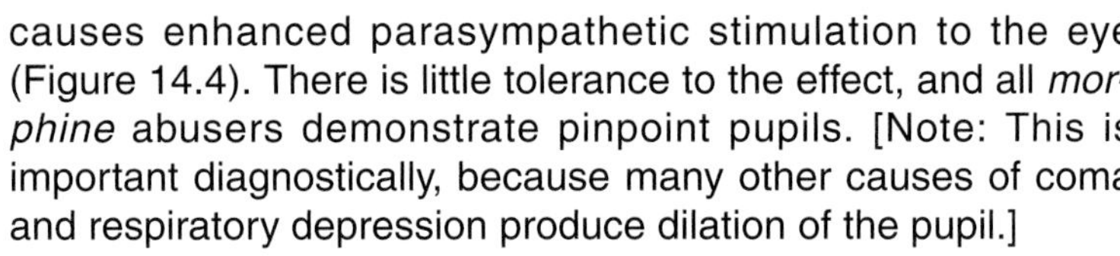

causes enhanced parasympathetic stimulation to the eye (Figure 14.4). There is little tolerance to the effect, and all *morphine* abusers demonstrate pinpoint pupils. [Note: This is important diagnostically, because many other causes of coma and respiratory depression produce dilation of the pupil.]

f. **Emesis:** *Morphine* directly stimulates the chemoreceptor trigger zone in the area postrema that causes vomiting. However, the emesis does not produce unpleasant sensations.

g. **Gastrointestinal tract:** *Morphine* relieves diarrhea and dysentery by decreasing the motility and increasing the tone of the intestinal smooth muscle. *Morphine* also increases the tone of the anal sphincter. Overall, *morphine* produces constipation, with little tolerance developing. It can also increase biliary tract pressure due to contraction of the gallbladder and constriction of the biliary sphincter.

h. **Cardiovascular:** *Morphine* has no major effects on the blood pressure or heart rate except at large doses, when hypotension and bradycardia may occur. Because of respiratory depression and carbon dioxide retention, cerebral vessels dilate and increase the cerebrospinal fluid (CSF) pressure. Therefore, *morphine* is usually contraindicated in individuals with severe brain injury.

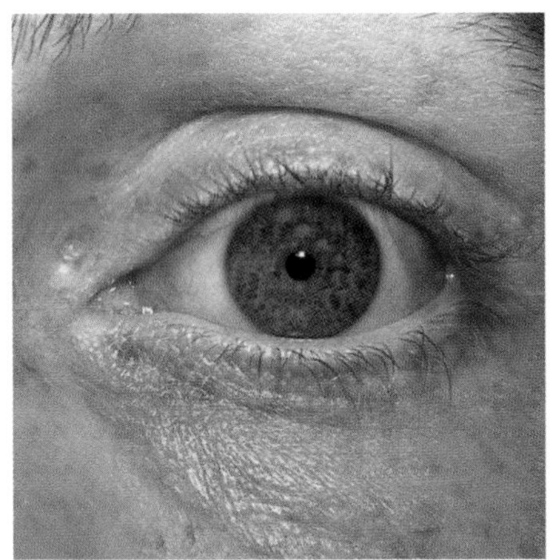

Figure 14.4
Morphine causes enhanced parasympathetic stimulation to the eye, resulting in pinpoint pupils.

i. **Histamine release:** *Morphine* releases histamine from mast cells, causing urticaria, sweating, and vasodilation. Because it can cause bronchoconstriction, asthmatics should not receive the drug.

j. **Hormonal actions:** *Morphine* inhibits release of gonadotropin-releasing hormone and corticotropin-releasing hormone, and it decreases the concentration of luteinizing hormone, follicle-stimulating hormone, adrenocorticotropic hormone, and β-endorphin. Testosterone and cortisol levels decrease. *Morphine* increases prolactin and growth hormone release by diminishing dopaminergic inhibition. It increases antidiuretic hormone and, thus, leads to urinary retention. [Note: It also can inhibit the urinary bladder voiding reflex; thus catheterization may be required.]

3. **Therapeutic uses:**

a. **Analgesia:** Despite intensive research, few other drugs have been developed that are as effective as *morphine* in the relief of pain. Opioids induce sleep, and in clinical situations when pain is present and sleep is necessary, opiates may be used to supplement the sleep-inducing properties of benzodiazepines, such as *flurazepam*. [Note: The sedative-hypnotic drugs are not usually analgesic, and may have diminished sedative effect in the presence of pain.]

b. **Treatment of diarrhea:** *Morphine* decreases the motility and increases the tone of intestinal smooth muscle. [Note: This can cause constipation.]

c. **Relief of cough:** *Morphine* suppresses the cough reflex; however, *codeine* or *dextromethorphan* are more widely used for this purpose. *Codeine* has greater antitussive action than *morphine*.

d. **Treatment of acute pulmonary edema:** Intravenous (IV) *morphine* dramatically relieves dyspnea caused by pulmonary edema associated with left ventricular failure—possibly by its vasodilatory effect.

4. **Pharmacokinetics:**

a. **Administration:** Absorption of *morphine* from the gastrointestinal tract is slow and erratic, and the drug is usually not given orally. *Codeine*, by contrast, is well absorbed when given by mouth. Significant first-pass metabolism of *morphine* occurs in the liver; therefore, intramuscular (IM), subcutaneous, or IV injections produce the most reliable responses. [Note: In cases of chronic pain associated with neoplastic disease, it has become common practice to use either the new slow-release tablets orally or pumps that allow the patient to control the pain through self-administration, Figure 14.5.] Opiates have been taken for nonmedical purposes by inhaling powders or smoke from burning crude opium, which provide a rapid onset of drug action.

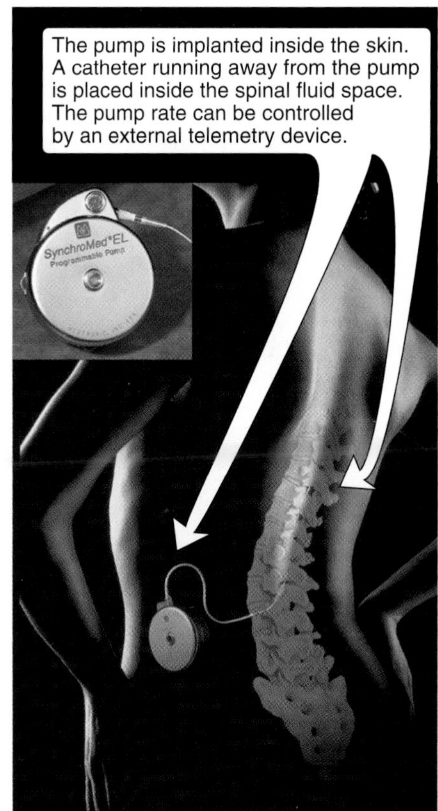

The pump is implanted inside the skin.
A catheter running away from the pump is placed inside the spinal fluid space.
The pump rate can be controlled by an external telemetry device.
SynchroMed®EL
Programmable Pump

Figure 14.5
Implanted pump for delivery of morphine.

b. **Distribution:** *Morphine* rapidly enters all body tissues, including the fetuses of pregnant women, and should not be used for analgesia during labor. Infants born of addicted mothers show physical dependence on opiates and exhibit withdrawal symptoms if opioids are not administered. Only a small percentage of *morphine* crosses the blood-brain barrier, because *morphine* is the least lipophilic of the common opioids. This contrasts with the more fat-soluble opioids, such as *fentanyl*, *methadone*, and *heroin*, which readily penetrate into the brain

c. **Fate:** *Morphine* is conjugated in the liver to glucuronic acid. Morphine-6-glucuronide is a very potent analgesic, whereas the conjugate at the 3-position is much less active. The conjugates are excreted primarily in the urine, with small quantities appearing in the bile. The duration of action of *morphine* is four to six hours when administered systemically to naïve individuals but considerably longer when injected epidurally, because its low lipophilicity prevents redistribution from the epidural space. [Note: A patient's age can influence the response to *morphine*. Elderly patients are more sensitive to the analgesic effects of the drug, possibly due to decreased metabolism or other factors, such as decreased lean body mass, renal function, etc. They should be treated with lower doses. Neonates should not receive *morphine* because of their low conjugating capacity.]

5. **Adverse effects:** Severe respiratory depression occurs and can result in death in acute opoid poisoning. A serious effect of the drug is stoppage of respiratory exchange in patients with emphysema or cor pulmonale. [Note: If employed in such individuals,

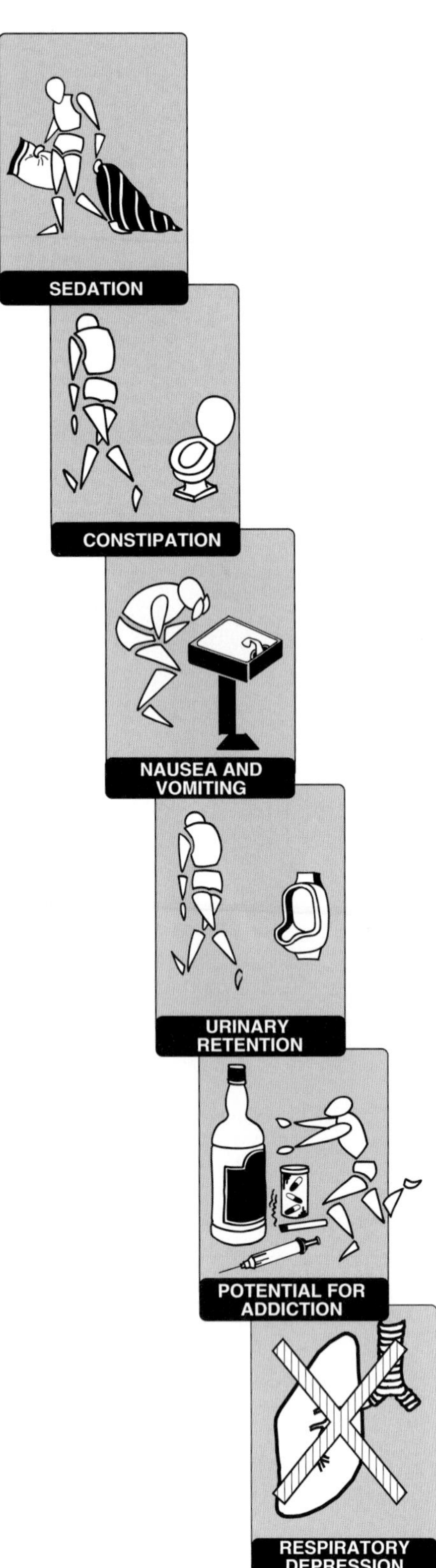

Figure 14.6
Adverse effects commonly observed in individuals treated with opioids.

respiration must be carefully monitored.] Other effects include vomiting, dysphoria, and allergy-enhanced hypotensive effects (Figure 14.6). The elevation of intracranial pressure, particularly in head injury, can be serious. *Morphine* enhances cerebral and spinal ischemia. In prostatic hypertrophy, *morphine* may cause acute urinary retention. Patients with adrenal insufficiency or myxedema may experience extended and increased effects from the opioids. *Morphine* should be used with caution in patients with bronchial asthma or liver failure.

6. **Tolerance and physical dependence:** Repeated use produces tolerance to the respiratory depressant, analgesic, euphoric, and sedative effects of *morphine*. However, tolerance usually does not develop to the pupil-constricting and constipating effects of the drug. Physical and psychological dependence readily occur with *morphine* and with some of the other agonists to be described (see Figure 14.3). Withdrawal produces a series of autonomic, motor, and psychological responses that incapacitate the individual and cause serious—almost unbearable—symptoms. However, it is very rare that the effects are so profound as to cause death. [Note: Detoxification of *heroin-* or *morphine*-dependent individuals is usually accomplished through the oral administration of *methadone* (see below) or *clonidine*.]

7. **Drug interactions:** The depressant actions of *morphine* are enhanced by phenothiazines, monoamine oxidase inhibitors, and tricyclic antidepressants (see Figure 14.7). Low doses of *amphetamine* inexplicably enhance analgesia, as does *hydroxyzine*.

B. Meperidine

Meperidine [me PER i deen] is a synthetic opioid structurally unrelated to *morphine*. It is used for acute pain.

1. **Mechanism of action:** *Meperidine* binds to opioid receptors, particularly μ receptors. However, it also binds well to κ receptors.

2. **Actions:** *Meperidine* causes a depression of respiration similar to that of *morphine*, but it has no significant cardiovascular action when given orally. On IV administration, *meperidine* produces a decrease in peripheral resistance and an increase in peripheral blood flow, and it may cause an increase in cardiac rate. As with *morphine*, *meperidine* dilates cerebral vessels, increases CSF pressure, and contracts smooth muscle (the latter to a lesser extent than does *morphine*). *Meperidine* does not cause pinpoint pupils but, rather, causes the pupils to dilate because of an *atropine*-like action.

3. **Therapeutic uses:** *Meperidine* provides analgesia for any type of severe pain. Unlike *morphine*, *meperidine* is not clinically useful in the treatment of diarrhea or cough. *Meperidine* produces less of an increase in urinary retention than does *morphine*. It is the opioid commonly employed in obstetrics (see below).

4. **Pharmacokinetics:** Unlike *morphine*, *meperidine* is well absorbed from the gastrointestinal tract, and is useful when an orally administered, potent analgesic is needed. However, *meperidine* is most often administered IM. The drug has a duration of action of two to four hours, which is shorter than that of *morphine* (Figure 14.8). *Meperidine* is N-demethylated to normeperidine in the liver and is excreted in the urine. [Note: Because of its shorter action and different route of metabolism, *meperidine* is preferred over *morphine* for analgesia during labor.]

5. **Adverse effects:** Large or repetitive doses of *meperidine* can cause anxiety, tremors, muscle twitches, and rarely, convulsions due to the accumulation of normeperidine. The drug differs from opioids in that when given in large doses, it dilates the pupil and causes hyperactive reflexes. Severe hypotension can occur when the drug is administered postoperatively. Due to its antimuscarinic action, patients may experience dry mouth and blurred vision. When used with major neuroleptics, depression is greatly enhanced. Administration to patients taking monoamine oxidase inhibitors can provoke severe reactions, such as convulsions and hyperthermia. *Meperidine* can cause dependence, and can substitute for *morphine* or *heroin* in opiate-dependent persons. Partial cross-tolerance with the other opioids occurs.

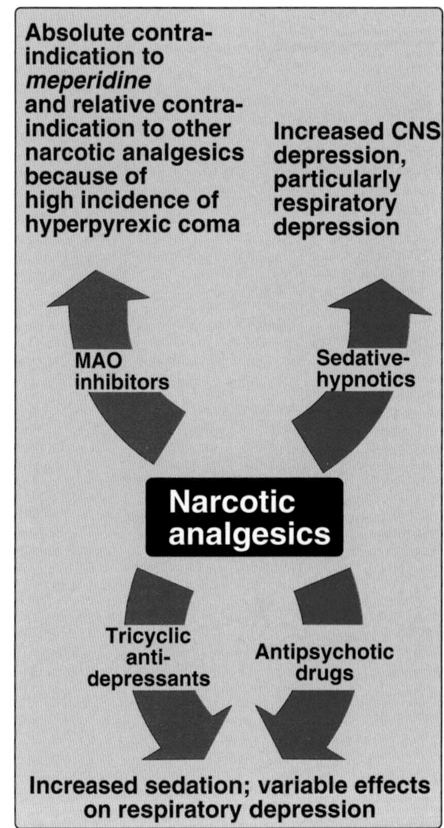

Figure 14.7
Drugs interacting with narcotic analgesics. CNS = central nervous system; MAO = monoamine oxidase.

C. Methadone

Methadone [METH a done] is a synthetic, orally effective opioid that is approximately equal in potency to *morphine* but induces less euphoria and has a somewhat longer duration of action.

1. **Mechanism of action:** The actions of *methadone* are mediated by the μ receptors.

2. **Actions:** The analgesic activity of *methadone* is equivalent to that of *morphine* (see Figure 14.3). *Methadone* is well-absorbed when administered orally, in contrast to *morphine*, which is only partially absorbed from the gastrointestinal tract. The miotic and respiratory-depressant actions of *methadone* have average half-lives of 24 hours. Like *morphine*, *methadone* increases biliary pressure and is also constipating.

3. **Therapeutic uses:** *Methadone* is used in the controlled withdrawal of dependent abusers from *heroin* and *morphine*. Orally administered, *methadone* is substituted for the injected opioid. The patient is then slowly weaned from *methadone*. *Methadone* causes a withdrawal syndrome that is milder but more protracted (days to weeks) than with other opioids

4. **Pharmacokinetics:** *Methadone* is readily absorbed following oral administration. It accumulates in tissues, where it remains bound to protein, from which it is slowly released. The drug is biotransformed in the liver and excreted in the urine, mainly as inactive metabolites.

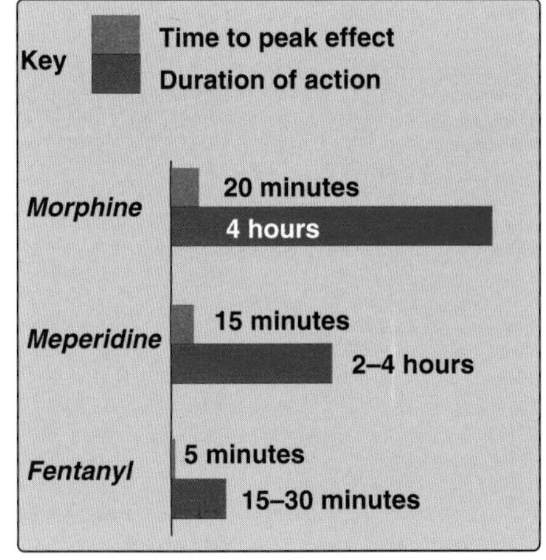

Figure 14.8
Time to peak effect and duration of action of several opioids administered intravenously.

5. **Adverse effects:** *Methadone* can produce physical dependence like that of *morphine*.

D. Fentanyl

Fentanyl [FEN ta nil], which is chemically related to *meperidine*, has 100-fold the analgesic potency of *morphine*, and is used in anesthesia. It has a rapid onset and short duration of action (fifteen to thirty minutes). It is usually injected IV, epidurally, or intrathecally. Epidural *fentanyl* is used for analgesia postoperatively and during labor. An oral transmucosal preparation and a transdermal patch are also available. The transmucosal preparation is used in the treatment of cancer patients with breakthrough pain who are tolerant to opioids. The transdermal patch must be used with caution, because death resulting from hypoventilation has been known to occur. [Note: The transdermal patch creates a reservoir of the drug in the skin. Hence, the onset is delayed twelve hours, and the offset is prolonged.] *Fentanyl* is metabolized to inactive metabolites by the cytochrome P4503A4 system, and drugs that inhibit this isozyme can potentiate the effect of *fentanyl*. Most of the drug and metabolites are eliminated through the urine. Adverse effects of *fentanyl* are similar to those of other μ receptor agonists. Because of life-threatening hypoventilation, the *fentanyl* patch is contraindicated in the management of acute and postoperative pain or pain that can be ameliorated with other analgesics. Unlike *meperidine*, it causes pupillary constriction.

E. Sufentanil, alfentanil, and remifentanil

Three drugs related to *fentanyl—sufentanil* [soo FEN ta nil], *alfentanil* (al FEN ta nil), and *remifentanil* [rem i FEN ta nil]—differ in their potency and metabolic disposition. *Sufentanil* is even more potent than *fentanyl*, whereas the other two are less potent but much shorter-acting.

F. Heroin

Heroin [HAIR o in] does not occur naturally. It is produced by diacetylation of *morphine*, which leads to a threefold increase in its potency. Its greater lipid solubility allows it to cross the blood-brain barrier more rapidly than *morphine*, causing a more exaggerated euphoria when the drug is taken by injection. *Heroin* is converted to *morphine* in the body, but its effects last about half as long. It has no accepted medical use in the United States.

IV. MODERATE AGONISTS

A. Codeine

Codeine [KOE deen] is a much less potent analgesic than *morphine*, but it has a higher oral effectiveness. *Codeine* shows good antitussive activity at doses that do not cause analgesia. The drug has a lower potential for abuse than *morphine*, and rarely produces dependence. *Codeine* produces less euphoria than *morphine*. *Codeine* is often used in combination with *aspirin* or *acetaminophen*. [Note: In most nonprescription cough preparations, *codeine* has been replaced by drugs such as *dextromethorphan*—a synthetic cough depressant that has no analgesic action and a low potential for abuse.] Figure 14.9 shows some of the actions of *codeine*.

B. Oxycodone

Oxycodone [ok see KOE done] is a semisynthetic derivative of *morphine*. It is orally active and is sometimes formulated with *aspirin* or *acetaminophen*. It is used to treat moderate to severe pain, and has many properties in common with *morphine*. *Oxycodone* is metabolized to products with lower analgesic activity. Excretion is via the kidney. Abuse of the sustained-release preparation (ingestion of crushed tablets) has been implicated in many deaths. It is important that the higher-dosage forms of the latter preparation be used only by patients who are tolerant to opioids.

C. Propoxyphene

Propoxyphene [proe POX i feen] is a derivative of *methadone*. The dextro isomer is used as an analgesic to relieve mild to moderate pain. The levo isomer is not analgesic, but it has antitussive action. *Propoxyphene* is a weaker analgesic than *codeine*, requiring approximately twice the dose to achieve an equivalent effect to that of *codeine*. *Propoxyphene* is often used in combination with *aspirin* or *acetaminophen* for an analgesia greater than that obtained with either drug alone. It is well absorbed orally, with peak plasma levels occurring in one hour, and it is metabolized in the liver. *Propoxyphene* can produce nausea, anorexia, and constipation. In toxic doses, it can cause respiratory depression, convulsions, hallucinations, and confusion. When toxic doses are taken, a very serious problem can arise in some individuals, with resultant cardiotoxicity and pulmonary edema. [Note: When used with alcohol and sedatives, a severe CNS depression is produced, and death by respiratory depression and cardiotoxicity can result. The respiratory depression and sedation can be antagonized by *naloxone*, but the cardiotoxicity cannot.]

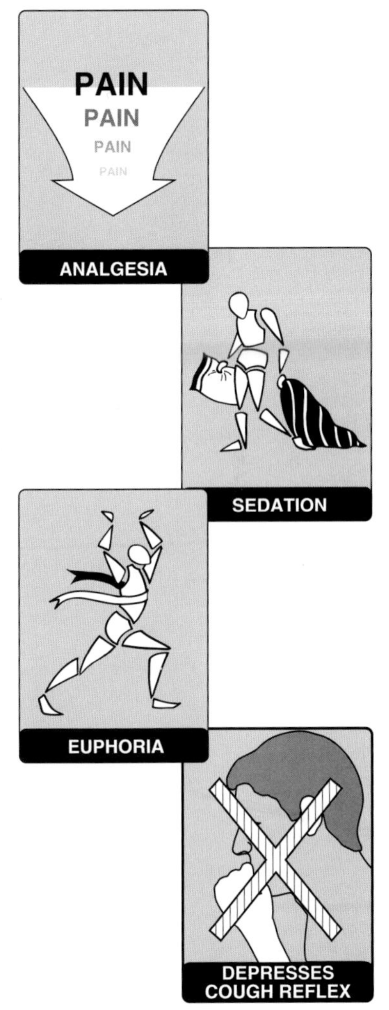

Figure 14.9
Some actions of *codeine*.

V. MIXED AGONIST-ANTAGONISTS AND PARTIAL AGONISTS

Drugs that stimulate one receptor but block another are termed mixed agonist-antagonists. The effects of these drugs depend on previous exposure to opioids. In individuals who have not recently received opioids, mixed agonist-antagonists show agonist activity and are used to relieve pain. In the patient with opioid dependence, the agonist-antagonist drugs may show primarily blocking effects—that is, produce withdrawal symptoms.

A. Pentazocine

Pentazocine [pen TAZ oh seen] acts as an agonist on κ receptors, and is a weak antagonist at μ and δ receptors. *Pentazocine* promotes analgesia by activating receptors in the spinal cord, and it is used to relieve moderate pain. It may be administered either orally or parenterally. *Pentazocine* produces less euphoria compared to *morphine*. In higher doses, the drug causes respiratory depression and decreases the activity of the gastrointestinal tract. High doses increase blood pressure and can cause hallucinations, nightmares, tachycardia, and dizziness. The latter properties have led to its decreased use. In angina, *pentazocine* increases the mean aortic pressure and pulmonary arterial pressure and, thus, increases the work of the heart. The drug decreases renal plasma flow. Despite its antagonist action, *pentazocine* does not antagonize the respiratory depression of *morphine*, but it can precipitate a withdrawal syndrome in a *morphine* abuser. Tolerance and dependence develop on repeated use.

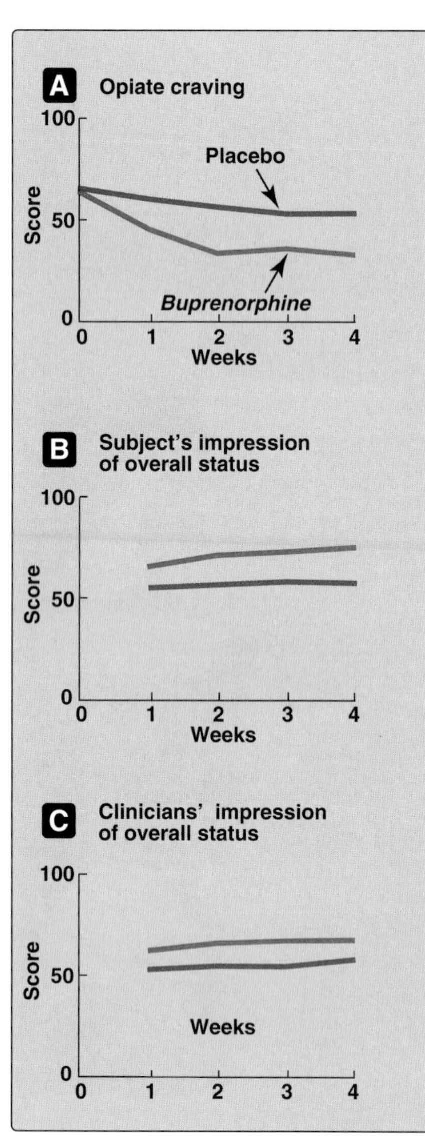

Figure 14.10
Scores for opiate craving and overall status in opioid-addicted patients assigned to office-based treatment with *buprenorphine* or placebo.

B. Buprenorphine

Buprenorphine [byoo pre NOR feen] is classified as a partial agonist, acting at the μ receptor. It acts like *morphine* in naïve patients, but it can also precipitate withdrawal in *morphine* users. A major use is in opiate detoxication, because it has a less severe and shorter duration of withdrawal symptoms compared to *methadone* (Figure 14.10). It causes little sedation, respiratory depression, and hypotension, even at high doses. In contrast to *methadone,* which is available only at specialized clinics, *buprenorphine* is approved for office-based detoxification or maintenance. *Buprenorphine* is administered sublingually or parenterally, and has a long duration of action because of its tight binding to the receptor. It is metabolized by the liver and excreted in the bile and urine. Adverse effects include respiratory depression that cannot be reversed by *naloxone*, decreased (or, rarely, increased) blood pressure, nausea, and dizziness.

C. Nalbuphine and butorphanol

Nalbuphine [NAL byoo feen] and *butorphanol* [byoo TOR fa nole], like *pentazocine*, play a limited role in the treatment of chronic pain. Neither is available for oral use. Their propensity to cause psychotomimetic effects is less than that of *pentazocine*. *Nalbuphine* does not affect the heart or increase blood pressure, in contrast to *pentazocine* and *butorphanol*. A benefit of all three medications is that they exhibit a ceiling effect for respiratory depression.

VI. OTHER ANALGESICS

A. Tramadol

Tramadol (TRA ma dole) is a centrally acting analgesic that binds to the μ-opioid receptor. In addition, it weakly inhibits re-uptake of norepinephrine and serotonin. It is used to manage moderate to moderately severe pain. Its respiratory-depressant activity is less than that of *morphine*. *Naloxone* (see below) can only partially reverse the analgesia produced by *tramadol* or its active metabolite. The drug undergoes extensive metabolism, and one metabolite is active. Concurrent use with *carbamazepine* results in increased metabolism, presumably by induction of the cytochrome P450 system 2D6. [Note: *Quinidine*, which inhibits this isozyme, increases levels of *tramadol* when taken concurrently.] Anaphylactoid reactions have been reported. Of concern are the seizures that can occur, especially in patients taking selective serotonin re-uptake inhibitors or tricyclic antidepressants. *Tramadol* should also be avoided in patients taking monoamine oxidase inhibitors.

VII. ANTAGONISTS

The opioid antagonists bind with high affinity to opioid receptors, but fail to activate the receptor-mediated response. Administration of opioid antagonists produces no profound effects in normal individuals. However, in patients dependent on opioids, antagonists rapidly reverse the effect of agonists, such as *heroin*, and precipitate the symptoms of opiate withdrawal.

A. Naloxone

Naloxone [nal OX one] is used to reverse the coma and respiratory depression of opioid overdose. It rapidly displaces all receptor-bound opioid molecules and, therefore, is able to reverse the effect of a *heroin* overdose (Figure 14.11). Within thirty seconds of IV injection of *naloxone*, the respiratory depression and coma characteristic of high doses of *heroin* are reversed, causing the patient to be revived and alert. *Naloxone* has a half-life of 60 to 100 minutes. [Note: Because of its relatively short duration of action, a depressed patient who has been treated and recovered may lapse back into respiratory depression.] *Naloxone* is a competitive antagonist at μ, κ, and δ, receptors, with a ten-fold higher affinity for μ receptors than for κ. This may explain why *naloxone* readily reverses respiratory depression with only minimal reversal of the analgesia that results from agonist stimulation of κ receptors in the spinal cord. *Naloxone* produces no pharmacologic effects in normal individuals, but it precipitates withdrawal symptoms in opioid abusers.

B. Naltrexone

Naltrexone [nal TREX one] has actions similar to those of *naloxone*. It has a longer duration of action than *naloxone*, and a single oral dose of *naltrexone* blocks the effect of injected *heroin* for up to 48 hours. *Naltrexone* in combination with *clonidine*—and, sometimes, with *bruprenorphine*—is employed for rapid opioid detoxification. It may also be beneficial in treating chronic alcoholism by an unknown mechanism, but benzodiazopines and *clonidine* are preferred. *Naltrexone* is hepatotoxic.

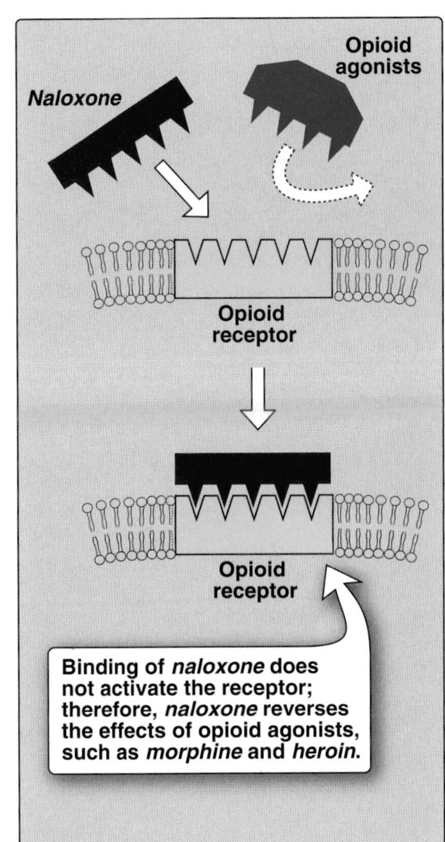

Opioid agonists
Naloxone
Opioid receptor
Opioid receptor
Binding of naloxone does not activate the receptor; therefore, naloxone reverses the effects of opioid agonists, such as morphine and heroin.

Figure 14.11
Competition of *naloxone* with opioid agonists.

Study Questions

Choose the ONE best answer.

14.1 A young man is brought into the emergency room. He is unconscious, and he has pupillary constriction and depressed respiration. You note needle marks on his legs. You administer naltrexone, and he awakens. This agent was effective because:

A. the patient was suffering from an overdose by an opioid.
B. naltrexone antagonizes opiates at the receptor site.
C. naltrexone is a stimulant of the CNS.
D. naltrexone binds to the opioid and inactivates it.

> Correct answer = B. The indications are that the patient is suffering from an overdose of an opioid, such as heroin. Naltrexone antagonizes the opioid by displacing it from the receptor. It is used in preference to naloxone, because it is longer acting and, thus, can act as long as the opiate is in the body.

14.2 A heroin addict has entered a rehabilatation program that requires she take methadone. Methadone is effective in this situation because it:

A. is an antagonist at the morphine receptors.
B. has less potent analgesic activity than heroin.
C. is longer acting than heroin; hence, the withdrawal is milder than with the latter drug.
D. does not cause constipation.
E. is nonaddictive.

> Correct answer = C. It is used in rehabilatation programs as a substitute for heroin. It has similar euphorigenic and analgetic activity, is orally active, and can be easily controlled. Most importantly, it is long acting, and the withdrawal the patient undergoes as she is being weaned off the drug is much milder than would be the case with heroin. Methadone is a synthetic orally effective opioid that acts at the μ receptors. Its analgetic activity is equal to that of morphine and similar to that of heroin. It does cause constipation and can be addictive.

14.3 Which of the following statements about morphine is correct?

A. It is used therapeutically to relieve pain caused by severe head injury.
B. Its withdrawal symptoms can be relieved by naloxone.
C. It causes diarrhea.
D. It is most effective by oral administration.
E. It rapidly enters all body tissues, including the fetus of a pregnant woman.

> Correct answer = E. Morphine causes increased cerebrospinal fluid pressure secondary to dilation of cerebral vasculature and is contraindicated in severe head injury. Naloxone is an opioid antagonist and can precipitate withdrawal symptoms in morphine-addicted individuals. Morphine is administered parenterally, because absorption from the gastrointestinal tract is unreliable. It causes constipation.

14.4 The pain of a patient with bone cancer has been managed with a morphine pump. However, he has become tolerant to morphine. Which of the following might be indicated to ameliorate his pain?

A. Meperidine
B. Codeine
C. Fentanyl
D. Methadone
E. Buprenorphine

> Correct Answer= C. Fentanyl is used in anesthesia. It produces analgesia and is usually injected epidurally. However, its analgetic action is also beneficial in cancer patients. It is available as a transdermal patch and an oral transmucosal preparation. Meperidine and codeine show cross-tolerance with morphine and, thus, would not be effective. Buprenorphine, like methadone, is used in opiate detoxication, and could precipitate withdrawal.

Drugs Used To Treat Epilepsy

15

I. OVERVIEW

Epilepsy is widespread among the general population, with more than 2.5 million affected individuals in the United States. It is the second most common neurologic disorder after stroke. Epilepsy is not a single entity but, instead, is a family of different recurrent seizure disorders that have in common the sudden, excessive, and synchronous discharge of cerebral neurons. This results in abnormal movements or perceptions that are of short duration but tend to recur. The site of the electric discharge determines the symptoms that are produced. For example, epileptic seizures may cause convulsions if the motor cortex is involved. The seizures may include visual, auditory, or olfactory hallucinations if the parietal or occipital cortex plays a role. Although drug therapy is the most widely effective mode for the treatment of epilepsy, it is not 100 percent effective in all patients. For example, it is frequently hindered by poor patient adherence, and it is often complicated by drug interactions. However, seizures can be controlled completely in approximately fifty percent of epileptic patients, and meaningful improvement is achieved in at least half of the remaining patients. A summary of antiepileptic drugs is shown in Figure 15.1.

A. Types of epilepsy

The neuronal discharge in epilepsy results from the firing of a small population of neurons in some specific area of the brain that is referred to as the primary focus. Anatomically, this focal area may appear to be perfectly normal. However, in some patients, brain abnormalities can be identified using neuroimaging techniques (Figure 15.2). Epilepsy usually has no identifiable cause, although the focal areas that are functionally abnormal may be triggered into activity by changes in any of a variety of environmental factors, including alteration in blood gases, pH, electrolytes, or glucose availability.

1. **Primary epilepsy:** When no specific anatomic cause for the seizure, such as trauma or neoplasm, is evident, the syndrome is called idiopathic or primary epilepsy. These seizures may be produced by an inherited abnormality in the central nervous system (CNS). Patients are treated chronically with antiepileptic drugs, often for life.

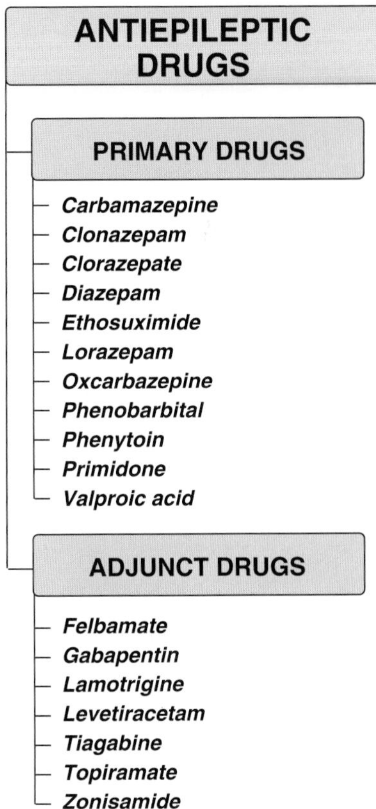

ANTIEPILEPTIC DRUGS
PRIMARY DRUGS
Carbamazepine
Clonazepam
Clorazepate
Diazepam
Ethosuximide
Lorazepam
Oxcarbazepine
Phenobarbital
Phenytoin
Primidone
Valproic acid
ADJUNCT DRUGS
Felbamate
Gabapentin
Lamotrigine
Levetiracetam
Tiagabine
Topiramate
Zonisamide

Figure 15.1
Summary of agents used in the treatment of epilepsy.

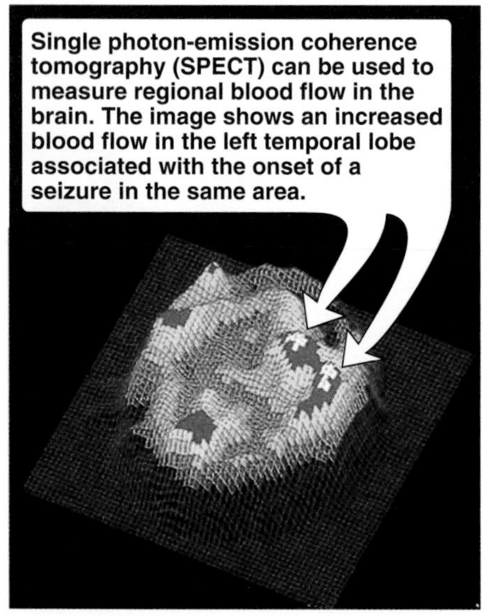

Figure 15.2
Region of the brain in an epileptic individual showing increased blood flow during a seizure.

2. **Secondary epilepsy:** A number of reversible disturbances, such as tumors, head injury, hypoglycemia, meningeal infection, or rapid withdrawal of alcohol from an alcoholic, can precipitate seizures. Antiepileptic drugs are given until the primary cause of the seizures can be corrected. Seizures secondary to stroke or trauma may cause irreversible CNS damage.

B. Classification of seizures

Seizures have been classified into two broad groups: partial (or focal), and generalized. Choice of drug treatment is based on the classification of the seizures being treated (Figure 15.3).

1. **Partial:** The symptoms of each seizure type depend on the site of neuronal discharge and on the extent to which the electrical activity spreads to other neurons in the brain. Partial seizures may progress, becoming generalized tonic-clonic seizures.

   a. **Simple partial:** These seizures are caused by a group of hyperactive neurons exhibiting abnormal electrical activity, which are confined to a single locus in the brain. The electrical discharge does not spread, and the patient does not lose consciousness. The patient often exhibits abnormal activity of a single limb or muscle group that is controlled by the region of the brain experiencing the disturbance. The patient may also show sensory distortions. Simple partial seizures may occur at any age.

   b. **Complex partial:** These seizures exhibit complex sensory hallucinations, mental distortion, and loss of consciousness. Motor dysfunction may involve chewing movements, diarrhea, and/or urination. Eighty percent of individuals with complex partial epilepsy experience their initial seizures before twenty years of age.

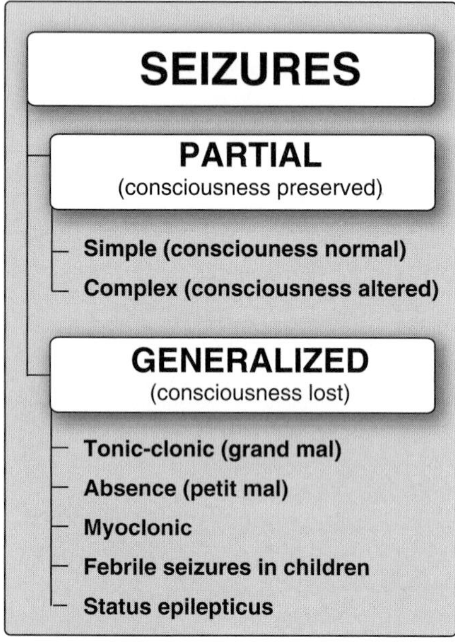

Figure 15.3
Classification of epilepsy.

2. **Generalized:** These seizures begin locally, but they rapidly spread, producing abnormal electrical discharges throughout both hemispheres of the brain. Generalized seizures may be convulsive or nonconvulsive, and the patient usually has an immediate loss of consciousness.

   a. **Tonic-clonic (grand mal):** This is the most commonly encountered—and the most dramatic—form of epilepsy. Seizures result in loss of consciousness, followed by tonic (continuous contraction) and then clonic (rapid contraction and relaxation) phases. The seizure is followed by a period of confusion and exhaustion due to the depletion of energy stores.

   b. **Absence (petit mal):** These seizures involve a brief, abrupt, and self-limiting loss of consciousness. The onset occurs in patients at three to five years of age and lasts until puberty. The patient stares and exhibits rapid eye-blinking, which lasts for three to five seconds.

c. **Myoclonic:** These seizures consist of short episodes of muscle contractions that may reoccur for several minutes. Myoclonic seizures are rare, occur at any age, and are often a result of permanent neurologic damage acquired as a result of hypoxia, uremia, encephalitis, or drug poisoning.

d. **Febrile seizures:** Young children (three months to five years of age) frequently develop seizures with illness accompanied by high fever. The febrile seizures consist of generalized tonic-clonic convulsions of short duration. Although febrile seizures may be frightening to observers, they are benign and do not cause death, neurologic damage, injury, or learning disorders, Febrile seizures rarely require medication.

e. **Status epilepticus:** These seizures are rapidly recurrent.

C. Mechanism of action of antiepileptic drugs

Drugs that are effective in seizure reduction can either block the initiation of the electrical discharge from the focal area or, more commonly, prevent the spread of the abnormal electrical discharge to adjacent brain areas. They accomplish this by a variety of mechanisms, including blockade of voltage-gated channels (Na^+ or Ca^{2+}), enhancement of inhibitory GABAergic impulses, or interference with excitatory glutamate transmission.

II. PRIMARY ANTIEPILEPTIC DRUGS

Initial drug treatment to suppress or reduce the incidence of seizures is based on the specific type of seizure. Thus, tonic-clonic (grand mal) seizures are treated differently than absence seizures (petit mal). Several drugs may be equally effective, and the toxicity of the agent is often a major consideration in drug selection. Monotherapy is instituted with a single agent until seizures are controlled or toxic signs occur. [Note: Compared to those receiving combination therapy, patients receiving monotherapy show better compliance and fewer side-effects. Thus, if seizures are not controlled with the first drug, monotherapy with an alternate antiepileptic drug that is indicated for the patient's seizuire type should be initiated before a combination of drugs is tried (Figure 15.4).] When therapy with a single drug is ineffective, a second drug may be added to the therapeutic regimen. Antiepileptic drugs developed over the last fifteen years are all approved as adjunct therapy, although a few of them are also employed as monotherapy. These agents are described later in this chapter. [Note: Antiepileptic therapy for tonic-clonic seizures should never be terminated abruptly; otherwise, seizures may result.] Therapeutic indications for the primary anticonvulsant drugs used to treat different types of epilepsy are shown in Figure 15.5.

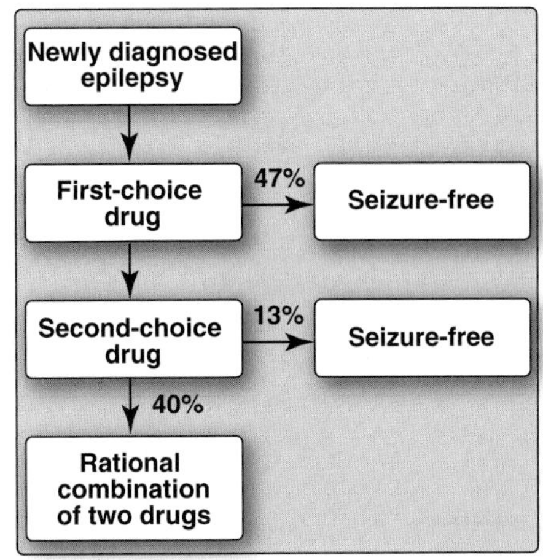

Figure 15.4
Therapeutic strategies for managing newly diagnosed epilepsy.

A. Phenytoin

Phenytoin [FEN i toin] (formerly called diphenylhydantoin) is effective in suppressing tonic-clonic and partial seizures, and is a drug of choice for initial therapy, particularly in treating adults.

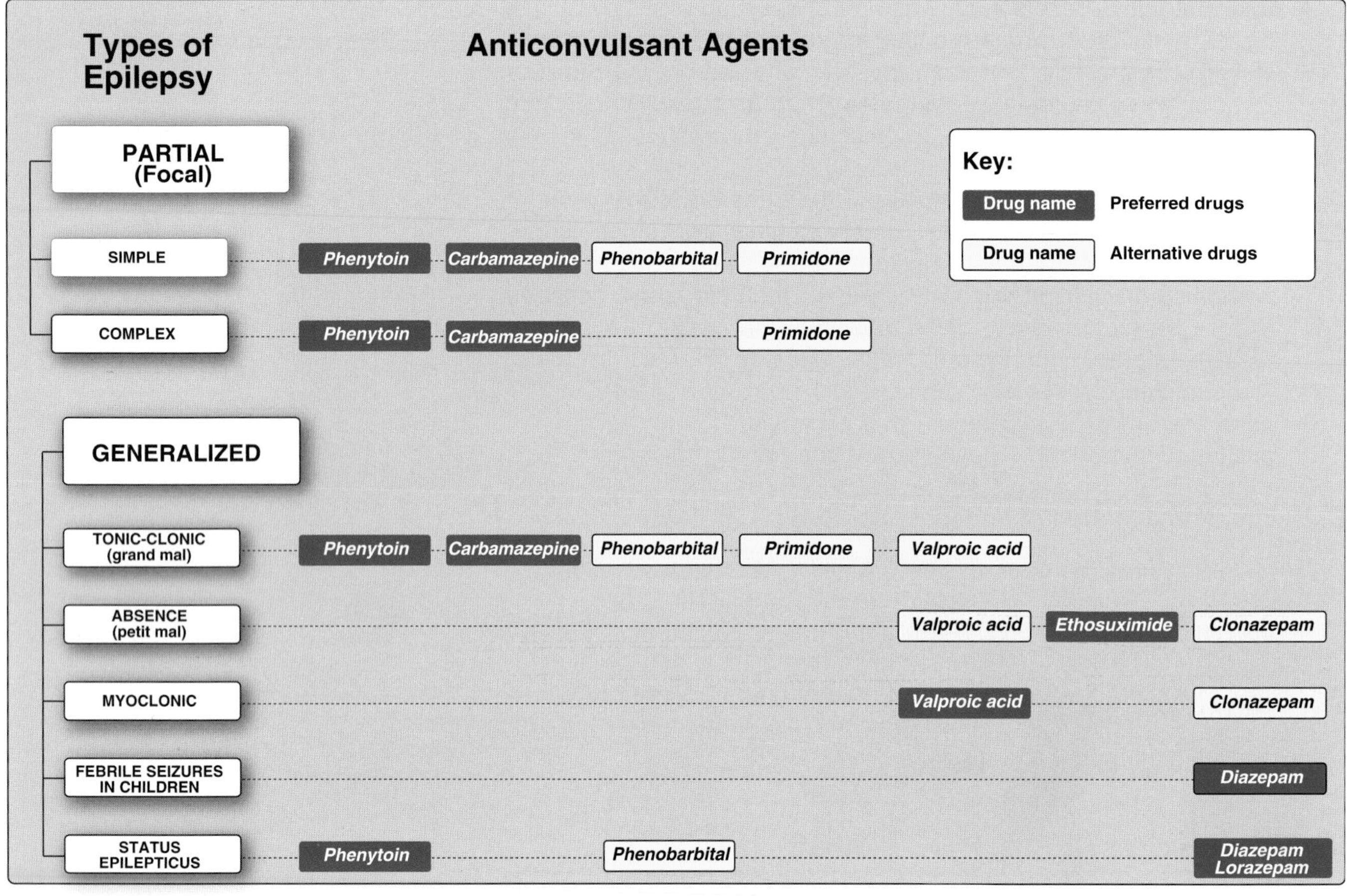

Figure 15.5
Therapeutic indications for the primary anticonvulsant agents.

1. **Mechanism of action:** *Phenytoin* blocks voltage-gated sodium channels by selectively binding to the channel in the inactive state and slowing its rate of recovery. Thus, depolarized and frequently firing neurons are particularly sensitive to the blockade. At much higher concentrations, *phenytoin* can block voltage-dependent calcium channels and interfere with the release of monoaminergic neurotransmitters.

2. **Actions:** *Phenytoin* is not a generalized CNS depressant like the barbiturates, but it does produce some degree of drowsiness and lethargy without progression to hypnosis. *Phenytoin* reduces the propagation of abnormal impulses in the brain.

3. **Therapeutic uses:** *Phenytoin* is highly effective for all partial seizures (simple and complex), for tonic-clonic seizures, and in the treatment of status epilepticus caused by recurrent tonic-clonic seizures (see Figure 15.5). *Phenytoin* is not effective for absence seizures, which often may worsen if treated with this drug.

4. **Absorption and fate:** Oral absorption of *phenytoin* is slow, but once it occurs, distribution is rapid and brain concentrations are high. Chronic administration of *phenytoin* is always oral. In status epilepticus, it should be given intravenously in the form of *fosphenytoin*, a prodrug of *phenytoin*. [Note: The trade name of *fosphenytoin* is Cerebyx, which is easily confused with Celebrex, the cyclooxygenase-2 inhibitor, and Celexa, the antidepressant.] The drug is largely bound to plasma albumin. Less than five percent of a given dose is excreted unchanged in the urine. *Phenytoin* is metabolized by the hepatic cytochrome P450 system to an inactive metabolite. At low doses, the drug has a half-life of 24 hours, but as the dosage increases, the hydroxylation system becomes saturated. Thus, relatively small increases in each dose can produce large increases in the plasma concentration, resulting in drug-induced toxicity (Figure 15.6). Furthermore, large genetic variations in the rate of the drug's metabolism occur.

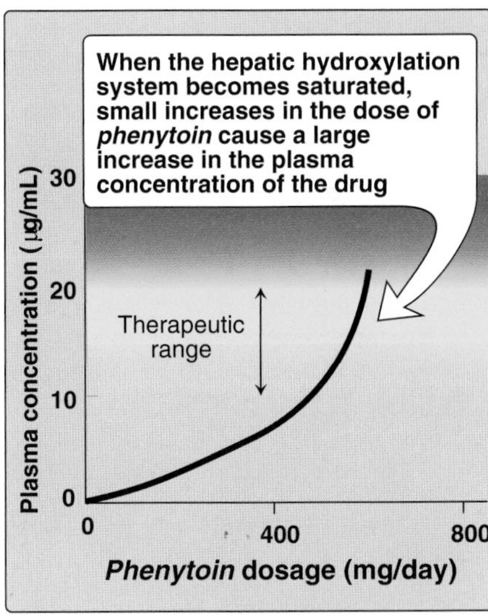

Figure 15.6
Nonlinear effect of *phenytoin* dosage on the plasma concentration of the drug.

5. **Adverse effects:** Depression of the CNS occurs particularly in the cerebellum and vestibular system, causing nystagmus and ataxia. Gastrointestinal problems (nausea and vomiting) are common. Gingival hyperplasia may cause the gums to grow over the teeth, particularly in children. This hyperplasia slowly regresses after termination of drug therapy. Coarsening of facial features occurs in children. Megaloblastic anemia occurs, because the drug interferes with reactions for which vitamin B_{12} is a cofactor. Behavioral changes, such as confusion, hallucination, and drowsiness, are common. Inhibition of antidiuretic hormone release occurs as well as hyperglycemia and glycosuria caused by inhibition of insulin secretion. *Phenytoin* is also an antiarrhythmic drug. Treatment with *phenytoin* should not be stopped abruptly.

6. **Teratogenic effects:** *Phenytoin* causes teratogenic effects in the offspring of mothers who are given the drug during pregnancy. "Fetal hydantoin syndrome" includes cleft lip, cleft palate, and congenital heart disease, as well as slowed growth and mental deficiency. Almost half of untreated epileptic women have an increased seizure frequency during pregnancy. These seizures can lead to anoxic episodes, which yield a higher incidence of congenital birth defects. Antiepileptic drugs are given at the lowest possible dose to control seizures.

7. **Drug interactions:**

   a. **Drugs that affect phenytoin metabolism:** Inhibition of the microsomal metabolism of *phenytoin* in the liver is caused by *chloramphenicol*, *dicumarol*, *cimetidine*, *sulfonamides*, and *isoniazid*. When used chronically, these drugs increase the concentration of *phenytoin* in plasma by preventing its metabolism. In contrast, *phenytoin* metabolism is enhanced by *carbamazepine*, resulting in a decrease in the plasma concentration of *phenytoin* (Figure 15.7).

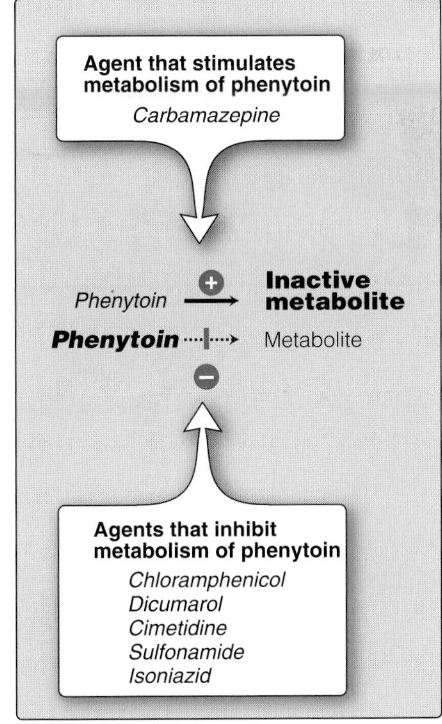

Figure 15.7
Drugs affecting the metabolism of *phenytoin*.

b. **Increased metabolism of other drugs caused by phenytoin:** *Phenytoin* induces the cytochrome P450 system, which leads to an increase in the metabolism of other antiepileptics, anticoagulants, oral contraceptives, *quinidine*, *doxycycline*, *cyclosporine*, *mexiletine*, *methadone*, and *levodopa*.

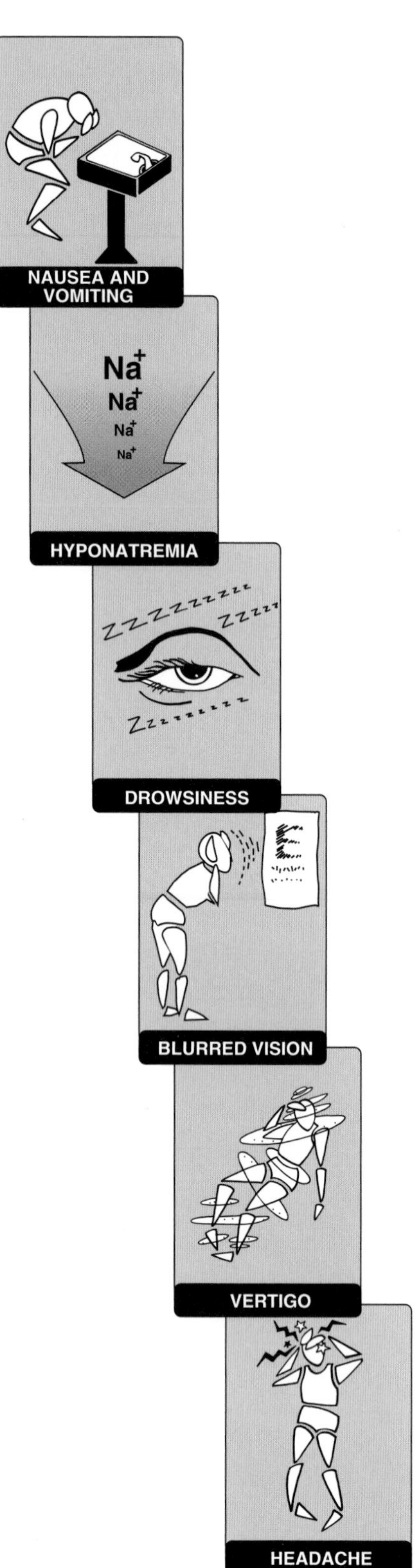

Figure 15.8
Some adverse effects of *carbamazepine* and *oxcarbazepine*.

B. Carbamazepine

1. **Actions:** *Carbamazepine* [kar ba MAZ a peen] reduces the propagation of abnormal impulses in the brain by blocking sodium channels, thereby inhibiting the generation of repetitive action potentials in the epileptic focus and preventing their spread.

2. **Therapeutic uses:** *Carbamazepine* is highly effective for all partial seizures (simple and complex) and is often the drug of first choice. In addition, the drug is highly effective for tonic-clonic seizures and is used to treat trigeminal neuralgia. It has occasionally been used in manic-depressive patients to ameliorate the symptoms.

3. **Absorption and fate:** *Carbamazepine* is absorbed slowly following oral administration. It enters the brain rapidly because of its high lipid solubility. *Carbamazepine* induces the drug metabolizing enzymes in the liver, and its half-life therefore decreases with chronic administration, requiring dosage adjustments during initiation of therapy. The enhanced hepatic cytochrome P450 system activity also increases the metabolism of many drugs including other antiepileptic drugs. *Carbamazepine* is an inducer of the cytochrome P450 isozyme CYP3A4, which decrease the effects of drugs that are metabolized by this enzyme.

4. **Adverse effects:** Chronic administration of *carbamazepine* can cause stupor, coma, and respiratory depression, along with drowsiness, vertigo, ataxia, blurred vision, and a characteristic rash (Figure 15.8). The drug is irritating to the stomach, and nausea and vomiting may occur. The 10,11-epoxide metabolite of the drug has been implicated in causing blood dyscrasias, including leukopenia and aplastic anemia, as well as inducing serious liver toxicity. Therefore, anyone being treated with *carbamazepine* should have frequent blood and liver function tests. Hyponatremia may occur, particularly in the elderly.

5. **Drug interactions:** The hepatic metabolism of *carbamazepine* is inhibited by several drugs (Figure 15.9). Toxic symptoms may arise if the dose is not adjusted.

C. Oxcarbazepine

Oxcarbazepine [ox car BAH e peen] is the 10-keto derivative of *carbamazepine*. In humans, *oxcarbazepine* depends on rapid reduction to the 10-monohydroxy metabolite for its anticonvulsant activity. Like *carbamazepine*, this active metabolite blocks sodium channels preventing the spread of the abnormal discharge. Its anticonvulsant spectrum and CNS toxicities are similar to that of *carbamazepine*. Hyponatremia may occur. There have been no reports of hepatic failure or bone marrow disorders. *Oxcarbazepine* is a less potent inducer of drug-metabolizing enzymes compared to *carbamazepine*, but reduced effectiveness of oral contraceptives has been reported.

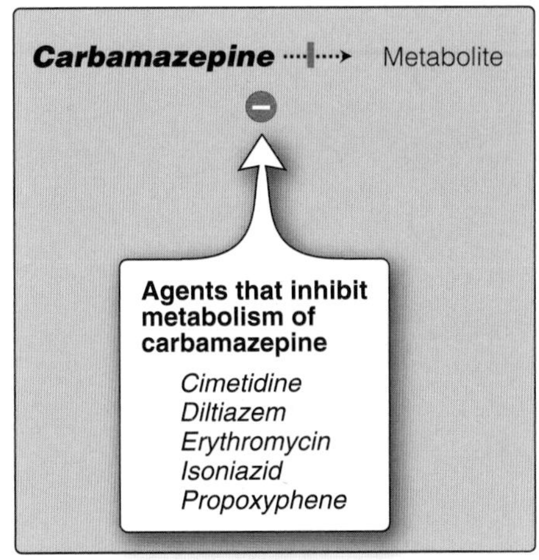

Figure 15.9
Drugs affecting the metabolism of *carbamazepine*.

D. Phenobarbital

1. **Actions:** *Phenobarbital* has antiepileptic activity, limiting the spread of seizure discharges in the brain and elevating the seizure threshold. Its mechanism of action is unknown, but may involve potentiation of the inhibitory effects of γ-aminobutyric acid (GABA)-mediated neurons. Doses required for antiepileptic action are lower than those that cause pronounced CNS depression.

2. **Therapeutic uses:** *Phenobarbital* provides a fifty-percent favorable response rate for simple partial seizures, but it is not very effective for complex partial seizures. The drug had been regarded as the first choice in treating recurrent seizures in children, including febrile seizures, although *diazepam* is also effective. Prophylaxis of infantile febrile seizures is no longer recommended. *Phenobarbital* is also used to treat recurrent tonic-clonic seizures, especially in patients who do not respond to *diazepam* plus *phenytoin*. *Phenobarbital* is also used as a mild sedative to relieve anxiety, nervous tension, and insomnia, although benzodiazepines are superior.

3. **Absorption and fate:** *Phenobarbital* is well absorbed orally. The drug freely penetrates the brain. Approximately 75 percent of the drug is inactivated by the hepatic microsomal system, whereas the remaining drug is excreted unchanged by the kidney. *Phenobarbital* is a potent inducer of the cytochrome P450 system, and when given chronically, it enhances the metabolism of other agents.

4. **Adverse effects:** Sedation, ataxia, nystagmus, vertigo, and acute psychotic reactions may occur with chronic use. Nausea and vomiting are seen as well as a morbilliform rash in sensitive individuals. Agitation and confusion occur at high doses. Rebound seizures can occur on discontinuance of *phenobarbital*.

E. Primidone

Primidone [PRIM i done] is structurally related to *phenobarbital*, and it resembles *phenobarbital* in its anticonvulsant activity. *Primidone* is an alternative choice in partial seizures and tonic-clonic seizures. Much of the efficacy of *primidone* comes from its metabolites *phenobarbital* and phenylethylmalonamide, which have longer half-lives than the parent drug. *Phenobarbital* is effective against tonic-clonic and simple partial seizures, and phenylethylmalonamide is effective against complex partial seizures. *Primidone* is often used with *carbamazepine* and *phenytoin*, allowing smaller doses of these agents to be used. It is ineffective in absence seizures (see Figure 15.5). *Primidone* is well absorbed orally. It exhibits poor protein binding. This drug has the same adverse effects as those seen with *phenobarbital*.

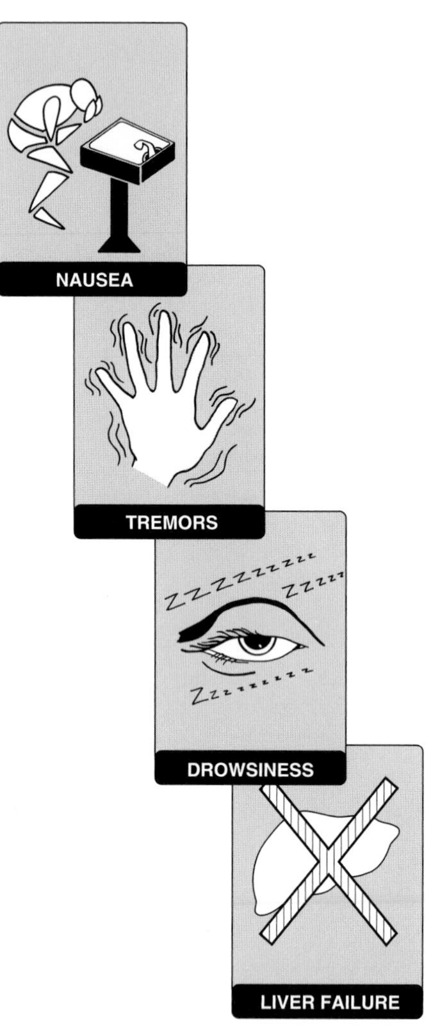

Figure 15.10
Some adverse effects of *valproic acid.*

F. Valproic acid

Valproic acid [val PROE ic] has multiple actions, including sodium-channel blockade and enhancement of GABAergic transmission. *Valproic acid* is a broad-spectrum anticonvulsant. It is the most effective agent available for treatment of myoclonic seizures. It also diminishes absence seizures, but because of its hepatotoxic potential, it is a second choice. *Valproic acid* also reduces the incidence and severity of tonic-clonic seizures (see Figure 15.5). The drug is effective orally and is rapidly absorbed. About ninety percent is bound to plasma proteins. Only three percent of the drug is excreted unchanged; the rest is converted to active metabolites by the liver. *Valproic acid* is metabolized by the cytochrome P450 system, but it does not induce P450 enzyme synthesis. The glucuronylated metabolites are excreted in the urine. *Valproic acid* can cause nausea and vomiting, and sedation, ataxia, and tremor are common (Figure 15.10). Rare hepatic toxicity may cause a rise in hepatic enzymes in plasma, which should be monitored frequently. In some individuals, a rash and alopecia may occur. Bleeding times may increase because of both thrombocytopenia and an inhibition of platelet aggregation. *Valproic acid* inhibits the metabolism of a number of antiepileptic drugs, including *phenobarbital*, *carbamazepine*, and *ethosuximide.*

G. Ethosuximide

Ethosuximide [eth oh SUX i mide] reduces propagation of abnormal electrical activity in the brain, most likely by inhibiting T-type calcium channels in a manner similar to the action of *phenytoin* on sodium channels. It is the first choice in absence seizures (see Figure 15.5). *Ethosuximide* is well absorbed orally and is not bound to plasma proteins. About 25 percent of the drug is excreted unchanged in the urine, and 75 percent is converted to inactive metabolites in the liver by the microsomal cytochrome P450 system. *Ethosuximide* does not induce P450 enzyme synthesis. The drug is irritating to the stomach, and nausea and vomiting may occur on chronic administration. Drowsiness, lethargy, dizziness, restlessness, agitation, anxiety, and the inability to concentrate are often observed. In sensitive individuals, a Stevens-Johnson syndrome or urticaria may occur, as well as leukopenia, aplastic anemia, and thrombocytopenia.

H. Benzodiazepines

Several of the benzodiazepines show antiepileptic activity. *Clonazepam* and *clorazepate* are used for chronic treatment, whereas *diazepam* and *lorazepam* are the drugs of choice in the acute treatment of status epilepticus. *Clonazepam* suppresses seizure spread from the epileptogenic focus and is effective in absence and myoclonic seizures (see Figure 15.5), but tolerance develops. *Clorazepate* is effective in partial seizures when used in conjunction with other drugs. *Diazepam* and *lorazepam* are both effective in interrupting the repetitive seizures of status epilepticus. *Lorazepam* has a longer duration of action and is preferred by some clinicians. Of all the antiepileptics, the benzodiazepines are the safest and most free from severe side effects. All benzodiazepines have sedative properties. Thus, drowsiness, somnolence, and fatigue can occur with higher dosage, as can ataxia, dizziness, and behavioral changes. Respiratory depression and cardiac depression may occur when given intravenously in acute situations.

III. ADJUNCT ANTIEPILEPTIC DRUGS

The following antiepileptic drugs have been developed over the last decade. All have demonstrated efficacy as add-on therapy in refractory epilepsies. Several of them are also effective as monotherapies. [Note: Most experts prefer to start therapy with a conventional or primary antiepilepsy drug but move quickly to a newer agent if necessary.] A number of the drugs have actions on the GABA-receptor complex or on glutamate-receptor complexes.

A. Felbamate

Felbamate [FEL ba mate] has a broad spectrum of anticonvulsant action. However, it is reserved for use in refractory epilepsies (particularly Lennox-Gestaut) because of the risk of aplastic anemia (about 1:4,000) and hepatic failure. *Felbamate* owes its broad spectrum of activity to its ability to 1) block voltage-dependent sodium channels, 2) compete with the glycine-coagonist binding site on the N-methyl-D-aspartate (NMDA) glutamate receptor, 3) prevent seizures induced by α-amino-3-hydroxy-5-methyl-4-isoxazolepropionic acid (AMPA) glutamate receptor stimulation, and 4) block calcium channels. Approximately half the administered dose appears in the urine as metabolites. Enzyme inducers, such as *carbamazepine* and *phenytoin*, may decrease the level of *felbamate*. One of the metabolites, an α,β-unsaturated aldehyde, 2-phenylpropenal, is chemically reactive, like acrolein, covalently linking proteins as well as DNA. It can cause liver and bone marrow toxicities. In most individuals, the aldehyde is conjugated with glutathione, but a small percentage of patients may become glutathione-depleted, allowing accumulation of the reactive metabolite.

B. Gabapentin

Gabapentin [GA ba pen tin] is an analog of GABA. Its precise mechanism of action is not known, although it may interfere with voltage-dependent calcium channels. [Note: It does not react at GABA receptors.] It is approved as adjunct therapy for partial seizures and secondary generalized tonic-clonic seizures. *Gabapentin* exhibits dose-dependent oral absorption, probably because it requires a saturable transport system for its uptake from the gut. *Gabapentin* does not bind to plasma proteins and is excreted unchanged through the kidneys. These properties minimize the potential for drug interactions, and explain the attractiveness of *gabapentin* as an adjunct drug for seizure control. Adverse effects are those that are common to anticonvulsant medications, including somnolence, dizziness, ataxia, nystagmus, and headache. There is a very low incidence of serious toxic reactions. *Gabapentin* has also been shown to alleviate both diabetic neuropathic pain and postherpetic pain.

C. Lamotrigine

Lamotrigine [la MOE tri jeen] blocks sodium channels as well as high voltage-dependent calcium channels. *Lamotrigine* is effective in a wide variety of seizure disorders, including partial seizures, generalized seizures, typical absence seizures, and the Lennox-Gestaut syndrome. It is approved as adjunctive therapy in children and adults and as monotherapy in adults. Oral absorption is nearly 100 percent and is not altered by meals. *Lamotrigine* is metabolized primarily to the N-2 glucuronide, and the parent drug and its metabolite are excreted in the urine. The half-life of *lamotrigine* (24–35 hours) is decreased by enzyme-inducing drugs (for example, *carbamazepine* and *phenytoin*) and increased by *valproic acid*. Adverse effects of *lamotrigine* include headache, dizziness, and ataxia. *Lamotrigine* also causes a rash, which in some patients may progress to a serious, life-threatening reaction. Because this risk is greater in children (younger than sixteen years), *lamotrigine* should only be used for Lennox-Gestaut syndrome in this age group.

D. Levetiracetam

Levetiracetam [lee ve tye RA se tam] is approved for adjunctive therapy of refractory partial seizures. Its mechanism of anticonvulsant action is unknown. The drug is well absorbed orally, and excretion is urinary, with most of the drug (66 percent) being unchanged. *Levetiracetam* is remarkably free of pharmacokinetic drug interactions, which makes it a good choice for adjunctive therapy. Side effects include dizziness, sleep disturbances, headache, and asthenia.

E. Tiagabine

Tiagabine [ty AG a been] blocks GABA uptake into presynaptic neurons, permitting more GABA to be available for receptor binding, thus causing enhanced inhibitory activity. In clinical trials, *tiagabine* is effective in decreasing the number of seizures in refractory patients with focal epileptic disorders. *Tiagabine* is well absorbed orally (its bioavailability is ninety percent), although food slows the rate, but not the extent, of absorption. Binding to plasma proteins is 95 percent, but it is not displaced by or displace *phenytoin*, *carbamazepine*, or *phenobarbital*. *Tiagabine* undergoes two major modifications, namely oxidation of the thiophene ring and glucuronylation. Only two percent is excreted unchanged. The majority of the excretion is biliary (65 percent), with some urinary excretion (25 percent). The half-life in healthy volunteers is seven to nine hours, which may be decreased in half by enzyme inducers. Decreased maintenance doses may be necessary in individuals with hepatic impairment. Adverse effects include tiredness, dizziness, and gastrointestinal upset.

F. Topiramate

Like many of the antiepileptic drugs, *topiramate* [toe PEER a mate] possesses several actions at therapeutic concentrations that contribute to its anticonvulsant activity. *Topiramate* blocks voltage-dependent, use-dependent sodium channels, much like the actions of *phenytoin* and *carbamazepine*. Additionally, *topiramate* has been shown to increase the frequency of chloride channel opening by binding to the GABA receptor. Evidence to date indicates that the binding site is distinct from the benzodiazepine site. High-voltage calcium currents (L type) are reduced by *topiramate*. Some evidence suggests *topiramate* binds to phosphorylation sites and prevents phosphorylation of a variety of proteins, including the antiepileptic targets. This delays channel conductance and may represent a unifying mechanism for its many effects. *Topiramate* is effective in both refractory partial seizures and secondary generalized seizures.

1. **Pharmacokinetics:** *Topiramate* is well absorbed, with an oral bioavailability of nearly 100 percent. Peak concentrations occur in about two hours. Some thirty percent of each dose is metabolized, with the remainder being excreted unchanged in the urine. The half-life of *topiramate* is about 20 to 25 hours.

2. **Adverse effects:** These are primarily CNS and gastrointestinal disturbances. They include impaired concentration, dizziness, ataxia, diplopia, somnolence, nervousness, and confusion, as well as nausea and weight loss. Renal stones have been reported in 1.5 percent of patients. There is a small risk of glaucoma. *Topiramate* is teratogenic in animals and should be avoided during pregnancy. Inducers of drug metabolism, such as *phenytoin* and *carbamazepine*, decrease *topiramate* serum concentrations by approximately fifty percent. *Topiramate* decreases the *ethinyl estradiol* concentration of oral contraceptive preparations, and individuals using these drugs should therefore supplement the amount of *ethinyl estradiol*.

G. Zonisamide

Zonisamide [zoe NIS a mide] is a sulfonamide derivative with antiseizure activity against both focal and generalized seizures. This broad spectrum of action resides in the compound's effects on multiple neuronal systems involved in seizure generation. These include the block of both voltage-gated sodium channels and T-type calcium currents as well as enhancement of GABA-receptor function. Like most sulfonamides, *zonisamide* is orally active and is well distributed throughout the body. It has a long half-life (50–60 hours) that may be shortened to from 25 to 30 hours if enzyme inducers are given concurrently. The parent compound (thirty percent), its N-acetyl metabolite (twenty percent), and its glucuronide (fifty percent) are excreted in the urine. Aside from the typical CNS adverse effects, *zonisamide* may cause kidney stones. Oligohidrosis has been reported in children; therefore, they should be monitored for increased body temperature and decreased sweating, particularly during the summer months.

Figure 15.11 sumarizes the therapeutic advantages and disadvantages of some of the antiepileptic drugs.

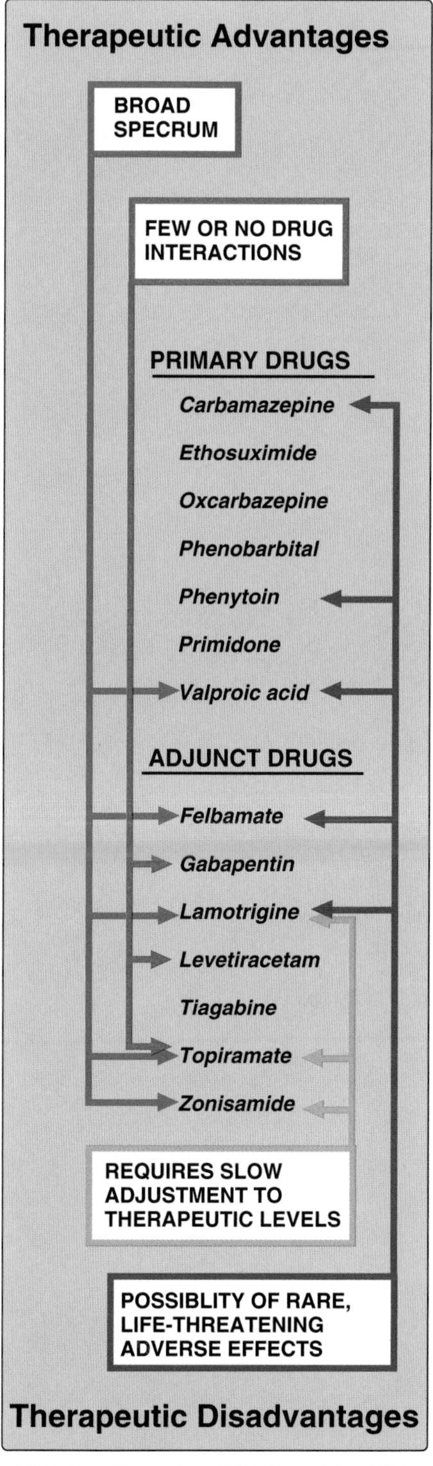

Figure 15.11
Summary of therapeutic advantages and disadvantages of some antiepileptic drugs.

Study Questions

Choose the ONE best answer.

15.1 A nine-year-old boy is sent for neurologic evaluation because of episodes of "confusion." Over the past year, the child has experienced episodes during which he develops a blank look on his face and fails to respond to questions. However, it appears to take several minutes before the boy recovers from the episodes. Which one the following best describes this patient's seizures?

A. Simple partial
B. Complex partial
C. Tonic-clonic
D. Absence
E. Myoclonic

Correct answer = B. The patient is exhibiting episodes of complex partial seizures. Complex partial seizures impair consciousness. and can occur in all age groups. Typically, staring is accompanied by impaired consciousness, and recall. If asked a question, the patient might respond with an inappropriate or unintelligible answer. Automatic movements are associated with most complex partial seizures and involve the mouth and face (lipsmacking, chewing, tasting, and swallowing movements), upper extremities (fumbling, picking, tapping, or clasping movements), vocal apparatus (grunts or repetition of words or phrases), or more complex acts (such as walking or mixing foods in a bowl), although subtle lateralizing signs (such as an asymmetric smile) may be present.

15.2 Which one of the following therapies would be most appropriate in the patient described in the above question?

A. Ethosuximide
B. Carbamazepine
C. Diazepam
D. Carbamazepine plus primidone
E. Watchful waiting

Correct answer = B. The patient has had many seizures, and the risks of not starting drug therapy would be substantially greater than the risks of treating his seizures. Because the child has impaired consciousness during the seizure, he is at substantial risk for injury during an attack. Monotherapy with primary agents is preferred for most patients. The advantages of monotherapy include reduced frequency of adverse effects, absence of interactions between antiepileptic drugs, lower cost, and improved compliance. Ethosuximide and diazepam are not indicated for complex partial sezures.

15.3 The patient described in question 15.1 was treated for six months with carbamazepine but, recently, has been experiencing breakthrough seizures on a more frequent basis. You are considering adding a second drug to this patient's antiseizure regimen. Which of the following drugs is least likely to have a pharmacokinetic interaction with carbamazepine?

A. Topiramate
B. Tiagabine
C. Levetiracetam
D. Lamotrigine
E. Zonisamide

Correct answer = C. Of the drugs listed, all of which are approved as adjunctive therapy for refractory complex partial seizures, only levetiracetam does not affect the pharmacokinetics of other antiepileptic drugs, and neither are its pharmacokinetic properties significantly altered by other drugs.

UNIT IV: Drugs Affecting the Cardiovascular System

Treatment of Heart Failure

16

I. OVERVIEW

Heart failure (HF) is a complex, progressive disorder in which the heart is unable to pump sufficient blood to meet the needs of the body. Its cardinal symptoms are dyspnea, fatigue, and fluid retention. HF is due to an impaired ability of the heart to adequately fill with or eject, blood. HF is often accompanied by abnormal increases in blood volume and interstitial fluid, hence the term "congestive" HF, because symptoms include dyspnea from pulmonary congestion in left HF, and peripheral edema in right HF. Underlying causes of HF include arteriosclerotic heart disease, mycardial infarction, hypertensive heart disease, valvular heart disease, dilated cardiomyopathy, and congenital heart disease. Left systolic dysfunction secondary to coronary artery disease is the most common cause of HF, accounting for nearly seventy percent of all cases. The number of newly diagnosed patients with HF is increasing, because more individuals now survive acute myocardial infarction.

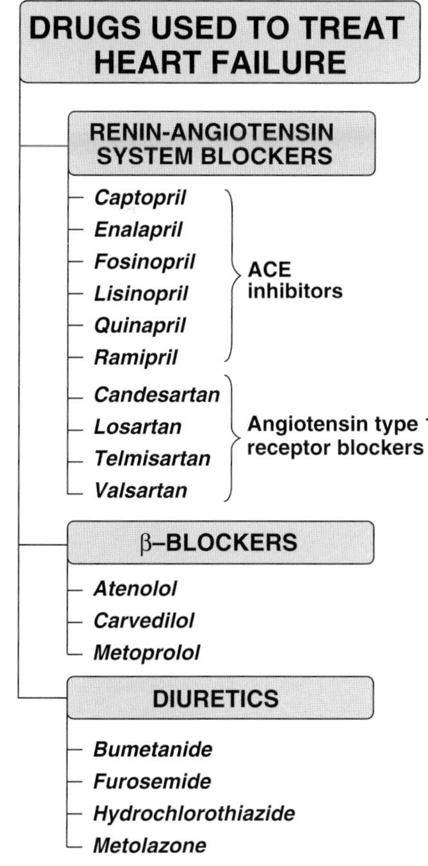

Figure 16.1
Summary of drugs used to treat heart failure. ACE = angiotensin-converting enzyme. (Continued on the next page.)

A. Role of physiologic compensatory mechanisms in the progression of HF

Chronic activation of the sympathetic nervous system and the renin-angiotensin-aldosterone axis is associated with remodeling of cardiac tissue, characterized by loss of myocytes, hypertrophy, and fibrosis. The geometry of the heart becomes more spherical, interfering with its ability to efficiently function as a pump. This prompts additional neurohumoral activation, creating a vicious cycle that, if left untreated, leads to death.

B. Goals of pharmacologic intervention in HF

The goals are to alleviate symptoms, slow disease progression, and improve survival. Accordingly, six classes of drugs have been shown to be effective: 1) inhibitors of the renin-angiotensin system, 2) β-adrenoreceptor blockers, 3) diuretics, 4) inotropic agents, 5) direct

Lippincott's Illustrated Reviews: Pharmacology, Third Edition,
by Richard D. Howland and Mary J. Mycek.

DRUGS USED TO TREAT HEART FAILURE

- **DIRECT VASODILATORS**
  - *Hydralazine*
  - *Isosorbide dinitrate*
  - *Sodium nitroprusside*
- **INOTROPIC AGENTS**
  - *Amrinone*
  - *Digitoxin*
  - *Digoxin*
  - *Dobutamine*
  - *Milrinone*
- **ALDOSTERONE ANTAGONISTS**
  - *Spironolactone*

Figure 16.1 (continued)
Summary of drugs used to treat heart failure.

vasodilators, and 6) aldosterone antagonists (Figure 16.1). Depending on the severity of cardiac failure and individual patient factors, one or more of these classes of drugs are administered. Beneficial effects of pharmacologic intervention include reduction of the load on the myocardium, decreased extracellular fluid volume, improved cardiac contractility, and slowing of the rate of cardiac remodeling. Knowledge of the physiology of cardiac muscle contraction is essential to an understanding of the compensatory responses evoked by the failing heart, as well as the actions of drugs used to treat HF.

II. PHYSIOLOGY OF MUSCLE CONTRACTION

The myocardium, like smooth and skeletal muscle, responds to stimulation by depolarization of the membrane, which is followed by shortening of the contractile proteins and ends with relaxation and return to the resting state. However, unlike skeletal muscle, which shows graded contractions depending on the number of muscle cells that are stimulated, the cardiac muscle cells are interconnected in groups that respond to stimuli as a unit, contracting together whenever a single cell is stimulated.

A. Action potential

Cardiac muscle cells are electrically excitable. However, unlike the cells of other muscles and nerves, the cells of cardiac muscle show a spontaneous, intrinsic rhythm generated by specialized "pacemaker" cells located in the sinoatrial and atrioventricular nodes. The cardiac cells also have an unusually long action potential, which can be divided into five phases (0–4). Figure 16.2 illustrates the major ions contributing to depolarization and polarization of cardiac cells. These ions pass through channels in the sarcolemmal membrane and, thus, create a current. The channels open and close at different times during the action potential. Some respond primarily to changes in ion concentration, whereas others are either adenosine triphosphate (ATP)– or voltage–sensitive.

B. Cardiac contraction

The contractile machinery of the myocardial cell is essentially the same as that in striated muscle. The force of contraction of the cardiac muscle is directly related to the concentration of free (unbound) cytosolic calcium. Therefore, agents that increase these calcium levels (or that increase the sensitivity of the contractile machinery to calcium) result in an increased force of contraction (inotropic effect). [Note: The inotropic agents increase the contractility of the heart by directly or indirectly altering the mechanisms that control the concentration of intracellular calcium.]

1. **Sources of free intracellular calcium:** Calcium comes from two sources. The first is from outside the cell, where opening of voltage-sensitive calcium channels causes an immediate rise in free cytosolic calcium. The second is the release of calcium from the sarcoplasmic reticulum and mitochondria, which further increases the cytosolic level of calcium (Figure 16.3).

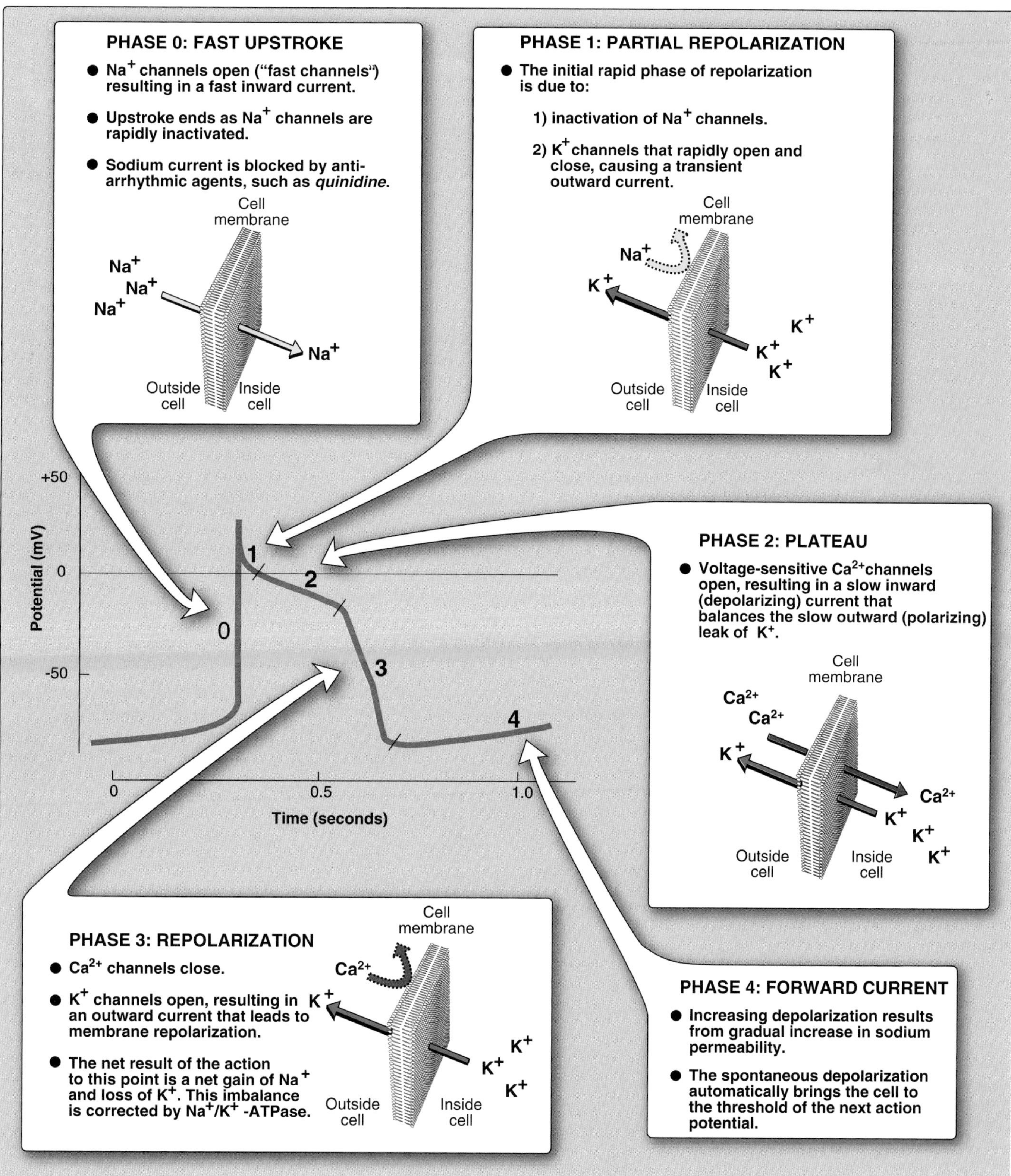
PHASE 0: FAST UPSTROKE
● Na+ channels open ("fast channels") resulting in a fast inward current.
● Upstroke ends as Na+ channels are rapidly inactivated.
● Sodium current is blocked by anti-arrhythmic agents, such as *quinidine*.
Cell membrane
Na+
Na+
Na+
Na+
Outside cell
Inside cell
PHASE 1: PARTIAL REPOLARIZATION
● The initial rapid phase of repolarization is due to:
1) inactivation of Na+ channels.
2) K+ channels that rapidly open and close, causing a transient outward current.
Cell membrane
Na+
K+
K+
K+
K+
Outside cell
Inside cell
+50
0
-50
Potential (mV)
0
1
2
3
4
0
0.5
1.0
Time (seconds)
PHASE 2: PLATEAU
● Voltage-sensitive Ca2+ channels open, resulting in a slow inward (depolarizing) current that balances the slow outward (polarizing) leak of K+.
Cell membrane
Ca2+
Ca2+
K+
Ca2+
K+
K+
K+
Outside cell
Inside cell
PHASE 3: REPOLARIZATION
● Ca2+ channels close.
● K+ channels open, resulting in an outward current that leads to membrane repolarization.
● The net result of the action to this point is a net gain of Na+ and loss of K+. This imbalance is corrected by Na+/K+ -ATPase.
Cell membrane
Ca2+
K+
K+
K+
K+
Outside cell
Inside cell
PHASE 4: FORWARD CURRENT
● Increasing depolarization results from gradual increase in sodium permeability.
● The spontaneous depolarization automatically brings the cell to the threshold of the next action potential.

Figure 16.2
Action potential of a Purkinje fiber. ATPase = adenosine triphosphatase.

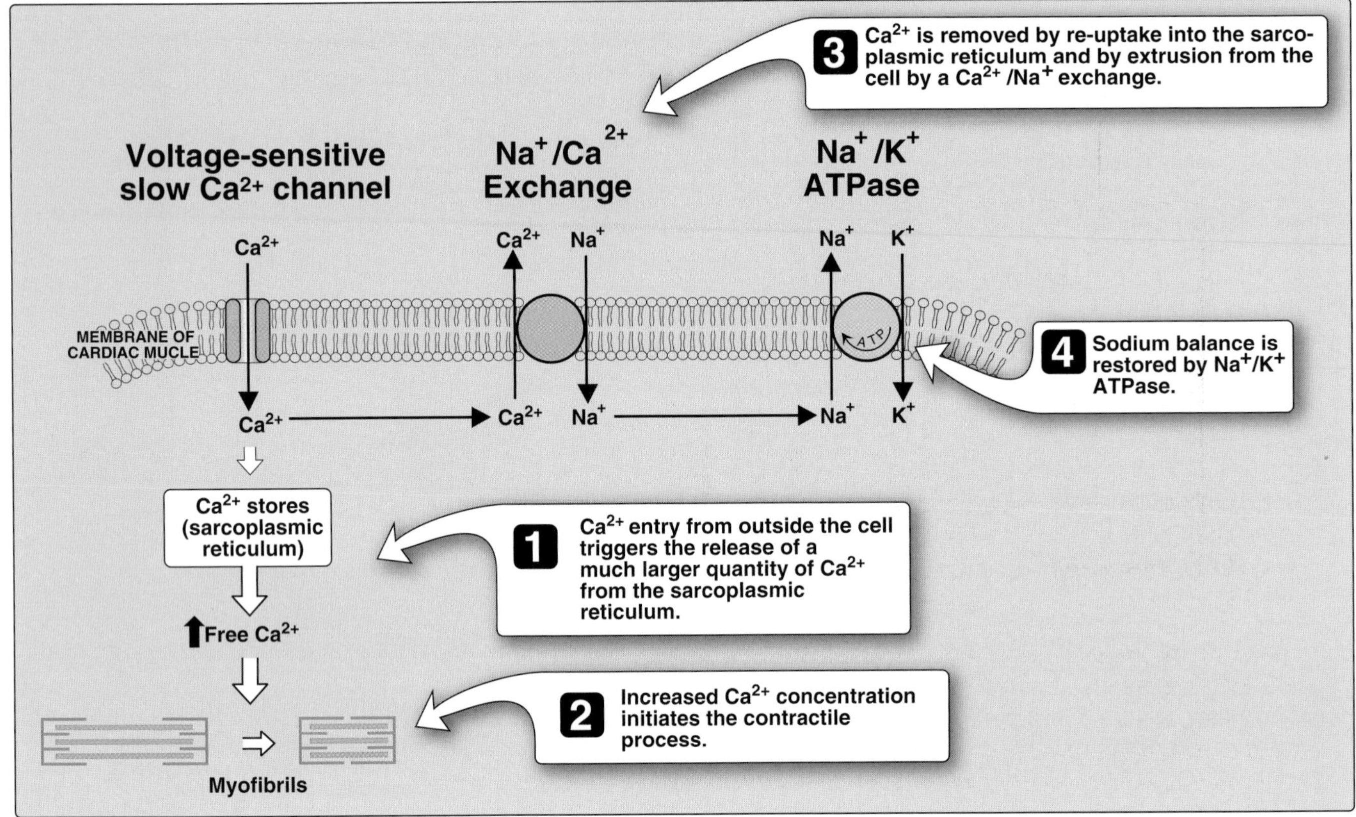

Figure 16.3
Ion movements during the contraction of cardiac muscle. ATPase = adenosine triphosphatase.

2. **Removal of free cytosolic calcium:** If free cytosolic calcium levels were to remain high the cardiac muscle would be in a constant state of contraction, rather than showing a periodic contraction. Mechanisms of removal include two alternatives.

   a. **Sodium-calcium exchange:** Calcium is removed by a sodium/calcium-exchange reaction that reversibly exchanges calcium ions for sodium ions across the cell membrane (see Figure 16.3). This interaction between the movement of calcium and sodium ions is significant, because changes in intracellular sodium can affect cellular levels of calcium.

   b. **Uptake of calcium by the sarcoplasmic reticulum and mitochondria:** Calcium is also recaptured by the sarcoplasmic reticulum and the mitochondria. More than 99 percent of the intracellular calcium is located in these organelles, and even a modest shift between these stores and free calcium can lead to large changes in the concentration of free cytosolic calcium.

C. Compensatory physiological responses in HF

The failing heart evokes three major compensatory mechanisms to enhance cardiac output (Figure 16.4). Although initially beneficial, these alterations ultimately result in further deterioration of cardiac function.

1. **Increased sympathetic activity:** Baroreceptors sense a decrease in blood pressure, and activate the sympathetic nervous system, which stimulates β-adrenergic receptors in the heart. This results in an increased heart rate and a greater force of contraction of the heart muscle (see Figure 16.4). In addition, vasoconstriction (α_1-mediated) enhances venous return and increases cardiac preload. These compensatory responses increase the work of the heart and, therefore, can contribute to further decline in cardiac function.

2. **Activation of the renin-angiotensin system:** A fall in cardiac output decreases blood flow to the kidney, prompting the release of renin, with a resulting increase in the formation of angiotensin II and release of aldosterone. This results in increased peripheral resistance and retention of sodium and water. Blood volume increases, and more blood is returned to the heart. If the heart is unable to pump this extra volume, venous pressure increases and peripheral edema and pulmonary edema occur (see Figure 16.4). These compensatory responses increase the work of the heart and, therefore, can contribute to further decline in cardiac function.

3. **Myocardial hypertrophy:** The heart increases in size, and the chambers dilate and become more globular. Initially, stretching of the heart muscle leads to a stronger contraction of the heart. However, excessive elongation of the fibers results in weaker contractions, and the geometry diminishes the ability to eject blood. This type of failure is termed systolic failure and is the result of a ventricle being unable to pump effectively. Less commonly, patients with HF may have diastolic dysfunction—a term applied when the ability of the ventricles to relax and accept blood is impaired by structural changes, such as hypertrophy. The thickening of the ventricular wall and subsequent decrease in ventricular volume decreases the ability of heart muscle to relax. In this case, the ventricle does not fill adequately, and the inadequacy of cardiac output is termed diastolic HF—a particularly common feature of HF in elderly women.

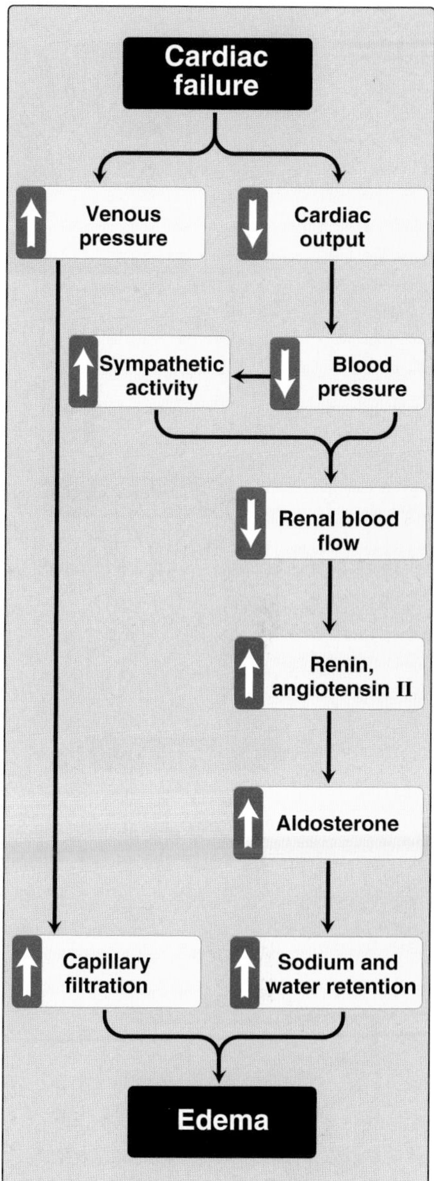

Figure 16.4
Cardiovascular consequences of heart failure.

D. Decompensated HF

If the mechanisms listed above adequately restore cardiac output, the HF is said to be compensated. However, these compensations increase the work of the heart and contribute to further decline in cardiac performance. If the adaptive mechanisms fail to maintain cardiac output, the HF is termed decompensated.

E. Therapeutic strategies in HF

Chronic HF is typically managed by a reduction in physical activity, low dietary intake of sodium (<1500 mg/day), treatment of comorbid conditions, and judicious use of diuretics, inhibitors of the renin-angiotensin system, and inotropic agents. Drugs that may precipitate or exacerbate HF, such as nonsteroidal anti-inflammatory drugs, alcohol, calcium channel blockers, and some antiarrhythmic drugs, should be avoided if possible. Patients with HF complain of dyspnea on exertion, orthopnea, paroxysmal nocturnal dyspnea, fatigue, and dependent edema.

III. INHIBITORS OF THE RENIN-ANGIOTENSIN SYSTEM

HF leads to activation of the renin-angiotensin system via two mechanisms: 1) increased renin release by juxtaglomerular cells in renal afferent arterioles occurs in response to the diminished renal perfusion pressure produced by the failing heart, and 2) renin release by the juxtaglomerular cells is promoted by sympathetic stimulation. The production of angiotensin II—a potent vasoconstrictor—and the subsequent stimulation of aldosterone release that causes salt and water retention lead to the increases in both preload and afterload that are characteristic of the failing heart.

A. Angiotensin-converting enzyme inhibitors

Angiotensin-converting enzyme (ACE) inhibitors are the agents of choice in HF. These drugs block the enzyme that cleaves angiotensin I to form the potent vasoconstrictor angiotensin II (Figure 16.5). These agents also diminish the rate of bradykinin inactivation. [Note: Vasodilation occurs as a result of the combined effects of lower vasoconstriction caused by diminished levels of angiotensin II and the potent vasodilating effect of increased bradykinin.] By reducing circulating angiotensin II levels, ACE inhibitors also decrease the secretion of aldosterone, resulting in decreased sodium and water retention.

1. **Actions on the heart:** ACE inhibitors decrease vascular resistance, venous tone, and blood pressure, resulting in an increased cardiac output (see Figure 16.5). ACE inhibitors also blunt the usual angiotensin II–mediated increase in epinephrine and aldosterone seen in HF. ACE inhibitors improve clinical signs and symptoms in patients also receiving thiazide or loop diuretics and/or *digoxin*. The use of ACE inhibitors in the treatment of HF has significantly decreased both morbidity and mortality. For example, Figure 16.6 shows that the ACE inhibitor *enalapril* [e NAL a pril] decreases the cumulative mortality in patients with congestive HF. [Note: Reduction in mortality is due primarily to a decrease in deaths caused by progressive HF.] Treatment with *enalapril* also reduces arrhythmic death, myocardial infarction, and strokes. Similar data have been obtained with other ACE inhibitors.

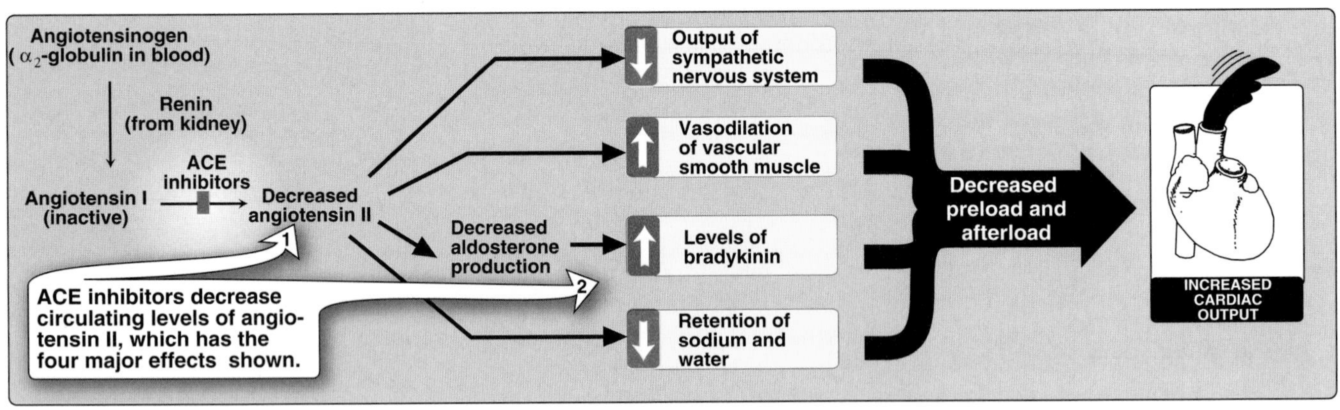

Figure 16.5
Effects of angiotensin-converting enzyme (ACE) inhibitors.

2. **Indications:** ACE inhibitors may be considered for single-agent therapy in patients who present with mild dyspnea on exertion and do not show signs or symptoms of volume overload. ACE inhibitors are useful in decreasing HF in asymptomatic patients with an ejection fraction of less than 35 percent (left ventricular dysfunction). Patients who have had a recent myocardial infarction also benefit from long-term ACE inhibitor therapy. Patients with the lowest ejection fraction show the greatest benefit. Early use of ACE inhibitors is indicated in patients with all stages of left-ventricular failure, with and without symptoms, and therapy should be initiated immediately after myocardial infarction. (See p. 219 for the use of ACE inhibitors in the treatment of hypertension.)

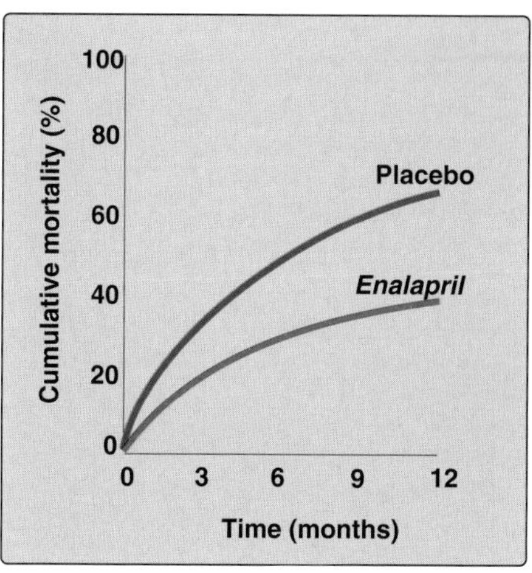

Figure 16.6
Effect of *enalapril* on the mortality of patients with congestive heart failure.

3. **Pharmacokinetics:** All ACE inhibitors are adequately but incompletely absorbed followed oral administration. The presence of food may decrease absorption, so they should be taken on an empty stomach. Except for *captopril*, ACE inhibitors are prodrugs that require activation by hydrolysis via hepatic enzymes. Renal elimination of the active moiety is important for most ACE inhibitors, an exception being *fosinopril*. Plasma half-lives of active compounds vary from two to twelve hours, although the inhibition of ACE may be much longer. The newer compounds such as *ramipril* and *fosinopril* only require once a day dosing.

4. **Adverse effects:** These include postural hypotension, renal insufficiency, hyperkalemia, angioedema, and a persistent dry cough. The potential for symptomatic hypotension with ACE inhibitor therapy requires careful monitoring. ACE inhibitors should not be used in pregnant women, because they are fetotoxic.

B. Angiotensin-receptor blockers

Angiotensin-receptor blockers (ARBs) are nonpeptide, orally active compounds that are extremely potent competitive antagonists of the angiotensin type 1 receptor. *Losartan* [loe SAR tan] is the prototype drug. ARBs have the theoretic advantage of more complete blockade of angiotensin action, because ACE inhibitors only inhibit one enzyme responsible for the production of angiotensin II and they do not affect bradykinin levels. Although ARBs have actions similar to those of ACE inhibitors, they are not therapeutically identical. Even so, ARBs are a substitute for ACE inhibitors in those patients who cannot tolerate the latter.

1. **Actions on the cardiovascular system:** All the ARBs are approved for treatment of hypertension based on their clinical efficacy in lowering blood pressure and reducing the morbidity and mortality associated with hypertension. As indicated above, their use in HF is as a substitute for ACE inhibitors in those patients with severe cough or angioedema.

2. **Pharmacokinetics:** All the drugs are orally active and require only once-a-day dosing. *Losartan*, the first approved member of the class, differs from the others in that it undergoes extensive first-pass hepatic metabolism, including conversion to its active metabolite. The other drugs have inactive metabolites. Elimination of

metabolites and parent compounds occurs in the urine and feces; the proportion is dependent on the individual drug. All are highly plasma protein–bound (greater than ninety percent) and, except for *candesartan* [kan des AR tan], have large volumes of distribution.

3. **Adverse effects:** ARBs have an adverse effect profile similar to that of ACE inhibitors. However, ARBs do not produce cough. ARBs are contraindicated in pregnancy.

IV. β-BLOCKERS

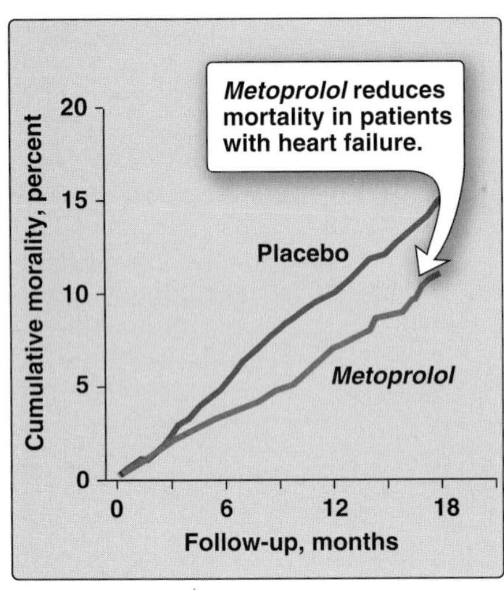

Figure 16.7
Cumulative mortality in patients with heart failure treated with placebo or *metoprolol*.

Although it may seem counterintuitive to administer drugs with negative inotropic activity to a patient with HF, several clinical studies have clearly demonstrated improved systolic functioning and reverse cardiac remodeling in patients receiving β-blockers. These benefits arise in spite of occasional initial exacerbation of symptoms. The benefit of β-blockers is attributed, in part, to their ability to prevent the changes that occur because of the chronic activation of the sympathetic nervous system, including decreasing the heart rate and inhibiting the release of renin. Two β-blockers have been approved for use in HF: *carvedilol* [KAR ve dil ol], and long-acting *metoprolol* [me TOE proe lol]. *Carvedilol* is a nonselective β-adrenoreceptor antagonist that also blocks α adrenoreceptors, whereas *metoprolol* is a β_1-selective antagonist. [Note: The pharmacology of β-blockers is described in detail in Chapter 7.] β-Blockade is recommended for all patients with heart disease except those who are at high risk but have no symptoms or those who are in acute HF. Obviously, the patient who also is hypertensive will obtain additional benefit from the β-blocker. Figure 16.7 shows the benefical effect of *metoprolol* treatment in patients with HF.

V. DIURETICS

Diuretics relieve pulmonary congestion and peripheral edema. These agents are also useful in reducing the symptoms of volume overload, including orthopnea and paroxysmal nocturnal dyspnea. Diuretics decrease plasma volume and, subsequently, decrease venous return to the heart (preload). This decreases the cardiac workload and the oxygen demand. Diuretics also decrease afterload by reducing plasma volume, thus decreasing blood pressure. Thiazide diuretics are relatively mild diuretics and lose efficacy if patient creatinine clearance is less than 50 mL/min. Loop diuretics are used for patients who require extensive diuresis and those with renal insufficiency. [Note: Overdoses of loop diuretics can lead to profound hypovolemia.]

VI. DIRECT VASODILATORS

Dilation of venous blood vessels leads to a decrease in cardiac preload by increasing the venous capacitance; arterial dilators reduce systemic arteriolar resistance and decrease afterload. Nitrates are commonly employed venous dilators for patients with congestive HF. If the patient is intolerant of ACE inhibitors or β-blockers, the combination of *hydralazine* and *isosorbide dinitrate* is most commonly used. [Note: Calcium channel blockers should be avoided in patients with HF.]

VII. INOTROPIC DRUGS

Positive inotropic agents enhance cardiac muscle contractility and, thus, increase cardiac output. Although these drugs act by different mechanisms, in each case the inotropic action is the result of an increased cytoplasmic calcium concentration that enhances the contractility of cardiac muscle.

A. Digitalis

The cardiac glycosides are often called *digitalis* or digitalis glycosides, because most of the drugs come from the digitalis (foxglove) plant. They are a group of chemically similar compounds that can increase the contractility of the heart muscle and, therefore, are widely used in treating HF. Like the antiarrhythmic drugs described in Chapter 17, the cardiac glycosides influence the sodium and calcium ion flows in the cardiac muscle, thereby increasing contraction of the atrial and ventricular myocardium (positive inotropic action). The digitalis glycosides show only a small difference between a therapeutically effective dose and doses that are toxic or even fatal. Therefore, the drugs have a low therapeutic index. The most widely used agent is *digoxin* [di JOX in].

1. Mechanism of action:

a. Regulation of cytosolic calcium concentration: Free cytosolic calcium concentrations at the end of contraction must be lowered for cardiac muscle to relax. The Na^+/Ca^{2+}-exchanger plays an important role in this process by extruding Ca^{2+} from the myocyte in exchange for Na^+ (Figure 16.8). The concentration gradient for both ions is a major determinant of the net movement of ions. By inhibiting the ability of the myocyte to actively pump Na^+ from the cell, cardiac glycosides decrease the Na^+ concentration gradient and, consequently, the ability of the Na^+/Ca^{2+}-exchanger to move calcium out of the cell. Because more Ca^{2+} is retained intracellularly, a small but physiologically important increase occurs in the free Ca^{2+} that

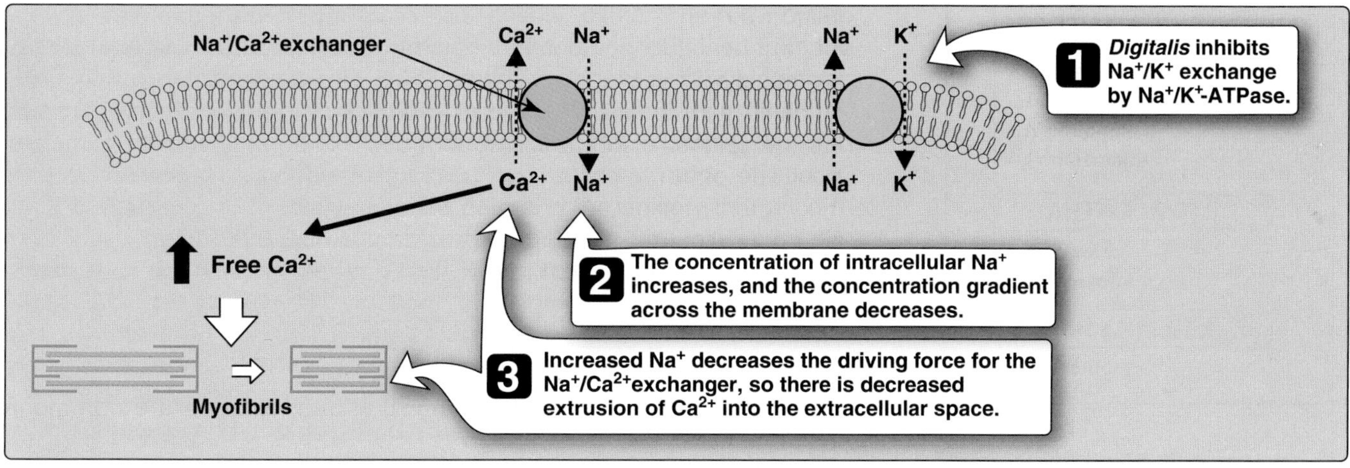

Figure 16.8
Mechanism of action of cardiac glycosides, or *digitalis*. ATPase = adenosine triphosphatase.

is available at the next contraction cycle of the cardiac muscle. It follows that if the Na^+/K^+–adenosine triphosphatase is extensively inhibited, the ionic gradient becomes so disturbed that dysrhythmias can occur.

b. **Increased contractility of the cardiac muscle:** Administration of digitalis glycosides increases the force of cardiac contractility, causing the cardiac output to more closely resemble that of the normal heart (Figure 16.9). An increased myocardial contraction leads to a decrease in end-diastolic volume, thus increasing the efficiency of contraction (increased ejection fraction). The resulting improved circulation leads to reduced sympathetic activity, which then reduces peripheral resistance. Together, these effects cause a reduction in heart rate. Vagal tone is also enhanced, so the heart rate decreases and myocardial oxygen demand diminishes. [Note: In the normal heart, the positive inotropic effect of *digitalis* is counteracted by compensatory autonomic reflexes.]

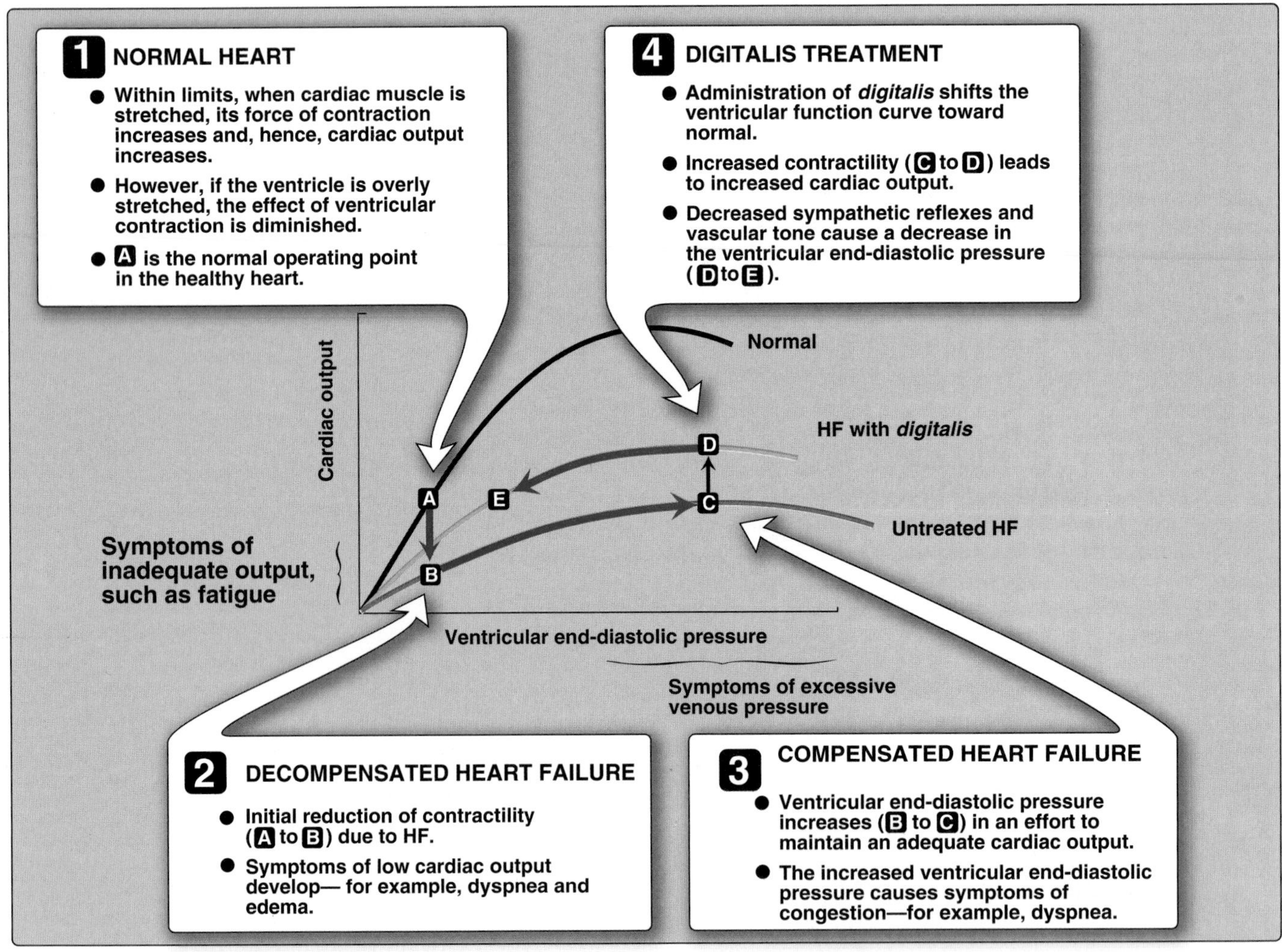

Figure 16.9
Ventricular function curves in the normal heart, in heart failure (HF), and in HF treated with *digitalis*.

2. **Therapeutic uses:** *Digoxin* therapy is indicated in patients with severe left-ventricular systolic dysfunction after initiation of diuretic, ACE inhibitor, and β-blocker therapy. *Digoxin* is not indicated in patients with diastolic or right-sided HF. *Dobutamine*, another inotropic agent, can be given intravenously in the hospital, but at present, no good oral inotropic agents exist other than *digoxin*. Patients with mild to moderate HF will often respond to treatment with ACE inhibitors and diuretics, and they do not require *digoxin*.

3. **Pharmacokinetics:** All digitalis glycosides possess the same pharmacologic actions, but they vary in potency and pharmacokinetics (Figure 16.10). *Digoxin* has the advantage of a relatively short half-life, which allows better treatment of toxic reactions. *Digoxin* also has a more rapid onset of action, making it useful in emergency situations. *Digoxin* is eliminated largely unchanged in the urine (see Figure 16.10). *Digitoxin* [DIJ i tox in] is extensively metabolized by the liver before excretion in the feces, and patients with hepatic disease may require decreased doses.

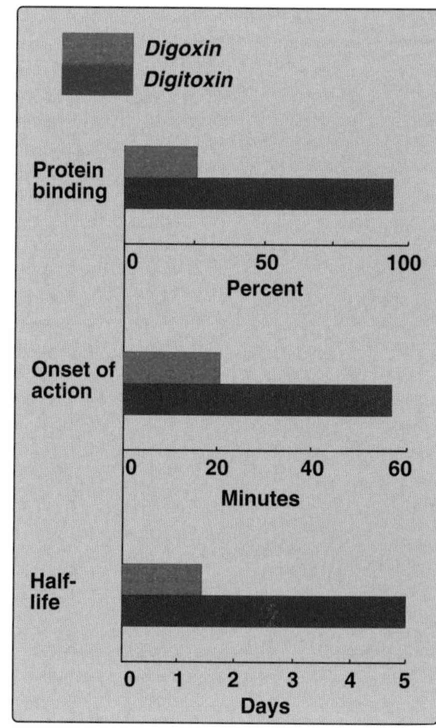

Figure 16.10
A comparison of the properties of *digoxin* and *digitoxin*.

4. **Adverse effects:** *Digitalis* toxicity is one of the most commonly encountered adverse drug reactions. Side effects often can be managed by discontinuing cardiac glycoside therapy, determining serum potassium levels, and if indicated, giving potassium supplements. In general, decreased serum levels of potassium predispose a patient to *digoxin* toxicity. *Digoxin* levels must be closely monitored in the presence of renal insufficiency, and dosage adjustment may be necessary. Severe toxicity resulting in ventricular tachycardia may require administration of antiarrhythmic drugs and the use of antibodies to *digoxin* (digoxin immune fab), which bind and inactivate the drug. Types of adverse effects include:

   a. **Cardiac effects:** The major effect is progressively more severe dysrhythmia, moving from decreased or blocked atrioventricular nodal conduction to paroxysmal supraventricular tachycardia, to the conversion of atrial flutter to atrial fibrillation, premature ventricular depolarization, ventricular fibrillation, and finally, to complete heart block. A decrease in intracellular potassium is the primary predisposing factor in these effects.

   b. **Gastrointestinal effects:** Anorexia, nausea, and vomiting are commonly encountered adverse effects.

   c. **Central nervous system effects:** These include headache, fatigue, confusion, blurred vision, alteration of color perception, and halos on dark objects.

5. **Factors predisposing to digitalis toxicity:**

   a. **Electrolytic disturbances:** Hypokalemia can precipitate serious arrhythmia. Reduction of serum potassium levels is most frequently observed in patients receiving thiazide or loop diuretics, and usually can be prevented by use of a potassium-sparing diuretic, or supplementation with potassium chloride. Hypercalcemia and hypomagnesemia also predispose to *digitalis* toxicity.

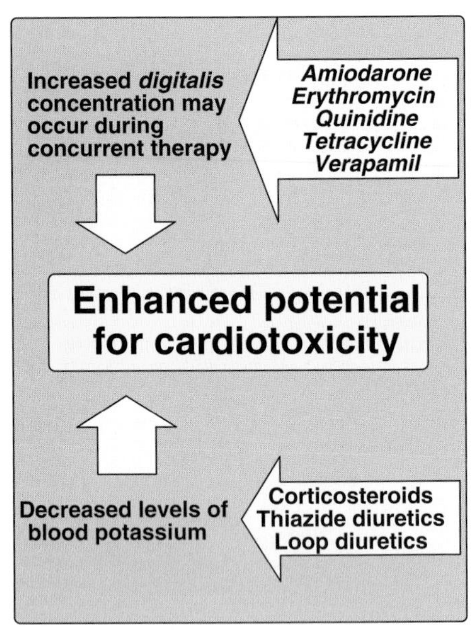

Figure 16.11
Drugs interacting with *digoxin* and other digitalis glycosides.

b. **Drugs:** *Quinidine*, *verapamil*, and *amiodarone*, to name a few, can cause *digoxin* intoxication, both by displacing *digoxin* from tissue protein binding sites, and by competing with *digoxin* for renal excretion. As a consequence, *digoxin* plasma levels may increase by 70 to 100 percent, requiring dosage reduction. Potassium-depleting diuretics, corticosteroids, and a variety of other drugs can also increase *digoxin* toxicity (Figure 16.11). Hypothyroidism, hypoxia, renal failure, and myocarditis are also predisposing factors to *digoxin* toxicity.

B. β-Adrenergic agonists

β-Adrenergic stimulation improves cardiac performance by causing positive inotropic effects and vasodilation. *Dobutamine* is the most commonly used inotropic agent other than *digitalis*. *Dobutamine* leads to an increase in intracellular cyclic adenosine monophosphate (cAMP), which results in the activation of protein kinase. Slow calcium channels are one important site of phosphorylation by protein kinase. When phosphorylated, the entry of calcium ion into the myocardial cells increases, thus enhancing contraction (Figure 16.12). *Dobutamine* must be given by intravenous infusion and is primarily used in the treatment of acute HF in a hospital setting.

C. Phosphodiesterase inhibitors

Amrinone [AM ri none] and *milrinone* [MIL ri none] are phosphodiesterase inhibitors that increase the intracellular concentration of cAMP (see Figure 16.12). This results in an increase of intracellular calcium and, therefore, cardiac contractility, as discussed above for

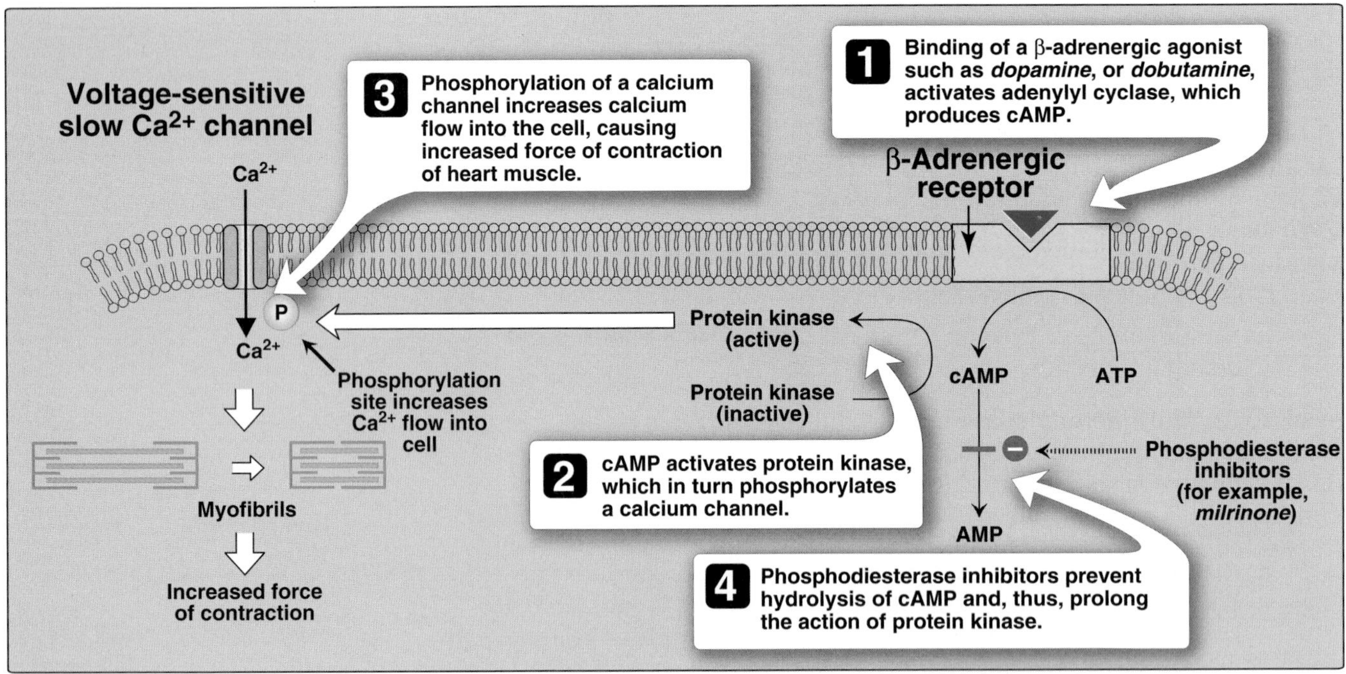

Figure 16.12
Sites of action by β-adrenergic agonists on heart muscle.

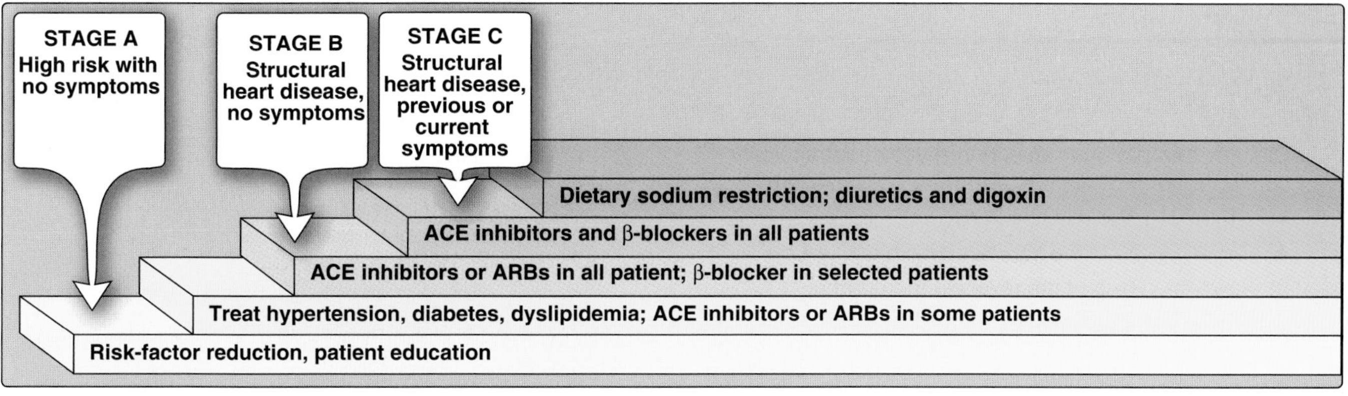

Figure 16.13
Treatment options for various stages of heart failure. ACE = Angiotensin-converting enzyme; ARB = angiotensin-receptor blockers. Stage D (refractory symptoms requiring special interventions) is not shown.

the β-adrenergic agonists. Long-term *amrinone* or *milrinone* therapy may be associated with a substantial increase in the risk of mortality However, short-term use of intravenous *milrinone* is not associated with increased mortality, and some symptomatic benefit may be obtained when it is used in patients with refractory HF.

VIII. SPIRONOLACTONE

Patients with advanced heart disease have elevated levels of aldosterone due to angiotensin II stimulation and reduced hepatic clearance of the hormone. *Spironolactone* is a direct antagonist of aldosterone, thereby preventing salt retention, myocardial hypertrophy, and hypokalemia. *Spironolactone* therapy should be reserved for the most advanced cases of HF. Because *spironolactone* promotes potassium retention, patients should not be taking potassium supplements. Adverse effects include gastric disturbances, such as gastritis and peptic ulcer; central nervous system effects, such as lethargy and confusion; and endocrine abnormalities, such as gynecomastia, decreased libido, and menstrual irregularities.

IX. ORDER OF THERAPY

Experts have classified HF into four stages, from least severe to most severe. Figure 16.13 shows a treatment strategy using this classification and the drugs described in this chapter. Note that as the disease progesses, polytherapy is initiated. For example, Figure 16.14 shows that treatment with *digoxin* plus a diuretic plus an ACE inhibitor in patients with HF is superior to treatment with diuretics alone or a diuretic plus either *digoxin* or an ACE inhibitor.

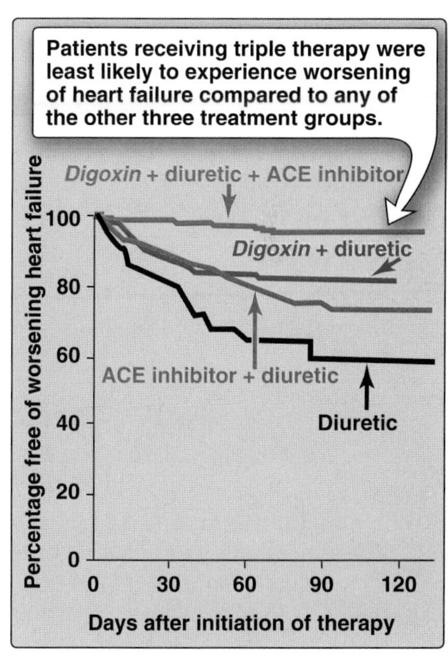

Figure 16.14
Use of multiple drugs in the treatment of heart failure. ACE = angiotensin-converting enzyme.

Study Questions

Choose the ONE best answer.

16.1 Digitalis has profound effect on myocyte intracellular concentrations of Na^+, K^+, and Ca^{2+}. These effects are caused by digitalis inhibiting:

A. Ca^{2+}-ATPase of the sarcoplasmic reticulum.
B. Na^+/K^+-ATPase of the myocyte membrane.
C. Cardiac phosphodiesterase.
D. Cardiac β_1 receptors.
E. Juxtaglomerular renin release.

Correct answer = B. The cardiac glycosides bind to and block the action of the Na^+/K^+-ATPase. This leads to increased intracellular sodium. The diminished sodium gradient results in less Ca^{2+} being extruded from the cell via the Na^+/Ca^{2+}-exchanger. Cardiac glycosides do not bind to the Ca^{2+}-ATPase. They have no direct effect on phosphodiesterase, β_1 receptors, or renin release.

16.2 Compensatory increases in heart rate and renin release that occur in heart failure may be alleviated by which of the following drugs?

A. Milrinone
B. Digoxin
C. Dobutamine
D. Enalapril
E. Metoprolol

Correct answer = E. Metoprolol, a β_1-selective antagonist, prevents the increased heart rate and renin release that result from sympathetic stimulation, which occurs as compensation for reduced cardiac output of heart failure. Enalapril is an ACE inhibitor that actually increases renin release. Dobutamine increases cardiac contractility but does not slow the heart rate or interfere with renin release. Digoxin decreases the heart rate because of its vagomimetic effects, but it does not decrease renin release.

16.3 A 58-year-old man is admitted to the hospital with acute heart failure and pulmonary edema. Which one of the following drugs would be most useful in treating the pulmonary edema?

A. Digoxin
B. Dobutamine
C. Furosemide
D. Minoxidil
E. Spironolactone

Correct answer = C. Furosemide has the ability to dilate vessels in the context of acute heart failure. It also mobilizes the edema fluid and promotes its excretion. Dobutamine increases contractility, but does not appreciably improve pulmonary edema. Digoxin acts too slowly and has no vasodilating effects. Minoxidil decreases arterial pressure and causes reflex tachycardia. Spironolactone does not alleviate acute pulmonary edema.

16.4 A 46-year-old man is admitted to the emergency department. He has taken more than ninety digoxin tablets (0.25 mg each), ingesting them about three hours before admission. His pulse is fifty to sixty beats per minute, and the electrocardiogram shows third-degree heart block. Which one of the following is the most important therapy to initiate in this patient?

A. Digoxin immune fab
B. Potassium salts
C. Lidocaine
D. Phenytoin
E. DC cardioversion

Correct answer = A. In the severely poisoned patient, reduction of digoxin plasma concentrations is paramount, and can be accomplished with administration of antidigoxin antibodies. Potassium concentrations, if low, can be increased, but to not much greater than 4 mM. Antiarrhythmics are useful if there is need, but not in this case. DC cardioversion is only used if ventricular fibrillation occurs.

Antiarrhythmic Drugs

17

I. OVERVIEW

In contrast to skeletal muscle, which contracts only when it receives a stimulus, the heart contains specialized cells that exhibit automaticity; that is, they can intrinsically generate rhythmic action potentials in the absence of external stimuli. These "pacemaker" cells differ from other myocardial cells in showing a slow, spontaneous depolarization during diastole (Phase 4), caused by an inward positive current carried by sodium- and calcium-ion flows. This depolarization is fastest in the sinoatrial (SA) node (the normal initiation site of the action potential), and decreases throughout the normal conduction pathway through the atrioventricular (AV) node to the bundle of His and the Purkinje system. Dysfunction of impulse generation or conduction at any of a number of sites in the heart can cause an abnormality in cardiac rhythm. Figure 17.1 summarizes the drugs used to treat cardiac arrhythmias.

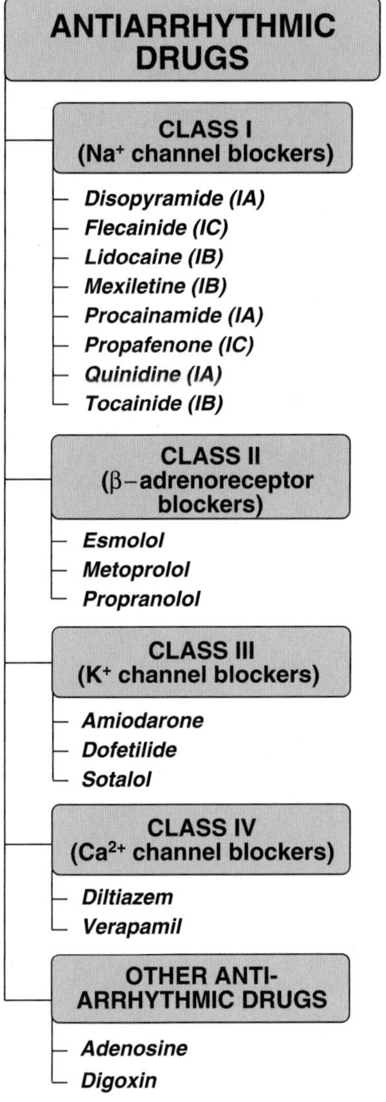

Figure 17.1
Summary of antiarrhythmic drugs.

II. INTRODUCTION TO THE ARRHYTHMIAS

The arrhythmias are conceptually simple—dysfunctions cause abnormalities in impulse formation and conduction in the myocardium. However, in the clinic, arrhythmias present as a complex family of disorders that show a variety of symptoms. For example, cardiac arrhythmias may cause the heart 1) to beat too slowly (sinus bradycardia), 2) to beat too rapidly (sinus or ventricular tachycardia, atrial or ventricular premature depolarization, atrial flutter), 3) to respond to impulses originating from sites other than the SA node, or 4) to respond to impulses traveling along accessory (extra) pathways that lead to deviant depolarizations (AV reentry, Wolff-Parkinson-White syndrome). To make sense of this large group of disorders, it is useful to organize the arrhythmias into groups according to the anatomic site of the the abnormality—the atria, the AV node, or the ventricles. Figure 17.2 summarizes several commonly occurring atrial, AV junction, or ventricular arrhythmias. Although not shown here, each of these abnormalities can be further divided into subgroups depending on the electrocardiogram findings.

Lippincott's Illustrated Reviews: Pharmacology, Third Edition,
by Richard D. Howland and Mary J. Mycek.
Lippincott Williams & Wilkins, Baltimore, MD © 2006.

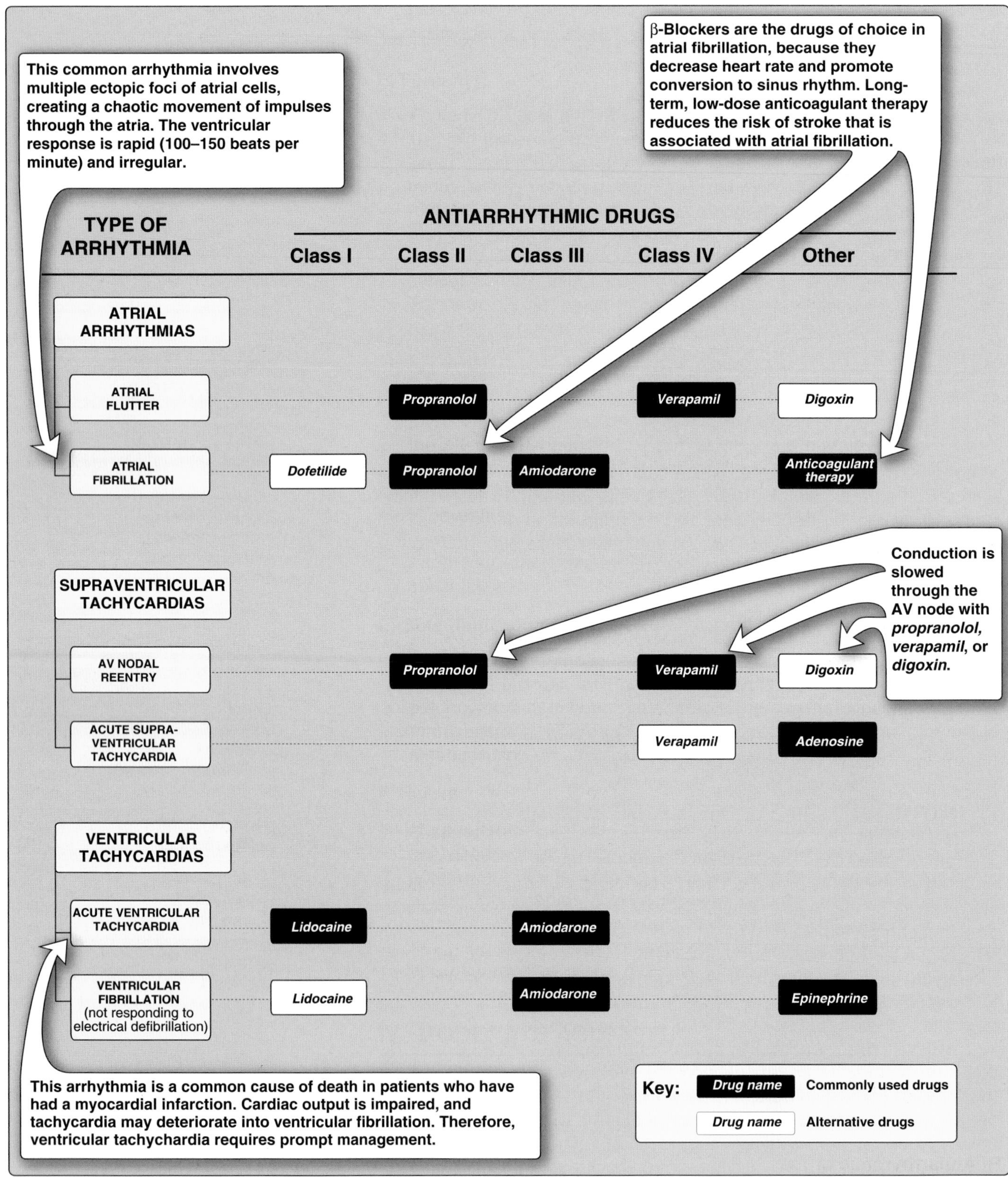

Figure 17.2
Therapeutic indications for some commonly encountered arrhythmias. AV = atrioventricular.

A. Causes of arrhythmias

Most arrhythmias arise either from aberrations in impulse generation (abnormal automaticity) or from a defect in impulse conduction.

1. **Abnormal automaticity:** The SA node shows the fastest rate of Phase 4 depolarization and, therefore, exhibits a higher rate of discharge than that occurring in other pacemaker cells exhibiting automaticity. Thus the SA node normally sets the pace of contraction for the myocardium, and latent pacemakers are depolarized by impulses coming from the SA node. However, if cardiac sites other than the SA node show enhanced automaticity, they may generate competing stimuli, and arrhythmias may arise. Abnormal automaticity may also occur if the myocardial cells are damaged (for example, by hypoxia or potassium imbalance). These cells may remain partially depolarized during diastole and, therefore, can reach the firing threshold earlier than normal cells. Abnormal automatic discharges may thus be induced.

2. **Effect of drugs on automaticity:** Most of the antiarrhythmic agents suppress automaticity by blocking either Na^+ or Ca^{2+} channels to reduce the ratio of these ions to K^+. This decreases the slope of Phase 4 (diastolic) depolarization and/or raises the threshold of discharge to a less negative voltage. Such drugs cause the frequency of discharge to decrease—an effect that is more pronounced in cells with ectopic pacemaker activity than in normal cells.

3. **Abnormalities in impulse conduction:** Impulses from higher pacemaker centers are normally conducted down pathways that bifurcate to activate the entire ventricular surface (Figure 17.3). A phenomenon called reentry can occur if a unidirectional block caused by myocardial injury or a prolonged refractory period results in an abnormal conduction pathway. Reentry is the most common cause of arrhythmias, and it can occur at any level of the cardiac conduction system. For example, consider a single Purkinje fiber with two conduction pathways to ventricular muscle. An impulse normally travels down both limbs of the conduction path. However, if myocardial injury results in a unidirectional block, the impulse may only be conducted down pathway 1 (see Figure 17.3). If the block in pathway 2 is in the forward direction only, the impulse may travel in a retrograde fashion through pathway 2 and reenter the point of bifurcation. This short-circuit pathway results in reexcitation of the ventricular muscle, causing premature contraction or sustained ventricular arrhythmia.

4. **Effects of drugs on conduction abnormalities:** Antiarrhythmic agents prevent reentry by slowing conduction and/or increasing the refractory period, thereby converting a unidirectional block into a bidirectional block.

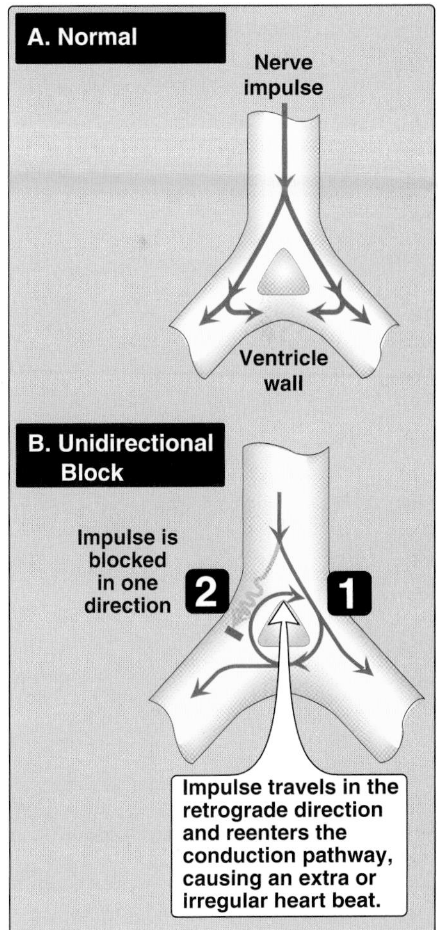

Figure 17.3
Schematic representation of reentry.

B. Antiarrhythmic drugs

As noted above, the antiarrhythmic drugs can modify impulse generation and conduction. More than a dozen such drugs that are potentially useful in treating arrhythmias are currently available. However, only a limited number of these agents are clinically beneficial in the treatment of selected arrhythmias. For example, the acute termination of ventricular tachycardia by *lidocaine* or of supraventricular tachycardia by *adenosine* or *verapamil* are examples in which antiarrhythmic therapy results in decreased morbidity. In contrast, many of the antiarrhythmic agents are now known to have dangerous proarrhythmic actions—that is, to cause arrhythmias. The efficacy of many antiarrhythmic agents remains unproven in placebo-controlled, random trials. [Note: Implantable cardioverter defibrolators are becoming more widely used to manage this condition.]

III. CLASS I ANTIARRHYTHMIC DRUGS

The antiarrhythmic drugs can be classified according to their predominant effects on the action potential (Figure 17.4). Although this classification is convenient, it is not entirely clear-cut, because many of the drugs have actions relating to more than one class or may have active metabolites with a different class of action. Class I antiarrhythmic drugs act by blocking voltage-sensitive sodium channels via the same mechanism as local anesthetics. The decreased rate of entry of sodium slows the rate of rise of Phase 0 of the action potential. [Note: At therapeutic doses, these drugs have little effect on the resting, fully polarized membrane because of their higher affinity for the active and inactive channels rather than for the resting channel.] Class I antiarrhythmic drugs therefore generally cause a decrease in excitability and conduction velocity. The use of sodium channel blockers has been declining continously due to their possible proarrhythmic effects, particularly in patients with reduced left ventricular function and ischemic heart disease.

A. Use-dependence

Class I drugs bind more rapidly to open or inactivated sodium channels than to channels that are fully repolarized following recovery from the previous depolarization cycle. Therefore, these drugs show a greater degree of blockade in tissues that are frequently depolarizing (for example, during tachycardia, when the sodium channels

CLASSIFICATION OF DRUG	MECHANISM OF ACTION	COMMENT
IA	Na^+ channel blocker	Slows Phase 0 depolarization
IB	Na^+ channel blocker	Shortens Phase 3 repolarization
IC	Na^+ channel blocker	Markedly slows Phase 0 depolarization
II	β-Adrenoreceptor blocker	Suppresses Phase 4 depolarization
III	K^+ channel blocker	Prolongs Phase 3 repolarization
IV	Ca^{2+} channel blocker	Shortens action potential

Figure 17.4
Actions of antiarrhythmic drugs.

open often). This property is called use-dependence (or state-dependence), and it enables these drugs to block cells that are discharging at an abnormally high frequency without interfering with the normal, low-frequency beating of the heart. The Class I drugs have been subdivided into three groups according to their effect on the duration of the action potential. Class IA agents slow the rate of rise of the action potential (thus slowing conduction), prolong the action potential, and increase the ventricular effective refractory period. They have an intermediate speed of association with activated/inactivated sodium channels and an intermediate rate of dissociation from resting channels. Class IB drugs have little effect on the rate of depolarization; rather, they decrease the duration of the action potential by shortening repolarization. They rapidly interact with sodium channels. Class IC agents markedly depress the rate of rise of the membrane action potential. Therefore, they cause marked conduction slowing but have little effect on the duration of the membrane action potential or the ventricular effective refractory period. They bind slowly to sodium channels.

B. Quinidine

Quinidine [KWIN i deen] is the prototype Class IA drug. At high doses, it can actually precipitate arrhythmias, which can lead to fatal ventricular fibrillation. Because of the toxic potential of *quinidine*, calcium antagonists, such as *verapamil*, are increasingly replacing this drug in clinical use.

1. **Mechanism of action:** *Quinidine* binds to open and inactivated sodium channels and prevents sodium influx, thus slowing the rapid upstroke during Phase 0 (Figure 17.5). It also decreases the slope of Phase 4 spontaneous depolarization.

2. **Actions:** *Quinidine* inhibits ectopic arrhythmias and ventricular arrhythmias caused by increased normal automaticity. *Quinidine* also prevents reentry arrhythmias by producing a bidirectional block. It does so by decreasing membrane responsiveness and prolonging the effective refractory period. The drug has little effect on normal automaticity. [Note: *Quinidine* can induce tachycardia in normal individuals because of its *atropine*-like (anticholinergic) effect.]

3. **Therapeutic uses:** *Quinidine* is used in the treatment of a wide variety of arrhythmias, including atrial, AV-junctional, and ventricular tachyarrhythmias. *Quinidine* is used to maintain sinus rhythm after direct-current cardioversion of atrial flutter or fibrillation and to prevent frequent ventricular tachycardia.

4. **Pharmacokinetics:** *Quinidine sulfate* is rapidly and almost completely absorbed after oral administration. It undergoes extensive metabolism by the hepatic cytochrome P450 enzymes, forming active metabolites. Excretion is through the kidney.

5. **Adverse effects:** A potential adverse effect of *quinidine* (or of any antiarrhythmic drug) is exacerbation of the arrhythmia. *Quinidine* may cause SA and AV block or asystole. At toxic levels, the drug may induce ventricular tachycardia. Cardiotoxic effects are

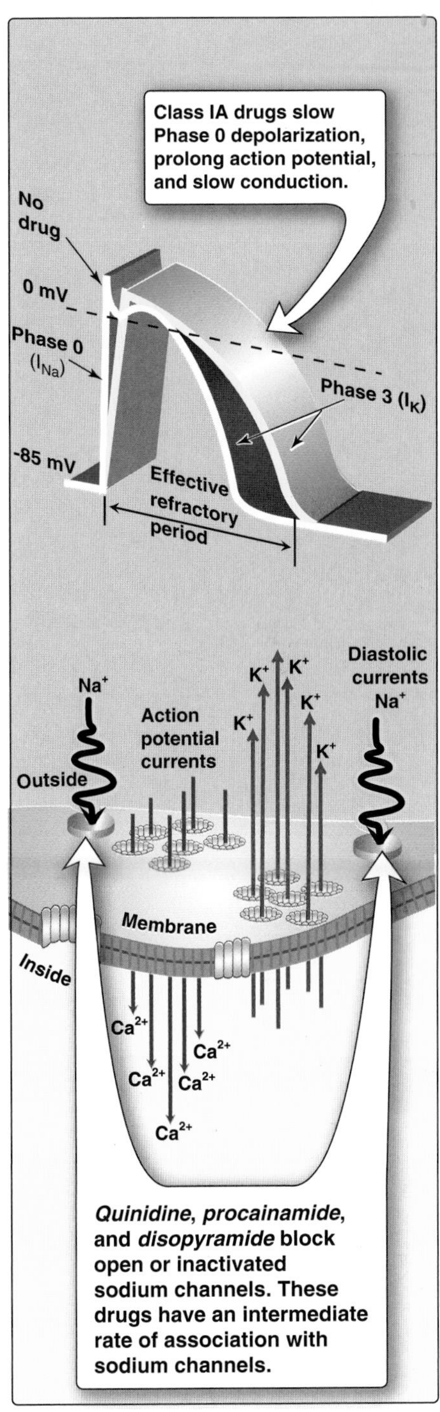

Figure 17.5
Schematic diagram of the effects of Class IA agents. I_{Na} and I_K are transmembrane currents due to the movement of Na^+ and K^+, respectively.

exacerbated by hyperkalemia. Nausea, vomiting, and diarrhea are commonly observed. Large doses of *quinidine* may induce the symptoms of cinchonism (for example, blurred vision, tinnitus, headache, disorientation, and psychosis). The drug has a mild α-adrenergic blocking action as well as an *atropine*-like effect. *Quinidine* can increase the steady-state concentration of *digoxin* by displacement of *digoxin* from tissue-binding sites (minor effect), and by decreasing *digoxin* renal clearance (major effect). Interactions with other drugs may occur. For example, patients taking *phenytoin* may require higher doses of *quinidine*.

C. Procainamide

1. **Actions:** This Class IA drug, a derivative of the local anesthetic *procaine*, shows actions similar to those of *quinidine*.

2. **Pharmacokinetics:** *Procainamide* [proe KANE a mide] is well-absorbed following oral administration. [Note: The intravenous route is rarely used, because hypotension occurs if the drug is infused too rapidly.] *Procainamide* has a relatively short half-life of two to three hours. A portion of the drug is acetylated in the liver to N-acetylprocainamide (NAPA), which has little effect on the maximum polarization of Purkinje fibers but prolongs the duration of the action potential. Thus, NAPA has properties of a Class III drug. NAPA is eliminated via the kidney, and dosages of *procainamide* may need to be adjusted in patients with renal failure.

3. **Adverse effects:** With chronic use, *procainamide* causes a high incidence of side effects, including a reversible lupus erythematosus-like syndrome that develops in 25 to 30 percent of patients. Toxic concentrations of *procainamide* may cause asystole or induction of ventricular arrhythmias. Central nervous system (CNS) side effects include depression, hallucination, and psychosis. With this drug, gastrointestinal intolerance is less frequent than with *quinidine*.

D. Disopyramide

1. **Actions:** This Class IA drug shows actions similar to those of *quinidine*. *Disopyramide* [dye soe PEER a mide] produces a negative inotropic effect that is greater than the weak effect exerted by *quinidine* and *procainamide*, and unlike the latter drugs, *disopyramide* causes peripheral vasoconstriction. The drug may produce a clinically important decrease in myocardial contractility in patients with preexisting impairment of left ventricular function. *Disopyramide* is used in the treatment of ventricular arrhythmias as an alternative to *procainamide* or *quinidine*.

2. **Pharmacokinetics:** Approximately half of the orally ingested drug is excreted unchanged by the kidneys. Approximately thirty percent of the drug is converted by the liver to the less active mono-N-dealkylated metabolite.

3. **Adverse effects:** *Disopyramide* shows effects of anticholinergic activity (for example, dry mouth, urinary retention, blurred vision,

and constipation). Because of frequent toxicity, *procainamide* and *disopyramide* are used less frequently than other Class IA drugs, and then mainly in patients who cannot tolerate the other agents. Its use is contraindicated in patients with heart failure.

E. Lidocaine

Lidocaine [LYE doe kane] is a Class IB drug. The Class IB agents rapidly associate and dissociate from sodium channels. Thus, the actions of Class IB agents are manifested when the cardiac cell is depolarized or firing rapidly. Class IB drugs are particularly useful in treating ventricular arrhythmias. *Lidocaine* is the drug of choice for emergency treatment of cardiac arrhythmias.

1. **Actions:** *Lidocaine*, a local anesthetic, shortens Phase 3 repolarization and decreases the duration of the action potential (Figure 17.6). Unlike *quinidine*, which suppresses arrhythmias caused by increased normal automaticity, *lidocaine* suppresses arrhythmias caused by abnormal automaticity. *Lidocaine*, like *quinidine*, abolishes ventricular reentry.

2. **Therapeutic uses:** *Lidocaine* is useful in treating ventricular arrhythmias arising during myocardial ischemia, such as that experienced during a myocardial infarction. The drug does not markedly slow conduction and, thus, has little effect on atrial or AV junction arrhythmias.

3. **Pharmacokinetics:** *Lidocaine* is given intravenously because of extensive first-pass transformation by the liver, which precludes oral administration. The drug is dealkylated and eliminated almost entirely by the liver; consequently, dosage adjustment may be necessary in patients with liver dysfunction, or those taking drugs that lower hepatic blood flow, such as *propranolol*.

4. **Adverse effects:** *Lidocaine* has a fairly wide toxic-to-therapeutic ratio. It shows little impairment of left ventricular function and has no negative inotropic effect. CNS effects include drowsiness, slurred speech, paresthesia, agitation, confusion, and convulsions. Cardiac arrhythmias may also occur.

F. Mexiletine and tocainide

These Class IB drugs have actions similar to those of *lidocaine*, and they can be administered orally. *Mexiletine* [MEX i le teen] is used for chronic treatment of ventricular arrhythmias associated with previous myocardial infarction. *Tocainide* [toe KAY nide] is used for treatment of ventricular tachyarrhythmias. *Tocainide* has pulmonary toxicity, which may lead to pulmonary fibrosis.

G. Flecainide

Flecainide [FLEK a nide] is a Class IC drug. These drugs slowly dissociate from resting sodium channels, and show prominent effects even at normal heart rates. They are approved only for refractory ventricular arrhythmias. However, recent data have cast serious doubts on the safety of the Class IC drugs.

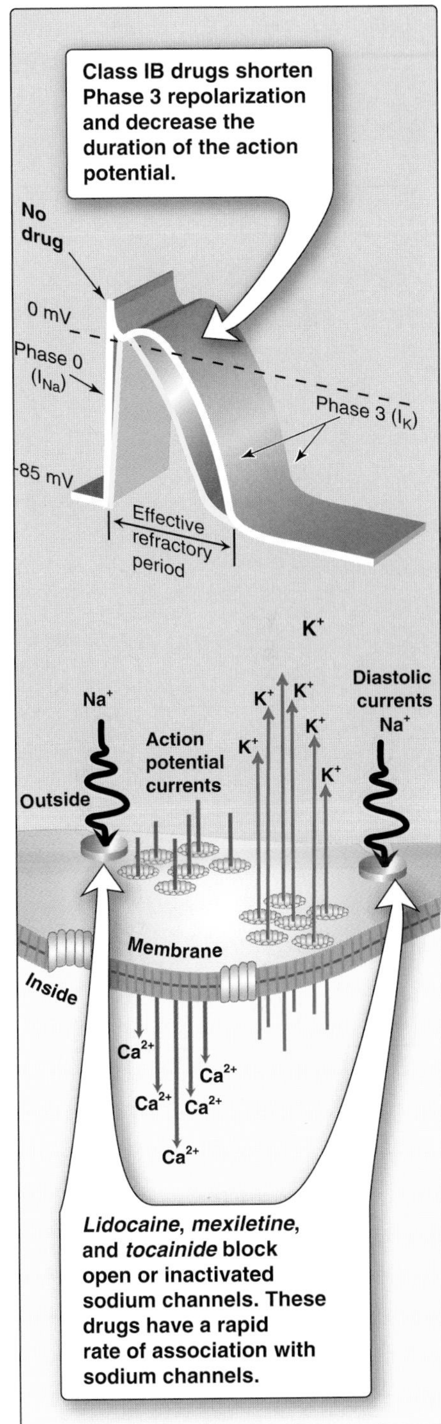

Figure 17.6
Schematic diagram of the effects of Class IB agents. I_{Na} and I_K are transmembrane currents due to the movement of Na^+ and K^+, respectively.

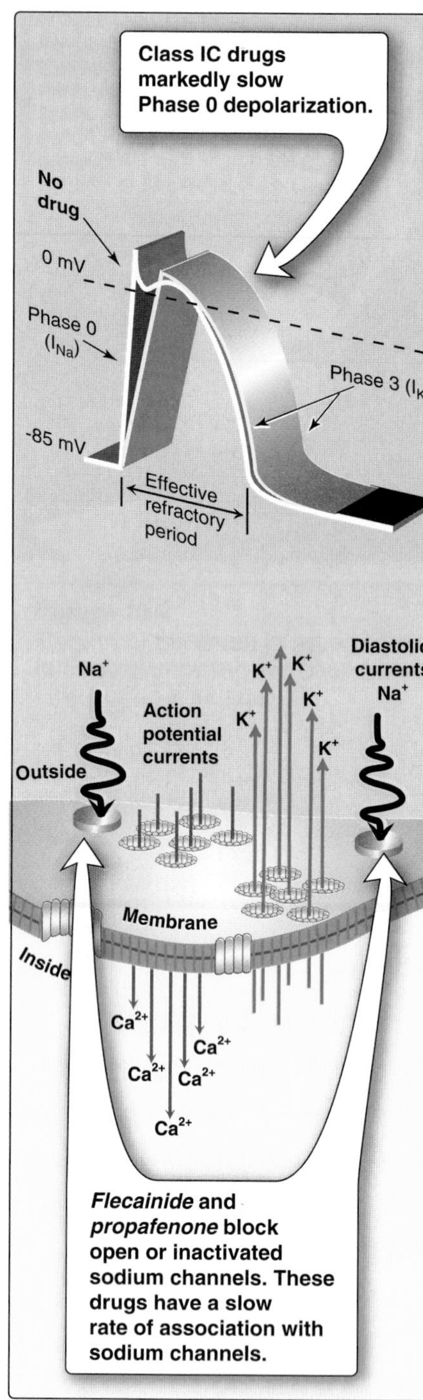

Figure 17.7
Schematic diagram of the effects of Class IC agents. I_{Na} and I_K are transmembrane currents due to the movement of Na^+ and K^+, respectively.

1. **Actions:** *Flecainide* suppresses Phase 0 upstroke in Purkinje and myocardial fibers (Figure 17.7). This causes marked slowing of conduction in all cardiac tissue, with a minor effect on the duration of the action potential and refractoriness. Automaticity is reduced by an increase in the threshold potential rather than a decrease in the slope of Phase 4 depolarization.

2. **Therapeutic uses:** *Flecainide* is useful in treating refractory ventricular arrhythmias. It is particularly useful in suppressing premature ventricular contraction. *Flecainide* has a negative inotropic effect and can aggravate congestive heart failure.

3. **Pharmacokinetics:** *Flecainide* is absorbed orally, undergoes minimal biotransformation, and has a half-life of sixteen to twenty hours.

4. **Adverse effects:** *Flecainide* can cause dizziness, blurred vision, headache, and nausea. Like other Class IC drugs, *flecainide* can aggravate preexisting arrhythmias or induce life-threatening ventricular tachycardia that is resistant to treatment.

H. Propafenone

This Class IC drug shows actions similar to those of *flecainide*. *Propafenone* [proe pa FEEN one], like *flecainide*, slows conduction in all cardiac tissues and is considered to be a broad-spectrum antiarrhythmic agent.

IV. CLASS II ANTIARRHYTHMIC DRUGS

Class II agents are β-adrenergic antagonists. These drugs diminish Phase 4 depolarization, thus depressing automaticity, prolonging AV conduction, and deÌcreasing heart rate and contractility. Class II agents are useful in treating tachyarrhythmias caused by increased sympathetic activity. They are also used for atrial flutter and fibrillation and for AV-nodal reentrant tachycardia. [Note: In contrast to the sodium channel blockers, β-blockers and class III compounds, such as *sotalol* and *amiodarone*, are increasing in use.]

A. Propranolol

Propranolol reduces the incidence of sudden arrhythmic death after myocardial infarction (the most common cause of death in this group of patients). The mortality rate in the first year after a heart attack is significantly reduced by *propranolol*, partly because of its ability to prevent ventricular arrhythmias.

B. Metoprolol

Propranolol is the β-adrenergic antagonist most widely used in the treatment of cardiac arrhythmias. However, β_1-specific drugs, such as *metoprolol*, reduce the risk of bronchospasm.

C. Esmolol

Esmolol [ESS moe lol] is a very short-acting β-blocker used for intravenous administration in acute arrhythmias that occur during surgery or emergency situations.

V. CLASS III ANTIARRHYTHMIC DRUGS

Class III agents block potassium channels and, thus, diminish the outward potassium current during repolarization of cardiac cells. These agents prolong the duration of the action potential without altering Phase 0 of depolarization or the resting membrane potential (Figure 17.8). Instead, they prolong the effective refractory period. All Class III drugs have the potential to induce arrhythmias.

A. Amiodarone

1. **Actions:** *Amiodarone* [a MEE oh da rone] contains iodine and is related structurally to thyroxine. It has complex effects, showing Class I, II, III, and IV actions. Its dominant effect is prolongation of the action potential duration and the refractory period. *Amiodarone* has antianginal as well as antiarrhythmic activity. Unlike the Class I antiarrhythmic drugs, *amiodarone* does not prolong the QT interval, and is the preferred antiarrhythmic in patients with moderate to severe heart failure.

2. **Therapeutic uses:** *Amiodarone* is effective in the treatment of severe refractory supraventricular and ventricular tachyarrhythmias. Its clinical usefulness is limited by its toxicity.

3. **Pharmacokinetics:** *Amiodarone* is incompletely absorbed after oral administration. The drug is unusual in having a prolonged half-life of several weeks. Full clinical effects may not be achieved until six weeks after initiation of treatment.

4. **Adverse effects:** *Amiodarone* shows a variety of toxic effects. After long-term use, more than half of patients receiving the drug show side effects that are severe enough to prompt its discontinuation. Some of the more common effects include interstitial pulmonary fibrosis, gastrointestinal tract intolerance, tremor, ataxia, dizziness, hyper- or hypothyroidism, liver toxicity, photosensitivity, neuropathy, muscle weakness, and blue skin discoloration caused by iodine accumulation in the skin. As noted earlier, recent clinical trials have shown that *amiodarone* does not reduce the incidence of sudden death or prolong survival in patients with congestive heart failure.

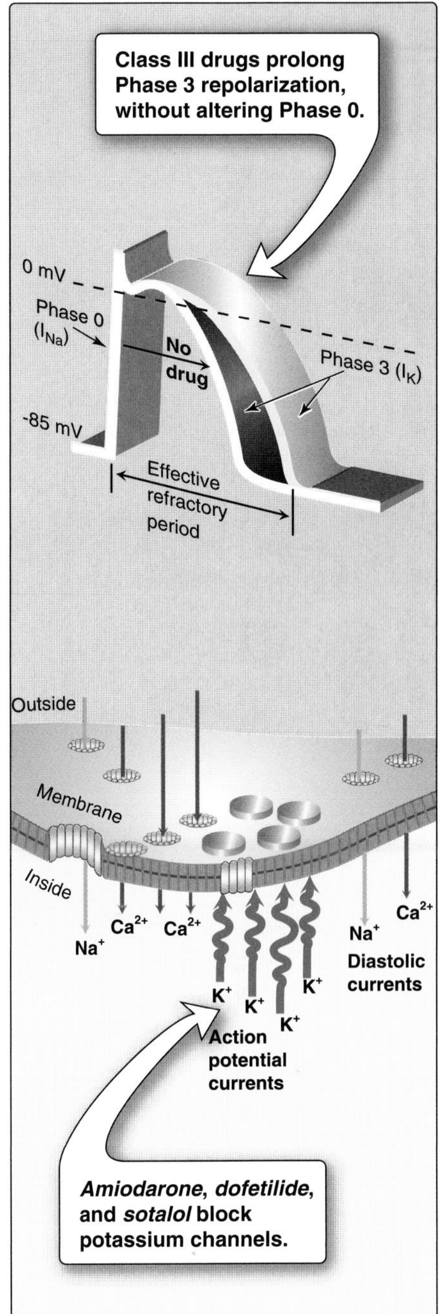

Figure 17.8
Schematic diagram of the effects of Class III agents. I_{Na} and I_K are transmembrane currents due to the movement of Na^+ and K^+, respectively.

B. Sotalol

Sotalol [SOE ta lol], although a class III antiarrhythmic agent, also has potent β-blocker activity. It is well established that β-blockers reduce mortality associated with acute myocardial infarction.

1. **Actions:** *Sotalol* blocks a rapid outward potassium current, known as the delayed rectifier. This blockade prolongs both repolarization and duration of the action potential, thus lengthening the effective refractory period.

2. **Therapeutic uses:** β-Blockers are used for long-term therapy to decrease the rate of sudden death following an acute myocardial infarction. β-Blockers have a modest ability to suppress ectopic beats and to reduce myocardial oxygen demand. They have

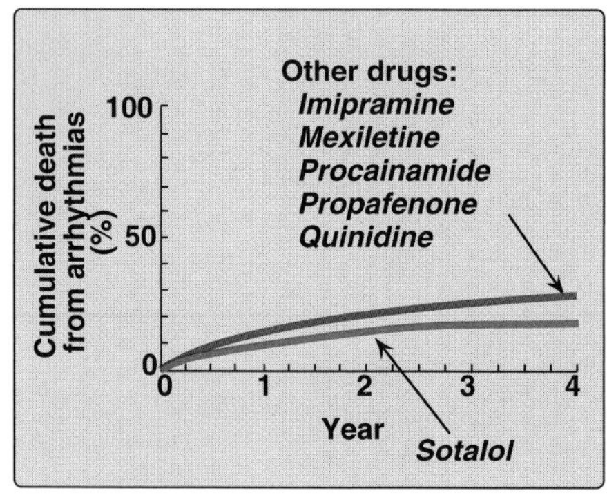

Figure 17.9
Comparison of *sotalol* with six other drugs with respect to deaths due to cardiac arrhythmias.

strong antifibrillary effects, particularly in the ischemic myocardium. *Sotalol* was more effective in preventing recurrence of arrhythmia and in decreasing mortality than *imipramine*, *mexiletine*, *procainamide*, *propafenone*, and *quinidine* in patients with sustained ventricular tachycardia (Figure 17.9).

3. **Adverse effects:** This drug also had the lowest rate of acute or long-term adverse effects. As with all drugs that prolong the QT interval, the syndrome of torsade de pointes is a serious potential adverse effect, typically seen in three to four percent of patients.

C. Dofetilide

Dofetilide [doh FET il ide] can be used as a first-line antiarrhythmic agent in patients with persistent atrial fibrillation and heart failure, or in those with coronary artery disease with impaired left ventricular function. Because of the risk of proarrhythmia, *dofetilide* initiation is limited to the inpatient setting and is restricted to prescribers who have completed a specific manufacturer's training session. Along with *amiodarone* and β-blockers, *dofetilide* is the only antiarrhythmic drug that is recommended by experts for the treatment of atrial fibrillation in a wide range of patients. The half-life is ten hours. Excretion is in the urine, with eighty percent as unchanged drug and twenty percent as inactive or minimally active metabolites.

VI. CLASS IV ANTIARRHYTHMIC DRUGS

Class IV drugs are calcium channel blockers (see p. 221). They decrease the inward current carried by calcium, resulting in a decreased rate of Phase 4 spontaneous depolarization. They also slow conduction in tissues that are dependent on calcium currents, such as the AV node (Figure 17.10). Although voltage-sensitive calcium channels occur in many different tissues, the major effect of calcium channel blockers is on vascular smooth muscle and the heart.

A. Verapamil and diltiazem

Verapamil [ver AP a mil] shows greater action on the heart than on vascular smooth muscle, whereas *nifedipine*, a calcium channel blocker used to treat hypertension (see p. 221), exerts a stronger effect on the vascular smooth muscle than on the heart. *Diltiazem* [dil TYE a zem] is intermediate in its actions.

1. **Actions:** Calcium enters cells by voltage-sensitive channels and by receptor-operated channels that are controlled by the binding of agonists, such as catecholamines, to membrane receptors. Calcium channel blockers, such as *verapamil* and *diltiazem*, are more effective against the voltage-sensitive channels, causing a decrease in the slow inward current that triggers cardiac contraction. *Verapamil* and *diltiazem* bind only to open, depolarized channels, thus preventing repolarization until the drug dissociates from the channel. These drugs are therefore use-dependent; that is, they block most effectively when the heart is beating rapidly, because in a normally paced heart, the calcium channels have

time to repolarize and the bound drug dissociates from the channel before the next conduction pulse. By decreasing the inward current carried by calcium, *verapamil* and *diltiazem* slow conduction and prolong the effective refractory period in tissues that are dependent on calcium currents, such as the AV node. These drugs are therefore effective in treating arrhythmias that must traverse calcium-dependent cardiac tissues.

2. **Therapeutic uses:** *Verapamil* and *diltiazem* are more effective against atrial than againstventricular dysrhythmias. They are useful in treating reentrant supraventricular tachycardia and in reducing the ventricular rate in atrial flutter and fibrillation. In addition, these drugs are used to treat hypertension and angina.

3. **Pharmacokinetics:** *Verapamil* and *diltiazem* are absorbed after oral administration. *Verapamil* is extensively metabolized by the liver; thus, care should be taken when administering this drug to patients with hepatic dysfunction.

4. **Adverse effects:** *Verapamil* and *diltiazem* have negative inotropic properties and, therefore, may be contraindicated in patients with preexisting depressed cardiac function. Both drugs can also produce a decrease in blood pressure because of peripheral vasodilation—an effect that is actually beneficial in treating hypertension.

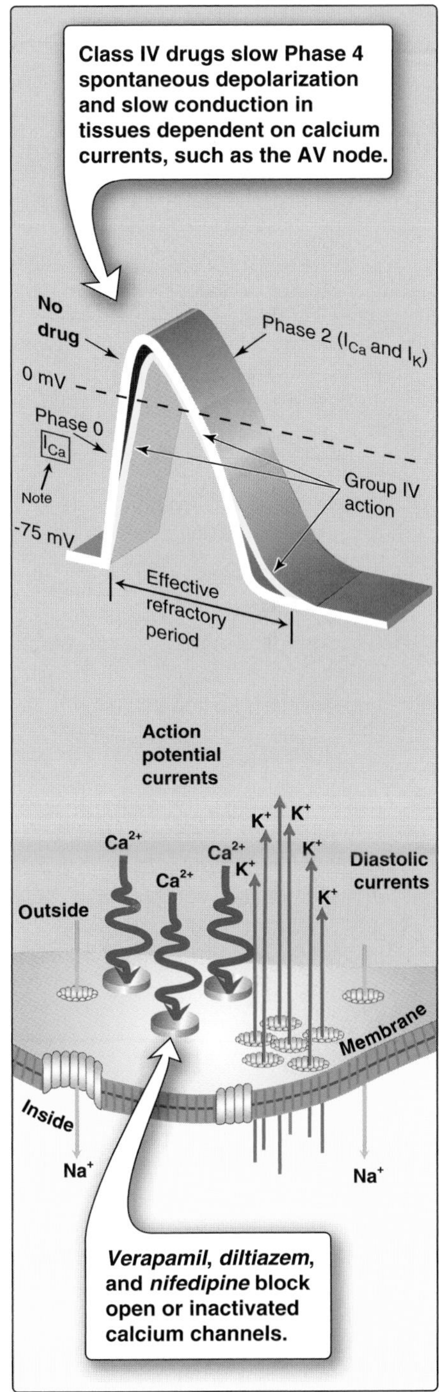

Figure 17.10
Schematic diagram of the effects of Class IV agents. I_{Ca} and I_K are transmembrane currents due to the movement of Ca^{2+} and K^+, respectively.

VII. OTHER ANTIARRHYTHMIC DRUGS

A. Digoxin

Digoxin shortens the refractory period in atrial and ventricular myocardial cells while prolonging the effective refractory period and diminishing conduction velocity in Purkinje fibers. *Digoxin* is used to control the ventricular response rate in atrial fibrillation and flutter. At toxic concentrations, *digoxin* causes ectopic ventricular beats that may result in ventricular tachycardia and fibrillation. [Note: This arrhythmia is usually treated with *lidocaine* or *phenytoin*.]

B. Adenosine

Adenosine [ah DEN oh zeen] is a naturally occurring nucleoside, but at high doses, the drug decreases conduction velocity, prolongs the refractory period, and decreases automaticity in the AV node. Intravenous *adenosine* is the drug of choice for abolishing acute supraventricular tachycardia. It has low toxicity but causes flushing, chest pain, and hypotension. *Adenosine* has an extremely short duration of action (approximately fifteen seconds).

Study Questions

Choose the ONE best answer.

17.1 A 66-year-old man had a myocardial infarct. Which one of the following would be appropriate prophylactic antiarrhythmic therapy?

A. Lidocaine
B. Metoprolol
C. Procainamide
D. Quinidine
E. Verapamil

Correct answer = B. β-Blockers, such as metoprolol, prevent cardiac arrhythmias that occur subsequent to a myocardial infarction. None of the other drugs has been shown to be particularly effective in preventing postinfarct arrhythmias.

17.2 Suppression of arrhythmias resulting from a reentry focus is most likely to occur if the drug:

A. has vagomimetic effects on the AV node.
B. is a β-blocker.
C. converts a unidirectional block to a bidirectional block.
D. slows conduction through the atria.
E. has atropine-like effects on the AV node.

Correct answer = C. Current theory holds that a reentrant arrhythmia is caused by damaged heart muscle such that conduction is slowed through the damaged area in only one direction. A drug that prevents conduction in either direction through the damaged area interrupts the reentrant arrhythmia. Class I antiarrhythmics, such as lidocaine, are capable of producing bidirectional block. The other choices do not have any direct effects on the direction of blockade of conduction through damaged cardiac muscle.

17.3 A 57-year-old man is being treated for an atrial arrhythmia. He complains of headache, dizziness, and tinnitus. Which one of the following antiarrhythmic drugs is the most likely cause?

A. Amiodarone
B. Procainamide
C. Propranolol
D. Quinidine
E. Verapamil

Correct answer = D. The clustered symptoms of headache, dizziness, and tinnitus are characteristic of cinchoism, which is caused by quinidine. The other drugs have characteristic adverse effects, but not this particular group.

17.4 A 58-year-old woman is being treated for chronic suppression of a ventricular arrhythmia. After two months of therapy, she complains about feeling tired all the time. Examination reveals a resting heart rate of ten beats per minute lower than her previous rate. Her skin is cool and clammy. Laboratory test results indicate low thyroxin and elevated thyroid-stimulating hormone levels. Which of the following antiarrhythmic drugs is the likely cause of these signs and symptoms?

A. Amiodarone
B. Procainamide
C. Propranolol
D. Quinidine
E. Verapamil

Correct answer = A. The patient is exhibiting symptoms of hypothyroidism, which is often associated with amiodarone therapy. Propranolol could slow the heart but would not produce the changes in thyroid function. None of the other antiarrhythmics is likely to cause hypothyroidism.

Antianginal Drugs

18

I. OVERVIEW

Angina pectoris is a characteristic sudden, severe, pressing chest pain radiating to the neck, jaw, back, and arms. It is caused by coronary blood flow that is insufficient to meet the oxygen demands of the myocardium, leading to ischemia. The imbalance between oxygen delivery and utilization may result during exertion, from a spasm of the vascular smooth muscle, or from obstruction of blood vessels caused by atherosclerotic lesions. These transient episodes (fifteen seconds to fifteen minutes) of myocardial ischemia do not cause cellular death, such as occurs in myocardial infarction. Three classes of drugs, used either alone or in combination, are effective in treating patients with stable angina: organic nitrates, β-blockers, and calcium channel blockers (Figure 18.1). These agents lower the oxygen demand of the heart by affecting blood pressure, heart rate, and contractility. Lifestyle and risk factor modifications, especially cessation of smoking, are also important in the treatment of angina. [Note: Options other than medications for treating angina include angioplasty and coronary artery bypass surgery.]

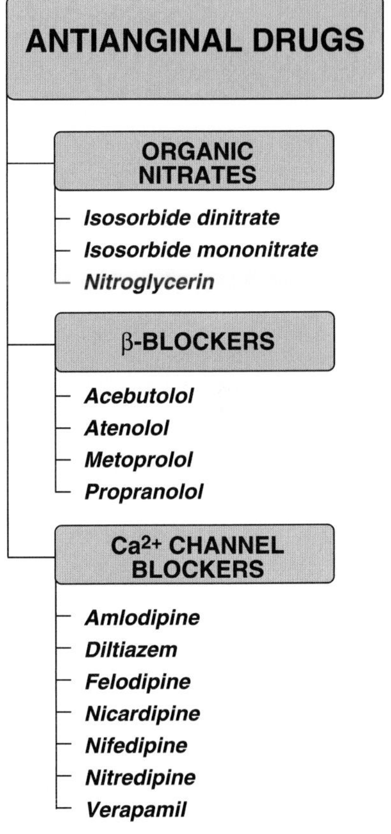

ANTIANGINAL DRUGS
ORGANIC NITRATES
Isosorbide dinitrate
Isosorbide mononitrate
Nitroglycerin
β-BLOCKERS
Acebutolol
Atenolol
Metoprolol
Propranolol
Ca2+ CHANNEL BLOCKERS
Amlodipine
Diltiazem
Felodipine
Nicardipine
Nifedipine
Nitredipine
Verapamil

Figure 18.1
Summary of antianginal drugs.

II. TYPES OF ANGINA

Angina pectoris has three overlapping patterns: 1) stable or typical angina, 2) unstable angina, and 3) Prinzmetal or variant angina. They are caused by varying combinations of increased myocardial demand and decreased myocardial perfusion.

A. Stable angina

Stable angina is the most common form of angina and, therefore, is called typical angina pectoris. It is characterized by a burning, heavy, or squeezing feeling in the chest. It is caused by the reduction of coronary perfusion due to coronary atherosclerosis. The heart becomes vulnerable to ischemia whenever there is increased demand, such as that produced by physical activity, emotional excitement, or any other cause of increased cardiac workload. Typical angina pectoris is promptly relieved by rest or *nitroglycerin* (a vasodilator).

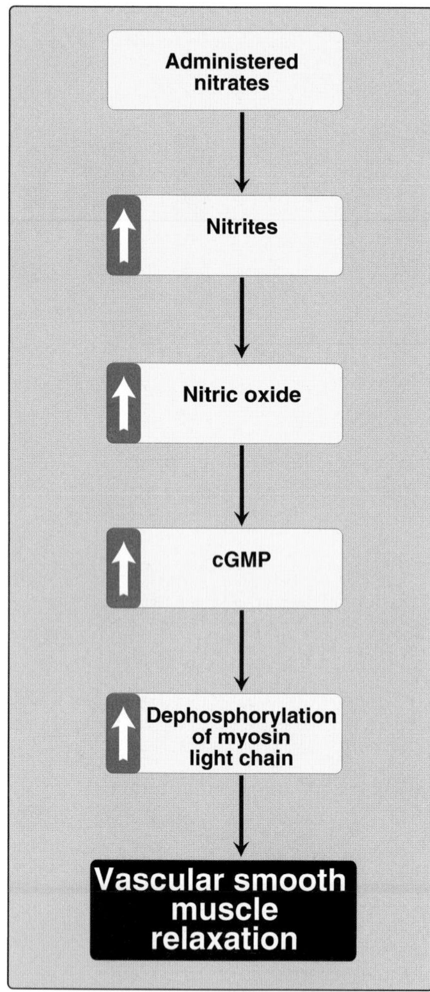

Figure 18.2
Effects of nitrates and nitrites on smooth muscle. cGMP = cyclic guanosine 3', 5'-monophosphate

B. Unstable angina

Unstable angina lies between stable angina on the one hand and myocardial infarction on the other. Unstable angina occurs with progressively increasing frequency and is precipitated with progressively less effort. It is often unrelated to exercise and occurs at rest. The symptoms are not relieved by rest or *nitroglycerin*. Unstable angina may require more aggressive therapy (for example, treatment of dyslipidemias, hypertension, or diabetes if present) to retard the progression to myocardial infarction.

C. Prinzmetal or variant angina

Prinzmetal angina is an uncommon pattern of episodic angina that occurs at rest and is due to coronary artery spasm. The symptoms are caused by decreased blood flow to the heart's muscle or by spasm of the coronary artery. Although individuals with this form of angina may well have significant coronary atherosclerosis, the anginal attacks are unrelated to physical activity, heart rate, or blood pressure. Prinzmetal angina generally responds promptly to vasodilators such as *nitroglycerin* and calcium channel blockers.

III. ORGANIC NITRATES

Organic nitrates (and nitrites) used in the treatment of angina pectoris are simple nitric and nitrous acid esters of glycerol. They differ in their volatility. For example, *isosorbide dinitrate* and *isosorbide mononitrate* are solids at room temperature, *nitroglycerin* is only moderately volatile, and *amyl nitrate* is extremely volatile. These compounds cause a rapid reduction in myocardial oxygen demand, followed by rapid relief of symptoms. They are effective in stable and unstable angina as well as in variant angina pectoris.

A. Mechanism of action

Nitrates decrease coronary vasoconstriction or spasm and increase perfusion of the myocardium by relaxing coronary arteries. Their potent venodilator activity decreases myocardial oxygen demand by reducing venous return to the heart. The organic nitrates, such as *nitroglycerin* [nye troe GLIS er in], which is also known as *glyceryl trinitrate*, are thought to relax vascular smooth muscle by their intracellular conversion to nitrite ions, and then to nitric oxide, which in turn activates guanylate cyclase and increases the cells' cyclic GMP.[1] Elevated cGMP ultimately leads to dephosphorylation of the myosin light chain, resulting in vascular smooth muscle relaxation (Figure 18.2).

B. Effects on the cardiovascular system

All these agents are effective, but they differ in their onset of action and rate of elimination. For prompt relief of an ongoing attack of angina precipitated by exercise or emotional stress, sublingual (or spray form) *nitroglycerin* is the drug of choice. At therapeutic doses, *nitroglycerin* has two major effects. First, it causes dilation of the large veins, resulting in pooling of blood in the veins. This diminishes preload (venous return to the heart) and reduces the work of the heart. Second, *nitroglycerin* dilates the coronary vasculature,

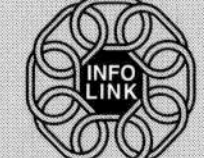

[1]See p. 149 in ***Lippincott's Illustrated Reviews: Biochemistry*** (3rd ed.) for a discussion of the role of nitric oxide in cyclic GMP production.

providing an increased blood supply to the heart muscle. *Nitroglycerin* decreases myocardial oxygen consumption because of decreased cardiac work.

C. Pharmacokinetics

The time to onset of action varies from one minute for *nitroglycerin* to more than one hour for *isosorbide mononitrate* (Figure 18.3). Significant first-pass metabolism of *nitroglycerin* occurs in the liver. Therefore, it is common to take the drug either sublingually or via a transdermal patch, thereby avoiding this route of elimination. *Isosorbide mononitrate* owes its improved bioavailability and long duration of action to its stability against hepatic breakdown. Oral *isosorbide dinitrate* undergoes denitration to two mononitrates, both of which possess antianginal activity.

D. Adverse effects

The most common adverse effect of *nitroglycerin*, as well as of the other nitrates, is headache. Thirty to sixty percent of patients receiving intermittent nitrate therapy with long-acting agents develop headaches. High doses of organic nitrates can also cause postural hypotension, facial flushing, and tachycardia. *Sildenafil* potentiates the action of the nitrates. To preclude the dangerous hypotension that may occur, an interval of at least six hours between the ingestion of the two drugs is recommended.

E. Tolerance

Tolerance to the actions of nitrates develops rapidly. The blood vessels become desensitized to the vasodilation. Tolerance can be overcome by providing a daily "nitrate-free interval" to restore sensitivity to the drug. This interval is typically ten to twelve hours, usually at night, because demand on the heart is decreased at that time. *Nitroglycerin* patches are worn for twelve hours then removed for twelve hours. However, variant angina worsens early in the morning, perhaps due to circadian catecholamine surges. Therefore, the nitrate-free interval in these patients should occur in the late afternoon. Patients who continue to have angina despite nitrate therapy may benefit by addition of another class of agent.

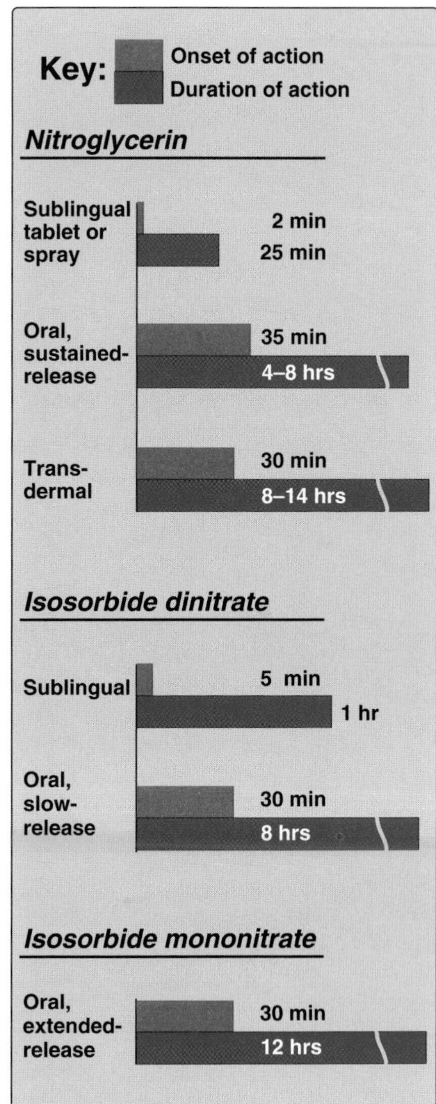

Figure 18.3
Time to peak effect and duration of action for some common organic nitrate preparations.

IV. β-ADRENERGIC BLOCKERS

The β-adrenergic blocking agents decrease the oxygen demands of the myocardium by lowering both the rate and the force of contraction of the heart (see p. 84). They suppress the activation of the heart by blocking β_1 receptors, and they reduce the work of the heart by decreasing cardiac output and blood pressure. The demand for oxygen by the myocardium is reduced both during exertion and at rest. *Propranolol* is the prototype for this class of compounds, but it is not cardioselective. Thus, other β-blockers, such as *metoprolol*, *acebutolol*, or *atenolol*, are preferred. [Note: All β-blockers are nonselective at high doses and can inhibit β_2 receptors. This is particularly important to remember in the case of asthmatics.] Agents with intrinsic sympathomimetic activity (for example, *pindolol*) are less effective and should be avoided. The β-blockers reduce the frequency and severity of angina attacks. These agents are particularly use-

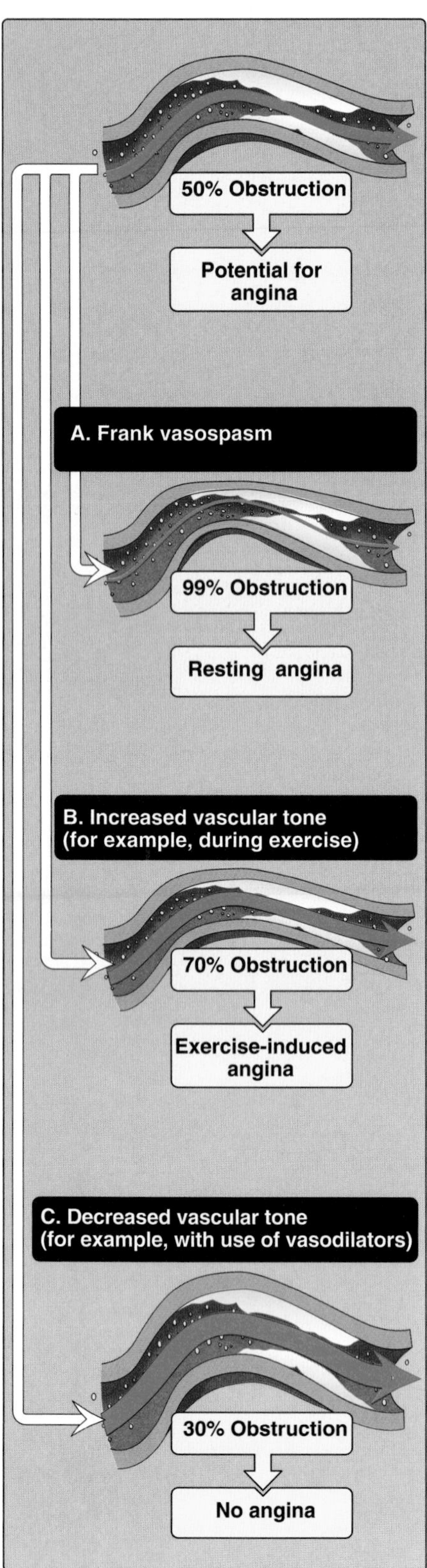

Figure 18.4
Blood flow in a coronary artery partially blocked with atherosclerotic plaques.

ful in the treatment of patients with myocardial infarction, and have been shown to prolong survival. The β-blockers can be used with nitrates to increase exercise duration and tolerance. They are, however, contraindicated in patients with asthma, diabetes, severe bradycardia, peripheral vascular disease, or chronic obstructive pulmonary disease. [Note: It is important not to discontinue β-blocker therapy abruptly. The dose should be gradually tapered off over five to ten days to avoid rebound angina or hypertension.]

V. CALCIUM CHANNEL BLOCKERS

Calcium is essential for muscular contraction. Calcium influx is increased in ischemia because of the membrane depolarization that hypoxia produces. In turn, this promotes the activity of several ATP-consuming enzymes, thereby depleting energy stores and worsening the ischemia. The calcium channel blockers protect the tissue by inhibiting the entrance of calcium into cardiac and smooth muscle cells of the coronary and systemic arterial beds. All calcium channel blockers are therefore vasodilators that cause a decrease in smooth muscle tone and vascular resistance. (See p. 204 for a description of the mechanism of action for this group of drugs.) At clinical doses, these agents affect primarily the resistance of vascular smooth muscle and the myocardium. [Note: *Verapamil* mainly affects the myocardium, whereas *nifedipine* exerts a greater effect on smooth muscle in the peripheral vasculature. *Diltiazem* is intermediate in its actions.] All calcium channel blockers lower blood pressure. They may worsen heart failure due to their negative inotropic effect. [Note: Variant angina caused by spontaneous coronary spasm (either at work or at rest, Figure 18.4) rather than by increased myocardial oxygen requirements is controlled by organic nitrates or calcium channel blockers; β-blockers are contraindicated.]

A. Nifedipine

Nifedipine [nye FED i peen], a dihydropyridine derivative, functions mainly as an arteriolar vasodilator. This drug has minimal effect on cardiac conduction or heart rate. Other members of this class, *amlodipine*, *nicardipine*, *felodipine*, and *nitrendipine*, have similar cardiovascular characteristics except for *amlodipine*, which does not affect heart rate or cardiac output. *Nifedipine* is administered orally, usually as extended-release tablets. It undergoes hepatic metabolism to products that are eliminated in both urine and the feces. The vasodilation effect of *nifedipine* is useful in the treatment of variant angina caused by spontaneous coronary spasm. *Nifedipine* can cause flushing, headache, hypotension, and peripheral edema as side effects of its vasodilation activity. As with all calcium channel blockers, constipation is a problem. Because it has little to no sympathetic antagonistic action, *nifedipine* may cause reflex tachycardia if peripheral vasodilation is marked, resulting in a substantial decrease in blood pressure. [Note: The general consensus is that short-acting dihydropyridines should be avoided in coronary artery disease.]

B. Verapamil

The diphenylalkylamine *verapamil* [ver AP a mil] slows cardiac conduction directly and, thus, decreases heart rate and oxygen

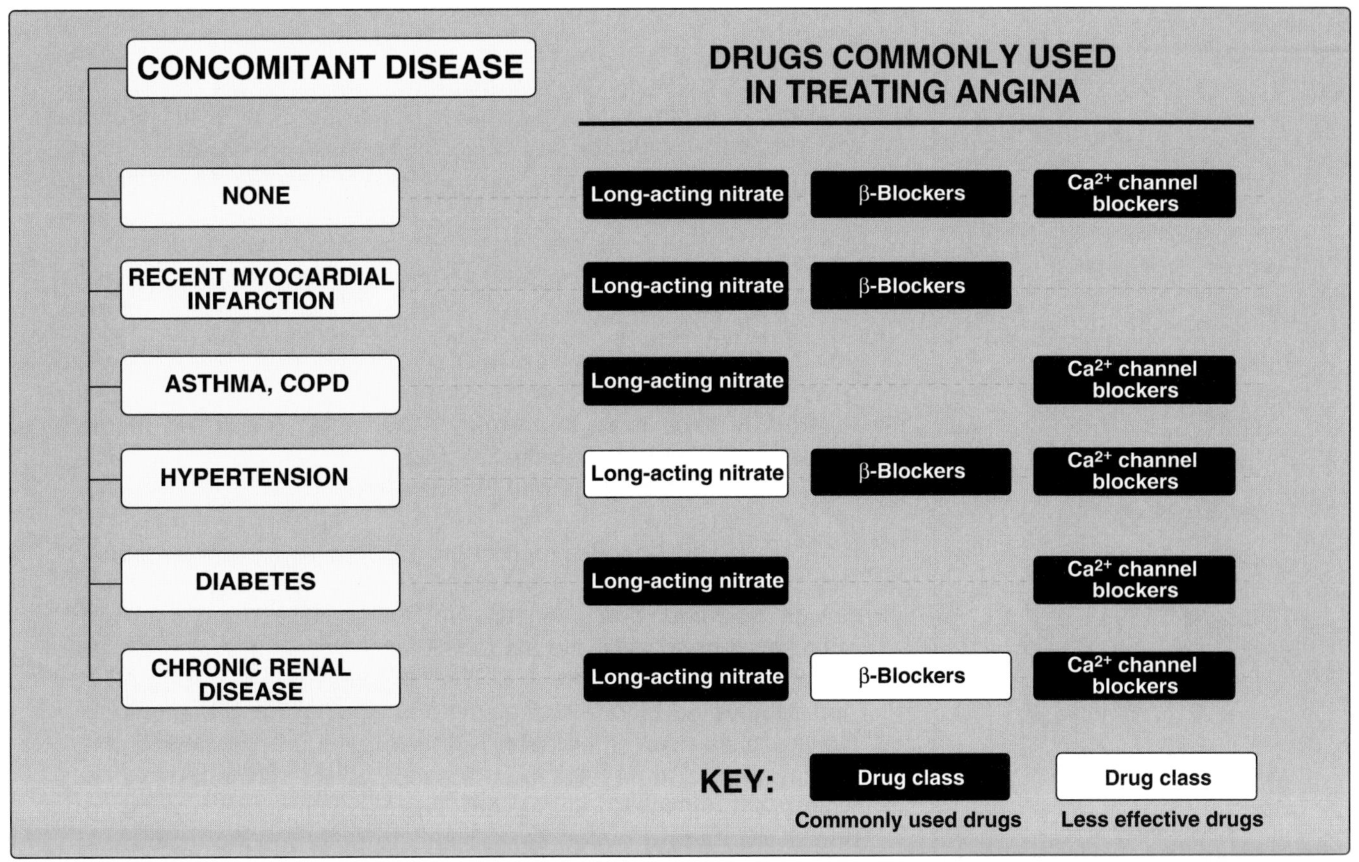

Figure 18.5
Treatment of angina in patients with concomitant diseases. COPD = chronic obstructive pulmonary disease.

demand. *Verapamil* causes greater negative inotropic effects than *nifedipine*, but it is a weaker vasodilator. The drug is extensively metabolized by the liver; therefore, care must be taken to adjust the dose in patients with liver dysfunction. *Verapamil* is contraindicated in patients with preexisting depressed cardiac function or atrioventricular (AV) conduction abnormalities. It also causes constipation. *Verapamil* should be used with caution in patients taking *digoxin* because *verapamil* increases *digoxin* levels.

C. Diltiazem

Diltiazem [dil TYE a zem] has cardiovascular effects that are similar to those of *verapamil*. Both drugs slow AV conduction and decrease the rate of firing of the sinus node pacemaker. *Diltiazem* reduces the heart rate, although to a lesser extent than *verapamil*, and also decreases blood pressure. In addition, *diltiazem* can relieve coronary artery spasm and, therefore, is particularly useful in patients with variant angina. It is extensively metabolized by the liver. The incidence of adverse side effects is low (the same as those for other calcium channel blockers). Interactions with other drugs are the same as those indicated for *verapamil*.

Figure 18.5 summarizes the treatment of angina in patients with concomitant diseases.

Study Questions

Choose the ONE best answer.

18.1 A 56-year-old patient complains of chest pain following any sustained exercise. He is diagnosed with atherosclerotic angina. He is prescribed sublingual nitroglycerin for treatment of acute chest pain. Which of the following adverse effects is likely to be experienced by this patient?

A. Hypertension
B. Throbbing headache
C. Bradycardia
D. Sexual dysfunction
E. Anemia

Correct answer = B. Nitroglycerin causes throbbing headache in thirty to sixty percent of patients who are taking the drug. The other choices are incorrect.

18.2 The patient described in question 18.1 is also prescribed propranolol to prevent episodes of angina. The β-blocker has the added benefit of preventing which of the following side effects of sublingual nitroglycerin?

A. Dizziness
B. Methemoglobinemia
C. Throbbing headache
D. Reflex tachycardia
E. Edema

Correct answer = D. Nitroglycerin can cause a reflex tachycardia because of its vasodilating properties. This reflex is blocked by propranolol. The other effects are either not prevented by propranolol or not caused by nitroglycerin (edema).

18.3 A 68-year-old man has been successfully treated for exercise-induced angina for several years. He recently has been complaining about being awakened at night with chest pain. Which of the following drugs would be useful in preventing this patient's nocturnal angina?

A. Amyl nitrite
B. Nitroglycerin (sublingual)
C. Nitroglycerin (transdermal)
D. Esmolol
E. Hydralazine

Correct answer = C. Transdermal nitroglycerin can sustain blood levels for as long as 24 hours. Because tolerance occurs, however, it is recommended that the patch be removed after eight to ten hours to allow recovery of sensitivity. Amyl nitrite, sublingual nitroglycerin, and esmolol all have short durations of actions. Hydralazine may actually precipitate an angina attack.

Antihypertensive Drugs

19

I. OVERVIEW

Hypertension requiring drug therapy is defined as either a sustained systolic blood pressure (SBP) of greater than 140 mm Hg or a sustained diastolic blood pressure (DBP) of greater than 90 mm Hg. Hypertension results from increased peripheral vascular smooth muscle tone, which leads to increased arteriolar resistance and reduced capacitance of the venous system. Elevated blood pressure is an extremely common disorder, affecting approximately fifteen percent of the population of the United States (sixty million people). Although many of these individuals have no symptoms, chronic hypertension—either systolic or diastolic—can lead to congestive heart failure, myocardial infarction, renal damage, and cerebrovascular accidents. The incidence of morbidity and mortality significantly decreases when hypertension is diagnosed early and is properly treated. In recognition of the progressive nature of hypertension, the Seventh Report of the Joint National Committee classifies hypertension into four categories for the purpose of treatment management. The categories are normal (SBP/DBP, <120/<80), prehypertension (SBP/DBP, 120–139/80–89), stage 1 hypertension (SBP/DBP, 140–159/90–99), and stage 2 hypertension (SBP/DBP $\geq$160/$\geq$100).

II. ETIOLOGY OF HYPERTENSION

Although hypertension may occur secondary to other disease processes, more than ninety percent of patients have essential hypertension, a disorder of unknown origin affecting the blood pressure regulating mechanism. A family history of hypertension increases the likelihood that an individual will develop hypertensive disease. Essential hypertension is four-fold more frequent among blacks than among whites, and it occurs more often among middle-aged males than among middle-aged females. Environmental factors, such as a stressful lifestyle, high dietary intake of sodium, obesity, and smoking, all further predispose an individual to the occurrence of hypertension. Figure 19.1 summarizes the drugs used to treat hypertension. [Note: Nonsteroidal anti-inflammatory drugs interfere with the hypotensive action of many antihypertensives.]

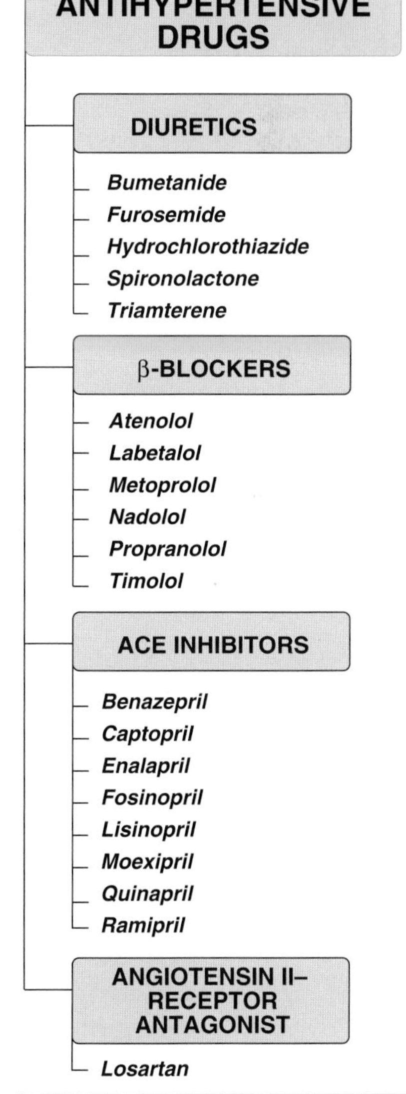

Figure 19.1
Summary of antihypertensive drugs. ACE = angiotensin-converting enzyme. (Continued on next page.)

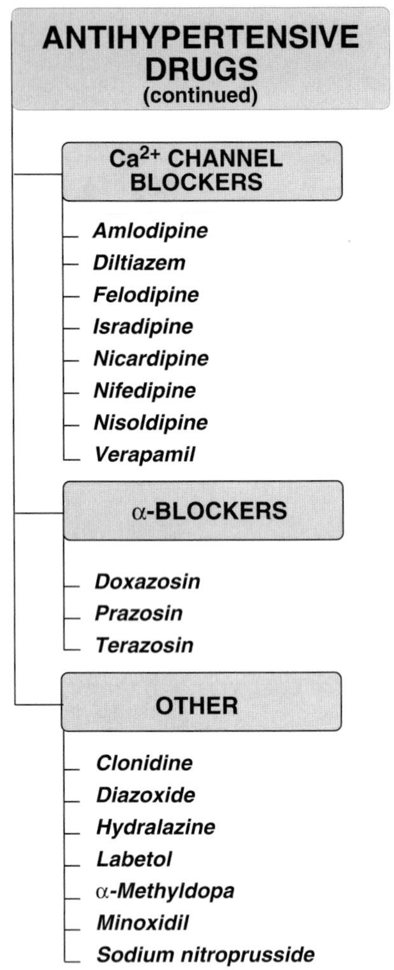

Figure 19.1
Summary of antihypertensive drugs.

III. MECHANISMS FOR CONTROLLING BLOOD PRESSURE

Arterial blood pressure is regulated within a narrow range to provide adequate perfusion of the tissues without causing damage to the vascular system, particularly the arterial intima. Arterial blood pressure is directly proportional to the product of the cardiac output and the peripheral vascular resistance (Figure 19.2). In both normal and hypertensive individuals, cardiac output and peripheral resistance are controlled mainly by two overlapping control mechanisms: the baroreflexes, which are mediated by the sympathetic nervous system, and the renin-angiotensin-aldosterone system (Figure 19.3). Most antihypertensive drugs lower blood pressure by reducing cardiac output and/or decreasing peripheral resistance.

A. Baroreceptors and the sympathetic nervous system

Baroreflexes involving the sympathetic nervous system are responsible for the rapid, moment-to-moment regulation of blood pressure. A fall in blood pressure causes pressure-sensitive neurons (baroreceptors in the aortic arch and carotid sinuses) to send fewer impulses to cardiovascular centers in the spinal cord. This prompts a reflex response of increased sympathetic and decreased parasympathetic output to the heart and vasculature, resulting in vasoconstriction and increased cardiac output. These changes result in a compensatory rise in blood pressure (see Figure 19.3).

B. Renin-angiotensin-aldosterone system

The kidney provides for the long-term control of blood pressure by altering the blood volume. Baroreceptors in the kidney respond to reduced arterial pressure (and to sympathetic stimulation of β adrenoceptors) by releasing the enzyme renin (see Figure 19.3). This peptidase converts angiotensinogen to angiotensin I, which is converted in turn to angiotensin II in the presence of angiotensin-converting enzyme (ACE). Angiotensin II is the body's most potent circulating vasoconstrictor, causing an increase in blood pressure. Furthermore, angiotensin II stimulates aldosterone secretion, leading to increased renal sodium reabsorption and increased blood volume, which contribute to a further increase in blood pressure.

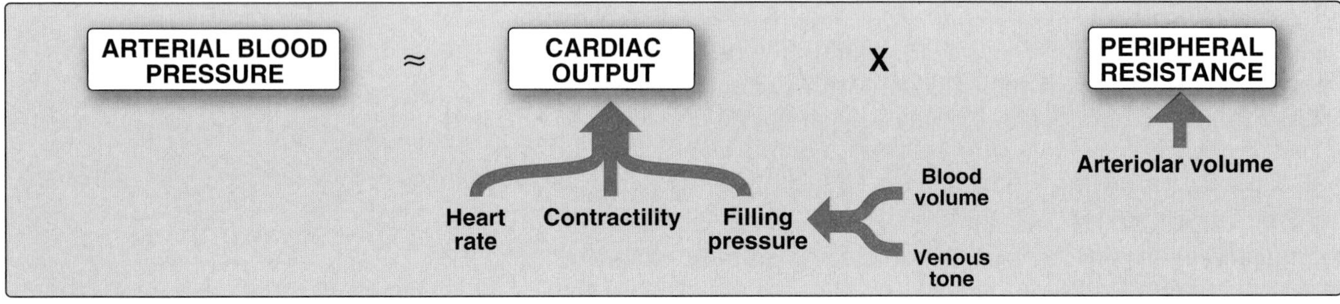

Figure 19.2
Major factors influencing blood pressure.

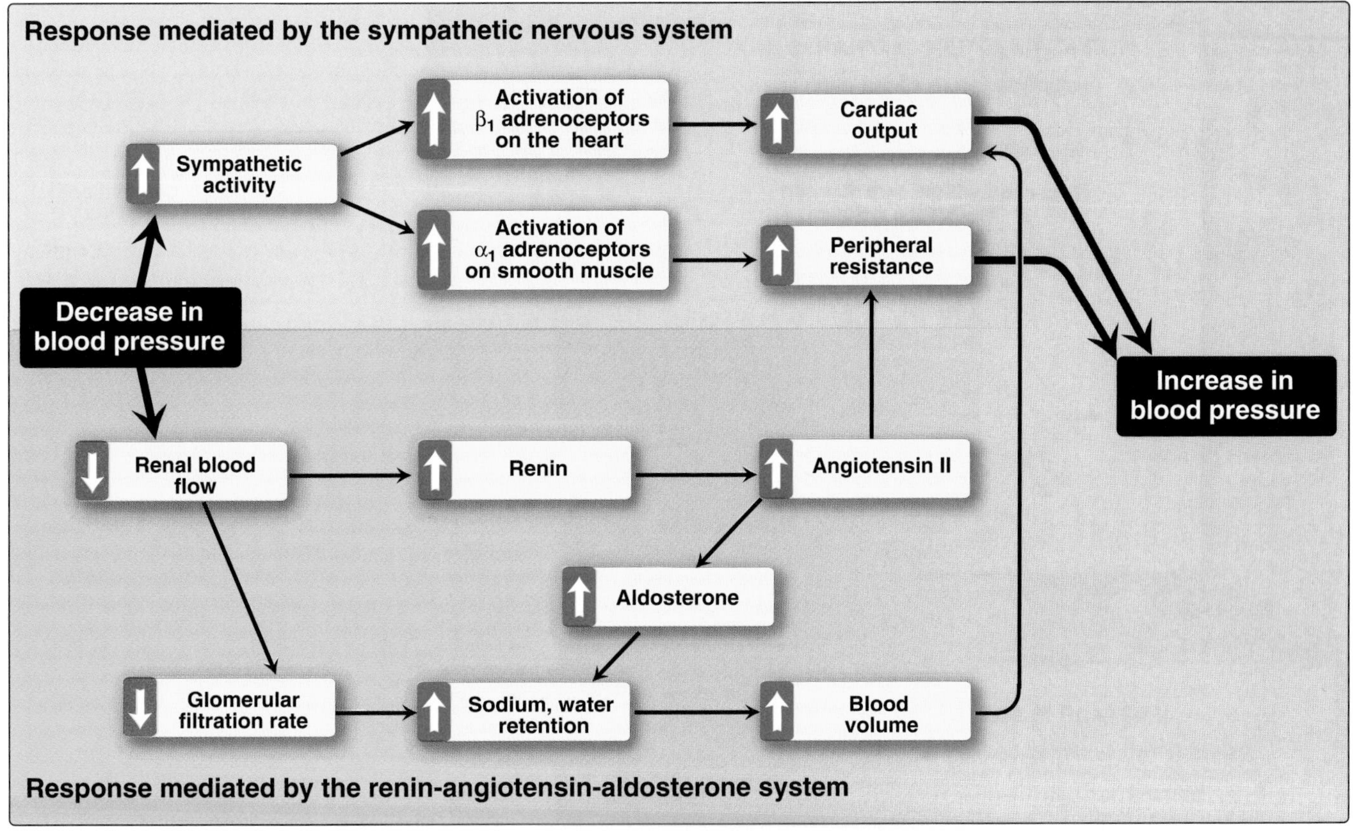

Figure 19.3
Response of the autonomic nervous system and the renin-angiotensin-aldosterone system to a decrease in blood pressure.

IV. TREATMENT STRATEGIES

The goal of antihypertensive therapy is to reduce cardiovascular and renal morbidity and mortality. The relationship between blood pressure and the risk of a cardiovascular event is continuous. The newly added classification of "prehypertension" recognizes this relationship and emphasizes the need for decreasing blood pressure in the general population by education and adoption of blood pressure–lowering behaviors. Mild hypertension can often be controlled with a single drug. Current treatment recommendations are to initiate therapy with a thiazide diuretic unless there are compelling reasons to employ other drug classes (Figure 19.4). If blood pressure is inadequately controlled, a second drug is added, with the selection based on minimizing the adverse effects of the combined regimen. A β-blocker is usually added if the initial drug was a diuretic, or a diuretic is usually added if the first drug was a β-blocker. A vasodilator can be added as a third step for those patients who still fail to respond.

A. Individualized care

Certain subsets of the hypertensive population respond better to one class of drug than they do to another. For example, black patients respond well to diuretics and calcium channel blockers, but therapy

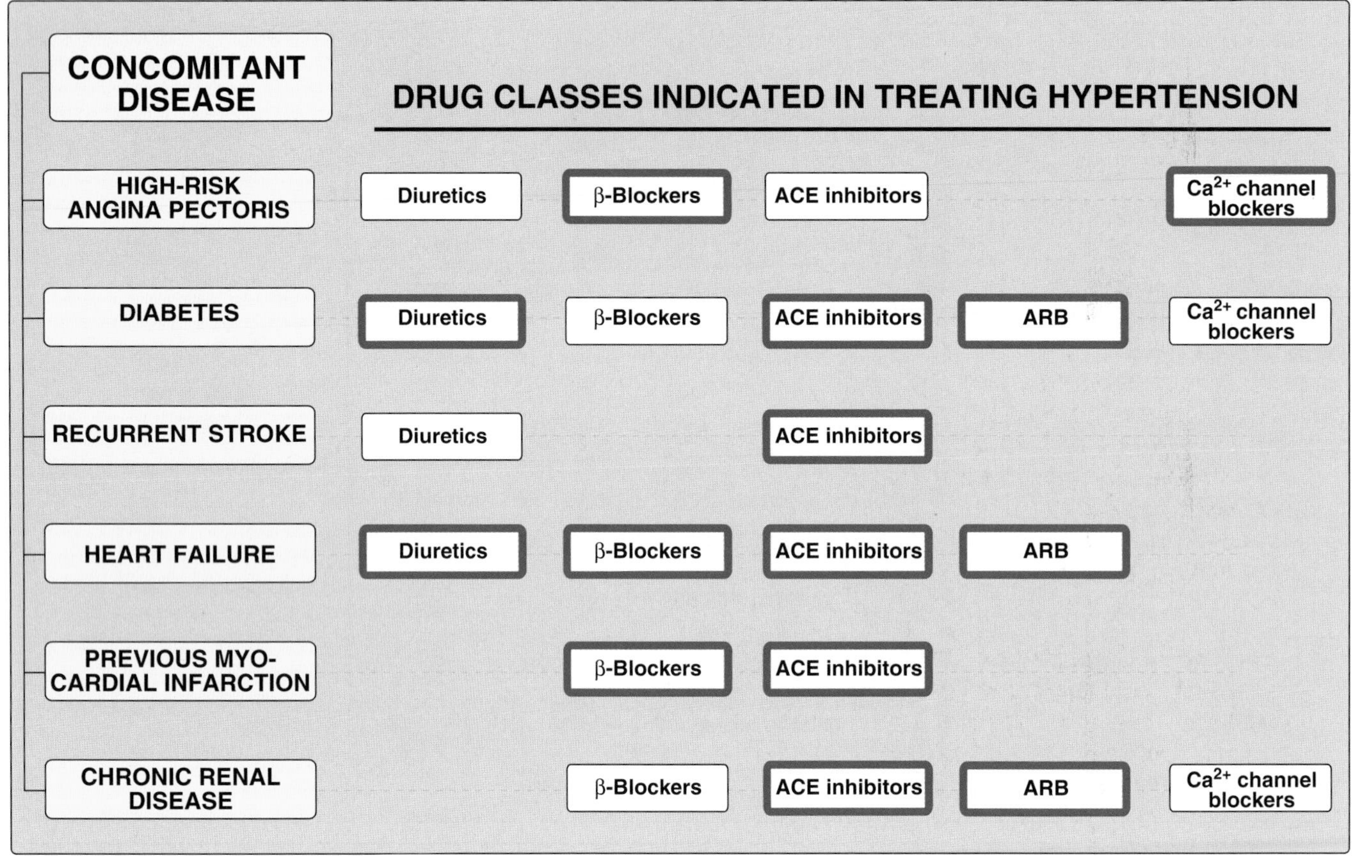

Figure 19.4
Treatment of hypertension in patients with concomitant diseases. Drug classes shown in blue boxes provide improvement in outcome independent of blood pressure. [Note: ARBs are an alternative to ACE inhibitors. No added benefit is gained if ARBs and ACE inhibitors are combined.] ACE = angiotensin-converting enzyme; ARB = angiotensin receptor blocker.

with β-blockers or ACE inhibitors is often less effective. Similarly, calcium channel blockers, ACE inhibitors, and diuretics are favored for treatment of hypertension in the elderly, whereas β-blockers and α-antagonists are less well tolerated. Furthermore, hypertension may coexist with other diseases that can be aggravated by some of the antihypertensive drugs. For example, Figure 19.4 shows the preferred therapy in hypertensive patients with various concomitant diseases. In such cases, it is important to match antihypertensive drugs to the particular patient. Figure 19.5 shows the frequency of concomitant disease in the hypertensive patient population.

B. Patient compliance in antihypertensive therapy

Lack of patient compliance is the most common reason for failure of antihypertensive therapy. The hypertensive patient is usually asymptomatic and is diagnosed by routine screening before the occurrence of overt end-organ damage. Thus, therapy is generally directed at preventing disease sequelae (that occur in the future), rather than in relieving the patient's present discomfort. The adverse effects associated with the hypertensive therapy may influence the patient more than the future benefits. For example, β-blockers can decrease libido and induce impotence in males, particularly middle-aged and elderly men. This drug-induced sexual dysfunction may prompt the patient to discontinue therapy. Thus, it is important to enhance compliance by carefully selecting a drug regimen that both reduces adverse effects and minimizes the number of doses required daily.

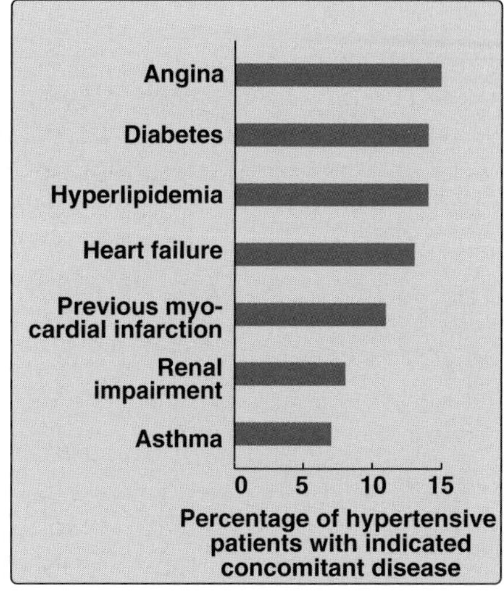

Figure 19.5
Frequency of occurrence of concomitant disease among the hypertensive patient population.

V. DIURETICS

Diuretics are currently recommended as the first-line drug therapy for hypertension unless there are compelling reasons to chose another agent. Low-dose diuretic therapy is safe and effective in preventing stroke, myocardial infarction, and congestive heart failure, all of which can cause mortality. Recent data suggest that diuretics are superior to β-blockers in older adults.

A. Thiazide diuretics

All oral diuretic drugs are effective in the treatment of hypertension, but the thiazides have found the most widespread use.

1. **Actions:** Thiazide diuretics, such as *hydrochlorothiazide* [hye droe klor oh THYE a zide], lower blood pressure initially by increasing sodium and water excretion. This causes a decrease in extracellular volume, resulting in a decrease in cardiac output and renal blood flow (Figure 19.6). With long-term treatment, plasma volume approaches a normal value, but peripheral resistance decreases. *Spironolactone* [speer on oh LAK tone], a potassium-sparing diuretic, is often used with thiazides. *Spironolactone* has the additional benefit of diminishing the cardiac remodeling that occurs in heart failure. (A complete discussion of diuretics is found in Chapter 22, p. 257.)

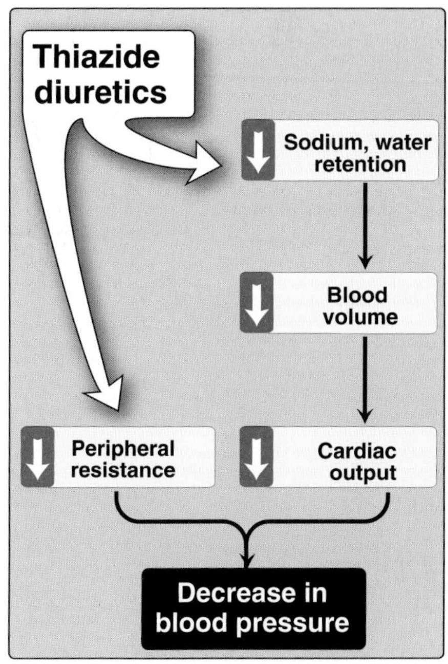

Figure 19.6
Actions of thiazide diuretics.

2. **Therapeutic uses:** Thiazide diuretics decrease blood pressure in both the supine and standing positions, and postural hypotension is rarely observed except in elderly, volume-depleted patients. These agents counteract the sodium and water retention observed with other agents used in the treatment of hypertension (for example, *hydralazine*). Thiazides are therefore useful in combination therapy with a variety of other antihypertensive agents, including β-blockers and ACE inhibitors. Thiazide diuretics are particularly useful in the treatment of black or elderly patients. They are not effective in patients with inadequate kidney function (creatinine clearance <50 mL/min). Loop diuretics may be required in these patients.

3. **Pharmacokinetics:** Thiazide diuretics are orally active. Absorption and elimination rates vary considerably, although no clear advantage is present for one agent over another. All thiazides are ligands for the organic acid secretory system of the nephron, and as such, they may compete with uric acid for elimination.

4. **Adverse effects:** Thiazide diuretics induce hypokalemia and hyperuricemia in seventy percent of patients and hyperglycemia in ten percent of patients. Hypomagnesemia may also occur. Serum

potassium levels should be monitored closely in patients who are predisposed to cardiac arrhythmias (particularly individuals with left-ventricular hypertrophy, ischemic heart disease, or chronic heart failure) and who are concurrently being treated with both thiazide diuretics and digitalis glycosides.

B. Loop diuretics

The loop diuretics act promptly, even in patients with poor renal function or who have not responded to thiazides or other diuretics. The loop diuretics cause decreased renal vascular resistance and increased renal blood flow. [Note: Loop diuretics increase the Ca^{2+} content of urine, whereas thiazide diuretics decrease the Ca^{2+} concentration of the urine.]

VI. β-ADRENOCEPTOR–BLOCKING AGENTS

β-Blockers are currently recommended as first-line drug therapy for hypertension when indicated—for example, with heart failure. These drugs are efficacious but have some contraindications.

A. Actions

The β-blockers reduce blood pressure primarily by decreasing cardiac output (Figure 19.7). They may also decrease sympathetic outflow from the CNS and inhibit the release of renin from the kidneys, thus decreasing the formation of angiotensin II and the secretion of aldosterone. The prototype β-blocker is *propranolol* [proe PRAN oh lol], which acts at both β_1 and β_2 receptors. Selective blockers of β_1 receptors, such as *metoprolol* [met OH pro lol] and *atenolol* [ah TEN oh lol], are among the most commonly prescribed β-blockers. The selective β-blockers may be administered cautiously to hypertensive

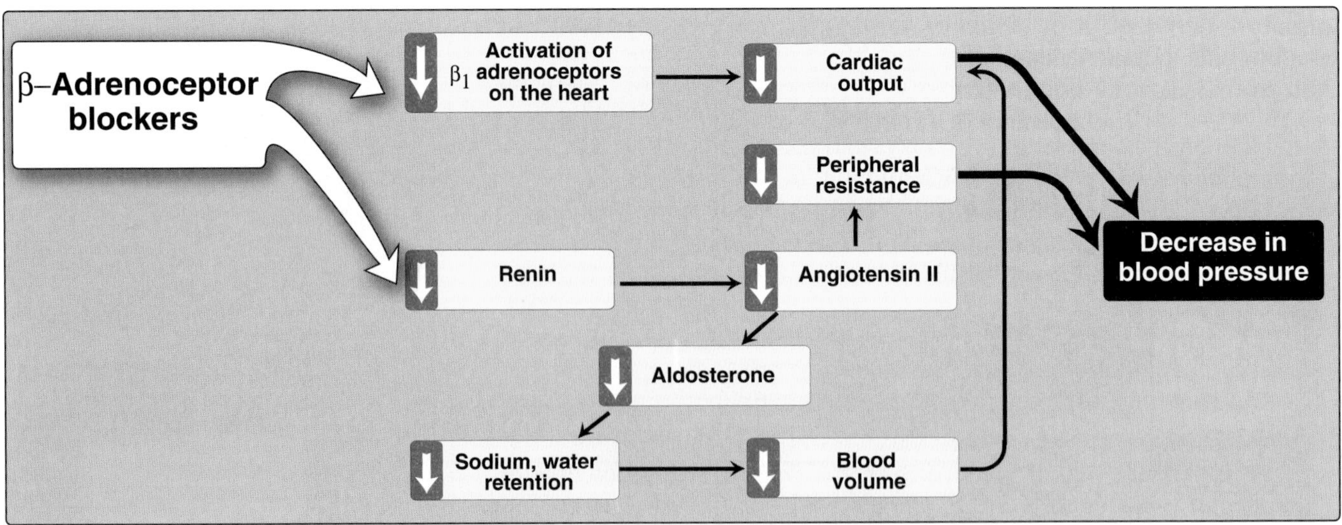

Figure 19.7
Actions of β-adrenoceptor blocking agents.

patients who also have asthma, for which *propranolol* is contraindicated due to its blockade of β_2-mediated bronchodilation. (See p. 218 for a discussion of the β-blockers.)

B. Therapeutic uses

1. **Subsets of the hypertensive population:** The β-blockers are more effective for treating hypertension in white than in black patients, and in young compared to elderly patients. [Note: Conditions that discourage the use of β-blockers (for example, severe chronic obstructive lung disease, chronic congestive heart failure, or severe symptomatic occlusive peripheral vascular disease) are more commonly found in the elderly and in diabetics.]

2. **Hypertensive patients with concomitant diseases:** The β-blockers are useful in treating conditions that may coexist with hypertension, such as supraventricular tachyarrhythmia, previous myocardial infarction, angina pectoris, chronic heart failure, and migraine headache.

C. Pharmacokinetics

The β-blockers are orally active. *Propranolol* undergoes extensive and highly variable first-pass metabolism. The β-blockers may take several weeks to develop their full effects.

D. Adverse effects

1. **Common effects:** The β-blockers may cause bradycardia, and CNS side effects such as fatigue, lethargy, insomnia, and hallucinations; these drugs can also cause hypotension (Figure 19.8). The β-blockers may decrease libido and cause impotence. [Note: Drug-induced sexual dysfunction can severely reduce patient compliance.]

2. **Alterations in serum lipid patterns:** The β-blockers may disturb lipid metabolism, decreasing high-density lipoprotein and increasing plasma triacylglycerol.

3. **Drug withdrawal:** Abrupt withdrawal may cause rebound hypertension, probably as a result of up-regulation of β receptors. Removal from β-blocker therapy should therefore be tapered to avoid precipitation of arrhythmias. The β-blockers should be employed cautiously in the treatment of patients with asthma, acute heart failure, or peripheral vascular disease.

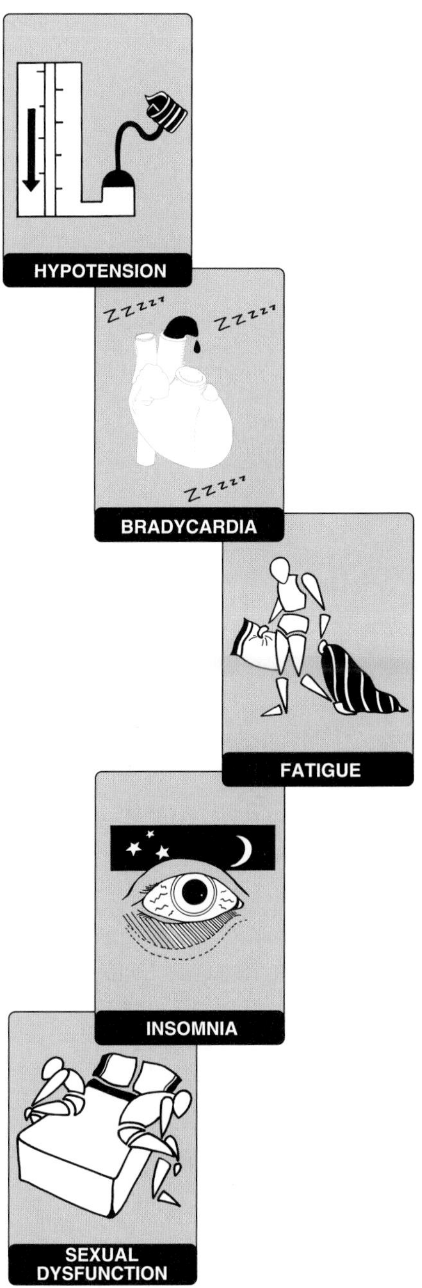

Figure 19.8
Some adverse effects of β-blockers.

VII. ACE INHIBITORS

The ACE inhibitors, such as *enalapril* [e NAL ah pril] or *lisinopril* [lye SIN oh pril], are recommended when the preferred first-line agents (diuretics or β-blockers) are contraindicated or ineffective. Despite their widespread use, it is not clear if antihypertensive therapy with ACE inhibitors increases the risk of other major diseases.

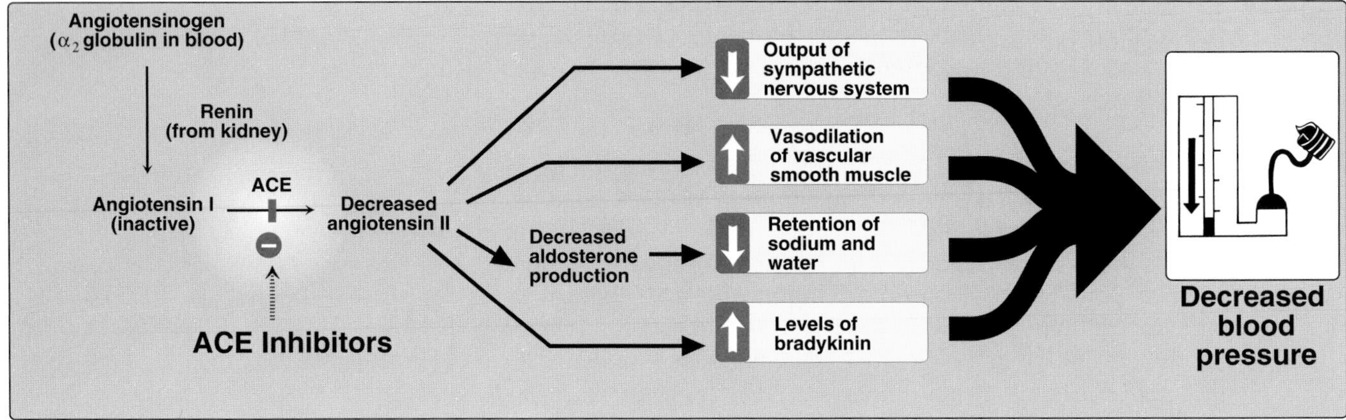

Figure 19.9
Effects of angiotensin-converting enzyme (ACE) inhibitors.

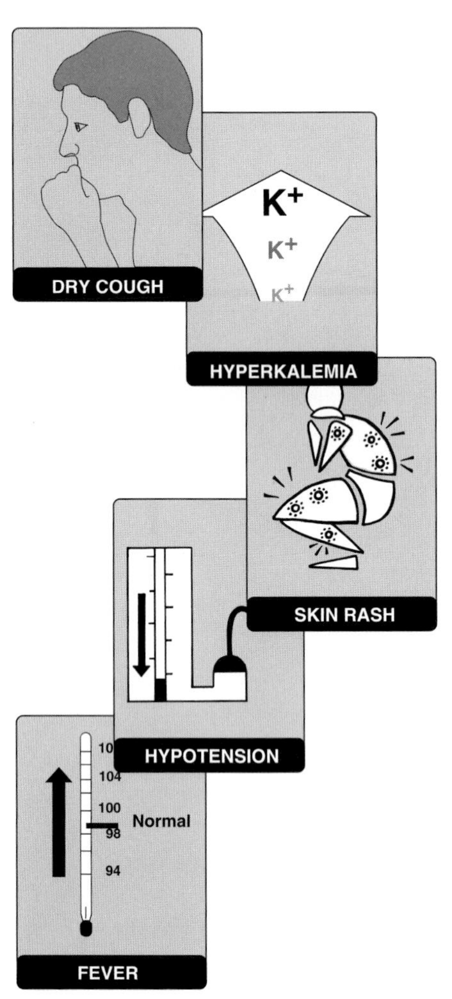

Figure 19.10
Some common adverse effects of the ACE inhibitors.

A. Actions

The ACE inhibitors lower blood pressure by reducing peripheral vascular resistance without reflexively increasing cardiac output, rate, or contractility. These drugs block the ACE that cleaves angiotensin I to form the potent vasoconstrictor angiotensin II (Figure 19.9). The converting enzyme is also responsible for the breakdown of bradykinin. Vasodilation occurs as a result of the combined effects of lower vasoconstriction caused by diminished levels of angiotensin II and the potent vasodilating effect of increased bradykinin. By reducing circulating angiotensin II levels, ACE inhibitors also decrease the secretion of aldosterone, resulting in decreased sodium and water retention.

B. Therapeutic uses

Like β-blockers, ACE inhibitors are most effective in hypertensive patients who are white and young. However, when used in combination with a diuretic, the effectiveness of ACE inhibitors is similar in white and black patients with hypertension. Along with the angiotensin receptor blockers, ACE inhibitors slow the progression of diabetic nephropathy and decrease albuminuria. ACE inhibitors are also effective in the management of patients with chronic heart failure. ACE inhibitors are a standard in the care of a patient following a myocardial infarction. Therapy is started 24 hours after the end of the infarction.

C. Adverse effects

Common side effects include dry cough, rash, fever, altered taste, hypotension (in hypovolemic states), and hyperkalemia (Figure 19.10). The dry cough, which occurs in about ten percent of patients, is thought to be due to increased levels of bradykinin in the pulmonary tree. Potassium levels must be monitored, and potassium supplements or *spironolactone* are contraindicated. Angioedema is a rare but potentially life-threatening reaction and may also be due to increased levels of bradykinin. Because of the risk of angioedema and first-dose syncope, ACE inhibitors are first administered in the physician's office with close observation. Reversible renal failure can occur in patients with severe renal artery stenosis. ACE inhibitors are fetotoxic and should not be used by women who are pregnant.

VIII. ANGIOTENSIN II–RECEPTOR ANTAGONISTS

The angiotensin II–receptor blockers (ARBs) are alternatives to the ACE inhibitors. *Losartan* [LOW sar tan], is the prototypic ARB; currently, there are six additional ARBs. Their pharmacologic effects are similar to those of ACE inhibitors in that they produce vasodilation and block aldosterone secretion, thus lowering blood pressure and decreasing salt and water retention. ARBs decrease the nephrotoxicity of diabetes, making them an attractive therapy in hypertensive diabetics. Their adverse effects are similar to those of ACE inhibitors, although the risks of cough and angioedema are significantly decreased. They are fetotoxic. [Note: The ARBs are discussed more fully in Chapter 16.]

IX. CALCIUM CHANNEL BLOCKERS

Calcium channel blockers are recommended when the preferred first-line agents are contraindicated or ineffective. They are effective in treating hypertension in patients with angina or diabetes. High doses of short-acting calcium channel blockers should be avoided because of increased risk of myocardial infarction.

A. Classes of calcium channel blockers

The calcium channel blockers are divided into three chemical classes, each with different pharmacokinetic properties and clinical indications (Figure 19.11).

1. **Diphenylalkylamines:** *Verapamil* [ver AP ah mil] is the only member of this class that is currently approved in the United States. *Verapamil* is the least selective of any calcium channel blocker, and has significant effects on both cardiac and vascular smooth-muscle cells. It is used to treat angina, supraventricular tachyarrhythmias, and migraine headache.

2. **Benzothiazepines:** *Diltiazem* [dil TYE ah zem] is the only member of this class that is currently approved in the United States. Like *verapamil*, *diltiazem* affects both cardiac and vascular smooth-muscle cells; however, it has a less pronounced negative inotropic effect on the heart compared to that of *verapamil*. *Diltiazem* has a favorable side-effect profile.

3. **Dihydropyridines:** This rapidly expanding class of calcium channel blockers includes the first-generation *nifedipine* [ni FED i peen] and five second-generation agents for treating cardiovascular disease: *amlodipine* [am LOE di peen], *felodipine* [fe LOE di peen], *isradipine* [iz RA di peen], *nicardipine* [nye KAR de peen], and *nisoldipine* [ni SOLD i peen]. These second-generation calcium channel blockers differ in pharmacokinetics, approved uses,

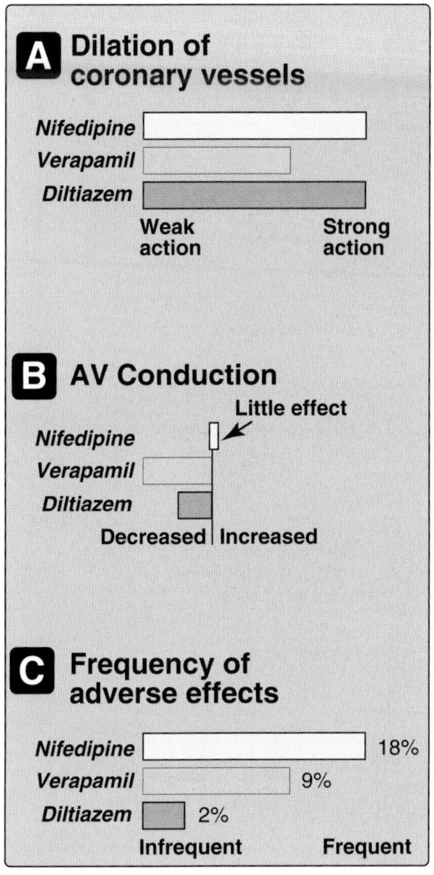

Figure 19.11
Actions of calcium channel blockers.

and drug interactions. All dihydropyridines have a much greater affinity for vascular calcium channels than for calcium channels in the heart. They are therefore particularly attractive in treating hypertension. Some of the newer agents, such as *amlodipine* and *nicardipine*, have the advantage that they show little interaction with other cardiovascular drugs, such as *digoxin* or *warfarin*, which are often used concomitantly with calcium channel blockers.

B. Actions

The intracellular concentration of calcium plays an important role in maintaining the tone of smooth muscle and in the contraction of the myocardium. Calcium enters muscle cells through special voltage-sensitive calcium channels. This triggers release of calcium from the sarcoplasmic reticulum and mitochondria, which further increases the cytosolic level of calcium. Calcium channel antagonists block the inward movement of calcium by binding to L-type calcium channels in the heart and in smooth muscle of the coronary and peripheral vasculature. This causes vascular smooth muscle to relax, dilating mainly arterioles.

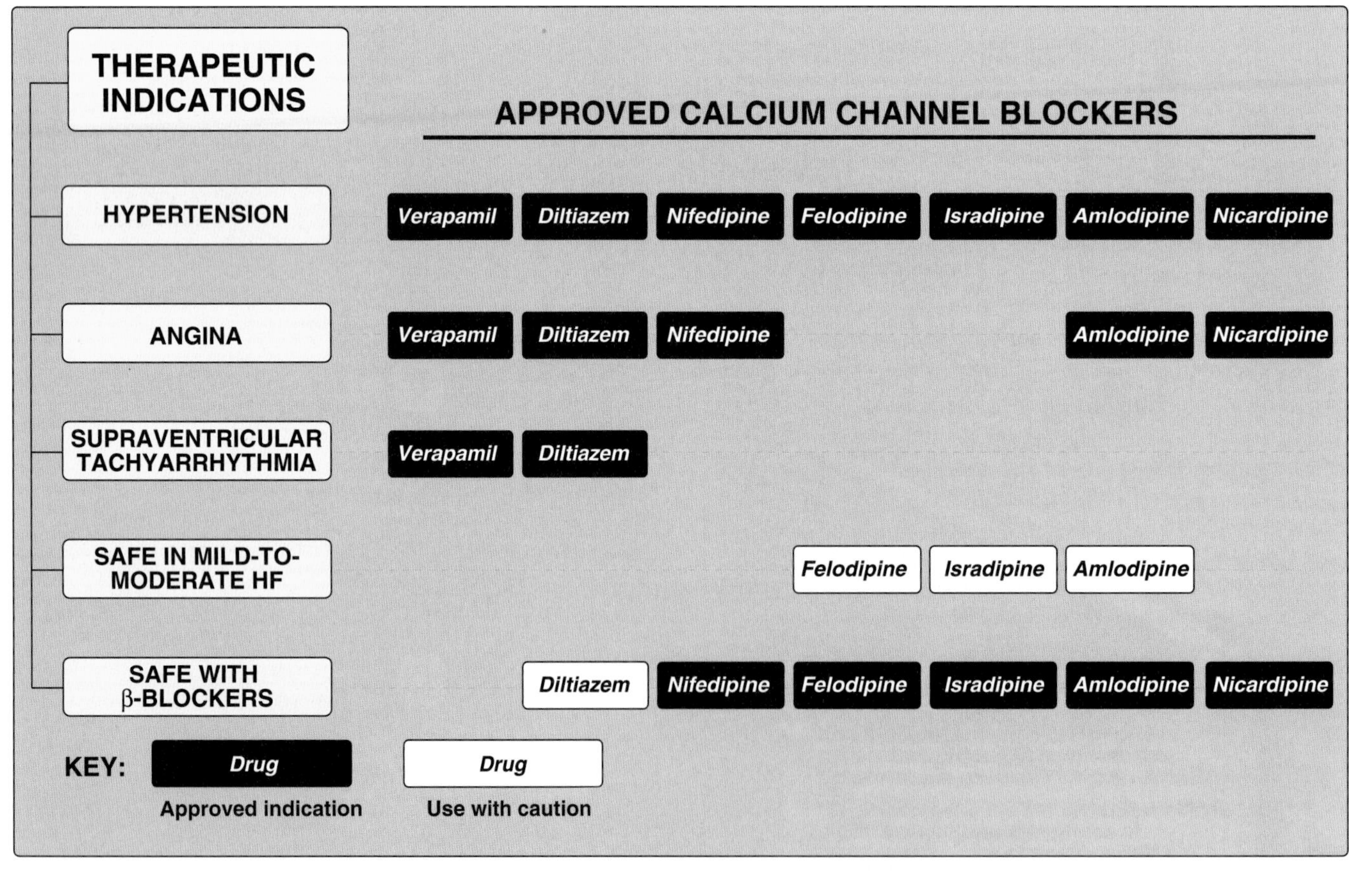

Figure 19.12
Some therapeutic applications of calcium channel blockers. HF = heart failure.

C. Therapeutic uses

Calcium channel blockers have an intrinsic natriuretic effect and, therefore, do not usually require the addition of a diuretic. These agents are useful in the treatment of hypertensive patients who also have asthma, diabetes, angina, and/or peripheral vascular disease (Figure 19.12). Black hypertensives respond well to calcium channel blockers.

D. Pharmacokinetics

Most of these agents have short half-lives (three to eight hours) following an oral dose. Treatment is required three times a day to maintain good control of hypertension. Sustained-release preparations permit less frequent dosing.

E. Adverse effects

Although infrequent, side effects include constipation in ten percent of patients, as well as dizziness, headache, and a feeling of fatigue caused by a decrease in blood pressure (Figure 19.13). *Verapamil* should be avoided in patients with congestive heart failure due to its negative inotropic effects.

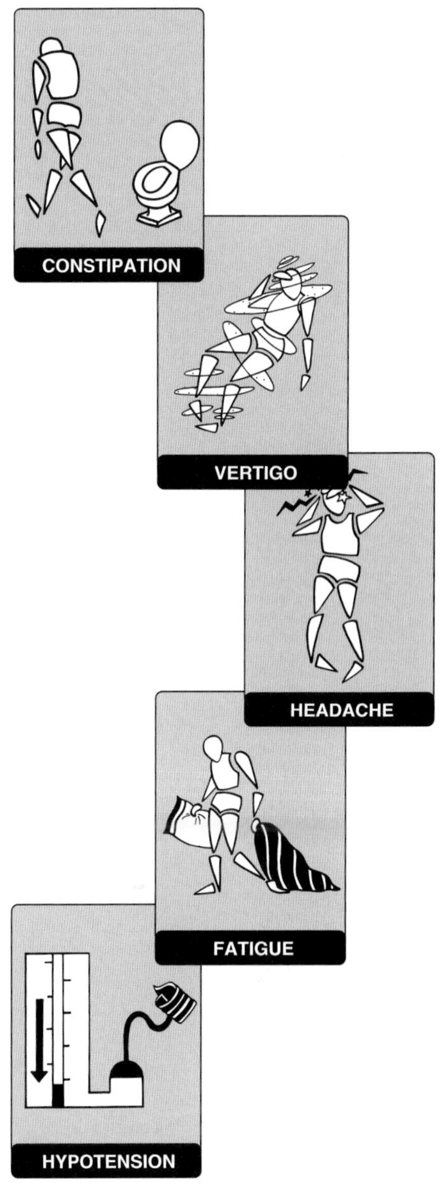

Figure 19.13
Some common adverse effects of the calcium channel blockers.

X. α-ADRENOCEPTOR–BLOCKING AGENTS

Prazosin, *doxazosin*, and *terazosin* produce a competitive block of α_1 adrenoceptors. They decrease the peripheral vascular resistance and lower the arterial blood pressure by causing relaxation of both arterial and venous smooth muscle. These drugs cause only minimal changes in cardiac output, renal blood flow, and glomerular filtration rate. Therefore, long-term tachycardia does not occur, but salt and water retention does. Postural hypotension may occur in some individuals. *Prazosin* is used to treat mild to moderate hypertension and is prescribed in combination with *propranolol* or a diuretic for additive effects. Reflex tachycardia and first-dose syncope are almost universal adverse effects. Concomitant use of a β-blocker may be necessary to blunt the short-term effect of reflex tachycardia. An increased rate of congestive heart failure occurs in patients taking *doxazosin* alone compared to those taking a thiazide diuretic alone.

XI. CENTRALLY ACTING ADRENERGIC DRUGS

A. Clonidine

This α_2 agonist diminishes central adrenergic outflow. *Clonidine* [KLOE ni deen] is used primarily for the treatment of mild to moderate hypertension that has not responded adequately to treatment with diuretics alone. *Clonidine* does not decrease renal blood flow or glomerular filtration and, therefore, is useful in the treatment of hypertension complicated by renal disease. *Clonidine* is absorbed well after oral administration and is excreted by the kidney. Because it causes sodium and water retention, *clonidine* is usually administered in combination with a diuretic. Adverse effects are generally mild, but the drug can produce sedation and drying of the nasal mucosa. Rebound hypertension occurs following abrupt withdrawal of *clonidine*. The drug should therefore be withdrawn slowly if the clinician wishes to change agents.

B. α-Methyldopa

This α_2 agonist is converted to methylnorepinephrine centrally to diminish the adrenergic outflow from the CNS. This leads to reduced total peripheral resistance and a decreased blood pressure. Cardiac output is not decreased, and blood flow to vital organs is not diminished. Because blood flow to the kidney is not diminished by its use, *α-methyldopa* [meth ill DOE pa] is especially valuable in treating hypertensive patients with renal insufficiency. The most common side effects of *α-methyldopa* are sedation and drowsiness.

XII. VASODILATORS

The direct-acting smooth muscle relaxants, such as *hydralazine* and *minoxidil*, have traditionally not been used as primary drugs to treat hypertension. Vasodilators act by producing relaxation of vascular smooth muscle, which decreases resistance and, therefore, blood pressure. These agents produce reflex stimulation of the heart, resulting in the competing reflexes of increased myocardial contractility, heart rate, and oxygen consumption. These actions may prompt angina pectoris, myocardial infarction, or cardiac failure in predisposed individuals. Vasodilators also increase plasma renin concentration, resulting in sodium and water retention. These undesirable side effects can be blocked by concomitant use of a diuretic and a β-blocker.

A. Hydralazine

This drug causes direct vasodilation, acting primarily on arteries and arterioles. This results in a decreased peripheral resistance, which in turn prompts a reflex elevation in heart rate and cardiac output. *Hydralazine* [hye DRAL ah zeen] is used to treat moderately severe hypertension. It is almost always administered in combination with a β-blocker, such as *propranolol* (to balance the reflex tachycardia), and a diuretic (to decrease sodium retention). Together, the three drugs decrease cardiac output, plasma volume, and peripheral vascular resistance. *Hydralazine* monotherapy is an accepted method of controlling blood pressure in pregnancy-induced hypertension. Adverse effects of *hydralazine* therapy include headache, nausea, sweating, arrhythmia, and precipitation of angina. A lupus-like syndrome can occur with high dosage, but it is reversible on discontinuation of the drug.

B. Minoxidil

This drug causes dilation of resistance vessels (arterioles) but not of capacitance vessels (venules). *Minoxidil* [mi NOX i dill] is administered orally for treatment of severe to malignant hypertension that is refractory to other drugs. Reflex tachycardia may be severe and require the concomitant use of a diuretic and a β-blocker. *Minoxidil* causes serious sodium and water retention, leading to volume overload, edema, and congestive heart failure. [Note: *Minoxidil* treatment also causes hypertrichosis (the growth of body hair). This drug is now used topically to treat male pattern baldness.]

XIII. HYPERTENSIVE EMERGENCY

Hypertensive emergency is a rare but life-threatening situation in which the DBP is either >150 mm Hg (with SBP >210 mm Hg) in an otherwise healthy person, or a DBP of 130 mm Hg in an individual with preexisting complications, such as encephalopathy, cerebral hemorrhage, left-ventricular failure, or aortic stenosis. The therapeutic goal is to rapidly reduce blood pressure.

A. Sodium nitroprusside

Nitroprusside [nye troe PRUSS ide] is administered intravenously, and causes prompt vasodilation with reflex tachycardia. It is capable of reducing blood pressure in all patients regardless of the cause of hypertension (Figure 19.14). The drug has little effect outside the vascular system, acting equally on arterial and venous smooth muscle. [Note: Because *nitroprusside* also acts on the veins, it can reduce cardiac preload.] *Nitroprusside* is metabolized rapidly (half-life of minutes) and requires continuous infusion to maintain its hypotensive action. *Sodium nitroprusside* exerts few adverse effects except for those of hypotension caused by overdose. *Nitroprusside* metabolism results in cyanide ion production. Although cyanide toxicity is rare, it can be effectively treated with an infusion of *sodium thiosulfate* to produce thiocyanate, which is less toxic and is eliminated by the kidneys. [Note: *Nitroprusside* is poisonous if given orally because of its hydrolysis to cyanide.]

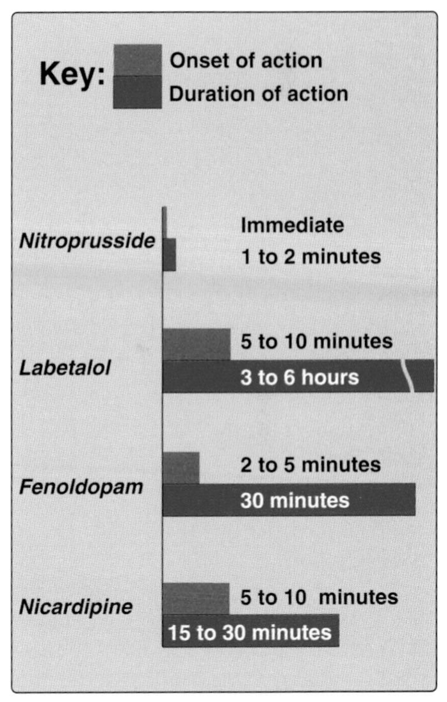

Figure 19.14
Time to peak effect and duration of action for some drugs used in hypertensive emergency.

B. Labetalol

Labetalol is both an α- and a β-blocker and is given as an intravenous bolus or infusion in hypertensive emergencies. *Labetalol* does not cause reflex tachycardia. *Labetalol* carries the contraindications of a nonselective β-blocker. The major limitation is a longer half-life, which precludes rapid titration (see Figure 19.14)

C. Fenoldopam

Fenoldopam [feh NOL doh pam] is a peripheral dopamine-1 receptor agonist that is given as an intravenous infusion. Unlike other parenteral antihypertensive agents, *fenoldopam* maintains or increases renal perfusion while it lowers blood pressure. *Fenoldopam* can be safely used in all hypertensive emergencies and may be particularly beneficial in patients with renal insufficiency. The drug is contraindicated in patients with glaucoma.

D. Nicardipine

Nicardipine, a calcium channel blocker, can be given as an intravenous infusion.

Study Questions

Choose the ONE best answer.

19.1 A 45-year-old man has recently been diagnosed with hypertension and started on monotherapy designed to reduce peripheral resistance and prevent NaCl and water retention. He has developed a persistent cough. Which of the following drugs would have the same benefits but would not cause cough?

A. Losartan
B. Nifedipine
C. Prazosin
D. Propranolol

Correct answer = A. The cough is an adverse effect of an ACE inhibitor. Losartan is an angiotensin-receptor blocker that will have the same beneficial effects as an ACE inhibitor but will not produce a cough. The other drugs also do not cause this side effect.

19.2 Which one of the following drugs may cause a precipitous fall in blood pressure and fainting on initial administration?

A. Atenolol
B. Hydrochlorothiazide
C. Nifedipine
D. Prazosin
E. Verapamil

Correct answer = D. Prazosin produces first-dose hypotension, presumably by blocking α_1 receptors. This effect is minimized by initially giving the drug in small, divided doses. The other agents do not have this adverse effect.

19.3 Which one of the following antihypertensive drugs can precipitate a hypertensive crisis following abrupt cessation of therapy?

A. Clonidine
B. Diltiazem
C. Enalapril
D. Losartan
E. Hydrochlorothiazide

Correct answer = A. Increased sympathetic nervous system activity occurs if clonidine therapy is abruptly stopped after prolonged administration. Uncontrolled elevation in blood pressure can occur. Patients should be slowly weaned from clonidine while other antihypertensive medications are initiated. The other drugs on the list do not produce this phenomenon.

19.4 A 48-year-old hypertensive patient has been successfully treated with a thiazide diuretic for the last five years. Over the last three months, his diastolic pressure has steadily increased, and he has been started on an additional hypertensive medication. He complains of several instances of being unable to achieve an erection and that he is no longer able to complete three sets of tennis. The second antihypertensive medication is most likely which one of the following?

A. Captopril
B. Losartan
C. Minoxidil
D. Metoprolol
E. Nifedipine

Correct answer = D. The side effect profile of β-blockers such as metoprolol, are characterized by interference with sexual performance and decreased exercise tolerance. None of the other drugs are likely to produce this combination of side effects.

Drugs Affecting The Blood

20

I. OVERVIEW

This chapter describes drugs that are useful in treating three important dysfunctions of blood: thrombosis, bleeding, and anemia. Thrombosis—the formation of an unwanted clot within a blood vessel—is the most common abnormality of hemostasis. Thrombotic disorders include acute myocardial infarction, deep-vein thrombosis, pulmonary embolism, and acute ischemic stroke. These are treated with drugs such as anticoagulants and fibrinolytics. Bleeding disorders involving the failure of hemostasis are less common than thromboembolic diseases. These disorders include hemophilia, which is treated with transfusion of factor VIII prepared by recombinant DNA techniques, and vitamin K deficiency, which is treated with dietary supplements of the vitamin. Anemias caused by nutritional deficiencies, such as the commonly encountered iron-deficiency anemia, can be treated with either dietary or pharmaceutical supplementation. However, individuals with anemias that have a genetic basis, such as sickle-cell disease, can benefit from additional treatment. See Figure 20.1 for a summary of drugs affecting the blood.

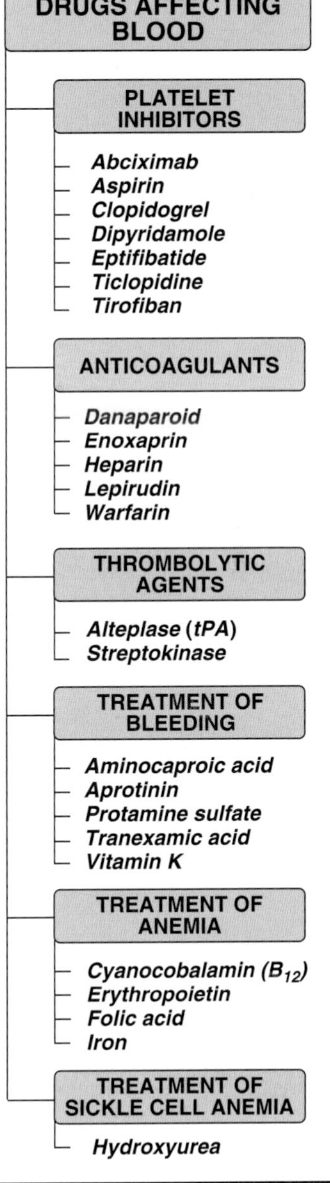

Figure 20.1
Summary of drugs used in treating dysfunctions of the blood.

II. THROMBUS VS. EMBOLUS

First, a few definitions to clarify the discussion of undesirable blood clots: A clot that adheres to a vessel wall is called a thrombus, whereas an intravascular clot that floats in the blood is termed an embolus. Thus, a detached thrombus becomes an embolus. Both thrombi and emboli are dangerous, because they may occlude blood vessels and deprive tissues of oxygen and nutrients. Arterial thrombosis most often occurs in medium-sized vessels rendered thrombogenic by surface lesions of endothelial cells caused by atherosclerosis. Arterial thrombosis usually consists of a platelet-rich clot. In contrast, venous thrombosis is triggered by blood stasis or inappropriate activation of the coagulation cascade, frequently as a result of a defect in the normal hemostatic defense mechanisms. Venous thrombosis typically involves a clot that is rich in fibrin, with fewer platelets than are observed with arterial clots.

III. PLATELET RESPONSE TO VASCULAR INJURY

Physical trauma to the vascular system, such as a puncture or a cut, initiates a complex series of interactions between platelets, endothelial cells, and the coagulation cascade. This results in the formation of a platelet-fibrin plug (clot) at the site of the puncture. The creation of an unwanted thrombus involves many of the same steps as normal clot formation, except that the triggering stimulus is a pathologic condition in the vascular system rather than an external physical trauma.

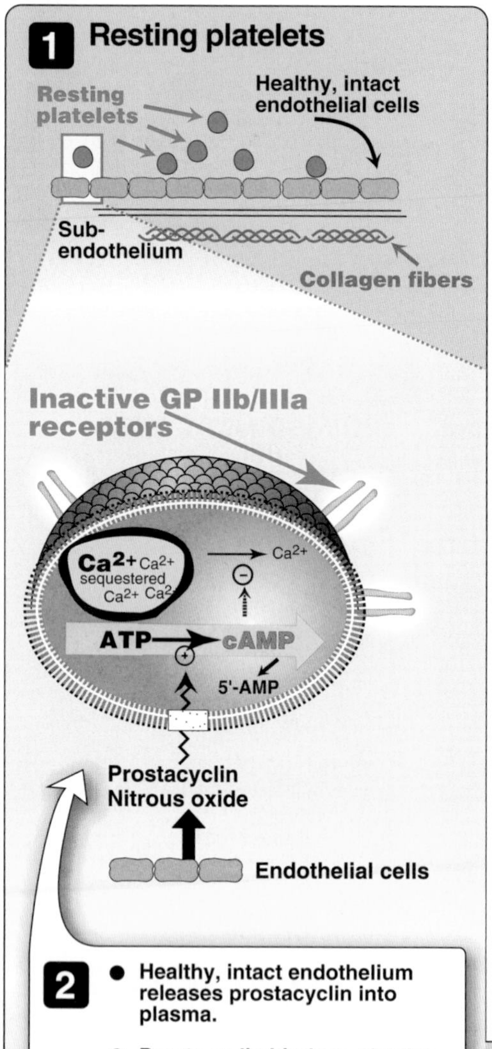

A. Resting platelets

Platelets act as vascular sentries, monitoring the integrity of the endothelium. In the absence of injury, resting platelets circulate freely, because the balance of chemical signals indicates that the vascular system is not damaged (Figure 20.2 **1**).

1. **Chemical mediators synthesized by endothelial cells:** Chemical mediators, such as prostacyclin and nitric oxide, are synthesized by intact endothelial cells and act as inhibitors of platelet aggregation. Prostacyclin (prostaglandin I_2) acts by binding to platelet membrane receptors that are coupled to the synthesis of cyclic adenosine monophosphate (cAMP, Figure 20.2 **2**)—an intracellular messenger.[1] Elevated levels of intracellular cAMP are associated with a decrease in intracellular Ca^{2+}. This leads to inhibition of platelet activation and of the subsequent release of platelet aggregation agents. [Note: The drug *dipyridamole* inhibits the enzyme phosphodiesterase, which inactivates cAMP, thus prolonging its active life.] Damaged endothelial cells synthesize less prostacyclin, resulting in a localized reduction in prostacyclin levels. The binding of prostacyclin to platelet receptors is decreased, resulting in lower levels of intracellular cAMP, which leads to platelet aggregation.

2. **Roles of thrombin, thromboxanes, and collagen:** The platelet membrane also contains receptors that can bind thrombin, thromboxanes,[2] and exposed collagen.[3] In the intact, normal vessel, circulating levels of thrombin and thromboxane are low, and the intact endothelium covers the collagen in the subendothelial layers. The

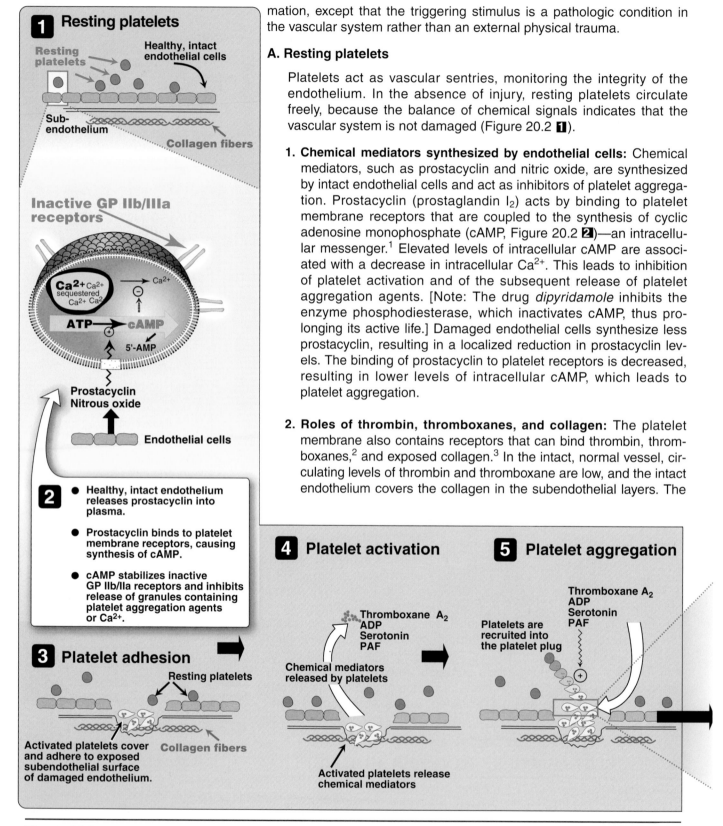

1 Resting platelets

Resting platelets
Healthy, intact endothelial cells
Sub-endothelium
Collagen fibers
Inactive GP IIb/IIIa receptors
Ca^{2+} Ca^{2+} sequestered Ca^{2+} Ca^{2+}
Ca^{2+}
ATP → cAMP
5'-AMP
Prostacyclin
Nitrous oxide
Endothelial cells

2
- Healthy, intact endothelium releases prostacyclin into plasma.
- Prostacyclin binds to platelet membrane receptors, causing synthesis of cAMP.
- cAMP stabilizes inactive GP IIb/IIa receptors and inhibits release of granules containing platelet aggregation agents or Ca^{2+}.

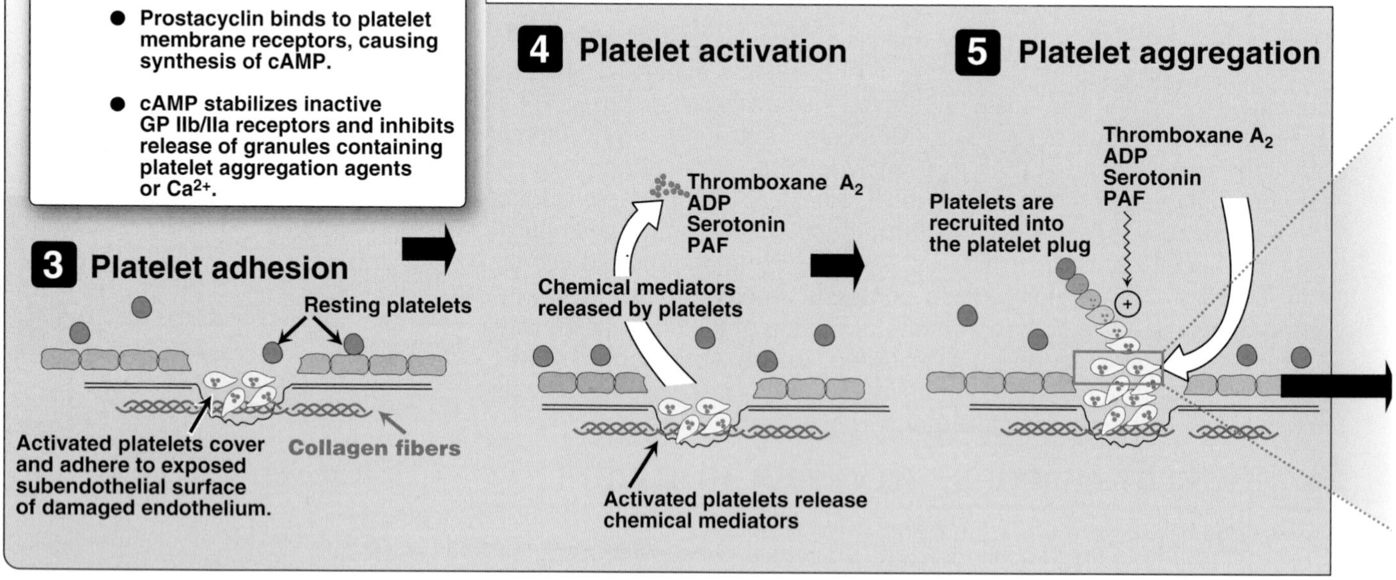

3 Platelet adhesion

Resting platelets
Activated platelets cover and adhere to exposed subendothelial surface of damaged endothelium.
Collagen fibers

4 Platelet activation

Thromboxane A_2
ADP
Serotonin
PAF
Chemical mediators released by platelets
Activated platelets release chemical mediators

5 Platelet aggregation

Thromboxane A_2
ADP
Serotonin
PAF
Platelets are recruited into the platelet plug

Figure 20.2
Formation of a hemostatic plug. (Continued on facing page.)

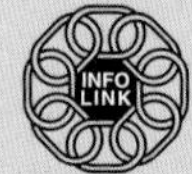

[1]See p. 92 in ***Lippincott's Illustrated Reviews: Biochemistry*** (3rd ed.) for a discussion of intracellular messages. [2]See p. 211 for a discussion of thromboxane synthesis. [3]See p. 43 in for a discussion of collagen.

corresponding platelet receptors are thus unoccupied and remain inactive; as a result, platelet activation and aggregation are not initiated. However, when occupied, each of these receptor types triggers a series of reactions leading to the release into the circulation of intracellular granules by the platelets. This ultimately stimulates platelet aggregation.

B. Platelet adhesion

When the endothelium is injured, platelets adhere to and virtually cover the exposed collagen of the subendothelium (Figure 20.2 **3**). This triggers a complex series of chemical reactions, resulting in platelet activation.

C. Platelet activation

Receptors on the surface of the adhering platelets are activated by the collagen of the underlying connective tissue. This causes morphologic changes in the platelets (Figure 20.3), and the release of platelet granules containing chemical mediators, such as adenosine diphosphate (ADP), thromboxane A_2, serotonin, platelet-activation factor, and thrombin (Figure 20.2 **4**). These signaling molecules bind to receptors in the outer membrane of resting platelets circulating nearby. These receptors function as sensors that are activated by the signals sent from the adhering platelets. The previously dormant platelets become activated and start to aggregate—actions mediated by several messenger systems that ultimately result in elevated levels of Ca^{2+} and a decreased concentration of cAMP within the platelet.

D. Platelet aggregation

The increase in cytosolic Ca^{2+} accompanying activation is due to a release of sequestered stores within the platelet (Figure 20.2 **5**).

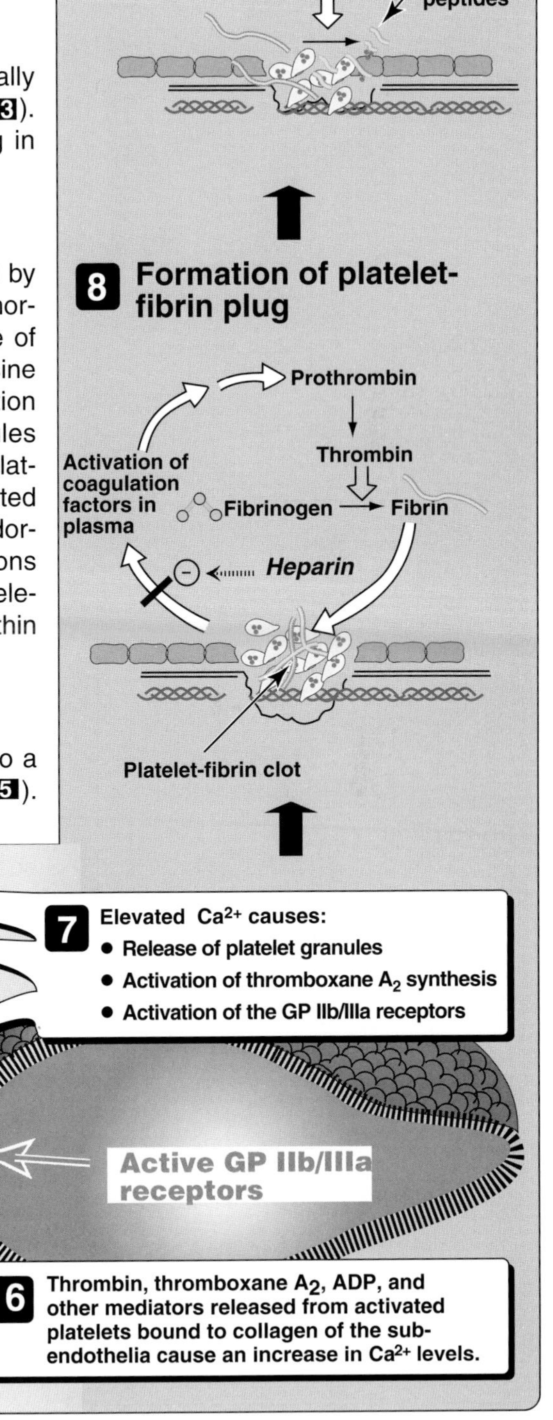

Figure 20.2 (continued)
Formation of a hemostatic plug. PAF = platelet-activation factor.

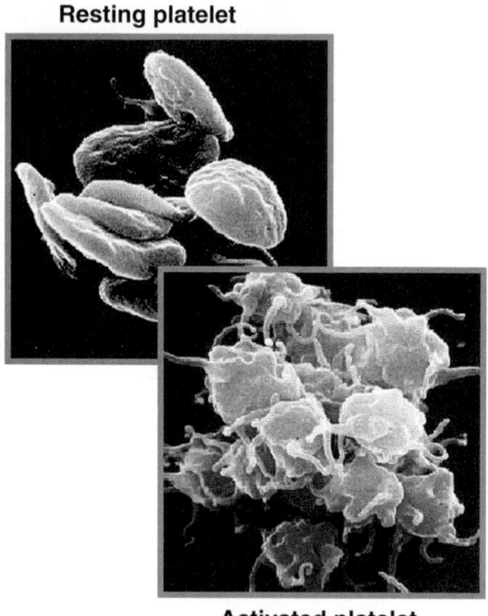

Figure 20.3
Scanning electron micrograph of platelets.

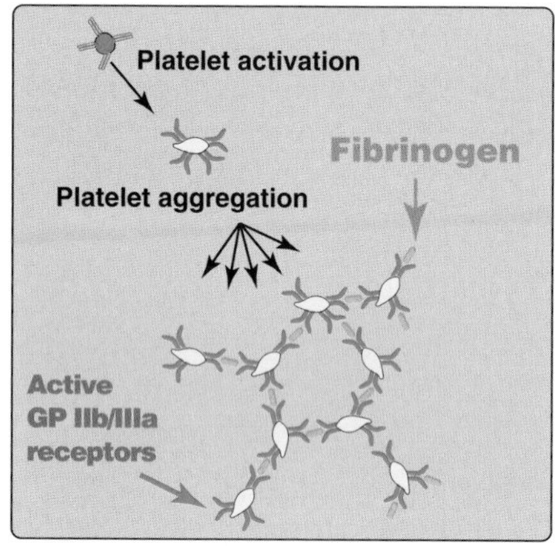

Figure 20.4
Activation and aggregation of platelets. GP = glycoprotein.

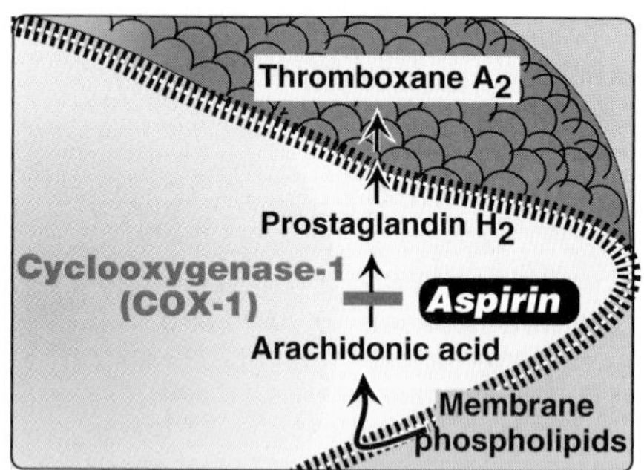

Figure 20.5
Aspirin irreversibly inhibits platelet cyclooxygenase-1.

This leads to 1) the release of platelet granules containing mediators, such as ADP and serotonin that activate other platelets; 2) activation of thromboxane A_2 synthesis; 3) activation of the glycoprotein (GP) IIb/IIIa receptors that bind fibrinogen and, ultimately, regulate platelet-platelet interaction and thrombus formation (Figure 20.2 6, 7). Fibrinogen, a soluble plasma glycoprotein, simultaneously binds to GP IIb/IIIa receptors on two separate platelets, resulting in platelet cross-linking and platelet aggregation. This leads to an avalanche of platelet aggregation, because each activated platelet can recruit other platelets (Figure 20.4).

E. Formation of a clot

Local stimulation of the coagulation cascade by tissue factors released from the injured tissue and by mediators on the surface of platelets results in the formation of thrombin (Factor IIa). In turn, thrombin—a serine protease—catalyzes the hydrolysis of fibrinogen to fibrin, which is incorporated into the plug . Subsequent cross-linking of the fibrin strands stabilizes the clot and forms a hemostatic platelet-fibrin plug (Figure 20.2 8).

F. Fibrinolysis

During plug formation, the fibrinolytic pathway is locally activated. Plasminogen is enzymatically processed to plasmin (fibrinolysin) by plasminogen activators in the tissue (Figure 20.2, 9). Plasmin limits the growth of the clot and dissolves the fibrin network as wounds heal. At present, a number of fibrinolytic enzymes are available for treatment of myocardial infarctions, pulmonary emboli, or ischemic stroke.

IV. PLATELET AGGREGATION INHIBITORS

Platelet aggregation inhibitors decrease the formation or the action of chemical signals that promote platelet aggregation. The last step in this response to vascular trauma depends on a family of membrane GP receptors that—after activation—can bind adhesive proteins, such as fibrinogen, von Willebrand factor, and fibronectin. The most important of these is the GP IIb/IIIa receptor that ultimately regulates platelet-platelet interaction and thrombus formation. Thus, platelet activation agents, such as thromboxane A_2, ADP, thrombin, serotonin, and collagen, all promote the conformational change necessary for the GP IIb/IIIa receptor to bind ligands, particularly fibrinogen. Fibrinogen simultaneously binds to GP IIb/IIIa receptors on two separate platelets, resulting in platelet cross-linking and aggregation (see Figure 20.4). The platelet aggregation inhibitors described below inhibit cyclooxygenase-1 (COX-1), or block GP IIb/IIIa or ADP receptors, thereby interfering in the signals that promote platelet aggregation. These agents are beneficial in the prevention and treatment of occlusive cardiovascular diseases, the maintenance of vascular grafts and arterial patency, and as adjuncts to thrombin inhibitors or thrombolytic therapy in myocardial infarction.

A. Aspirin

Stimulation of platelets by thrombin, collagen and ADP results in activation of platelet membrane phospholipases that liberate arachidonic acid from membrane phospholipids.[4] Arachidonic acid is first converted to prostaglandin H_2 by COX-1 (Figure 20.5); prostaglandin H_2 is further metabolized to thromboxane A_2, which is released into plasma. Thromboxane A_2 produced by the aggregating platelets further promotes the clumping process that is essential to the rapid formation of a hemostatic plug. *Aspirin* [AS pir in] inhibits thromboxane A_2 synthesis from arachidonic acid in platelets by irreversible acetylation of a serine, resulting in a blockade of arachidonate to the active site and, thus, inhibition of COX-1 (Figure 20.6). This shifts the balance of chemical mediators to favor the anti-aggregatory effects of prostacyclin (PGI_2), thus impeding platelet aggregation. The inhibitory effect is rapid, apparently occurring in the portal circulation. The *aspirin*-induced suppression of thromboxane A_2 synthetase and the resulting suppression of platelet aggregation last for the life of the anucleate platelet—approximately seven to ten days. *Aspirin* is currently employed in the prophylactic treatment of transient cerebral ischemia, to reduce the incidence of recurrent myocardial infarction, and to decrease mortality in pre– and post–myocardial infarct patients. A single loading oral dose of 325 mg of *aspirin* followed by a daily dose of 81 to 165 mg, is recommended. Bleeding time is prolonged by *aspirin* treatment, causing complications that include an increased incidence of hemorrhagic stroke as well as gastrointestinal bleeding, especially at higher doses of the drug. *Aspirin* is frequently used in combination with other drugs having anticlotting properties, for example, *heparin* or *clopidogrel*. Non-steroidal antiinflammatory drugs, such as *ibuprofen* and *acetaminophen* inhibit COX-1 by transiently competing at the catalytic site. *Ibuprofen*, if taken concomittantly or two hours prior to *aspirin*, can obstruct the access of *aspirin* to the serine residue and, thereby, antagonize the platelet inhibition by *aspirin*. Although selective COX-2 inhibitors (see Chapter 39) do not interfere in the antiaggregation activity of *aspirin*, there is some evidence that they may contribute to cardiovascular events by shifting the balance of chemical mediators in favor of thromboxane A_2.

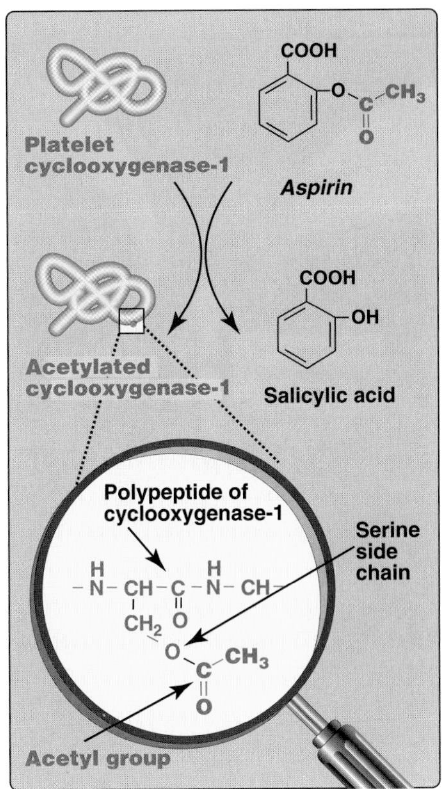

Figure 20.6
Acetylation of cyclooxygenase-1 by *aspirin*.

B. Ticlopidine and clopidogrel

Ticlopidine [ti KLOE pi deen] and *clopidogrel* (kloh PID oh grel) are closely related thienopyridines that also block platelet aggregation, but by a mechanism different from that of *aspirin*.

1. **Mechanism of action:** These drugs interfere with the binding of ADP to its receptors on platelets and, thus, inhibit the activation of the GP IIb/IIIa receptors required for platelets to bind to fibrinogen and to each other (Figure 20.7).

2. **Therapeutic use:** Both drugs have been shown to be effective in preventing cerebrovascular and cardiovascular as well as peripheral vascular disease, and are now routinely used in stent insertion during a myocardial infarction.

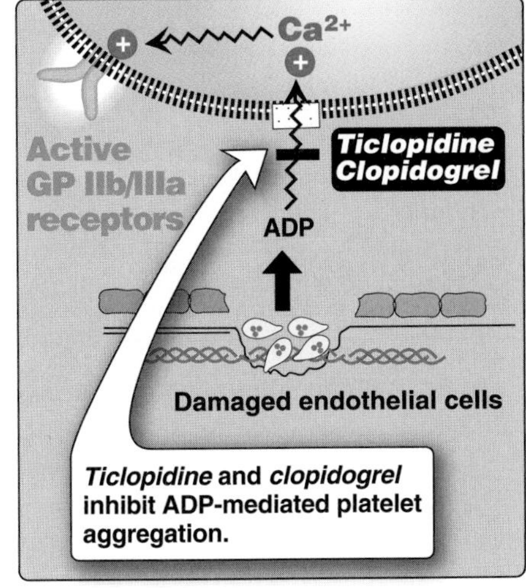

Figure 20.7
Mechanism of action of *ticlopidine* and *clopidogrel*. GP = glycoprotein.

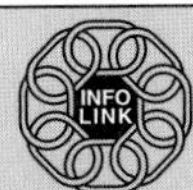

[4]See p. 211 in ***Lippincott's Illustrated Reviews: Biochemistry*** (3rd ed.) for a discussion of the function of membrane-bound phsoholipase.

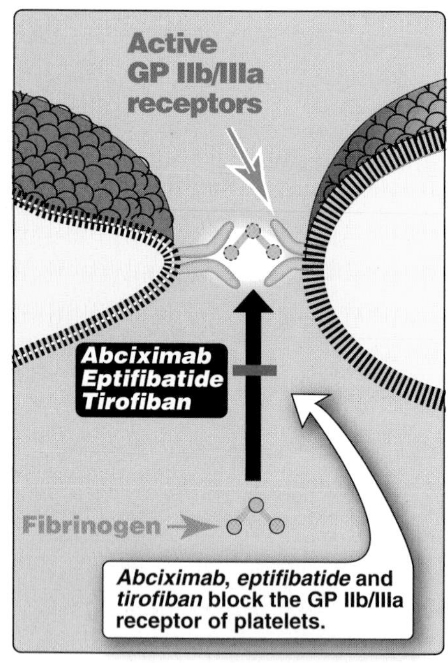

Figure 20.8
Mechanism of action of glycoprotein (GP) IIb/IIIa–receptor blockers.

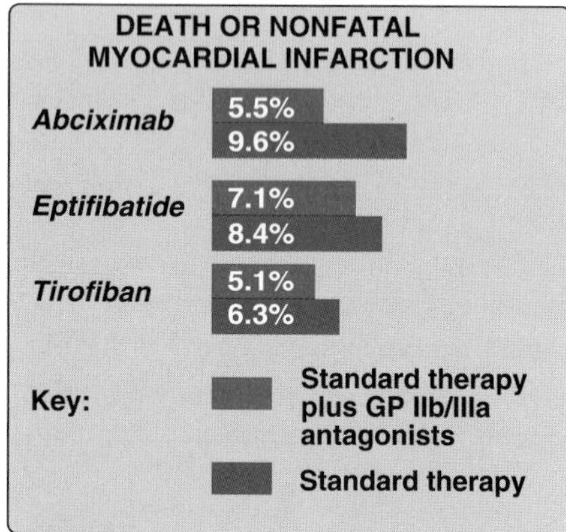

Figure 20.9
Effects of glycoprotein (GP) IIb/IIIa–receptor antagonists on the incidence of death or nonfatal myocardial infarction following percutaneous transluminal coronary angioplasty. [Note: Data are from several studies; thus, reported incidence of complications with standard therapy, such as as heparin, is not the same for each drug.]

3. **Pharmacokinetics:** Food interferes with the absorption of *ticlopidine* but not of *clopidogrel*. After oral ingestion, both drugs are extensively bound to plasma proteins. They undergo hepatic metabolism by the cytochrome P450 system to active metabolite that are yet to be identified. The maximum effect is achieved in three to five days; suspension of treatment delays recovery of the platelet system. Elimination of the drugs and metabolites occurs by both the renal and fecal routes. Both drugs can cause prolonged bleeding for which there is no antidote. The most serious adverse effect of *ticlopidine* is neutropenia, requiring frequent blood monitoring. *Clopidogrel* causes fewer adverse reactions, and the incidence of neutropenia is lower. Thrombocytopenic purpura has been reported as an adverse effect for both drugs. Because these drugs can inhibit cytochrome P450, they may interfere with the metabolism of drugs such as *phenytoin*, *tolbutamide*, *warfarin*, *fluvastatin*, and *tamoxifen* if taken concomitantly. Indeed, *phenytoin* toxicity has been reported when taken with *ticlopidine*.

C. Abciximab

Realization of the key role of the platelet GP IIb/IIIa receptor in stimulating platelet aggregation directed attempts to block this receptor on activated platelets. This led to the development of a chimeric monoclonal antibody, *abciximab* [ab SIKS eh mab], which is composed of the constant regions of human immunoglobulin joined to the Fab fragments of a murine monoclonal antibody directed against the GP IIb/IIIa complex. By binding to GP IIb/IIIa, the antibody blocks the binding of fibrinogen and von Willebrand factor; consequently, aggregation does not occur (Figure 20.8). *Abciximab* is given intravenously along with *heparin* or *aspirin* as an adjunct to percutaneous coronary intervention for the prevention of cardiac ischemic complications. After cessation of infusion, platelet function gradually returns to normal, with the antiplatelet effect persisting for 24 to 48 hours.The major adverse effect of *abciximab* therapy is the potential for bleeding, especially if the drug is used with anticoagulants or if the patient has a clinical hemorrhagic condition.

D. Eptifibatide and tirofiban

These two antiplatelet drugs act similarly to *abciximab*—namely blocking the GP IIb/IIIa receptor (see Figure 20.8). *Eptifibatide* [ep ti FIB ih tide] is a cyclic peptide that binds to GP IIb/IIIa at the site that interacts with the arginine-glycine-aspartic acid sequence of fibrinogen. *Tirofiban* [tye roe FYE ban] is not a peptide, but blocks the same site as *eptifibatide*. These compounds, like *abciximab*, can decrease the incidence of thrombotic complications associated with acute coronary syndromes. When intravenous infusion is stopped, these agents are rapidly cleared from the plasma, but their effect can persist for as long as four hours. [Note: Oral preparations of GP IIb/IIIa blockers are too toxic.] *Eptifibatide* and its metabolites are excreted by the kidney. *Tirofiban* is excreted unchanged by the kidney. The major adverse effect of both drugs is bleeding. Figure 20.9 summarizes the effects of the GP IIb/IIIa receptor antagonists on death and myocardial infarction.

E. Dipyridamole

Dipyridamole [dye peer ID a mole], a coronary vasodilator, is employed prophylactically to treat angina pectoris. It is usually given in combination with *aspirin*; it is ineffective when used alone. *Dipyridamole* increases intracellular levels of cAMP by inhibiting cyclic nucleotide phosphodiesterase, resulting in decreased thromboxane A_2 synthesis. It may potentiate the effect of PGI_2 to antagonize platelet stickiness and, therefore, decrease platelet adhesion to thrombogenic surfaces (see Figure 20.2 5). The meager data available suggest that *dipyridamole* makes only a marginal contribution to the antithrombotic action of *aspirin*. In combination with *warfarin*, however, *dipyridamole* is effective for inhibiting embolization from prosthetic heart valves.

V. BLOOD COAGULATION

The coagulation process that generates thrombin consists of two interrelated pathways—the extrinsic and the intrinsic systems. The extrinsic system, which is probably the more important in vivo, is initiated by the activation of clotting Factor VII by a tissue factor, thromboplastin—a phospholipid and protein mixture. The intrinsic system is triggered by the activation of clotting Factor XII, following its contact in vitro with glass or highly charged surfaces. Both systems involve a cascade of enzyme reactions that sequentially transform various plasma factors (proenzymes) to their active (enzymatic) forms. They ultimately produce Factor Xa, which converts prothrombin (Factor II) to thrombin (Figure 20.10). Thrombin plays a key role in coagulation, because it is responsible for generation of fibrin, the glycoprotein that forms the mesh-like matrix of the blood clot. If thrombin is not formed or if its function is impeded (for example, by antithrombin III), coagulation is inhibited.

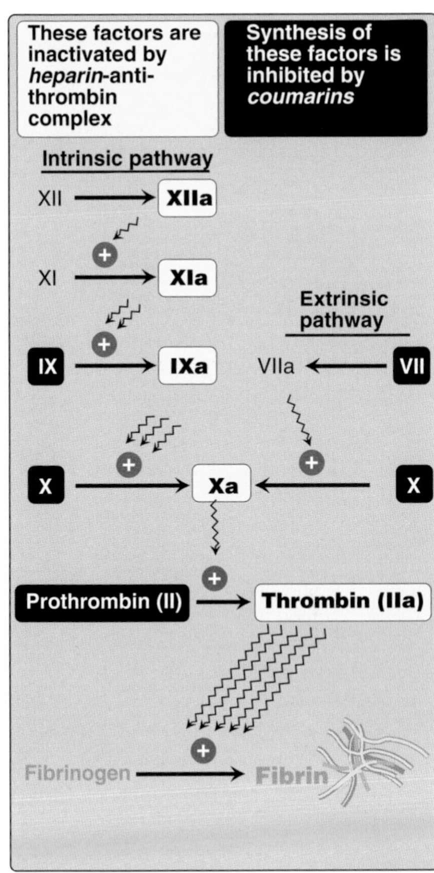

Figure 20.10
Formation of fibrin clot .

VI. ANTICOAGULANTS

The anticoagulant drugs either inhibit the action of the coagulation factors (the thrombin inhibitors, such as *heparin* and *heparin*-related agents) or interfere with the synthesis of the coagulation factors (the vitamin K antagonists, such as *warfarin*).

A. Thrombin inhibitors: heparin and low-molecular-weight heparins

Heparin [HEP a rin] is an injectable, rapidly acting anticoagulant that is often used acutely to interfere with the formation of thrombi. *Heparin* normally occurs as a macromolecule complexed with histamine in mast cells, where its physiologic role is unknown. It is extracted for commercial use from porcine intestine or bovine lung. Unfractionated *heparin* is a mixture of straight-chain, anionic glycosaminoglycans with a wide range of molecular weights (Figure 20.11). It is strongly acidic because of the presence of sulfate and carboxylic acid groups (Figure 20.12). [Note: In this discussion, the term *heparin* will indicate the unfractionated form of the drug.] The realization that low-molecular-weight forms of *heparin* (*LMWHs*) can also act as anticoagulants led to the isolation of *enoxaparin* [e NOX a par in], the first *LMWH* (<6000) available in the United States. The *LMWHs* are heterogeneous compounds produced by the chemical or

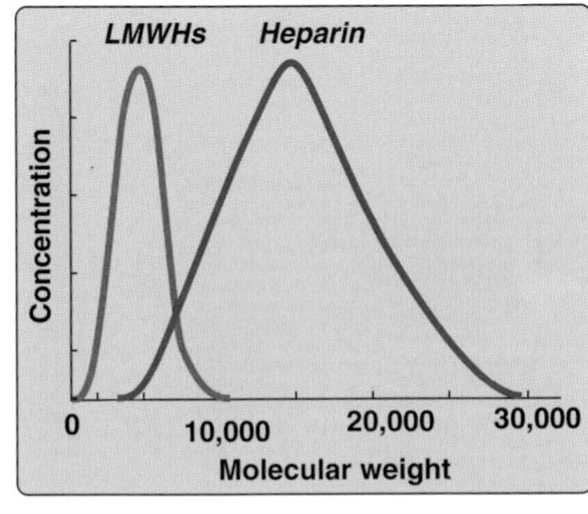

Figure 20.11
Typical molecular weight distributions of *low-molecular-weight heparins* (*LMWHs*) and *heparin*.

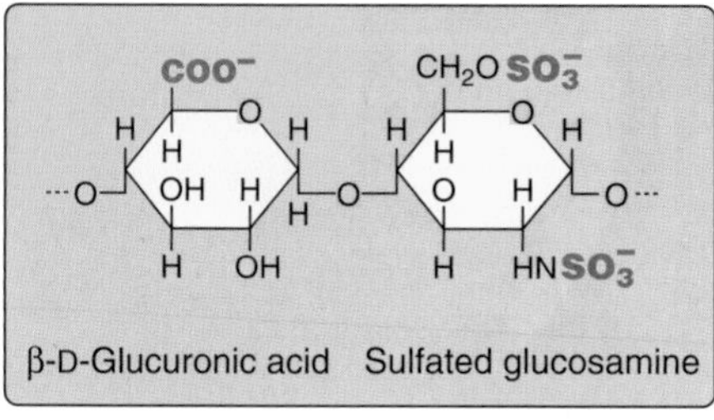

Figure 20.12
Disaccharide component of *heparin* showing negative charges due to carboxyl and sulfate groups.

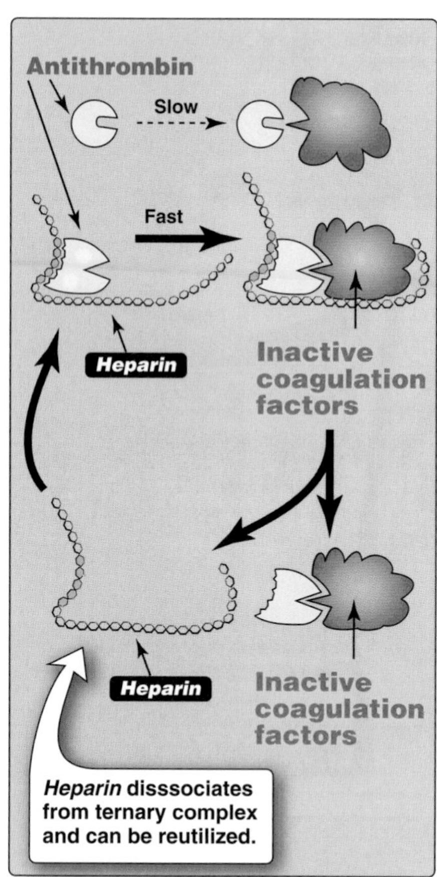

Figure 20.13
Heparin accelerates inactivation of coagulation factors by antithrombin.

enzymatic depolymerization of unfractionated *heparin*. Because they are free of some of the drawbacks associated with the polymer, they are replacing the use of *heparin* in many clinical situations. *Heparin* is used in the prevention of venous thrombosis and the treatment of a variety of thrombotic diseases, such as pulmonary embolism and acute myocardial infarction.

1. **Mechanism of action:** *Heparin* acts at a number of molecular targets, but its anticoagulant effect is a consequence of binding to antithrombin III, with the subsequent rapid inactivation of coagulation factors (Figure 20.13). Antithrombin III is an α-globulin. It inhibits serine proteases, including several of the clotting factors—most importantly, thrombin (Factor IIa) and Factor Xa (see Figure 20.10). In the absence of *heparin*, antithrombin III interacts very slowly with thrombin and Factor Xa. In the presence of *heparin*, antithrombin III changes conformation, allowing the antithrombin to rapidly combine with and inhibit circulating thrombin and Factor Xa (Figure 20.14). In contrast, *LMWH* complexes with antithrombin and inactivates Factor Xa—including that located on platelet surfaces—but does not bind as avidly to thrombin. Indeed, *LMWHs* are less likely than *heparin* to activate resting platelets. [Note: A unique pentasaccharide sequence contained in *heparin* and *LMWH* permits their binding to antithrombin III (see Figure 20.14).]. A synthetic pentasaccharide presently undergoing clinical trials shows the promise of being another antithrombin agent that selectively inhibits Factor Xa. This drug has the advantage of being a pure, defined compound, rather than a heterogenous mixture of polysaccharides.

2. **Therapeutic uses:** *Heparin* and the *LMWHs* limit the expansion of thrombi by preventing fibrin formation. *Heparin* has been the major antithrombotic drug for the treatment of deep-vein thrombosis and pulmonary embolism. The incidence of recurrent thromboembolic episodes is also decreased. Clinically, *heparin* is used prophylactically to prevent postoperative venous thrombosis in patients undergoing elective surgery (for example, hip replacement) and those in the acute phase of myocardial infarction. Coronary artery rethrombosis after thrombolytic treatment is reduced with *heparin*. The drug is also used in extracorporeal devices (for example, dialysis machines) to prevent thrombosis. *Heparin* and *LMWHs* are the anticoagulants of choice for treating pregnant women with prosthetic heart valves or venous thromboembolism, because these agents do not cross the placenta. *Heparin* has the advantage of speedy onset of action, which is rapidly terminated on suspension of therapy. However, it is being supplanted by the *LMWHs*, such as *enoxaparin* and *dalteparin*, because they can be conveniently injected subcutaneously on a patient weight–adjusted basis, and they have predictable therapeutic effects (Figure 20.15). They are therefore useful in outpatient therapy.

3. **Pharmacokinetics:**

   a. **Absorption:** Whereas the anticoagulant effect with *heparin* occurs within minutes of intravenous administration (or one to

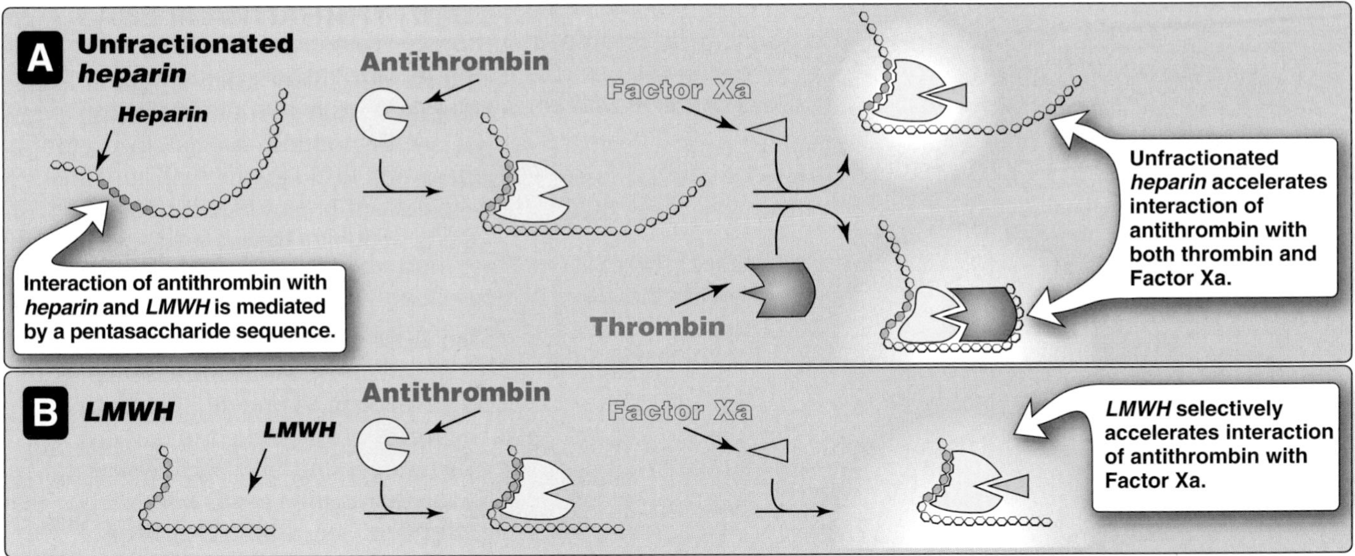

Figure 20.14
Heparin- and *low-molecular-weight heparin* (*LMWH*)–mediated inactivation of thrombin or Factor Xa.

two hours after subcutaneous injection), the maximum anti–Factor Xa activity of the *LMWHs* occurs about four hours after subcutaneous injection. (This is in comparison to the vitamin K–antagonist anticoagulants, such as *warfarin*, the maximum activity of which requires eight to twelve hours.) *Heparin* must be given parenterally, either in a deep subcutaneous site or intravenously, because the drug does not readily cross membranes (Figure 20.16). The *LMWHs* are administered subcutaneously. [Note: Intramuscular administration of either agent is contraindicated because of hematoma formation.] *Heparin* is often administered intravenously in a bolus to achieve immediate anticoagulation. This is followed by lower doses or continuous infusion of *heparin* for seven to ten days, titrating the dose so that the activated partial thromboplastin time (aPTT) is 1.5- to 2.5-fold that of the normal control. It is usually not necessary to obtain such an index with the *LMWHs,* because the plasma levels and pharmacokinetics of these drugs are predictable, except in cases of abnormal renal function or pregnancy.

b. Fate: In the blood, *heparin* binds to many proteins that neutralize its activity, thereby causing resistance to the drug. Although generally restricted to the circulation, *heparin* is taken up by the monocyte/macrophage system, and it undergoes depolymerization and desulfation to inactive products. [Note: *Heparin* therefore has a longer half-life in patients with hepatic cirrhosis.] The inactive metabolites as well as some of the parent *heparin* and *LMWHs* are excreted into the urine. Therefore, renal insufficiency also prolongs the half-life. Neither *heparin* nor the *LMWHs* cross the placental barrier. The half-life of *heparin* increases with dose; the half-life of the *LMWHs* is about four hours—double that of the larger species.

DRUG CHARACTERISTIC	*HEPARIN*	*LMWHs*
Intravenous half-life	Two hours	Four hours
Anticoagulant response	Variable	Predicable
Bioavailability:	Twenty %	Ninety %
Major adverse effect	Frequent bleeding	Less frequent bleeding
Setting for therapy	Hospital	Hospital and outpatient

Figure 20.15
Some properties of *heparin* and *low-molecular-weight heparins* (*LMWHs*)

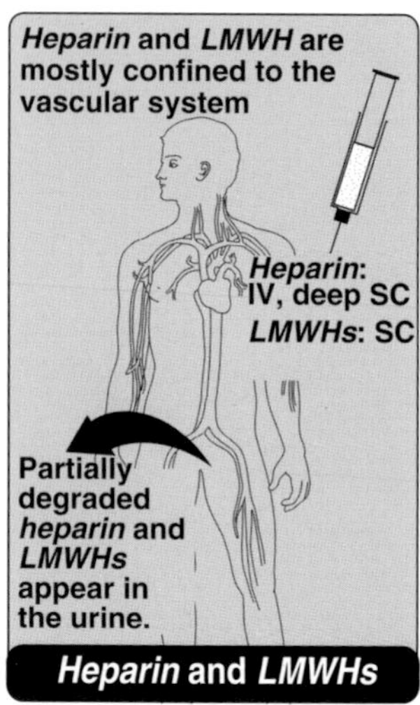

Figure 20.16
Administration and fate of *heparin* and *low-molecular-weight heparins* (*LMWHs*).

4. **Adverse effects:** Despite early hopes of fewer side effects with *enoxaprin*, complications have proven to be similar to those seen with *heparin*. Exceptions are thromboembolic problems, which are less common with the *LMWHs*.

   a. **Bleeding complications:** The chief complication of *heparin* therapy is hemorrhage (Figure 20.17). Careful monitoring of the bleeding time is required to minimize this problem. Excessive bleeding may be managed by ceasing administration of the drug, or by treating with *protamine sulfate*. Infused slowly, the latter combines ionically with *heparin* to form a stable, inactive complex.

   b. **Hypersensitivity reactions:** Because *heparin* preparations are obtained from animal sources and, therefore, may be antigenic. Possible adverse reactions include chills, fever, urticaria, or anaphylactic shock.

   c. **Thrombosis:** Chronic or intermittent administration of *heparin* can lead to a reduction in antithrombin III activity, thus decreasing the inactivation of coagulation factors and, thereby, increasing the risk of thrombosis. To minimize this risk, low-dose *heparin* therapy is usually employed.

   d. **Thrombocytopenia:** This condition, in which circulating blood contains an abnormally small number of platelets, is a common abnormality among hospital patients and can be caused by a variety of factors. One of these is associated with the use of *heparin* and is called *heparin*-induced thrombocytopenia (HIT). Two types of this abnormality have been identified. Type I is common and involves a mild decrease in platelet number due to nonimmunologic mechanisms. Type I usually occurs within the first five days of treatment, and is not serious. In Type II, platelets are activated by an immunoglobulin G-mediated reaction with a *heparin*–platelet Factor 4 complex, causing platelet aggregation and release of platelet contents. This can result in thrombocytopenia and thrombosis—dangerous complications of *heparin* therapy occurring between the fifth and fourteenth days of treatment—that range from mild to life-threatening. Platelet counts can drop fifty percent or more, and thromboembolic complications can develop. Although Type II is relatively rare, the wide use of *heparin* has resulted in a greater recognition of its role in thrombocytopenia. It is imperative that *heparin* therapy be discontinued in such patients. *Heparin* can be replaced by another anticoagulant, such as *lepirudin* (see below).

   e. **Contraindications:** *Heparin* is contraindicated for patients who are hypersensitive to it, have bleeding disorders, are alcoholics, or are having or have had surgery of the brain, eye, or spinal cord.

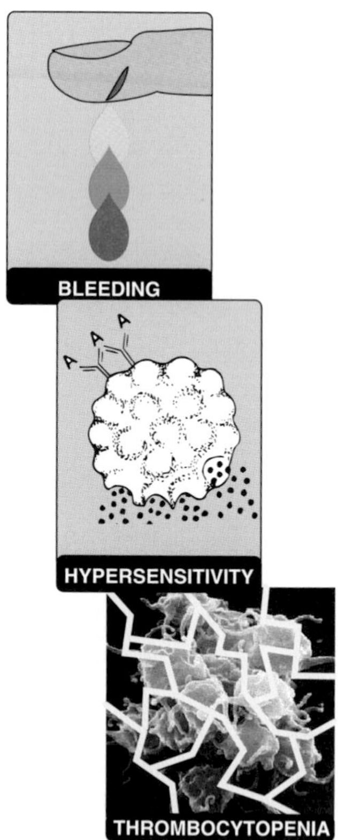

Figure 20.17
Adverse effects of *heparin*.

B. Other thrombin inhibitors

1. **Lepirudin:** A highly specific, direct thrombin antagonist, *lepirudin* [leh PEE roo din] is a polypeptide that is closely related to

hirudin—a thrombin inhibitor from the leech. *Lepirudin* is produced in yeast cells by recombinant DNA technology. One molecule of *lepirudin* binds to one molecule of thrombin, resulting in blockade of the thrombogenic activity of thrombin. It has little effect on platelet aggregation. Administered intravenously (Figure 20.18), *lepirudin* is effective in the treatment of *heparin*-induced thrombocytopenia and other thromboembolic disorders, and it can prevent further thromboembolic complications. *Lepirudin* has a half-life of about one hour, and it undergoes hydrolysis. The parent drug and its fragments are eliminated in the urine. Bleeding is the major adverse effect of treatment with *lepirudin*, and can be exacerbated by concommitant thrombolytic therapy, such as treatment with *streptokinase* or *alteplase*. About half the patients receiving *lepirudin* develop antibodies. However, the drug-antibody complex retains anticoagulant activity. Because renal elimination of the complex is slower than that of the free drug, the anticoagulant effect may be increased. It is important to monitor the aPTT when a patient is receiving *lepirudin* for a prolonged time.

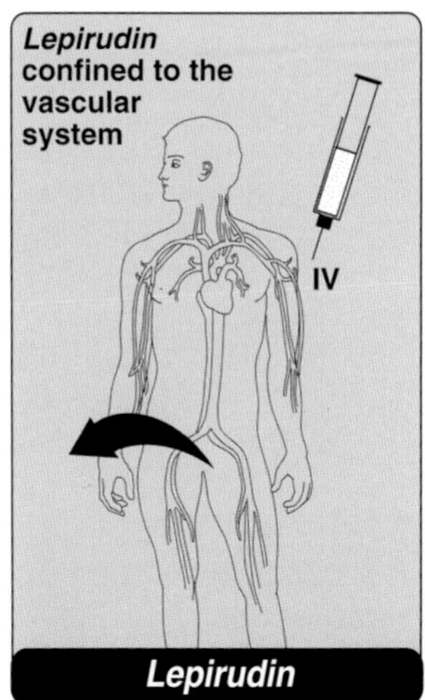

Figure 20.18
Administration of *lepirudin*.

2. **Danaparoid:** Another anti–Factor Xa and antithrombin inhibitor is the heparinoid agent *danaparoid* (da NAP a roid), which is isolated from porcine mucosa. It consists of a mixture of the sulfates of *heparin*, dermatan, and chondroitin.[5] Its anti–Factor Xa activity far exceeds its antithrombin activity. *Danaparoid* is administered subcutaneously and undergoes renal elimination. It has been approved for the prophylaxis of deep-vein thrombosis in hip replacement surgery, and has been shown to be effective in the treatment of HIT Type II. Patients who are allergic to pork or sulfites may develop allergies to *danaparoid*, and hemorrhage is also possible.

C. Vitamin K antagonists

The coumarin anticoagulants, which include *warfarin* [WAR far in], and *dicumarol* [dye KOO ma role] (formerly *bishydroxycoumarin*) owe their action to their ability to antagonize the cofactor functions of vitamin K. Initially used as a rodenticide, *warfarin* is now widely employed clinically as an oral anticoagulant. With the availability of the *LMWHs* and platelet aggregate inhibitors, however, use of the vitamin K antagonists is decreasing. The potential morbidity associated with the use of these agents makes it important to identify those patients who are truly at risk for thrombosis. Even careful monitoring to keep the prothrombin time at 1.5- to 2.5-fold longer than normal values does not prevent bleeding complications in about twenty percent of the patients.

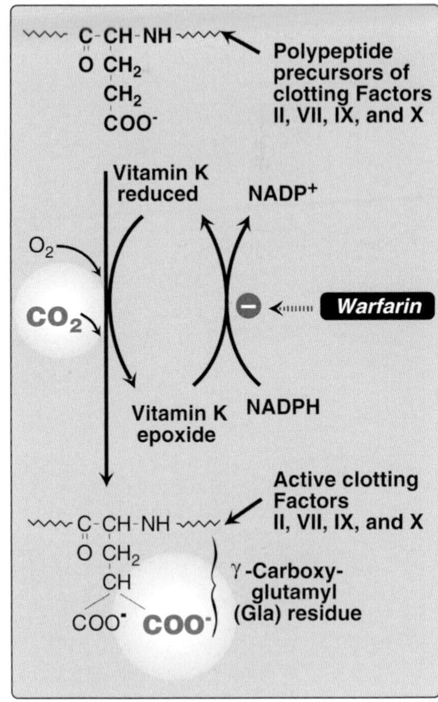

Figure 20.19
Mechanism of action of *warfarin*. NADP+ = oxidized form of nicotinamide-adenine dinucleotide phosphate; NADPH = reduced form of nicotinamide-adenine dinucleotide phosphate.

1. **Mechanism of action:** Several of the protein factors (including Factors II, VII, IX, and X; see Figure 20.10) that are involved in coagulation reactions require vitamin K as a cofactor for their synthesis by the liver. These factors undergo vitamin K–dependent posttranslational modification, whereby a number of their glutamic acid residues are carboxylated to form γ-carboxyglutamic acid residues (Figure 20.19). The γ-carboxyglutamyl residues bind calcium ions, which are essential for interaction between the coagulation factors and platelet membranes. In the carboxylation

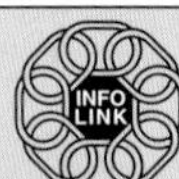

[5]See p. 157 ***Lippincott's Illustrated Reviews: Biochemistry*** (3rd ed.) for a discussion of the structure of heparin, dermatan and chondroitin.

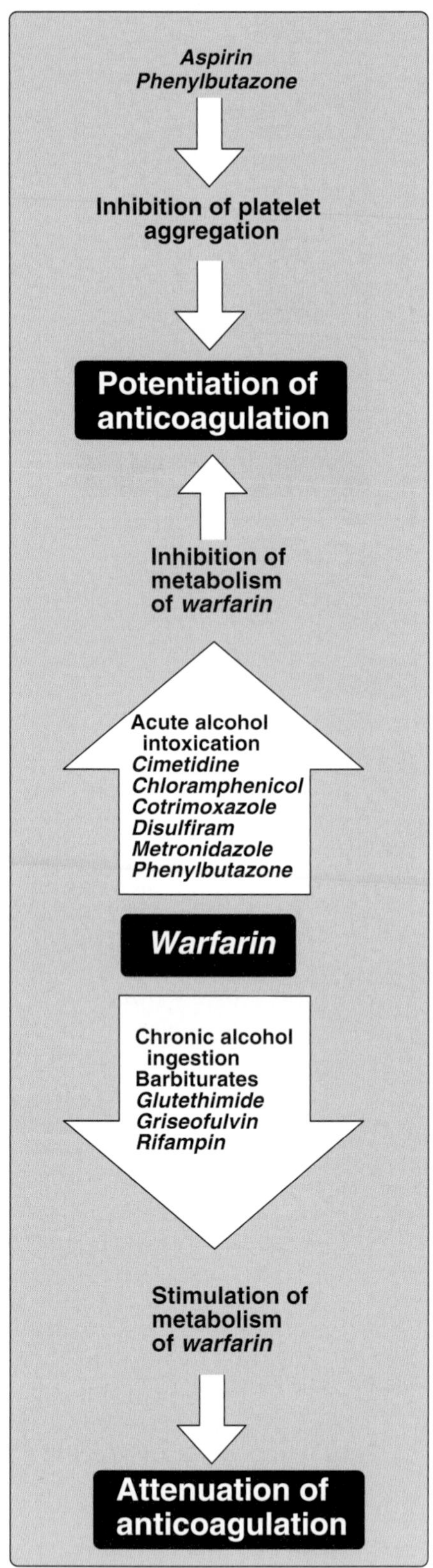

Figure 20.20
Drugs affecting the anticoagulant effect of *warfarin.*

reactions, the vitamin K–dependent carboxylase fixes CO_2 to form the new COOH group on glutamic acid. The reduced vitamin K cofactor is converted to vitamin K epoxide during the reaction. Vitamin K is regenerated from the epoxide by vitamin K epoxide reductase—the enzyme that is inhibited by *warfarin. Warfarin* or *dicumarol* treatment results in the production of inactive clotting factors, because they lack the γ-carboxyglutamyl side chains. Unlike *heparin*, the anticoagulant effects of *warfarin* are not observed until eight to twelve hours after drug administration. The anticoagulant effects of *warfarin* can be overcome by the administration of vitamin K. However, reversal following administration of vitamin K takes approximately 24 hours.

2. Pharmacokinetics

a. Absorption: *Warfarin* is rapidly and completely absorbed after oral administration. Although food may delay absorption, it does not affect the extent of absorption of the drug. *Warfarin* is 99 percent bound to plasma albumin, which prevents its diffusion into the cerebrospinal fluid, urine, and breast milk. However, drugs that have a greater affinity for the albumin binding site, such as sulfonamides, can displace the anticoagulant and lead to a transient, elevated activity. *Warfarin* readily crosses the placental barrier.

b. Fate: The products of *warfarin* metabolism, catalyzed by the cytochrome P450 system, are inactive. After conjugation to glucuronic acid, they are excreted in the urine and stool.

3. Adverse effects

a. Bleeding disorders: The principal untoward reaction caused by *warfarin* treatment is hemorrhage. Therefore, it is important to frequently monitor and adjust the anticoagulant effect. Minor bleeding may be treated by withdrawal of the drug and administration of oral vitamin K_1; severe bleeding requires that greater doses of the vitamin be given intravenously. Whole blood, frozen plasma, or plasma concentrates of the blood factors may also be employed to arrest hemorrhaging.

b. Drug interactions: A number of drug interactions that potentiate or attenuate the anticoagulant effects of *warfarin* have been identified. A summary of the most important of these interactions is shown in Figure 20.20.

c. Disease states: Vitamin K deficiency, hepatic disease that impairs synthesis of the clotting factors, and hypermetabolic states that increase catabolism of the vitamin K–dependent clotting factors can all influence the hypoprothrombinemic state of the patient and augment the response to the oral anticoagulants.

d. Contraindications: *Warfarin* should never be used during pregnancy, because it is teratogenic and can cause abortion.

VII. THROMBOLYTIC DRUGS

Acute thromboembolic disease in selected patients may be treated by the administration of agents that activate the conversion of plasminogen to plasmin—a serine protease that hydrolyzes fibrin and, thus, dissolves clots (Figure 20.21). *Streptokinase*, one of the first such agents to be approved, causes a systemic fibrinolytic state that can lead to bleeding problems. *Alteplase* acts more locally on the thrombotic fibrin to produce fibrinolysis. Figure 20.22 compares these commonly used thrombolytic agents. Clinical experience has shown about equal efficacy between *streptokinase* and *alteplase*. Unfortunately, thrombolytic therapy is unsuccessful in about twenty percent of infarcted arteries, and about fifteen percent of the arteries that are opened will later close again. In the case of acute myocardial infarction, the thrombolytic drugs are reserved for those instances when angioplasty is not an option or until the patient can be taken to a facility where it is.

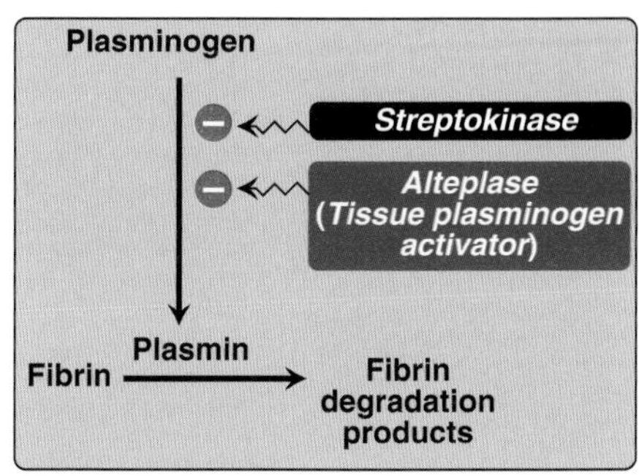

Figure 20.21
Activation of plasminogen by fibrinolytic agents.

A. Common characteristics of thrombolytic agents

1. **Mechanism of action:** The thrombolytic agents share some common features. All act either directly or indirectly to convert plasminogen to plasmin, which in turn cleaves fibrin, thus lysing thrombi (see Figure 20.21). Clot dissolution and reperfusion occur with a higher frequency when therapy is initiated early after clot formation, because clots become more resistant to lysis as they age. Unfortunately, increased local thrombi may occur as the clot dissolves, leading to enhanced platelet aggregability and thrombosis. Strategies to prevent this include administration of antiplatelet drugs, such as *aspirin*, or antithrombotics, such as *heparin*.

2. **Therapeutic uses:** Originally used for the treatment of deep-vein thrombosis and serious pulmonary embolism, thrombolytic drugs are now being used with less frequency for these conditions or to treat acute myocardial infarction or peripheral arterial thrombosis and emboli, because of the ability of these drugs to cause bleeding. Thrombolytic agents are helpful for unclotting catheters and shunts.

3. **Pharmacokinetics:** For myocardial infarction, intracoronary delivery of the drugs is the most reliable in terms of achieving recanalization. However, cardiac catheterization may not be possible in the two- to six-hour "therapeutic window," beyond which significant myocardial salvage becomes less likely. Thus, thrombolytic agents are usually administered intravenously, because this route is rapid, inexpensive, and does not have the risks of catheterization.

4. **Adverse effects:** The thrombolytic agents do not distinguish between the fibrin of an unwanted thrombus and the fibrin of a beneficial hemostatic plug. Thus, hemorrhage is a major side effect. For example, a previously unsuspected lesion, such as a peptic ulcer, may hemorrhage following injection of a thrombolytic agent (Figure 20.23). These drugs are contraindicated in patients with healing wounds, pregnancy, history of cerebrovascular accident, or metastatic cancer. Continued presence of thrombogenic stimuli may cause rethrombosis after lysis of the initial clot.

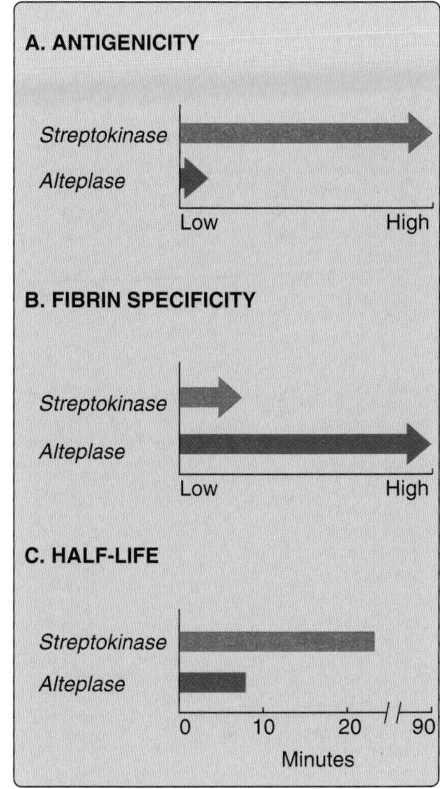

Figure 20.22
A comparison of *streptokinase* and *alteplase*.

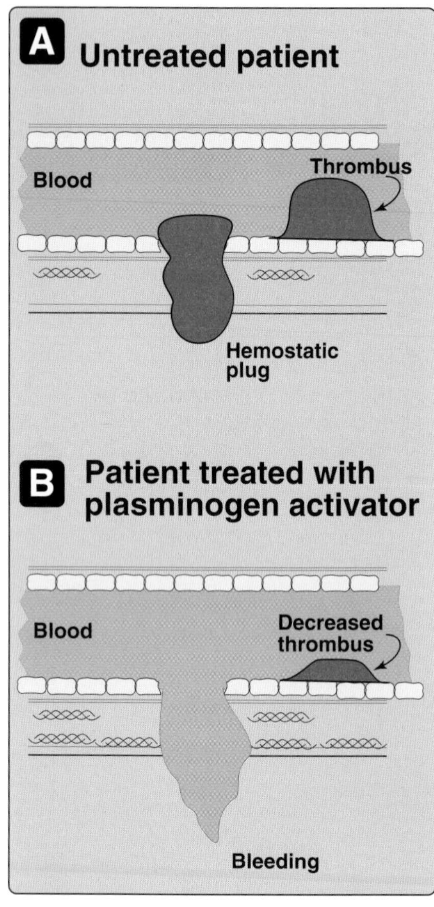

Figure 20.23
Degradation of an unwanted thrombus and a beneficial hemostatic plug by plasminogen activators.

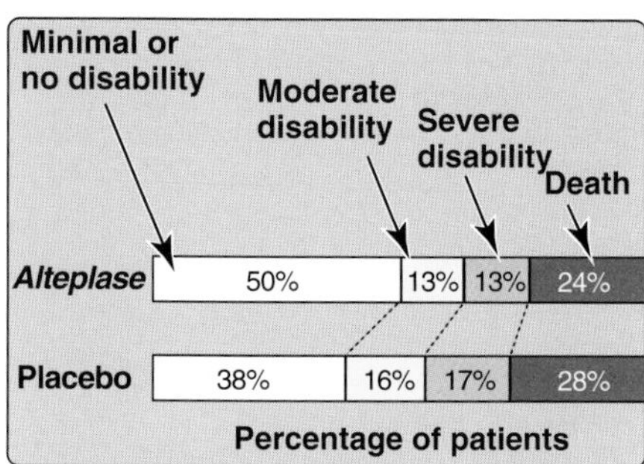

Figure 20.24
Outcome at 12 months of stroke patients treated with *alteplase* within 3 hours of the onset of symptoms compared to those treated with placebo.

B. Alteplase

Alteplase [AL te place] (formerly known as *tissue-type plasminogen activator*, or *tPA*) is a serine protease originally derived from cultured human melanoma cells. It is now obtained as a product of recombinant DNA technology.

1. **Mechanism of action:** *Alteplase* has a low affinity for free plasminogen in the plasma, but it rapidly activates plasminogen that is bound to fibrin in a thrombus or a hemostatic plug. Thus, *alteplase* is said to be "fibrin selective," and at low doses it has the advantage of lysing only fibrin, without unwanted degradation of other proteins—notably fibrinogen. This contrasts with *streptokinase*, which acts on free plasminogen and induces a general fibrinolytic state. [Note: At dose levels of *alteplase* currently in use clinically, circulating plasminogen may be activated, resulting in hemorrhage.]

2. **Therapeutic uses:** *Alteplase* is approved for the treatment of myocardial infarction, massive pulmonary embolism, and acute ischemic stroke. *Alteplase* seems to be superior to *streptokinase* in dissolving older clots and, ultimately, may be approved for other applications. *Alteplase,* administered within three hours of the onset of ischemic stroke, significantly improves clinical outcome—that is, the patient's ability to perform activites of daily living (Figure 20.24).

3. **Pharmacokinetics:** *Alteplase* has a very short half-life (about five minutes) and, therefore, is administered as a 100 mg dose, with 10 mg injected intravenously as a bolus and the remaining drug administered over ninety minutes.

4. **Adverse effects:** Bleeding complications, including gastrointestinal and cerebral hemorrhages, may occur.

C. Streptokinase

Streptokinase [strep toe KYE nase] is an extracellular protein purified from culture broths of Group C β-hemolytic streptococci.[6]

1. **Mechanism of action:** *Streptokinase* has no enzymic activity. Instead, it forms an active one-to-one complex with plasminogen. This enzymatically active complex converts uncomplexed plasminogen to the active enzyme plasmin (Figure 20.25). In addition to the hydrolysis of fibrin plugs, the complex also catalyzes the degradation of fibrinogen as well as clotting Factors V and VII (Figure 20.26).

2. **Therapeutic uses:** *Streptokinase* is approved for use in acute pulmonary embolism, deep-vein thrombosis, acute myocardial infarction, arterial thrombosis, and occluded access shunts.

3. **Pharmacokinetics:** *Streptokinase* therapy is instituted within four hours of a myocardial infarction and is infused for one hour. Its half-life is less than half an hour. Thromboplastin time is monitored and maintained at two- to five-fold the control value. On dis-

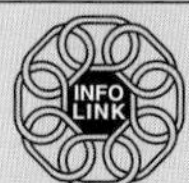

[6]See p. 145 in ***Lippincott's Illustrated Reviews: Microbiology*** for a discussion of the streptococci.

continuation of treatment, either *heparin* or oral anticoagulants may be administered.

4. Adverse effects

a. Bleeding disorders: Activation of circulating plasminogen by *streptokinase* leads to elevated levels of plasmin, which may precipitate bleeding by dissolving hemostatic plugs (see Figure 20.23). In the rare instance of life-threatening hemorrhage, *aminocaproic acid* may be administered.

b. Hypersensitivity: *Streptokinase* is a foreign protein and is antigenic. Rashes, fever, and rarely, anaphylaxis occur. Because most individuals have had a streptococcal infection sometime in their lives, circulating antibodies against *streptokinase* are likely to be present in most patients. These antibodies can combine with *streptokinase* and neutralize its fibrinolytic properties. Therefore, sufficient quantities of *streptokinase* must be administered to overwhelm the antibodies and provide a therapeutic concentration of plasmin. Fever, allergic reactions, and therapeutic failure may be associated with the presence of antistreptococcal antibodies in the patient. The incidence of allergic reactions is approximately three percent.

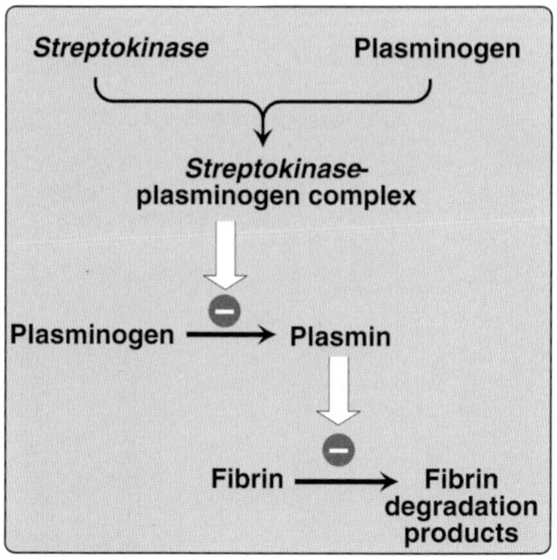

Figure 20.25
Mechanism of action of *streptokinase*.

VIII. DRUGS USED TO TREAT BLEEDING

Bleeding problems may have their origin in naturally occurring pathologic conditions, such as hemophilia, or as a result of fibrinolytic states that may arise after gastrointestinal surgery or prostatectomy. The use of anticoagulants may also give rise to hemorrhaging. Certain natural proteins and *vitamin K*, as well as synthetic antagonists, are effective in controlling this bleeding. For example, hemophilia is a consequence of a deficiency in plasma coagulation factors, most frequently Factors VIII and IX. Concentrated preparations of these factors are available from human donors. However, these preparations carry the risk of transferring viral infections. Blood transfusion is also an option for treating severe hemorrhage.

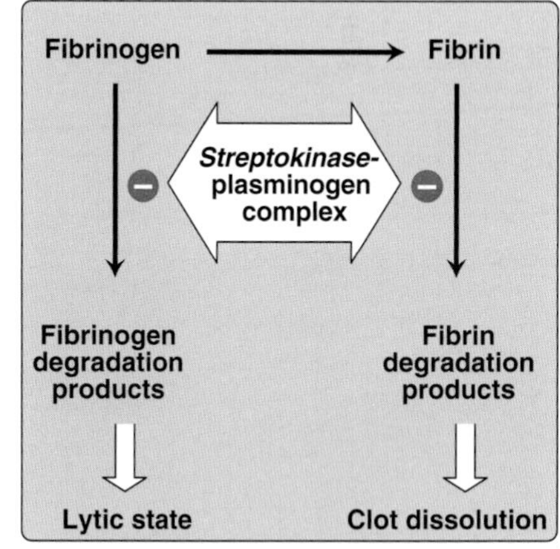

Figure 20.26
Streptokinase degrades both fibrin and fibrinogen.

A. Aminocaproic acid and tranexamic acid

Fibrinolytic states can be controlled by the administration of *aminocaproic acid* [a mee noe ka PROE ic] or *tranexamic acid* [tran ex AM ic]. Both agents are synthetic, inhibit plasminogen activation, are orally active, and are excreted in the urine. A potential side effect of treatment with one of these drugs is intravascular thrombosis.

B. Protamine sulfate

Protamine sulfate [PROE ta meen] antagonizes the anticoagulant effects of *heparin*. This protein is derived from fish sperm or testes and is high in arginine content, which explains its basicity. The positively charged *protamine* interacts with the negatively charged *heparin*, forming a stable complex without anticoagulant activity. Adverse effects of drug administration include hypersensitivity as well as dyspnea, flushing, bradycardia, and hypotension when rapidly injected.

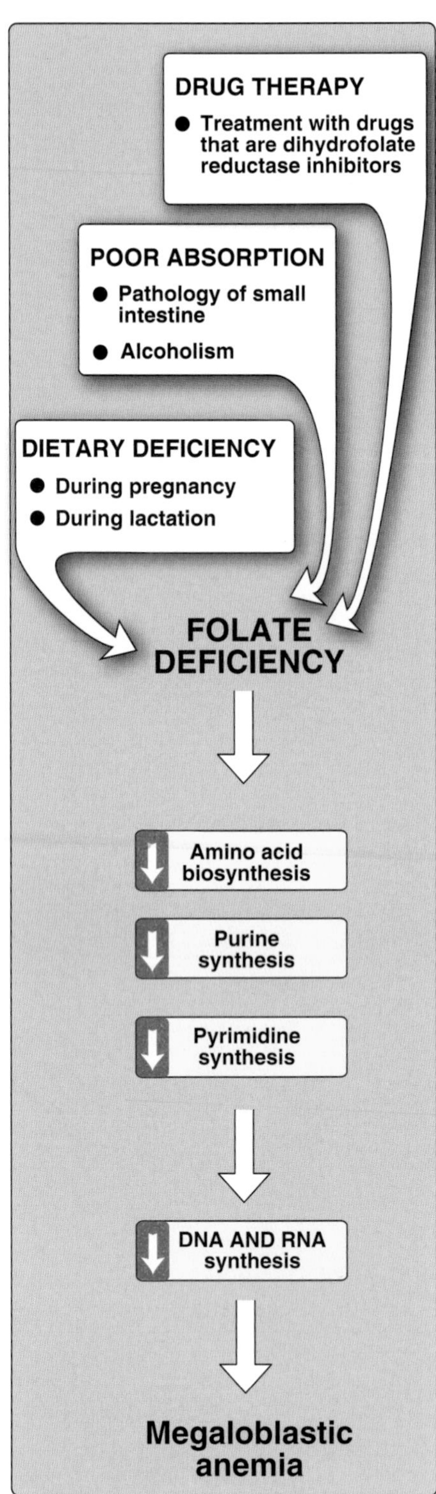

Figure 20.27
Causes and consequences of folic acid depletion.

C. Vitamin K

That *vitamin K_1* (*phytonadione*) administration can stem bleeding problems due to the oral anticoagulants is not surprising, because those substances act by interfering with the action of the vitamin (see Figure 20.19). The response to *vitamin K* is slow, requiring about 24 hours. Thus, if immediate hemostasis is required, fresh-frozen plasma should be infused. [Note: *Vitamin K* supplementation is required for patients receiving the cephalosporins *cefamandole*, *cefoperazone*, and *moxalactam*.]

D. Aprotinin

Aprotinin [ah PRO ti nin] is a serine protease inhibitor that stops-bleeding by blocking plasmin. It can inhibit the *streptokinase*. It is approved for prophylactic use to reduce perioperative blood loss and the need for blood transfusion in patients undergoing cardiopulmonary bypass surgery. The drug also attenuates an inflammatory response. Its adverse effects appear to be minimal.

IX. AGENTS USED TO TREAT ANEMIA

Anemia is defined as a below-normal plasma hemoglobin concentration resulting from a decreased number of circulating red blood cells or an abnormally low total hemoglobin content per unit of blood volume. Anemia can be caused by chronic blood loss, bone marrow abnormalities, increased hemolysis, infections, malignancy, endocrine deficiencies, and a number of other disease states. Anemia can be at least temporarily corrected by transfusion of whole blood. A large number of drugs cause toxic effects on blood cells, hemoglobin production, or erythropoietic organs, which in turn may cause anemia. In addition, nutritional anemias are caused by dietary deficiencies of substances such as iron, folic acid, or vitamin B_{12} (cyanocobalamin) that are necessary for normal erythropoiesis.

A. Iron

Iron is stored in intestinal mucosal cells as ferritin (an iron-protein complex) until needed by the body. Iron deficiency results from acute or chronic blood loss, from insufficient intake during periods of accelerated growth in children, or in heavily menstruating or pregnant women. Thus, iron deficiency results from a negative iron balance due to depletion of iron stores and/or inadequate intake, culminating in hypochromic microcytic anemia. Supplementation with *ferrous sulfate* is required to correct the deficiency. Gastrointestinal disturbances caused by local irritation are the most common adverse effects of iron supplements.

B. Folic acid

The primary use of *folic acid* is in treating deficiency states that arise from inadequate levels of the vitamin. Folate deficiency may be caused by 1) increased demand (for example, pregnancy and lactation), 2) poor absorption caused by pathology of the small intestine, 3) alcoholism, or 4) treatment with drugs that are dihydrofolate reductase inhibitors (for example, *methotrexate* or *trimethoprim*). A primary result of folic acid deficiency is megaloblastic anemia, which is caused by diminished synthesis of purines and pyrimidines that leads to an inability of erythropoietic tissue to make DNA and, thereby, proliferate[7] (Figure 20.27). [Note: It is important to evaluate the basis of the megaloblastic anemia prior to instituting therapy, because vitamin B_{12} deficiency indirectly causes symptoms of this disorder (see below).] *Folic acid* is well absorbed in the jejunum unless pathology is present. If excessive amounts of the vitamin are ingested, they are excreted in the urine and feces. *Folic acid* administered orally has no known toxicity.

C. Cyanocobalamin (vitamin B_{12})

Deficiencies of vitamin B_{12} can result from either low dietary levels or, more commonly, poor absorption of the vitamin due to the failure of gastric parietal cells to produce intrinsic factor (as in pernicious anemia) or a loss of activity of the receptor needed for intestinal uptake of the vitamin.[8] Nonspecific malabsorption syndromes or gastric resection can also cause vitamin B_{12} deficiency. The vitamin may be administered orally (for dietary deficiencies) or intramuscularly or deep subcutaneously (for pernicious anemia). [Note: *Folic acid* administration alone reverses the hematologic abnormality and, thus, masks the B_{12} deficiency, which can then proceed to severe neurologic dysfunction and disease. Therefore, megaloblastic anemia should not be treated with *folic acid* alone but, rather, with a combination of *folate* and *vitamin B_{12}*.] Therapy must be continued for the remainder of the life of a patient suffering from pernicious anemia. There are no known adverse effects of this vitamin.

D. Erythropoietin

Erythropoietin [ee rith ro POI eh tin] is a glycoprotein, normally made by the kidney, that regulates red cell proliferation and differentiation in bone marrow. Human *erythropoietin*, produced by recombinant DNA technology, is effective in the treatment of anemia caused by end-stage renal disease, anemia associated with HIV-infected patients, and anemia in some cancer patients. Supplementation with iron may be required to assure an adequate response. The protein is usually administered intravenously in renal dialysis patients, but in others, the subcutaneous route is preferred. Side effects, such as iron deficiency and an elevation in blood pressure, occur. [Note: The latter may be due to increases in peripheral vascular resistance and/or blood viscosity.]

X. AGENTS USED TO TREAT SICKLE-CELL DISEASE

Clinical trials have shown that *hydroxyurea* can relieve the painful clinical course of sickle-cell disease (Figure 20.28). *Hydroxyurea* is currently also being used to treat chronic myelogenous leukemia and polycythemia vera. In sickle-cell disease, the drug apparently increases fetal hemoglobin levels, thus diluting the abnormal hemoglobin S (HbS).[9] This process takes several months. Polymerization of HbS is delayed in the treated patients so that painful crises are not caused by sickled cells blocking capillaries and causing tissue anoxia. The optimal dose of *hydroxyurea*, and its safety over the long run, remain to be determined.

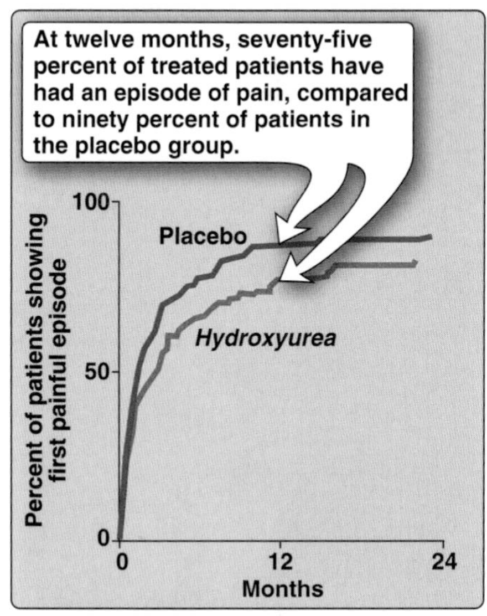

Figure 20.28
Effect of treatment with *hydroxyurea* on the percentage of sickle-cell patients experiencing first painful episode.

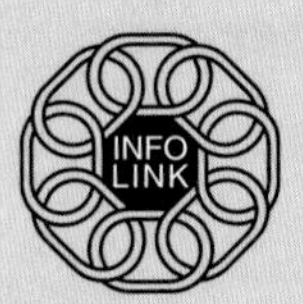

[7]See p. 372 in ***Lippincott's Illustrated Reviews: Biochemistry*** (3rd ed.) for a discussion of folic acid deficiency and DNA replication.

[8]See p. 375 in ***Lippincott's Illustrated Reviews: Biochemistry*** (3rd ed.) for a discussion of Vitamin B_{12} and its deficiency state.

[9]See p. 35 in ***Lippincott's Illustrated Reviews: Biochemistry*** (3rd ed.) for a discussion of sickle-cell diseases and hemoglobin.

Study Questions

Choose the ONE best answer.

20.1 A 22-year-old woman who experienced pain and swelling in her right leg presented at the emergency room. An ultrasound study showed thrombosis in the popliteal vein. The patient, who was in her second trimester of pregnancy, was treated for seven days with intravenous unfractionated heparin. The pain resolved during the course of therapy, and the patient was discharged on day eight. Which one of the following drugs would be most appropriate outpatient follow-up therapy for this patient, who lives 100 miles from the nearest hospital?

A. Warfarin
B. Aspirin
C. Alteplase
D. Unfractionated heparin
E. Low-molecular-weight heparin (LMWH)

Correct answer = E. LMWH has a reliable dose response and can be administered subcutaneously by selected patients who have been taught home injection technique. LMWHs do not cross the placenta and show no teratogenic effects. By contrast, warfarin is teratogenic and is contraindicated in pregnant patients. Aspirin, which inhibits platelet aggregation, has little effect on venous thrombosis, which is composed of fibrin with only a few platelets. Alteplase is not indicated for deep-vein thrombosis.

20.2 A 60-year-old man is diagnosed with deep-vein thrombosis. The patient was treated with a bolus of heparin, and a heparin drip was started. One hour later, he was bleeding profusely from the intravenous site. The heparin therapy was suspended, but the bleeding continued. Protamine was administered intravenously and the bleeding resolved. The protamine:

A. degraded the heparin.
B. inactivates antithrombin.
C. activates the coagulation cascade.
D. activates tissue-plasminogen activator.
E. ionically combines with heparin.

Correct answer = E. Excessive bleeding may be managed by ceasing administration of the drug or by treating with protamine sulfate. Infused slowly, protamine combines ionically with heparin to form a stable, inactive complex.

20.3 A 54-year-old male with a prosthetic aortic valve replacement complained to his family physician of black and tarry stools. Physical examination and vital signs were unremarkable except for subconjunctivial hemorrhages and bleeding gums. Stools tested positive for heme and hematuria was observed. The patient has been receiving oral warfarin since his valve replacement one year earlier. Prothrombin time was found to be significantly elevated. Which one of the following therapies would provide the most rapid recovery from the observed bleeding secondary to warfarin treatment?

A. Intravenous vitamin K
B. Transfusion of fresh-frozen plasma
C. Intravenous protamine
D. Immediate withdrawal of warfarin treatment
E. Intravenous administration of anti-warfarin antibodies

Correct answer = B. Whole blood, frozen plasma, or plasma concentrates of the blood factors may be employed to rapidly arrest hemorrhaging. Minor bleeding may be treated by withdrawal of the drug and administration of oral vitamin K_1; severe bleeding requires greater doses of the vitamin given intravenously. However, reversal by following administration of vitamin K takes approximately 24 hours. Protamine is used to neutralize an overdose of heparin, not an overdose of warfarin. Immediate withdrawal of warfarin treatment will not have an immediate effect, because the anticoagulant effects of warfarin last between five and seven days.

Antihyperlipidemic Drugs

21

I. OVERVIEW

Coronary heart disease (CHD) is the cause of about half of all deaths in the United States. The incidence of CHD is correlated with elevated levels of low-density lipoprotein (LDL) cholesterol and triacylglycerols and with low levels of high-density lipoprotein (HDL) cholesterol. Other risk factors for CHD incude cigarette smoking, hypertension, obesity, and diabetes. Cholesterol levels may be elevated as a result of an individual's lifestyle (for example, by lack of exercise and consumption of a diet containing excess saturated fatty acids). Hyperlipidemias can also result from a single inherited gene defect in lipoprotein metabolism or, more commonly, by a combination of genetic and lifestyle factors. Appropriate lifestyle changes in combination with drug therapy can lead to a decline in the progression of coronary plaque, regression of preexisting lesions, and reduction in mortality due to CHD by thirty to forty percent. Antihyperlipidemic drugs must be taken indefinitely; when therapy is terminated, plasma lipid levels return to pretreatment levels. The antihyperlipidemic drugs are listed in Figure 21.1. Figure 21.2 illustrates the normal metabolism of serum lipoproteins and the characteristics of the major genetic hyperlipidemias.

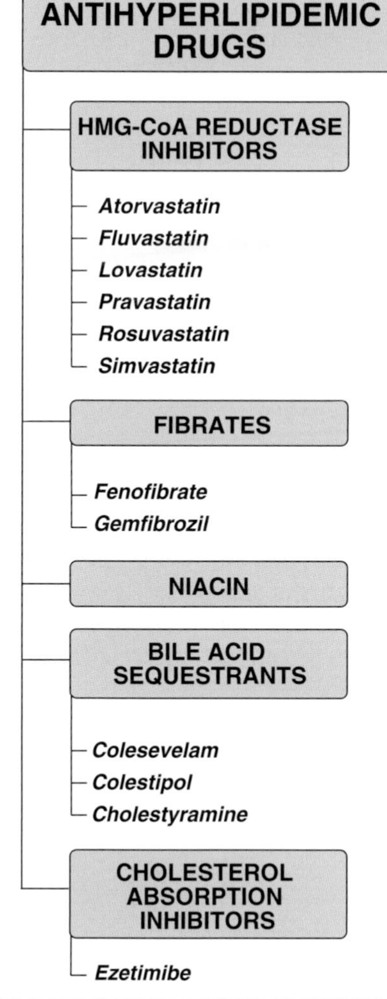

Figure 21.1
Summary of antihyperlipidemic drugs. HMG-CoA = 3-hydroxy-3-methylglutaryl coenzyme A.

II. TREATMENT GOALS

Plasma lipids consist mostly of lipoproteins—spherical macromolecular complexes of lipids and specific proteins (apolipoproteins). The clinically important lipoproteins, listed in decreasing order of atherogenicity, are LDL, very-low-density lipoprotein (VLDL) and chylomicrons, and HDL. The occurence of CHD is positively associated with high total cholesterol, and even more strongly with elevated LDL cholesterol in the blood. In contrast to LDL, high levels of HDL cholesterol, have been associated with a decreased risk for heart disease (Figure 21.3). Reduction of the LDL level is the primary goal of cholesterol-lowering therapy. Figure 21.4 shows the current goals in the teatment of hyperlipidemia. Recommendations for the reduction of LDL cholesterol to specific target levels are influenced by the coexistence of CHD and the number of other cardiac risk factors. The higher the overall risk of heart disease, the more aggressive the recommended LDL-lowering therapy.

Lippincott's Illustrated Reviews: Pharmacology, Third Edition,
by Richard D. Howland and Mary J. Mycek.

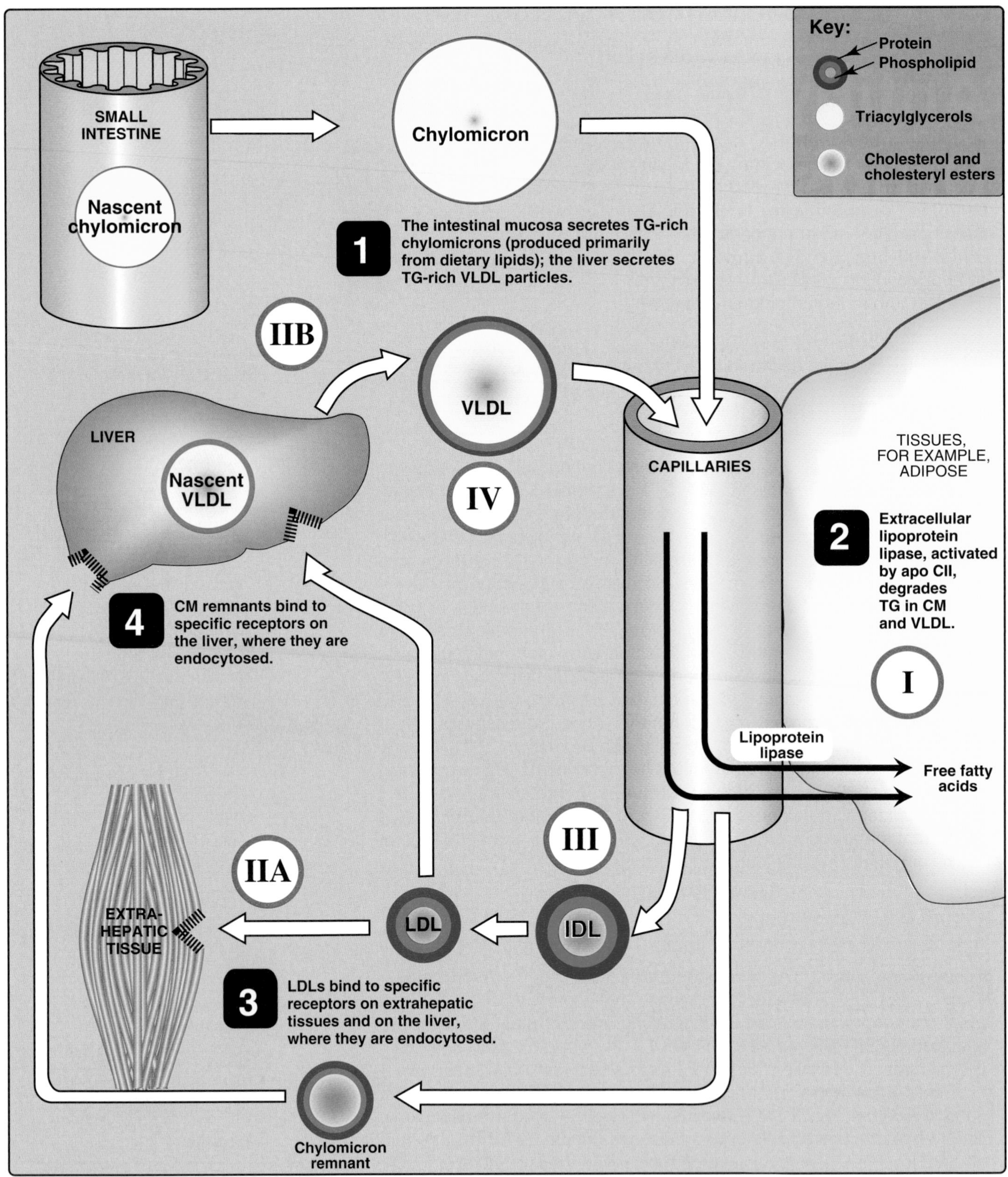

Figure 21.2
Metabolism of plasma lipoproteins and related genetic diseases. The Roman numerals in the white circles refer to specific genetic types of hyperlipidemias summarized on the facing page. CM=chylomicron, TG = triacylglycerol; VLDL=very-low density lipoprotein, LDL=low-density lipoprotein, IDL=intermediate-density lipoprotein, apo CII= apolipoprotein CII found in chylomicrons and VLDL.

Type I [FAMILIAL HYPERCHYLOMICRONEMIA]

- Massive fasting hyperchylomicronemia, even following normal dietary fat intake, resulting in greatly elevated serum TG levels.
- Deficiency of lipoprotein lipase or deficiency of normal apolipoprotein CII (rare).
- Type I is not associated with an increase in coronary heart disease.
- Treatment: Low-fat diet. No drug therapy is effective for Type I hyperlipidemia.

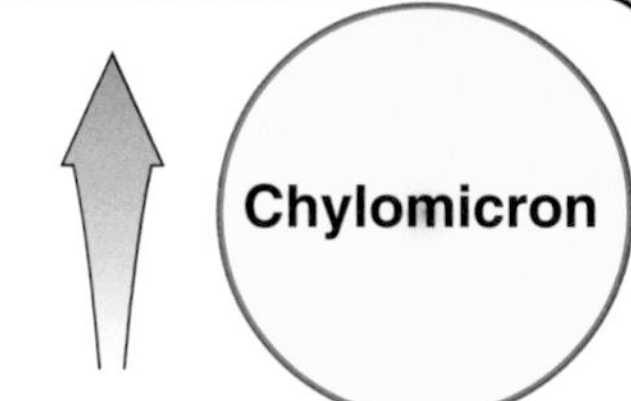

Type IIA [FAMILIAL HYPERCHOLESTEROLEMIA]

- Elevated LDL with normal VLDL levels due to a block in LDL degradation. This results in increased serum cholesterol but normal TG levels.
- Caused by defects in the synthesis or processing of LDL receptors.
- Ischemic heart disease is greatly accelerated.
- Treatment: Diet. Heterozygotes: *Cholestyramine* and *niacin*, or a statin.

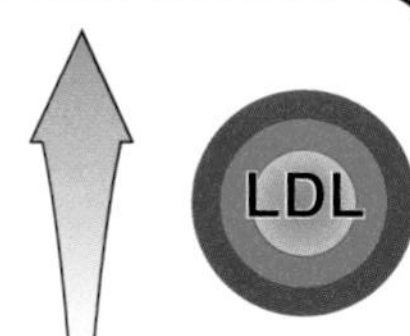

Type IIB [FAMILIAL COMBINED (MIXED) HYPERLIPIDEMIA]

- Similar to IIA except that VLDL is also increased, resulting in elevated serum TG as well as cholesterol levels.
- Caused by overproduction of VLDL by the liver.
- Relatively common.
- Treatment: Diet. Drug therapy is similar to that for Type IIA .

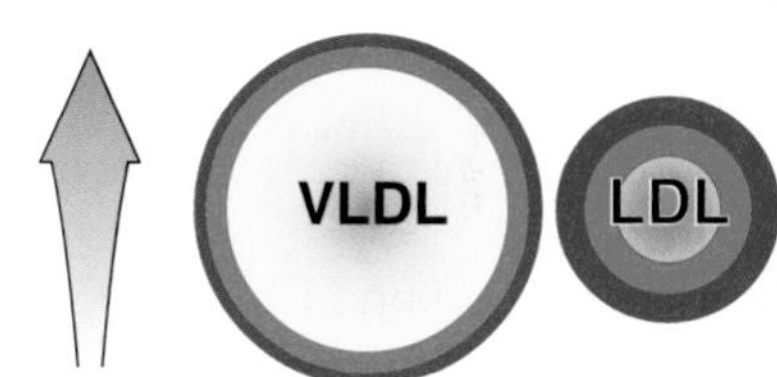

Type III [FAMILIAL DYSBETALIPOPROTEINEMIA]

- Serum concentrations of IDL are increased, resulting in increased TG and cholesterol levels.
- Cause is either overproduction or underutilization of IDL due to mutant apolipoprotein E.
- Xanthomas and accelerated vascular disease develop in patients by middle age.
- Treatment: Diet. Drug therapy includes *niacin* and *fenofibrate*, or a statin.

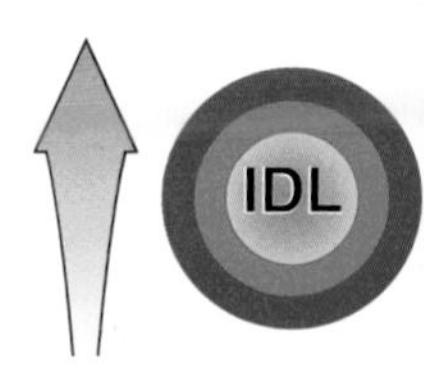

Type IV [FAMILIAL HYPERTRIGLYCERIDEMIA]

- VLDL levels are increased, whereas LDL levels are normal or decreased, resulting in normal to elevated cholesterol, and greatly elevated circulating TG levels.
- Cause is overproduction and/or decreased removal of VLDL TG in serum.
- This is a relatively common disease. It has few clinical manifestations other than accelerated ischemic heart disease. Patients with this disorder are frequently obese, diabetic, and hyperuricemic.
- Treatment: Diet. If necessary, drug therapy includes *niacin* and/or *fenofibrate*.

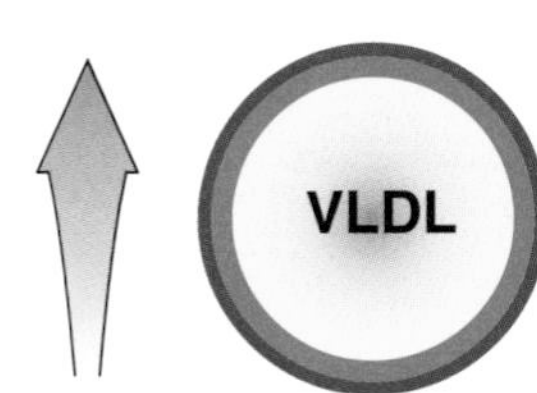

Type V [FAMILIAL MIXED HYPERTRIGLYCERIDEMIA]

- Serum VLDL and chylomicrons are elevated. LDL is normal or decreased. This results in elevated cholesterol and greatly elevated TG levels.
- Cause is either increased production or decreased clearance of VLDL and chylomicrons. Usually, it is a genetic defect.
- Occurs most commonly in adults who are obese and/or diabetic.
- Treatment: Diet. If necessary, drug therapy includes *niacin*, and/or *fenofibrate*, or a statin.

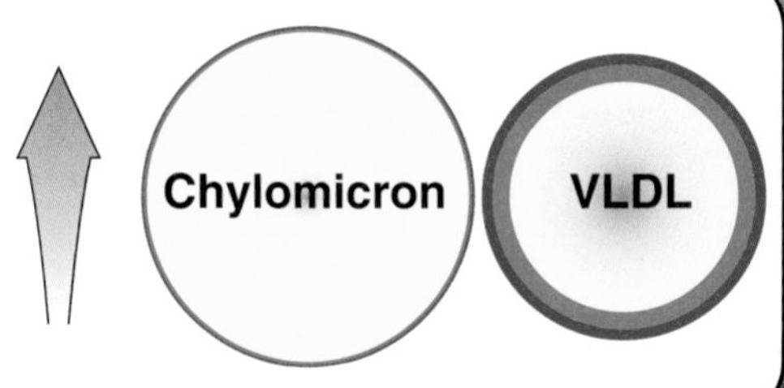

Figure 21.2 (continued).

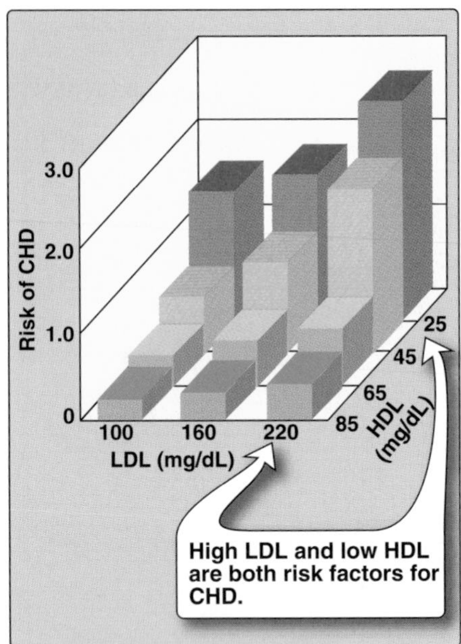

Figure 21.3
Effect of circulating LDL and HDL on the risk of coronary heart disease (CHD).

A. Treatment options for hypercholesterolemia

In patients with moderate hyperlipidemia, lifestyle changes, such as diet, exercise, and weight reduction, can lead to modest decreases in LDL and increases in HDL levels. However, most patients are unwilling to modify their lifestyle sufficiently to achieve LDL treatment goals, and drug therapy may be required. Patients with LDL levels higher than 160 mg/dL and with one other major risk factor such as hypertension, diabetes, smoking, or a family history of early CHD, are candidates for drug therapy. Patients with two or more additional risk factors should be treated aggressively, with the aim of reducing their LDL level to less than 130 mg/dL.

B. Treatment options for hypertriacylglycerolemia

Elevated triacylglycerol levels are independently associated with increased risk of CHD. Diet and exercise are the primary modes of treating hypertriacylglycerolemia. If indicated, *niacin* and fibric acid derivatives are the most efficacious in lowering triacylglycerol levels. Triacylglycerol reduction is a secondary benefit of the statin drugs (the primary benefit being LDL cholesterol reduction). [Note: The major lipid component of VLDL is composed of triacylglycerol.]

III. DRUGS THAT LOWER THE SERUM LIPOPROTEIN CONCENTRATION

Antihyperlipidemic drugs target the problem of elevated serum lipids with complementary strategies. Some of these agents decrease production of the lipoprotein carriers of cholesterol and triacylglycerol, whereas others increase the degradation of lipoprotein. Still others decrease cholesterol absorption or directly increase cholesterol removal from the body. These drugs may be used singly or in combination.

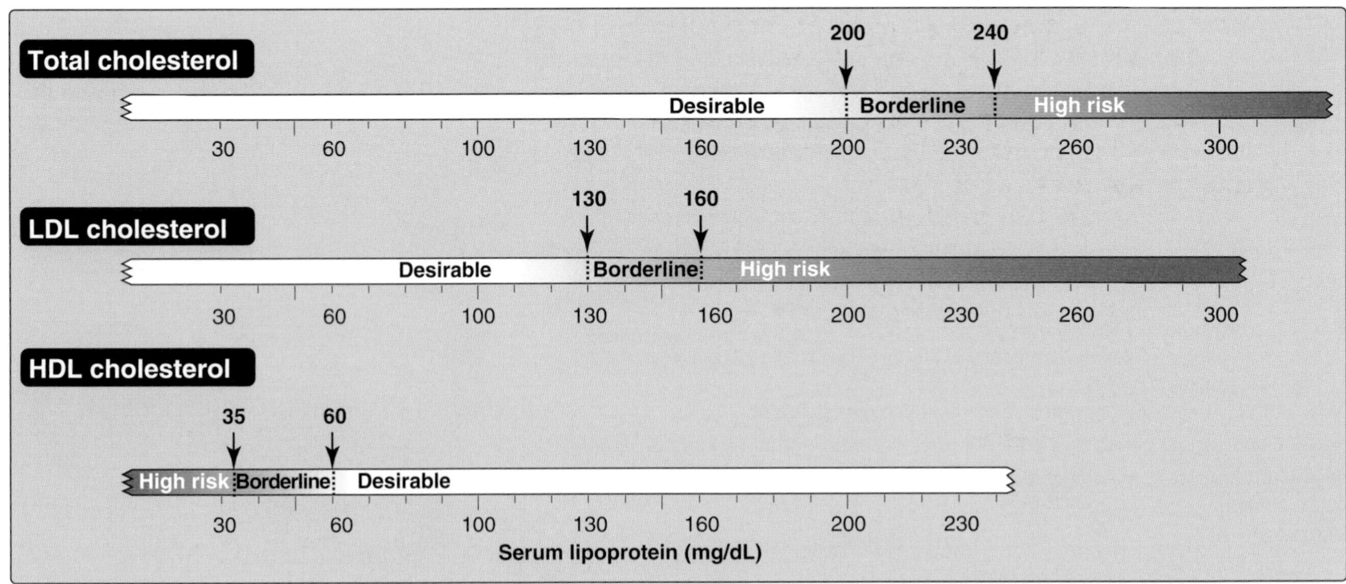

Figure 21.4
Goal lipoprotein levels achieved with dietary or drug therapy for the prevention of coronary heart disease. [Note: Lower goals for total and LDL cholesterol are recommended for patients with a history of heart disease.]

However, they are always accompanied by the requirement that dietary saturated and trans-fats[1] be low, and the caloric content of the diet must be closely monitored.

A. HMG CoA reductase inhibitors

3-Hydroxy-3-methylglutaryl (HMG) coenzyme A reductase inhibitors (commonly known as statins) lower elevated LDL cholesterol levels, resulting in a substantial reduction in coronary events and death from CHD. This group of antihyperlipidemic agents inhibits the first committed enzymatic step of cholesterol synthesis. Therapeutic benefits include plaque stabilization, improvement of coronary endothelial function, inhibition of platelet thrombus formation, and anti-inflammatory activity. The value of lowering the level of cholesterol with statin drugs has now been demonstrated in 1) patients with CHD, with or without hyperlipidemia; 2) men with hyperlipidemia but no known CHD; and 3) men and women with average total and LDL cholesterol levels and no known CHD.

1. Mechanism of action:

a. Inhibition of HMG CoA reductase: *Lovastatin* [LOE vah stat in] *simvastatin* [sim vah STAT in], *pravastatin* [PRAH vah stat in], *atorvastatin* (a TOR vah stat in), *fluvastatin* [FLOO vah stat in], and *rosuvastatin* [roe SOO va sta tin] are analogs of 3-hydroxy-3-methylglutarate, the precursor of cholesterol. *Lovastatin* and *simvastatin* are lactones that are hydrolyzed to the active drug. *Pravastatin* and *fluvastatin* are active as such. Because of their strong affinity for the enzyme, all compete effectively to inhibit HMG CoA reductase, the rate-limiting step in cholesterol synthesis. By inhibiting de novo cholesterol synthesis, they deplete the intracellular supply of cholesterol (Figure 21.5). *Rosuvastatin* and *atorvastatin* are the most potent LDL cholesterol–lowering statin drugs, followed by *pravastatin* and *fluvastatin* and then *lovastatin* and *simvastatin*.

b. Increase in LDL receptors: Depletion of intracellular cholesterol causes the cell to increase the number of specific cell-surface LDL receptors that can bind and internalize circulating LDLs. Thus, the end result is a reduction in plasma cholesterol, both by lowered cholesterol synthesis and by increased catabolism of LDL. [Note: Because these agents undergo a marked first-pass extraction by the liver, their dominant effect is on that organ.] The HMG CoA reductase inhibitors, like the bile acid sequesterant *cholestyramine*, can increase plasma HDL levels in some patients, resulting in an additional lowering of risk for CHD. Decreases in triacylglycerol also occur.

2. Therapeutic uses: These drugs are effective in lowering plasma cholesterol levels in all types of hyperlipidemias (Figure 21.6). However, patients who are homozygous for familial hypercholesterolemia lack LDL receptors and, therefore, benefit much less from treatment with these drugs. [Note: These drugs are often given in combination with other antihyperlipidemic drugs, see

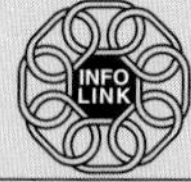

[1]See p. 362 in ***Lippincott's Illustrated Reviews: Biochemistry*** (3rd ed.) for a discussion of trans fatty acids.

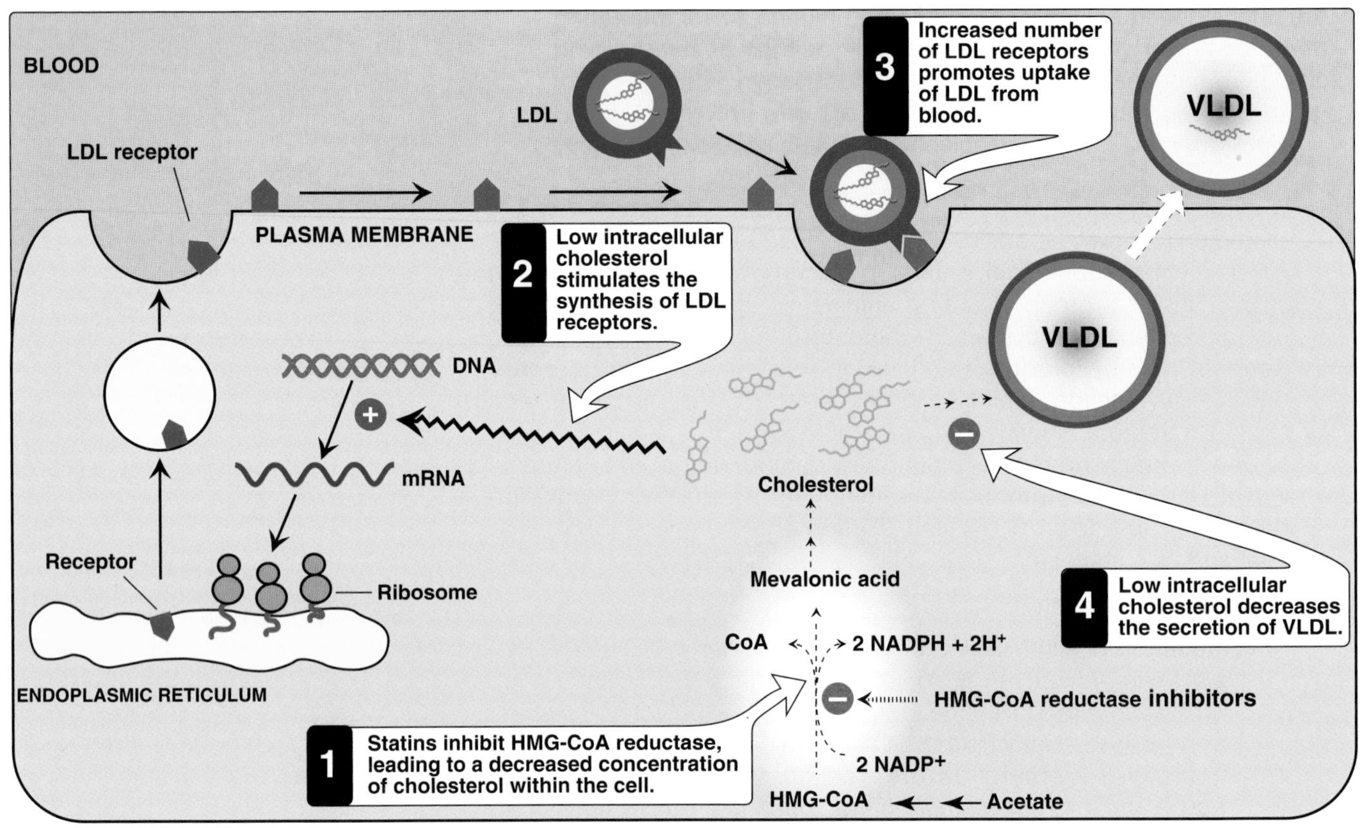

Figure 21.5
Inhibition of HMG-CoA reductase by the statin drugs.

below.] It should be noted that in spite of the protection afforded by cholesterol lowering, about one-fourth of the patients treated with these drugs still presente with coronary events. Thus, additional strategies, such as diet, exercise, or additional agents, may be warranted.

3. **Pharmacokinetics:** *Pravastatin* and *fluvastatin* are almost completely absorbed after oral administration; oral doses of *lovastatin* and *simvastatin* are absorbed from thirty to fifty percent. Similarly, *pravastatin* and *fluvastatin* are active as such, whereas *lovastatin* and *simvastatin* must be hydrolyzed to their acid forms. Due to first-pass extraction, the primary action of these drugs is on the liver. All are biotransformed, with some of the products retaining activity. Excretion takes place principally through the bile and feces, but some urinary elimination also occurs. Their half-lives range from 1.5 to 2 hours. Some characteristics of the statins are summarized in Figure 21.7

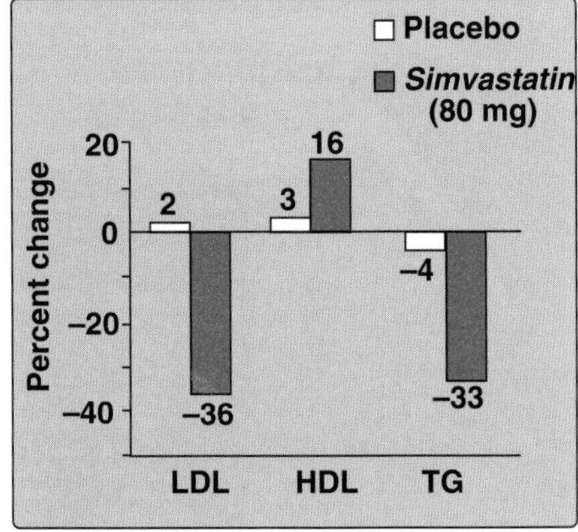

Figure 21.6
Effect of *simvastatin* on serum lipids of 130 patients with Type 2 diabetes treated for six weeks. HDL = high-density lipoprotein; LDL = low-density lipoprotein; TG = triacylglycerol.

4. **Adverse effects:** It is noteworthy that during the five-year trials of *simvastatin* and *lovastatin*, only a few adverse effects, related to liver and muscle function, were reported (Figure 21.8).

   a. **Liver:** Biochemical abnormalities in liver function have occurred with the HMG CoA reductase inhibitors. Therefore, it

Characteristic	*Atorvastatin*	*Fluvastatin*	*Lovastatin*	*Pravastatin*	*Rosuvastatin*	*Simvastatin*
Serum LDL cholesterol reduction produced (%)	50	24	34	34	50	41
Serum triacylglycerol reduction produced (%)	29	10	16	24	18	18
Serum HDL cholesterol increase produced (%)	6	8	9	12	8	12
Plasma half-life (hr)	14	1–2	2	1–2	19	1–2
Penetration of central nervous system	No	No	Yes	No	No	Yes
Renal excretion of absorbed dose (%)	2	<6	10	20	10	13

Figure 21.7
Summary of 3-hydroxy-3-methylglutaryl–coenzyme (HMG-CoA) reductase inhibitors.

is prudent to evaluate liver function and measure serum transaminase levels periodically. These return to normal on suspension of the drug. [Note: Hepatic insufficiency can cause drug accumulation.]

b. Muscle: Myopathy and rhabdomyolysis (disintegration or dissolution of muscle) have been reported only rarely. In most of these cases, patients usually suffered from renal insufficiency, or were taking drugs such as *cyclosporine*, *itraconazole*, *erythromycin*, *gemfibrozil*, or *niacin*. Plasma creatine kinase levels should be determined regularly.

c. Drug interactions: The HMG CoA reductase inhibitors also increase *warfarin* levels. Thus, it is important to evaluate prothrombin times frequently.

d. Contraindications: These drugs are contraindicated during pregnancy and in nursing mothers. They should not be used in children or teenagers.

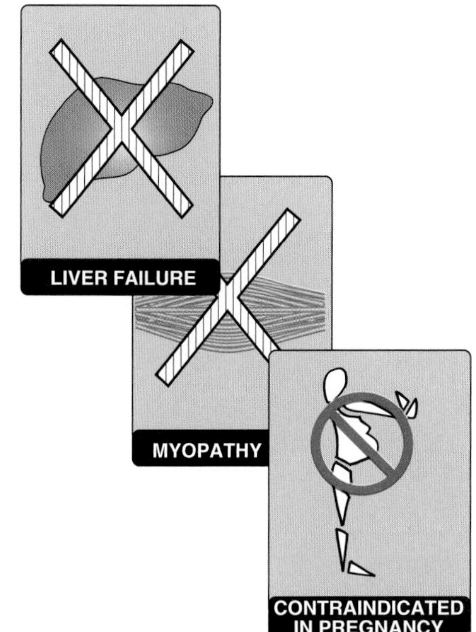

Figure 21.8
Some adverse effects and precautions associated with 3-hydroxy-3-methylglutaryl–coenzyme (HMG-CoA) reductase inhibitors.

B. Niacin (nicotinic acid)

Niacin[2] [NYE a sin] can reduce LDL (the "bad" cholesterol carrier) levels by ten to twenty percent and is the most effective agent for increasing HDL (the "good" cholesterol carrier) levels. *Niacin* can be used in combination with statins, and a fixed-dose combination of lovastatin and long-acting *niacin* is available.

1. **Mechanism of action:** At gram doses, *niacin* strongly inhibits lipolysis in adipose tissue—the primary producer of circulating free fatty acids. The liver normally utilizes these circulating fatty acids as a major precursor for triacylglycerol synthesis. Thus, *niacin* causes a decrease in liver triacylglycerol synthesis, which

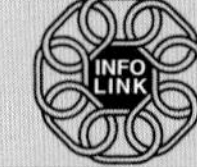

[2]See p. 377 in ***Lippincott's Illustrated Reviews: Biochemistry*** (3rd ed.) for a discussion of niacin as a vitamin.

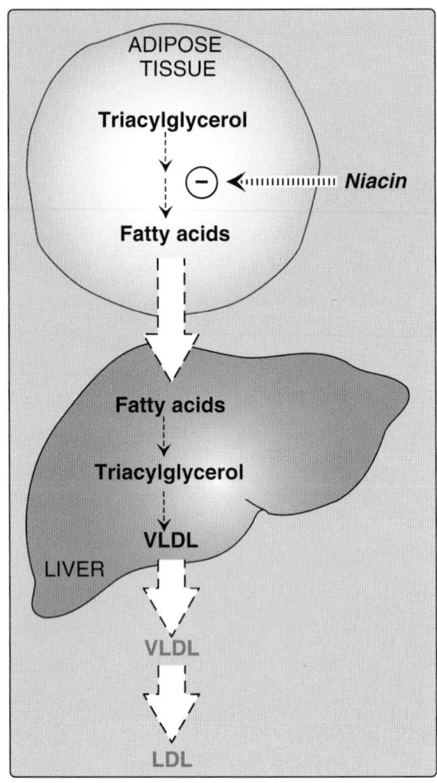

Figure 21.9
Niacin inhibits lipolysis in adipose tissue, resulting in decreased hepatic VLDL synthesis and production of LDLs in the plasma.

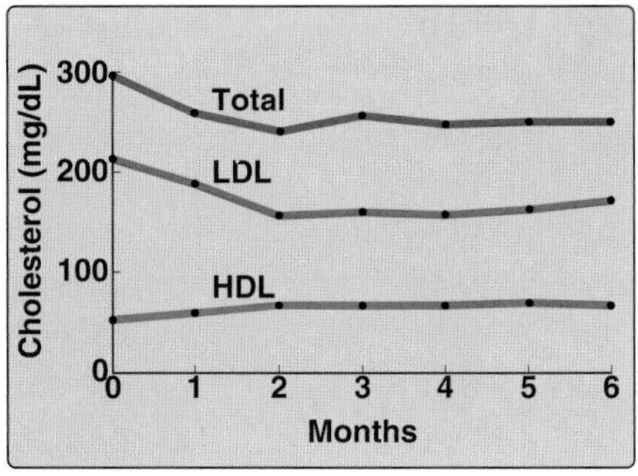

Figure 21.10
Plasma levels of cholesterol in hyperlipidemic patients during treatment with *niacin*.

is required for VLDL production (Figure 21.9). LDL (the cholesterol-rich lipoprotein) is derived from VLDL in the plasma. Therefore, a reduction in the VLDL concentration also results in a decreased plasma LDL concentration. Thus, both plasma triacylglycerol (in VLDL) and cholesterol (in VLDL and LDL) are lowered (Figure 21.10). Furthermore, *niacin* treatment increases HDL cholesterol levels. Moreover, by boosting secretion of tissue-plasminogen activator and lowering the level of plasma fibrinogen, *niacin* can reverse some of the endothelial cell dysfunction contributing to thrombosis associated with hypercholesterolemia and atherosclerosis.

2. **Therapeutic uses:** *Niacin* lowers plasma levels of both cholesterol and triacylglycerol. Therefore, it is particularly useful in the treatment of familial hyperlipidemias. *Niacin* is also used to treat other severe hypercholesterolemias, often in combination with other antihyperlipidemic agents. In addition, it is the most potent antihyperlipidemic agent for raising plasma HDL levels.

3. **Pharmacokinetics:** *Niacin* is administered orally. It is converted in the body to nicotinamide, which is incorporated into the cofactor nicotinamide adenine dinucleotide (NAD^+). *Niacin*, its nicotinamide derivative, and other metabolites are excreted in the urine. [Note: Nicotinamide alone does not decrease plasma lipid levels.]

4. **Adverse effects:** The most common side effects of *niacin* therapy are an intense cutaneous flush (accompanied by an uncomfortable feeling of warmth) and pruritus. Administration of *aspirin* prior to taking *niacin* decreases the flush, which is prostaglandin-mediated. The sustained-release formulation of *niacin*, which is taken once daily at bedtime, reduces bothersome initial adverse effects. Some patients also experience nausea and abdominal pain. *Niacin* inhibits tubular secretion of uric acid and, thus, predisposes to hyperuricemia and gout. Impaired glucose tolerance and hepatotoxicity have also been reported.

C. The fibrates: Fenofibrate and gemfibrozil

Fenofibrate and *gemfibrozil* are derivatives of fibric acid that lower serum triacylglycerols and increase HDL levels. Both have the same mechanism of action. However, *fenofibrate* is more effective than *gemfibrozil* in lowering plasma LDL cholesterol and triacylglycerol levels.

1. **Mechanism of action:** The peroxisome proliferator–activated receptors (PPARs) are members of the nuclear receptor supergene family that regulates lipid metabolism. PPAR functions as a ligand-activated transcription factor. Upon binding to its natural ligand (fatty acids or eicosanoids) or hypolipidemic drugs, PPARs are activated. They then bind to peroxisome proliferator response elements, which are localized in numerous gene promoters. In particular, PPAR regulates the expression of genes encoding for proteins involved in lipoprotein structure and function. Fibrate-mediated gene expression ultimately leads to decreased triacyl-

glycerol concentrations by increasing the expression of lipoprotein lipase (Figure 22.11) and decreasing apo C-II concentration. Fibrates also increase the level of HDL cholesterol by increasing the expression of apo A-I and apo A-II. *Fenofibrate* is a prodrug, producing an active metabolite, fenofibric acid, which is responsible for the primary effects of the drug.

2. **Therapeutic uses:** The fibrates are used in the treatment of hypertriacylglycerolemias, causing a significant decrease in plasma triacylglycerol levels. *Fenofibrate* and *gemfibrozil* are particularly useful in treating Type III hyperlipidemia (dysbetalipoproteinemia), in which intermediate density lipoproteins particles accumulate. Patients with hypertriacylglycerolemia [Type IV (elevated VLDL) or Type V (elevated VLDL plus chylomicron) disease] who do not respond to diet or other drugs may also benefit from treatment with these agents.

3. **Pharmacokinetics:** Both drugs are completely absorbed after an oral dose. *Gemfibrozil* and *fenofibrate* distribute widely, bound to albumin. Both drugs undergo extensive biotransformation and are excreted in the urine as their glucuronide conjugates.

4. **Adverse effects**

   a. **Gastrointestinal effects:** The most common adverse effects are mild gastrointestinal disturbances. These lessen as the therapy progresses.

   b. **Lithiasis:** Because these drugs increase biliary cholesterol excretion, there is a predisposition to the formation of gallstones.

   c. **Muscle:** Myositis (inflammation of a voluntary muscle) can occur with both drugs; thus, muscle weakness or tenderness should be evaluated. Patients with renal insufficiency may be at risk. Myopathy and rhabdomyolysis have been reported in a few patients taking *gemfibrozil* and *lovastatin* together.

   d. **Drug interactions:** Both fibrates compete with the *coumarin* anticoagulants for binding sites on plasma proteins, thus transiently potentiating anticoagulant activity. Prothrombin levels should therefore be monitored when a patient is taking both drugs. Similarly, these drugs may transiently elevate the levels of sulfonylureas.

   e. **Contraindications:** The safety of these agents in pregnant or lactating women has not been established. They should not be used in patients with severe hepatic and renal dysfunction or in patients with preexisting gallbladder disease.

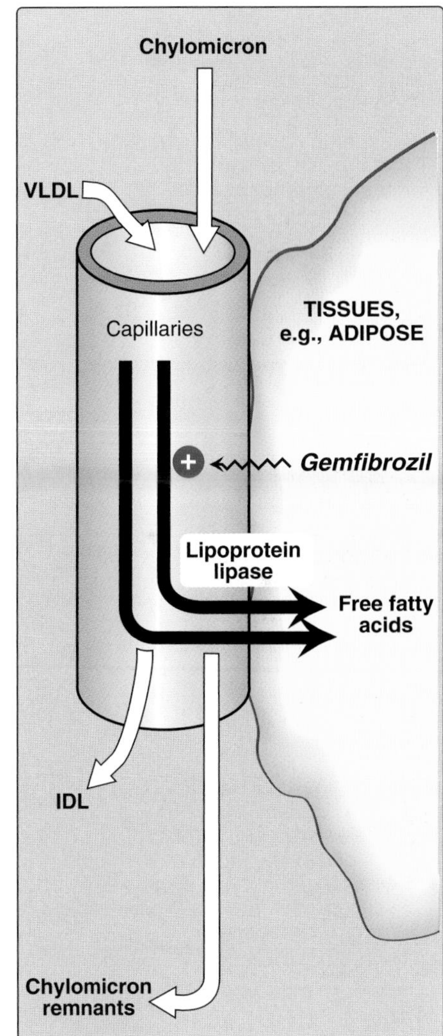

Figure 21.11
Activation of lipoprotein lipase by *gemfibrozil*.

D. Bile acid–binding resins

Bile acid sequestrants (resins) have significant LDL cholesterol–lowering effects, although the benefits are less than those observed with statins.

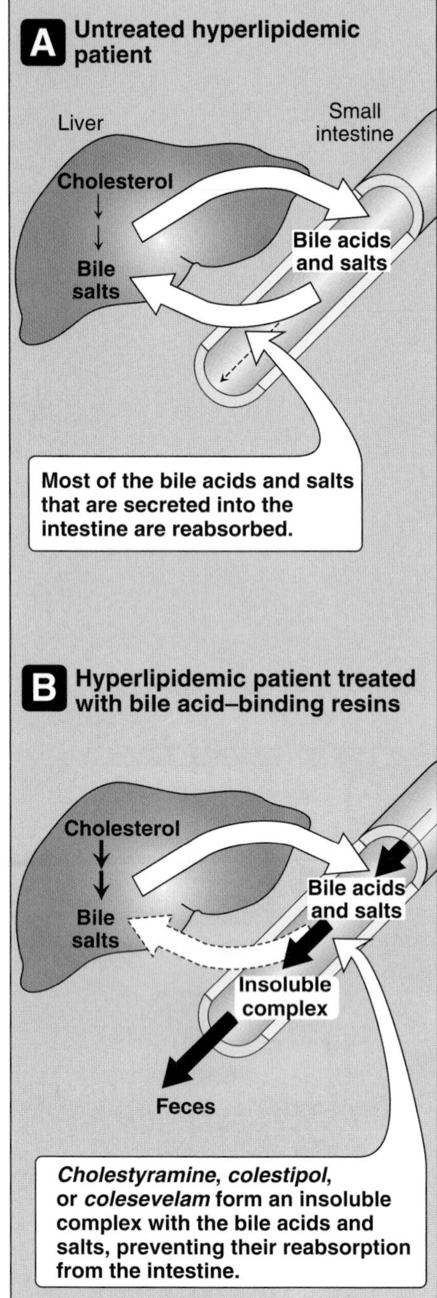

Figure 21.12
Mechanism of bile acid–binding resins.

1. **Mechanism of action:** *Cholestyramine* [koe LES tir a meen], *colestipol* [koe LES tih pole], and *colesevelam* [koh le SEV e lam] are anion-exchange resins that bind negatively charged bile acids and bile salts in the small intestine (Figure 21.12). The resin/bile acid complex is excreted in the feces, thus preventing the bile acids from returning to the liver by the enterohepatic circulation. Lowering the bile acid concentration causes hepatocytes to increase conversion of cholesterol to bile acids, resulting in a replenished supply of these compounds, which are essential components of the bile. Consequently, the intracellular cholesterol concentration decreases, which activates an increased hepatic uptake of cholesterol-containing LDL particles, leading to a fall in plasma LDL. [Note: This increased uptake is mediated by an up-regulation of cell-surface LDL receptors.] In some patients, a modest rise in plasma HDL levels is also observed. The final outcome of this sequence of events is a decreased total plasma cholesterol concentration.

2. **Therapeutic uses:** The bile acid–binding resins are the drugs of choice (often in combination with diet or *niacin*) in treating Type IIa and Type IIb hyperlipidemias. [Note: In those rare individuals who are homozygous for Type IIa—that is, for whom functional LDL receptors are totally lacking—these drugs have little effect on plasma LDL levels.] *Cholestyramine* can also relieve pruritus caused by accumulation of bile acids in patients with biliary obstruction.

3. **Pharmacokinetics:** *Cholestyramine*, *colestipol*, and *colesevelam* are taken orally. Because they are insoluble in water and are very large (molecular weights are greater than 10^6), they are neither absorbed nor metabolically altered by the intestine. Instead, they are totally excreted in the feces.

4. **Adverse effects:**

   a. **Gastrointestinal effects:** The most common side effects are gastrointestinal disturbances, such as constipation, nausea, and flatulence. *Colesevelam* has fewer gastrointestinal side effects than other bile acid sequestrants.

   b. **Impaired absorptions:** At high doses, *cholestyramine* and *colestipol* (but not *colesevelam*) impair the absorption of the fat-soluble vitamins (A, D, E, and K).

   c. **Drug interactions:** *Cholestyramine* and *colestipol* interfere with the intestinal absorption of many drugs—for example, *tetracycline*, *phenobarbital*, *digoxin*, *warfarin*, *pravastatin*, *fluvastatin*, *aspirin*, and thiazide diuretics. Therefore, drugs should be taken at least one to two hours before, or four to six hours after, the bile acid–binding resins.

E. Cholesterol absorption inhibitors

Ezetimibe [eh ZEH teh mib] selectively inhibits intestinal absorption of dietary and biliary cholesterol in the small intestine, leading to a decrease in the delivery of intestinal cholesterol to the liver. This causes a reduction of hepatic cholesterol stores and an increase in clearance of cholesterol from the blood. *Ezetimibe* lowers LDL cholesterol by 17 percent and triacylglycerols by 6 percent, and it increases HDL cholesterol by 1.3 percent. *Ezetimibe* is primarily metabolized in the small intestine and liver via glucuronide conjugation (a Phase II reaction), with subsequent biliary and renal excretion. Both *ezetimibe* and *ezetimibe*-glucuronide are slowly eliminated from plasma, with a half-life of approximately 22 hours. *Ezetimibe* has no clinically meaningful effect on the plasma concentrations of the fat-soluble vitamins A, D, and E. Patients with moderate to severe hepatic insufficiency should not be treated with *ezetimibe*. [Note: A formulation of *ezetimibe* and *simvastin* has been shown to lower LDL levels more effectively than the statin alone.]

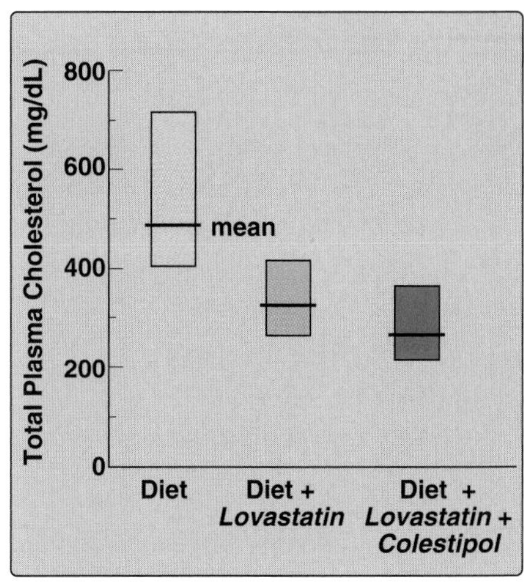

Figure 21.13
Response of total plasma cholesterol in patients with heterozygous familial hypercholesterolemia to a diet (low in cholesterol, low in saturated fat) and antihyperlipidemic drugs.

F. Combination Drug Therapy

It is sometimes necessary to employ two antihyperlipidemic drugs to achieve treatment goals in plasma lipid levels. For example, in Type II hyperlipidemias, patients are commonly treated with a combination of *niacin* plus a bile acid–binding agent, such as cholestyramine. [Note: Remember that cholestyramine causes an increase in LDL receptors that clears the plasma of circulating LDL, whereas *niacin* decreases synthesis of VLDL and, therefore, also the synthesis of LDL.] The combination of an HMG CoA reductase inhibitor with a bile acid–binding agent has also been shown to be useful in lowering LDL cholesterol levels (Figure 21.13).

Figure 21.14 summarizes some actions of the antihyperlipidemia drugs.

TYPE OF DRUG	EFFECT ON LDL	EFFECT ON HDL	EFFECT ON TRIACYLGLYCEROLS
HMG-CoA reducatase inhibitors (statins)	↓↓↓↓	↑↑	↓↓
Fibrates	↓	↑↑↑	↓↓↓↓
Niacin	↓↓	↑↑↑↑	↓↓↓
Bile acid sequestrants	↓↓↓	↑	Minimal
Cholesterol absorption inhibitor	↓	↑	↓

Figure 21.14
Characteristics of hyperlipidemic drug families. HDL = high-density lipoprotein; HMG-CoA = 3-hydroxy-3-methylglutaryl–coenzyme A; LDL = low-density lipoprotein.

Study Questions

Choose the ONE best answer.

21.1 Which one of the following is the most common side effect of antihyperlipidemic drug therapy?

A. Elevated blood pressure
B. Gastrointestinal disturbance
C. Neurologic problems
D. Heart palpitations
E. Migraine headaches

Correct answer = B. Gastrointestinal disturbances frequently occur as a side effect of antihyperlipidemic drug therapy.

21.2 Which one of the following hyperlipidemias is characterized by elevated plasma levels of chylomicrons and has no drug therapy available to lower the plasma lipoprotein levels?

A. Type I
B. Type II
C. Type III
D. Type IV
E. Type V

Correct answer = A. Type I hyperlipidemia (hyperchylomicronemia) is treated with a low-fat diet. No drug therapy is effective for this disorder.

21.3 Which one of the following drugs decreases de novo cholesterol synthesis by inhibiting the enzyme 3-hydroxy-3-methylglutaryl CoA reductase?

A. Fenofibrate
B. Niacin
C. Cholestyramine
D. Lovastatin
E. Gemfibrozil

Correct answer = D. Fenofibrate and gemfibrozil increase the activity of lipoprotein lipase, thereby increasing the removal of VLDL from plasma. Niacin inhibits lipolysis in adipose tissue, thus eliminating the building blocks needed by the liver to produce triacylglycerol and, therefore, VLDL. Cholestyramine lowers the amount of bile acids returning to the liver via the enterohepatic circulation.

21.4 Which one of the following drugs causes a decrease in liver triacylglycerol synthesis by limiting available free fatty acids needed as building blocks for this pathway?

A. Niacin
B. Fenofibrate
C. Cholestyramine
D. Probucol
E. Lovastatin

Correct answer = A. Niacin.

21.5 Which one of the following drugs binds bile acids in the intestine, thus preventing their return to the liver via the enterohepatic circulation?

A. Niacin
B. Fenofibrate
C. Cholestyramine
D. Probucol

Correct answer = C. Cholestyramine..

Diuretic Drugs

22

I. OVERVIEW

Drugs inducing a state of increased urine flow are called diuretics. These agents are inhibitors of renal ion transporters that decrease the reabsorption of Na^+ at different sites in the nephron. As a result, Na^+ and other ions, such as Cl^-, enter the urine in greater than normal amounts along with water, which is carried passively to maintain osmotic equilibrium. Diuretics thus increase the volume of both urine, and often change its pH as well as the ionic composition of the urine and blood. The efficacy of the different classes of diuretics varies considerably, with the increase in Na^+ secretion varying from less than two percent for the weak, potassium-sparing diuretics to over twenty percent for the potent loop diuretics. In addition to these ion-transport inhibitors, there are osmotic diuretics that prevent water reabsorption, as well as aldosterone antagonists, and a carbonic anhydrase inhibitor. The major clinical uses of diuretics are in managing disorders involving abnormal fluid retention (edema) or treating hypertension in which their diuretic action causes a decreased blood volume, leading to reduced blood pressure. In this chapter, the diuretic drugs (Figure 22.1) are discussed according to the frequency of their use.

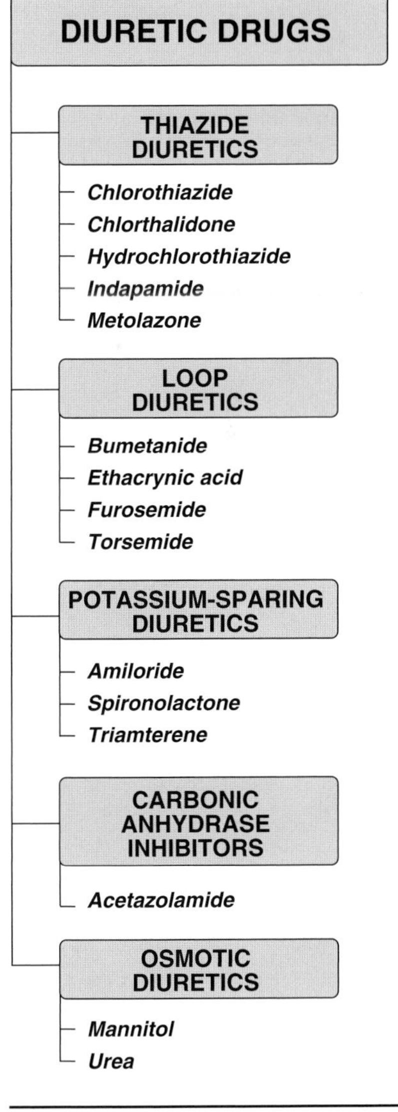

Figure 22.1
Summary of diuretic drugs.

II. NORMAL REGULATION OF FLUID AND ELECTROLYTES BY THE KIDNEYS

Approximately sixteen to twenty percent of the blood plasma entering the kidneys is filtered from the glomerular capillaries into the Bowman capsule. The filtrate, although normally free of proteins and blood cells, does contain most low-molecular-weight plasma components in approximately the same concentrations as are found in the plasma. These include glucose, sodium bicarbonate, amino acids, and other organic solutes, as well as electrolytes, such as Na^+, K^+, and Cl^-. The kidney regulates the ionic composition and volume of urine by the active reabsorption or secretion of ions and/or the passive reabsorption of water at five functional zones along the nephron, namely the proximal convoluted tubule, the descending loop of Henle, the ascending loop of Henle, the distal convoluted tubule, and the collecting duct (Figure 22.2).

Lippincott's Illustrated Reviews: Pharmacology, Third Edition,
by Richard D. Howland and Mary J. Mycek.

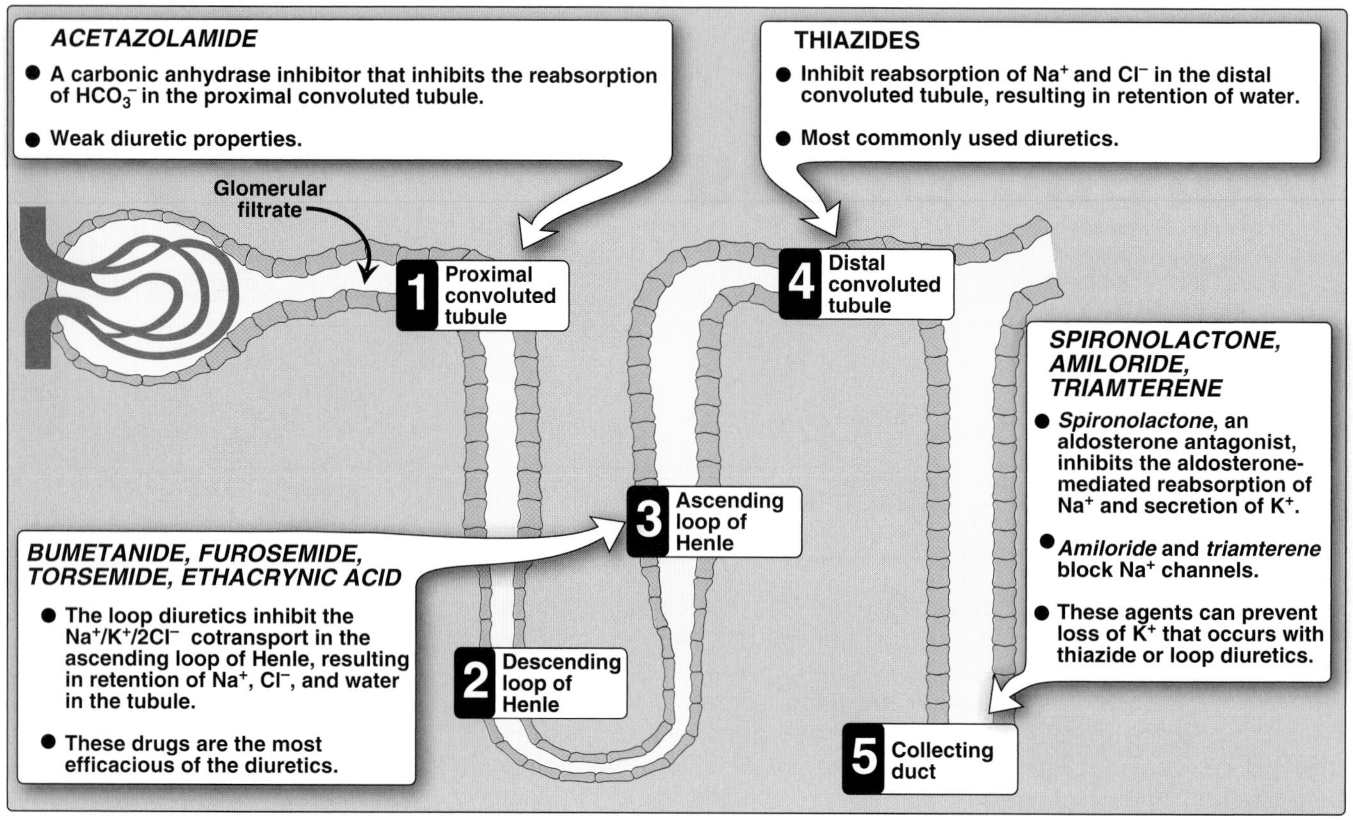

Figure 22.2
Major locations of ion and water exchange in the nephron, showing sites of action of the diuretic drugs.

A. Proximal convoluted tubule

In the extensively convoluted proximal tubule located in the cortex of the kidney, almost all the glucose, bicarbonate, amino acids, and other metabolites are reabsorbed. Approximately two-thirds of the Na^+ is also reabsorbed. Chloride enters in exchange for a base anion, such as formate or oxalate, as well as paracellularly through the lumen. Water follows passively to maintain osmolar equality. If not for the extensive reabsorption of solutes and water in the proximal tubule, the mammalian organism would rapidly become dehydrated and lose its normal osmolarity. The Na^+ that is reabsorbed is pumped into the interstitium by Na^+/K^+–adenosine triphosphatase (ATPase), thereby maintaining normal levels of Na^+ and K^+ in the cell. Carbonic anhydrase in the luminal membrane and cell of the proximal tubule modulates the reabsorption of bicarbonate (see *acetazolamide* below). Water follows salt reabsorption; thus, the presence of sustances like mannitol and glucose would tend to become concentrated. This condition results in a higher osmolarity of the tubular fluid and prevents further water reabsorption, resulting in osmotic diuresis.

1. **Acid and base secretory systems:** The proximal tubule is the site of the organic acid and base secretory systems (Figure 22.3). The organic acid secretory system, located in the middle-third segment, secretes a variety of organic acids, such as uric acid,

some antibiotics, and diuretics, from the bloodstream into the proximal tubule's lumen. Most diuretic drugs are delivered to the tubular fluid via this system. The organic acid secretory system is saturable, and diuretic drugs in the bloodstream compete for transfer with endogenous organic acids, such as uric acid. This explains the hyperuricemia seen with certain of the diuretic drugs, such as *furosemide* or *chlorothiazide*. A number of other interactions can also occur; for example, *probenecid* interferes with *penicillin* secretion. The organic base secretory system is responsible for the secretion of creatinine, choline, and so on, and it is found in the upper and middle segments of the proximal tubule.

B. Descending loop of Henle

The remaining filtrate, which is isotonic, next enters the descending limb of the loop of Henle and passes into the medulla of the kidney. The osmolarity increases along the descending portion of the loop of Henle because of the countercurrent mechanism that is responsible for water reabsorption. This results in a tubular fluid with a threefold increase in salt concentration. Osmotic diuretics exert part of their action in this region (see Figure 22.2).

C. Ascending loop of Henle

The cells of the ascending tubular epithelium are unique in being impermeable to water. Active reabsorption of Na^+, K^+ and Cl^- is mediated by a $Na^+/K^+/2Cl^-$ cotransporter. Both Mg^{2+} and Ca^{2+} enter the interstitial fluid via the paracellular pathway. The ascending loop is thus a diluting region of the nephron. Approximately 25 to 30 percent of the tubular sodium chloride returns to the interstitial fluid, thus helping to maintain the fluid's high osmolarity. Because the ascending loop of Henle is a major site for salt reabsorption, drugs affecting this site, such as loop diuretics (see Figure 22.2), are the most efficacious of all the diuretic classes.

D. Distal convoluted tubule

The cells of the distal convoluted tubule are also impermeable to water. About ten percent of the filtered sodium chloride is reabsorbed via a Na^+/Cl^- transporter that is sensitive to thiazide diuretics. Calcium reabsorption is mediated by passage through a channel and then transported by a Na^+/Ca^{2+} exchanger into the interstitial fluid. The mechanism thus differs from that in the loop of Henle. Additionally, Ca^{2+} excretion is regulated by parathyroid hormone in this portion of the tubule.

E. Collecting tubule and duct

The principal cells of the collecting tubule are responsible for Na^+, K^+, and water transport, whereas the intercalated cells effect H^+ secretion. The sodium enters the principal cells through channels but relies on a Na^+/K^+-ATPase to be transported into the blood. Aldosterone receptors in the principal cells influence Na^+ reabsorption and K^+ secretion. Antidiuretic hormone (ADH; vasopressin) receptors promote the reabsorption of water from the collecting tubules and ducts (see Figure 22.3). This action is mediated by cyclic adenosine monophosphate (cAMP).

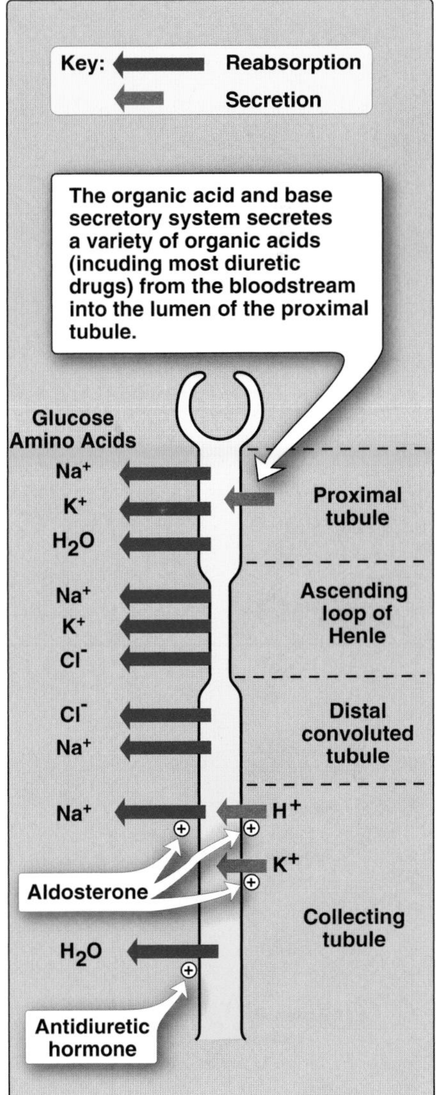

Figure 22.3
Sites of transport of solutes and water along the nephron.

III. KIDNEY FUNCTION IN DISEASE

A. Edematous states

In many diseases, the amount of sodium chloride reabsorbed by the kidney tubules is abnormally high. This leads to the retention of water, an increase in blood volume, and expansion of the extravascular fluid compartment, resulting in edema of the tissues. Several commonly encountered causes of edema include the following.

1. **Heart failure:** The decreased ability of the failing heart to sustain adequate cardiac output causes the kidney to respond as if there were a decrease in blood volume (hypovolemia). The kidney, as part of the normal compensatory mechanism, retains more salt and water as a means of raising blood volume and increasing the amount of blood that is returned to the heart. However, the diseased heart cannot increase its output, and the increased vascular volume results in edema (see p. 181 for causes and treatment of heart failure). Loop diuretics are commonly used.

2. **Hepatic ascites:** Ascites, the accumulation of fluid in the abdominal cavity, is a common complication of cirrhosis of the liver.

   a. **Increased portal blood pressure:** Blood flow in the portal system is often obstructed in cirrhosis, resulting in an increased portal blood pressure. Furthermore, the colloidal osmotic pressure of the blood is decreased as a result of impaired synthesis of plasma proteins by the diseased liver. Increased portal blood pressure and low osmolarity of the blood cause fluid to escape from the portal vascular system and collect in the abdomen.

   b. **Secondary hyperaldosteronism:** Fluid retention is also promoted by elevated levels of circulating aldosterone due to decreased blood volume. This secondary hyperaldosteronism results from the decreased ability of the liver to inactivate the steroid hormone and leads to increased Na^+ and water reabsorption, increased vascular volume, and exacerbation of fluid accumulation (see Figure 22.3). The potassium-sparing diuretic *spironolactone* is effective in this condition, but the loop diuretics are usually not.

3. **Nephrotic syndrome:** When damaged by disease, the glomerular membranes allow plasma proteins to enter the glomerular ultrafiltrate. The loss of protein from the plasma reduces the colloidal osmotic pressure, resulting in edema. The low plasma volume stimulates aldosterone secretion through the renin-angiotensin-aldosterone system. This leads to retention of Na^+ and fluid, further aggravating the edema.

4. **Premenstrual edema:** Edema associated with menstruation is the result of imbalances in hormones, such as estrogen excess, which facilitates the loss of fluid into the extracellular space. Diuretics can reduce the edema.

B. Nonedematous states

Diuretics also find wide usage in the treatment of nonedematous diseases.

1. **Hypertension:** Thiazides have been widely used in the treatment of hypertension, because of their ability to not only reduce blood volume but also to dilate arterioles (see p. 217).

2. **Hypercalcemia:** The seriousness of this condition requires a fast response. Usually, loop diuretics are employed, because they promote calcium excretion. However, it is important to understand that hypovolemia may counteract the desired effect; therefore, normal saline must also be infused to maintain blood volume.

3. **Diabetes insipidus:** When patients suffer from polyuria and polydipsia associated with this condition, they usually respond to thiazide diuretics. This seemingly paradoxic treatment depends on the ability of the thiazide to reduce plasma volume, thus causing a drop in glomerular filtration rate and promoting the reabsorption of Na^+ and water. The volume of urine entering the diluting segment and the subsequent urine flow are both decreased.

IV. THIAZIDES AND RELATED AGENTS

The thiazides are the most widely used of the diuretic drugs. They are sulfonamide derivatives and, as such, are related in structure to the carbonic anhydrase inhibitors. However, the thiazides have significantly greater diuretic activity than *acetazolamide* (see below), and they act on the kidney by different mechanisms. All thiazides affect the distal tubule, and all have equal maximum diuretic effects, differing only in potency (expressed on a per milligram basis). [Note: They are sometimes called "ceiling diuretics" because increasing the dose above normal does not promote a further diuretic response.] Like the actions of the loop diuretics, the thiazides partly depend on renal prostaglandin synthesis by a mechanism that is not yet understood.

A. Chlorothiazide and hydrochlorothiazide

Chlorothiazide [klor oh THYE ah zide] was the first modern diuretic that was active orally, and was capable of affecting the severe edema of cirrhosis and heart failure with a minimum of side effects. Its properties are representative of the thiazide group, although newer derivatives, such as *hydrochlorothiazide* [hi dro klor oh THYE ah zide] or *chlorthalidone*, are now used more commonly. *Hydrochlorothiazide* has far less ability to inhibit carbonic anhydrase compared to *chlorothiazide*. It is also more potent, so that the required dose is considerably lower than that of *chlorothiazide*. On the other hand, the efficacy is exactly the same as that of the parent drug. In all other aspects it resembles *chlorothiazide*. [Note: *Chlorthalidone*, *indapamide*, and *metolazone* are referred to as thiazide-like diuretics, because they contain the sulfonamide residue in their chemical structures and their mechanism of action is similar. However, they are not truly thiazides.]

1. **Mechanism of action:** The thiazide derivatives act mainly in the distal tubule to decrease the reabsorption of Na^+—apparently by inhibition of a Na^+/Cl^- cotransporter on the luminal membrane of the distal convoluted tubule (see Figure 22.2). They have a lesser effect in the proximal tubule. As a result, these drugs increase the concentration of Na^+ and Cl^- in the tubular fluid. The acid-base balance is not usually affected. [Note: Because the site of action of the thiazide derivatives is on the luminal membrane, these drugs must be excreted into the tubular lumen to be effective. Therefore, with decreased renal function, thiazide diuretics lose efficacy.]

2. **Actions:**

   a. **Increased excretion of Na^+ and Cl^-:** *Chlorothiazide* causes diuresis with increased Na^+ and Cl^- excretion, which can result in the excretion of a very hyperosmolar urine. This latter effect is unique; the other diuretic classes are unlikely to produce a hyperosmolar urine. The diuretic action is not affected by the acid-base status of the body, nor does *chlorothiazide* change the acid-base status of the blood. The relative changes in the ionic composition of the urine during therapy with thiazide diuretics are given in Figure 22.4.

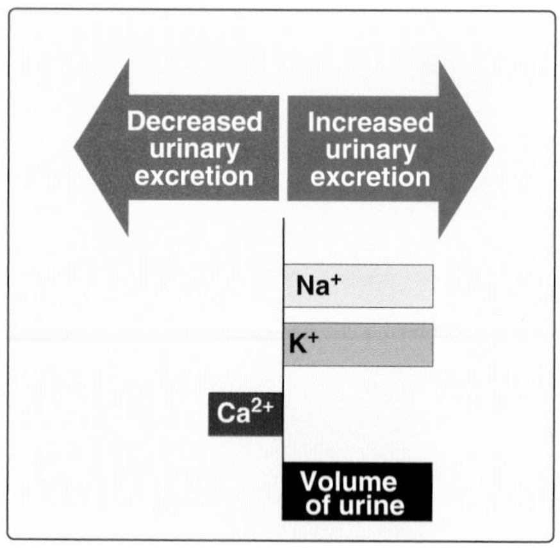

Figure 22.4
Relative changes in the composition of urine induced by thiazide diuretics.

   b. **Loss of K^+:** Because thiazides increase the Na^+ in the filtrate arriving at the distal tubule, more K^+ is also exchanged for Na^+, resulting in a continual loss of K^+ from the body with prolonged use of these drugs. Therefore, it is imperative to measure serum K^+ often (more frequently at the beginning of therapy) to assure that hypokalemia does not develop.

   c. **Loss of Mg^{2+}:** Magnesium deficiency requiring supplementation can occur with chronic use of thiazide diuretics, particularly in the elderly. The mechanism for the magnesuria is not understood.

   d. **Decreased urinary calcium excretion:** Thiazide diuretics decrease the Ca^{2+} content of urine by promoting the reabsorption of Ca^{2+}. This contrasts with the loop diuretics, which increase the Ca^{2+} concentration of the urine. [Note: There is evidence from epidemiologic studies that use of thiazides preserves bone mineral density at the hip and spine and that the risk for hip fracture is reduced by a third.]

   e. **Reduced peripheral vascular resistance:** An initial reduction in blood pressure results from a decrease in blood volume and, therefore, a decrease in cardiac output. With continued therapy, volume recovery occurs. However, there are continued hypotensive effects, resulting from reduced peripheral vascular resistance caused by relaxation of arteriolar smooth muscle. This usually occurs prior to the diuretic effect.

3. **Therapeutic uses:**

   a. **Hypertension:** Clinically, the thiazides have long been the mainstay of antihypertensive medication, because they are inexpensive, convenient to administer, and well tolerated. They are effective in reducing systolic and diastolic blood pressure for extended periods in the majority of patients with mild to moderate essential hypertension (see p. 215 for details on the treatment of hypertension). After three to seven days of treatment, the blood pressure stabilizes at a lower level and can be maintained indefinitely by a daily-dosage level of the drug, which causes lower peripheral resistance without having a major diuretic effect. Many patients can be continued for years on the thiazides alone, although a small percentage of patients require additional medication, such as β-adrenergic blockers. [Note: The hypotensive actions of angiotensin-converting enzyme inhibitors are enhanced when given in combination with the thiazides.]

b. **Heart failure:** Thiazides can be the diuretic of choice in reducing extracellular volume in mild to moderate heart failure. If the thiazide fails, loop diuretics may be useful.

c. **Hypercalciuria:** The thiazides can be useful in treating idiopathic hypercalciuria, because they inhibit urinary Ca^{2+} excretion. This is particularly beneficial for patients with calcium oxalate stones in the urinary tract.

d. **Diabetes insipidus:** Thiazides have the unique ability to produce a hyperosmolar urine. Thiazides can substitute for antidiuretic hormone in the treatment of nephrogenic diabetes insipidus. The urine volume of such individuals may drop from 11 L/day to about 3 L/day when treated with the drug.

4. **Pharmacokinetics:** The drugs are effective orally. Most thiazides take one to three weeks to produce a stable reduction in blood pressure, and they exhibit a prolonged biologic half-life (forty hours). All thiazides are secreted by the organic acid secretory system of the kidney (see Figure 22.3).

5. **Adverse effects:** Most of the adverse effects involve problems in fluid and electrolyte balance.

a. **Potassium depletion:** Hypokalemia is the most frequent problem encountered with the thiazide diuretics, and it can predispose patients who are taking digitalis to ventricular arrhythmias (Figure 22.5). Often, K^+ can be supplemented by diet alone, such as by increasing the intake of citrus fruits, bananas, and prunes. In some cases, K^+ salt supplementation may be necessary. Activation of the renin-angiotensin-aldosterone system by the decrease in intravascular volume contributes significantly to urinary K^+ losses. Under these circumstances, the K^+ deficiency can be overcome by *spironolactone*, which interferes with aldosterone action, or by administering *triamterene*, which acts to retain K^+. Low-sodium diets blunt the potassium depletion caused by thiazide diuretics.

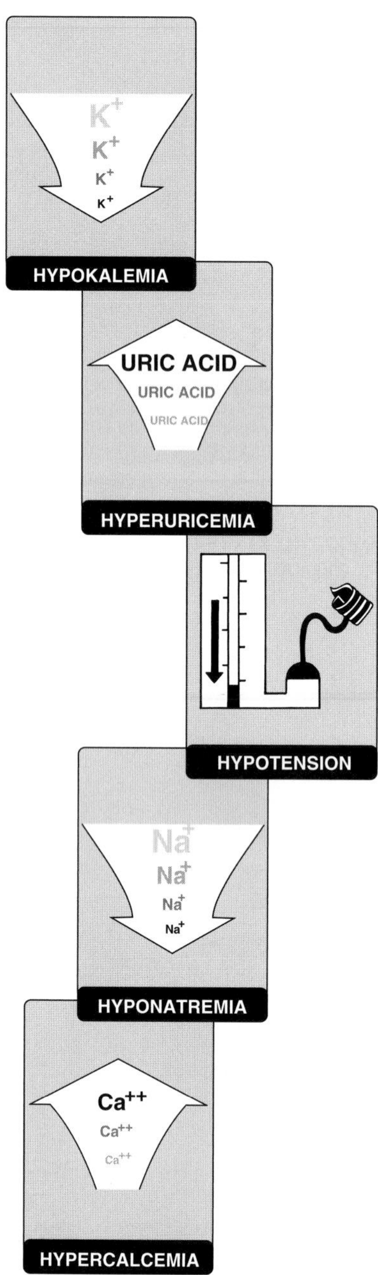

Figure 22.5
Summary of some adverse effects commonly observed with thiazide diuretics.

b. **Hyponatremia:** This serious adverse effect may develop due to elevation of ADH as a result of hypovolemia, as well as diminished diluting capacity of the kidney and increased thirst. Limiting water intake and lowering the dose of diuretic can prevent this condition.

c. **Hyperuricemia:** Thiazides increase serum uric acid by decreasing the amount of acid excreted by the organic acid secretory system. Being insoluble, the uric acid deposits in the joints, and a full-blown attack of gout may result in individuals who are predisposed to gouty attacks. It is important, therefore, to perform periodic blood tests for uric acid levels. [Note: *Probenecid*, a drug sometimes used in the treatment of gout, can interfere in the excretion of the thiazides, and increase serum uric acid levels.]

d. **Volume depletion:** This can cause orthostatic hypotension or light-headedness.

e. **Hypercalcemia:** The thiazides inhibit the secretion of Ca^{2+}, sometimes leading to elevated levels of Ca^{2+} in the blood.

f. **Hyperglycemia:** Patients with diabetes mellitus who are taking thiazides for hypertension may become hyperglycemic and have difficulty in maintaining appropriate blood sugar levels. This is due to impaired release of insulin and tissue uptake of glucose.

g. **Hyperlipidemia:** The thiazides can cause a five- to fifteen-percent increase in serum cholesterol as well as increased serum low-density lipoproteins. Lipid levels, however, may return to normal with long-term therapy.

h. **Hypersensitivity:** Bone marrow suppression, dermatitis, necrotizing vasculitis, and interstitial nephritis are very rare. Individuals who are hypersensitive to sulfa drugs may also be allergic to the thiazide diuretics.

B. Thiazide-like analogs

These compounds lack the thiazide structure, but like the thiazides they have the unsubstituted sulfonamide group and share their mechanism of action.

1. **Chlorthalidone:** *Chlorthalidone* [klor THAL i done] is a nonthiazide derivative that behaves pharmacologically like *hydrochlorothiazide.* It has a very long duration of action and, therefore, is often used to treat hypertension. It is given once per day for this indication.

2. **Metolazone:** *Metolazone* [me TOL ah zone] is more potent than the thiazides and, unlike the thiazides, causes Na^{+} excretion in advanced renal failure.

3. **Indapamide:** *Indapamide* [in DAP a mide] is a lipid-soluble, nonthiazide diuretic that has a long duration of action. At low doses, it shows significant antihypertensive action with minimal diuretic effects. *Indapamide* is metabolized and excreted by the gastrointestinal tract and the kidneys. It is therefore less likely to accumulate in patients with renal failure, and may be useful in their treatment.

V. LOOP OR HIGH-CEILING DIURETICS

Bumetanide [byoo MET ah nide], *furosemide* [fu RO se mide], *torsemide* [TOR se myde], and *ethacrynic acid* [eth a KRIN ik] are four diuretics that have their major action on the ascending limb of the loop of Henle (see Figure 22.2). Compared to all other classes of diuretics, these drugs have the highest efficacy in mobilizing Na^+ and Cl^- from the body. They produce copious amounts of urine. *Furosemide* is the most commonly used of these drugs. *Ethacrynic acid* has a steeper dose-response curve than *furosemide*, but it shows greater side effects than those seen with the other loop diuretics, and its use is therefore limited. *Bumetanide* is much more potent than *furosemide*, and its use is increasing. *Bumetanide* and *furosemide* are sulfonamide derivatives.

A. Bumetanide, furosemide, torsemide, and ethacrynic acid

1. **Mechanism of action:** Loop diuretics inhibit the cotransport of $Na^+/K^+/2Cl^-$ in the luminal membrane in the ascending limb of the loop of Henle. Therefore, reabsorption of these ions is decreased (Figure 22.6). The loop diuretics are the most efficacious of the diuretic drugs, because the ascending limb accounts for the reabsorption of 25 to 30 percent of filtered NaCl and downstream sites are not able to compensate for this increased Na^+ load.

2. **Actions:** The loop diuretics act promptly, even among patients who have poor renal function or have not responded to thiazides or other diuretics. Changes in the composition of the urine induced by loop diuretics are shown in Figure 22.6. [Note: Loop diuretics increase the Ca^{2+} content of urine, whereas thiazide diuretics decrease the Ca^{2+} concentration of the urine. In patients with normal serum Ca^{2+} concentrations, hypocalcemia does not result, because Ca^{2+} is reabsorbed in the distal convoluted tubule. However, hypomagnesemia can occur due to loss of Mg^{2+}.] The loop diuretics cause decreased renal vascular resistance and increased renal blood flow. In addition, loop diuretics increase prostaglandin synthesis. The prostaglandins have a role in their diuretic action, and substances such as *indomethacin* that interfere in prostaglandin synthesis can reduce the diuretic action of these agents.

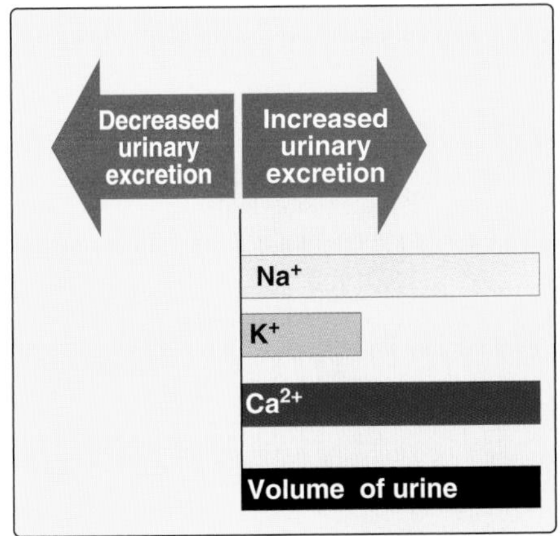

Figure 22.6
Relative changes in the composition of urine induced by loop diuretics.

3. **Therapeutic uses:** The loop diuretics are the drugs of choice for reducing the acute pulmonary edema of heart failure. Because of their rapid onset of action, particularly when given intravenously, the drugs are useful in emergency situations, such as acute pulmonary edema, which calls for a rapid, intense diuresis. Loop

diuretics (along with hydration) are also useful in treating hypercalcemia, because they stimulate tubular Ca^{2+} excretion. They also are useful in the treatment of hyperkalemia.

4. **Pharmacokinetics:** Loop diuretics are administered orally or parenterally. Their duration of action is relatively brief—two to four hours. They are secreted into the urine.

5. **Adverse effects:** The adverse effects of the loop diuretics are summarized in Figure 22.7.

    a. **Ototoxicity:** Hearing can be affected adversely by the loop diuretics, particularly when used in conjunction with the aminoglycoside antibiotics. Permanent damage may result with continued treatment. *Ethacrynic acid* is the most likely to cause deafness. Vestibular function is less likely to be disturbed, but it, too, may be affected by combined treatment with the antibiotic.

    b. **Hyperuricemia:** *Furosemide* and *ethacrynic acid* compete with uric acid for the renal and biliary secretory systems, thus blocking its secretion and, thereby, causing or exacerbating gouty attacks.

    c. **Acute hypovolemia:** Loop diuretics can cause a severe and rapid reduction in blood volume, with the possibility of hypotension, shock, and cardiac arrhythmias. Hypercalcemia may occur under these conditions.

    d. **Potassium depletion:** The heavy load of Na^+ presented to the collecting tubule results in increased exchange of tubular Na^+ for K^+, with the possibility of inducing hypokalemia. The loss of K^+ from cells in exchange for H^+ leads to hypokalemic alkalosis. Potassium depletion can be averted by use of potassium-sparing diuretics or dietary supplementation with K^+.

    e. **Hypomagnesemia:** A combination of chronic use of loop diuretics and low dietary intake of Mg^{2+} can lead to hypomagnesemia, particularly in the elderly. This can be corrected by oral supplementation.

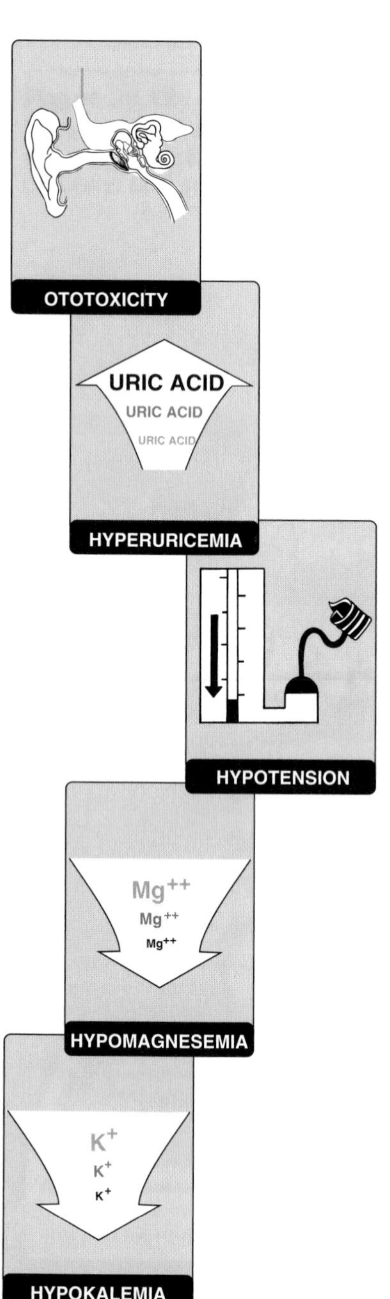

Figure 22.7
Summary of some adverse effects commonly observed with loop diuretics.

VI. POTASSIUM-SPARING DIURETICS

Potassium-sparing diuretics act in the collecting tubule to inhibit Na^+ reabsorption and K^+ excretion (Figure 22.8). Potassium-sparing diuretics are used alone primarily when aldosterone is present in excess. The major use of potassium-sparing agents is in the treatment of hypertension, most often in combination with a thiazide. It is extremely important that patients who are treated with any potassium-sparing diuretic be closely monitored for potassium levels. Exogenous potassium supplementation is usually discontinued when potassium-sparing diuretic therapy is instituted.

A. Spironolactone

1. **Mechanism of action:** *Spironolactone* [spear oh no LAK tone] is a synthetic steroid that antagonizes aldosterone at intracellular cytoplasmic receptor sites. The *spironolactone*-receptor complex is inactive. That is, it prevents translocation of the receptor complex into the nucleus of the target cell; thus, it cannot bind to DNA. This results in a failure to produce proteins that are normally synthesized in response to aldosterone. These mediator proteins normally stimulate the Na^+/K^+-exchange sites of the collecting tubule. Thus, a lack of mediator proteins prevents Na^+ reabsorption and, therefore, K^+ and H^+ secretion.

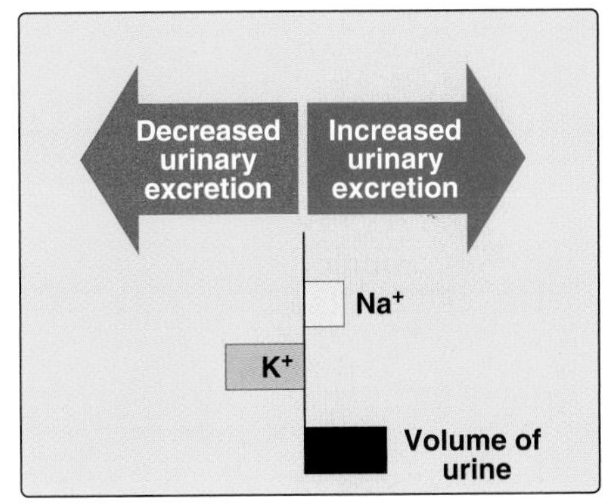

Figure 22.8
Relative changes in the composition of urine induced by potassium-sparing diuretics.

2. **Actions:** In most edematous states, blood levels of aldosterone are high, which is instrumental in retaining Na^+. When *spironolactone* is given to a patient with elevated circulating levels of aldosterone, the drug antagonizes the activity of the hormone, resulting in retention of K^+ and excretion of Na^+ (see Figure 22.8). In patients who have no significant circulating levels of aldosterone, such as those with Addison disease (primary adrenal insufficiency), no diuretic effect of the drug occurs. In common with the thiazides and loop diuretics, the effect of *spironolactone* depends on renal prostaglandin synthesis.

3. **Therapeutic uses:**

   a. **Diuretic:** Although *spironolactone* has a low efficacy in mobilizing Na^+ from the body in comparison with the other drugs, it has the useful property of causing the retention of K^+. Because of this latter action, *spironolactone* is often given in conjunction with a thiazide or loop diuretic to prevent the K^+ excretion that would otherwise occur with these drugs. It is the diuretic of choice in patients with hepatic cirrhosis.

   b. **Secondary hyperaldosteronism:** *Spironolactone* is the only potassium-sparing diuretic that is routinely used alone to induce a net negative salt balance. It is particularly effective in clinical situations associated with secondary hyperaldosteronism.

   c. **Heart failure:** *Spironolactone* prevents the remodeling that occurs as compensation for the progressive failure of the heart.

4. **Pharmacokinetics:** *Spironolactone* is completely absorbed orally and is strongly bound to proteins. It is rapidly converted to an active metabolite, canrenone. The action of *spironolactone* is largely due to the effect of canrenone, which has mineralocorticoid-blocking activity. *Spironolactone* induces hepatic cytochrome P450.

5. **Adverse effects:** *Spironolactone* frequently causes gastric upsets and can cause peptic ulcers. Because it chemically resembles some of the sex steroids, *spironolactone* may act at receptors in other organs to induce gynecomastia in males and menstrual

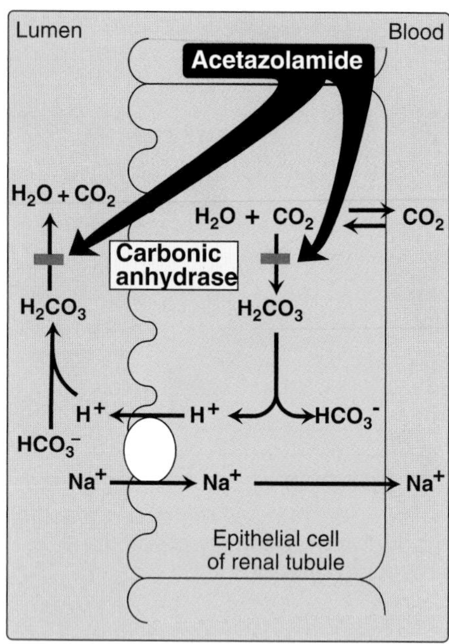

Figure 22.9
Role of carbonic anhydrase in sodium retention by epithelial cells of renal tubule.

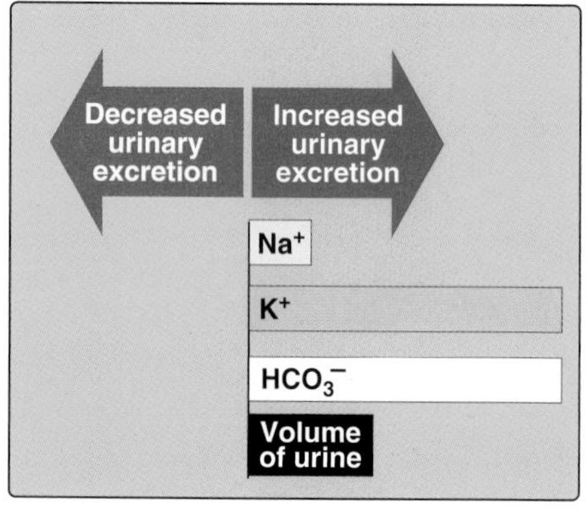

Figure 22.10
Relative changes in the composition of urine induced by *acetazolamide*.

irregularities in females; therefore, the drug should not be given at high doses on a chronic basis. It is most effectively employed in mild edematous states for which it is given for a few days at a time. At low doses, *spironolactone* can be used chronically with few side effects. Hyperkalemia, nausea, lethargy, and mental confusion can occur.

B. Triamterene and amiloride

Triamterene [trye AM ter een] and *amiloride* [a MIL oh ride] block Na^+ transport channels, resulting in a decrease in Na^+/K^+ exchange. Although they have a K^+-sparing diuretic action similar to that of *spironolactone*, their ability to block the Na^+/K^+-exchange site in the collecting tubule does not depend on the presence of aldosterone. Thus, they have diuretic activity even in individuals with Addison disease. Like *spironolactone*, they are not very efficacious diuretics. Both *triamterene* and *amiloride* are frequently used in combination with other diuretics, usually for their potassium-sparing properties. For example, much like *spironolactone*, they prevent the loss of K^+ that occurs with thiazides and *furosemide*. The side effects of *triamterene* are leg cramps and the possibility of increased blood urea nitrogen, as well as uric acid and K^+ retention.

VII. CARBONIC ANHYDRASE INHIBITORS

Acetazolamide [ah set a ZOLE a mide] inhibits the enzyme carbonic anhydrase in the proximal tubular epithelial cells. Carbonic anhydrase inhibitors are more often used for their other pharmacologic actions rather than for their diuretic effect, because they are much less efficacious than the thiazides or loop diuretics.

A. Acetazolamide

1. **Mechanism of action:** *Acetazolamide* inhibits carbonic anhydrase located intracellularly (cytoplasm) and on the apical membrane of the proximal tubular epithelium (Figure 22.9). [Note: Carbonic anhydrase catalyzes the reaction of CO_2 and H_2O, leading to H_2CO_3, which spontaneously ionizes to H^+ and HCO_3^- (bicarbonate)]. The decreased ability to exchange Na^+ for H^+ in the presence of *acetazolamide* results in a mild diuresis. Additionally, HCO_3^- is retained in the lumen, with marked elevation in urinary pH. The loss of HCO_3^- causes a hyperchloremic metabolic acidosis and decreased diuretic efficacy following several days of therapy. Changes in the composition of urinary electrolytes induced by *acetazolamide* are summarized in Figure 22.10. Phosphate excretion is increased by an unknown mechanism.

2. **Therapeutic uses:**

   a. **Treatment of glaucoma:** The most common use of *acetazolamide* is to reduce the elevated intraocular pressure of open-angle glaucoma. *Acetazolamide* decreases the production of aqueous humor, probably by blocking carbonic anhydrase in the ciliary body of the eye. It is useful in the chronic treatment of glaucoma but should not be used for an acute attack; *pilocarpine* is preferred for an acute attack because of its immediate action. Topical carbonic anhydrase inhibitors, such as *dorzolamide* and *brinzolamide*, have the advantage of not causing any systemic effects.

b. **Mountain sickness:** Less commonly, *acetazolamide* can be used in the prophylaxis of acute mountain sickness among healthy, physically active individuals who rapidly ascend above 10,000 feet. *Acetazolamide* given nightly for five days before the ascent prevents the weakness, breathlessness, dizziness, nausea, and cerebral as well as pulmonary edema characteristic of the syndrome.

3. **Pharmacokinetics:** *Acetazolamide* is given orally once a day. It is secreted by the proximal tubule.

4. **Adverse effects:** Metabolic acidosis (mild), potassium depletion, renal stone formation, drowsiness, and paresthesia may occur. The drug should be avoided in patients with hepatic cirrhosis, because it could lead to a decreased excretion of NH_4^+.

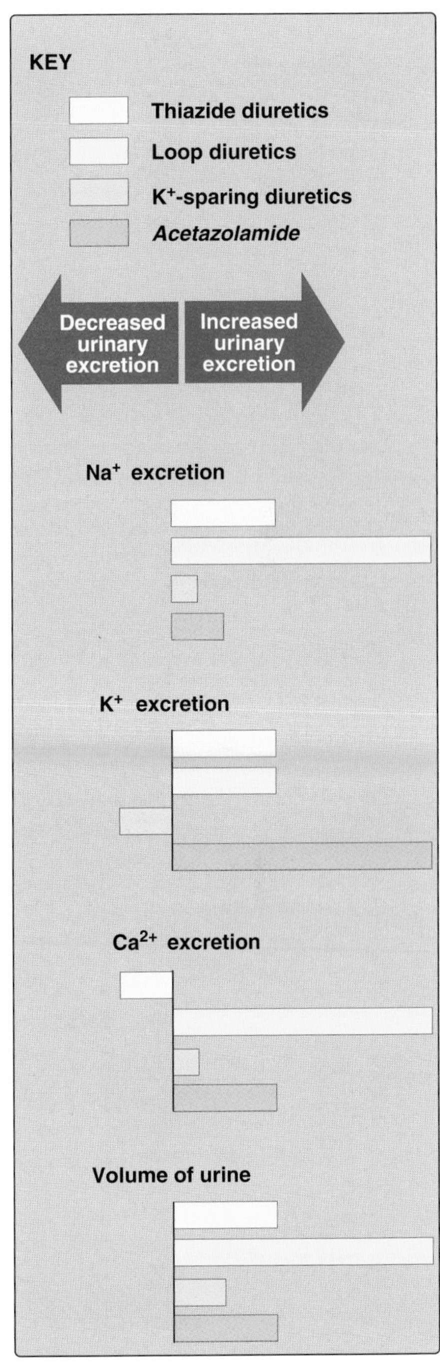

Figure 22.11
Summary of relative changes in urinary composition induced by diuretic drugs

VIII. OSMOTIC DIURETICS

A number of simple, hydrophilic chemical substances that are filtered through the glomerulus, such as *mannitol* [MAN i tol] and *urea* [yu REE ah], result in some degree of diuresis. This is due to their ability to carry water with them into the tubular fluid. If the substance that is filtered subsequently undergoes little or no reabsorption, then the filtered substance will cause an increase in urinary output. Only a small amount of additional salt may also be excreted. Because osmotic diuretics are used to effect increased water excretion rather than Na^+ excretion, they are not useful for treating conditions in which Na^+ retention occurs. They are used to maintain urine flow following acute toxic ingestion of substances capable of producing acute renal failure. Osmotic diuretics are a mainstay of treatment for patients with increased intracranial pressure or acute renal failure due to shock, drug toxicities, and trauma. Maintaining urine flow preserves long-term kidney function and may save the patient from dialysis. [Note: *Mannitol* is not absorbed when given orally, and should only be given intravenously.] Adverse effects include extracellular water expansion and dehydration, as well as hypernatremia. The expansion of extracellular water results because the presence of *mannitol* in the extracellular fluid extracts water from the cells and causes hyponatremia until diuresis occurs. Dehydration, on the other hand, can occur if water is not replaced adequately.

Figure 22.11 summarizes the relative changes in urinary composition induced by diuretic drugs.

Study Questions

Choose the ONE best answer.

22.1 An elderly patient with a history of heart disease and who is having difficulty breathing is brought into the emergency room. Examination reveals that she has pulmonary edema. Which of the following treatments is indicated?

A. Spironolactone
B. Furosemide
C. Acetazolamide
D. Chlorthalidone
E. Hydrochlorothiazide

Correct choice = B. This is a potentially fatal situation. It is important to administer a diuretic that will reduce fluid accumulation in the lungs and, thus, improve oxygenation and heart function. The loop diuretics are most effective in removing large fluid volumes from the body, and are the treatment of choice in this situation. Furosemide is usually administered intravenously. The other choices are inappropriate.

22.2 A group of college students is planning a mountain climbing trip to the Andes. Which of the following drugs would be appropriate for them to take to prevent mountain sickness?

A. A thiazide diuretic
B. An anti-cholinergic
C. A carbonic anhydrase inhibitor
D. A loop diuretic
E. A β-blocker

Correct choice = C. Acetazolamide is used prophylactically for several days before an ascent above 10,000 feet. This treatment prevents the cerebral and pulmonary problems associated with the syndrome as well as other difficulties, such as nausea.

22.3 An alcoholic male has developed hepatic cirrhosis. In order to control the ascites and edema, he is prescribed which one of the following?

A. Hydrochlorothiazide
B. Acetazolamide
C. Spironolactone
D. Furosemide
E. Chlorthalidone

Correct choice = C. Spironolactone is very effective in the treatment of hepatic edema. These patients are frequently resistant to the diuretic action of loop diuretics, although a combination with spironolactone may be beneficial. The other agents are not indicated.

2.4 A 55-year-old male with kidney stones has been placed on a diuretic to decrease calcium excretion. However, after a few weeks, he develops an attack of gout. Which diuretic was he taking?

A. Furosemide
B. Hydrochlorothiazide
C. Spironolactone
D. Triamterene

Correct choice = B. Hydrochlorothiazide is effective in increasing calcium reabsorption and, thus, decreasing the amount excreted, which often causes kidney stones that contain calcium phosphate or calcium oxalate. However, hydrochlorothiazide can also inhibit the excretion of uric acid and cause its accumulation, leading to an attack of gout in some individuals. Furosemide increases the excretion of calcium, whereas the K^+-sparing diuretics, spironolactone and triamterene, do not have an effect.

2.5 An 75-year-old woman with hypertension is being treated with a thiazide. Her blood pressure responds and reads at 120/76 mm Hg. After several months on the medication, she complains of being tired and weak. An analysis of the blood indicates low values for which of the following ?

A. Calcium
B. Uric acid
C. Potassium
D. Sodium
E. Glucose

Correct choice = C. Hypokalemia is a common adverse effect of the thiazides, and causes fatigue and lethargy in the patient. Supplementation with potassium chloride or with foods high in K^+ corrects the problem. Alternatively, one may add a potassium-sparing diuretic like spironolactone. Calcium, uric acid, and glucose are usually elevated by thiazide diuretics. The sodium loss does not weaken the patient.

UNIT V:

Drugs Affecting the Endocrine System

Hormones of the Pituitary and Thyroid

23

I. OVERVIEW

The neuroendocrine system, which is controlled by the pituitary and hypothalamus, coordinates body functions by transmitting messages between individual cells and tissues. The nervous system communicates locally by electrical impulses and neurotransmitters directed through neurons to other neurons or to specific target organs, such as muscle or glands. Nerve impulses generally act within milliseconds. In contrast, the endocrine system releases hormones into the bloodstream, which carries these chemical messengers to target cells throughout the body. Hormones have a much broader range of response time than do nerve impulses, requiring from seconds to days, or longer, to cause a response that may last for weeks or months. The two regulatory systems are closely interrelated. For example, in several instances, the release of hormones is stimulated or inhibited by the nervous system, and some hormones can stimulate or inhibit nerve impulses. Chapters 24 to 26 focus on drugs that affect the synthesis and/or secretion of specific hormones and their actions. In this chapter, the central role of the hypothalamic and pituitary hormones in regulating body functions is briefly presented (Figure 23.1). In addition, drugs affecting thyroid hormone synthesis and/or secretion are discussed.

HYPOTHALAMIC AND ANTERIOR PITUITARY HORMONES

- *Chorionic gonadotropin*
- *Cosyntropin*
- *Follitropin beta*
- *Gonadorellin*
- *Goserelin*
- *Histrelin*
- *Leuprolide*
- *Menotropins*
- *Nafarelin*
- *Somatotropin*
- *Somatostatin*
- *Somatrem*
- *Urofollitropin*

HORMONES OF THE POSTERIOR PITUITARY

- *Desmopressin*
- *Oxytocin*
- *Vasopressin (ADH)*

DRUGS AFFECTING THE THYROID

- *Iodide*
- *Levothyronine*
- *Methimazole*
- *Propylthiouracil*
- *Thyroxine*
- *Triiodothyronine*

Figure 23.1
Some of the hormones and drugs affecting the hypothalamus, pituitary, and thyroid.

II. HYPOTHALAMIC AND ANTERIOR PITUITARY HORMONES

The hormones secreted by the hypothalamus and the pituitary are all peptides or low-molecular-weight proteins that act by binding to specific receptor sites on their target tissues. The hormones of the anterior pituitary are regulated by neuropeptides that are called either "releasing" or "inhibiting" factors or hormones. These are produced in cell bodies in the hypothalamus, and they reach the cells of the pituitary by the

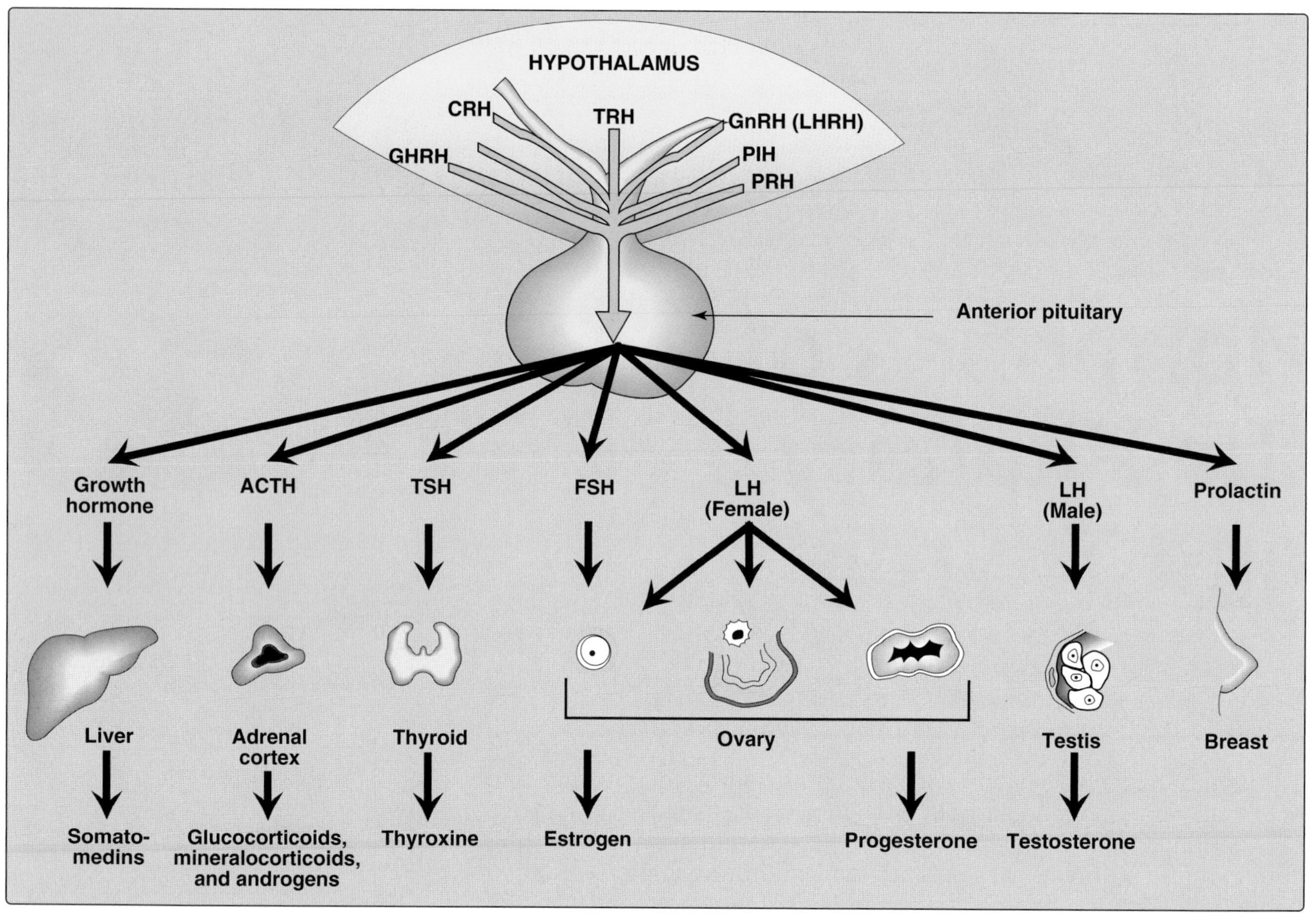

Figure 23.2
Hypothalamic-releasing hormones and actions of anterior pituitary hormones. GHRH= growth hormone-releasing hormone; TRH= thyrotropin-releasing hormone; CRH= corticotropin-releasing hormone; GnRH (LHRH)=gonadotropin-releasing hormone (luteinizing hormone-releasing hormone); PIH= prolactin-inhibiting hormone (dopamine); and PRH= prolactin-releasing hormone; ACTH= adrenocorticotropic hormone; TSH= thyrotropin-stimulating hormone; FSH= follicle-stimulating hormone; LH= luteinizing hormone

hypophysial portal system (Figure 23.2). The interaction of the releasing hormones with their receptors results in the activation of genes that promote the synthesis of protein precursors. These are then processed posttranslationally to the hormones and are released into the circulation. [Note: Unlike those of the posterior pituitary, the hormones of the anterior pituitary are not stored in granules prior to release.] Each hypothalamic regulatory hormone controls the release of a specific hormone from the anterior pituitary. The hypothalamic-releasing hormones are primarily used for diagnostic purposes (that is, to determine pituitary insufficiency). [Note: The hypothalamus also synthesizes the precursor proteins of the hormones vasopressin and oxytocin, which are transported to the posterior pituitary, where they are stored until released.] Although a number of pituitary hormone preparations are currently used therapeutically for specific hormonal deficiencies (examples of which follow), most of these agents have limited therapeutic applications. Hormones of the anterior and posterior pituitary are administered either intramuscularly (IM), subcutaneously, or intranasally, but not orally, because their peptidic nature makes them susceptible to destruction by the proteolytic enzymes of the digestive tract.

A. Adrenocorticotropic hormone (corticotropin)

Corticotropin-releasing hormone (CRH) is responsible for the synthesis and release of the peptide proopiomelanocortin by the hypothalamus (Figure 23.3). Adrenocorticotropic hormone (ACTH) or corticotropin [kor ti koe TROE pin] is a product of the posttranslational processing of this precursor polypeptide. [Note: CRH is used diagnostically to differentiate between Cushing syndrome and ectopic ACTH-producing cells.] Other products are γ-melanocyte–stimulating hormone, and β-lipotropin, the latter being the precursor of the endorphins. Normally, ACTH is released from the pituitary in pulses with an overriding diurnal rhythm, with the highest concentration occurring at approximately 6 AM, and the lowest in the evening. Stress stimulates its secretion, whereas cortisol suppresses its release.

1. **Mechanism of action:** The target organ of ACTH is the adrenal cortex, where it binds to specific receptors on the cell surfaces. The occupied receptors activate G protein–coupled processes to increase cyclic adenosine monophosphate (cAMP), which in turn stimulates the rate-limiting step in the adrenocorticosteroid synthetic pathway (cholesterol to pregnenolone). This pathway ends with the synthesis and release of the adrenocorticosteroids and the adrenal androgens (see Figure 23.3).

2. **Therapeutic uses:** The availability of synthetic adrenocorticosteroids with specific properties has limited the use of *corticotropin* to serving as a diagnostic tool for differentiating between primary adrenal insufficiency (Addison disease, associated with adrenal atrophy) and secondary adrenal insufficiency (caused by the inadequate secretion of ACTH by the pituitary). Therapeutic *corticotropin* preparations are extracts from the anterior pituitaries of domestic animals or synthetic human ACTH. The latter, *cosyntropin* [ko sin TROE pin], which consists of the amino-terminal 24 amino acids of the hormone, is preferred for the diagnosis of adrenal insufficiency.

3. **Adverse effects:** Toxicities are similar to those of glucocorticoids. Antibodies can form against ACTH derived from animal sources.

B. Growth hormone (somatotropin)

Somatotropin [soe mah toe TROE pin] is a large polypeptide that is released by the anterior pituitary in response to growth hormone–releasing hormone produced by the hypothalamus (see Figure 23.2). Secretion of growth hormone (GH) is inhibited by another pituitary hormone, *somatostatin* (see below). GH is released in a pulsatile manner, with the highest levels occurring during sleep. With increasing age, GH secretion decreases, being accompanied by a decrease in lean muscle mass. Human GH is produced synthetically by recombinant DNA technology. GH from

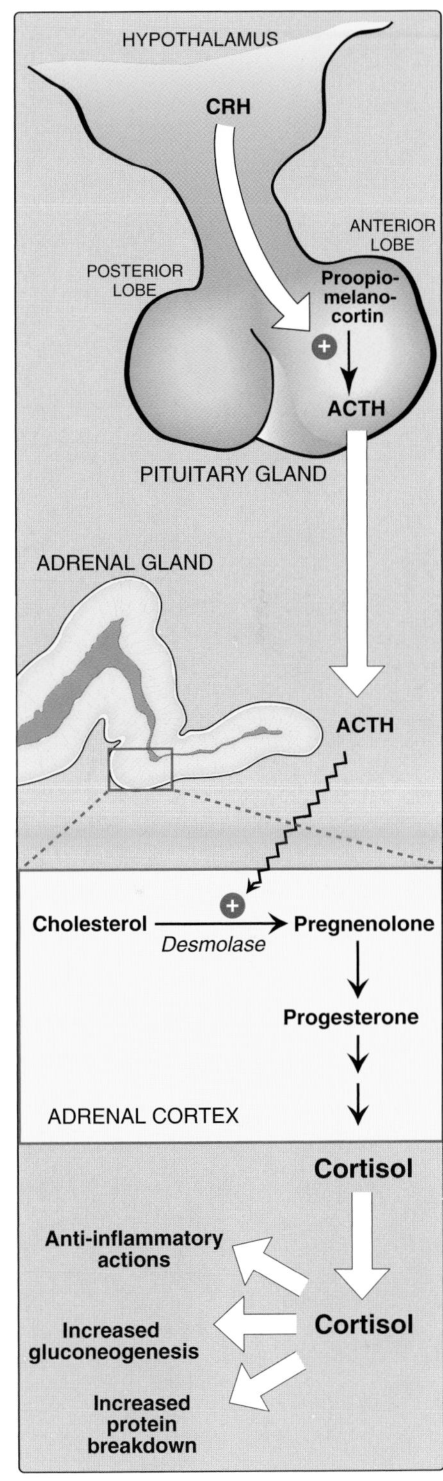

Figure 23.3
Secretion and actions of adrenocorticotropic hormone (ACTH). CRH = corticotropin-releasing hormone.

animal sources is ineffective in humans. *Somatotropin* influences a wide variety of biochemical processes; for example, through stimulation of protein synthetic processes, cell proliferation and bone growth are promoted. Increased formation of hydroxyproline from proline boosts cartilage synthesis.

1. **Mechanism of action:** Although many physiologic effects of GH are exerted directly at its targets, others are mediated through the somatomedins—insulin-like growth factors I and II (IGF-I and IGF-II). [Note: In acromegaly, IGF-I levels are consistently high, reflecting elevated GH.]

2. **Therapeutic uses:** *Somatotropin* is used in the treatment of GH deficiency in children. It is important to establish whether the GH deficit is actually due to hypopituitarism, because other factors, such as normal thyroid status, are essential for successful *somatotropin* therapy. [Note: After a study published in 1990 indicated that GH administered to men over sixty years of age for six months increased their lean body mass, bone density, and skin thickness, whereas adipose tissue mass decreased, many started to call GH the antiaging hormone. This has led to abuse by some athletes seeking to enhance their performance. GH is not approved for this purpose, and some who have taken it have developed diabetes.] A therapeutically equivalent drug, *somatrem* [SOE ma trem], contains an extra terminal methionyl residue not found in *somatotropin*. Although the half-lives of these drugs are short (approximately 25 minutes), they induce the release from the liver of IGF-I (formerly somatomedin C), which is responsible for subsequent GH-like actions. *Somatotropin* and *somatrem* should not be used in individuals with closed epiphyses or an enlarging intracranial mass.

C. Growth hormone–inhibiting hormone (somatostatin)

In the pituitary, *somatostatin* [SOE ma toe STAT in] binds to distinct receptors, SSTR2 and SSTR5, which suppress GH and thyroid-stimulating hormone release. Originally isolated from the hypothalamus, *somatostatin* is a small polypeptide that is also found in neurons throughout the body as well as in the intestine and pancreas. *Somatostatin* therefore has a number of actions. For example, it not only inhibits the release of GH but, also, of insulin, glucagon, and gastrin. *Octreotide* [ok TREE oh tide] is a synthetic octapeptide analog of *somatostatin*. Its half-life is longer than the natural compound, and a depot form is also available. The two forms suppress GH and IGF-I for twelve hours and six weeks, respectively. They have found use in the treatment of acromegaly caused by hormone-secreting tumors and in secretory diarrhea associated with tumors producing the vasoactive intestinal peptide. Adverse effects of *octreotide* treatment are flatulence, nausea, and steatorrhea. Gallbladder emptying is delayed, and asymptomatic cholesterol gallstones can occur with long-term treatment. [Note: An analog of human GH that has polyethylene glycol (PEG) polymers attached, *pegvisomant* [peg VI soe mant], is being employed in the treatment of acromegaly that is refractory to other modes of surgical, radiologic, or pharmacologic intervention. It acts as an antagonist at one of the GH receptors and results in the normalization of IGF-I levels.

D. Gonadotropin-releasing hormone/luteinizing hormone–releasing hormone

Gonadotropin-releasing hormone (GnRH), also called *gonadorelin* [go nad oh RELL in], is a decapeptide obtained from the hypothalamus. Pulsatile secretion of GnRH is essential for the release of follicle-stimulating hormone (FSH) and luteinizing hormone (LH) from the pituitary, whereas continuous administration inhibits gonadotropin release. GnRH is employed to stimulate gonadal hormone production in hypogonadism. A number of synthetic analogs, such as *leuprolide* [loo PROE lide], *goserelin* [GOE se rel in], *nafarelin* [naf A rel in], and *histrelin* [his TREL in], act as inhibitors of GnRH (Figure 23.4). These are effective in suppressing production of the gonadal hormones and, thus, are effective in the treatment of prostatic cancer, endometriosis, and precocious puberty. Adverse effects of *gonadorelin* include hypersensitivity, dermatitis, and headache. In women, the analogs may cause hot flushes and sweating, as well as diminished libido, depression, and ovarian cysts. They are contraindicated in pregnancy and breast-feeding. In men, they initially cause a rise in testosterone that can result in bone pain; hot flushes, edema, gynecomastia, and diminished libido also occur.

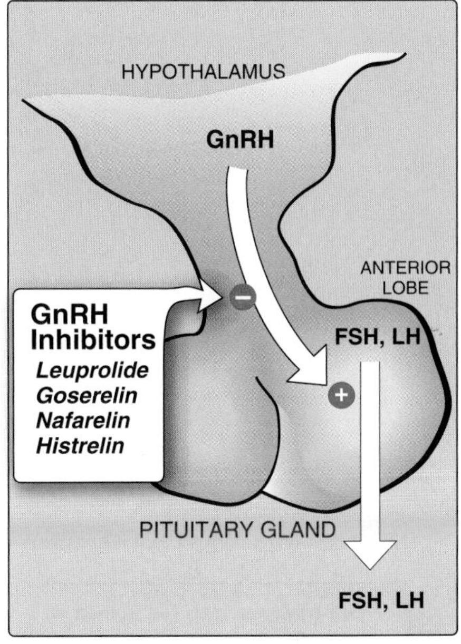

Figure 23.4
Secretion of follicle-stimulating hormone (FSH) and lutenizing hormone (LH). GnRH = gonadotropin-releasing hormone.

E. Gonadotropins: human menopausal gonadotropin, follicle-stimulating hormone, and human chorionic gonadoptropin

The gonadotropins are glycoproteins that are produced in the anterior pituitary. The regulation of gonadal steroid hormones depends on these agents. They find use in the treatment of infertility in men and women. *Menotropins* [men oh TROE pin] (*human menopausal gonadotropins*, *hMG*) are obtained from the urine of menopausal women and contain *follicle-stimulating hormone* (*FSH*) and *luteinizing hormone* (*LH*). *Chorionic gonadotropin* (*hCG*) is a placental hormone and an *LH* agonist, to which it is structurally related. It is also excreted in the urine. *Urofollitropin* [yoor oh fol li TROE pin] is *FSH* obtained from menopausal women and is devoid of *LH*. *Follitropin beta* [fol ih TROE pin] is human *FSH* manufactured by recombinant DNA technology. All of these hormones are injected IM. Injection of *hMG* or *FSH* over a period of five to twelve days causes ovarian follicular growth and maturation, and with subsequent injection of *hCG*, ovulation occurs. In men who are lacking gonadotropins, treatment with *hCG* causes external sexual maturation, and with the subsequent injection of *hMG*, spermatogenesis occurs. Adverse effects include ovarian enlargement and possible hypovolemia. Multiple births are not uncommon. Men may develop gynecomastia.

F. Prolactin

Prolactin is a peptide hormone similar in structure to GH, and is also secreted by the anterior pituitary. Its secretion is inhibited by dopamine. Its primary function is to stimulate and maintain lactation. In addition, it decreases sexual drive and reproductive function. The hormone enters a cell, where it activates a tyrosine kinase to pro-

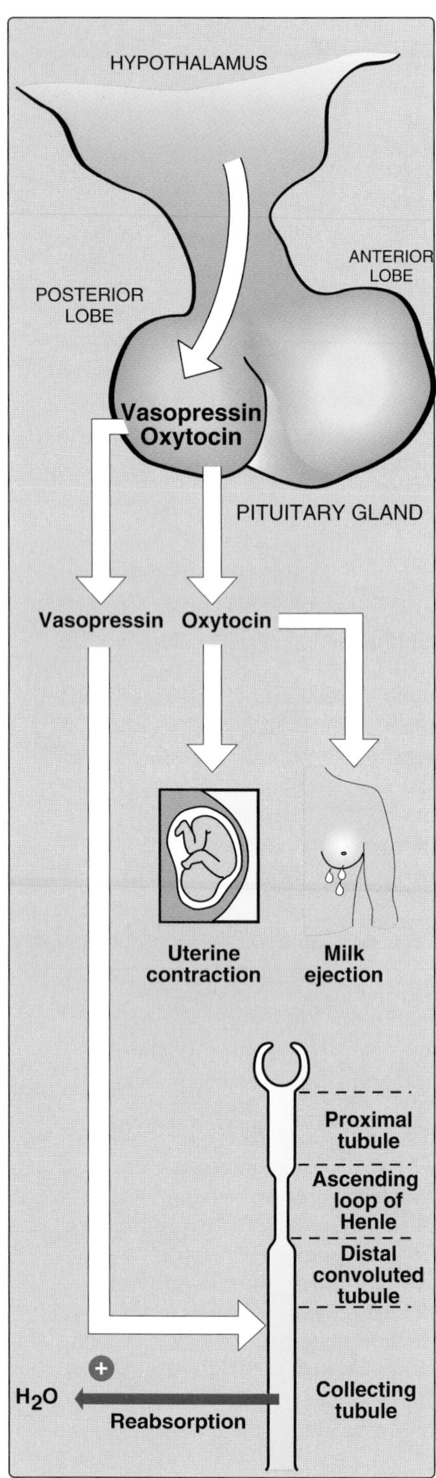

Figure 23.5
Actions of oxytocin and vasopressin. ACTH = adrenocorticotropic hormone.

mote tyrosine phosphorylation and gene activation. There is no preparation available for hypoprolactinemic conditions. On the other hand, hyperprolactinemia, which is associated with galactorrhea and hypogonadism, is usually treated with dopamine agonists, such as *bromocriptine* and *cabergoline*. Both of these agents also find use in the treatment of microadenomas and macroprolactinomas. They not only act at the dopamine receptor to inhibit prolactin secretion but also cause increased hypothalamic dopamine by decreasing its turnover. Among their adverse effects are nausea, headache, and sometimes, psychiatric problems.

III. HORMONES OF THE POSTERIOR PITUITARY

In contrast to the hormones of the anterior lobe of the pituitary, those of the posterior lobe, vasopressin and oxytocin, are not regulated by releasing hormones. Instead, they are synthesized in the hypothalamus, transported to the posterior pituitary, and released in response to specific physiologic signals, such as high plasma osmolarity or parturition. Each is a nonapeptide with a circular structure due to a disulfide bridge. Reduction of the disulfide inactivates these hormones. They are susceptible to proteolytic cleavage and, thus, are given parenterally. Both hormones have very short half-lives. Their actions are summarized in Figure 23.5.

A. Oxytocin

Oxytocin [ok se TOE sin], originally extracted from animal posterior pituitaries, is now chemically synthesized. Its only use is in obstetrics, where it is employed to stimulate uterine contraction to induce or reinforce labor or to promote ejection of breast milk. [Note: The sensitivity of the uterus to *oxytocin* increases with the duration of pregnancy when it is under estrogenic dominance.] To induce labor, the drug is administered intravenously. However, when used to induce "milk let-down," it is given as a nasal spray. *Oxytocin* causes milk ejection by contracting the myoepithelial cells around the mammary alveoli. Although toxicities are uncommon when the drug is used properly, hypertensive crises, uterine rupture, water retention, and fetal death have been reported. Its antidiuretic and pressor activities are very much lower than those of *vasopressin*. [Note: *Oxytocin* is contraindicated in abnormal fetal presentation, fetal distress, and premature births.]

B. Vasopressin

Vasopressin [vas oh PRESS in] (antidiuretic hormone), is structurally related to *oxytocin*. The chemically synthesized nonapeptide has replaced that extracted from animal posterior pituitaries. *Vasopressin* has both antidiuretic and vasopressor effects (see Figure 23.5). In the kidney, it binds to the V_2 receptor to increase water permeability and resorption in the collecting tubules. Thus, the major use of *vasopressin* is to treat diabetes insipidus. It also finds use in controlling bleeding due to esophageal varices or colonic diverticula. Other effects of *vasopressin* are mediated by the V_1 receptor, which is found in liver, vascular smooth muscle (where it causes constriction), and other tissues. As might be expected, the major toxicities are water intoxication and hyponatremia. Headache, bronchoconstriction, and tremor can also occur. Caution must be used when treating patients with coronary artery disease, epilepsy, and asthma.

C. Desmopressin

Because of its pressor properties, *vasopressin* has been modified to *desmopressin* [des moe PRESS in] (1-desamino-8-D-arginine vasopressin), which has minimal activity at the V_1 receptor, making it largely free of pressor effects. This analog is now preferred for diabetes insipidus and nocturnal enuresis and is longer-acting than *vasopressin*. *Desmopressin* is conveniently administered intranasally. However, local irritation may occur.

IV. THYROID HORMONES

The thyroid gland facilitates normal growth and maturation by maintaining a level of metabolism in the tissues that is optimal for their normal function. The two major thyroid hormones are *triiodothyronine* (*T_3*; the most active form), and *thyroxine* (*T_4*). Although the thyroid gland is not essential for life, inadequate secretion of thyroid hormone (hypothyroidism) results in bradycardia, poor resistance to cold, and mental and physical slowing (in children, this can cause mental retardation and dwarfism). If, however, an excess of thyroid hormones is secreted (hyperthyroidism), then tachycardia and cardiac arrhythmias, body wasting, nervousness, tremor, and excess heat production can occur. [Note: The thyroid gland also secretes the hormone calcitonin—a serum calcium-lowering hormone.]

A. Thyroid hormone synthesis and secretion

The thyroid gland is made up of multiple follicles that consist of a single layer of epithelial cells surrounding a lumen filled with colloid (thyroglobulin), which is the storage form of thyroid hormone. A summary of the steps in thyroid hormone synthesis and secretion is shown in Figure 23.6.

1. **Regulation of synthesis:** Thyroid function is controlled by a tropic hormone, thyroid-stimulating hormone (TSH; thyrotropin). TSH is a glycoprotein, structurally related to *LH* and *FSH*, which is synthesized by the anterior pituitary (see Figure 23.2). TSH generation is governed by the hypothalamic thyrotropin-releasing hormone (TRH). TSH action is mediated by cAMP and leads to stimulation of iodide (I^-) uptake. Oxidation to iodine (I_2) by a peroxidase is followed by iodination of tyrosines on thyroglobulin. [Note: Antibodies to thyroid peroxide are diagnostic for Hashimoto thyroiditis.] Condensation of two diiodotyrosine residues gives rise to *T_4* or *T_3*, which is still bound to the protein. The hormones are released following proteolytic cleavage of the thyroglobulin.

2. **Regulation of secretion:** Secretion of TSH by the anterior pituitary is stimulated by the hypothalamic TRH. Feedback inhibition of TRH occurs with high levels of circulating thyroid hormone. [Note: At pharmacologic doses, *dopamine*, *somatostatin*, or glucocorti-

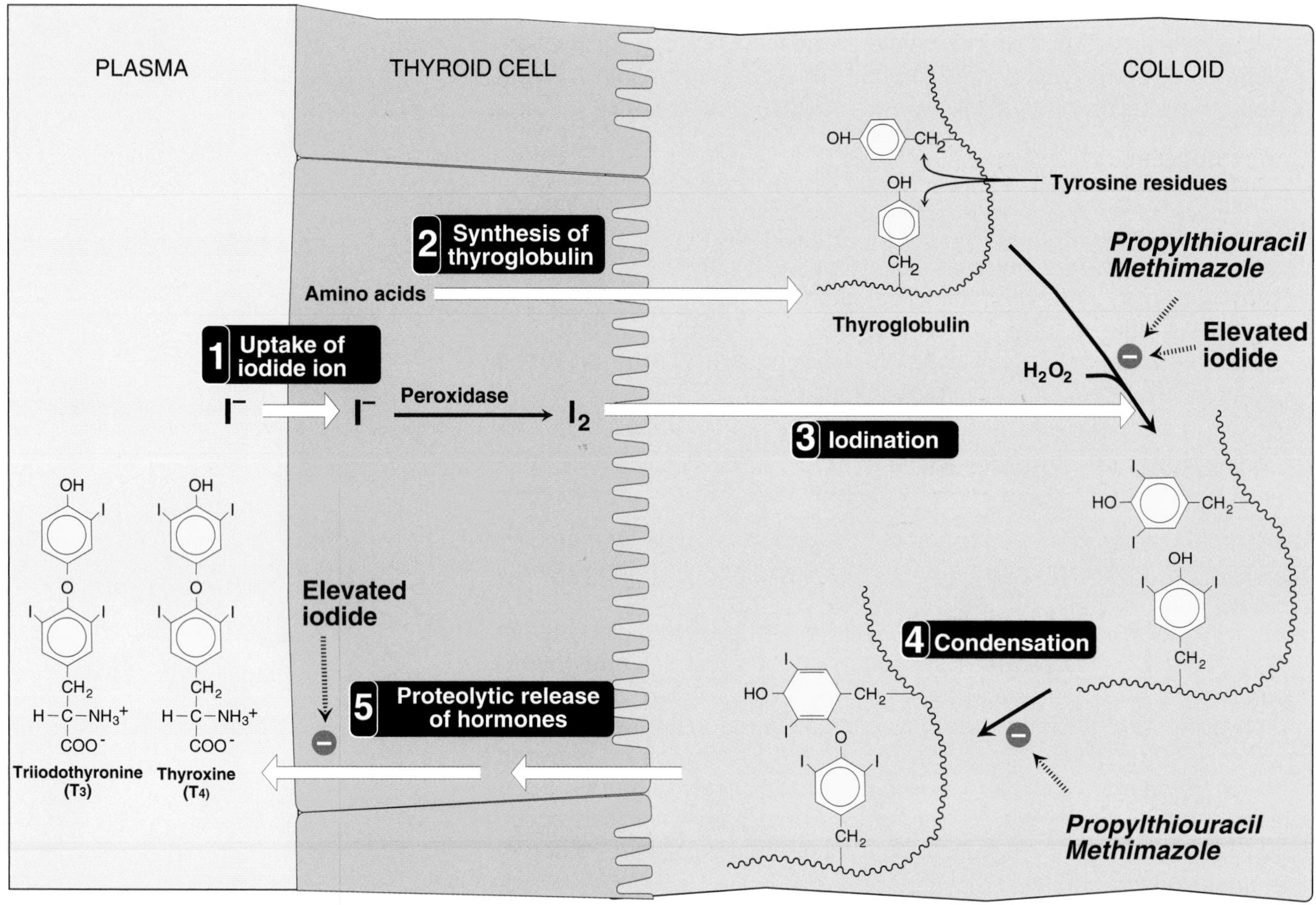

Figure 23.6
Biosynthesis of thyroid hormones.

coids can also suppress TSH secretion.] Most of the hormone (T_3 and T_4) is bound to thyroxine-binding globulin in the plasma.

B. Mechanism of action

Both T_4 and T_3 must dissociate from thyroxine-binding plasma proteins prior to entry into cells, either by diffusion or by active transport. In the cell, T_4 is enzymatically deiodinated to T_3, which enters the nucleus and attaches to specific receptors. The activation of these receptors promotes the formation of RNA and subsequent protein synthesis, which is responsible for the effects of T_4.

C. Pharmacokinetics

Both T_4 and T_3 are absorbed after oral administration. Food, calcium preparations, and aluminum-containing antacids can decrease the absorption of T_4 but not T_3. T_4 is converted to T_3 by one of two distinct deiodinases, depending on the tissue. The hormones are metabolized through the microsomal P450 system. Drugs that induce the P450 enzymes, such as *phenytoin*, *rifampin*, and *phenobarbital*, accelerate metabolism of the thyroid hormones (Figure 23.7).

D. Treatment of hypothyroidism

Hypothyroidism usually results from autoimmune destruction of the gland or the peroidase and is diagnosed by elevated TSH. It is treated with *levothyroxine* (*T_4*) [leh vo thye ROK sin]. The drug is given once daily because of its long half-life. Steady state is achieved in six to eight weeks. Toxicity is directly related to *T_4* levels, and manifests itself as nervousness, heart palpitations and tachycardia, intolerance to heat, and unexplained weight loss.

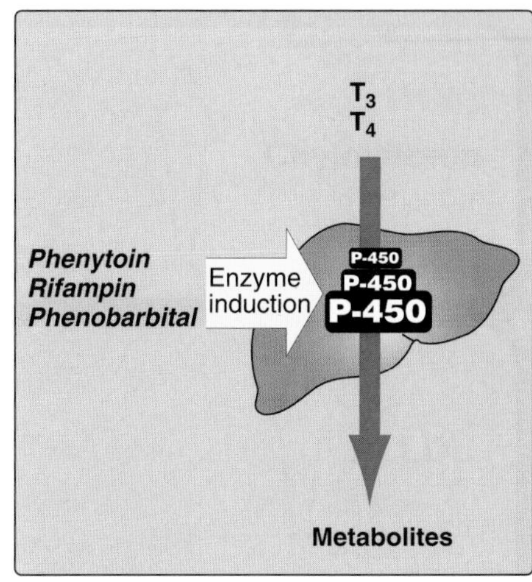

Figure 23.7
Enzyme induction can increase the metabolism of the thydroid hormones. T_3 = triiodothyronine; T_4 = thyroxine.

E. Treatment of hyperthyroidism (thyrotoxicosis)

Excessive amounts of thyroid hormones in the circulation are associated with a number of disease states, including Graves disease, toxic adenoma, and goiter. In these situations, TSH levels are reduced. The goal of therapy is to decrease synthesis and/or release of additional hormone. This can be accomplished by removing part or all of the thyroid gland, by inhibiting synthesis of the hormones, or by blocking release of the hormones from the follicle.

1. **Removal of part or all of the thyroid:** This can be accomplished either surgically or by destruction of the gland by beta particles emitted by radioactive iodine (^{131}I), which is selectively taken up by the thyroid follicular cells. Younger patients are treated with the isotope without prior pretreatment with *methimazole* (see below), whereas the opposite is the case in elderly patients. Most patients become hypothyroid as a result of this drug and require treatment with *levothyroxine*.

2. **Inhibition of thyroid hormone synthesis:** The thioamides, *propylthiouracil* [proe pil thye oh YOOR ah sil] (*PTU*) and *methimazole* [meth IM ah zole], are concentrated in the thyroid, where they inhibit both the oxidative processes required for iodination of tyrosyl groups and the coupling of iodotyrosines to form *T_3* and *T_4* (see Figure 23.6). *PTU* can also block the conversion of *T_4* to *T_3*. [Note: These drugs have no effect on the thyroglobulin already stored in the gland; therefore, observation of any clinical effects of these drugs may be delayed until thyroglobulin stores are depleted.] The thioamides are well absorbed from the gastrointestinal tract, but they have short half-lives. Several doses of *PTU* are required per day, whereas a single dose of *methimazole* suffices due to the duration of its antithyroid effect. The effects of these drugs are slow in onset; thus, they are not effective in the treatment of thyroid storm (see below). Relapse may occur. Relatively rare adverse effects include agranulocytosis, rash, and edema.

3. **Thyroid storm:** β-Blockers that lack sympathomimetic activity, such as *propranolol*, are effective in blunting the widespread sympathetic stimulation that occurs in hyperthyroidism. Intravenous administration is effective in treating thyroid storm. An alternative in patients suffering from severe heart failure or asthma is the calcium channel blocker, *diltiazem*.

4. **Blockade of hormone release:** A pharmacologic dose of *iodide* inhibits the iodination of tyrosines, thus decreasing the supply of stored thyroglobulin. *Iodide* also inhibits release of thyroid hormone by mechanisms not yet understood. Today, *iodide* is rarely used as the sole therapy. However, it is employed to treat potentially fatal thyrotoxic crisis (thyroid storm) or prior to surgery, because it decreases the vascularity of the thyroid gland. *Iodide* is not useful for long-term therapy, because the thyroid ceases to respond to the drug after a few weeks. *Iodide* is administered orally. Adverse effects are relatively minor and include sore mouth and throat, rashes, ulcerations of mucous membranes, and a metallic taste in the mouth.

Study Questions

Choose the ONE best answer.

23.1 Symptoms of hyperthyroidism include all of following EXCEPT:

A. tachycardia.
B. nervousness.
C. poor resistance to cold.
D. body wasting.
E. tremor.

Correct answer = C. An individual with hyperthyroidism often experiences excess heat production.

23.2 Which of the following best describes the effect of propylthiouracil on thyroid hormone production?

A. It blocks the release of thyrotropin-releasing hormone.
B. It inhibits uptake of iodide by thyroid cells.
C. It prevents the release of thyroid hormone from thyroglobulin.
D. It blocks iodination and coupling of tyrosines in thyroglobulin to form thyroid hormones.
E. It blocks the release of hormones from the thyroid gland.

Correct answer = D. Propylthiouracil blocks the synthesis of the thyroid hormones, but it does not affect the uptake of iodide, proteolytic cleavage of thyroglobulin, or release of hormones from the thyroid gland. The thyroid hormones inhibit the secretion of thyroid-stimulating hormone from the anterior pituitary.

23.3 Hyperthyroidism can be treated by all but which one of the following?

A. Triiodothyronine
B. Surgical removal of the thyroid gland
C. Iodide
D. Propylthiouracil
E. Methimazole

Correct answer = A. Triiodothyronine is a thyroid hormone that is overproduced in hyperthyroidism.

Insulin and Oral Hypoglycemic Drugs

24

I. OVERVIEW

The pancreas is both an endocrine gland that produces the peptide hormones *insulin*, glucagon, and somatostatin, and an exocrine gland that produces digestive enzymes. The peptide hormones are secreted from cells located in the islets of Langerhans (β or B-cells produce *insulin*, α_2 or A-cells produce glucagon, and α_1 or D-cells produce somatostatin). These hormones play an important role in regulating the metabolic activities of the body, particularly the homeostasis of blood glucose.[1] Hyperinsulinemia (due, for example, to an insulinoma) can cause severe hypoglycemia. More commonly, a relative or absolute lack of *insulin*, such as in diabetes mellitus, can cause serious hyperglycemia, which, if left untreated, can result in retinopathy, nephropathy, neuropathy, and cardiovascular complications. Administration of *insulin* preparations or oral hypoglycemic agents (Figure 24.1) can prevent morbidity and reduce mortality associated with diabetes.

HYPOGLYCEMIC DRUGS

INSULIN
- *Aspart insulin*
- *Extended zinc insulin*
- *Glargine insulin*
- *Glulisine insulin*
- *Insulin zinc suspension*
- *Lispro insulin*
- *NPH insulin suspension*
- *Protamine zinc insulin*
- *Semilente insulin*
- *Ultralente insulin*

ORAL HYPOGLYCEMIC DRUGS
- *Glipizide*
- *Glimepiride*
- *Glyburide*
- *Metformin*
- *Nateglinide*
- *Pioglitazone*
- *Repaglinide*
- *Rosiglitazone*
- *Tolbutamide*
- *Troglitazone*

α-GLUCOSIDASE INHIBITORS
- *Acarbose*
- *Miglitol*

GASTROINTESTINAL HORMONES
- *Exenatide*

Figure 24.1
Summary of hypoglycemic agents.

II. DIABETES MELLITUS

The incidence of diabetes is growing rapidly both in the United States and worldwide; for example, it is estimated that 135 million people worldwide are afflicted with the most common form, Type 2. In the United States, 20 million people are estimated to suffer from this type of diabetes, and it is a major cause of morbidity and mortality. Diabetes is not a single disease. Rather, it is a heterogeneous group of syndromes characterized by an elevation of blood glucose caused by a relative or absolute deficiency of *insulin*. [Note: Frequently, the inadequate release of *insulin* is aggravated by an excess of glucagon.] Diabetics can be divided into two main groups based on their requirements for *insulin*: *insulin*-dependent diabetes mellitus (Type 1), and non–*insulin*-dependent diabetes mellitus (Type 2).[2] Figure 24.2 summarizes the characteristics of Type 1 and Type 2 diabetes. Other types of diabetes have also been identified. For example, maturity-onset diabetes of the young

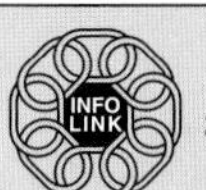

[1]See p. 308 in ***Lippincott's Illustrated Reviews: Biochemistry*** (3rd ed.) for a discussion of insulin in glucose homestasis.
[2]See p. 335 in ***Lippincott's Illustrated Reviews: Biochemistry*** (3rd ed.) for a discussion of Type 1 and Type 2 diabetes.

	Type 1 (Insulin-dependent diabetes)	**Type 2** (Non–insulin-dependent diabetes)
Age of onset	Usually during childhood or puberty	Frequently over age 35
Nutritional status at time of onset	Frequently undernourished	Obesity usually present
Prevalence	10 to 20 percent of diagnosed diabetics	80 to 90 percent of diagnosed diabetics
Genetic predisposition	Moderate	Very strong
Defect or deficiency	β Cells are destroyed, eliminating the production of insulin	Inability of β cells to produce appropriate quantities of insulin; insulin resistance; other defects

Figure 24.2
Comparison of Type 1 and Type 2 diabetes.

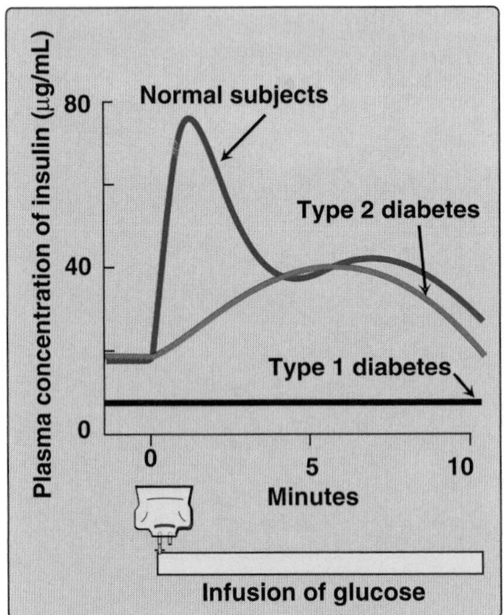

Figure 24.3
Release of insulin that occurs in response to the constant infusion of glucose in normal subjects and diabetic patients.

(MODY), also known as a Type 3 diabetes, is a heterogeneous group of disorders in which dysregulation of glucose sensing or *insulin* secretion is due to mutations of particular genes. It is inherited in an autosomally dominant fashion, is nonketotic, and occurs before 25 years of age. Unlike those with Type 2, patients with Type 3 are not obese, and *insulin* resistance and hypertriacylglycerolemia are absent. It is estimated that MODY may account for one to five percent of all diabetes cases. Treatment varies with the type of MODY. Gestational diabetes, classified as Type 4, is defined as glucose intolerance associated with pregnancy. It is important to maintain tight glycemic control close to the normal range during pregnancy, because hyperglycemia can lead to congenital abnormalities in the fetus. Diet, exercise, and/or *insulin* administration are effective in this condition.

A. Type 1 diabetes (insulin-dependent diabetes mellitus)

Insulin-dependent diabetes mellitus most commonly afflicts individuals around the time of puberty but can occur at any age. The disease is characterized by an absolute deficiency of *insulin* caused by massive β-cell necrosis. Loss of β-cell function is usually ascribed to autoimmune-mediated processes directed against the β-cell, and it may be triggered by an invasion of viruses or the action of chemical toxins. As a result of the destruction of these cells, the pancreas fails to respond to glucose, and the Type 1 diabetic shows classic symptoms of *insulin* deficiency (polydipsia, polyphagia, polyuria, and weight loss). Type 1 diabetics require exogenous *insulin* to avoid the catabolic state that results from and is characterized by hyperglycemia and life-threatening ketoacidosis.

1. **Cause of Type 1 diabetes:** In the postabsorptive period of a normal individual, low, basal levels of circulating *insulin* are maintained through constant β-cell secretion. This suppresses lipolysis, proteolysis, and glycogenolysis. A burst of *insulin* secretion occurs within two minutes after ingesting a meal, in response to transient increases in the levels of circulating glucose and amino acids. This lasts for up to fifteen minutes, and is followed by the postprandial secretion of *insulin*. However, having virtually no functional β-cells, the Type 1 diabetic can neither maintain a basal secretion level of *insulin* nor respond to variations in circulating fuels (Figure 24.3). The development and progression of neuropathy, nephropathy, and retinopathy are directly related to the extent of glycemic control (measured as blood levels of glucose and/or hemoglobin A_{1c}).[3]

2. **Treatment:** A Type 1 diabetic must rely on exogenous (injected) *insulin* to control hyperglycemia, avoid ketoacidosis, and maintain acceptable levels of glycosylated hemoglobin (HbA_{1c}). [Note: The rate of formation of HbA_{1c} is proportional to the average blood glucose concentration over the previous several months; thus, HbA_{1c} provides a measure of how well treatment has normalized blood glucose in diabetics.] The goal in administering *insulin* to Type 1 diabetics is to maintain blood glucose concentrations as close to normal as possible, and to avoid wide swings in their levels that

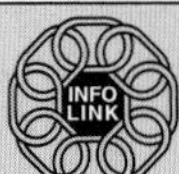

[3]See p. 34 in ***Lippincott's Illustrated Reviews: Biochemistry*** (3rd ed.) for a discussion of hemoglobin A_{1C}.

may contribute to long-term complications. The use of portable blood glucose analyzers facilitates frequent self-monitoring and treatment by injection of the hormone. Continuous subcutaneous *insulin* infusion—sometimes called the *insulin* pump—is also being used. This method of administration not only is more convenient, eliminating the multiple daily injections of the hormone, it is programmed to deliver the basal rate of *insulin* secretion. It also allows the patient to control delivery of a bolus of the hormone to compensate for high blood glucose or in anticipation of postprandial needs. Inhaled forms of *insulin* are presently in trial and may be available in the near future. Diabetics with autonomic insufficiency have difficulty controlling blood glucose levels. They may benefit from pancreas transplantation, often in conjunction with kidney transplantation. Transplantation of islet cells is also under investigation. [Note: The primary disadvantage of these transplant procedures is the subsequent requirement for immunosuppressant therapy with drugs such as *tacrolimus* to prevent transplant rejection.]

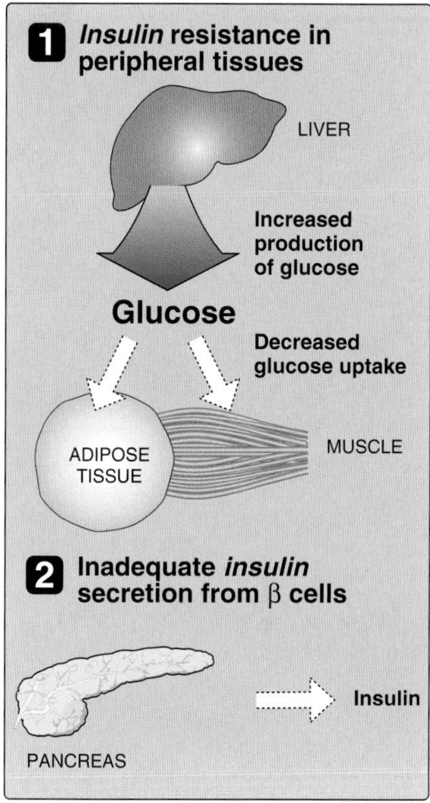

Figure 24.4
Major factors contributing to hyperglycemia observed in Type 2 diabetes.

B. Type 2 diabetes (non–insulin-dependent diabetes mellitus)

Most diabetics are Type 2. The disease is influenced by genetic factors, aging, obesity, and peripheral *insulin* resistance rather than by autoimmune processes or viruses. The metabolic alterations observed are milder than those described for Type 1 (for example, Type 2 patients typically are not ketotic), but the long-term clinical consequences can be just as devastating (for example, vascular complications and subsequent infection can lead to amputation of the lower limbs).

1. **Cause:** In non-*insulin*-dependent diabetes mellitus the pancreas retains some β-cell function, but variable *insulin* secretion is insufficient to maintain glucose homeostasis (see Figure 24.3). The β-cell mass may become gradually reduced in Type 2 diabetes. In contrast to patients with Type 1, those with Type 2 diabetes are often obese. [Note: Not all obese individuals become diabetic.] Type 2 diabetes is frequently accompanied by the lack of sensitivity of target organs to either endogenous or exogenous *insulin* (Figure 24.4). This resistance to *insulin* is considered to be a major causation of this type of diabetes, which is sometimes referred to as "metabolic syndrome."

2. **Treatment:** The goal in treating Type 2 diabetes is to maintain blood glucose concentrations within normal limits and to prevent the development of long-term complications of the disease. Weight reduction, exercise, and dietary modification decrease *insulin* resistance and correct the hyperglycemia of Type 2 diabetes in some patients. However, most are dependent on pharmacologic intervention with oral hypoglycemic agents. As the disease progresses, β-cell function declines, and *insulin* therapy is often required to achieve satisfactory serum glucose levels (Figure 24.5).

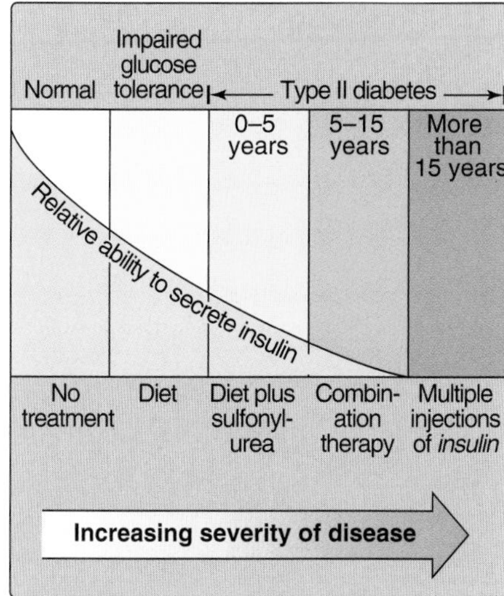

Figure 24.5
Duration of non–insulin-dependent (Type 2) diabetes mellitus, sufficiency of endogenous insulin, and recommended sequence of therapy.

III. INSULIN AND ITS ANALOGS

Insulin [IN su lin] is a polypeptide hormone consisting of two peptide chains that are connected by disulfide bonds. It is synthesized as a precursor (pro-insulin) that undergoes proteolytic cleavage to form *insulin* and peptide C, both of which are secreted by the β-cells of the pancreas.[4] [Note: Normal individuals secrete less pro-insulin than *insulin*, whereas Type 2 patients secrete high levels of the prohormone. Because radioimmunoassays do not distinguish between these two types of *insulin*, Type 2 patients may have lower levels of the active hormone than the assay indicates. Thus, measurement of circulating C peptide provides a better index of *insulin* levels.]

A. Insulin secretion

Insulin secretion is regulated not only by blood glucose levels but also by certain amino acids, other hormones (see gastrointestinal hormones below), and autonomic mediators. Secretion is most commonly triggered by high blood glucose, which is taken up by the glucose transporter into the β-cells of the pancreas. There, it is phosphorylated by glucokinase, which acts as a glucose sensor. The products of glucose metabolism enter the mitochondrial respiratory chain and generate adenosine triphosphate (ATP). The rise in ATP levels causes a block of K^+ channels, leading to membrane depolarization and an influx of Ca^{2+}, which results in pulsatile *insulin* exocytosis. The sulfonylureas and meglitinides owe their hypoglycemic effect to the inhibition of the K^+ channels. [Note: Glucose given by injection has a weaker effect on *insulin* secretion than does glucose taken orally, because orally, glucose stimulates production of digestive hormones by the gut, which in turn stimulate *insulin* secretion by the pancreas.]

B. Sources of insulin

Human *insulin* has largely replaced that isolated from beef or pork pancreas for therapeutic use. Human *insulin* is produced by recombinant DNA technology using special strains of Escherichia coli or yeast that have been genetically altered to contain the gene for human *insulin*. Modifications of the amino acid sequence of human *insulin* have produced *insulins* with different pharmacokinetic properties. For example, three such *insulins—lispro*, *aspart*, and *glulisine*—have a faster onset and shorter duration of action than regular *insulin*, because they do not aggregate or form complexes. On the other hand, *insulin glargine* and *insulin detimir* are long-acting *insulin*s and show prolonged, flat levels of the hormone following a single injection. [Note: *Insulin detimir* has received an "Approvable Letter" from the FDA but has not been approved as of this writing.]

C. Insulin administration

Because *insulin* is a polypeptide, it is degraded in the gastrointestinal tract if taken orally. It therefore is generally administered by subcutaneous injection. [Note: In a hyperglycemic emergency, regular *insulin*

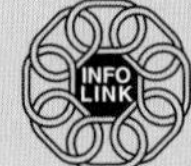

[4]See p. 306 in ***Lippincott's Illustrated Reviews: Biochemistry*** (3rd ed.) for a discussion of insulin synthesis and secretion.

is injected intravenously.] Continuous subcutaneous *insulin* infusion has become popular, because it does not require multiple injections. In an effort to eliminate the need for injections, an aerosol preparation that is inhaled and absorbed in the deep lung is undergoing trials, as is an oral spray that is absorbed through the buccal mucosa. *Insulin* preparations vary primarily in their times of onset of activity and in their durations of activity. This is due to the size and composition of the *insulin* crystals in the preparations as well as to the amino acid sequences of the polypeptides. [Note: The less soluble an *insulin* preparation, the longer it acts.] Dose, site of injection, blood supply, temperature, and physical activity can affect the duration of action of the various preparations. *Insulin* is inactivated by the reducing enzyme, insulinase, which is found mainly in the liver and kidney.

D. Adverse reactions to insulin

The symptoms of hypoglycemia are the most serious and common adverse reactions to an overdose of *insulin* (Figure 24.6). Long-term diabetics often do not produce adequate amounts of the counter-regulatory hormones (glucagon, epinephrine, cortisol, and growth hormone), which normally provide an effective defense against hypoglycemia. Other adverse reactions include lipodystrophy (less common with human *insulin*) and allergic reactions. Diabetics with renal insufficiency must have their doses of *insulin* adjusted.

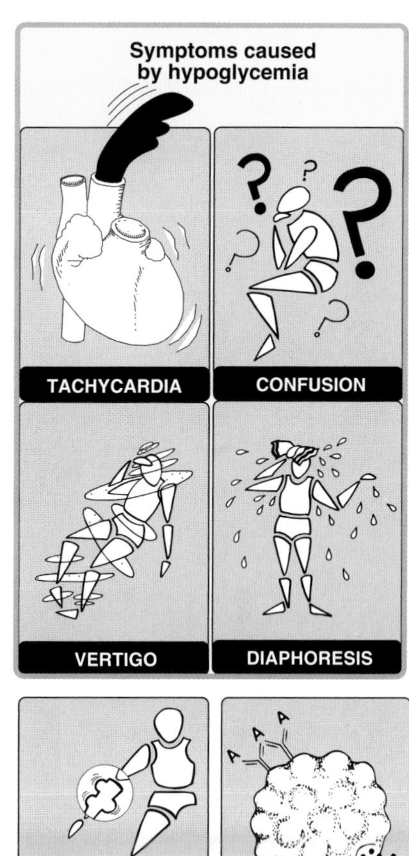

Figure 24.6
Adverse effects observed with *insulin*; Note: Lipodystrophy is a local atrophy or hypertrophy of subcutaneous fatty tissue at the site of injections.

IV. INSULIN PREPARATIONS AND TREATMENT

It is important that any change in *insulin* treatment be made cautiously by the clinician, with strict attention paid to the dose. Figure 24.7 summarizes the various types of *insulins* that are currently in use, their onsets of action, when their peak levels occur, and their durations.

A. Rapid-onset and ultrashort-acting insulin preparations

Four *insulin* preparations fall into this category: *regular insulin, insulin lispro, insulin aspart* and *insulin glulisine. Regular insulin* is a short-acting, soluble, crystalline *zinc insulin.* It is usually given subcutaneously (or intravenously in emergencies), and it rapidly lowers

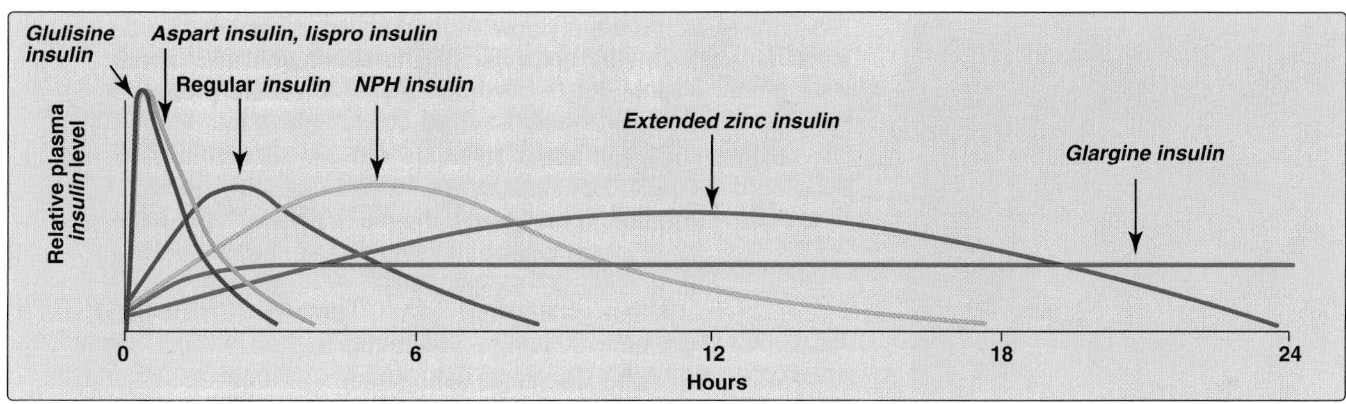

Figure 24.7
Onset and duration of action of human *insulin* and *insulin* analogs.

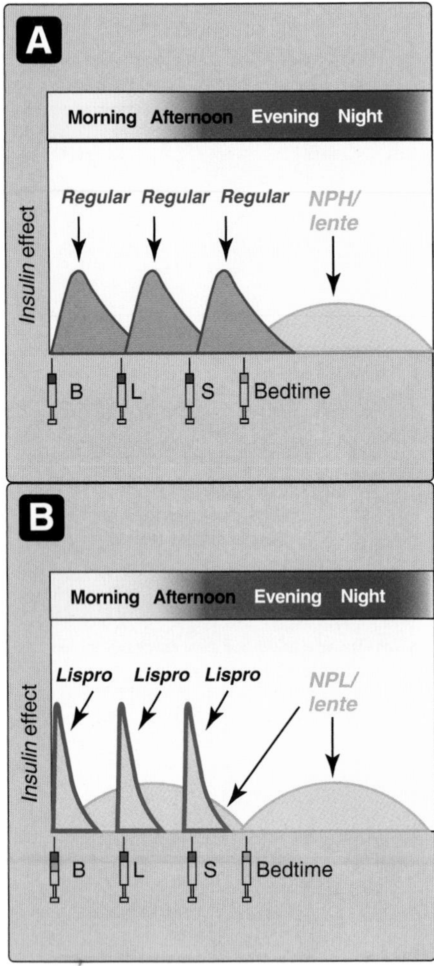

Figure 24.8
Examples of two regimens that provide both prandial and basal *insulin* replacement. B = breakfast; L = lunch; S = supper.

blood sugar (Figure 24.8). It is safely used in pregnancy, whereas use of the other three preparations is advised in pregnancy only if clearly needed. Because of their rapid onset and short duration of action, the *lispro* [LIS proe], *aspart* [AS part], and *glulisine* [gloo LYSE een] forms of *insulin* are classified as ultrashort-acting *insulins*. These agents offer more flexible treatment regimens and lower the risk of hypoglycemia. *Lispro insulin* differs from *regular insulin* in that lysine and proline at positions 28 and 29 in the B chain are reversed. This results in more rapid absorption after subcutaneous injection than is seen with *regular insulin*; as a consequence, *lispro insulin* acts more rapidly. *Lispro insulin* is usually administered fifteen minutes prior to a meal, whereas *glulisine* can be taken either fifteen minutes before a meal or within twenty minutes after starting a meal. Peak levels of *lispro insulin* are seen at 30 to 90 minutes after injection, as compared with 50 to 120 minutes for *regular insulin*. *Lispro insulin* also has a shorter duration of activity. *Aspart insulin* and *glulisine insulin* have pharmacokinetic and pharmacodynamic properties similar to those of *lispro*. They are administered to mimic the prandial (mealtime) release of *insulin*, and they are usually not used alone but, rather, along with a longer-acting *insulin* to assure proper glucose control. Like *regular insulin*, they are administered subcutaneously, although *lispro insulin* is also suitable for intravenous administration. [Note: *Lispro insulin* is preferred for external *insulin* pumps over the buffered form of *regular insulin*, because it does not form hexamers. There have, however, been reports of precipitation of the *lispro insulin* in infusion catheters, resulting in fluctuations in glucose control.]

B. Intermediate-acting insulin preparations

1. **Lente insulin:** This is an amorphous precipitate of *insulin* with zinc ion in acetate buffer combined with seventy percent *ultralente insulin*. Its onset of action and peak effect are somewhat slower than those of *regular insulin*, but are sustained for a longer period. It is not suitable for intravenous administration.

2. **Isophane NPH insulin suspension:** *Neutral protamine Hagedorn* (*NPH*) *insulin* is a suspension of crystalline *zinc insulin* combined at neutral pH with a positively charged polypeptide, protamine. [Note: Another name for this preparation is *isophane insulin*.] Its duration of action is intermediate. This is due to delayed absorption of the *insulin* because of its conjugation with protamine, forming a less-soluble complex. *NPH insulin* should only be given subcutaneously (never intravenously) and is useful in treating all forms of diabetes except diabetic ketoacidosis or emergency hyperglycemia. It is usually given along with *regular insulin*. [Note: A similar compound called *neutral protamine lyspro* (*NPL*) *insulin*, has been prepared that is used only in combination with *lispro insulin* (see below).] Figure 24.8 shows two of many regimens that use combinations of *insulins*.

C. Prolonged-acting insulin preparations

1. **Ultralente insulin:** Sometimes referred to as *extended zinc insulin*, this is a suspension of *zinc insulin* crystals in acetate buffer. This

produces large particles that are slow to dissolve, resulting in a slow onset of action and a long-lasting hypoglycemic effect (see Figure 24.7).

2. **Insulin glargine:** The isoelectric point of *insulin glargine* (GLAR geen) is lower than that of *human insulin*, leading to precipitation at the injection site, thereby extending its action. It is slower in onset than *NPH insulin* and has a flat, prolonged hypoglycemic effect—that is, it has no peak (see Figure 24.7). Like the other *insulins*, it must be given subcutaneously. *Insulin detimir* (deh TEE meer), which is presently in clinical trials, has a fatty-acid side chain. It associates with tissue-bound albumin at the injection site, and has properties similar to those of *insulin glargine*.

D. Insulin combinations

Various premixed combinations of human *insulins*, such as seventy-percent *NPH insulin* plus thirty-percent *regular insulin*, fifty percent of each of these, or 75-percent *NPL insulin* plus 25-percent *lispro insulin*, are also available.

E. Standard treatment versus intensive treatment

Standard treatment of patients with diabetes mellitus involves injection of *insulin* twice daily. This results in mean blood glucose levels in the range of 225 to 275 mg/dL, with HbA_{1c} of eight to nine percent of total hemoglobin. In contrast, intensive treatment seeks to normalize blood glucose through more frequent injections of *insulin* (three or more times daily in response to monitoring blood glucose levels). Mean blood glucose levels of 150 mg/dL can be achieved with intensive treatment, with an HbA_{1c} of approximately seven percent of total hemoglobin. [Note: Normal mean blood glucose is approximately 110 mg/dL or less, with an HbA_{1c} of six percent or less.] Thus, total normalization of blood glucose levels is not achieved, and the frequency of hypoglycemic episodes, coma, and seizures due to excessive *insulin* is particularly high with intensive treatment regimens (Figure 24.9A). Nonetheless, patients on intensive therapy show a sixty-percent reduction in the long-term complications of diabetes—retinopathy, nephropathy, and neuropathy—compared to patients receiving standard care (Figure 24.9B).

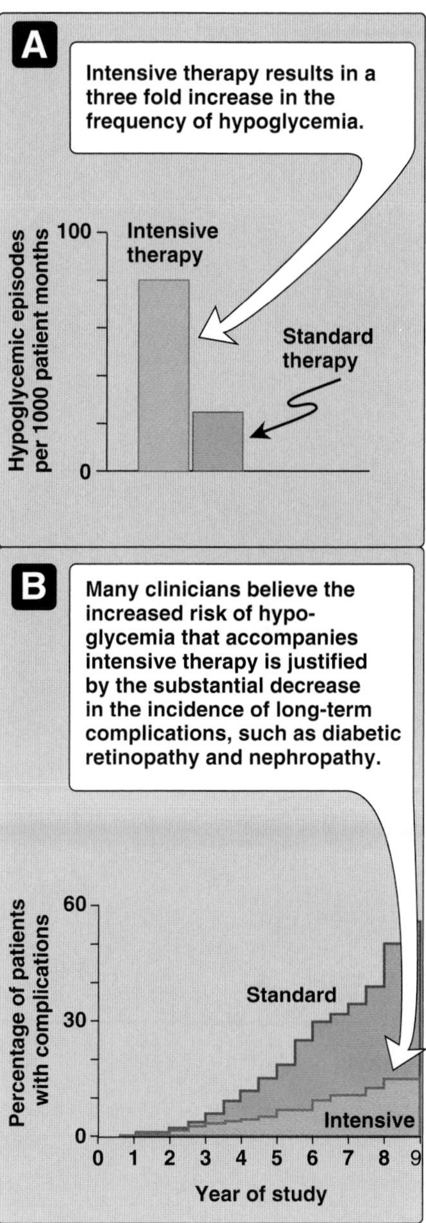

Figure 24.9
A. Effect of tight glucose control on hypoglycemic episodes in a population of patients receiving intensive or standard therapy.
B. Effect of standard and intensive care on the long-term complications of diabetes.

V. ORAL HYPOGLYCEMIC AGENTS: INSULIN SECRETAGOGUES

These agents are useful in the treatment of patients who have Type 2 (non–*insulin*-dependent) diabetes but cannot be managed by diet alone. The patient most likely to respond well to oral hypoglycemic agents is one who develops diabetes after age forty and has had diabetes less than five years. Patients with long-standing disease may require a combination of hypoglycemic drugs with or without *insulin* to control their hyperglycemia. The hormone is added because of the progressive decline in β-cells that occurs due to the disease or aging. Oral hypoglycemic agents should not be given to patients with Type 1 diabetes.

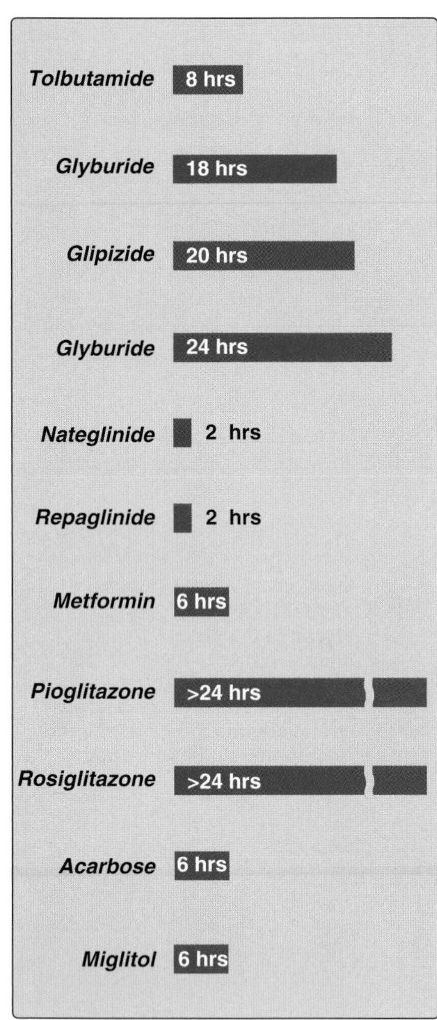

Figure 24.10
Duration of action of some oral hypoglycemic agents.

Figure 24.10 summarizes the duration of action of some of the oral hypoglycemic drugs, and Figure 24.11 illustrates some of the common adverse effects of these agents.

A. Sulfonylureas

These agents are classified as *insulin* secretagogues, because they promote *insulin* release from the β-cells of the pancreas. The primary drugs used today are *tolbutamide* [tole BYOO ta mide] and the second-generation derivatives, *glyburide* [GLYE byoor ide], *glipizide* [GLIP i zide], and *glimepiride* [GLYE me pih ride].

1. **Mechanisms of action of the sulfonylureas:** These include 1) stimulation of *insulin* release from the β-cells of the pancreas by blocking the ATP-sensitive K^+ channels, resulting in depolarization and Ca^{2+} influx; 2) reduction of serum glucagon levels; and 3) increasing binding of *insulin* to target tissues and receptors.

2. **Pharmacokinetics and fate:** Given orally, these drugs bind to serum proteins, are metabolized by the liver, and are excreted by the liver or kidney. *Tolbutamide* has the shortest duration of action (six to twelve hours), whereas the second-generation agents last about 24 hours.

3. **Adverse effects:** Shortcomings of the sulfonylureas are their propensity to cause weight gain, hyperinsulinemia, and hypoglycemia. These drugs are contraindicated in patients with hepatic or renal insufficiency, because delayed excretion of the drug—resulting in its accumulation—may cause hypoglycemia. Renal impairment is a particular problem in the case of those agents that are metabolized to active compounds, such as *glyburide* and *glimepiride*. The sulfonylureas traverse the placenta, and can deplete *insulin* from the fetal pancreas; therefore pregnant women with Type 2 diabetes should be treated with *insulin*. Figure 24.12 summarizes some of the interactions of the sulfonylureas with other drugs.

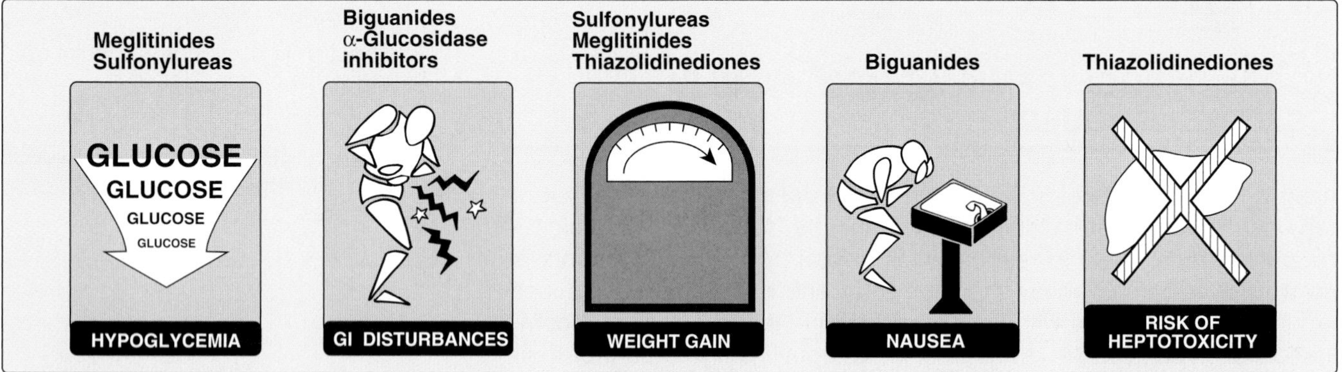

Figure 24.11
Some adverse effects observed with oral hypoglycemic agents.

B. Meglitinide analogs

This class of agents includes *repaglinide* [re PAG lin ide] and *nateglinide* [nuh TAY gli nide]. Although they are not sulfonylureas, they have common actions.

1. **Mechanism of action:** Like the sulfonylureas, their action is dependent on functioning pancreatic β-cells. They bind to a distinct site on the sulfonylurea receptor of ATP-sensitive potassium channels, thereby initiating a series of reactions culminating in the release of *insulin*. However, in contrast to the sulfonylureas, the meglitinides have a rapid onset and short duration of action. They are particularly effective in the early release of *insulin* that occurs after a meal and, thus, are categorized as postprandial glucose regulators. Combined therapy of these agents with *metformin* or the glitazones has been shown to be better than monotherapy with either agent in improving glycemic control.

2. **Pharmacokinetics and fate:** These drugs are well absorbed orally after being taken one to thirty minutes before meals. Both meglitinides are metabolized to inactive products by CYP3A4 (see p. 14) in the liver and are excreted through the bile.

3. **Adverse effects:** Although these drugs can cause hypoglycemia, the incidence of this adverse effect appears to be lower than with the sulfonylureas. [Note: Drugs that inhibit CYP3A4, like *ketoconazole*, *itraconazole*, *fluconazole*, *erythromycin*, and *clarithromycin*, may enhance the glucose-lowering effect of *repaglinide*, whereas drugs that increase levels of this enzyme, such as barbiturates, *carbamazepine*, and *rifampin*, may have the opposite effect.] *Repaglinide* has been reported to cause severe hypoglycemia in patients who are also taking the lipid-lowering drug *gemfibrozil*. Weight gain is less of a problem with the meglitinides than with the sulfonylureas. These agents must be used with caution in patients with hepatic impairment.

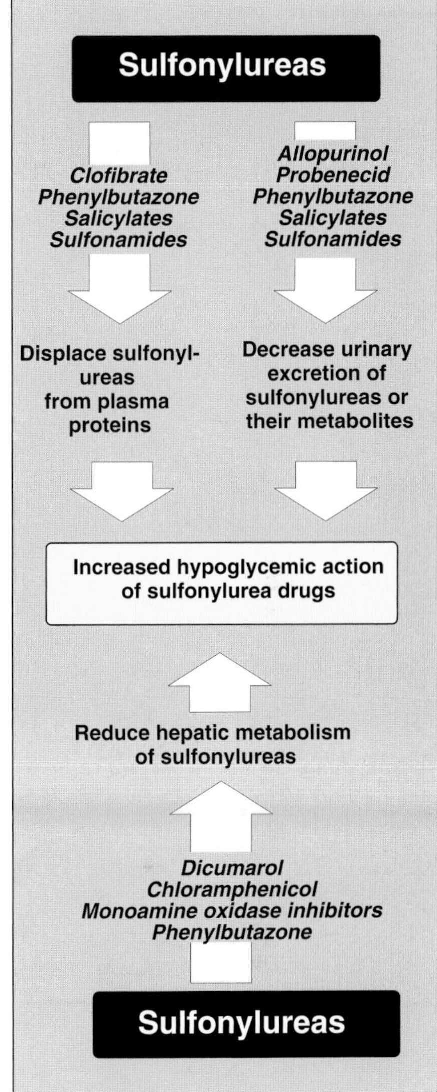

Figure 24.12
Drugs interacting with sulfonylurea drugs.

VI. ORAL HYPOGLYCEMIC AGENTS: INSULIN SENSITIZERS

Two classes of oral hypoglycemic drugs—the biguanides and thiazolidinediones—improve *insulin* action. These agents lower blood sugar by improving target-cell response to *insulin* without increasing pancreatic *insulin* secretion.

A. Biguanides

Metformin [met FOR min], the only currently available biguanide, is classed as an *insulin* sensitizer; that is, it increases glucose uptake and utilization by target tissues, thereby decreasing *insulin* resistance. Like the sulfonylureas, *metformin* requires *insulin* for its action, but it differs from the sulfonylureas in that it does not promote *insulin* secretion. Hyperinsulinemia is not a problem. Thus, the risk of hypoglycemia is far less than with sulfonylurea agents, and it may only occur if caloric intake is not adequate or exercise is not compensated for calorically.

1. **Mechanism of action:** *Metformin* reduces hepatic glucose output, largely by inhibiting hepatic gluconeogenesis. [Note: Excess glucose produced by the liver is the major source of high blood sugar in Type 2 diabetes, accounting for the high blood sugars on waking in the morning.] It also slows intestinal absorption of sugars. A very important property of this drug is its ability to modestly reduce hyperlipidemia (LDL and VLDL cholesterol concentrations fall, and HDL cholesterol rises). These effects may not be apparent until four to six weeks of use. The patient often loses weight because of loss of appetite. Some experts consider *metformin* to be the drug of choice for newly diagnosed Type 2 diabetics. It is the only oral hypoglycemic agent proven to decrease cardiovascular mortality. *Metformin* may be used alone or in combination with one of the other agents, as well as with *insulin*. Hypoglycemia has occurred when *metformin* was taken in combination. [Note: If used with *insulin*, the dose of the hormone must be adjusted, because *metformin* decreases the production of glucose by the liver.]

2. **Pharmacokinetics and fate:** *Metformin* is well absorbed orally, is not bound to serum proteins, and is not metabolized. The highest concentrations are in the saliva and intestinal wall. Excretion is via the urine.

3. **Adverse effects:** These are largely gastrointestinal. *Metformin* is contraindicated in diabetics with renal and/or hepatic disease, cardiac or respiratory insufficiency, a history of alcohol abuse, severe infection, or pregnancy. The drug should be discontinued in patients undergoing diagnosis requiring intravenous radiographic contrast agents. Rarely, potentially fatal lactic acidosis has occurred. [Note: Diabetics being treated with heart-failure medications should not be given *metformin* because of an increased risk in lactic acidosis.] Long-term use may interfere with vitamin B_{12} absorption. A number of drug-drug interactions have been identified; the effects of *metformin* may be enhanced by *cimetidine*, *furosemide*, *nifedipine*, and other agents.

4. **Other uses:** In addition the treatment of Type 2 diabetes, *metformin* is effective in the treatment of polycystic ovary disease. Its ability to lower *insulin* resistance in these women can result in ovulation and, possibly, pregnancy.

B. Thiazolidinediones or glitazones

Another group of agents that are *insulin* sensitizers are the thiazolidinediones (TZDs) or, more familiarly, glitazones. Although *insulin* is required for their action, these drugs do not promote its release from the pancreatic β cells; thus, hyperinsulinemia does not result. *Troglitazone* [TROE glit a zone] was the first of these to be approved for the treatment of Type 2 diabetic patients but was withdrawn after a number of deaths due to hepatotoxicity were reported. Presently, two members of this class are available, *pioglitazone* [pye oh GLI ta zone] and *rosiglitazone* [roe si GLI ta zone].

1. **Mechanism of action:** Although the exact mechanism by which the TZDs lower *insulin* resistance remains to be elucidated, they are known to target the peroxisome proliferator–activated receptor-γ (PPARγ)—a nuclear hormone receptor. Ligands for PPARγ regulate adipocyte production and secretion of fatty acids as well as glucose metabolism, resulting in increased *insulin* sensitivity in adipose tissue, liver, and skeletal muscle. Hyperglycemia, hyperinsulinemia, hypertriacylglycerolemia, and elevated HbA_{1c} levels are improved. Interestingly, LDL levels are not affected by *pioglitazone* monotherapy or when the drug is used in combination with other agents, whereas LDL levels have increased with *rosiglitazone*. HDL levels increase with both drugs. The TZDs lead to an expansion of subcutaneous fat. [Note: Whether the adipogenic effects can be separated from those of increased *insulin* sensitivity is the subject of much research, particularly because of the role of obesity in this disease.] *Pioglitazone* can be used as monotherapy or in combination with other hypoglycemics or with *insulin*. The dose of *insulin* required for adequate glucose control in these circumstances may have to be lowered. *Rosiglitazone* may also be used in combination with other hypoglycemics but not with *insulin*, because edema occurs with higher frequency. For example, in Type 2 diabetics who do not achieve glycemic control with a combination of *glyburide/* and *metformin*, the addition of *rosiglitazone* to the treatment regimine improves glycemic control and lowers HbA_{1C} levels.

2. **Pharmacokinetics:** Both *pioglitazone* and *rosiglitazone* are absorbed very well after oral administration and are extensively bound to serum albumin. Both undergo extensive metabolism by different cytochrome P450 isozymes (see p. 14). Some metabolites of *pioglitazone* have activity. The metabolites are primarily excreted in the urine, but the parent agent leaves via the bile. No dosage adjustment is required in renal impairment. It is recommended that these agents not be used in nursing mothers.

3. **Adverse effects:** Because there have been deaths from hepatotoxicity in patients taking *troglitazone*, it is strongly recommended that liver enzyme levels of patients on these medications be measured initially, then every two months for a year, and periodically thereafter. Weight increase can occur, possibly through the ability of TZDs to increase subcutaneous fat or due to fluid retention. [Note: The latter can lead to or worsen heart failure.] Other adverse effects include headache and anemia. Women taking oral contraceptives and TZDs may become pregnant, because the latter have been shown to reduce plasma concentrations of the estrogen-containing contraceptives.

4. **Other uses:** As with *metformin*, the relief of *insulin* resistance with the TZDs can cause ovulation to resume in premenopausal women with polycystic ovarian syndrome.

VII. ORAL HYPOGLYCEMIC AGENTS: α-GLUCOSDASE INHIBITORS

A. Acarbose and miglitol

Acarbose [AY car bose] and *miglitol* [MIG li tol] are orally active drugs used for the treatment of patients with Type 2 diabetes.

1. **Mechanism of action:** These drugs are taken at the beginning of meals. They act by delaying the digestion of carbohydrates, thereby decreasing glucose absorption. Both drugs exert their effects by reversibly inhibiting membrane-bound α-glucosidase in the intestinal brush border. This enzyme is responsible for the hydrolysis of oligosaccharides to glucose and other sugars. [Note: *Acarbose* also inhibits pancreatic α-amylase, thus interfering with the breakdown of starch to oligosaccharides.] Consequently, the postprandial rise of blood glucose is blunted. Unlike the other oral hypoglycemic agents, these drugs do not stimulate *insulin* release, nor do they increase *insulin* action in target tissues. Thus, as monotherapy, they do not cause hypoglycemia. However, when used in combination with the sulfonylureas or with *insulin*, hypoglycemia may develop. [Note: It is important that the hypoglycemic patient be treated with glucose rather than sucrose, because sucrase is also inhibited by these drugs.]

2. **Pharmacokinetics:** *Acarbose* is poorly absorbed. It is metabolized primarily by intestinal bacteria, and some of the metabolites are absorbed and excreted into the urine. On the other hand, *miglitol* is very well absorbed but has no systemic effects. It is excreted unchanged by the kidney.

3. **Adverse effects:** The major side effects are flatulence, diarrhea, and abdominal cramping. Patients with inflammatory bowel disease, colonic ulceration, or intestinal obstruction should not use these drugs. They also decrease the bioavailability of *metformin*; concurrent use should be avoided.

VIII. GASTROINTESTINAL HORMONES

Oral glucose results in a higher secretion of *insulin* than occurs when an equal load of glucose is given intravenously. This effect is referred to as the “incretin effect,” and is apparently reduced in Type 2 diabetes. It demonstrates the important role of the gastrointestinal hormones—notably glucagon-like peptide-1(GLIP-1) and gastric inhibitory polypeptide—in the digestion and absorption of nutrients including glucose. A new drug, *exenatide* [EX e nah tide], with a polypeptide sequence about fifty-percent homologous to GLIP-1, has been introduced. It apparently mediates its effect through the GLIP-1 receptor, and it not only improves *insulin* secretion but also slows gastric emptying time, decreases food intake, increases glucose suppression of glucagon secretion, and promotes β cell regeneration or decreased apoptosis. Consequently, weight gain, postprandial hyperglycemia, and loss of β cells are reduced, and HbA_{1c} levels decline. Being a polypeptide, *exenatide* must be administered parenterally. A drawback to its use is its short duration of action, requiring frequent injections. Research to find longer-acting agents with similar effects is being actively pursued. *Exenatide* is well tolerated, with a small number of patients reporting nausea.

A summary of the oral antidiabetic agents is presented in Figure 24.13.

	MECHANISM OF ACTION	EFFECT ON PLASMA INSULIN	RISK OF HYPO-GLYCEMIA	COMMENTS
First-generation sulfonylureas				
Tolbutamide	Stimulates insulin secretion	↑	Yes	Well-established history of effectiveness. Weight gain can occur.
Second-generation sulfonylureas				
Glipizide *Glyburide* *Glimepiride*	Stimulates insulin secretion	↑	Yes	Well-established history of effectiveness. Weight gain can occur.
Meglitinide analogs				
Nateglinide *Repaglinide*	Stimulates insulin secretion	↑	Yes (rarely)	Short action with less hypoglycemia either at night or with missed meal. Post-prandial effect.
Biguanides				
Metformin	Decreased endogenous hepatic production of glucose	↓	No	Well-established history of effectiveness. Weight loss may occur. Convenient daily dosing. Decreases micro- and macro-vascular disease risk. Many contraindications. Not metabolized; excreted by kidneys; may be used either alone or in combination with sulfonylureas
Thiazolidinediones (glitazones)				
Pioglitazone *Rosiglitazone*	Binds to peroxisome proliferator–activated receptor-γ in muscle, fat and liver to decrease insulin resistance.	↓↓	No	Effective in highly insulin-resistant patients. Once-daily dosing.
α-Glucosidase inhibitors				
Acarbose *Miglitol*	Decreased glucose absorption	⇔	No	Taken with meals. Adverse gastro-intestinal effects.

Figure 24.13
Summary of oral hypoglycemic agents. ⇔ = little or no change.

Study Questions

Choose the ONE best answer.

24.1 A fifty-year-old woman has just been diagnosed as a Type 2 diabetic and given a prescription for metformin. Which of the following statements is characteristic of this medication?

A. Hypoglycemia is a common adverse effect.
B. Metformin undergoes metabolism to an active compound.
C. Many drug-drug interactions have been identified.
D. t increases peripheral glucose uptake and utilization in target tissues.
E. The patient often gains weight.

Correct answer = D. Metformin is classified as an insulin sensitizer. Hypoglycemia is not a problem with metformin, because it does not release insulin from the pancreas. B and C are incorrect, because metformin is not metabolized and no drug-drug interactions occur. Unlike the sulfonylureas and thiazolidinediones, metformin causes the patient to lose appetite and, thus, to lose weight.

24.2 Which of the following statements is true for therapy with insulin glargine?

A. It is primarily used to control prandial hyperglycemia.
B. It should not be combined with any other insulin.
C. It is now used preferentially in Type 1 diabeticswho are pregnant.
D. Pharmacokinetically, there is no peak activity, and the activity lasts about 24 hours.
E. It is effective by inhalation.

Correct answer = D. Insulin glargine is a long-acting insulin. It is slowly released from subcutaneous sites and exhibits no peak. Because of its low levels and prolonged action, insulin glargine best mimics basal secretion of insulin. It is used in combination with other insulins—for example, lispro. It is not used in the treatment of pregnant diabetics, because insulin-like growth factor-I increases—a change that has been implicated in some tumors. E is incorrect, because there are no insulins that are effective by this route at present.

24.3 The ability to reduce insulin resistance is associated with which one of the following classes of hypoglycemic agents?

A. Meglitinides
B. Sulfonylureas
C. α-Glucosidase inhibitors
D. Thiazolidinediones
E. Gastrointestinal hormones

Correct answer = D. Insulin resistance is lowered by insulin sensitizers, which include the thiazolidinediones as well as metformin. The other agents do not have an effect.

24.4 A 64-year-old woman with a history of Type 2 diabetes is diagnosed with heart failure. Which of the following drugs would be a poor choice in controlling her diabetes?

A. Metformin
B. Exenatide
C. Glyburide
D. Glipizide
E. Pioglitazone

Correct answer = E. Edema is an adverse effect of pioglitazone, and so it would not be a good choice. Metformin, which is an insulin sensitizer, or the sulfonamides, glyburide and glipizide, could be used. Exenatide is a new agent that acts as an analog of GLIP-1. It has the ability to improve insulin secretion, lowers postprandial hyperglycemia, decreases body weight, and is well tolerated.

Estrogens and Androgens

25

I. OVERVIEW

Sex hormones produced by the gonads are necessary for conception, embryonic maturation, and development of primary and secondary sexual characteristics at puberty. Their activity in target cells is modulated by receptors. The gonadal hormones are used therapeutically in replacement therapy, for contraception, management of menopausal symptoms, and osteoporosis. Several antagonists are effective in cancer chemotherapy. All gonadal hormones are synthesized from the precursor, cholesterol, in a series of steps that include shortening of the hydrocarbon sidechain and hydroxylation of the steroid nucleus. Aromatization is the last step in estrogen synthesis.[1] Figure 25.1 lists the steroid hormones referred to in this chapter.

SEX HORMONES

ESTROGENS
- ***Diethylstilbestrol***
- ***Estradiol***
- ***Estriol***
- ***Estrone***
- ***Ethinyl estradiol***
- ***Mestranol***

SELECTIVE ESTROGEN MODULATORS
- ***Clomiphene***
- ***Raloxifene***
- ***Tamoxifen***
- ***Toremifene***

PROGESTINS
- ***Hydroxyprogesterone***
- ***Medroxyprogesterone***
- ***Norethindrone***
- ***Norgestrel***

ANTIPROGESTIN
- ***Mifepristone***

Figure 25.1
Summary of sex hormones. (Figure continued on next page.)

II. ESTROGENS

Estradiol [ess tra DYE ole], also known as *17-β-estradiol*, is the most potent estrogen produced and secreted by the ovary. The other major estrogens, *estrone* [ESS trone] and *estriol* [essTRI ole], are formed in other tissues, such as the liver and adrenal gland, and have about one tenth the potency of *estradiol*. A preparation of conjugated estrogens containing sulfate esters of *estrone* and *equilin*—obtained from pregnant mare's urine—is a widely used oral preparation. Synthetic estrogens, such as *ethinyl estradiol* [ETH ih nil ess tra DYE ole], undergo less first-pass metabolism than naturally-occurring steroids and, thus, are effective when administered orally at lower doses. Nonsteroidal compounds that bind to estrogen receptors and exert either estrogenic or antiestrogenic effects on target tissues are called selective estrogen-receptor modulators. These include *tamoxifen* and *raloxifene*, among others.

A. Mechanism of action

After dissociation from their binding sites on sex hormone–binding globulin or albumin in the plasma, steroid hormones diffuse across the cell membrane and bind with high affinity to specific nuclear-receptor proteins. [Note: These receptors belong to a large, nuclear hormone–receptor family that includes those for thyroid hormones

INFO LINK [1]See p. 235 in ***Lippincott's Illustrated Reviews: Biochemistry*** (3rd ed.) for a discussion of steroid hormone synthesis.

Lippincott's Illustrated Reviews: Pharmacology, Third Edition, by Richard D. Howland and Mary J. Mycek.

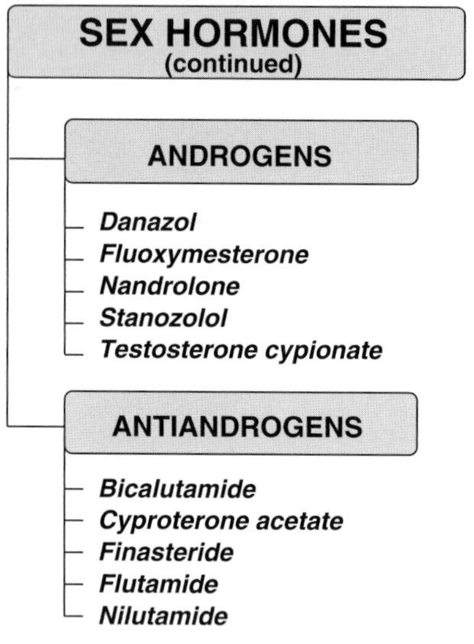

Figure 25.1 (continued)
Summary of sex hormones.

and vitamin D.] Two estrogen-receptor subtypes, α and β, mediate the effects of the hormone; the α receptor may be considered as the classic estrogen receptor. The β receptor is highly homologous to the α receptor. However, the N-terminal portion of the α receptor contains a region that promotes transcription activation, whereas the β receptor contains a repressor domain. As a result, the transcriptional properties of the α and β estrogen receptors are different. Affinity for the receptor type varies with the particular estrogen. These receptor isoforms vary in structure, chromosomal location, and tissue distribution. The activated steroid-receptor complex interacts with nuclear chromatin to initiate hormone-specific RNA synthesis. The attachment of two estrogen-linked receptors to the genome is required for a response. This results in the synthesis of specific proteins that mediate a number of physiologic functions. [Note: The steroid hormones may elicit the synthesis of different RNA species in diverse target tissues and, therefore, are both receptor- and tissue-specific.] Other pathways that require these hormones have been identified that lead to more rapid results. For example, activation of an estrogen receptor in the membranes of hypothalamic cells has been shown to couple to a G-protein, thereby initiating a second messenger cascade.[2] In addition, estrogen-mediated dilation of coronary arteries occurs by the increased formation and release of nitric oxide and prostacyclin in endothelial cells.

B. Therapeutic uses of estrogens

The most frequent uses of estrogens are for contraception, postmenopausal hormone therapy, and osteoporosis. Estrogens are also used extensively for replacement therapy in premonopausal patients who are deficient in this hormone. Such a deficiency can be due to lack of development of the ovaries, menopause, castration. The American College of Obstetrics and Gynecology has stated that the risks of using hormone replacement therapy for postmenopausal women outweigh the benefits, and it recommends that the hormone be prescribed at the lowest effective dose for the shortest possible time to relieve vasomotor symptoms and vaginal atrophy.

1. **Postmenopausal hormone therapy:** Estrogen therapy is generally reserved for menopausal women who are experiencing vasomotor symptoms (for example, "hot flashes"), postmenopausal atrophy, and for women wishing to reduce the risk of osteoporosis (Figure 25.2). For women who have not undergone a hysterectomy, a progestin is always included with the estrogen therapy, because the combination reduces the risk of endometrial carcinoma associated with estrogen treatment alone. For women whose uterus has been surgically removed, unopposed estrogen therapy is recommended, because progestins may unfavorably alter the high-density/low-density lipoprotein (HDL/LDL) ratio.[3] [Note: The amount of estrogen used in replacement therapy is substantially less than the doses used in oral contraception. Thus, the adverse effects of estrogen replacement therapy tend to be less severe than the side effects seen in women who are taking estrogen for contraceptive purposes.] Delivery of *estradiol* by transdermal patch is also effective in treating postmenopausal

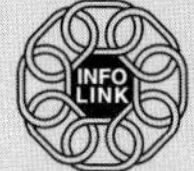

[2]See p. 93 in ***Lippincott's Illustrated Reviews: Biochemistry*** (3rd ed.) for a discussion of the role of G-proteins and second messengers.
[3]See p. 358 in ***Lippincott's Illustrated Reviews: Biochemistry*** (3rd ed.) for a discussion of LDLs, HDLs, and health.

symptoms. Osteoporosis is effectively treated with estrogen; however, other drugs, such as *alendronate*, are also beneficial. (See p. 337 for a summary of some of the agents that are useful in the treatment of osteoporosis.)

2. **Primary hypogonadism:** Estrogen therapy mimicking the natural cyclic pattern, and usually in combination with progestins, is instituted to stimulate development of secondary sex characteristics in young women (eleven to thirteen years of age) with hypogonadism. Continued treatment is required after growth is completed.

C. Pharmacokinetics

1. **Naturally occurring estrogens:** These agents and their esterified or conjugated derivatives are readily absorbed through the gastrointestinal tract, skin, and mucous membranes. *Estrogen* is also quickly distributed when administered intramuscularly. Taken orally, *estradiol* is rapidly metabolized (and partially inactivated) by the microsomal enzymes of the liver. Micronized estradiol is now available and has better bioavailability. Although there is some first-pass metabolism, it is not sufficient to lessen the effectiveness when taken orally.

2. **Synthetic estrogen analogs:** These compounds, such as *ethinyl estradiol* and *mestranol* [MES trah nole]), are well absorbed after oral administration or through the skin or mucous membranes. *Mestranol* is quickly oxidized to *ethinyl estradiol*, which is metabolized more slowly than the naturally occurring estrogens by the liver and peripheral tissues. Being fat soluble, they are stored in adipose tissue, from which they are slowly released. Therefore, the synthetic estrogen analogs have a prolonged action and a higher potency compared to those of natural estrogens.

3. **Metabolism:** Estrogens are transported in the blood while bound to serum albumin or sex hormone–binding globulin. As mentioned above, bioavailability of *estrogen* taken orally is low due to first-pass metabolism in the liver. To reduce first-pass metabolism, the drugs may be administered by transdermal patch, intravaginally, or by injection. They are hydroxylated in the liver to derivatives that are subsequently glucuronidated or sulfated. The parent drugs and their metabolites undergo excretion into the bile and are then reabsorbed through the enterohepatic circulation. Inactive products are excreted in the urine. [Note: In individuals with liver damage, serum estrogen levels may increase due to reduced metabolism, causing feminization in males or signs of estrogen excess in females.]

D. Adverse effects

Nausea and vomiting are the most common adverse effects of *estrogen* therapy. Postmenopausal uterine bleeding can occur. In addition, thromboembolic problems, myocardial infarction, as well as breast and endometrial cancer occur. Other effects of *estrogen* therapy are shown in Figure 25.3. *Diethylstilbestrol* has been implicated

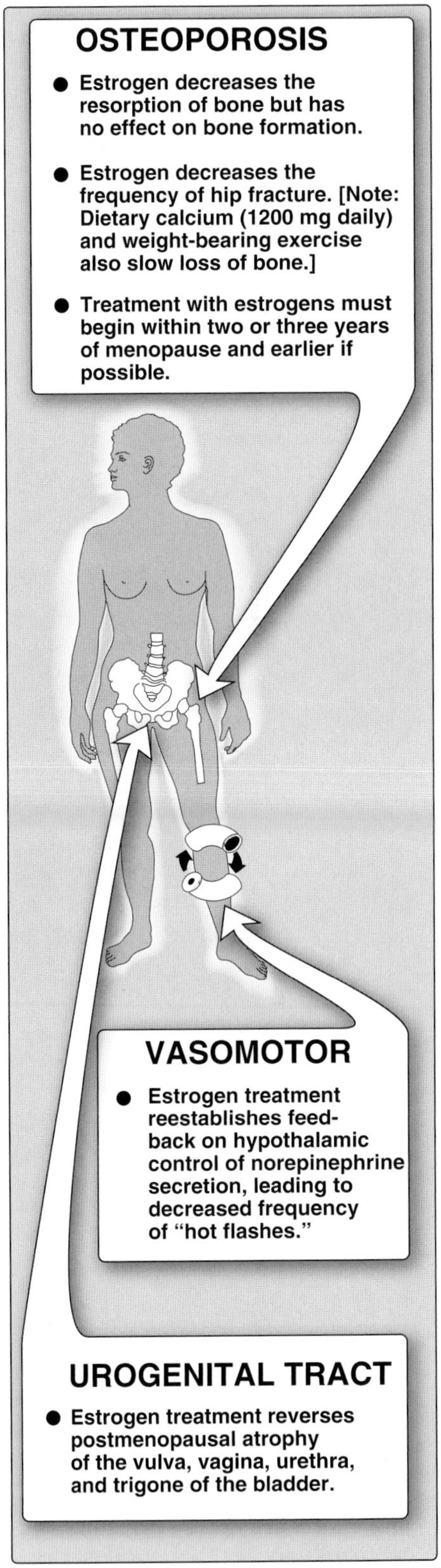

OSTEOPOROSIS

- **Estrogen decreases the resorption of bone but has no effect on bone formation.**
- **Estrogen decreases the frequency of hip fracture. [Note: Dietary calcium (1200 mg daily) and weight-bearing exercise also slow loss of bone.]**
- **Treatment with estrogens must begin within two or three years of menopause and earlier if possible.**

VASOMOTOR

- **Estrogen treatment reestablishes feedback on hypothalamic control of norepinephrine secretion, leading to decreased frequency of "hot flashes."**

UROGENITAL TRACT

- **Estrogen treatment reverses postmenopausal atrophy of the vulva, vagina, urethra, and trigone of the bladder.**

Figure 25.2
Benefits associated with postmenopausal estrogen replacement.

as the possible cause of a rare, clear-cell cervical or vaginal adenocarcinoma observed among the daughters of women who took the drug during early pregnancy.

III. SELECTIVE ESTROGEN RECEPTOR MODULATORS

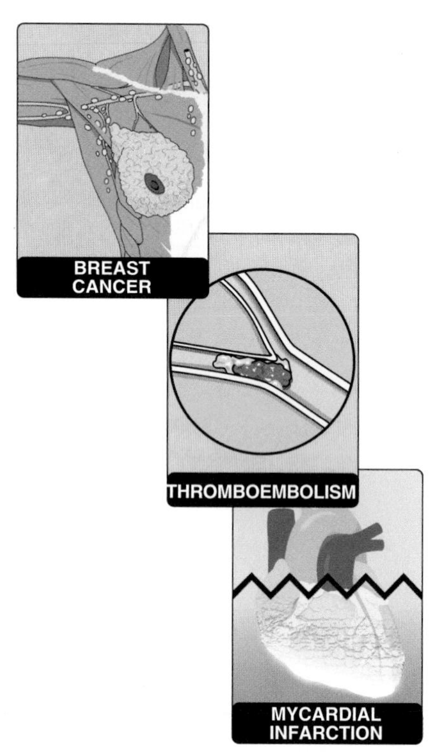

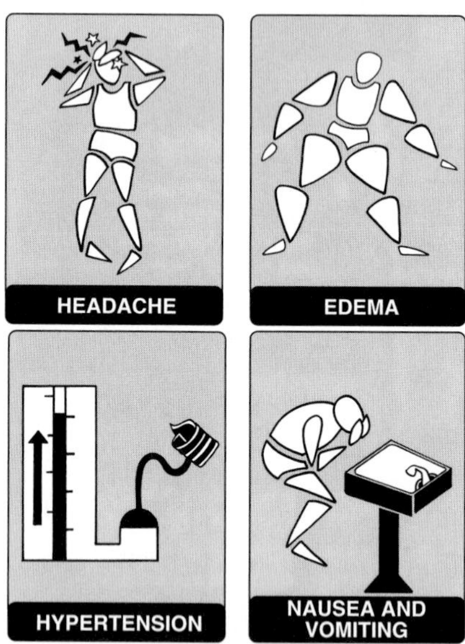

Figure 25.3
Some adverse effects associated with estrogen therapy.

Selective estrogen receptor modulators (SERMs) are a new class of estrogen-related compounds. In the past, a number of these agents had been categorized as antiestrogens, and consequently, there is some confusion. The term SERM is now reserved for compounds that interact at estrogen receptors but have different effects on different tissues; that is, they display selective agonism or antagonism according to the tissue type. For example, *tamoxifen* is an estrogen antagonist in breast cancer tissue but can cause endometrial hyperplasia by acting as a partial agonist in the uterus. Other SERMs are *toremifene* and *raloxifene*. *Clomiphene* is also sometimes designated as a SERM.

A. Tamoxifen

This drug, considered to be the first SERM, competes with the natural hormone for binding to the estrogen receptor and is currently used in the palliative treatment of advanced breast cancer in postmenopausal women. [Note: Normal breast growth is stimulated by estrogens. It is therefore not surprising that some breast tumors regress following treatment with antiestrogens.] The most frequent adverse effects of *tamoxifen* teatment are hot flashes, nausea, and vomiting. Menstrual irregularities and vaginal bleeding can also occur. Due to its estrogenic activity in the endometrium, hyperplasia and malignancies have been reported in women who have been maintained on *tamoxifen*. This has led to limiting the length of time they remain on the drug.

B. Raloxifene

Raloxifene [rah LOX ih feen] is a second generation SERM that is related to *tamoxifen*. Its clinical use is based on its ability to decrease bone resorption and overall bone turnover. Bone density is increased, and vertebral fractures are decreased (Figure 25.4). Unlike *estrogen* and *tamoxifen*, it apparently has little to no effect on the endometrium and, therefore, may not predispose to uterine cancer. *Raloxifene* lowers total cholesterol and LDL in the serum, but it has no effect on HDL or triacylclycerol levels. Whether the latter protects against cardiovascular problems remains to be ascertained. [Note: *Raloxifene* has been reported to increase the risk of thromboembolic episodes, but the benefits are believed to outweigh the risks.] The drug is currently approved only for the preventive treatment of osteoporosis in postmenopausal women, especially those who would prefer not to take *estrogen*. *Raloxifene* reduces the incidence of breast cancer in postmenopausal women. [Note: At the present time, *raloxifene* is not approved for the treatment of breast cancer.]

1. **Pharmacokinetics:** The drug is readily absorbed orally and is rapidly converted to glucuronide conjugates through first-pass metabolism. More than 95 percent of *raloxifene* is bound to

plasma proteins. Both the parent drug and the conjugates undergo enterohepatic cycling. The primary route of excretion is through the bile into the feces.

2. **Adverse effects:** As with the estrogens and *tamoxifen*, the use of *raloxifene* has an increased risk of deep-vein thrombosis, pulmonary embolism, and retinal-vein thrombosis. *Raloxifene* should be avoided in women who are or may become pregnant. In addition, women who have a past or active history of venous thromboembolic events should not take the drug. Coadministration with *cholestyramine* can reduce the absorption of *raloxifene* by sixty percent; therefore, these drugs should not be taken together. In one study, *raloxifene* caused a ten-percent drop in prothrombin time in patients taking *warfarin*. Thus, it is prudent to monitor prothrombin time in these individuals.

C. Toremifene

Toremifene [tor EH mih feen] is a relatively new SERM with properties and side effects similar to those of *tamoxifen*. Unlike the latter, however, *toremifene* does not increase the risk of endometrial cancer. The use of *toremifene* is restricted to postmenopausal women with metastatic breast cancer.

D. Clomiphene

By acting as a partial estrogen agonist and interfering with the negative feedback of estrogens on the hypothalamus and pituitary, *clomiphene* [KLOE mi feen] increases the secretion of gonadotropin-releasing hormone (Gn-RH) and gonadotropins, leading to a stimulation of ovulation. The drug has been used successfully to treat infertility associated with anovulatory cycles, but it is not effective in women whose ovulatory dysfunction is due to pituitary or ovarian failure. Adverse effects are dose-related and include ovarian enlargement, vasomotor flushes, and visual disturbances.

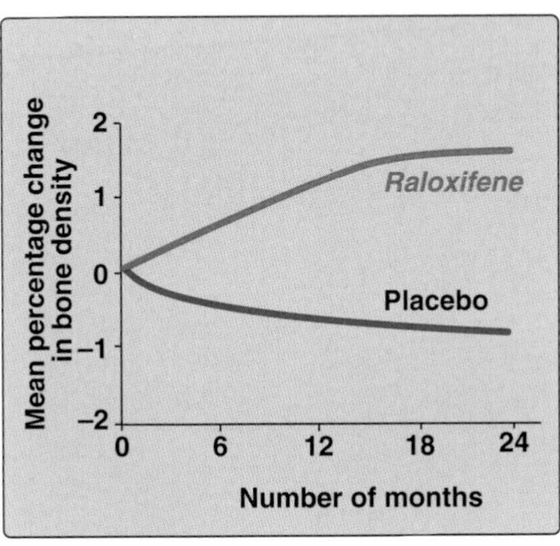

Figure 25.4
Hip bone density increases with *raloxifene* in postmenopausal women.

IV. PROGESTINS

Progesterone, the natural progestin, is produced in response to luteinizing hormone (LH) by both females (secreted by the corpus luteum, primarily during the second half of the menstrual cycle, and by the placenta) and by males (secreted by the testes). It is also synthesized by the adrenal cortex in both sexes. In females, progesterone promotes the development of a secretory endometrium that can accommodate implantation of a newly forming embryo. The high levels of progesterone that are released during the second half of the menstrual cycle (the luteal phase) inhibit the production of gonadotropin and, therefore, further ovulation. If conception takes place, progesterone continues to be secreted, maintaining the endometrium in a favorable state for the continuation of the pregnancy and reducing uterine contractions. If conception does not take place, the release of progesterone from the corpus luteum ceases abruptly. This decline stimulates the onset of menstruation. (Figure 25.5 summarizes the hormones produced during the menstrual cycle.) Progestins exert their mechanism of action in a

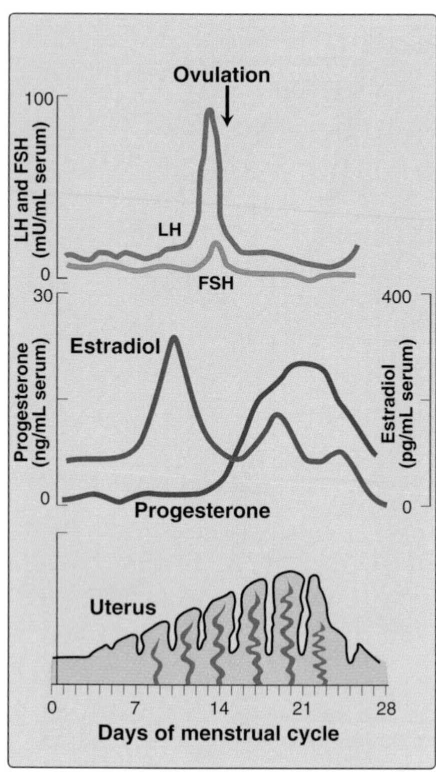

Figure 25.5
The menstrual cycle with plasma levels of pituitary and ovarian hormones and a schematic representation of changes in the morphology of the uterine lining. FSH = follicle-stimulating hormone; LH = luteinizing hormone.

manner analogous to that of the other steroid hormones. They cause: 1) an increase in hepatic glycogen—probably through an insulin-mediated mechanism; 2) a decrease in Na^+ reabsorption in the kidney due to competition with aldosterone at the mineralocorticoid receptor; 3) an increase in body temperature through an unknown mechanism; 4) a decrease in some plasma amino acids; and 5) an increase in excretion of urinary nitrogen.

A. Therapeutic uses of progestins

The major clinical uses of progestins are to rectify a hormonal deficiency and for contraception, in which they are generally used with estrogens, either in combination or in a sequential manner. Progesterone by itself is not used widely as a therapy because of its rapid metabolism, resulting in low bioavailability. Synthetic progestins used in contraception are more stable to first-pass metabolism, allowing for lower doses when administered orally. These agents include *medroxyprogesterone acetate* [me DROK see proe JES ter one], *hydroxyprogesterone acetate* [hye DROK see proe JES ter one], *norethindrone* [nor ETH in drone], and *norgestrel* [nor JES trel]. [Note: *Norethindrone* and *norgestrel* are sometimes called the nortestosterone progestins because of their structural similarity to the androgen. They also possess some androgenic activity.] Other clinical uses of the progestins are in the control of dysfunctional uterine bleeding, treatment of dysmenorrhea, suppression of postpartum lactation, and management of endometriosis. They are also used to treat endometrial carcinomas.

B. Pharmacokinetics

A micronized preparation of *progesterone* is rapidly absorbed after its administration by any route. It has a short half-life in the plasma and is almost completely metabolized by the liver. The glucuronidated metabolite (pregnanediol glucuronide) is excreted by the kidney. Synthetic progestins are less rapidly metabolized. The *hydroxy-* and *medroxyprogesterone* derivatives are injected intramuscularly and have a duration of action of one to two weeks and one to three months, respectively. The other progestins last from one to three days.

C. Adverse effects

The major adverse effects associated with the use of progestins are edema and depression. The androgen-like progestins (the 19-nortestosterone derivatives) can increase the ratio of LDL to HDL cholesterol and cause thrombophlebitis and pulmonary embolism as well as acne, hirsutism, and weight gain. Recent evidence suggests that the incidence of breast cancer increases in women taking an estrogen along with a progestin. However, an increased incidence of breast cancer has not been observed with oral contraceptives.

D. Antiprogestin

Mifepristone [mih feh PRIH stone] (also designated as RU 486) is a progestin antagonist with partial agonist activity. [Note: *Mifepristone* is also a potent antiglucocorticoid.] Administration of this drug to females early in pregnancy results, in most cases (85 percent), in abortion of the fetus due to the interference with progesterone and the decline in human chorionic gonadotropin. The major adverse effects are significant uterine bleeding and the possibility of an incomplete abortion. However, administration of *prostaglandin* E_1 intravaginally, or of *misoprostol* orally, after a single oral dose of *mifepristone* effectively terminates gestation. *Mifepristone* can also be used as a contraceptive, given once a month during the midluteal phase of the cycle, when progesterone is normally high (see Figure 25.5).

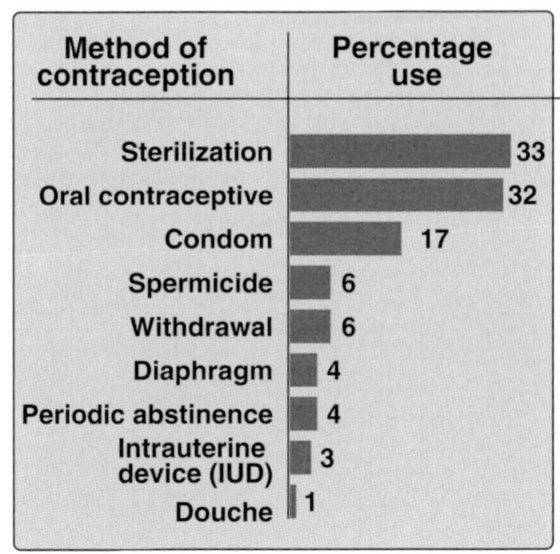

Figure 25.6
Comparison of contraceptive use among United States women ages 15 to 44 years.

V. ORAL AND IMPLANTABLE CONTRACEPTIVES

Drugs are available that decrease fertility by a number of different mechanisms, such as preventing ovulation, impairing gametogenesis or gamete maturation, or interfering with gestation. Currently, interference with ovulation is the most common pharmacologic intervention for preventing pregnancy (Figure 25.6).

A. Major classes of oral contraceptives

1. **Combination pills:** Products containing a combination of an estrogen and a progestin are the most common type of oral contraceptives. Combination pills contain a constant low dose of estrogen given over 21 days, plus a concurrent low but increasing dose of progestin given over three successive seven-day periods (called the "triphasic regimen"). The pills are taken for 21 days followed by a seven day withdrawal period to induce menses. [Note: Estrogens that are commonly present in the combination pills are *ethinyl estradiol* and *mestranol*. The preponderant progestin in these preparations is *norethindrone*.] These preparations are highly effective in achieving contraception (Figure 25.7).

2. **Progestin pills:** Products containing a progestin only, usually *norethindrone* or *norgestrel* (called a "mini-pill"), are taken daily on a continuous schedule. Progestin-only pills deliver a low, continuous dosage of drug. These preparations are less effective than the combination pill (see Figure 25.7), and may produce irregular menstrual cycles more frequently than the combination product. The progestin-only pill has limited patient acceptance, because of anxiety over the increased possibility of pregnancy and the frequent occurrence of menstrual irregularities.

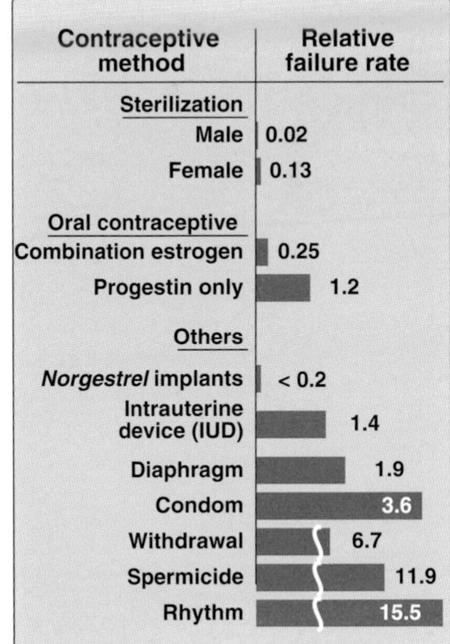

Figure 25.7
Comparison of failure rate for various methods of contraception. Longer bars indicate a higher failure rate—that is, more pregnancies.

3. **Progestin implants:** Subdermal capsules containing *levonorgestrel* offer long-term contraception. Six capsules, each the size of a matchstick, are placed subcutaneously in the upper arm. The progestin is slowly released from the capsules, providing contraceptive protection for approximately five years. The implant is cheaper than oral contraceptives, nearly as reliable as sterilization, and totally reversible if the implants are surgically removed. Once the progestin-containing capsules are implanted, this method of contraception does not rely on patient compliance. This may, in part, explain the low failure rate for this method. For example, Figure 25.8 shows that use of *levonorgestrel* implants by ado-

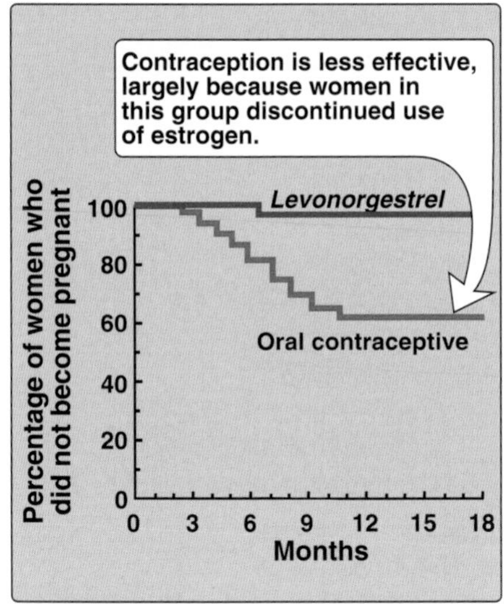

Figure 25.8
Superiority of *levonorgestrel* for preventing pregnancy in adolescent mothers.

lescent mothers results in significantly lower rates of new pregnancies when compared to women using oral contraceptives. Principal side effects of the implants are irregular menstrual bleeding and headaches.

4. **Postcoital contraception:** A fourth type of contraceptive strategy uses estrogen (for example, *ethinyl estradiol* or *mestranol*) administered within 72 hours of coitus and continued twice daily for five days (the "morning-after" pill). Alternatively, two doses of *ethinyl estradiol* plus *norgestrel* are given within 72 hours of coitus, followed by another two doses twelve hours later. A single dose of *mifepristone* has also been used.

B. Mechanism of action

The mechanism of action for these contraceptives is not completely understood. It is likely that the combination of estrogen and progestin administered over an approximately three-week period inhibits ovulation. [Note: The estrogen provides a negative feedback on the release of LH and follicle-stimulating hormone (FSH) by the pituitary gland, thus preventing ovulation. The progestin stimulates normal bleeding at the end of the menstrual cycle and thickens the cervical mucus, thus preventing access by sperm.]

C. Adverse effects

Most adverse effects are believed to be due to the estrogen component, but cardiovascular effects reflect the action of both estrogen and progestin. The incidence of side effects with oral contraceptives is relatively low and is determined by the specific compounds and combinations used.

1. **Major adverse effects:** The major side effects are breast fullness, depression, dizziness, edema, headache, nausea, and vomiting .

2. **Cardiovascular:** The most serious side effect of oral contraceptives is cardiovascular disease, including thromboembolism, thrombophlebitis, hypertension, increased incidences of myocardial infarction, and cerebral and coronary thrombosis. These adverse effects are most common among women who smoke and who are older than 35 years, although they may affect women of any age.

3. **Carcinogenicity:** Oral contraceptives have been shown to decrease the incidence of endometrial and ovarian cancer. Their ability to induce other neoplasms is controversial. The production of benign tumors of the liver that may rupture and hemorrhage is rare.

4. **Metabolic:** Decreased dietary carbohydrate absorption by the intestine is sometimes associated with oral contraceptives, along with an increased incidence of abnormal glucose tolerance tests (similar to the changes seen in pregnancy). Weight gain is common in women who are taking the *nortestosterone* derivatives.

5. **Serum lipids:** The combination pill causes a change in the serum lipoprotein profile: estrogen causes an increase in HDL and a decrease in LDL (a desirable occurrence), whereas progestins have the opposite effect. [Note: The potent progestin *norgestrel* causes the greatest increase in the LDL/HDL ratio. Therefore, estrogen-dominant preparations are best for individuals with elevated serum cholesterol.] Cholestatic jaundice, cholecystitis, and cholangitis are also encountered.

6. **Contraindications:** Oral contraceptives are contraindicated in the presence of cerebrovascular and thromboembolic disease, estrogen-dependent neoplasms, liver disease, and migraine headache.

VI. ANDROGENS

The androgens are a group of steroids that have anabolic and/or masculinizing effects in both males and females. Testosterone [tess TOSS te rone], the most important androgen in humans, is synthesized by Leydig cells in the testes and, in smaller amounts, by cells in the ovary of the female and by the adrenal gland. Other androgens secreted by the testis are 5-α-dihydrotestosterone (DHT), androstenedione, and dehydroepiandrosterone (DHEA) in small amounts. In adult males, testosterone secretion by Leydig cells is controlled by gonadotropin-releasing hormone from the hypothalamus, which stimulates the anterior pituitary gland to secrete FSH and LH. [Note: LH stimulates steroidogenesis in the Leydig cells, whereas FSH is necessary for spermatogenesis.] Testosterone or its active metabolite, DHT, inhibits production of these specific trophic hormones and, thus, regulates testosterone production (Figure 25.9). The androgens are required for 1) normal maturation in the male, 2) sperm production, 3) increased synthesis of muscle proteins and hemoglobin, and 4) decreased bone resorption. Synthetic modifications of the androgen structure are designed to modify solubility and susceptibility to enzymatic breakdown (thus prolonging the half-life of the hormone) and separate anabolic and androgenic effects.

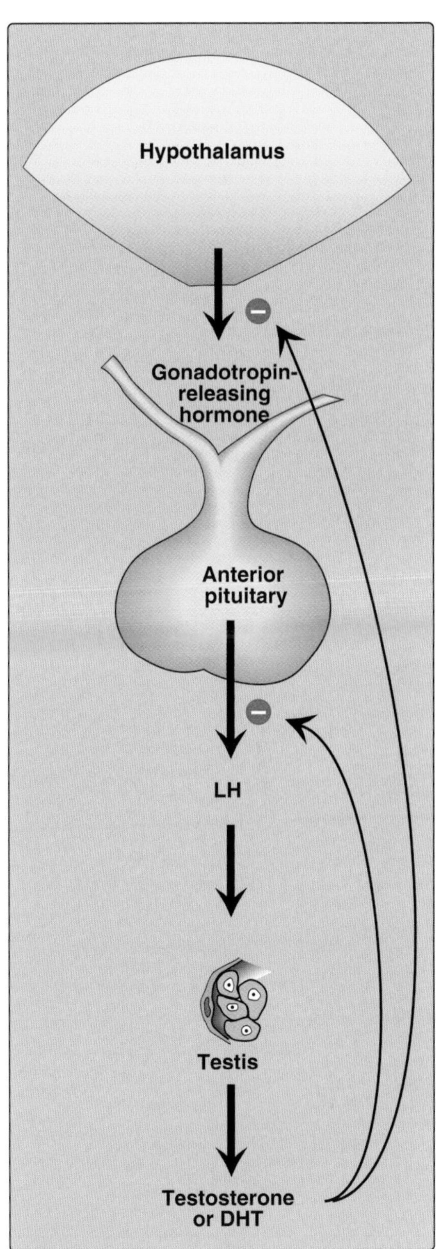

Figure 25.9
Regulation of secretion of testosterone. DHT = 5-α-dihydro testosterone; LH = luteinizing hormone.

A. Mechanism of action

Like the estrogens and progestins, androgens bind to a specific nuclear receptor in a target cell. Although testosterone itself is the active ligand in muscle and liver, in other tissues it must be metabolized to derivatives such as DHT. For example, after diffusing into the cells of the prostate, seminal vesicles, epididymis, and skin, testosterone is converted by 5-α-reductase to DHT, which binds to the receptor. In the brain, liver, and adipose tissue, testosterone is biotransformed to estradiol by cytochrome P450 aromatase. The hormone-receptor complex binds to DNA and stimulates the synthesis of specific RNAs and proteins. [Note: Testosterone analogs that cannot be converted to DHT have less effect on the reproductive system than they do on the skeletal musculature.]

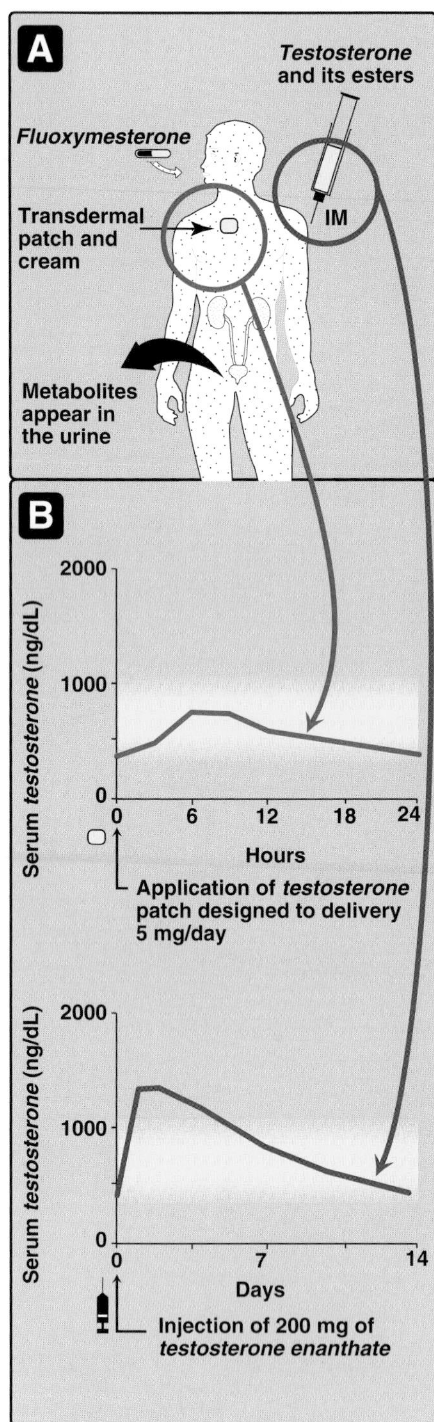

Figure 25.10
A. Administration and fate of androgens. B. Serum testosterone concentrations after administration by injection or transdermal patch to hypogonadal men. Yellow indicates the upper and lower limits of normal range.

B. Therapeutic uses

1. **Androgenic effects:** Androgenic steroids are used for males with inadequate androgen secretion. [Note: Hypogonadism can be due to Leydig cell dysfunction or, secondarily, to failure of the hypothalamic-pituitary unit. In each instance, androgen therapy is indicated.]

2. **Anabolic effects:** Anabolic steroids can be used to treat senile osteoporosis and severe burns, to speed recovery from surgery or chronic debilitating diseases, and to counteract the catabolic effects of externally administered adrenal cortical hormones. [Note: Therapy is combined with proper diet and exercise.]

3. **Growth:** Androgens are used in conjunction with other hormones to promote skeletal growth in prepubertal boys with pituitary dwarfism.

4. **Endometriosis:** *Danazol* [DAH nah zole], a mild androgen, is used in the treatment of endometriosis (ectopic growth of the endometrium). It inhibits several of the enzymes in the hormone synthetic pathway but has no effect on the aromatase. Weight gain, acne, decreased breast size, deepening voice, increased libido, and increased hair growth are among the adverse effects. *Danazole* has been reported occasionally to suppress adrenal function.

5. **Unapproved use:** Androgenic steroids are used to increase lean body mass, muscle strength, and aggressiveness in athletes and body builders (see below). In some popular publications, *DHEA* (a precursor of testosterone and estrogen) has been touted as the anti-aging hormone as well as a "performance enhancer." With its ready availability in health food stores, the drug has been abused. There is no definitive evidence that it slows aging, however, or that it improves performance at normal therapeutic doses.

C. Pharmacokinetics

1. **Testosterone:** This agent is ineffective orally because of inactivation by first-pass metabolism. As with the other sex steroids, *testosterone* is rapidly absorbed by the liver and other tissues, and is metabolized to relatively or completely inactive compounds that are excreted primarily in the urine but also in the feces. *Testosterone* and its C_{17}-esters (for example, *testosterone cypionate* or *enanthate*) are administered intramuscularly. [Note: The addition of the esterified lipid makes the hormone more lipid-soluble, thereby increasing its duration of action.] Transdermal patches, topical gels, and buccal tablets of *testosterone* are also available. Figure 25.10 shows serum levels of testosterone achieved by injection and by a transdermal patch in hypgonadal men. *Testosterone* and its esters demonstrate a 1:1 relative ratio of androgenic to anabolic activity.

2. **Testosterone derivatives:** Agents such as *fluoxymesterone* [floo ox ee MESS teh rone] also have a longer half-life in the body than

that of the naturally occurring androgen. *Fluoxymesterone* is effective when given orally, and it has a 1:2 androgenic to anabolic ratio. Because it is not readily converted to DHT, it is less active than *testosterone* in the reproductive system and does not induce puberty. It has a longer half-life than that of *testosterone*.

D. Adverse effects

1. **In females:** Androgens can cause masculinization, with acne, growth of facial hair, deepening of the voice, male pattern baldness, and excessive muscle development. Menstrual irregularities may also occur. *Testosterone* should not be used by pregnant women because of possible virilization of the female fetus.

2. **In males:** Excess androgens can cause priapism, impotence, decreased spermatogenesis, and gynecomastia. Cosmetic changes such as those described for females may also occur. Androgens can also stimulate growth of the prostate.

3. **In children:** Androgens can cause abnormal sexual maturation and growth disturbances resulting from premature closing of the epiphyseal plates.

4. **General effects:** Androgens increase serum LDL and lower serum HDL levels; therefore, they increase the LDL/HDL ratio and potentially increase the risk for premature coronary heart disease. Androgens can also cause fluid retention leading to edema.

5. **In athletes:** Use of anabolic steroids, (for example, *DHEA*, *nandrolone* NAN dro lone], or *stanozolol* [stan OH zoe lol] by athletes can cause premature closing of the epiphysis of the long bones, which stunts growth and interrupts development. The high doses taken by these young athletes may result in reduction of testicular size, hepatic abnormalities, increased aggression ("roid rage"), and psychotic episodes, and the other adverse effects described above.

E. Antiandrogens

Antiandrogens counter male hormonal action by interfering with the synthesis of androgens or by blocking their receptors. For example, at high doses, the antifungal drug *ketoconazole* inhibits several of the cytochrome P450 enzymes involved in steroid synthesis. *Finasteride* [fin AS ter ide], the steroid-like drug approved for the treatment of benign prostatic hypertrophy, inhibits 5-α-reductase. The resulting decrease in formation of DHT in the prostate leads to a reduction in prostate size. Antiandrogens, such as *cyproterone acetate* [SYE proe te rone] and *flutamide* [FLOO tah mide], act as competitive inhibitors of androgens at the target cell. *Cyproterone acetate* has been used to treat hirsutism in females, whereas *flutamide* is used in the treatment of prostatic carcinoma in males. Two other potent antiandrogens, *bicalutamide* [bye ka LOO ta mide] and *nilutamide* [nye LOO tah mide], are effective orally for the treatment of metastatic prostate cancer.

α_1-Adrenergic antagonists

- ***Terazosin, doxazosin, tamsulosin,*** **and *alfuzosin* relieve outlet obstruction of the bladder by reducing the tension of prostatic smooth muscle in the prostate, prostate capsule, and bladder neck.**
- **The most important side effects are orthostatic hypotension and dizziness.**

5-α-Reductase inhibitors

- ***Finasteride*** **and *dutasteride* act by reducing the size of the prostate gland. Treatment for 6 to 12 months is generally needed before prostate size is sufficiently reduced to improve symptoms.**
- **The major side effects of the α_1-adrenergic antagonists are decreased libido and ejaculatory or erectile dysfunction.**

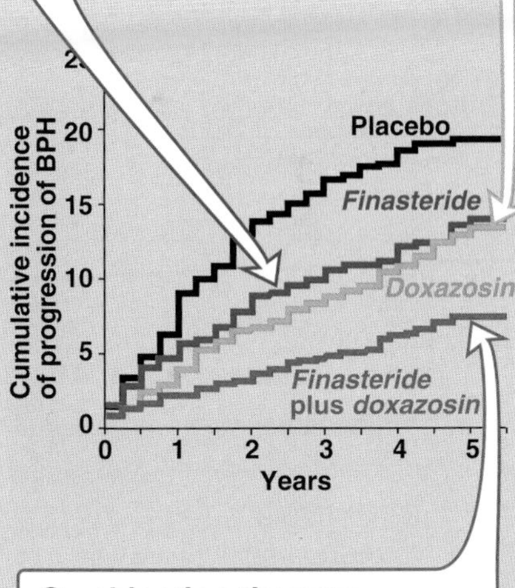

Combination therapy

- **Combination therapy with an α_1-adrenergic antagonist plus a 5-α-reductase inhibitor produces the greatest reduction in the symptoms of BPH, such as acute urinary retention, urinary incontinence, renal insufficiency, or recurrent urinary tract infections.**

Figure 25.11
Therapy for benign prostatic hyperplasia (BPH).

Study Questions

Choose the ONE best answer.

25.1 Young athletes who abuse androgens should be made aware of the side effects of these drugs. Which one of the following is, however, not of concern?

A. Increased muscle mass
B. Anemia due to bone marrow failure
C. Overly aggressive behavior
D. Decreased spermatogenesis
E. Stunted growth

Correct answer = B. Anabolic steroids stimulate the bone marrow and have been used in the treatment of anemia. Erythropoietin has largely replaced them in this regard. All the others are possible problems stemming from androgen abuse.

25.2 A 70-year-old woman is being treated with raloxifene for osteoporosis. There is an increased risk of her developing:

A. breast cancer.
B. uterine cancer.
C. vein thrombosis.
D. atrophic vaginitis.
E. hypercholesterolemia.

Correct answer = C. Unlike estrogen and tamoxifen, raloxifene does not result in an increased incidence of breast or uterine cancer. It lowers cholesterol, and the incidence of vaginitis is essentially the same as that in patients taking a placebo.

25.3 A 23-year-old woman has failed to become pregnant after two years of unprotected intercourse. Which of the following would be effective in treating infertility due anovulatory cycles?

A. A combination of an estrogen and progestin
B. Estrogen alone
C. Clomiphene
D. Raloxifene

Correct answer = C. Clomiphene is a SERM that increases the secretion of gonadotropin-releasing hormone and gonadotropins by inhibiting the negative feedback caused by estrogens. The other treatments would have the opposite effect.

25.4 Treatment with which of the following is inappropriate for treating osteoporosis?

A. Dehydroepiandrosterone
B. Estradiol
C. Tamoxifen
D. Norethindrone
E. Mestranol

Correct answer = D. Norethindrone is a progestin and has no effect on bone resorption. Estradiol, tamoxifen, and mestranol (a synthetic estrogen) can decrease bone resorption, as can the synthetic androgen DHEA, which is converted to testosterone in the body.

25.5 Estrogen replacement therapy in menopausal women:

A. restores bone loss accompanying osteoporosis.
B. may induce “hot flashes.”
C. may cause atrophic vaginitis.
D. is most effective if instituted at the first signs of menopause.
E. requires higher doses of estrogen than with oral contraceptive therapy.

Correct answer = D. Estrogens decrease, but do not restore, the age-related loss of bone. Vasomotor symptoms of menopause, such as hot flashes, are decreased with estrogen replacement therapy. Symptoms of menopause, such as atrophic vaginitis, are decreased with estrogen replacement therapy. Oral contraceptives contain higher doses of estrogen than are used with estrogen replacement therapy.

Adrenocorticosteroid Hormones

26

I. OVERVIEW

The adrenal gland consists of the cortex and the medulla. The latter secretes epinephrine, whereas the cortex, the subject of this chapter, synthesizes and secretes two major classes of steroid hormones—the adrenocorticosteroids (glucocorticoids and mineralocorticoids; Figure 26.1), and the adrenal androgens. The adrenal cortex is divided into three zones that synthesize various steroids from cholesterol and then secrete them (Figure 26.2). The outer zona glomerulosa produces mineralocorticoids (for example, aldosterone), which are responsible for regulating salt and water metabolism. Production of aldosterone is regulated primarily by the renin-angiotensin system (see p. 214). The middle zona fasciculata synthesizes glucocorticoids (for example, cortisol), which are involved with normal metabolism and resistance to stress. The inner zona reticularis secretes adrenal androgens (for example, dehydroepiandrosterone). Secretion by the two inner zones and, to some extent, the outer zone is controlled by pituitary corticotropin (ACTH), which is released in response to the hypothalamic corticotropin-releasing hormone (CRH; also called corticotropin-releasing factor). Glucocorticoids serve as feedback inhibitors of corticotropin and CRH secretion. Hormones of the adrenal cortex are used in replacement therapy; in the treatment and management of asthma as well as other inflammatory diseases, such as rheumatoid arthritis; in the treatment of severe allergic reactions; and in the treatment of some cancers.

ADRENAL CORTICOSTEROIDS

CORTICOSTEROIDS

- ***Beclomethasone***
- ***Betamethasone***
- ***Cortisone***
- ***Desoxycorticosterone***
- ***Dexamethasone***
- ***Fludrocortisone***
- ***Hydrocortisone***
- ***Methylprednisolone***
- ***Paramethasone***
- ***Prednisolone***
- ***Prednisone***
- ***Triamcinolone***

INHIBITORS OF ADRENOCORTICOID BIOSYNTHESIS OR FUNCTION

- ***Aminoglutethimide***
- ***Eplerenone***
- ***Ketoconazole***
- ***Metyrapone***
- ***Mifepristone***
- ***Spironolactone***
- ***Trilostane***

Figure 26.1
Summary of adrenal corticosteroids.

II. ADRENOCORTICOSTEROIDS

The adrenocorticoids bind to specific intracellular cytoplasmic receptors in target tissues. [Note: The glucocorticoid receptor is widely distributed throughout the body, whereas the mineralocorticoid receptor is confined to excretory organs, such as the kidney, colon, and salivary and sweat glands.] After dimerizing, the receptor-hormone complex translocates into the nucleus, where it attaches to gene promoter elements, acting

Lippincott's Illustrated Reviews: Pharmacology, Third Edition,
by Richard D. Howland and Mary J. Mycek.

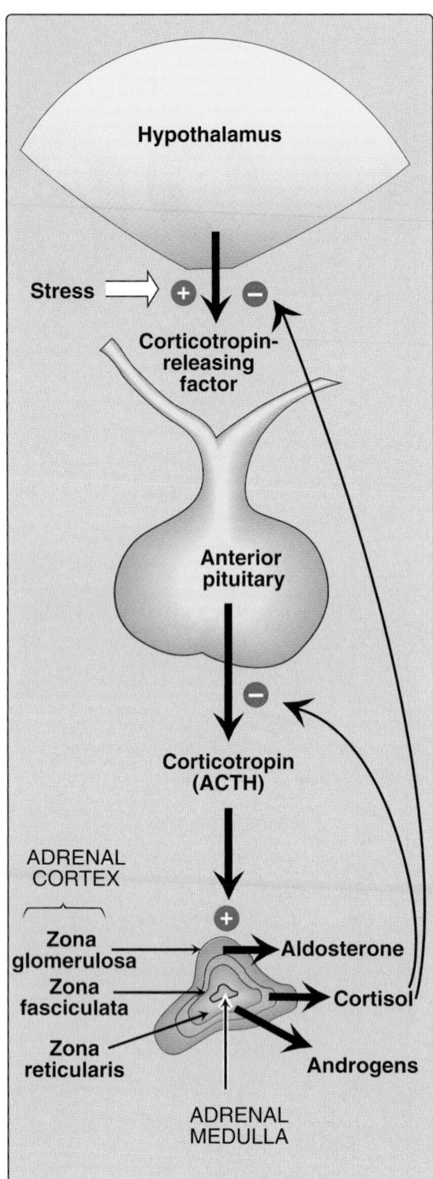

Figure 26.2
Regulation of corticosteroid secretion.

as a transcription factor to turn genes on or off, depending on the tissue (Figure 26.3). This mechanism requires time to produce an effect, but other glucocorticoid effects, such as their interaction with catecholamines to mediate dilation of vascular and bronchial musculature or lipolysis, have effects that are immediate. Some normal actions and some selected mechanisms of adrenocorticoids are described in this section. Understanding these actions aids the reader in better comprehending the results of adrenal insufficiency and the uses of adrenocorticoids as therapeutic agents in a variety of disorders.

A. Glucocorticoids

Cortisol is the principal human glucocorticoid. Normally, its production is diurnal, with a peak early in the morning followed by a decline and then a secondary, smaller peak in the late afternoon. Factors such as stress and levels of the circulating steroid influence secretion. The effects of cortisol are many and diverse. In general, all glucocorticoids:

1. **Promote normal intermediary metabolism:** Glucocorticoids favor gluconeogenesis through increasing amino acid uptake by the liver and kidney and elevating activities of gluconeogenic enzymes. They stimulate protein catabolism (except in the liver) and lipolysis, thereby providing the building blocks and energy that are needed for glucose synthesis. [Note: Glucocorticoid insufficiency may result in hypoglycemia (for example, during stressful periods or fasting).] Lipolysis results as a consequence of the glucocorticoid augmenting the action of growth hormone on adipocytes, causing an increase in the activity of hormone-sensitive lipase.

2. **Increase resistance to stress:** By raising plasma glucose levels, glucocorticoids provide the body with the energy it requires to combat stress caused, for example, by trauma, fright, infection, bleeding, or debilitating disease. Glucocorticoids can cause a modest rise in blood pressure, apparently by enhancing the vasoconstrictor action of adrenergic stimuli on small vessels. [Note: Individuals with adrenal insufficiency may respond to severe stress by becoming hypotensive.]

3. **Alter blood cell levels in plasma:** Glucocorticoids cause a decrease in eosinophils, basophils, monocytes, and lymphocytes by redistributing them from the circulation to lymphoid tissue. In contrast to this effect, they increase the blood levels of hemoglobin, erythrocytes, platelets, and polymorphonuclear leukocytes. [Note: The decrease in circulating lymphocytes and macrophages compromises the body's ability to fight infections. However, this property is important in the treatment of leukemia (see p. 473).]

4. **Have anti-inflammatory action:** The most important therapeutic property of the glucocorticoids is their ability to dramatically reduce the inflammatory response and to suppress immunity. The exact mechanism is complex and incompletely understood. However, the lowering and inhibition of peripheral lymphocytes

and macrophages is known to play a role. Also involved is the indirect inhibition of phospholipase A_2 (due to the steroid-mediated elevation of lipocortin), which blocks the release of arachidonic acid—the precursor of the prostaglandins and leukotrienes—from membrane-bound phospholipid. Cyclooxygenase-II synthesis in inflammatory cells is further reduced, lowering the availability of prostaglandins. In addition, interference in mast cell degranulation results in decreased histamine and capillary permeability.

5. **Affect other components of the endocrine system:** Feedback inhibition of corticotropin production by elevated glucocorticoids causes inhibition of further glucocorticoid synthesis as well as further production of thyroid-stimulating hormone. In contrast, growth hormone production is increased.

6. **Effects on other systems:** Adequate cortisol levels are essential for normal glomerular filtration. However, the effects of corticosteroids on other systems are mostly associated with the adverse effects of the hormones. High doses of glucocorticoids stimulate gastric acid and pepsin production and may exacerbate ulcers. Effects on the central nervous system that influence mental status have been identified. Chronic glucocorticoid therapy can cause severe bone loss. Myopathy leads patients to complain of weakness.

B. Mineralocorticoids

Mineralocorticoids help to control the body's water volume and concentration of electrolytes, especially sodium and potassium. Aldosterone acts on kidney tubules and collecting ducts, causing a reabsorption of sodium, bicarbonate, and water. Conversely, aldosterone decreases reabsorption of potassium, which, with H^+, is then lost in the urine. Enhancement of sodium reabsorption by aldosterone also occurs in gastrointestinal mucosa and in sweat and salivary glands. [Note: Elevated aldosterone levels may cause alkalosis and hypokalemia, whereas retention of sodium and water leads to an increase in blood volume and blood pressure. Hyperaldosteronism is treated with *spironolactone*.] Target cells for aldosterone action contain mineralocorticoid receptors that interact with the hormones in a manner analogous to that of the glucocorticoid receptor (see above).

C. Therapeutic uses of the adrenal corticosteroids

Several semisynthetic derivatives of the glucocorticoids have been developed that vary in their anti-inflammatory potency, degree to which they cause sodium retention, and duration of action. These are summarized in Figure 26.4.

1. **Replacement therapy for primary adrenocortical insufficiency (Addison disease):** This disease is caused by adrenal cortex dysfunction (as diagnosed by the lack of patient response to *corticotropin* administration). *Hydrocortisone* [hye droe KOR ti sone], which is identical to the natural cortisol, is given to correct the deficiency. Failure to do so results in death. The dosage of *hydrocortisone* is divided so that two-thirds of the normal daily dose is

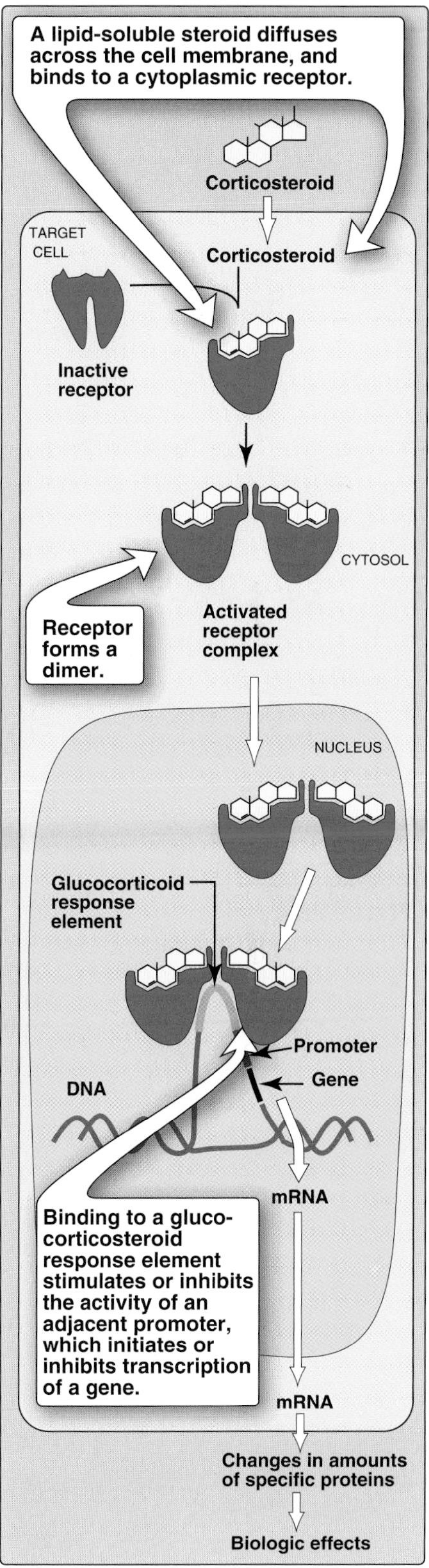

Figure 26.3
Gene regulation by glucocorticoids.

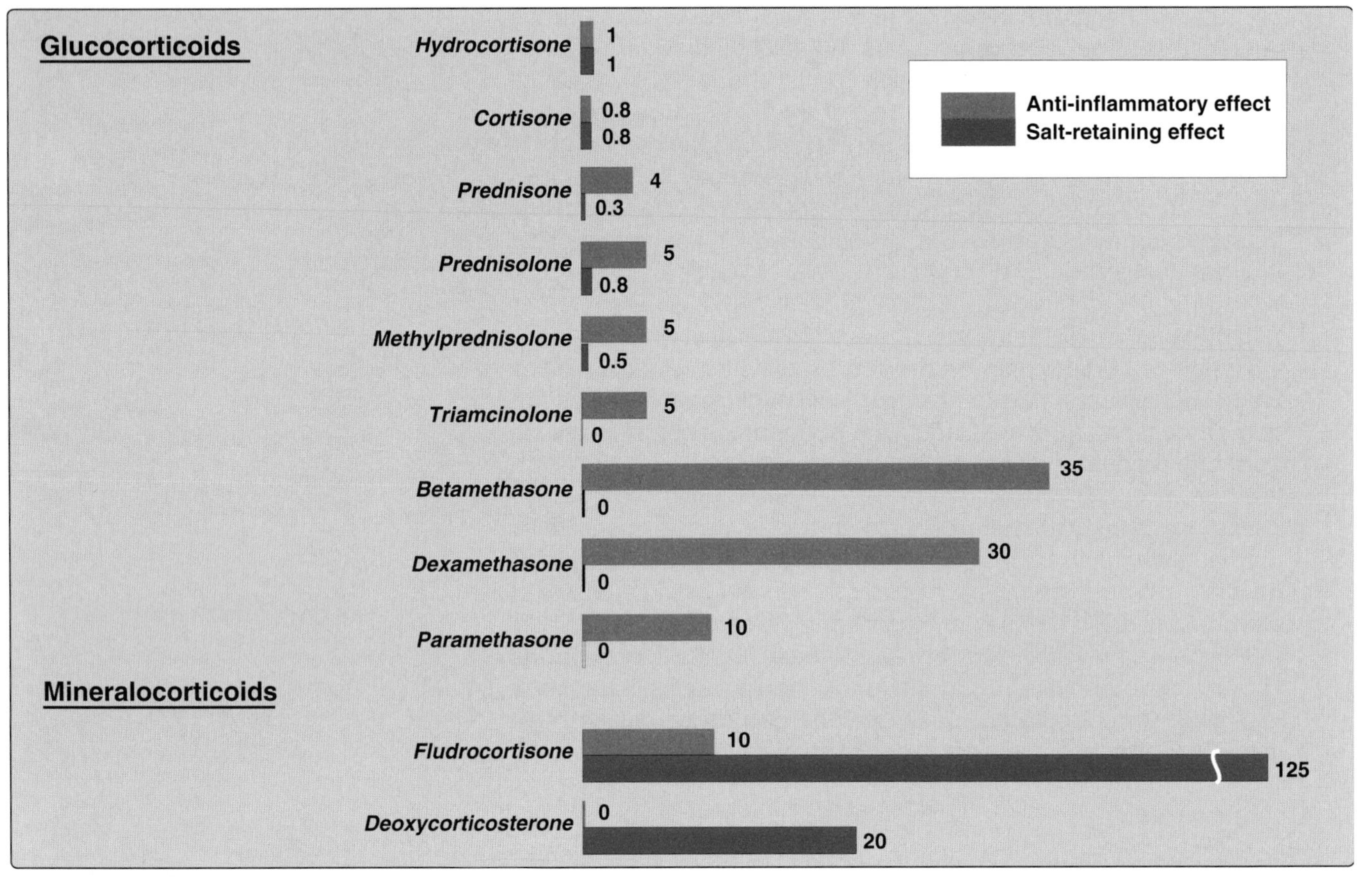

Figure 26.4
Pharmacologic effects and duration of action of some commonly used natural and synthetic corticosteroids. Activities are all relative to *hydrocortisone*, which is considered to be 1. Time refers to duration of action.

given in the morning and one-third is given in the afternoon. [Note: The goal of this regimen is to approximate the daily hormone levels resulting from the circadian rhythm exhibited by cortisol, which causes plasma levels to be maximal around 8 AM, and then to decrease throughout the day to their lowest level around 1 AM] Administration of *fludrocortisone* [floo droe KOR tih sone], a synthetic mineralocorticoid with some glucocorticoid activity, may also be necessary to raise the mineralocorticoid activity to normal levels.

2. **Replacement therapy for secondary or tertiary adrenocortical insufficiency:** These deficiencies are caused by a defect either in CRH production by the hypothalamus or in corticotropin production by the pituitary. [Note: Under these conditions, the synthesis of mineralocorticoids in the adrenal cortex is less impaired than that of glucocorticoids.] The adrenal cortex responds to corticotropin administration by synthesizing and releasing the adrenal corticosteroids. *Hydrocortisone* is also used for these deficiencies.

3. **Diagnosis of Cushing syndrome:** Cushing syndrome is caused by a hypersecretion of glucocorticoids that results either from excessive release of corticotropin by the anterior pituitary or an adrenal

tumor. The *dexamethasone* suppression test is used to diagnose the cause of an individual's case of Cushing syndrome. This synthetic glucocorticoid suppresses cortisol release in individuals with pituitary-dependent Cushing syndrome, but it does not suppress glucocorticoid release from adrenal tumors. [Note: Chronic treatment with high doses of glucocorticoid is a frequent cause of Cushing syndrome.]

4. **Replacement therapy for congenital adrenal hyperplasia:** This is a group of diseases resulting from an enzyme defect in the synthesis of one or more of the adrenal steroid hormones. This condition may lead to virilization in females due to overproduction of adrenal androgens (see below). Treatment of this condition requires administration of sufficient corticosteroids to normalize the patient's hormone levels by suppressing release of CRH and ACTH. This decreases production of adrenal androgens. Choice of replacement hormone depends on the specific enzyme defect.

5. **Relief of inflammatory symptoms:** Glucocorticoids dramatically reduce the manifestations of inflammations (for example, rheumatoid and osteoarthritic inflammations, and inflammatory conditions of the skin), including the redness, swelling, heat, and tenderness that are commonly present at the inflammatory site. The effect of glucocorticoids on the inflammatory process is the result of a number of actions, including the redistribution of leukocytes to other body compartments, thereby lowering their blood concentration; their function is also compromised. Other effects include an increase in the concentration of neutrophils; a decrease in the concentration of lymphocytes (T and B cells), basophils, eosinophils, and monocytes; and an inhibition of the ability of leukocytes and macrophages to respond to mitogens and antigens. The decreased production of prostaglandins and leukotrienes is believed to be central to the anti-inflammatory action. Glucocorticoids also influence the inflammatory response by their ability to reduce the amount of histamine that is released from basophils and mast cells to inhibit kinin activity. [Note: The ability of glucocorticoids to inhibit the immune response is also a result of the other actions described above.]

6. **Treatment of allergies:** Glucocorticoids are beneficial in the treatment of the symptoms of bronchial asthma, allergic rhinitis, and drug, serum, and transfusion allergic reactions. These drugs are not, however, curative. [Note: *Beclomethasone dipropionate* [bek loe METH ah sone], *triamcinolone* [tri am SIN o lone], and others (see Figure 26.4) are applied topically to the respiratory tract through inhalation from a metered-dose dispenser. This minimizes systemic effects and allows the patient to significantly reduce or eliminate the use of oral steroids.]

7. **Acceleration of lung maturation:** Respiratory distress syndrome is a problem in premature infants. Fetal cortisol is a regulator of lung maturation. Consequently, a dose of *beclomethasone* is administered intramuscularly to the mother 48 hours prior to birth followed by a second dose 24 hours before delivery.

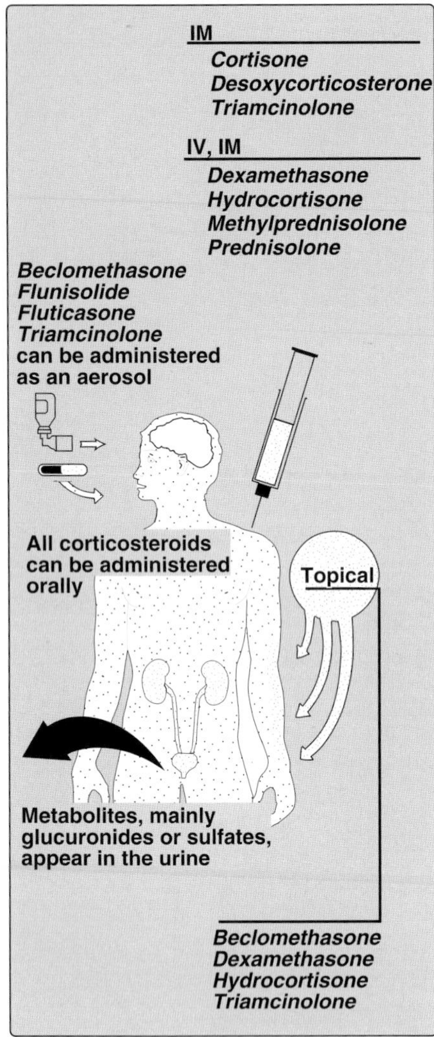

Figure 26.5
Routes of administration and elimination of corticosteriods.

D. Pharmacokinetics

1. **Absorption and fate:** Synthetic glucocorticoid preparations with unique pharmacokinetic characteristics are used therapeutically. Those that are administered orally are readily absorbed from the gastrointestinal tract. Selected compounds can also be administered intravenously, intramuscularly, intra-articularly (for example, into arthritic joints), topically, or as an aerosol for inhalation (Figure 26.5). Greater than ninety percent of the absorbed glucocorticoids are bound to plasma proteins—most to corticosteroid-binding globulin, and the remainder to albumin. Corticosteroids are metabolized by the liver microsomal oxidizing enzymes. The metabolites are conjugated to glucuronic acid or sulfate, and the products are excreted by the kidney. [Note: The half-life of adrenal steroids may increase dramatically in individuals with hepatic dysfunction.] The only glucocorticoid that has no affect on the fetus in pregnancy is *prednisone*. It is a prodrug that is not converted to the active compound, *prednisolone*, in the fetal liver. Any *prednisolone* formed in the mother is biotransformed to *prednisone* by the fetus.

2. **Dosage:** In determining the dosage of adrenocortical steroids, many factors need to be considered, including glucocorticoid versus mineralocorticoid activity, duration of action, type of preparation, and time of day that the steroid is administered. For example, when large doses of the hormone are required over an extended period of time (more than two weeks), suppression of the hypothalamic-pituitary-adrenal (HPA) axis occurs. To prevent this adverse effect, a regimen of alternate-day administration of the adrenocortical steroid may be useful. This schedule allows the HPA axis to recover/function on the days the hormone is not taken.

E. Adverse effects

The common side effects of long-term corticosteroid therapy are summarized in Figure 26.6. Osteoporosis is the most common adverse effect due to the ability of glucocorticoids to suppress intestinal Ca^{2+} absorption, inhibit bone formation, and decrease sex hormone synthesis. Alternate-day dosing does not prevent osteoporosis. Patients are advised to take calcium and vitamin D supplements. Drugs that are effective in treating osteoporosis may also be beneficial. [Note: Increased appetite is not necessarily an adverse effect. In fact, it is one of the reasons for the use of *prednisone* in cancer chemotherapy.] The classic Cushing-like syndrome—redistribution of body fat, puffy face, increased body hair growth, acne, insomnia, and increased appetite—are observed when excess corticosteroids are present. Increased frequency of cataracts also occurs with long-term corticosteroid therapy. Hyperglycemia may develop and lead to diabetes mellitus. Diabetics should monitor their blood glucose and adjust their medications accordingly. Hypokalemia caused by corticosteroid therapy can be counteracted by potassium supplementation. Coadministration of medications that induce or inhibit the hepatic mixed-function oxidases may require adjustment of the glucocorticoid dose.

F. Withdrawal

Withdrawal from these drugs can be a serious problem, because if the patient has experienced HPA suppression, abrupt removal of the corticosteroids causes an acute adrenal insufficiency syndrome that can be lethal. This, coupled with the possibility of psychologic dependence on the drug and the fact that withdrawal might cause an exacerbation of the disease, means the dose must be tapered according to the individual and may be based on trial and error. The patient must be monitored carefully.

G. Inhibitors of adrenocorticoid biosynthesis

Several substances have proven to be useful as inhibitors of the synthesis of adrenal steroids: *metyrapone*, *aminoglutethimide*, *ketoconazole*, *trilostane*, *spironolactone*, and *eplerenone*. *Mifepristone* competes with glucocorticoids for the receptor.

1. **Metyrapone:** *Metyrapone* [me TEER ah pone] is used for tests of adrenal function and can be used for the treatment of pregnant women with Cushing syndrome. [Note: *Dexamethasone* suppression is now used more commonly for diagnosis.] *Metyrapone* interferes with corticosteroid synthesis by blocking the final step (11-hydroxylation) in glucocorticoid synthesis, leading to an increase in 11-deoxycortisol as well as adrenal androgens and the potent mineralocorticoid 11-deoxycorticosterone. The adverse effects encountered with *metyrapone* include salt and water retention, hirsutism, transient dizziness, and gastrointestinal disturbances.

2. **Aminoglutethimide:** This drug acts by inhibiting the conversion of cholesterol to pregnenolone. As a result, the synthesis of all hormonally active steroids is reduced. *Aminoglutethimide* [ah mee noe glu TETH ih mide] has been used therapeutically in the treatment of breast cancer to reduce or eliminate androgen and estrogen production. [Note: *Tamoxifen* has largely replaced *aminoglutethimide* in the treatment of breast cancer.] In these cases, it is used in conjunction with *dexamethasone*. However, it increases the clearance of *dexamethasone*. *Aminoglutethimide* may also be useful in the treatment of malignancies of the adrenal cortex to reduce the secretion of steroids. Recent studies indicate it is an aromatase inhibitor.

3. **Ketoconazole:** *Ketoconazole* [kee toe KON ah zole] is an antifungal agent that strongly inhibits all gonadal and adrenal steroid hormone synthesis. It is used in the treatment of patients with Cushing syndrome.

4. **Trilostane:** *Trilostane* [TRYE loe stane] reversibly inhibits 3-β-hydroxysteroid dehydrogenase and, thus, affects aldosterone, cortisol, and gonadal hormone synthesis. Its side effects are gastrointestinal.

5. **Mifepristone:** At high doses, *mifepristone* is a potent glucocorticoid antagonist as well as an antiprogestin. It forms a complex

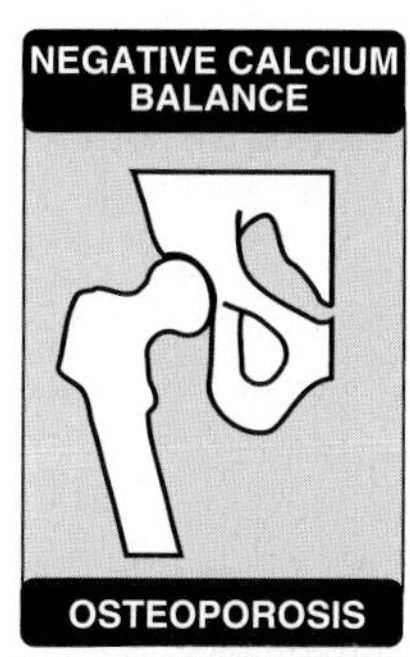

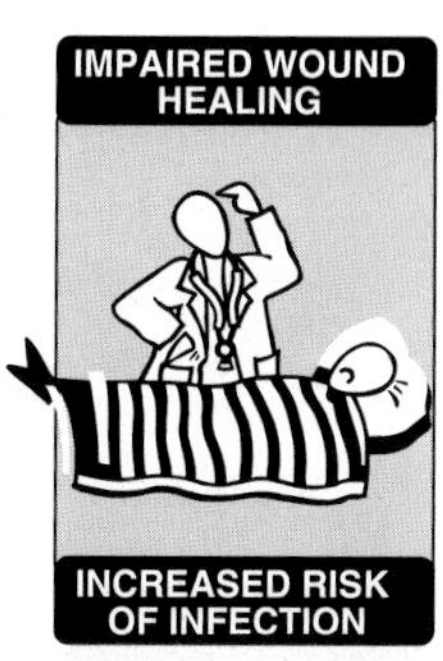

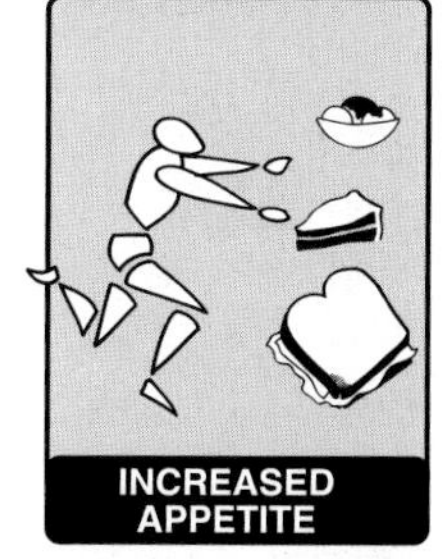

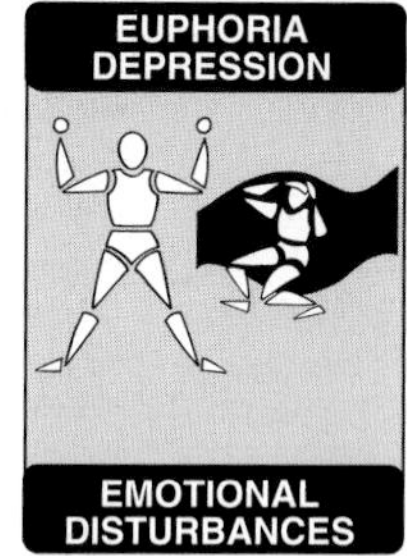

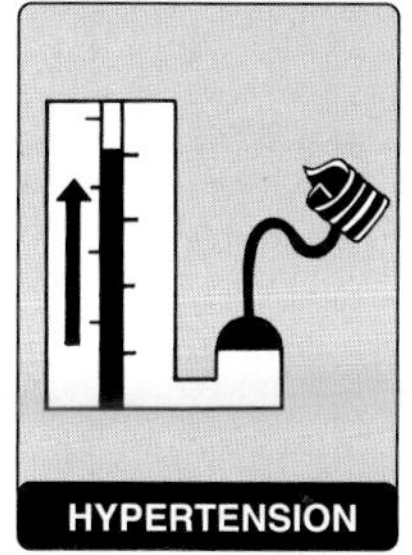

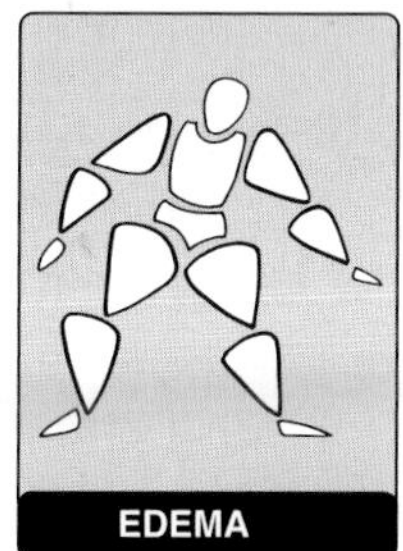

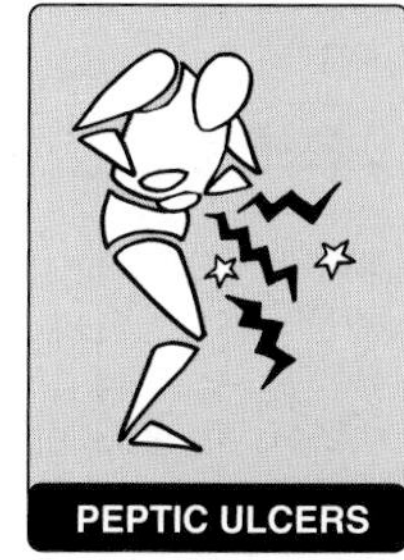

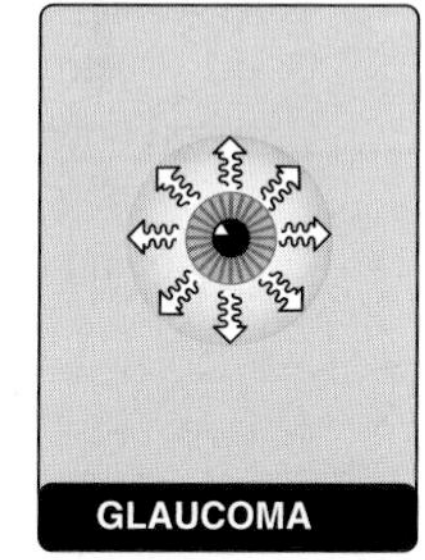

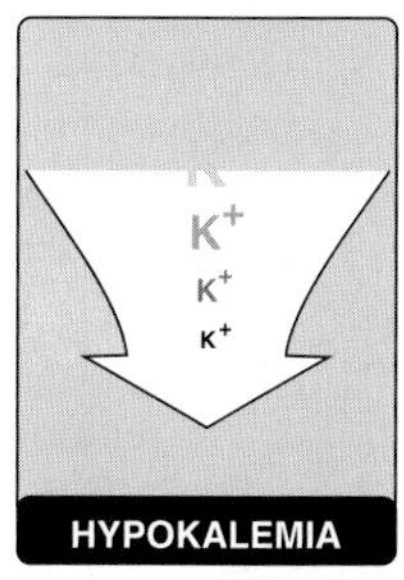

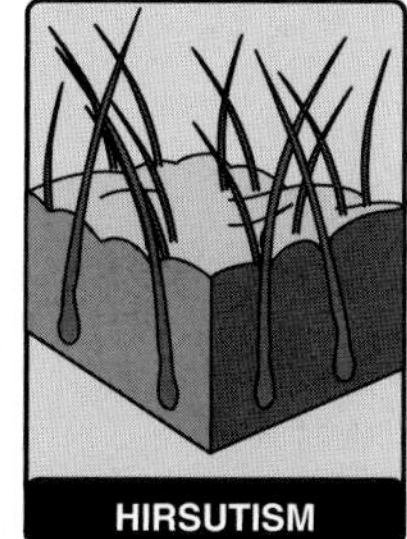

Figure 26.6
Some commonly observed effects of long-term corticosteroid therapy.

with the glucocorticoid receptor, but the rapid dissociation of the drug from the receptor leads to a faulty translocation into the nucleus. Its use is presently limited to treatment of inoperable patients with ectopic ACTH syndrome.

6. **Spironolactone:** This antihypertensive drug competes for the mineralocorticoid receptor and, thus, inhibits sodium reabsorption in the kidney. It can also antagonize aldosterone and testosterone synthesis. It is effective against hyperaldosteronism. *Spironolactone* is also useful in the treatment of hirsutism in women, probably due to interference at the androgen receptor of the hair follicle. Adverse effects include hyperkalemia, gynecomastia, menstrual irregularities, and skin rashes.

7. **Eplerenone:** *Eplerenone* [e PLER en one] specifically binds to the mineralocorticoid receptor, where it acts as an aldosterone antagonist. This specificity avoids the unwanted side effects of *spironolactone.* It is approved as an antihypertensive.

Study Questions

Choose the ONE best answer.

26.1 Measurements of cortisol precursors and plasma dehydroepiandrosterone sulfate confirm the diagnosis of congenital adrenal hyperplasia in a child. This condition can be effectively treated by:

A. suppressing the release of ACTH.
B. administering an androgen antagonist.
C. administering metapyrone to decrease cortisol synthesis.
D. removing the adrenal gland surgically.

Correct answer = A. CAH is the most common disorder of infancy and childhood. Because cortisol synthesis is decreased, feedback inhibition of ACTH formation and release is also decreased, resulting in enhanced ACTH formation. This in turn leads to increased levels of adrenal androgens and/or mineralocorticoids. The treatment is to administer a glucocorticoid, such as hydrocortisone (in infants) or prednisone, which would restore the feedback inhibition. The other options are inappropriate.

26.2 Osteoporosis is a major adverse effect caused by the glucocorticoids. It is due to their ability to:

A. increase the excretion of calcium.
B. inhibit absorption of calcium.
C. stimulate the hypothalamic-pituitary-adrenal axis.
D. decrease production of prostaglandins.

Correct answer = B. Glucocorticoid-induced osteoporosis is attributed to inhibition of calcium absorption as well as bone formation. Increased intake of calcium plus vitamin D or calcitonin, or of other drugs that are effective in this condition, is indicated. Glucocorticoids suppress rather than stimulate the hypothalamic-pituitary-adrenal axis. The decreased production of prostaglandins does not play a role in bone formation.

26.3 A child with asthma is being treated effectively with an inhaled preparation of beclomethasone dipropionate. Which of the following adverse effects is of particular concern?

A. Hypoglycemia
B. Hirsutism
C. Growth suppression
D. Cushing syndrome
E. Cataract formation

Correct answer = C. Growth hormone may be decreased by this treatment. Chronic treatment with the medication therefore may lead to growth suppression, so linear growth should be monitored periodically. Hyperglycemia, not hypoglycemia, is a possible adverse effect. Hirsutism, Cushing syndrome and cataract formation are unlikely with the dose that the child would receive by inhalation.

UNIT V: Drugs Affecting Other Organ Systems

Drugs Affecting the Respiratory System

27

DRUGS AFFECTING THE RESPIRATORY SYSTEM

DRUGS USED TO TREAT ASTHMA

- β_2-Adrenergic agonists
- Corticosteroids
- *Cromolyn* and *nedocromil*
- *Ipratropium*
- *Montelukast, zafirlukast, zileuton*
- *Omalizumab*
- *Theophylline*

DRUGS USED TO TREAT ALLERGIC RHINITIS

- α-Adrenergic agonists
- Antihistamines
- Corticosteroids
- *Cromolyn*

DRUGS USED TO TREAT CHRONIC OBSTRUCTIVE PULMONARY DISEASES

- β-Adrenergic agonists
- Corticosteroids
- *Ipratropium*

DRUGS USED TO TREAT COUGH

- *Dextromethorphan*
- Opiates

Figure 27.1
Summary of drugs affecting the respiratory system.

I. OVERVIEW

Asthma, chronic obstructive pulmonary disease (COPD; also called emphysema), and allergic rhinitis are commonly encountered respiratory diseases. Asthma is a chronic disease that affects ten million patients (four to five percent of the United States population), resulting annually in two million emergency room visits, 500,000 hospitalizations, and 5000 deaths. COPD affects approximately thirty million people in the United States, and is the fourth most common cause of death. Allergic rhinitis is an extremely common condition, affecting approximately twenty percent of the population. Drugs used to treat respiratory diseases can be delivered to the lungs by inhalation, or by oral or parenteral routes. Inhalation is often preferred, because the drug is delivered directly to the target tissue—the airways—and is effective in doses that do not cause significant systemic side effects. Clinically useful drugs act by various mechanisms, such as by relaxing bronchial smooth muscle or modulating the inflammatory response. Drugs used to treat asthma, rhinitis, COPD, and cough—commonly encountered respiratory disorders—are summarized in Figure 27.1.

II. FIRST-LINE DRUGS USED TO TREAT ASTHMA

Asthma is characterized by episodes of acute bronchoconstriction causing shortness of breath, cough, chest tightness, wheezing, and rapid respiration. These acute symptoms may resolve spontaneously or, more often, require therapy, such as a β_2-adrenergic agonist (see p. 72). Asthma, unlike chronic bronchitis, cystic fibrosis, or bronchiectasis, is usually not a progressive disease; that is, it does not inevitably lead to crippling COPD. Rather, the clinical course of asthma is characterized by exacerbations and remissions. Deaths due to asthma are

Lippincott's Illustrated Reviews: Pharmacology, Third Edition,
by Richard D. Howland and Mary J. Mycek.

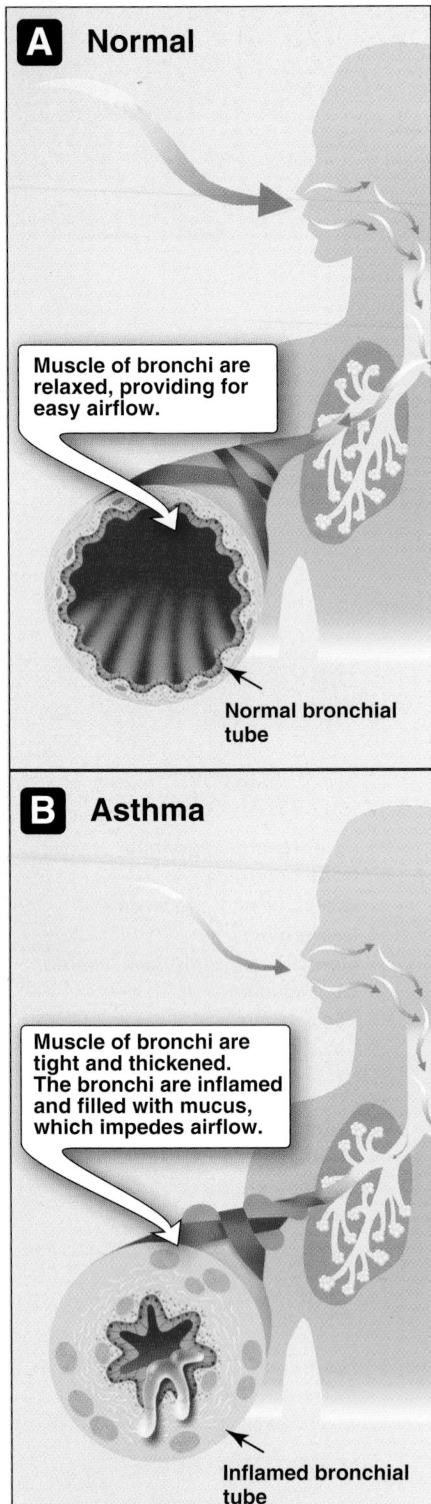

Figure 27.2
Comparison of bronchi of normal and asthmatic individuals.

infrequent, but morbidity results in significant outpatient costs and numerous hospitalizations. The goal of therapy is to relieve symptoms and, if possible, to prevent the recurrence of asthmatic attacks.

A. Role of inflammation in asthma

Airflow obstruction in asthma is due to bronchoconstriction that results from contraction of bronchial smooth muscle, inflammation of the bronchial wall, and increased mucous secretion (Figure 27.2). Asthmatic attacks may be related to recent exposure to allergens or inhaled irritants, leading to bronchial hyperactivity and inflammation of the airway mucosa. The symptoms of asthma may be effectively treated by several drugs, but no agent provides a cure for this obstructive lung disease.

B. Adrenergic agonists

Inhaled adrenergic agonists with β_2 activity are the drugs of choice for mild asthma—that is, in patients showing only occasional, intermittent symptoms (Figure 27.3). Direct-acting β_2 agonists are potent bronchodilators that relax airway smooth muscle.

1. **Short-acting drugs:** Most clinically useful β_2 agonists have a rapid onset of action (fifteen to thirty minutes) and provide relief for four to six hours. They are used for symptomatic treatment of bronchospasm and as "rescue agents" to combat acute bronchoconstriction. [Note: *Epinephrine* is the drug of choice for treatment of acute anaphylaxis.] β_2 Agonists have no anti-inflammatory effects, and they should never be used as the sole therapeutic agents for patients with chronic asthma. The direct-acting β_2-selective agonists, such as *pirbuterol*, *terbutaline*, and *albuterol*, offer the advantage of providing maximally attainable bronchodilation with little of the undesired effect of α or β_1 stimulation. (See p. 69 for the receptor-specific actions of adrenergic agonists.) The β_2 agonists are not catecholamines and, thus, are not inactivated by catechol-*O*-methyltransferase. Toxic side effects, such as tachycardia, hyperglycemia, hypokalemia, and hypomagnesemia are minimized when the drugs are delivered by inhalation rather than by systemic routes. Although tolerance to the effects of β_2 agonists on nonairway tissues occurs, it is uncommon with normal dosages.

2. **Long-acting drugs:** *Salmeterol xinafoate* [sal ME te rol] and *formoterol* [for MOH ter ol] are β_2-adrenergic selective, long-acting bronchodilators. They are chemical analogs of *albuterol* but differ by having a lipophilic side chain that increases the affinity of the drug for the β_2 adrenoceptor. *Salmeterol* and *formoterol* have a long duration of action, providing bronchodilation for at least twelve hours. *Salmeterol* has a slow onset of action and should not be used in acute asthmatic attacks; it should be prescribed only for administration at regular intervals and not to relieve acute symptoms. Doubling the dosage of inhaled corticosteriods or adding alternative drugs, such as the anti-leukotriene drugs *theophylline* or *cromolyn*, improves the course of the disease, but not as substantially as the combination of an inhaled corticosteroid and a long-acting β_2 agonist. Long-acting β_2 agonists are not substitutes for

CLASSIFICATION	BRONCHO-CONSTRICTIVE EPISODES	RESULTS OF PEAK FLOW OR SPIROMETRY	LONG-TERM CONTROL	QUICK RELIEF OF SYMPTOMS
Mild intermittent	Less than two per week	Near normal*	No daily medication	Short-acting β_2 agonist
Mild persistent	More than two per week	Near normal*	Low-dose inhaled corticosteroids	Short-acting β_2 agonist
Moderate persistent	Daily	60 to 80 percent of normal	Low- to medium-dose inhaled corticosteroids and a long-acting β_2 agonist	Short-acting β_2 agonist
Severe persistent	Continual	Less than 60 percent of normal	High-dose inhaled corticosteroids and a long-acting β_2 agonist	Short-acting β_2 agonist

Figure 27.3
Treatment of asthma. In all asthmatic patients, quick relief is provided by a short-acting β_2 agonist as needed for symptoms. *Eighty percent or more of predicted function.

anti-inflammatory therapy.

C. Corticosteroids

Inhaled glucocorticoids are the drugs of first choice in patients with moderate to severe asthma who require inhalation of β_2-adrenergic agonists more than two times per week (see Figure 27.3). Severe asthma may also require systemic glucocorticoids, usually for a short time. No other medications are as effective as inhaled corticosteroids in the longer-term control of asthma in children and adults. Inhaled glucocorticoids often reduce (or eliminate) the need for oral glucocorticoids in patients with severe asthma. To be effective in controlling inflammation, glucocorticoids must be taken continuously. (See p. 307 for a summary of the mechanism of action of corticosteroids.)

1. **Actions on lung:** Steroids have no direct effect on the airway smooth muscle. Instead, inhaled glucocorticoids decrease the number and activity of cells involved in airway inflammation—macrophages, eosinophils, and T lymphocytes. Prolonged (several months) inhalation of steroids reduces the hyperresponsiveness of the airway smooth muscle to a variety of bronchoconstrictor stimuli, such as allergens, irritants, cold air, and exercise. Anti-inflammatory steroids reduce inflammation by reversing mucosal edema, decreasing the permeability of capillaries, and inhibiting the release of leukotrienes.

2. **Pharmacokinetics**

   a. **Inhaled drugs:** The development of inhaled steroids has markedly reduced the need for systemic corticosteroid treatment. However, a few precautions are required for successful inhalation therapy. A large fraction (typically eighty to ninety percent) of inhaled glucocorticoids is either deposited in the mouth and pharynx, or is swallowed (Figure 27.4). These glucocorticosteroids are absorbed from the gut and enter the systemic circulation through the liver. [Note: Many of the clinically useful corticosteroids, such as *beclomethasone*, *triamcinolone*, and *flunisolide* [floo NISS oh lide], undergo extensive first-pass metabolism in the liver so that only a small amount of these

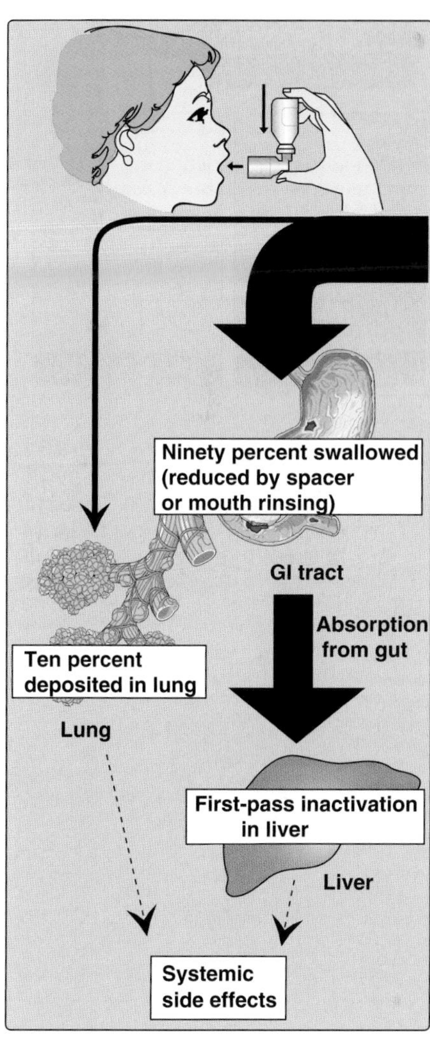

Figure 27.4
Pharmacokinetics of inhaled glucocorticoids.

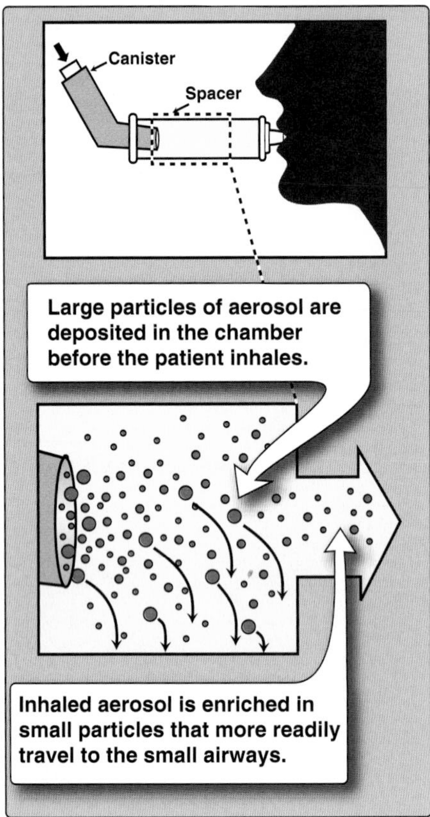

Canister
Spacer
Large particles of aerosol are deposited in the chamber before the patient inhales.
Inhaled aerosol is enriched in small particles that more readily travel to the small airways.

Figure 27.5
Effect of a spacer on the delivery of an inhaled aerosol.

drugs reaches the systemic circulation.] The ten to twenty percent of the metered dose of inhaled glucocorticoids that is not swallowed is deposited in the airway.

b. **Systemic steroids:** Patients with severe exacerbation of asthma (status asthmaticus) may require intravenous administration of *methylprednisolone* or oral *prednisone*. Once the patient has improved, the dose of drug is gradually reduced, leading to discontinuance in one to two weeks.

c. **Spacers:** A spacer is a large-volume chamber that is attached to a metered-dose inhaler, and is used to decrease the deposition of drug in the mouth (Figure 27.5). The chamber serves to reduce the velocity of the injected aerosol before it enters the mouth, and allows large drug particles to be deposited in the device. The smaller, higher-velocity drug particles are less likely to be deposited in the mouth and more likely to reach the target airway tissue. Spacers improve delivery of inhaled glucocorticoids and are advised for virtually all patients. [Note: Rinsing the mouth after inhalation can also decrease systemic absorption and the possibility of oropharyngeal candidiasis.]

3. **Adverse effects:** Oral or parenteral glucocorticoids have a variety of potentially serious side effects. However, inhaled glucocorticoids, particularly if used with a spacer, have few systemic effects. The risk of coriticosteroid-induced growth reduction in children is negligible, and it is far outweighed by the positive effects of inhaled steroid use. Oropharyngeal candidiasis—sometimes called thrush—may be a problem in patients who inhale glucocorticoids, particularly immunosuppressed patients. Spacers minimize the problem of adrenal suppression by reducing the amount of glucocorticoid deposited in the oropharynx.

III. ALTERNATIVE DRUGS USED TO TREAT ASTHMA

These drugs are useful for treatment of moderate to severe allergic asthma in patients who are poorly controlled by conventional therapy or experience adverse effects secondary to high-dose or prolonged corticosteroid treatment.

A. Antileukotriene drugs

Leukotriene B_4 (LTB_4) and the cysteinyl leukotrienes, LTC_4, LTD_4, and LTE_4, are products of the 5-lipoxygenase pathway of arachidonic acid metabolism.[1] 5-Lipoxygenase is found in cells of myeloid origin, such as mast cells, basophils, eosinophils, and neutrophils. LTB_4 is a potent chemoattractant for neutrophils and eosinophils, whereas the cysteinyl leukotrienes constrict bronchiolar smooth muscle, increase endothelial permeability, and promote mucus secretion. *Zileuton* [zye LOO ton] is a selective and specific inhibitor of 5-lipoxygenase, preventing the formation of both LTB_4 and the cysteinyl leukotrienes. *Zafirlukast* [za FIR loo kast] and *montelukast* [mon tee LOO kast] are selective, reversible inhibitors of the cysteinyl leukotriene-1

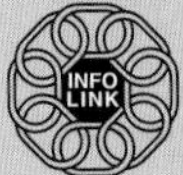

[1]See p. 212 in ***Lippincott's Illustrated Reviews: Biochemistry*** (3rd ed.) for a discussion of leukotriene synthesis.

receptor, thereby blocking the effects of cysteinyl leukotrienes (Figure 27.6). All three drugs are approved for the prophylaxis of asthma. However, they are not effective in situations where immediate bronchodilation is required. Modest reductions in the doses of β_2-adrenergic agonists and corticosteroids, as well as improved respiratory function, are among the therapeutic benefits.

1. **Pharmacokinetics:** All three drugs are orally active, although food impairs the absorption of *zafirlukast*. Greater than ninety percent of each drug is bound to plasma protein. The drugs are extensively metabolized. *Zileuton* and its metabolites are excreted in the urine, whereas *zafirlukast* and *montelukast* and their metabolites undergo biliary excretion.

2. **Adverse effects:** Elevations in serum hepatic enzymes have occurred with all three agents, requiring periodic monitoring and discontinuation when enzymes exceed normal levels by threefold. Although rare, eosinophilic vasculitis (Churg-Strauss syndrome) has been reported with all agents, particularly when the dose of concurrent glucocorticoids is reduced. Other effects include headache and dyspepsia. Both *zafirlukast* and *zileuton* are inhibitors of cytochrome P450. Both drugs can increase serum levels of *warfarin*. Figure 27.6 summarizes the drugs that modify the action of leukotrienes.

B. Cromolyn and nedocromil

Cromolyn [KROE moe lin] and *nedocromil* [ne doe KROE mil] are effective prophylactic anti-inflammatory agents. However, they are not useful in managing an acute asthmatic attack, because they are not direct bronchodilators. These agents can block the initiation of immediate and delayed asthmatic reactions. For use in asthma, *cromolyn* is administered either by inhalation of a microfine powder or as an aerosolized solution. Because it is poorly absorbed, only minor adverse effects are associated with it. Pretreatment with *cromolyn* blocks allergen- and exercise-induced bronchoconstriction. *Cromolyn* is also useful in reducing the symptoms of allergic rhinitis. A four- to six-week trial is required to determine efficacy. Given its safety, an initial trial of *cromolyn* is often recommended, particularly in children and pregnant women. Toxic reactions are mild and include a bitter taste and irritation of the pharynx and larynx.

C. Cholinergic antagonists

Anticholinergic agents are generally less effective than β_2-adrenergic agonists. They block the vagally mediated contraction of airway smooth muscle and mucus secretion. Inhaled *ipratropium* [i pra TROE pee um], a quaternary derivative of *atropine*, is useful in patients who are unable to tolerate adrenergic agonists. *Ipratropium* is slow in onset and nearly free of side-effects.

D. Theophylline

Theophylline [thee OFF i lin] is a bronchodilator that relieves airflow obstruction in chronic asthma and decreases its symptoms. Previously the mainstay of asthma therapy, *theophylline* has been

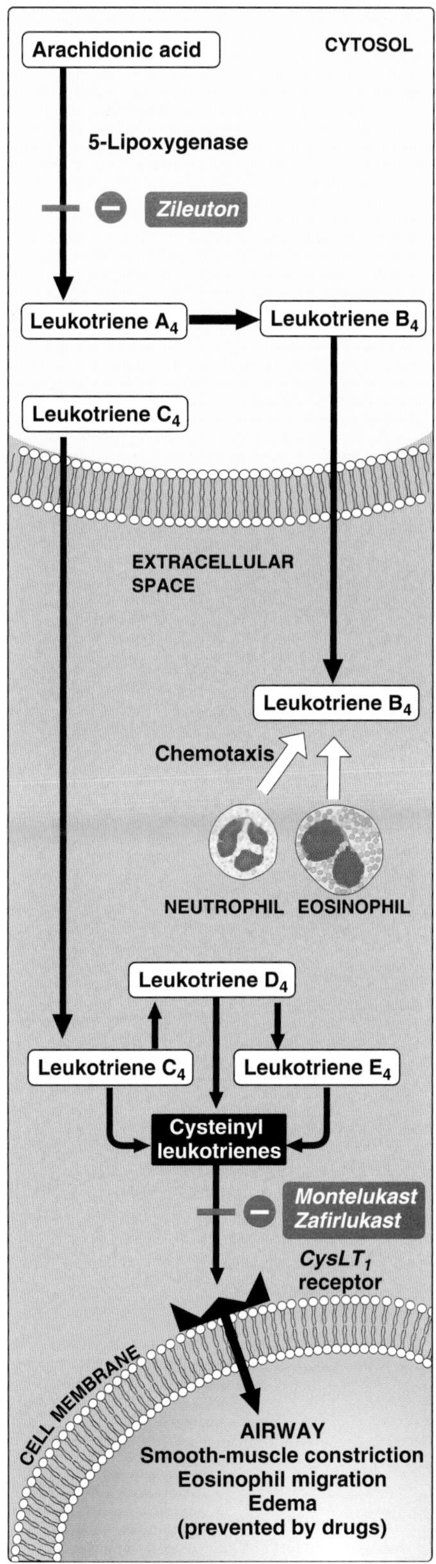

Figure 27.6
Sites of action of leukotriene-modifying drugs. $CysLT_1$ = cysteinyl leukotriene-1.

largely replaced with β_2 agonists and corticosteroids. *Theophylline* is well absorbed by the gastrointestinal tract, and several sustained-release preparations are available. The drug has a narrow therapeutic window, and an overdose of the drug may cause seizures or potentially fatal arrhythmias. Furthermore, *theophylline* interacts adversely with many drugs.

E. Omalizumab

Omalizumab [oh mah lye ZOO mab] is a recombinant DNA-derived monoclonal antibody that selectively binds to human immunoglobulin E (IgE). This leads to decreased binding of IgE to the high-affinity IgE receptor on the surface of mast cells and basophils. Reduction in surface-bound IgE limits the degree of release of mediators of the allergic response. *Omalizumab* may be particularly useful for treatment of moderate to severe allergic asthma in patients who are poorly controlled with conventional therapy. However, due to the high cost of the drug, limitations on dosage, and available clinical trial data, it is not presently used as first-line therapy.

IV. DRUGS USED TO TREAT CHRONIC OBSTRUCTIVE PULMONARY DISEASE

Chronic obstructive pulmonary disease (COPD) is a chronic, irreversible obstruction of airflow. Smoking is the greatest risk factor for COPD. Inhaled bronchodilators, such as anticholinergic agents and β_2-adrenergic agonists, are the foundation of therapy for COPD (Figure 27.7). These drugs increase airflow, alleviate symptoms, and decrease exacerbation of disease. Combination of an anticholinerrgic agent plus a β_2 agonist may be helpful in patients for whom a single inhaled bronchodilator has failed to provide an adequate response. For example, the combination of *albuterol* and *ipratroprium* provides greater brochodilation than with either drug alone. Longer-acting drugs, such as *salmeterol* and *tiotropium* [tee oh TROE pee um], have the advantage of less frequent dosing. Inhaled anti-inflammatory steroids should be restricted to patients with moderate to severe reduction in airflow for whom optimal brochodilator therapy has failed to improve symptoms. Addition of a long-acting β_2 agonist, such as *salmeterol*, improves lung function compared to either β_2 agonist or steroid alone.

STAGE	CHARACTERISTICS	LONG-TERM CONTROL
I: Mild COPD	FEV_1 greater than eighty percent predicted	Short-acting bronchodilator when needed
II: Moderate COPD	FEV_1 fifty to eighty percent predicted	Regular treatment with one or more bronchodilators Inhaled glucocorticosteroid
III: Severe COPD	FEV_1 less than thirty percent predicted	Regular treatment with one or more bronchodilators Inhaled glucocorticosteroid Antibiotics for acute exacerbations of COPD characterized by increased volume and purulence of secretions Long-term oxygen therapy

Figure 27.7
Treatment of stable chronic obstructive pulmonary disease (COPD). FEV_1 = forced expiratory volume in one second.

V. DRUGS USED TO TREAT ALLERGIC RHINITIS

Rhinitis is an inflammation of the mucous membranes of the nose, and is characterized by sneezing, nasal itching, watery rhinorrhea, and congestion. An attack may be precipitated by inhalation of an allergen (such as dust, pollen, or animal dander). The foreign material interacts with mast cells that are coated with IgE generated in response to a previous exposure to the allergen (Figure 27.8). The mast cells release mediators, such as histamine, leukotrienes, and chemotactic factors, which promote bronchiolar spasm and mucosal thickening from edema and cellular infiltration. Combinations of oral antihistamines with decongestants are the first-line therapy for allergic rhinitis. However, the systemic effects sometimes associated with these oral preparations (sedation, insomnia, and rarely, cardiac arrhythmias) have prompted interest in topical intranasal delivery of drugs.

A. Antihistamines (H_1-receptor blockers)

Antihistamines are the most frequently used agents in the treatment of sneezing and watery rhinorrhea associated with allergic rhinitis. H_1-histamine–receptor blockers, such as *diphenhydramine*, *chlorpheniramine, loratadine, and fexofenadine*, are useful in treating the symptoms of allergic rhinitis caused by histamine release. Combinations of antihistamines with decongestants (see below) are effective when congestion is a feature of rhinitis. Antihistamines differ in their ability to cause sedation and in their duration of action.

B. α-Adrenergic agonists

α-Adrenergic agonists ("nasal decongestants"), such as *phenylephrine*, constrict dilated arterioles in the nasal mucosa and reduce airway resistance. Long-acting *oxymetazoline* [ok see met AZ oh leen] is also available. When administered as an aerosol, these drugs have a rapid onset of action and show few systemic effects. Oral administration results in longer duration of action but also increased systemic effects. Combinations of these agents with antihistamines are frequently used. However, they should be used no longer than several days, because rebound nasal congestion often occurs on discontinuance of these drugs. Therefore, α-adrenergic agents have no place in the long-term treatment of allergic rhinitis.

C. Corticosteroids

Corticosteroids, such as *beclomethasone*, *fluticasone*, *flunisolide,* and *triamcinolone*, are effective when administered as nasal sprays. [Note: Systemic absorption is minimal, and side effects of intranasal corticosteroid treatment are localized. These include nasal irritation, nosebleed, sore throat, and rarely, candidiasis.] Topical steroids may be more effective than systemic antihistamines in relieving the nasal symptoms of both allergic and nonallergic rhinitis. The effects of long-term usage are unknown, but are considered to be generally safe. Periodic assessment of the patient is advised. Treatment of chronic rhinitis may not result in improvement until one to two weeks after starting therapy.

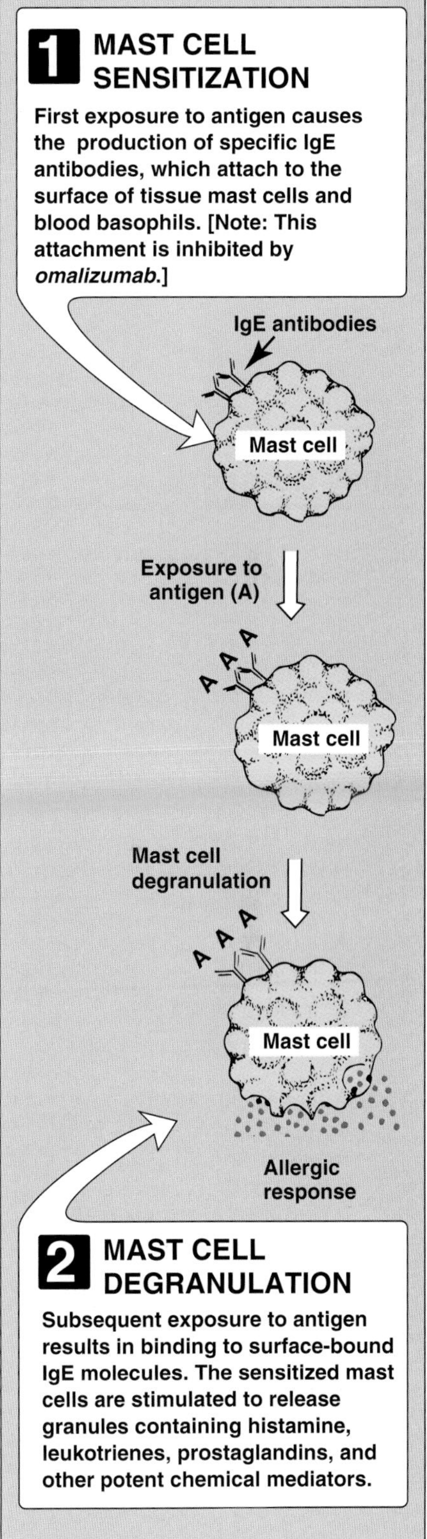

1 MAST CELL SENSITIZATION
First exposure to antigen causes the production of specific IgE antibodies, which attach to the surface of tissue mast cells and blood basophils. [Note: This attachment is inhibited by omalizumab.]
IgE antibodies
Mast cell
Exposure to antigen (A)
Mast cell
Mast cell degranulation
Mast cell
Allergic response
2 MAST CELL DEGRANULATION
Subsequent exposure to antigen results in binding to surface-bound IgE molecules. The sensitized mast cells are stimulated to release granules containing histamine, leukotrienes, prostaglandins, and other potent chemical mediators.

Figure 27.8
Hypersensitivity reactions mediated by immunoglobulin E (IgE) molecules can cause rhinitis.

D. Cromolyn

Intranasal *cromolyn* may be useful, particularly when administered before contact with an allergen.

VI. DRUGS USED TO TREAT COUGH

Codeine, *hydrocodone* [hy dro KO doan] and *hydromorphone* [hy dro MOR fone] decrease the sensitivity of cough centers in the central nervous system to peripheral stimuli and decrease mucosal secretion. These actions occur at doses lower than those required for analgesia. (See p. 158 for a more complete discussion of the opiates.) *Dextromethorphan* [dek stroe METH or fan], a synthetic derivative of *morphine*, suppresses the response of the cough center. It has no analgesic or addictive potential and is less constipating than *codeine*.

Study Questions

Choose the ONE best answer.

27.1 A 12-year-old girl with a childhood history of asthma complained of cough, dyspnea, and wheezing after visiting a riding stable. Her symptoms became so severe that her parent brought her to the emergency room. Physical examination revealed diaphoresis, dyspnea, tachycardia, and tachypnea. Her respiratory rate was 42 breaths per min, pulse rate 110 beats per minute, and blood pressure 132/65 mm Hg. Which of the following is the most appropriate drug to rapidly reverse her bronchoconstriction?

A. Inhaled cromolyn
B. Inhaled beclomethasone
C. Inhaled albuterol
D. Intravenous propranolol

Correct answer = C. Inhalation of a rapid-acting β_2 agonist, such as albuterol, usually provides immediate bronchodilation. An acute asthmatic crisis often requires intravenous corticosteroids, often methylprednisolone. Inhaled beclomethasone will not deliver enough steroid to fully combat airway inflammation. Propranolol is a β-blocker and would aggravate the patient's bronchoconstriction. Cromolyn can be used prophylactically to reduce the inflammatory response but is ineffective in relieving acute symptoms.

27.2 A 9-year-old girl has severe asthma which required three hospitalizations in the last year. She is now receiving therapy that has greatly reduced the frequency of these severe attacks. Which of the following therapies is most likely responsible for this benefit?

A. Albuterol by aerosol
B. Cromolyn by inhaler
C. Fluticasone by aerosol
D. Theophylline orally
E. Zafirlukast orally

Correct answer = C. Administration of a corticosteroid directly to the lung significantly reduces the frequency of severe asthma attacks. This benefit is accomplished with minimal risk of the severe systemic adverse effects of corticosteroid therapy. Albuterol is only used to treat acute asthmatic episodes. The other agents may reduce the severity of attacks but not to the same degree or consistency as fluticasone (or other corticosteroid).

Gastrointestinal and Antiemetic Drugs

28

I. OVERVIEW

This chapter describes drugs used to treat three common medical conditions involving the gastrointestinal tract: peptic ulcers and gastroesophageal reflux disease (GERD), chemotherapy-induced emesis, and diarrhea and constipation. Many drugs described in other chapters also find application in the treatment of gastrointestinal disorders. For example, the morphine derivative *diphenoxylate*, which decreases peristaltic activity of the gut, is useful in the treatment of severe diarrhea, and the corticosteroid *dexamethasone* has excellent antiemetic properties. Other drugs, (for example, H_2-receptor antagonists and proton-pump inhibitors employed to heal peptic ulcers, as well as the selective inhibitors of the serotonin receptors, such as *ondansetron* or *granisetron*, which prevent vomiting) are used almost exclusively to treat gastrointestinal tract disorders.

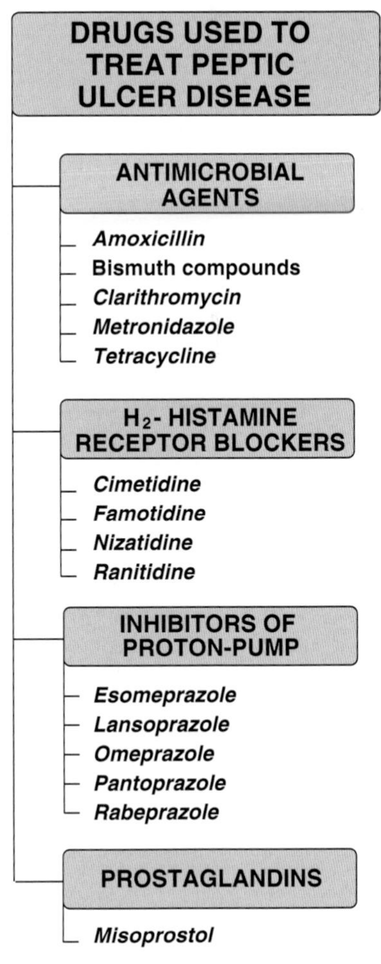

DRUGS USED TO TREAT PEPTIC ULCER DISEASE
ANTIMICROBIAL AGENTS
Amoxicillin
Bismuth compounds
Clarithromycin
Metronidazole
Tetracycline
H2- HISTAMINE RECEPTOR BLOCKERS
Cimetidine
Famotidine
Nizatidine
Ranitidine
INHIBITORS OF PROTON-PUMP
Esomeprazole
Lansoprazole
Omeprazole
Pantoprazole
Rabeprazole
PROSTAGLANDINS
Misoprostol

Figure 28.1
Summary of drugs used to treat peptic ulcer disease.
(Figure continues on next page.)

II. DRUGS USED TO TREAT PEPTIC ULCER DISEASE

Although the pathogenesis of peptic ulcer disease is not fully understood, three major causative factors are recognized: infection with gram-negative Helicobacter pylori, increased hydrochloric acid secretion, and inadequate mucosal defense against gastric acid. Treatment approaches include 1) eradicating the H. pylori infection, 2) reducing secretion of gastric acid or neutralizing the acid after it is released, and/or 3) providing agents that protect the gastric mucosa from damage. Figure 28.1 summarizes agents that are effective in treating peptic ulcer disease.

A. Antimicrobial agents

Optimal therapy for patients with peptic ulcer disease (both duodenal and gastric ulcers) who are infected with H. pylori requires antimicrobial treatment. To document infection with H. pylori, endoscopic biopsy of the gastric mucosa or various noninvasive methods are available, including serologic tests and breath tests for urea. Figure 28.2 shows a biopsy sample in which H. pylori is closely associated

Lippincott's Illustrated Reviews: Pharmacology, Third Edition,
by Richard D. Howland and Mary J. Mycek.

DRUGS USED TO TREAT PEPTIC ULCER DISEASE (continued)

ANTIMUSCARINIC AGENTS
- ***Dicyclomine***

ANTACIDS
- ***Aluminum hydroxide***
- ***Calcium carbonate***
- ***Magnesium hydroxide***
- ***Sodium bicarbonate***

MUCOSAL PROTECTIVE AGENTS
- ***Colloidal bismuth***
- ***Sucralfate***

Figure 28.1 (continued)
Summary of drugs used to treat peptic ulcer disease.

with the gastric mucosa. Eradication of H. pylori results in rapid healing of active peptic ulcers, and low recurrence rates (less than 15 percent compared with 60 to 100 percent per year for patients with initial ulcers healed by traditional antisecretory therapy). Successful eradication of H. pylori (eighty to ninety percent) is possible with various combinations of antimicrobial drugs. Currently, either triple therapy consisting of a proton-pump inhibitor (PPI) with either *metronidazole* or *amoxicillin* plus *clarithromycin*, or quadruple therapy of *bismuth subsalicylate* and *metronidazole* plus *tetracycline* plus a histamine H_2-receptor antagonist (see below) or a PPI, are administered for a two-week course. This usually results in a ninety percent or greater eradication rate. Bismuth salts do not neutralize stomach acid, but they inhibit pepsin and increase the secretion of mucus, thus helping to form a barrier against the diffusion of acid in the ulcer. Treatment with a single antimicrobial drug is less effective (twenty to forty percent eradication rates). [Note: GERD (that is, a heartburn-like sensation) is not associated with H. pylori infection and does not respond to treatment with antibiotics.]

B. Regulation of gastric acid secretion

Gastric acid secretion by parietal cells of the gastric mucosa is stimulated by acetylcholine, histamine, and gastrin (Figure 28.3). The receptor-mediated binding of acetylcholine, histamine, or gastrin results in the activation of protein kinases, which in turn stimulates the H^+/K^+-adenosine triphosphatase (ATPase) proton pump to secrete hydrogen ions in exchange for K^+ into the lumen of the stomach. A Cl^- channel couples chloride efflux to the release of H^+. In contrast, receptor binding of prostaglandin E_2 and somatostatin diminish gastric acid production. [Note: Histamine binding causes activation of adenylyl cyclase, whereas binding of prostaglandin E_2 inhibits this enzyme. Gastrin and acetylcholine act by inducing an increase in intracellular calcium levels.]

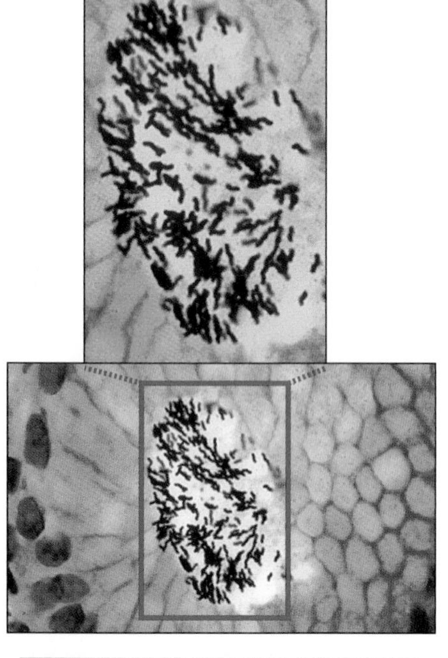

Figure 28.2
Helicobacter pylori in association with gastric mucosa.

C. H_2-receptor antagonists

Although antagonists of the histamine H_2 receptor block the actions of histamine at all H_2 receptors, their chief clinical use is to inhibit gastric acid secretion, being particularly effective against nocturnal acid secretion. By competitively blocking the binding of histamine to H_2 receptors, these agents reduce the intracellular concentrations of cyclic adenosine monophosphate (cAMP) and, thereby, secretion of gastric acid. The four drugs used in the United States—*cimetidine* [si MET ih deen], *ranitidine* [ra NI tih deen], *famotidine* [fa MOE ti deen], and *nizatidine* [nye ZA ti deen]—potently inhibit (greater than ninety percent) basal, food-stimulated, and nocturnal secretion of gastric acid after a single dose. *Cimetidine* is the prototype histamine H_2-receptor antagonist.

1. **Actions:** The histamine H_2-receptor antagonists—*cimetidine*, *ranitidine*, *famotidine*, and *nizatidine*—act selectively on H_2 receptors in the stomach, blood vessels, and other sites, but they have no effect on H_1 receptors. They are competitive antagonists of histamine and are fully reversible. These agents completely inhibit gastric acid secretion induced by histamine or gastrin. However, they only partially inhibit gastric acid secretion induced by acetylcholine or *bethanechol*.

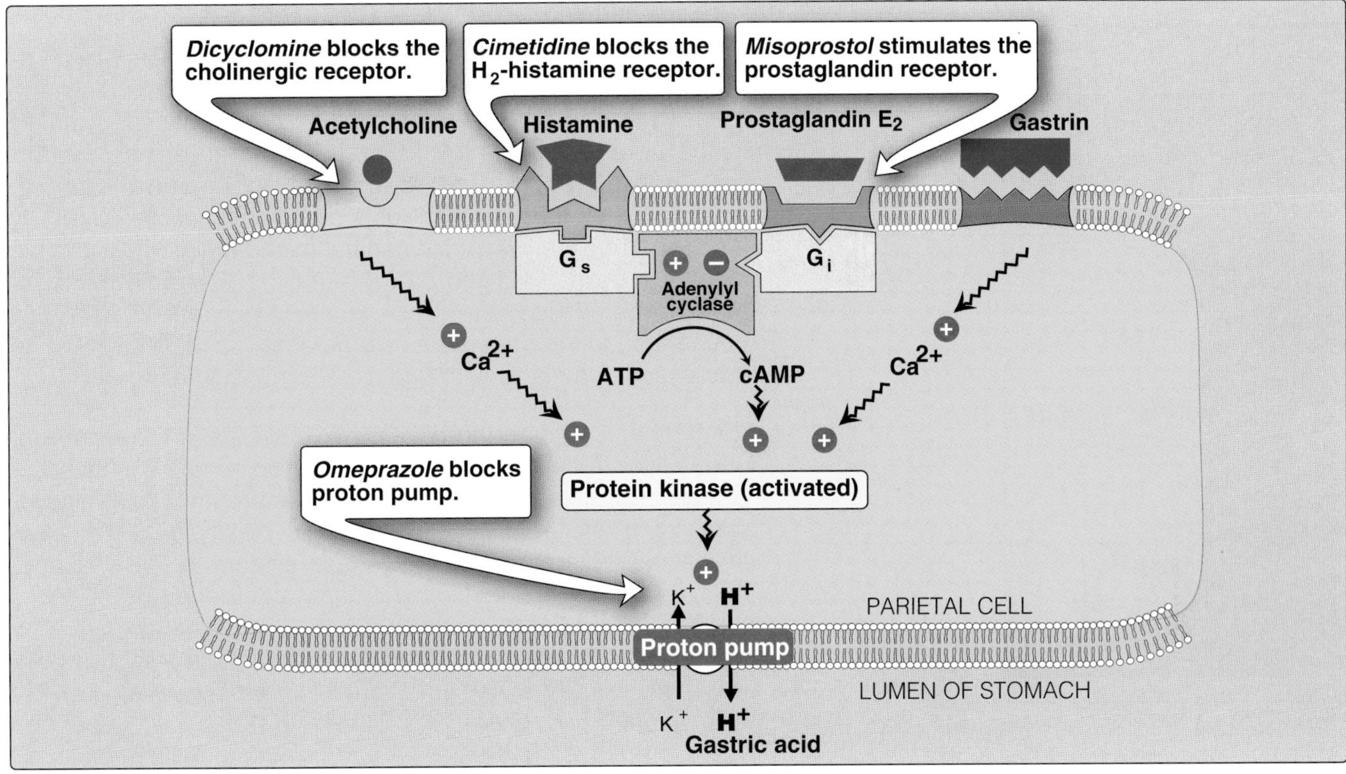

Figure 28.3
Effects of acetylcholine, histamine, prostaglandin E_2, and gastrin on gastric acid secretion by the parietal cells of stomach. G_s and G_i are membrane proteins that mediate the stimulatory or inhibitory effect of receptor coupling to adenylyl cyclase.

2. **Therapeutic uses:** The use of these agents has decreased with the advent of the PPIs.

   a. **Peptic ulcers:** All four agents are equally effective in promoting healing of duodenal and gastric ulcers. However, recurrence is common after treatment with H_2 antagonists is stopped (60 to 100 percent per year). This can be effectively prevented by eradication of H. pylori, and H_2 antagonists continue to be widely used in peptic ulcer therapy in combination with antimicrobial drugs.

   b. **Acute stress ulcers:** These drugs are useful in managing acute stress ulcers associated with major physical trauma in high-risk patients in intensive care units. They are usually injected intravenously.

   c. **GERD:** Low doses of H_2 antagonists, recently released for over-the-counter sale, appear to be effective for prevention and treatment of heartburn (gastroesophageal reflux). However, about fifty percent of patients do not find benefit, and PPIs are now used preferentially in the treatment of this disorder. Because H_2-receptor antagonists act by stopping acid secretion, they may not relieve symptoms for at least 45 minutes. Antacids more efficiently neutralize secreted acid already in the stomach, but their effects are shorter lasting.

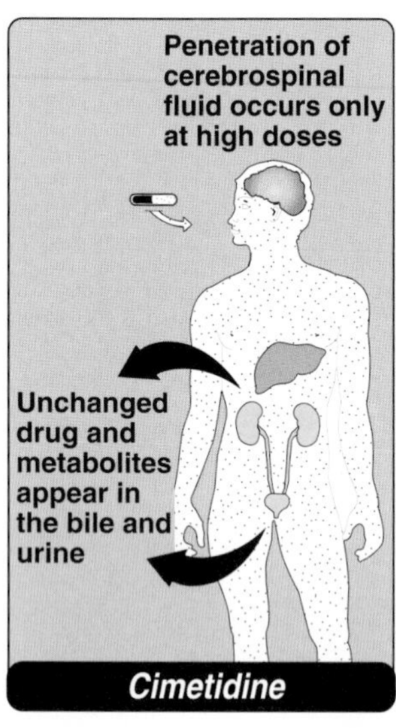

Figure 28.4
Administration and fate of *cimetidine*.

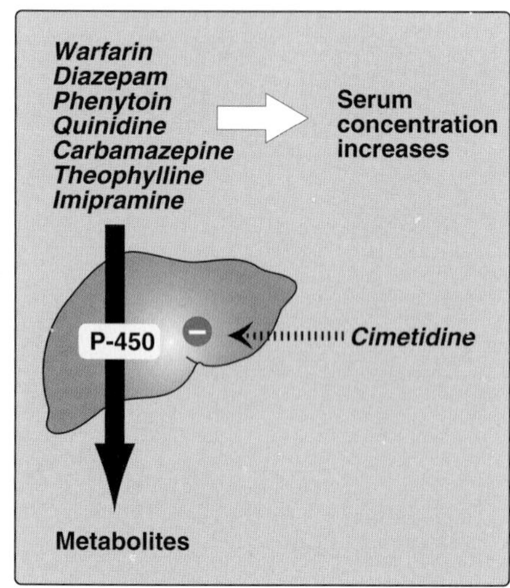

Figure 28.5
Drug interactions with *cimetidine*.

3. **Pharmacokinetics:**

   a. **Cimetidine:** *Cimetidine* and the other H_2 antagonists are given orally, distribute widely throughout the body (including into breast milk and across the placenta), and are excreted mainly in the urine (Figure 28.4). *Cimetidine* normally has a short serum half-life, which is increased in renal failure. Approximately thirty percent of a dose of *cimetidine* is slowly inactivated by the liver's microsomal mixed-function oxygenase system (see p. 14), and can interfere in the metabolism of many other drugs; the other seventy percent is excreted unchanged in the urine. The dosage of all these drugs must be decreased in patients with hepatic or renal failure.

   b. **Ranitidine:** Compared to *cimetidine*, *ranitidine* is longer acting, and is five- to tenfold more potent. *Ranitidine* has minimal side effects and does not produce the antiandrogenic or prolactin-stimulating effects of *cimetidine*. Unlike *cimetidine*, it does not inhibit the mixed-function oxygenase system in the liver and, thus, does not affect the concentrations of other drugs.

   c. **Famotidine:** *Famotidine* is similar to *ranitidine* in its pharmacologic action, but it is twenty to fifty times more potent than *cimetidine*, and three to twenty times more potent than *ranitidine*.

   d. **Nizatidine:** *Nizatidine* is similar to *ranitidine* in its pharmacologic action and potency. In contrast to *cimetidine*, *ranitidine*, and *famotidine*, which are metabolized by the liver, *nizatidine* is eliminated principally by the kidney. Because little first-pass metabolism occurs with *nizatidine*, its bioavailability is nearly 100 percent. No intravenous preparation is available.

4. **Adverse effects:** The adverse effects of *cimetidine* are usually minor and are associated mainly with the major pharmacologic activity of the drug—namely reduced gastric acid production. Side effects occur only in a small number of patients and generally do not require discontinuation of the drug. The most common side effects are headache, dizziness, diarrhea, and muscular pain. Other central nervous system effects (confusion, hallucinations) occur primarily in elderly patients or after intravenous administration. *Cimetidine* can also have endocrine effects, because it acts as a nonsteroidal antiandrogen. These effects include gynecomastia, galactorrhea (continuous release/discharge of milk), and reduced sperm count. *Cimetidine* inhibits cytochrome P450 and can slow metabolism (and, thus, potentiate the action) of several drugs (for example, *warfarin*, *diazepam*, *phenytoin*, *quinidine*, *carbamazepine*, *theophylline*, and *imipramine*; Figure 28.5), sometimes resulting in serious adverse clinical effects. Except for *famotidine*, all these agents inhibit the gastric first-pass metabolism of ethanol. Drugs such as *ketoconazole*, which depend on an acidic medium for gastric absorption, will not be efficiently absorbed if taken with one of these antagonists.

D. Inhibitors of the H^+/K^+-ATPase proton pump

Omeprazole [oh MEH pra zole] is the first of a class of drugs that bind to the H^+/K^+-ATPase enzyme system (proton pump) of the parietal cell, thereby suppressing secretion of hydrogen ions into the gastric lumen. The membrane-bound proton pump is the final step in the secretion of gastric acid (see Figure 28.3). Four additional PPIs are now available: *lansoprazole* [lan SO pra zole], *rabeprazole* [rah BEH pra zole], *pantoprazole* [pan TOE pra zole], and *esomeprazole* [es oh MEH pra zole].

1. **Actions:** All of these agents are prodrugs with an acid-resistant enteric coating to protect them from premature activation by gastric acid.. The coating is removed in the alkaline duodenum, and the prodrug, a weak base, is absorbed and transported to the parietal cell canaliculus. There, it is converted to the active form, which reacts with a cysteine residue of the H^+/K^+-ATPase, forming a stable covalent bond. It takes about eighteen hours for the enzyme to be resynthesized. At standard doses, all PPIs inhibit both basal and stimulated gastric acid secretion more than ninety percent. Acid suppression begins within one to two hours after the first dose of *lansoprazole* and slightly earlier with *omeprazole*.

2. **Therapeutic uses:** The superiority of the PPIs over the H_2 antagonists for suppressing acid production and healing peptic ulcers have made them the preferred drugs for treating erosive esophagitis and active duodenal ulcer and for long-term treatment of pathologic hypersecretory conditions (for example, Zollinger-Ellison syndrome, in which a gastrin-producing tumor causes hypersecretion of HCl). They are approved for the treatment of GERD. Clinical studies have shown that PPIs reduce the risk of bleeding from an ulcer caused by *aspirin* and other nonsteroidal anti-inflammatory agents (NSAIDS). They are also successfully used with antimicrobial regimens to eradicate H. pylori.

3. **Pharmacokinetics:** All these agents are delayed-release formulations and are effective orally. [Note: *Pantoprazole* is also available for intravenous injection.] Metabolites of these agents are excreted in urine and feces.

4. **Adverse effects:** The PPIs are generally well tolerated, but concerns about long-term safety have been raised due to the increased secretion of gastrin. In animal studies, the incidence of gastric carcinoid tumors increased, possibly related to the effects of prolonged hypochlorhydria and secondary hypergastrinemia. However, this has not been found in humans. Increased concentrations of viable bacteria in the stomach have been reported with continued use of these drugs. *Omeprazole* interferes in the oxidation of *warfarin*, *phenytoin*, *diazepam*, and *cyclosporine*. However, drug interactions are not a problem with the other PPIs. Prolonged therapy with agents that suppress gastric acid, such as the PPIs and H_2 antagonists, may result in low vitamin B_{12}, because acid is required for its absorption.

E. Prostaglandins

Prostaglandin E_2, produced by the gastric mucosa, inhibits secretion of HCl and stimulates secretion of mucus and bicarbonate (cytoprotective effect). A deficiency of prostaglandins is thought to be involved in the pathogenesis of peptic ulcers. *Misoprostol* [mye soe PROST ole], a stable analog of prostaglandin E_1, as well as *lansoprazole*, a proton pump inhibitor, are approved for prevention of gastric ulcers induced by NSAIDs (Figure 28.6). It is less effective than H_2 antagonists and the PPIs for acute treatment of peptic ulcers. Although *misoprostol* has cytoprotective actions, it is clinically effective only at higher doses that diminish gastric acid secretion. Routine prophylactic use of *misoprostol* may not be justified except in patients who are taking NSAIDs and are at high risk of NSAID-induced ulcers, such as the elderly or patients with ulcer complications. Like other prostaglandins, *misoprostol* produces uterine contractions and is contraindicated during pregnancy. Dose-related diarrhea and nausea are the most common adverse effects.

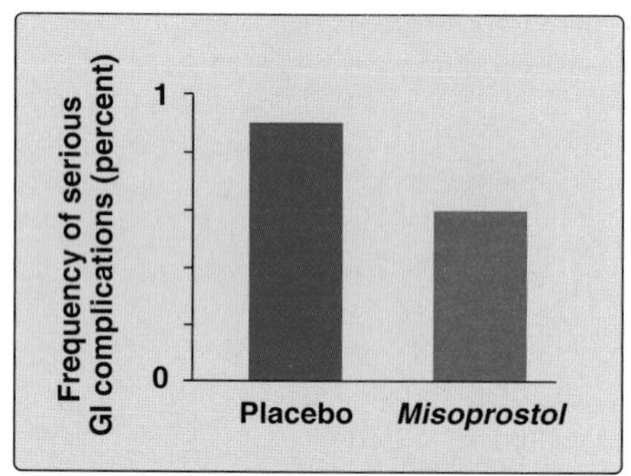

Figure 28.6
Misoprostol reduces serious gastrointestinal (GI) complications in patients with rheumatoid arthritis receiving nonsteroidal anti-inflammatory drugs.

F. Antimuscarinic agents

Muscarinic receptor stimulation increases gastrointestinal motility and secretory activity. A cholinergic antagonist, such as *dicyclomine* [dye SYE kloe meen], can be used as an adjunct in the management of peptic ulcer disease and Zollinger-Ellison syndrome, particularly in patients who are refractory to standard therapies. However, its many side effects (for example, cardiac arrhythmias and urinary retention) limit its use.

G. Antacids

Antacids are weak bases that react with gastric acid to form water and a salt, thereby diminishing gastric acidity. Because pepsin is inactive at a pH greater than 4, antacids also reduce peptic activity. They may have other actions as well, such as reduction of H. pylori colonization and stimulation of prostaglandin synthesis.

1. **Chemistry of antacids:** Antacid products vary widely in their chemical composition, acid-neutralizing capacity, sodium content, palatability, and price. The acid-neutralizing ability of an antacid depends on its capacity to neutralize gastric HCl and on whether the stomach is full or empty (food delays stomach emptying, allowing more time for the antacid to react). Commonly used antacids are salts of aluminum and magnesium, such as *aluminum hydroxide* (usually a mixture of $Al(OH)_3$ and aluminum oxide hydrates) or *magnesium hydroxide* [$Mg(OH)_2$], either alone or in combination. *Calcium carbonate* [$CaCO_3$] reacts with HCl to form CO_2 and $CaCl_2$ and is a commonly used preparation. Systemic absorption of *sodium bicarbonate* [$NaHCO_3$] can produce transient metabolic alkalosis; this antacid is not recommended for long-term use.

2. **Therapeutic uses:** Aluminum- and magnesium-containing antacids can promote healing of duodenal ulcers, but the evidence for efficacy in the treatment of acute gastric ulcers is less compelling. [Note: *Calcium carbonate* preparations are also used as calcium supplements for the treatment of osteoporosis.]

3. **Adverse effects:** *Aluminum hydroxide* may be constipating, and *magnesium hydroxide* may produce diarrhea. Preparations that combine these agents aid in normalizing bowel function. The

binding of phosphate by aluminum-containing antacids can lead to hypophosphatemia. In addition to the potential for systemic alkalosis, *sodium bicarbonate* liberates CO_2, causing belching and flatulence. Absorption of the cations from antacids (Mg^{2+}, Al^{3+}, Ca^{2+}) is usually not a problem in patients with normal renal function, but the sodium content of antacids can be an important consideration in patients with hypertension or congestive heart failure. Excessive intake of *calcium carbonate* along with calcium foods can result in hypercalcemia.

H. Mucosal protective agents

These compounds, known as cytoprotective compounds, have several actions that enhance mucosal protection mechanisms, thereby preventing mucosal injury, reducing inflammation, and healing existing ulcers.

1. **Sucralfate:** This complex of *aluminum hydroxide* and sulfated sucrose binds to positively charged groups in proteins of both normal and necrotic mucosa. By forming complex gels with epithelial cells, *sucralfate* [soo KRAL fate] creates a physical barrier that impairs diffusion of HCl and prevents degradation of mucus by pepsin and acid. It also stimulates prostaglandin release as well as mucus and bicarbonate output, and it inhibits peptic digestion. By these and other mechanisms, *sucralfate* effectively heals duodenal ulcers and is used in long-term maintenance therapy to prevent their recurrence. Because it requires an acidic pH for activation, *sucralfate* should not be administered with H_2 antagonists or antacids. Little of the drug is absorbed systemically. It is very well tolerated, but it can interfere with the absorption of other drugs by binding to them.

2. **Colloidal bismuth:** Preparations of this compound effectively heal peptic ulcers. In addition to their antimicrobial actions, they inhibit the activity of pepsin, increase secretion of mucus, and interact with glycoproteins in necrotic mucosal tissue to coat and protect the ulcer crater.

III. DRUGS USED TO CONTROL CHEMOTHERAPY-INDUCED EMESIS

Although nausea and vomiting may occur in a variety of conditions (for example, motion sickness, pregnancy, or hepatitis) and are always unpleasant for the patient, it is the nausea and vomiting produced by many chemotherapeutic agents that demand effective management. Nearly seventy to eighty percent of all patients who undergo chemotherapy experience nausea or vomiting. Several factors influence the incidence and severity of chemotherapy-induced emesis (Figure 28.7), including the specific chemotherapeutic drug, dose, route, and schedule of administration, as well as patient variables. For example, the young and women are more susceptible than older patients and men, and ten to forty percent of patients experience nausea or vomiting in anticipation of their chemotherapy (anticipatory vomiting). Emesis not only affects the quality of life but can lead to rejection of potentially curative antineoplas-

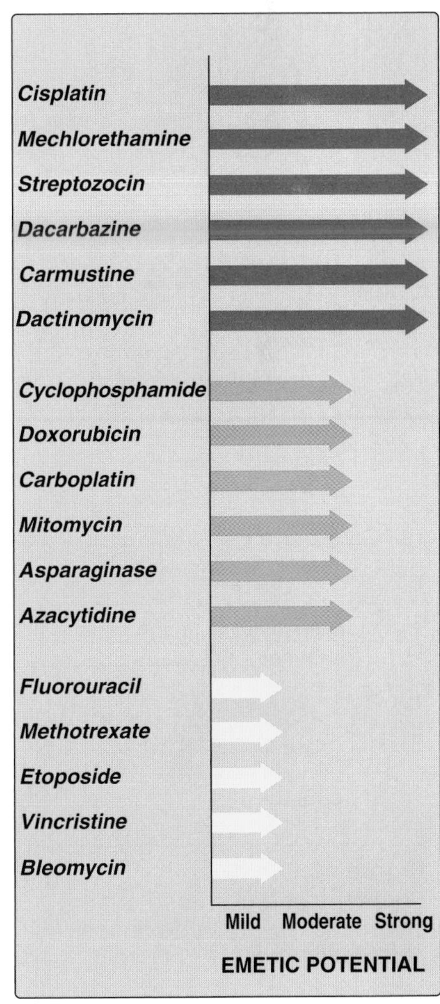

Figure 28.7
Comparison of emetic potential of anticancer drugs.

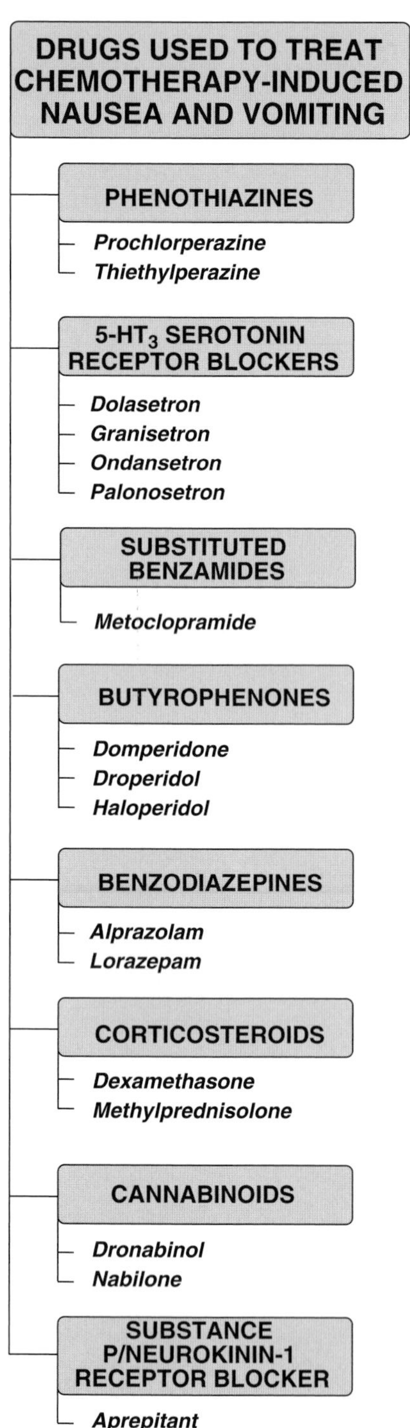

DRUGS USED TO TREAT CHEMOTHERAPY-INDUCED NAUSEA AND VOMITING
PHENOTHIAZINES
Prochlorperazine
Thiethylperazine
5-HT3 SEROTONIN RECEPTOR BLOCKERS
Dolasetron
Granisetron
Ondansetron
Palonosetron
SUBSTITUTED BENZAMIDES
Metoclopramide
BUTYROPHENONES
Domperidone
Droperidol
Haloperidol
BENZODIAZEPINES
Alprazolam
Lorazepam
CORTICOSTEROIDS
Dexamethasone
Methylprednisolone
CANNABINOIDS
Dronabinol
Nabilone
SUBSTANCE P/NEUROKININ-1 RECEPTOR BLOCKER
Aprepitant

Figure 28.8
Summary of drugs used to treat chemotherapy-induced nausea and vomiting. 5-HT_3 = serotonin type 3.

tic treatment. In addition, uncontrolled vomiting can produce dehydration, profound metabolic imbalances, and nutrient depletion.

A. Mechanisms that trigger vomiting

Two brainstem sites have key roles in the vomiting reflex pathway. The chemoreceptor trigger zone, which is located in the area postrema (a circumventricular structure at the caudal end of the fourth ventricle) is outside the blood-brain barrier. Thus, it can respond directly to chemical stimuli in the blood or cerebrospinal fluid. The second important site, the vomiting center, which is located in the lateral reticular formation of the medulla, coordinates the motor mechanisms of vomiting. The vomiting center also responds to afferent input from the vestibular system, the periphery (pharynx and gastrointestinal tract), and higher brainstem and cortical structures. The vestibular system functions mainly in motion sickness.

B. Emetic actions of chemotherapeutic agents

Chemotherapeutic agents (or their metabolites) can directly activate the medullary chemoreceptor trigger zone or vomiting center; several neuroreceptors, including dopamine receptor type 2 and serotonin type 3 (5-HT_3), play critical roles. Often, the color or smell of chemotherapeutic drugs (and even stimuli associated with chemotherapy, such as cues in the treatment room or the physician or nurse who administers the therapy) can activate higher brain centers and trigger emesis. Chemotherapeutic drugs can also act peripherally by causing cell damage in the gastrointestinal tract and releasing serotonin from the enterochromaffin cells of the small intestinal mucosa. The released serotonin activates 5-HT_3 receptors on vagal and splanchnic afferent fibers, which then carry sensory signals to the medulla, leading to the emetic response.

C. Antiemetic drugs

Considering the complexity of the mechanisms involved in emesis, it is not surprising that antiemetics represent a variety of classes (Figure 28.8) and offer a range of efficacies (Figures 28.9). Anticholinergic drugs, especially the muscarinic receptor antagonist, *scopolamine*, and H_1-receptor antagonists, such as *dimenhydrinate*, *meclizine*, and *cyclizine*, are very useful in motion sickness but are ineffective against substances that act directly on the chemoreceptor trigger zone. The major categories of drugs used to control chemotherapy-induced nausea and vomiting include the following.

1. **Phenothiazines:** The first group of drugs shown to be effective antiemetic agents, phenothiazines, such as *prochlorperazine* [proe klor PER ah zeen] and *thiethylperazine* [thye eth il PER a zeen], act by blocking dopamine receptors. They are effective against low or moderately emetogenic chemotherapeutic agents (for example, *fluorouracil* and *doxorubicin*; see Figure 28.7). Although increasing the dose improves antiemetic activity, side effects, including hypotension and restlessness, are dose-limiting. Other adverse reactions include extrapyramidal symptoms and sedation.

2. **5-HT_3 serotonin-receptor blockers:** This class of agents commands an important place in treating emesis linked with

chemotherapy. They have the advantage of a long duration of action. The specific antagonists of the 5-HT_3 receptor—*ondansetron* [on DAN seh tron], *granisetron* [gra NI seh tron], palonosetron [pa low NO seh tron] and *dolasetron* [dol A se tron]—selectively block 5-HT_3 receptors in the periphery (visceral vagal afferent fibers) and in the brain (chemoreceptor trigger zone). These drugs can be administered as a single dose prior to chemotherapy (intravenously or orally) and are efficacious against all grades of emetogenic therapy. One trial reported *ondansetron* and *granisetron* prevented emesis in fifty to sixty percent of *cisplatin*-treated patients. These agents are extensively metabolized by the liver, with hydroxydolasetron being an active metabolite of *dolasetron*. Thus, doses of these agents should be adjusted in patients with hepatic insufficiency. Elimination is through the urine. Headache is a common side effect. Electrocardiographic changes, such as prolongation of the QT interval, can occur with *dolasetron*; therefore, patients who may be at risk should receive this medication with caution. These drugs are costly.

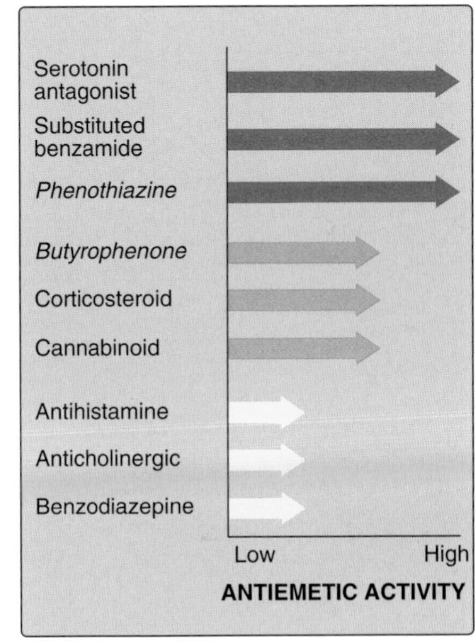

Figure 28.9
Potencies of of antiemetic drugs.

3. **Substituted benzamides:** One of several substituted benzamides with antiemetic activity, *metoclopramide* [met oh kloe PRAH mide] is highly effective at high doses against the highly emetogenic *cisplatin*, preventing emesis in thirty to forty percent of patients and reducing emesis in the majority. Antidopaminergic side effects, including sedation, diarrhea, and extrapyramidal symptoms, limit its high-dose use. These adverse reactions are most common in younger patients.

4. **Butyrophenones:** *Droperidol*, *domperidone*, and *haloperidol* act by blocking dopamine receptors. The butyrophenones are moderately effective antiemetics. *Droperidol* had been used most often for sedation in endoscopy and surgery, usually in combination with opiates or benzodiazepines. However, it may prolong the QT interval, and current practice reserves it for patients whose response to other agents is inadequate. High-dose *haloperidol* was found to be nearly as effective as high-dose *metoclopramide* in preventing *cisplatin*-induced emesis.

5. **Benzodiazepines:** The antiemetic potency of *lorazepam* and *alprazolam* is low. Their beneficial effects may be due to their sedative, anxiolytic, and amnesic properties. These same properties make benzodiazepines useful in treating anticipatory vomiting.

6. **Corticosteroids:** *Dexamethasone* and *methylprednisolone*, used alone, are effective against mildly to moderately emetogenic chemotherapy. Most frequently, however, they are used in combination with other agents. Their antiemetic mechanism is not known, but it may involve blockade of prostaglandins. These drugs can cause insomnia, and hyperglycemia in patients with diabetes mellitus.

7. **Cannabinoids:** Marijuana derivatives, including *dronabinol* [droe NAB i nol] and *nabilone* , are effective against moderately emetogenic chemotherapy. However, they are seldom first-line antiemet-

ics because of their serious side effects, including dysphoria, hallucinations, sedation, vertigo, and disorientation. In spite of their psychotropic properties, the antiemetic action of cannabinoids may not involve the brain, because synthetic cannabinoids, which have no psychotropic activity, nevertheless are antiemetic.

8. **Substance P/neurokinin-1–receptor blocker:** *Aprepitant* [ah PRE pih tant] belongs to a new family of antiemetic agents. It targets the neurokinin receptor in the brain, and blocks the actions of the natural substance. *Aprepitant* is usually administered orally with *dexamethasone* and *palonosetron*. It undergoes extensive metabolism, primarily by CYP3A4. Thus, as would be expected, it can affect the metabolism of other drugs that are metabolized by this enzyme. *Aprepitant* can also induce this enzyme and, thus, affect responses to other agents; for example, concomitant use with *warfarin* can shorten the half-life of the anticoagulant. Constipation and fatigue appear to be the major side effects.

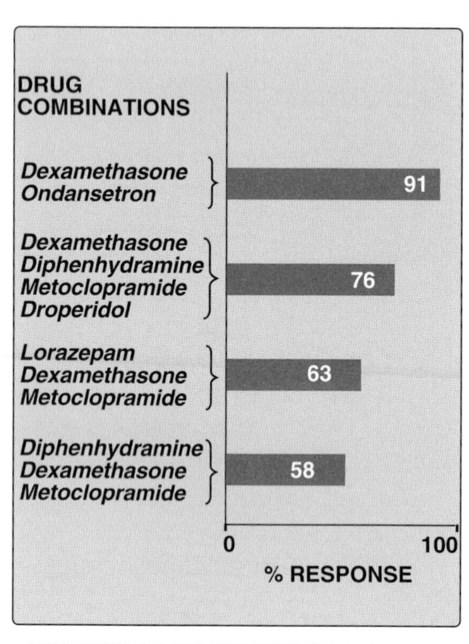

Figure 28.10
Effectiveness of antiemetic activity of some drug combinations against emetic episodes in the first 24 hours after *cisplatin* chemotherapy.

9. **Combination regimens:** Antiemetic drugs are often combined to increase antiemetic activity or decrease toxicity (Figure 28.10). Corticosteroids, most commonly *dexamethasone*, increase antiemetic activity when given with high-dose *metoclopramide*, a 5-HT_3 antagonist, *phenothiazine*, *butyrophenone*, a cannabinoid, or a benzodiazepine. Antihistamines, such as *diphenhydramine*, are often administered in combination with high-dose *metoclopramide* to reduce extrapyramidal reactions, or with corticosteroids to counter *metoclopramide*-induced diarrhea. Supplementing a cannabinoid regimen with *prochlorperazine* diminishes dysphoria.

IV. ANTIDIARRHEALS

Increased motility of the gastrointestinal tract and decreased absorption of fluid are major factors in diarrhea. Antidiarrheal drugs include antimotility agents, adsorbents, and drugs that modify fluid and electrolyte transport (Figure 28.11).

A. Antimotility agents

Two drugs that are widely used to control diarrhea are *diphenoxylate* [dye fen OX see late] and *loperamide* [loe PER ah mide]. Both are analogues of *meperidine* and have opioid-like actions on the gut, activating presynaptic opioid receptors in the enteric nervous system to inhibit acetylcholine release and decrease peristalsis. At the usual doses, they lack analgesic effects. Side effects include drowsiness, abdominal cramps, and dizziness. Because these drugs can cause toxic megacolon, they should not be used in young children or in patients with severe colitis.

B. Adsorbents

Adsorbent agents, such as *kaolin*, *pectin*, *methylcellulose*, *activated attapulgite*, and *magnesium aluminum silicate*, are widely used to control diarrhea, although their efficacy has not been documented by controlled clinical trials. Presumably, these agents act by adsorbing intestinal toxins or microorganisms and/or by coating or protecting the intestinal mucosa. They are much less effective than antimotility agents. In addition to causing constipation, they can interfere with the absorption of other drugs.

C. Agents that modify fluid and electrolyte transport

Experimental and clinical observations indicate that NSAIDs, such as *aspirin* and *indomethacin*, are effective in controlling diarrhea. This antidiarrheal action is probably due to inhibition of prostaglandin synthesis. *Bismuth subsalicylate*, used for traveler's diarrhea, decreases fluid secretion in the bowel. Its action may be due to its salicylate component.

V. LAXATIVES

Laxatives are commonly used to accelerate the movement of food through the gastrointestinal tract. These drugs can be classified on the basis of their mechanism of action as irritants or stimulants of the gut, bulking agents, and stool softeners.

A. Irritants and stimulants

Castor oil is broken down in the small intestine to ricinoleic acid, which is very irritating to the gut, and promptly increases peristalsis. *Cascara*, *senna*, and *aloe* contain emodin, which stimulates colonic activity. Onset of activity is delayed for six to eight hours, because emodin is excreted into the colon after these agents are absorbed. Emodin may pass into breast milk. *Bisacodyl* is a potent stimulant of the colon. Adverse effects include abdominal cramps and the potential for atonic colon with prolonged use.

B. Bulking agents

The bulk laxatives include hydrophilic colloids (from indigestible parts of fruits and vegetables). They form gels in the large intestine, causing water retention and intestinal distension, thereby increasing peristaltic activity. Similar actions are produced by *agar*, *methylcellulose*, *psyllium seeds*, and *bran*. Saline cathartics, such as *magnesium sulfate* and *magnesium hydroxide*, are nonabsorbable salts that hold water in the intestine by osmosis and distend the bowel, increasing intestinal activity and producing defecation in about one hour. Isosmotic electrolyte solutions containing *polyethylene glycol* are used as colonic lavage solutions to prepare the gut for radiologic or endoscopic procedures. *Lactulose* is a semisynthetic disaccharide (fructose and galactose) that also acts as an osmotic laxative.

C. Stool softeners

Surface-active agents that become emulsified with the stool produce softer feces and ease passage. These include *docusate sodium*, *mineral oil*, and *glycerin suppositories*.

DRUGS USED TO TREAT DIARRHEA AND CONSTIPATION

ANTIDIARRHEALS

- ***Activated attapulgite***
- ***Aspirin***
- ***Bismuth subsalicylate***
- ***Diphenoxylate***
- ***Indomethacin***
- ***Kaolin***
- ***Loperamide***
- ***Magnesium aluminum silicate***
- ***Methylcellulose***
- ***Pectin***

LAXATIVES

- ***Aloe***
- ***Bisacodyl***
- ***Bran***
- ***Castor oil***
- ***Docusate sodium***
- ***Glycerin suppositories***
- ***Hydrophilic colloids***
- ***Lactulose***
- ***Magnesium hydroxide***
- ***Magnesium sulfate***
- ***Methylcellulose***
- ***Mineral oil***
- ***Polyethylene glycol***
- ***Psyllium seeds***
- ***Senna***

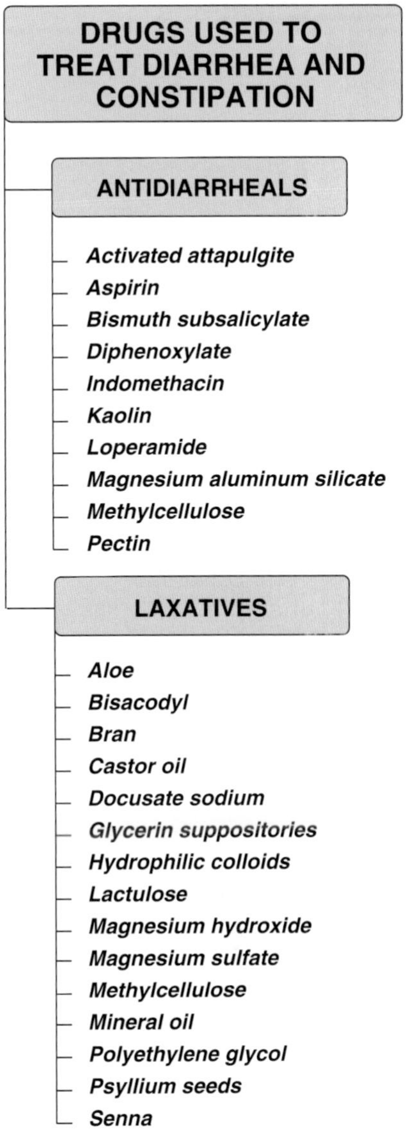

Figure 28.11
Summary of drugs used to treat diarrhea and constipation.

Study Questions

Choose the ONE best answer.

28.1 A 68-year-old patient with cardiac failure is diagnosed with ovarian cancer. She is started on cisplatin but becomes nauseous and suffers from severe vomiting. Which of the following medications would be most effective to counteract the emesis in this patient without exacerbating her cardiac problem?

A. Droperidol
B. Dolasetron
C. Prochlorperazine
D. Dronabinol
E. Ondansetron

Correct answer = E. Ondansetron is a 5-HT_3 antagonist that is effective against drugs with high emetogenic activity, such as cisplatin. Although dolasetron is also in this category, its propensity to have effects on the heart makes it a poor choice for this patient. Droperidol also has effects on the heart and now is generally a second-line drug used in combination with opiates or benzodiazepines. The antiemetic effect of prochloperazine, a phenothiazine, and dronabinol, a cannabinoid, are most beneficial against anticancer drugs with moderate to low emetogenic properties.

28.2 A 45-year-old woman is distressed by the dissolution of her marriage. She has been drinking heavily and overeating. She complains of persitent heartburn and an unpleasant, acid-like taste in her mouth. The clinician suspects gastrointestinal reflux disease and advises her to raise the head of her bed six to eight inches, not to eat several hours before retiring, to avoid alcohol, and to eat smaller meals. Two weeks later, she returns and says the symptoms have subsided slightly but still are a concern. The clinician prescribes:

A. an antacid such as aluminum hydroxide.
B. dicyclomine.
C. an antianxiety agent such as alprazolam.
D. esomeprazole.

Correct answer = D. It is appropriate to treat this patient with a proton-pump inhibitor (PPI). Acid production would be reduced and healing promoted. An H_2-receptor antagonist might also be effective, but the PPIs are preferred. An antacid would decrease acid production, but its effects are short-lived compared to those of the PPIs and H_2-receptor inhibitors. Dicyclomine is an antimuscarinic drug and would decrease acid production, but it is not as effective as the PPIs or the H_2 receptor inhibitors. An antianxiety agent might have antiemetic action but would have no effect on the acid production.

28.3 Which of the following agents interferes with most of the cytochrome P450 enzymes and, thus, leads to many drug-drug interactions?

A. Famotidine
B. Omeprazole
C. Cimetidine
D. Sucralfate
E. Ondansetron

Correct answer = C. Cimetidine interferes in the metabolism of many drugs that are metabolized by the cytochrome P450 enzymes. These include warfarin, phenytoin, metoprolol, propranolol, calcium channel blockers, and many others. Famotidine, another H_2-receptor antagonist, does not have this property, nor do the other drugs listed.

28.4 A couple celebrating their fortieth wedding anniversary is given a trip to Peru to visit Machu Picchu. Due to past experiences while travelling, they ask their doctor to prescribe an agent for diarrhea. Which of the following would be effective?

A. Omeprazole
B. Loperamide
C. Famotidine
D. Lorazepam

Correct answer = B. Loperamide is the only drug in this set that has antidiarrheal activity. Omeprazole is a PPI, famotidine antagonizes the H_2 receptor, and lorazepam is a benzodiazepine that is a sedative and anxiolytic agent.

Erectile Dysfunction, Osteoporosis, and Obesity

29

I. DRUGS USED TO TREAT ERECTILE DYSFUNCTION

Erectile dysfunction (ED)—that is, the inability to maintain penile erection for the successful performance of sexual activity—has both organic and psychogenic causes, including medications and sequelae to prostatic surgery. ED is estimated to affect up to thirty million men in the United States. Previous therapies have included penile implants, intrapenile injections of *alprostadil*, and intraurethral suppositories of *alprostadil*. However, because of their efficacy, ease of use, and safety, oral phosphodiesterase (PDE) inhibitors are now considered to be first-line therapy for men with ED. Three PDE-5 inhibitors, *sildenafil* [sil DEN a fil], *vardenafil* [var DEN na fil], and *tadalafil* [ta DAL a fil], are approved for the treatment of ED (Figure 29.1).

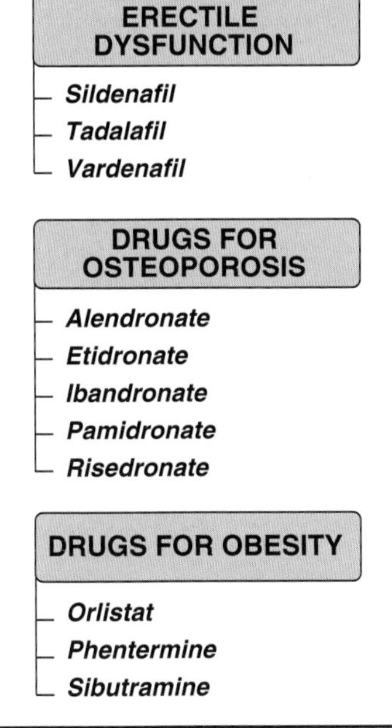

DRUGS FOR ERECTILE DYSFUNCTION
Sildenafil
Tadalafil
Vardenafil
DRUGS FOR OSTEOPOROSIS
Alendronate
Etidronate
Ibandronate
Pamidronate
Risedronate
DRUGS FOR OBESITY
Orlistat
Phentermine
Sibutramine

Figure 29.1
Summary of drugs used in the treatment of erectile dysfunction, osteoporosis, and obesity.

A. PDE-5 inhibitors

All three PDE-5 inhibitors are equally effective in treating ED, and the side-effect profiles of the drugs are similar. However, the duration of action of PDE-5 inhibitors differ, as do the effects of food on the rates of drug absorption.

1. **Mechanism of penile erection:** Sexual stimulation results in smooth muscle relaxation of the corpus cavernosum, increasing the inflow of blood (Figure 29.2). The mediator of this response is nitric oxide (NO). NO activates guanylyl cyclase, which forms cyclic guanosine monophosphate (cGMP) from guanosine triphosphate. cGMP produces smooth muscle relaxation through a reduction in the intracellular Ca^{2+} concentration. The duration of action of cyclic nucleotides is controlled by the action of PDE. At least eleven isozymes of PDE have been characterized. *Sildenafil*, *vardenafil*∏, and *tadalafil* inhibit PDE-5, the isozyme responsible for termination of cGMP in the corpus cavernosum. The action of PDE-5 inhibitors is to increase the flow of blood into the corpus cavernosum at any given level of sexual stimulation (Figure 29.3). At recommended doses, PDE-5 inhibitors have no effect in the

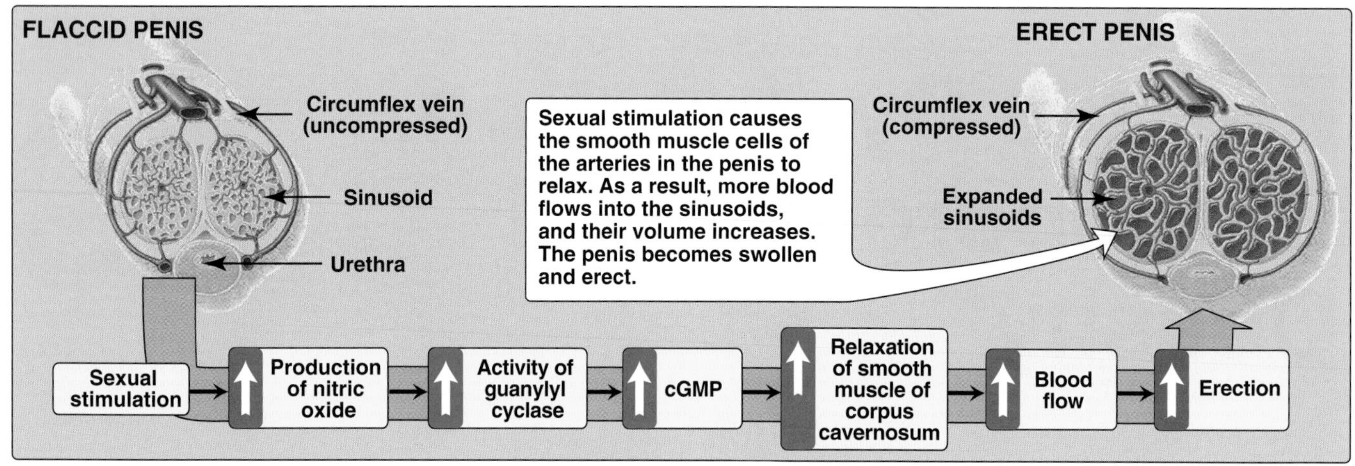

Figure 29.2
Mechanism of penile erection. cGMP = cyclic guanosine monophosphate.

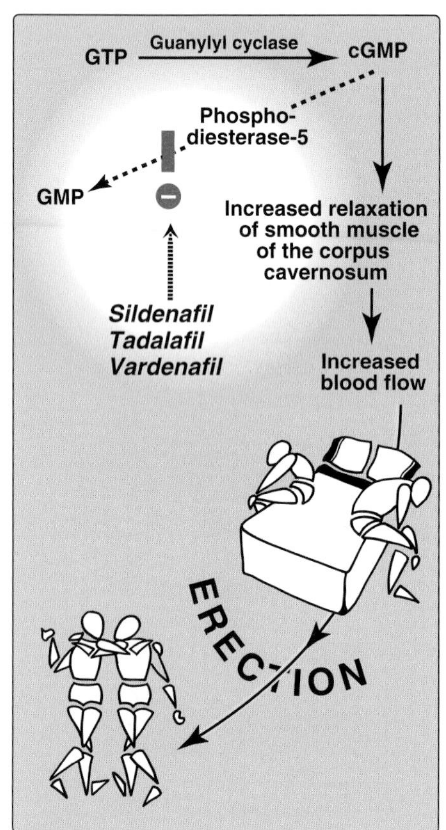

Figure 29.3
Effect of phosphodiesterase inhibitors on cyclic guanosine monophosphate (cGMP) levels in the smooth muscle of the corpus cavernosum. GTP = guanosine triphosphate.

absence of sexual stimulation. PDE-5 inhibitors are indicated for the treatment of ED due to organic or psychogenic causes.

2. **Pharmacokinetics:** *Sildenafil* and *vardenafil* have similar pharmacokinetic properties. Both drugs should be taken approximately one hour prior to anticipated sexual activity, with erectile enhancement observed up to four hours after administration. Thus, administration of *sildenafil* and *vardenafil* must be timed so that sexual activity occurs within one to six hours. The absorption of both drugs is delayed by consumption of food, particularly high-fat meals. By contrast, *tadalafil* has a slower onset of action (Figure 29.4) but a significantly longer half-life of approximately 18 hours, resulting in enhanced erectile function for at least 36 hours. Furthermore, the pharmacokinetics of *tadalafil* is not clinically influenced by food or alcohol intake. The timing of sexual activity is less critical for *tadalafil* because of its prolonged duration of effect. All three PDE-5 inhibitors are metabolized by the cytochrome P450 3A4 enzyme

3. **Adverse effects:** The most frequent adverse effects reported for PDE inhibitors are headache, flushing, dyspepsia, and nasal congestion. These effects are generally mild, and men with ED rarely discontinue treatment because of side effects. Disturbances in color vision (loss of blue/green discrimination) occur with *sildenafil*, probably because of inhibition of PDE-6 (a PDE found in the retina that is important in color vision). *Tadalafil* does not appear to disrupt PDE-6, and blue vision has not been reported with this medication. The incidence of these reactions appears to be dose-dependent. Treatment with a PDE does not increase the incidence of myocardial infarction. PDE-5 inhibitors should not be used more than once per day.

4. **Drug interactions:** Because of the ability of PDE inhibitors ability to potentiate the activity of NO, there is an absolute contraindication against the use of concurrent organic nitrates in any form.

Concomitant treatment with α-adrenergic antagonists (used to alleviate symptoms associated with benign prostatic hyperplasia) is contraindicated (due to potential hypotension with combination therapy) with the exception of *tamsulosin* (see p. 83), which may be used safely with *tadalafil.*

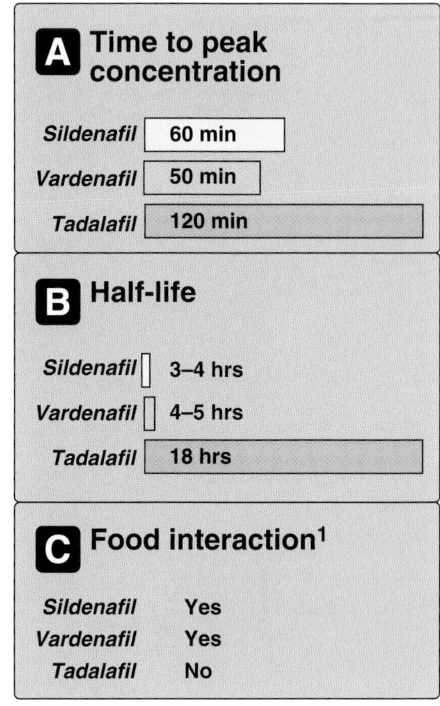

Figure 29.4
Some properties of phophodiesterase inhibitors. [1]Delay in time to reach peak drug concentration when taken with high-fat foods.

II. DRUGS USED TO TREAT OSTEOPOROSIS

Osteoporosis is a condition of skeletal fragility due to progressive loss of bone mass. It occurs in the elderly of both sexes but is most pronounced in postmenopausal women. Osteoporosis is characterized by frequent bone fractures, which are a major cause of disability among the elderly. Nondrug strategies to reduce bone loss in postmenopausal women include a diet adequate in calcium and vitamin D, weight-bearing exercise, and cessation of smoking. In addition, patients at risk for osteoporosis should avoid drugs that increase bone loss, such as glucocorticoids. Figure 29.5 shows the changes in bone morphology seen in osteoporosis.

A. Bisphosphonates

These analogs of pyrophosphate, including *etidronate* [e TID row nate], *risedronate* [rih SED row nate], *alendronate* [a LEND row nate], and *pamidronate* [pah MID row nate], comprise an important drug group used for the treatment of disorders of bone remodeling, such as osteoporosis and Paget disease, as well as for treatment of metastatic bone cancers. In addition, *alendronate* and *risedronate* have been approved for the prevention of osteoporosis. The beneficial effects of *alendronate* persist over several years of therapy, but bone loss occurs after treatment is stopped. The bisphosphonates decrease osteoclastic bone resorption via several mechanisms, including 1) inhibition of the osteoclastic proton pump necessary for dissolution of hydroxyapatite, 2) decrease in osteoclastic formation/activation, and 3) increased osteoclastic apoptosis (programmed cell death). The relative importance of the mechanisms may differ among the individual bisphosphonates, and it is not known if they are due to a single molecular activity. The decrease in osteoclastic bone resorption results in a small but significant net gain in bone mass in osteoporotic patients, because the bone-forming osteoblasts are not inhibited. The therapeutic effects of *alendronate* are sustained over a ten-year period (Figure 29.6). Discontinuation of *alendronate* results in a gradual loss of its effects. Decreased rates of bone fracture have been reported in patients with osteoporosis and those with Paget disease patients who are treated with bisphosphonates. In addition, bisphosphonates have been shown to decrease the number of bone and visceral metastases in patients with breast cancer.

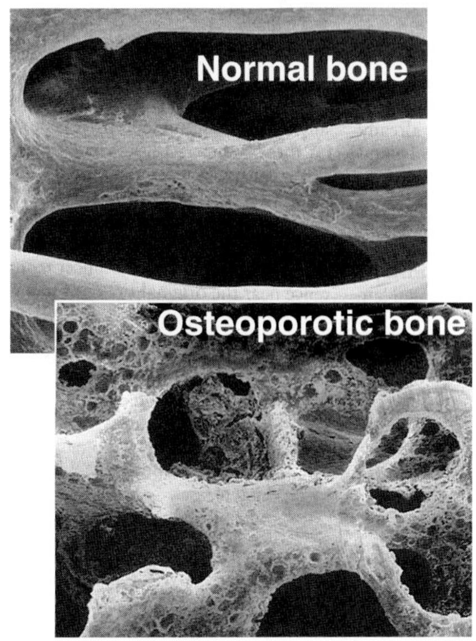

Figure 29.5
Changes in bone morphology seen in osteoporosis.

1. **Pharmacokinetics:** *Pamidronate* is administered intravenously. All of the other bisphosphonates are orally active, although less than ten percent of the administered dose is absorbed. Food significantly interferes with absorption. Bisphosphonates should be administered with six to eight ounces of water at least one hour before eating breakfast. The bisphosphonates are rapidly cleared

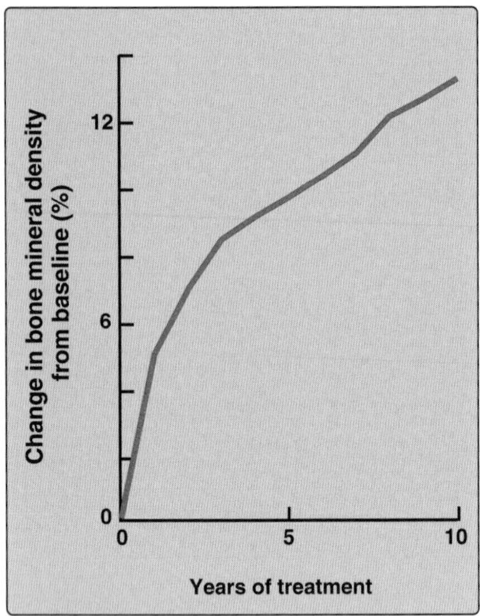

Figure 29.6
Effect of *alendronate* therapy on the bone mineral density of the lumbar spine.

from the plasma, primarily because they avidly bind to the hydroxyapatite mineral of bone. Once bound to bone, they are cleared over a period of months to years. Elimination from the body is solely through renal clearance, and the bisphosphonates should not be given to individuals with severe renal impairment.

2. **Adverse effects:** These include diarrhea, nausea, and abdominal pain. *Alendronate*, *etidronate*, and *risedronate* are associated with esophageal ulcers. *Etidronate* is the only member of the class that causes osteomalacia following long-term, continuous administration. Figure 29.7 shows the relative potencies of the bisphosphonates.

B. Teriparatide

Teriparatide [ter ih PAR a tide] is a recombinant segment of human parathyroid hormone for the parenteral treatment of osteoporosis. It increases spinal bone density and decreases the risk of vertebral fracture. [Note: In a comparison of *teriparatide* versus *alendronate*, *teriparatide* therapy resulted in a greater increase in spine density and a greater reduction in risk of nonvertebral fractures than with *alendronate* therapy.] *Teriparatide* is the first approved treatment for osteoporosis that stimulates bone formation. Other drugs approved for this indication inhibit bone resorption. Parathyroid hormone given continuously leads to dissolution of bone, but when it is given subcutaneously once daily, bone formation is the predominant effect. *Teriparatide* is also effective the treatment of glucocorticoid-induced osteoporosis. It is rapidly degraded, mostly in the liver and kidneys.

C. Selective estrogen-receptor modulators (SERMs)

Estrogen replacement is the most effective therapy for the prevention of postmenopausal bone loss. When initiated in the immediate postmenopausal period, estrogen therapyprevents osteoporosis and reduces the risk of hip fracture. *Raloxifene* is approved for the prevention and treatment of osteoporosis. It increases women's bone density without increasing the risk of endometrial cancer. In addition, *raloxifene* may reduce the the risk of estrogen receptor–positive breast cancer. *Raloxifene* reduces serum total and low-density lipoprotein (LDL) cholesterol concentrations. The risk of venous thromboembolism appears to be comparable to that with estrogen. [Note: Estrogen-progestin therapy is no longer the therapy of choice for the treatment of osteoporosis in postmenopausal women because of increased risk of breast cancer, stroke, venous thromboembolism, and perhaps, coronary disease.]

Bisphosphonate	Antiresorptive activity
Etidronate	1
Pamidronate	100
Alendronate	100–1000
Risedronate	1000–10,000

Figure 29.7
Structure and antiresorptive activity of some bisphosphonates.

D. Calcitonin

Salmon *calcitonin* [cal SIH toe nin], administered intranasally, is effective and well tolerated in postmenopausal women at risk of developing osteoporosis. The drug reduces bone resorption and improves bone architecture, relieves pain, and increases function. Unfortunately, tolerance occurs with continuous use.

III. DRUGS USED TO TREAT OBESITY

Two classes of drug are used in treating obesity: the anorexiants (appetite suppressants) *phentermine* or *sibutramine*, and a lipase inhibitor, *orlistat*.

A. Phentermine and sibutramine

These agents have many properties in common. Both are sympathomimetic amines that exert their pharmacologic action by interfering in the reuptake of serotonin and norepinephrine into the presynaptic nerve terminal, thereby increasing their brain levels. In the case of *phentermine* [FEN ter meen], there is an increased release of dopamine, whereas with *sibutramine* [si BYOO tra meen], the reuptake into the presynaptic nerve terminal of serotonin, norepinephrine, and to a lesser extent, dopamine is hindered. Figure 29.8 shows the effect of *sibutramine* treatment.

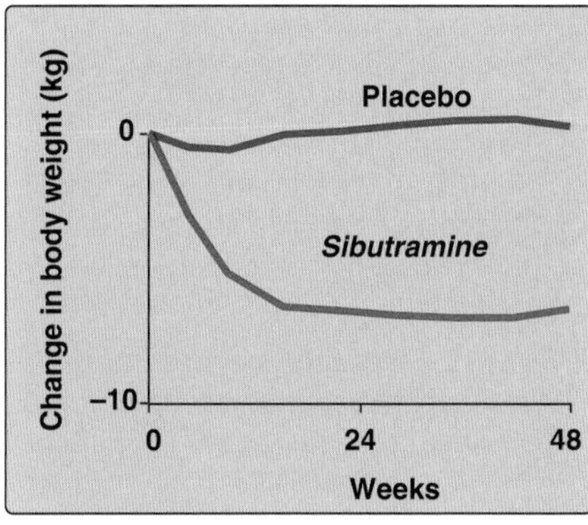

Figure 29.8
Effect of *sibutramine* treatment on body weight.

1. **Pharmacokinetics:** *Sibutramine* undergoes first-pass demethylation to active metabolites, which are biotransformed further in the liver and excreted primarily in the urine. The half-life is about fifteen hours.

2. **Adverse effects and contraindications:** These are similar for both drugs. For example, they are both controlled as Schedule IV agents (they have a low liability for dependence or abuse). Heart rate and blood pressure may be increased, and dry mouth, headache, insomnia, and constipation are common problems. *Sibutramine* should be avoided in patients who are taking monoamine oxidase inhibitors, selective serotonin inhibitors such as *fluoxetine*, serotonin agonists for migraine such as *sumatriptan*, as well as *lithium*, *dextromethorphan*, or *pentazocine*. Drug interactions can occur when *sibutramine* is administered with drugs that inhibit CYP3A4, such as *ketoconazole*, *erythromycin*, and *cimetidine*. The clinical releance of these interactions is not known.

B. Orlistat

Orlistat [OR lih stat] is the first drug in a new class of nonsystemically acting antiobesity drugs know as lipase inhibitors. *Orlistat* is a pentanoic acid ester that inhibits gastric and pancreatic lipases, thus decreasing the breakdown of dietary fat into smaller molecules. Fat absorption is decreased by about thirty percent. The loss of calories is the main cause of weight loss, but adverse gastrointestinal effects associated with the drug may also contribute to a decreased intake of food. In clinical trials, individuals treated with *orlistat* lost an average of ten percent of their body weight (compared to six percent for the placebo group) within one year (Figure 29.9). Total and LDL cholesterol decreased more in the treatment group than in the placebo group. The most common side effects associated with *orlistat* are gastrointestinal symptoms, such as oily spotting, flatulence with discharge, fecal urgency, and increased defecation. *Orlistat* interferes with the absorption of the fat-soluble vitamins, β-carotene, and carotenoids. *Orlistat* is contraindicated in patients with chronic malabsorption syndrome or cholestasis.

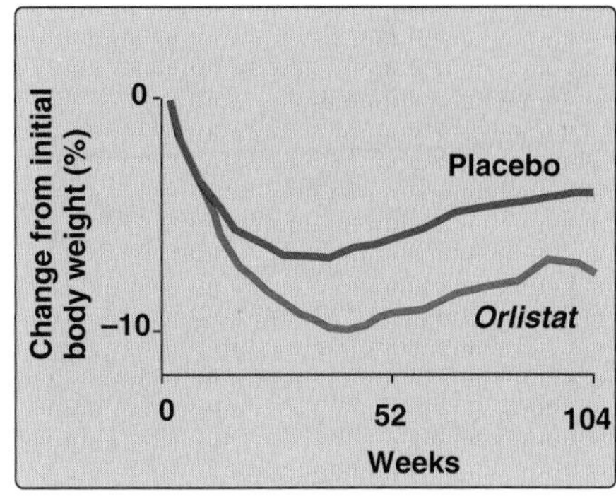

Figure 29.9
Effect of *orlistat* treatment on body weight.

Study Questions

Choose the ONE best answer.

29.1 A 66-year-old man complained of decreased libido and difficulty maintaining an erection. He is currently taking tamsulosin for benign prostatic hyperplasia. He is concerned about the use of drugs to restore sexual function, particularly about the need to time therapy with anticipated sexual activity. Which one of the following therapeutic options is indicated for this patient?

A. PDE-5 inhibitors are contraindicated because of treatment with tamsulosin.
B. Sildenafil is indicated because of its long duration of action.
C. Vardenafil is indicated because its absorption is not affected by food.
D. Tadalafil is indicated because it can be used concomitantly with tamsulosin.
E. Tadalafil is not indicated because of its short duration of action.

Correct answer = D. Concomitant treatment with α-adrenergic antagonists (used to alleviate symptoms associated with benign prostatic hyperplasia) is contraindicated with PDE inhbitiors (due to potential hypotension with combination therapy) with the exception of tamsulosin, which may be used safely with tadalafil. Tadalafil has a slow onset of action but a longer half-life of approximately 18 hours, resulting in enhanced erectile function for at least 36 hours. The timing of sexual activity is less critical for tadalafil because of its prolonged duration of effect.

29.2 Which of the following drugs causes osteomalacia and bone pain when administered chronically?

A. Risedronate
B.Calcitonin
C. Teriparatide
D. Calcitriol
E. Etidronate

Correct answer = E. The older bisphosphonates, such as etidronate, are not as potent inhibitors of osteoclast activity as the newer agents. Long-term therapy with etidronate also interferes with osteoblast activity resulting in bone malformations and pain. The other drugs do not cause this problem.

29.3 A 58-year-old male has been effectively treated for Paget disease for approximately six months. He is now beginning to experience renewed bone pain and radiologic evidence of advancing disease. Which of the following drugs is most likely to have resulted in this failure of therapy?

A. Alendronate
B. Calcitonin
C. Dihydrotachysterol
D.Ergocalciferol
E. Raloxifene

Correct answer = B. Paget disease can be treated effectively with either a bisphosphonate or calcitonin. Calcitonin therapy is complicated by the fact that tolerance develops to the action of the hormone when administration is continuous over a long period of time. The other drugs are not effective in the treatment of Paget disease.

UNIT VII:
Chemotherapeutic Drugs

Principles of Antimicrobial Therapy

30

I. OVERVIEW

Antimicrobial therapy takes advantage of the biochemical differences that exist between microorganisms and human beings. Antimicrobial drugs are effective in the treatment of infections because of their selective toxicity; that is, they have the ability to injure or kill an invading microorganism without harming the cells of the host. In most instances, the selective toxicity is relative rather than absolute, requiring that the concentration of the drug be carefully controlled to attack the microorganism while still being tolerated by the host.

II. SELECTION OF ANTIMICROBIAL AGENTS

Selection of the most appropriate antimicrobial agent requires knowledge of 1) the organism's identity, 2) its susceptibility to a particular agent, 3) the site of the infection, 4) patient factors, 5) the safety of the agent, and 6) the cost of therapy. However, some critically ill patients require empiric therapy—that is, immediate administration of drug(s) prior to bacterial identification and susceptibility testing.

A. Identification of the infecting organism

Characterization of the organism is central to selection of the proper drug. A rapid assessment of the nature of the pathogen can sometimes be made on the basis of the Gram stain, which is particularly useful in identifying the presence and morphologic features of microorganisms in body fluids that are normally sterile (cerebrospinal fluid, pleural fluid, synovial fluid, peritoneal fluid, and urine). However, it is generally necessary to culture the infective organism to arrive at a conclusive diagnosis and to determine the susceptibility of the bacteria to antimicrobial agents. Thus, it is essential to obtain a sample culture of the organism prior to initiating treatment. Definitive identification of the infecting organism may require other laboratory techniques, such as

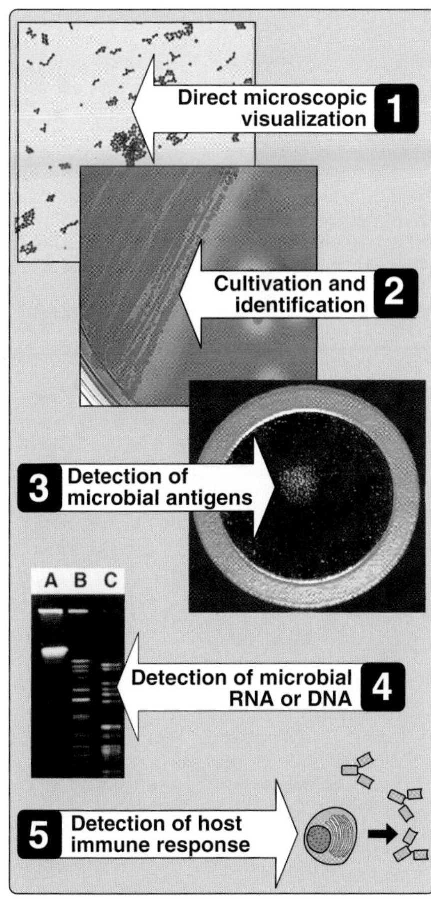

Figure 30.1
Some laboratory techniques that are useful in diagnosis of microbial diseases.

Lippincott's Illustrated Reviews: Pharmacology, Third Edition, by Richard D. Howland and Mary J. Mycek.
Lippincott Williams & Wilkins, Baltimore, MD © 2006.

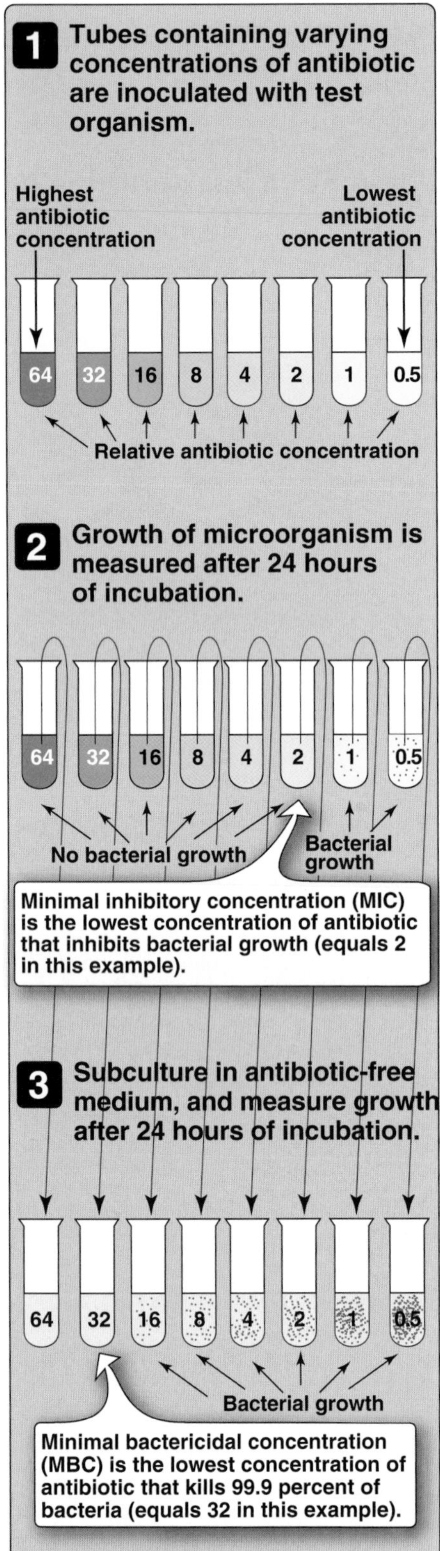

1 Tubes containing varying concentrations of antibiotic are inoculated with test organism.
Highest antibiotic concentration
Lowest antibiotic concentration
64
32
16
8
4
2
1
0.5
Relative antibiotic concentration
2 Growth of microorganism is measured after 24 hours of incubation.
No bacterial growth
Bacterial growth
Minimal inhibitory concentration (MIC) is the lowest concentration of antibiotic that inhibits bacterial growth (equals 2 in this example).
3 Subculture in antibiotic-free medium, and measure growth after 24 hours of incubation.
Bacterial growth
Minimal bactericidal concentration (MBC) is the lowest concentration of antibiotic that kills 99.9 percent of bacteria (equals 32 in this example).

Figure 30.2
Determination of minimum inhibitory concentration (MIC) and minimum bactericidal concentration (MBC) of an antibiotic.

detection of microbial antigens, microbial DNA or RNA, or detection of an inflammatory or host immune response to the microorganism (Figure 30.1).[1]

B. Empiric therapy prior to identification of the organism

Ideally, the antimicrobial agent used to treat an infection is selected after the organism has been identified and its drug susceptibility established. However, in the critically ill patient, such a delay could prove fatal, and immediate empiric therapy is indicated.

1. **The acutely ill patient:** Acutely ill patients with infections of unknown origin—for example, a neutropenic patient (one who has a reduction in neutrophil count, possibly indicating bacterial infection), or a patient with severe headache, a rigid neck, and sensitivity to bright lights (symptoms characteristic of meningitis)—require immediate treatment. Therapy is initiated after specimens for laboratory analysis have been obtained but before the results of the culture are available.

2. **Selecting a drug:** The choice of drug in the absence of susceptibility data is influenced by the site of infection, and the patient's history (for example, whether the infection was hospital- or community-acquired, whether the patient is immunocompromised, as well as the patient's travel record and age). Broad-spectrum therapy may be needed initially for serious infections when the identity of the organism is unknown or the site makes a polymicrobial infection likely. The choice of agents may also be guided by known association of particular organisms with infection in a given clinical setting. For example, a gram-positive coccus in the spinal fluid of a newborn infant is unlikely to be Streptococcus pneumoniae (pneumococcus) but most likely to be Streptococcus agalactiae (Group B). This organism is sensitive to *penicillin G*. By contrast, a gram-positive coccus in the spinal fluid of a forty-year-old patient is most likely to be S. pneumoniae. This organism is frequently resistant to *penicillin G*, and often requires treatment with a third-generation cephalosporin (such as *cefotaxime* or *ceftriaxone*) or *vancomycin*.

C. Determination of antimicrobial susceptibility of infective organisms

After a pathogen is cultured, its susceptibility to specific antibiotics serves as a guide in choosing antimicrobial therapy. Some pathogens, such as Streptococcus pyogenes and Neisseria meningitidis, usually have predictable susceptibility patterns to certain antibiotics. In contrast, most gram-negative bacilli, enterococci, and staphylococcal species often show unpredictable susceptibility patterns to various antibiotics, and require susceptibility testing to determine appropriate antimicrobial therapy. The minimum inhibitory and bactericidal concentrations of a drug can be experimentally determined (Figure 30.2).

1. **Bacteriostatic vs. bactericidal drugs:** Antimicrobial drugs are classified as either bacteriostatic or bactericidal. Bacteriostatic

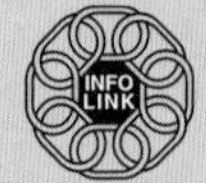

[1]See Chapter 4 in ***Lippincott's Illustrated Reviews: Microbiology*** for a more detailed presentation of the techniques used in diagnostic microbiology.

drugs arrest the growth and replication of bacteria at serum levels achievable in the patient, thus limiting the spread of infection while the body's immune system attacks, immobilizes, and eliminates the pathogens. If the drug is removed before the immune system has scavenged the organisms, enough viable organisms may remain to begin a second cycle of infection. Bactericidal drugs kill bacteria at drug serum levels achievable in the patient. Because of their more aggressive antimicrobial action, these agents are often the drugs of choice in seriously ill patients. Figure 30.3 shows a laboratory experiment in which the growth of bacteria is arrested by the addition of a bacteriostatic agent. Note that viable organisms remain even in the presence of the bacteriostatic drug. By contrast, addition of a bactericidal agent kills bacteria, and the total number of viable organisms decreases. Although practical, this classification may be too simplistic, because it is possible for an antibiotic to be bacteriostatic for one organism and bactericidal for another. For example, *chloramphenicol* is static against gram-negative rods and is cidal against other organisms, such as S. pneumoniae.

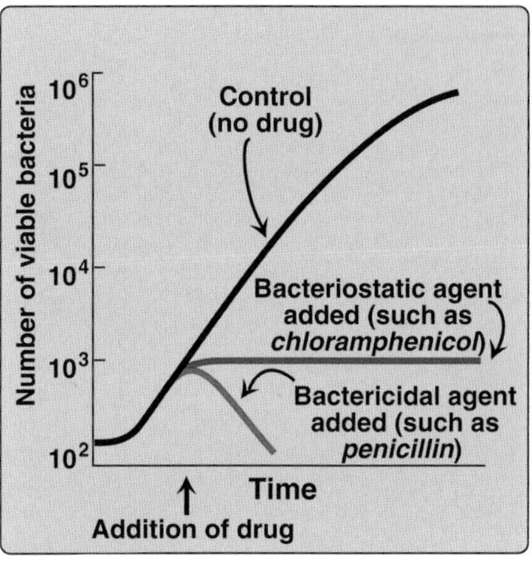

Figure 30.3
Effects of bactericidal and bacteriostatic drugs on the growth of bacteria in vitro.

2. **Minimum inhibitory concentration:** To determine the minimum inhibitory concentration (MIC), tubes containing serial dilutions of an antibiotic are inoculated with the organism whose susceptibility is to be tested (see Figure 30.2). The tubes are incubated and later observed to determine the MIC—that is, the lowest concentration of antibiotic that inhibits bacterial growth. To provide effective antimicrobial therapy, the clinically obtainable antibiotic concentration in body fluids should be greater than the MIC. [Note: This assay is now done automatically using microtiter plates.]

3. **Minimum bactericidal concentration:** This quantitative assay determines the minimal concentration of antibiotic that kills the bacteria under investigation. The tubes that show no growth in the MIC assay are subcultured into antibiotic-free media. The minimum bactericidal concentration (MBC) is the lowest concentration of antimicrobial agent that results in a 99.9 percent decline in colony count after overnight broth dilution incubations (see Figure 30.2).

D. Effect of the site of infection on therapy: The blood-brain barrier

Adequate levels of an antibiotic must reach the site of infection for the invading microorganisms to be effectively eradicated. Capillaries with varying degrees of permeability carry drugs to the body tissues. For example, the endothelial cells comprising the walls of capillaries of many tissues have fenestrations (openings that act like windows) that allow most drugs not bound by plasma proteins to penetrate. However, natural barriers to drug delivery are created by the structures of the capillaries of some tissues, such as the prostate, the vitreous body of the eye, and the central nervous system (CNS). Of particular significance are the capillaries in the brain, which help to create and maintain the blood-brain barrier. This barrier is formed by the single layer of tile-like endothelial cells fused by tight junctions that impede entry from the blood to the brain of virtually all molecules, except those that are small and lipophilic (Figure 30.4). This barrier can be demonstrated by injecting dyes into laboratory ani-

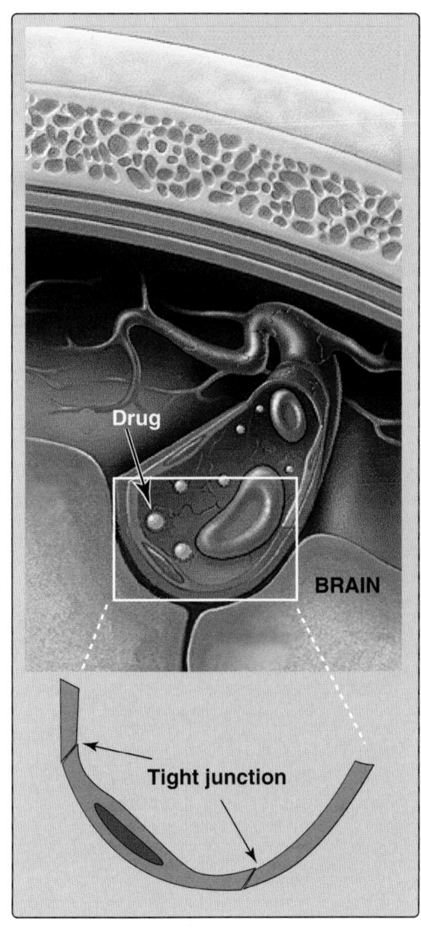

Figure 30.4
Essential features of the blood-brain barrier.

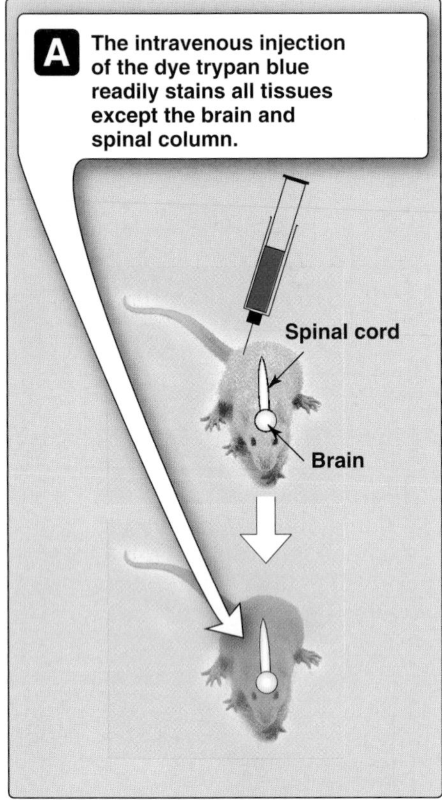

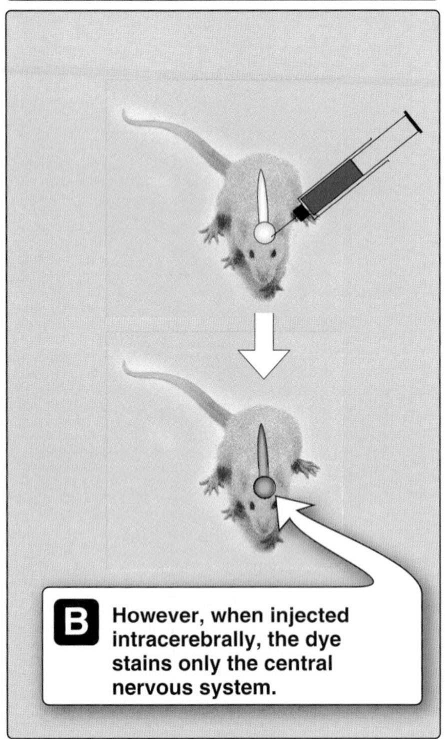

B
However, when injected intracerebrally, the dye stains only the central nervous system.

Figure 30.5
Schematic representation of the blood-brain barrier.

mals. Dyes injected into the circulation stain all tissues except brain. However, the same dyes injected into cerebral spinal fluid (CSF) stain only the cells of the CNS (Figure 30.5). The blood-brain barrier prevents the dye from escaping from the blood vessels in the brain, although they readily leak from the vessels throughout the rest of the body. The penetration and concentration of an antibacterial agent in the CSF is particularly influenced by the following:

1. **Lipid solubility of the drug:** All compounds without a specific transporter must pass intracellularly from the blood to the CSF (through two endothelial cell membranes, see Figure 30.5). The lipid solubility of a drug is therefore a major determinant of its ability to penetrate into the brain. For example, lipid-soluble drugs, such as the quinolones and *metronidazole*, have significant penetration into the CNS. In contrast, β-lactam antibiotics, such as *penicillin*, are ionized at physiologic pH and have low solubility in lipids. They therefore have limited penetration through the intact blood-brain barrier under normal circumstances. In infections such as meningitis, in which the brain becomes inflamed, the barrier does not function effectively, and local permeability is increased. Some β-lactam antibiotics can then enter the CSF in therapeutic amounts.

2. **Molecular weight of the drug:** A compound with a low molecular weight has an enhanced ability to cross the blood-brain barrier, whereas compounds with a high molecular weight (for example, *vancomycin*) penetrate poorly, even in the presence of meningeal inflammation.

3. **Protein binding of the drug:** A high degree of protein binding of a drug in the serum restricts its entry into the CSF. It therefore is the amount of free (unbound) drug in serum, rather than the total amount of drug present, that is important for CSF penetration.

E. Patient factors

In selecting an antibiotic, attention must be paid to the condition of the patient. For example, the status of the patient's immune system, kidneys, liver, circulation, and age must be considered. In women, pregnancy or breast-feeding an infant also affects selection of the antimicrobial agent.

1. **Immune system:** Elimination of infecting organisms from the body depends on an intact immune system. Antibacterial drugs decrease the microbial population (bactericidal) or inhibit further bacterial growth (bacteriostatic), but the host defense system must ultimately eliminate the invading organisms. Alcoholism, diabetes, infection with the human immunodeficiency virus, malnutrition, or advanced age can affect a patient's immunocompetency, as can therapy with immunosuppressive drugs. Higher-than-usual doses of bactericidal agents or longer courses of treatment are required to eliminate infective organisms in these individuals.

2. **Renal dysfunction:** Poor kidney function (ten percent or less of normal) causes accumulation in the body of antibiotics that ordinarily

are eliminated by this route. This may lead to serious adverse effects unless drug accumulation is controlled by adjusting the dose or the dosage schedule of the antibiotic. Serum creatinine levels are frequently used as an index of renal function for adjustment of drug regimens.[2] However, direct monitoring of serum levels of some antibiotics (for example, aminoglycosides) is preferred to identify maximum and minimum values. Rising minimum values alert the physician to potential toxicity. [Note: The number of functioning nephrons decreases with age. Thus, elderly patients are particularly vulnerable to accumulation of drugs eliminated by the kidneys. Antibiotics that undergo extensive metabolism or are excreted via the biliary route may be favored in such patients.]

3. **Hepatic dysfunction:** Antibiotics that are concentrated or eliminated by the liver (for example, *erythromycin* and *tetracycline*) are contraindicated in treating patients with liver disease.

4. **Poor perfusion:** Decreased circulation to an anatomic area, such as the lower limbs of a diabetic, reduces the amount of antibiotic that reaches that area, and makes infections notoriously difficult to treat.

5. **Age:** Renal or hepatic elimination processes are often poorly developed in newborns, making neonates particularly vulnerable to the toxic effects of *chloramphenicol* and sulfonamides. Young children should not be treated with tetracyclines, which affect bone growth.

6. **Pregnancy:** All antibiotics cross the placenta. Adverse effects to the fetus are rare, except for tooth dysplasia and inhibition of bone growth encountered with the tetracyclines. However, some anthelmintics are embryotoxic and teratogenic. Aminoglycosides should be avoided in pregnancy because of their ototoxic effect on the fetus. Figure 30.6 summarizes the United States Food and Drug Administration categories of antibiotic use during pregnancy.

7. **Lactation:** Drugs administered to a lactating mother may enter the nursing infant via the breast milk. Although the concentration of an antibiotic in breast milk is usually low, the total dose to the infant may be enough to cause problems.

CATEGORY	DESCRIPTION	DRUG
A	No human fetal risk or remote possibility of fetal harm	
B	No controlled studies show human risk; animal studies suggest potential toxicity	β-Lactams β-Lactams with inhibitors Cephalosporins *Aztreonam* *Clindamycin* *Erythromycin* *Azithromycin* *Metronidazole* *Nitrofurantoin* Sulfonamides
C	Animal fetal toxicity demonstrated; human risk undefined	*Chloramphenicol* Fluoroquinolones *Clarithromycin* *Trimethoprim* *Vancomycin* *Gentamicin* *Trimethoprim-sulfamethoxazole*
D	Human fetal risk present, but benefits outweigh risks	Tetracyclines Aminoglycosides (except *gentamicin*)
X	Human fetal risk present but does not outweigh benefits; contraindicated in pregnancy	

Figure 30.6
United States Food and Drug Administration categories of antimicrobials and fetal risk.

F. Safety of the agent

Many of the antibiotics, such as the penicillins, are among the least toxic of all drugs, because they interfere with a site unique to the growth of microorganisms. Other antimicrobial agents (for example, *chloramphenicol*) are less microorganism-specific, and are reserved for life-threatening infections because of the drug's potential for serious toxicity to the patient. [Note: As discussed above, safety is related not only to the inherent nature of the drug, but also to patient factors that can predispose to toxicity.]

INFO LINK [2]See Chapter 285 in ***Lippincott's Illustrated Reviews: Biochemistry*** (3rd ed.) for a discussion of creatinine.

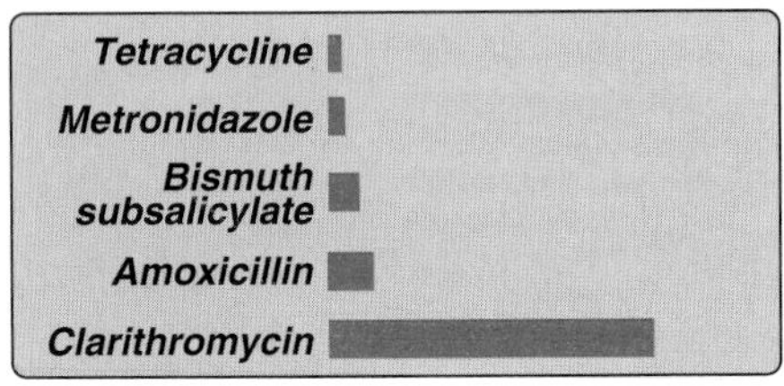

Figure 30.7
Relative cost of some drugs used for the treatment of peptic ulcers caused by Helicobacter pylori.

G. Cost of therapy

Often, several drugs may show similar efficacy in treating an infection but vary widely in cost. Figure 30.7 illustrates the cost of some antibacterial agents showing similar efficacy in eradicating the gram-negative bacillus Helicobacter pylori from the gastric mucosa. None of these agents shows a clear therapeutic superiority; thus, a combination of *metronidazole* with *bismuth subsalicylate* plus one other antibiotic is usually employed in the treatment of H. pylori-induced peptic ulcers. Selecting *clarithromycin* instead as the drug of choice would clearly make a considerable cost impact.

III. ROUTE OF ADMINISTRATION

The oral route of administration is chosen for infections that are mild and can be treated on an outpatient basis. In addition, economic pressures have prompted the use of oral antibiotic therapy in all but the most serious infectious diseases. In patients requiring a course of intravenous therapy initially, the switch to oral agents occurs as soon as possible. However, some antibiotics, such as *vancomycin*, the aminoglycosides, and *amphotericin* are so poorly absorbed from the gastrointestinal tract that adequate serum levels cannot be obtained by oral administration. Parenteral administration is used for drugs that are poorly absorbed from the the gastrointestinal tract, and for treatment of patients with serious infections, for whom it is necessary to maintain higher serum concentrations of antimicrobial agents than can be reliably obtained by the oral route.

IV. DETERMINANTS OF RATIONAL DOSING

Rational dosing of antimicrobial agents is based on their pharmacodynamics (the relationship of drug concentrations to antimicrobial effects) as well as their pharmacokinetic properties (the absorption, distribution, and elimination of the drug by the body). Two important pharmacodynamic properties that have a significant influence on the frequency of dosing are concentration-dependent killing and post-antibiotic effect.

A. Concentration-dependent killing

Certain antimicrobial agents, including aminoglycosides and fluoroquinolones, show a significant increase in the rate of bacterial killing as the concentration of antibiotic increases from 4- to 64-fold the MIC of the drug for the infecting organism. (Figure 30.8A). Giving drugs that exhibit this concentration-dependent killing by a once-a-day bolus infusion achieves high peak levels, favoring rapid killing of the infecting pathogen. By contrast, β-lactams, glycopeptides, macrolides, and *clindamycin* do not exhibit this property; that is, increasing the concentration of antibiotic to higher multiples of the MIC does not significantly increase the rate of kill (Figure 30.8B). The clinical efficacy of antimicrobials that have a nonsignificant, dose-dependent killing effect is best predicted by the percentage of time that blood concentrations of a drug remain above the MIC. This effect is sometimes called concentration-independent or time-dependent killing. For example, for the penicillins and cephalosporins, dosing schedules that ensure blood levels greater than the

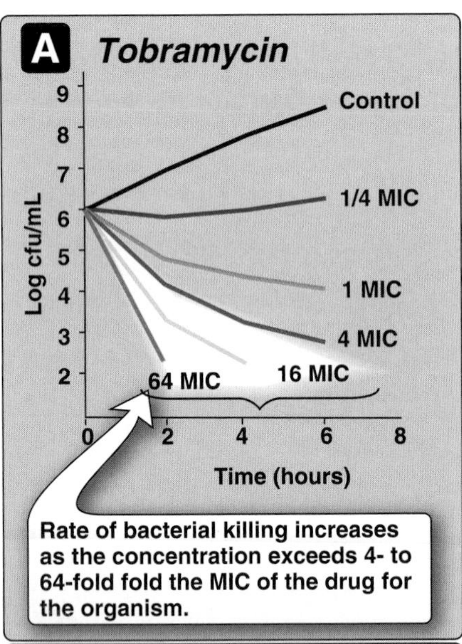

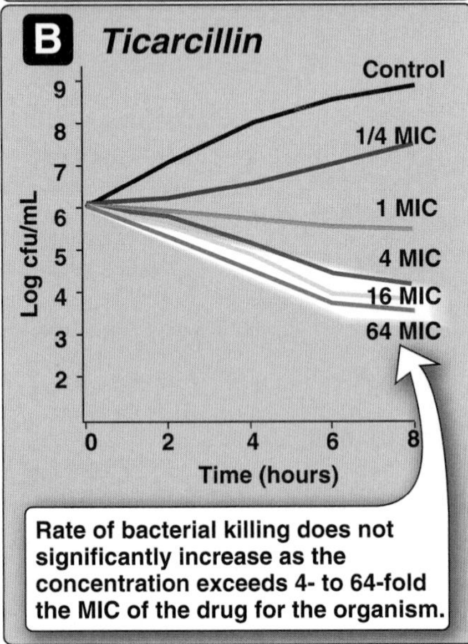

Figure 30.8
A. Significant dose-dependent killing effect shown by *tobramycin*.
B. Nonsignificant dose-dependent killing effect shown by *ticarcillin*.
Cfu = colony forming units; MIC = minimum inhibitory concentration.

MIC sixty to seventy percent of the time have been demonstrated to be clinically effective. Some experts therefore suggest that some severe infections are best treated by continuous infusion of these agents rather than by intermittent dosing.

B. Post-antibiotic effect

The post-antibiotic effect (PAE) is a persistent suppression of microbial growth that occurs after levels of antibiotic have fallen below the MIC. To measure the PAE of an antibiotic, a test culture is first incubated in antibiotic-containing medium and then transferred to antibiotic-free medium. The PAE is defined as the length of time it takes (after the transfer) for the culture to achieve log phase growth.[3] Antimicrobial drugs exhibiting a long PAE (several hours) often require only one dose per day. For example, antimicrobials such as aminoglycosides and fluoroquinolones exhibit a long PAE, particularly against gram-negative bacteria.

V. AGENTS USED IN BACTERIAL INFECTIONS

In this book, the clinically useful antibacterial drugs are organized into six families—penicillins, cephalosporins, tetracyclines, aminoglycosides, macrolides, and fluoroquinolones—plus a seventh group labeled "Other" that is used to represent any drug not included in one of the other six drug families (Figure 30.9A). Here and throughout this book, these seven groups are graphically presented as a bar chart (as a "drug stack"). The drug(s) of choice within each family that is/are used for treating a specific bacterial infection are shown in bold print, as illustrated for Staphylococcus aureus in Figure 30.9B. A key to additional antibiotic symbols used in this book is shown in Figure 30.9C.

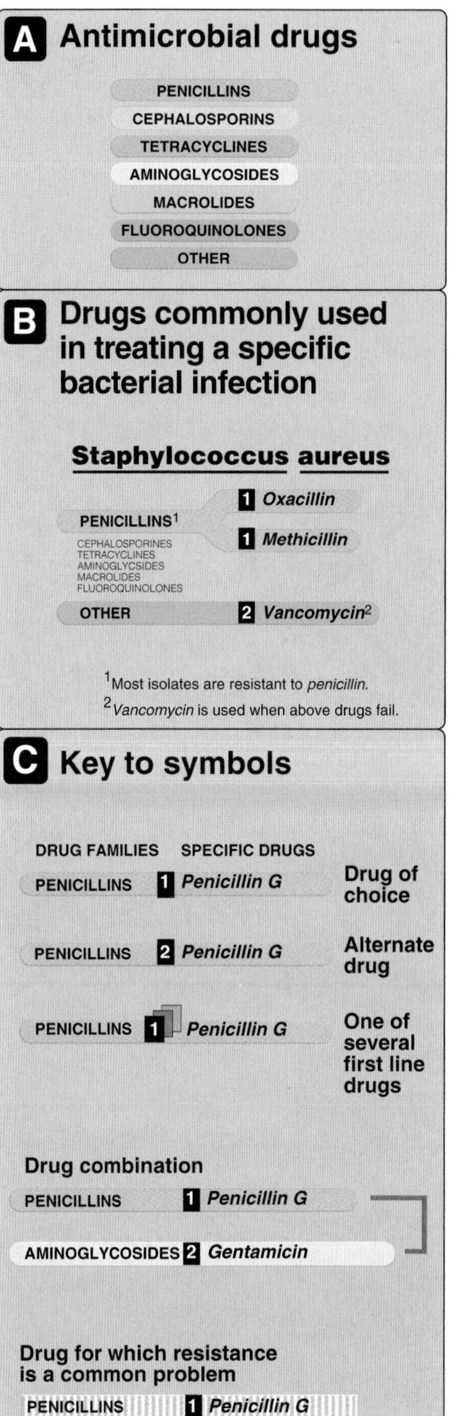

Figure 30.9
A. Bar chart showing the six most commonly used drug families. B. An example of the bar chart with the drugs of choice for the treatment of Staphylococcus aureus shown in bold print. C. Key to symbols used in this book.

VI. CHEMOTHERAPEUTIC SPECTRA

In this book, the clinically important bacteria have been organized into eight groups based on Gram stain, morphology, and biochemical or other characteristics, and they are represented as wedges of a "pie chart" (Figure 30.10A). The ninth section of the bacterial pie chart is labeled "Other," and is used to represent any organism not included in one of the other eight categories. In this chapter, the pie chart is used to illustrate the spectra of bacteria for which a particular class of antibiotics is therapeutically effective.

A. Narrow-spectrum antibiotics

Chemotherapeutic agents acting only on a single or a limited group of microorganisms are said to have a narrow spectrum. For example, *isoniazid* is active only against mycobacteria (Figure 30.10B).

B. Extended-spectrum antibiotics

Extended spectrum is the term applied to antibiotics that are effective against gram-positive organisms and also against a significant number of gram-negative bacteria. For example, *ampicillin* is consid-

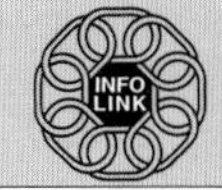

[3]See p. 109 in ***Lippincott's Illustrated Reviews: Microbiology*** for a discussion of the log phase of a bacterial growth curve.

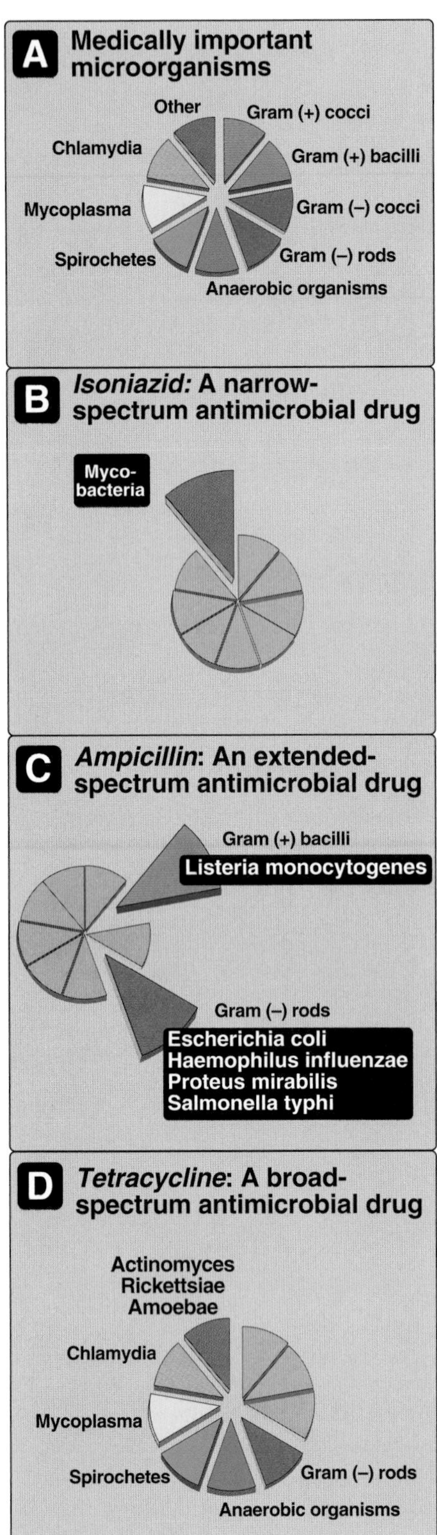

Figure 30.10
A. Color-coded representation of medically important microorganisms. B. *Isoniazid*, a narrow-spectrum antimicrobial agent. C. *Ampicillin*, an extended-spectrum antimicrobial agent. D. *Tetracycline*, a broad-spectrum antimicrobial agent.

ered to have an extended spectrum, because it acts against gram-positive and some gram-negative bacteria.

C. Broad-spectrum antibiotics

Drugs such as *tetracycline* and *chloramphenicol* affect a wide variety of microbial species and are referred to as broad-spectrum antibiotics (Figure 30.10C). Administration of broad-spectrum antibiotics can drastically alter the nature of the normal bacterial flora, and precipitate a superinfection of an organism such as Candida albicans, the growth of which is normally kept in check by the presence of other microorganisms.[4]

VII. COMBINATIONS OF ANTIMICROBIAL DRUGS

It is therapeutically advisable to treat patients with the single agent that is most specific for the infecting organism. This strategy reduces the possibility of superinfection, decreases the emergence of resistant organisms (see below), and minimizes toxicity. However, situations in which combinations of drugs are employed do exist. For example, the treatment of tuberculosis benefits from drug combinations.

A. Advantages of drug combinations

Certain combinations of antibiotics, such as β-lactams and aminoglycosides, show synergism; that is, the combination is more effective than either of the drugs used separately. Because such synergism among antimicrobial agents is rare, multiple drugs used in combination are only indicated in special situations—for example, when an infection is of unknown origin.

B. Disadvantages of drug combinations

A number of antibiotics act only when organisms are multiplying. Thus, coadministration of an agent that causes bacteriostasis plus a second agent that is bactericidal may result in the first drug interfering with the action of the second.

VIII. DRUG RESISTANCE

Bacteria are said to be resistant to an antibiotic if their growth is not halted by the maximal level of that antibiotic that can be tolerated by the host. Some organisms are inherently resistant to an antibiotic. For example, gram-negative organisms are inherently resistant to *vancomycin*. However, microbial species that are normally responsive to a particular drug may develop more virulent, resistant strains through spontaneous mutation or acquired resistance and selection. Some of these strains may even become resistant to more than one antibiotic.

A. Genetic alterations leading to drug resistance

Acquired antibiotic resistance requires the temporary or permanent gain or alteration of bacterial genetic information. Resistance develops due to the ability of DNA to undergo spontaneous mutation or to move from one organism to another (Figure 30.11).

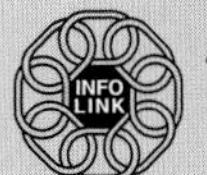

[4]See p. 125 in ***Lippincott's Illustrated Reviews: Microbiology*** for a discussion of beneficial functions of normal flora.

1. **Spontaneous mutations of DNA:** Chromosomal alteration may occur by insertion, deletion, or substitution of one or more nucleotides within the genome.[5] The resulting mutation may persist, be corrected by the organism, or be lethal to the cell. If the cell survives, it can replicate and transmit its mutated properties to progeny cells. Some spontaneous mutations have little or no effect on the susceptibility of the organism to antimicrobial agents. However, mutations that produce antibiotic-resistant strains can result in organisms that may proliferate under certain selective pressures. An example is the emergence of *rifampin*-resistant Mycobacterium tuberculosis when *rifampin* is used as a single antibiotic.

2. **DNA transfer of drug resistance:** Of particular clinical concern is resistance acquired due to DNA transfer from one bacterium to another. Resistance properties are usually encoded in extrachromosomal **R factors** (**resistance plasmids**). In fact, most resistance genes are plasmid mediated, although plasmid-mediated traits can become incorporated into host bacterial DNA. Plasmids may enter cells by processes such as transduction (phage mediated), transformation, or bacterial conjugation.[6]

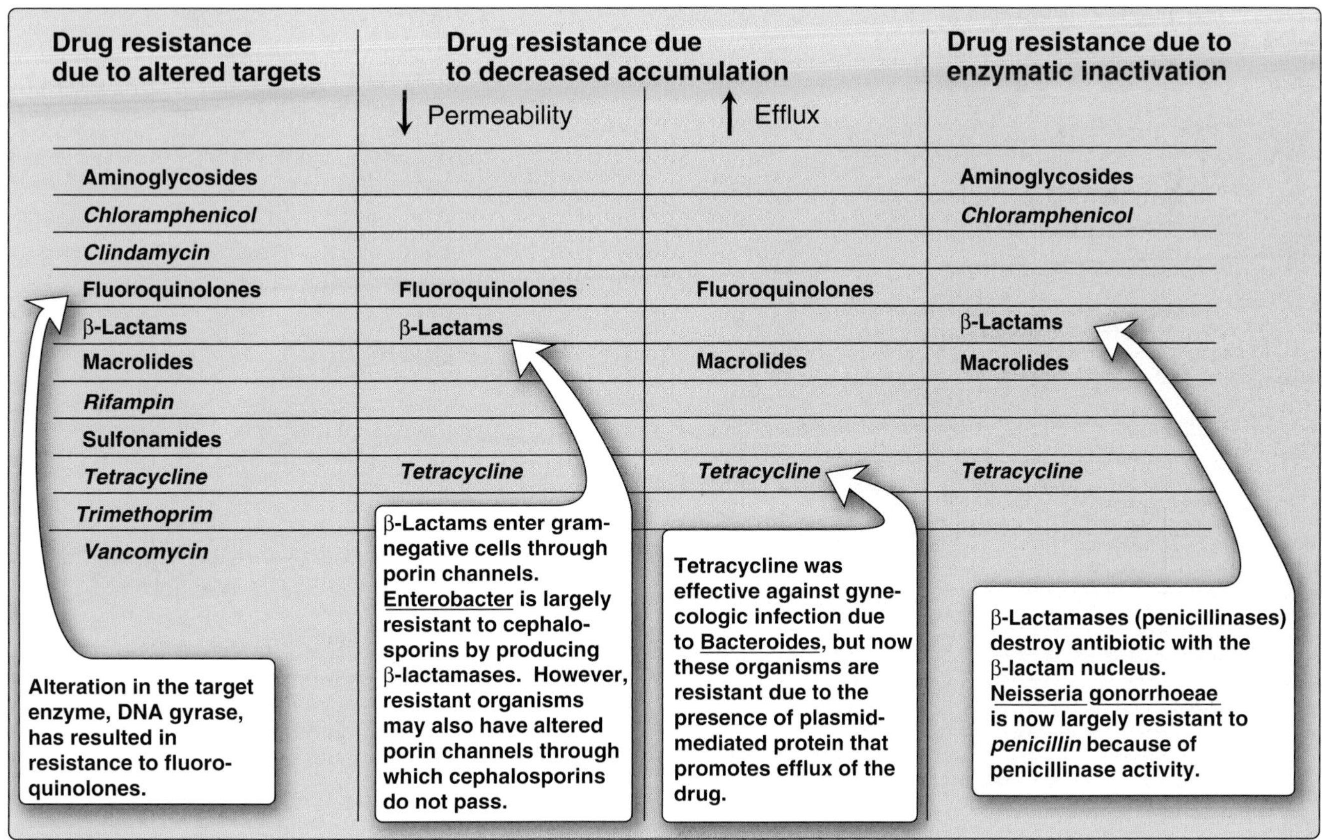

Drug resistance due to altered targets	Drug resistance due to decreased accumulation: ↓ Permeability	↑ Efflux	Drug resistance due to enzymatic inactivation
Aminoglycosides			Aminoglycosides
Chloramphenicol			*Chloramphenicol*
Clindamycin			
Fluoroquinolones	Fluoroquinolones	Fluoroquinolones	
β-Lactams	β-Lactams		β-Lactams
Macrolides		Macrolides	Macrolides
Rifampin			
Sulfonamides			
Tetracycline	*Tetracycline*	*Tetracycline*	*Tetracycline*
Trimethoprim			
Vancomycin			

Figure 30.11
Some mechanisms of resistance to antibiotics.

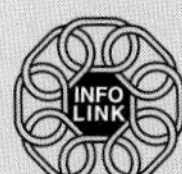

[5]See p. 125 in ***Lippincott's Illustrated Reviews: Microbiology*** for a discussion of DNA mutation.
[6]See p. 131 in ***Lippincott's Illustrated Reviews: Microbiology*** for a discussion of the integration of plasmid DNA into a host chromosome

Prevention of streptococcal infections in patients with a history of rheumatic heart disease. Patients may require years of treatment.

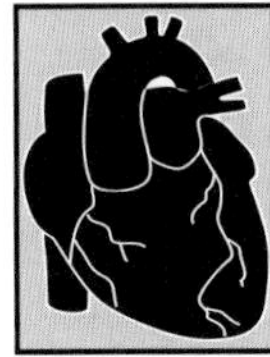

2

Pretreatment of patients undergoing dental extractions who have implanted prosthetic devices, such as artificial heart valves, to prevent seeding of the prosthesis.

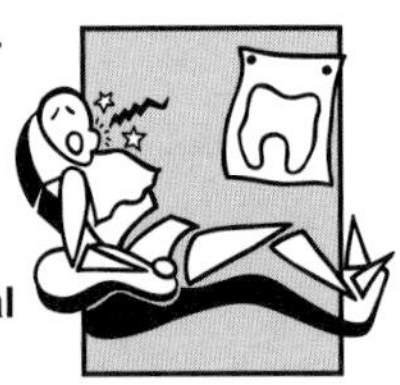

3

Prevention of tuberculosis or meningitis among individuals who are in close contact with infected patients.

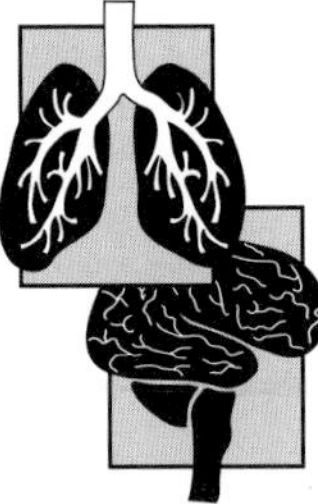

4

Treatment prior to certain surgical procedures (such as bowel surgery, joint replacement, and some gynecologic interventions) to prevent infection.

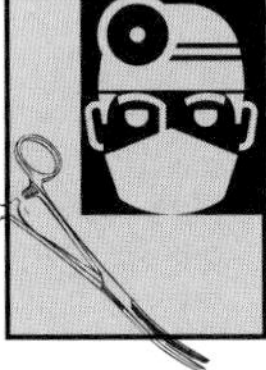

5

Treatment of the mother with *zidovudine* to protect the fetus in the case of an HIV-infected, pregnant woman.

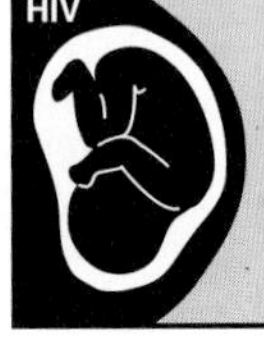

Figure 30.12
Some clinical situations in which prophylactic antibiotics are indicated.

B. Altered expression of proteins in drug-resistant organisms

Drug resistance may be mediated by a variety of mechanisms, such as a lack of or an alteration in an antibiotic target site, lowered penetrability of the drug due to decreased permeability, increased efflux of the drug, or presence of antibiotic-inactivating enzymes (see Figure 30.11).

1. **Modification of target sites:** Alteration of an antibiotic's target site through mutation can confer organismal resistance to one or more related antibiotics. For example, S. pneumoniae resistance to β-lactam antibiotics involves alterations in one or more of the major bacterial *penicillin*-binding proteins, resulting in decreased binding of the antibiotic to its target.

2. **Decreased accumulation:** Decreased uptake or increased efflux of an antibiotic can confer resistance, because the drug is unable to attain access to the site of its action in sufficient concentrations to injure or kill the organism. For example, gram-negative organisms can limit the penetration of certain agents, including β-lactam antibiotics, tetracyclines, and *chloramphenicol*, as a result of an alteration in the number and structure of porins (channels) in the outer membrane. Also, the presence of an efflux pump can limit levels of a drug in an organism.

3. **Enzymic inactivation:** The ability to destroy or inactivate the antimicrobial agent can also confer resistance on microorganisms. Examples of antibiotic-inactivating enzymes include 1) β-lactamases ("penicillinases") that hydrolytically inactivate the β-lactam ring of penicillins, cephalosporins, and related drugs; 2) acetyltransferases that transfer an acetyl group to the antibiotic, inactivating chloramphenicol or aminoglycosides; and 3) esterases that hydrolyze the lactone ring of macrolides.

IX. PROPHYLACTIC ANTIBIOTICS

Certain clinical situations require the use of antibiotics for the prevention rather than the treatment of infections (Figure 30.12). Because the indiscriminate use of antimicrobial agents can result in bacterial resistance and superinfection, prophylactic use is restricted to clinical situations in which the benefits outweigh the potential risks. The duration of prophylaxis is dictated by the duration of the risk of infection.

X. COMPLICATIONS OF ANTIBIOTIC THERAPY

Because the mechanism of action of a particular antibiotic is selectively toxic to an invading organism does not insure the host against adverse effects. For example, the drug may produce an allergic response or be toxic in ways unrelated to the drug's antimicrobial activity.

A. Hypersensitivity

Hypersensitivity reactions to antimicrobial drugs or their metabolic products frequently occur. For example, the penicillins, despite their almost absolute selective microbial toxicity, can cause serious hypersensitivity problems, ranging from urticaria (hives) to anaphylactic shock.

B. Direct toxicity

High serum levels of certain antibiotics may cause toxicity by directly affecting cellular processes in the host. For example, aminoglycosides can cause ototoxicity by interfering with membrane function in the hair cells of the organ of Corti.

C. Superinfections

Drug therapy, particularly with broad-spectrum antimicrobials or combinations of agents, can lead to alterations of the normal microbial flora of the upper respiratory, intestinal, and genitourinary tracts, permitting the overgrowth of opportunistic organisms, especially fungi or resistant bacteria. These infections are often difficult to treat.

XI. SITES OF ANTIMICROBIAL ACTIONS

Antimicrobial drugs can be classified in a number of ways. These include 1) by their chemical structure (for example, β-lactams or aminoglycosides), 2) by their mechanism of action (for example, cell wall synthesis inhibitors), or 3) by their activity against particular types of organisms (for example, bacteria, fungi, or viruses). Chapters 31 through 33 are organized by the mechanisms of action of the drug, and Chapters 34 through 38 are organized according to the type of organisms affected by the drug (Figure 30.13).

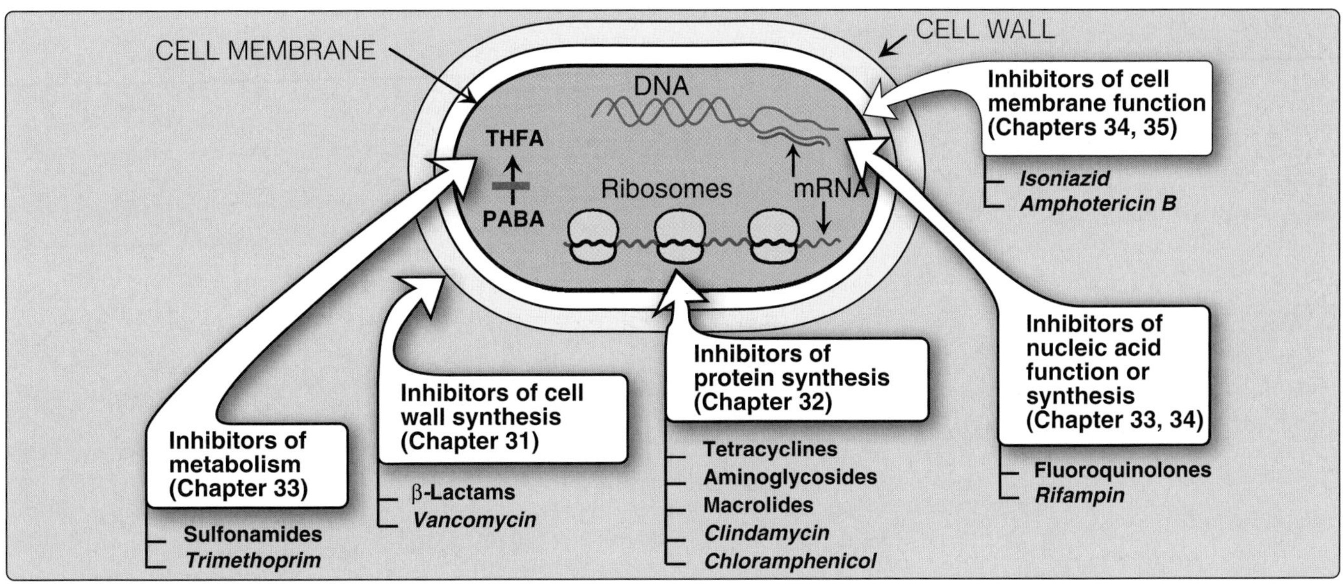

Figure 30.13
Classification of some antibacterial agents by their sites of action. (THFA = tetrahydrofolic acid; PABA = *p*-aminobenzoic acid)

Study Questions

Choose the ONE best answer.

30.1 Which one of the following patients is least likely to require antimicrobial treatment tailored to the individual's condition?

A. Patient undergoing cancer chemotherapy
B. Patient with kidney disease
C. Elderly patient
D. Patient with hypertension
E. Patient with liver disease

Correct answer = D. Elevated blood pressure would not be expected to markedly influence the type of antimicrobial treatment employed. Anticancer drugs often suppress the immune function, and these patients require additional antibiotics to eradicate infections. Impaired renal function may lead to accumulation of toxic levels of antimicrobial drugs. Renal and hepatic function are often decreased among the elderly. Impaired liver function may lead to the accumulation of toxic levels of antimicrobial drugs.

30.2 In which one of the following clinical situations is the prophylactic use of antibiotics NOT warranted?

A. Prevention of meningitis among individuals in close contact with infected patients.
B. Patient with a hip prosthesis who is having a tooth removed.
C. Presurgical treatment for implantation of a hip prosthesis.
D. Patient who complains of frequent respiratory illness.
E. Presurgical treatment in gastrointestinal procedures.

Correct answer = D. Respiratory illness may be of viral origin; furthermore, consequences of a chronic disorder may not warrant prophylactic use of antibiotics. Meningitis is a sufficiently contagious and serious disease to warrant prophylactic use of antibiotics. Following a tooth extraction, bacteria of the oral cavity can readily enter the circulation and colonize on a prosthesis, causing a serious and often fatal infection. Infection following implantation of a hip prosthesis is such a serious complication that prophylactic antibiotics are warranted. Infection is such a serious complication of gastrointestinal surgery that prophylactic antibiotics are warranted.

30.3 Which one of the following is the best route of administration/dosing schedule for treatment with aminoglycosides based on the drug's concentration-dependent killing property?

A. Oral every 8 hours
B. Oral every 24 hours
C. Parenterally by continuous intravenous infusion
D. Parenterally every 8 hours
E. Parenterally every 24 hours

Correct answer = E. Giving a drug that exhibits concentration-dependent killing by once-a-day bolus infusion achieves high peak levels favoring rapid killing of the infecting pathogen. The highly polar, polycationic structure of the aminoglycosides prevents adequate absorption after oral administration. Therefore, all aminoglycosides (except *neomycin*) must be given parenterally to achieve adequate serum levels.

Inhibitors of Cell Wall Synthesis

31

I. OVERVIEW

Some antimicrobial drugs selectively interfere with synthesis of the bacterial cell wall—a structure that mammalian cells do not possess. The cell wall is a polymer called peptidoglycan that consists of glycan units joined to each other by peptide cross-links. To be maximally effective, inhibitors of cell wall synthesis require actively proliferating microorganisms; they have little or no effect on bacteria that are not growing and dividing. The most important members of this group of drugs are the β-lactam antibiotics (named after the β-lactam ring that is essential to their activity) and *vancomycin*. Figure 31.1 shows the classification of agents affecting cell wall synthesis.

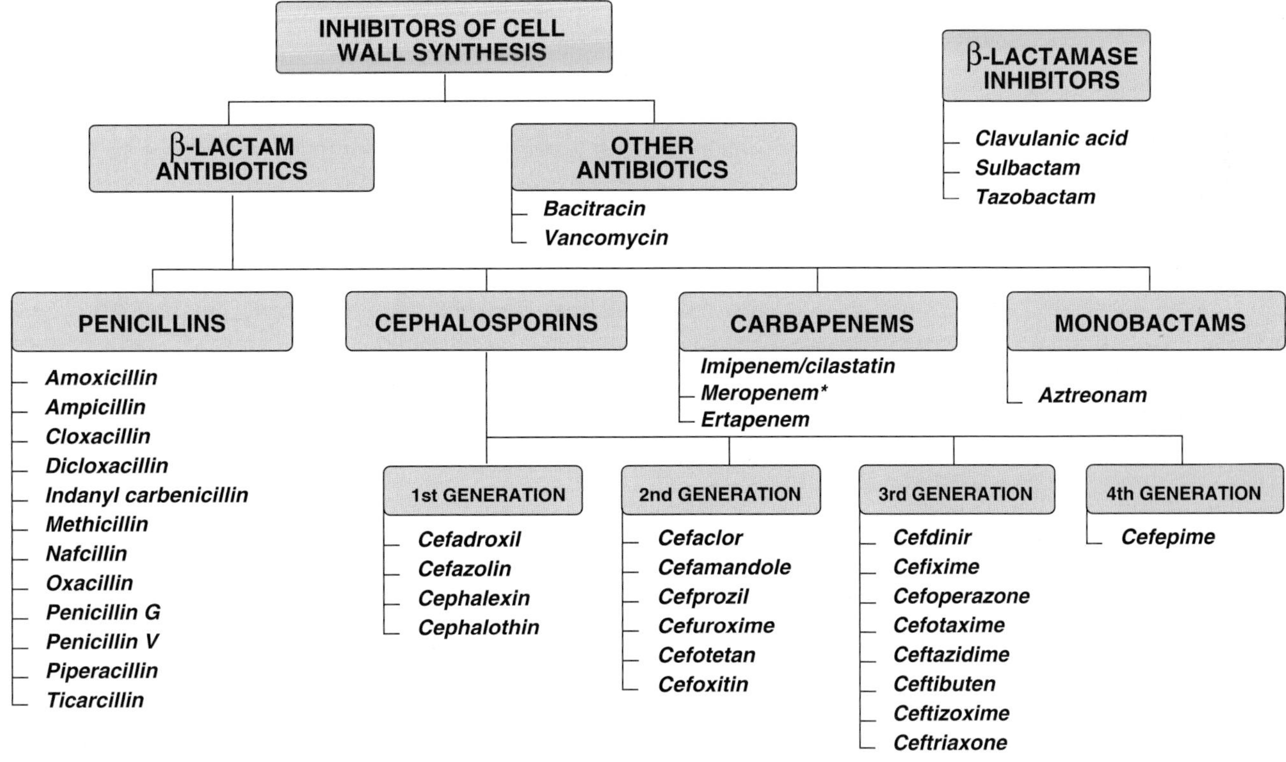

Figure 31.1
Summary of antimicrobial agents affecting cell wall synthesis **Cilastatin* is not an antibiotic but a peptidase inhibitor that protects *imipenem* from degradation.

Lippincott's Illustrated Reviews: Pharmacology, Third Edition,
by Richard D. Howland and Mary J. Mycek.
Lippincott Williams & Wilkins, Baltimore, MD © 2006.

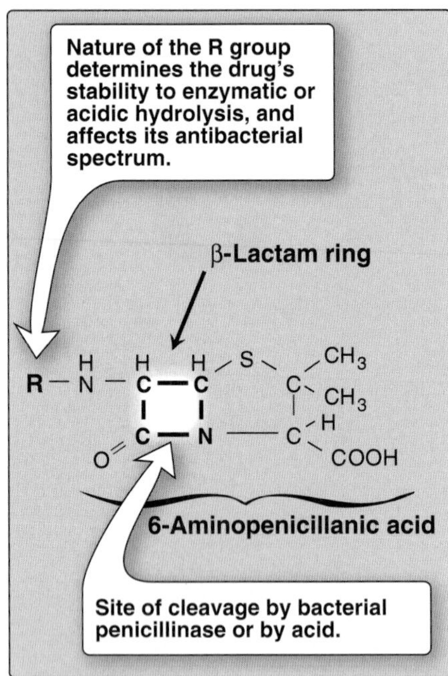

Figure 31.2
Structural features of β-lactam antibiotics.

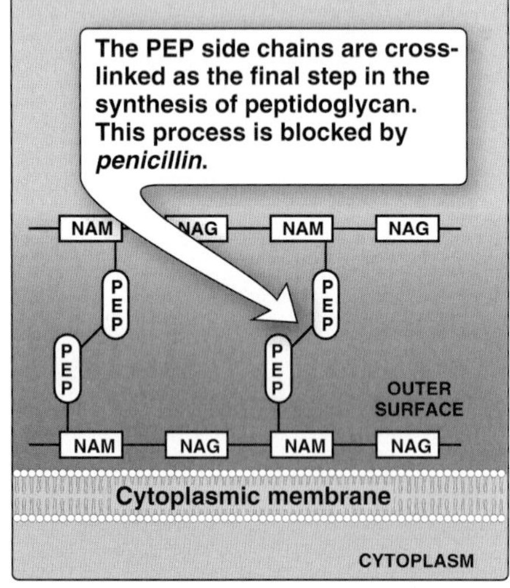

Figure 31.3
Bacterial cell wall of gram-positive bacteria. NAM = N-acetylmuramic acid; NAG = N-acetylglucosamine; PEP = cross-linking peptide.

II. PENICILLINS

The penicillins [pen i SILL in] are among the most widely effective antibiotics and also the least toxic drugs known, but increased resistance has limited their use. Members of this family differ from one another in the R substituent attached to the 6-aminopenicillanic acid residue (Figure 31.2). The nature of this side chain affects the antimicrobial spectrum, stability to stomach acid, and susceptibility to bacterial degradative enzymes (β-lactamases).

A. Mechanism of action

The penicillins interfere with the last step of bacterial cell wall synthesis (transpeptidation or cross-linkage[1]), resulting in exposure of the osmotically less stable membrane. Cell lysis can then occur, either through osmotic pressure or through the activation of autolysins. These drugs are thus bactericidal. The success of a penicillin antibiotic in causing cell death is related to the antibiotic's size, charge, and hydrophobicity. Penicillins are only effective against rapidly growing organisms that synthesize a peptidoglycan cell wall. Consequently, they are inactive against organisms devoid of this structure, such as mycobacteria, protozoa, fungi, and viruses.

1. **Penicillin-binding proteins:** Penicillins inactivate numerous proteins on the bacterial cell membrane. These penicillin-binding proteins (PBPs) are bacterial enzymes involved in the synthesis of the cell wall and in the maintenance of the morphologic features of the bacterium. Exposure to these antibiotics can therefore not only prevent cell wall synthesis, but also lead to morphologic changes or lysis of susceptible bacteria. The number of PBPs varies with the type of organism. Alterations in some of these target molecules provide the organism with resistance to the penicillins. [Note: *Methicillin*-resistant Staphylococcus aureus (MRSA) apparently arose because of such an alteration.]

2. **Inhibition of transpeptidase:** Some PBPs catalyze formation of the cross-linkages between peptidoglycan chains (Figure 31.3). Penicillins inhibit this transpeptidase-catalyzed reaction, thus hindering the formation of cross-links essential for cell wall integrity. As a result of this blockade of cell wall synthesis, the "Park nucleotide" (formerly called the "Park peptide"), UDP-acetylmuramyl-L-Ala-D-Gln-L-Lys-D-Ala-D-Ala, accumulates.

3. **Production of autolysins:** Many bacteria, particularly the gram-positive cocci, produce degradative enzymes (autolysins) that participate in the normal remodeling of the bacterial cell wall. In the presence of a penicillin, the degradative action of the autolysins proceeds in the absence of cell wall synthesis. [Note: The exact autolytic mechanism is unknown, but it may be due to a disinhibition of the autolysins.] Thus, the antibacterial effect of a penicillin is the result of both inhibition of cell wall synthesis and destruction of existing cell wall by autolysins.

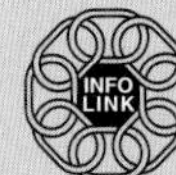

[1]See p. 111 in ***Lippincott's Illustrated Reviews: Microbiology*** for a discussion of bacterial cell wall synthesis.

B. Antibacterial spectrum

The antibacterial spectrum of the various penicillins is determined, in part, by their ability to cross the bacterial peptidoglycan cell wall to reach the PBPs in the periplasmic space. Factors that determine the susceptibility of PBPs to these antibiotics include the size, charge, and hydrophobicity of the particular β-lactam antibiotic. In general, gram-positive microorganisms have cell walls that are easily traversed by penicillins and, therefore, in the absence of resistance are susceptible to these drugs. Gram-negative microorganisms have an outer lipopolysaccharide membrane surrounding the cell wall that presents a barrier to the water-soluble penicillins. However, gram-negative bacteria have proteins inserted in the lipopolysaccharide layer that act as water-filled channels (called porins) that permit transmembrane entry. [Note: Pseudomonas aeruginosa lacks porins, making these organisms intrinsically resistant to many antimicrobial agents.]

1. **Natural penicillins:** These penicillins, which include those listed as antistaphylococcal, are obtained from fermentations of the mold Penicillium chrysogenum. Other penicillins, such as *ampicillin*, are called semisynthetic, because the different R groups are attached chemically to the 6-aminopenicillanic acid nucleus obtained from fermentation broths of the mold. *Penicillin G* (*benzylpenicillin*) is the cornerstone of therapy for infections caused by a number of gram-positive and gram-negative cocci, gram-positive bacilli, and spirochetes (Figure 31.4). *Penicillin G* is susceptible to inactivation by β-lactamases (penicillinases).

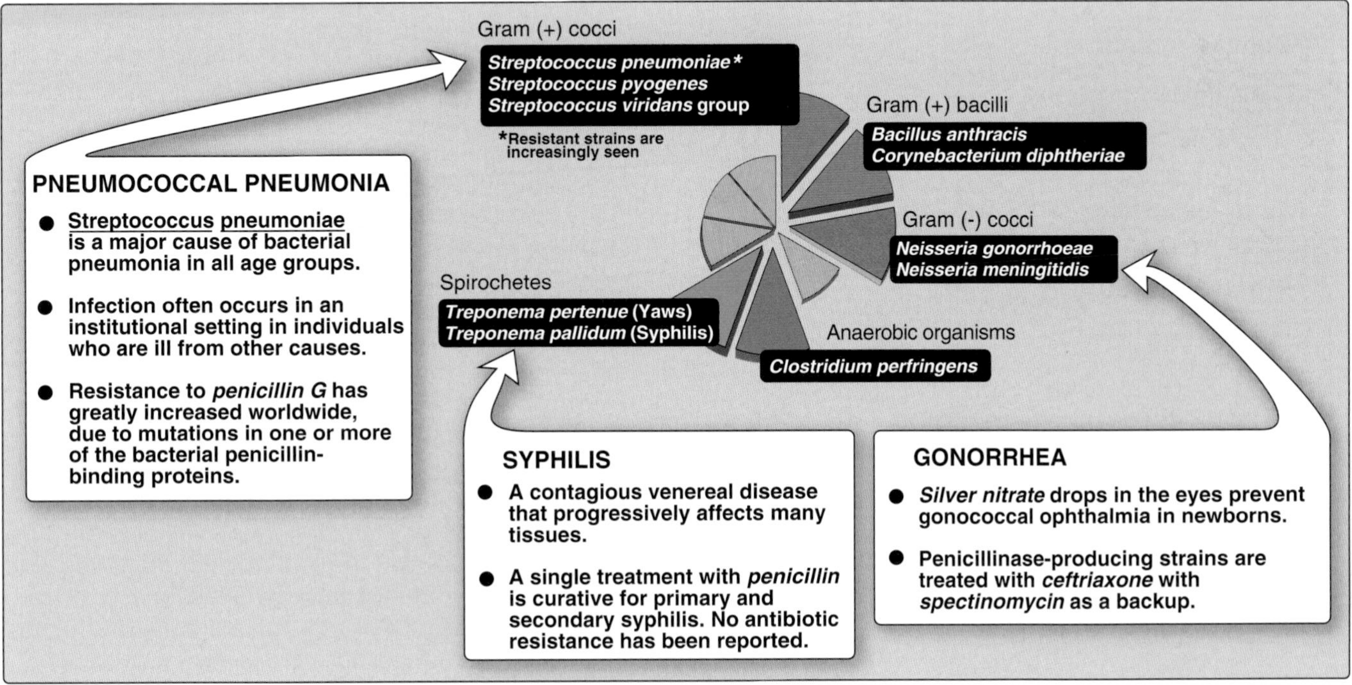

Figure 31.4
Typical therapeutic applications of *penicillin G*.

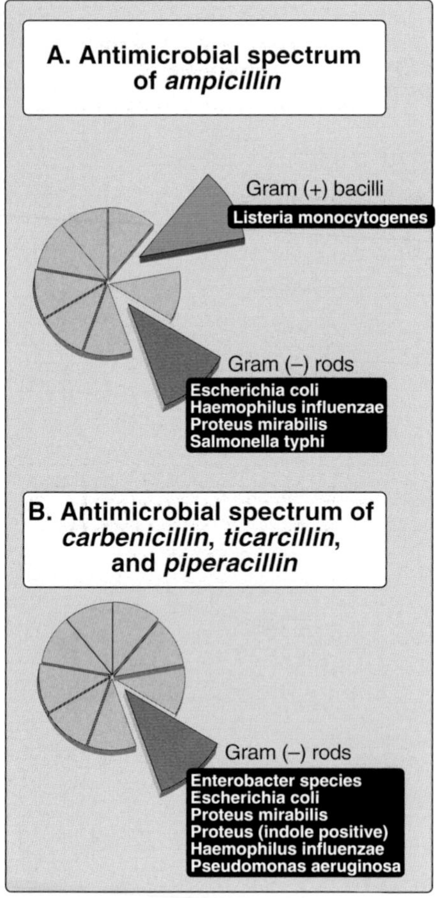

Figure 31.5
Typical therapeutic applications of *ampicillin* (A) and the antipseudomonal penicillins (B).

Penicillin V has a spectrum similar to that of penicillin G, but it is not used for treatment of bacteremia because of its higher minimum bactericidal concentration (the minimum amount of the drug needed to eliminate the infection, see p. 343). *Penicillin V* is more acid-stable than *penicillin G*. It is often employed in the treatment of oral infections, where it is effective against some anaerobic organisms.

2. **Antistaphylococcal penicillins:** *Methicillin* [meth i SILL in], *nafcillin* [naf SILL in], *oxacillin* [ox a SILL in], *cloxacillin* [klox a SILL in], and *dicloxacillin* [dye klox a SILL in] are penicillinase-resistant penicillins. Their use is restricted to the treatment of infections caused by penicillinase-producing staphylococci. [Note: Because of its toxicity, *methicillin* is not used except to identify resistant strains of S. aureus.] Currently a serious source of nosocomial (hospital-acquired) infections, MRSA are usually susceptible to *vancomycin* and, rarely, to *ciprofloxacin* or *rifampin*.

3. **Extended-spectrum penicillins:** *Ampicillin* [am pi SILL in] and *amoxicillin* [a mox i SILL in] have an antibacterial spectrum similar to that of *penicillin G*, but are more effective against gram-negative bacilli. They are therefore referred to as extended-spectrum penicillins (Figure 31.5A). *Ampicillin* is the drug of choice for the gram-positive bacillus Listeria monocytogenes. These agents are also widely used in the treatment of respiratory infections, and *amoxicillin* is employed prophylactically by dentists for patients with abnormal heart valves who are to undergo extensive oral surgery. Resistance to these antibiotics is now a major clinical problem because of inactivation by plasmid-mediated penicillinase. [Note: Escherichia coli and Haemophilus influenzae are frequently resistant.] Formulation with a β-lactamase inhibitor, such as *clavulanic acid* or *sulbactam*, protects *amoxicillin* or *ampicillin*, respectively, from enzymatic hydrolysis and extends their antimicrobial spectrum.

4. **Antipseudomonal penicillins:** *Indanyl carbenicillin* [kar ben i SILL in], *ticarcillin* [tye kar SILL in], and *piperacillin* [pip er a SILL in] are called antipseudomonal penicillins because of their activity against Pseudomonas aeruginosa (Figure 31.5B). *Piperacillin* is the most potent of these antibiotics. They are effective against many gram-negative bacilli, but not against klebsiella, because of its constitutive penicillinase. Formulation of *ticarcillin* or *piperacillin* with *clavulanic acid* or *tazobactam*, respectively, extends the antimicrobial spectrum of these antibiotics to include penicillinase-producing organisms. *Mezlocillin* [mez loe SILL in] (sometimes referred to as an acylureido penicillin) is also effective against P. aeruginosa as well as a large number of gram-negative organisms. It is susceptible to breakdown by β-lactamase. (Figure 31.6 summarizes of the stability of the penicillins to acid or the action of penicillinase.)

5. **Penicillins and aminoglycosides:** The antibacterial effects of all the β-lactam antibiotics are synergistic with the aminoglycosides. Because cell wall synthesis inhibitors alter the permeability of

bacterial cells, these drugs can facilitate the entry of other antibiotics (such as aminoglycosides) that might not ordinarily gain access to intracellular target sites. This can result in enhanced antimicrobial activity. [Note: Although the combination of a penicillin plus an aminoglycoside is used clinically, these drug types should never be placed in the same infusion fluid, because on prolonged contact, the positively charged aminoglycosides form an inactive complex with the negatively charged penicillins.]

C. Resistance

Natural resistance to the penicillins occurs in organisms that either lack a peptidoglycan cell wall (for example, the mycoplasma) or have cell walls that are impermeable to the drugs. Acquired resistance to the penicillins by plasmid transfer has become a significant clinical problem, because an organism may become resistant to several antibiotics at the same time due to acquisition of a plasmid that encodes resistance to multiple agents. Multiplication of such an organism will lead to increased dissemination of the resistance genes. By obtaining a resistance plasmid, bacteria may acquire one or more of the following properties, thus allowing it to withstand β-lactam antibiotics.

1. **β-Lactamase activity:** This family of enzymes hydrolyzes the cyclic amide bond of the β-lactam ring, which results in loss of bactericidal activity (see Figure 31.2). They are the major cause of resistance to the penicillins, and are an increasing problem. β-Lactamases are either constitutive or, more commonly, are acquired by the transfer of plasmids. Some of the β-lactam antibiotics are poor substrates for β-lactamases and resist cleavage, thus retaining their activity against β-lactamase-producing organisms. [Note: Certain organisms may have chromosome-associated β-lactamases that are inducible by β-lactam antibiotics (for example, *cefoxitin*).] Gram-positive organisms secrete β-lactamases extracellularly, whereas gram-negative bacteria have the enzymes in the periplasmic space between the inner and outer membranes.

2. **Decreased permeability to the drug:** Decreased penetration of the antibiotic through the outer cell membrane prevents the drug from reaching the target PBPs. The presence of an efflux pump can also reduce the amount of intracellular drug.

3. **Altered PBPs:** Modified PBPs have a lower affinity for β-lactam antibiotics, requiring clinically unattainable concentrations of the drug to effect inhibition of bacterial growth. This mechanism may explain MRSA, although it does not explain its resistance to non-β-lactam antibiotics like *erythromycin*, to which they are also refractory.

D. Pharmacokinetics

1. **Administration:** The route of administration of a β-lactam antibiotic is determined by the stability of the drug to gastric acid and by the severity of the infection.

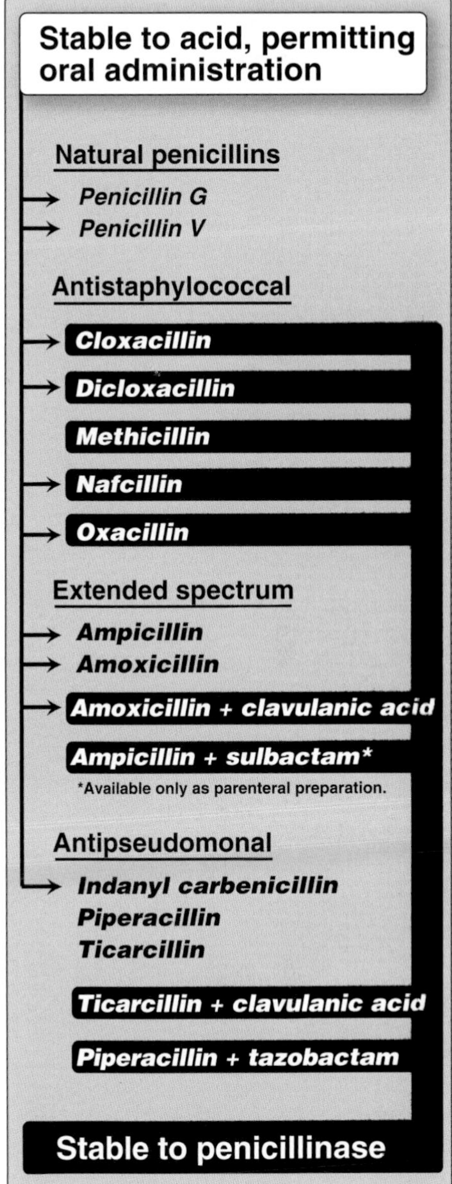

Figure 31.6
Stability of the penicillins to acid or the action of penicillinase.

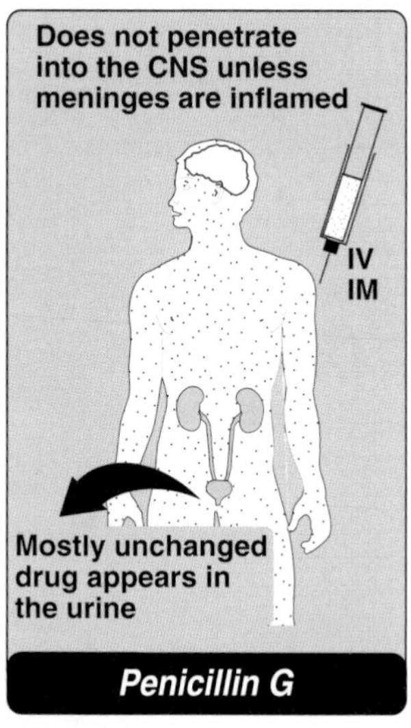

Figure 31.7
Administration and fate of *penicillin*.

a. **Routes of administration:** *Ticarcillin*, *carbenicillin*, *piperacillin*, and the combinations of *ampicillin* with *sulbactam*, *ticarcillin* with *clavulanic acid*, and *piperacillin* with *tazobactam* must be administered intravenously (IV) or intramuscularly (IM). *Penicillin V*, *amoxicillin*, *amoxicillin* combined with *clavulanic acid*, and *indanyl carbenicillin* (for treatment of urinary tract infections) are only available as oral preparations. Others are effective by the oral, IV, or IM routes (see Figure 31.6).

b. **Depot forms:** *Procaine penicillin G* and *benzathine penicillin G* are administered IM and serve as depot forms. They are slowly absorbed into the circulation and persist at low levels over a long time period.

2. **Absorption:** Most of the penicillins are incompletely absorbed after oral administration, and they reach the intestine in sufficient amounts to affect the composition of the intestinal flora. However, *amoxicillin* is almost completely absorbed. Consequently, it is not appropriate therapy for the treatment of shigella- or salmonella-derived enteritis, because therapeutically effective levels do not reach the organisms in the intestinal crypts. Absorption of all the penicillinase-resistant penicillins is decreased by food in the stomach, because gastric emptying time is lengthened, and the drugs are destroyed in the acidic environment. Therefore, they must be administered thirty to sixty minutes before meals or two to three hours postprandially. Other penicillins are less affected by food.

3. **Distribution:** Distribution of the β-lactam antibiotics throughout the body is good. All the penicillins cross the placental barrier, but none has been shown to be teratogenic. However, penetration into certain sites, such as bone or cerebrospinal fluid (CSF), is insufficient for therapy unless these sites are inflamed (Figures 31.7 and 31.8). [Note: During the acute phase of infection, the inflamed meninges are more permeable to the penicillins, resulting in an increased ratio of the amount of drug in the central nervous system compared to the amount in the serum. As the infection abates, inflammation subsides, and permeability barriers are reestablished.] Levels in the prostate are insufficient to be effective against infections.

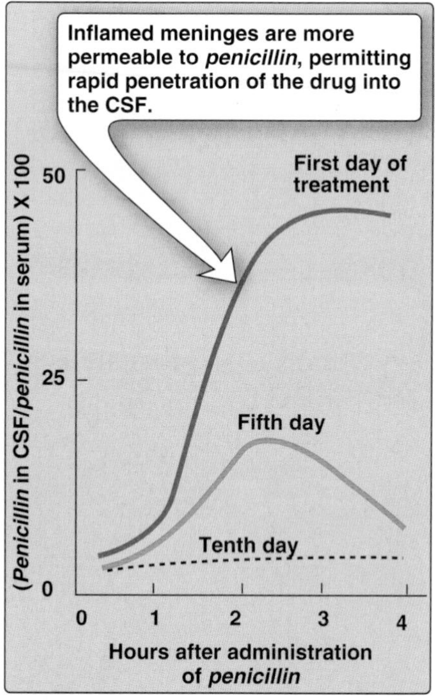

Figure 31.8
Enhanced penetration of *penicillin* into the cerebral spinal fluid (CSF) during inflammation.

4. **Metabolism:** Host metabolism of the β-lactam antibiotics is usually insignificant, but some metabolism of *penicillin G* has been shown to occur in patients with impaired renal function.

5. **Excretion:** The primary route of excretion is through the organic acid (tubular) secretory system of the kidney as well as by glomerular filtration. Patients with impaired renal function must have dosage regimens adjusted. Thus, the half-life ($t_{1/2}$) of *penicillin G* can increase from a normal of one-half to one hour, to ten hours in individuals with renal failure. *Probenecid* inhibits the secretion of penicillins and, thus, can increase blood levels. *Nafcillin* is eliminated primarily through the biliary route. [Note: This is also the preferential route for the acylureido penicillins in cases of renal failure.] The penicillins are also excreted into breast milk and into saliva.

E. Adverse reactions

Penicillins are among the safest drugs, and blood levels are not monitored. However, the following adverse reactions may occur (Figure 31.9).

1. **Hypersensitivity:** This is the most important adverse effect of the penicillins. The major antigenic determinant of penicillin hypersensitivity is its metabolite, penicilloic acid, which reacts with proteins and serves as a hapten to cause an immune reaction. Approximately five percent of patients have some kind of reaction, ranging from maculopapular rash (the most common rash seen with *ampicillin* hypersensitivity) to angioedema (marked swelling of the lips, tongue, and periorbital area) and anaphylaxis. Among patients with mononucleosis who are treated with *ampicillin*, the incidence of maculopapular rash approaches 100 percent. Cross-allergic reactions do occur among the β-lactam antibiotics.

2. **Diarrhea:** This effect, which is caused by a disruption of the normal balance of intestinal microorganisms, is a common problem. It occurs to a greater extent with those agents that are incompletely absorbed and have an extended antibacterial spectrum. As with some other antibiotics, pseudomembranous colitis[2] may occur.

3. **Nephritis:** All penicillins, but particularly *methicillin*, have the potential to cause acute interstitial nephritis. [Note: *Methicillin* is therefore no longer available.]

4. **Neurotoxicity:** The penicillins are irritating to neuronal tissue, and they can provoke seizures if injected intrathecally or if very high blood levels are reached. Epileptic patients are particularly at risk.

5. **Hematologic toxicities:** Decreased agglutination may be observed with the antipseudomonal penicillins (*carbenicillin* and *ticarcillin*) and, to some extent, with *penicillin G*. It is generally a concern when treating patients who are predisposed to hemorrhage (for example, uremics) or those receiving anticoagulants. Additional toxicities include eosinophilia.

6. **Cation toxicity:** Penicillins are generally administered as the sodium or potassium salt. Toxicities may be caused by the large quantities of sodium or potassium that accompany the penicillin. Sodium excess may result in hypokalemia. This can be avoided by using the most potent antibiotic, which permits lower doses of drug and accompanying cations.

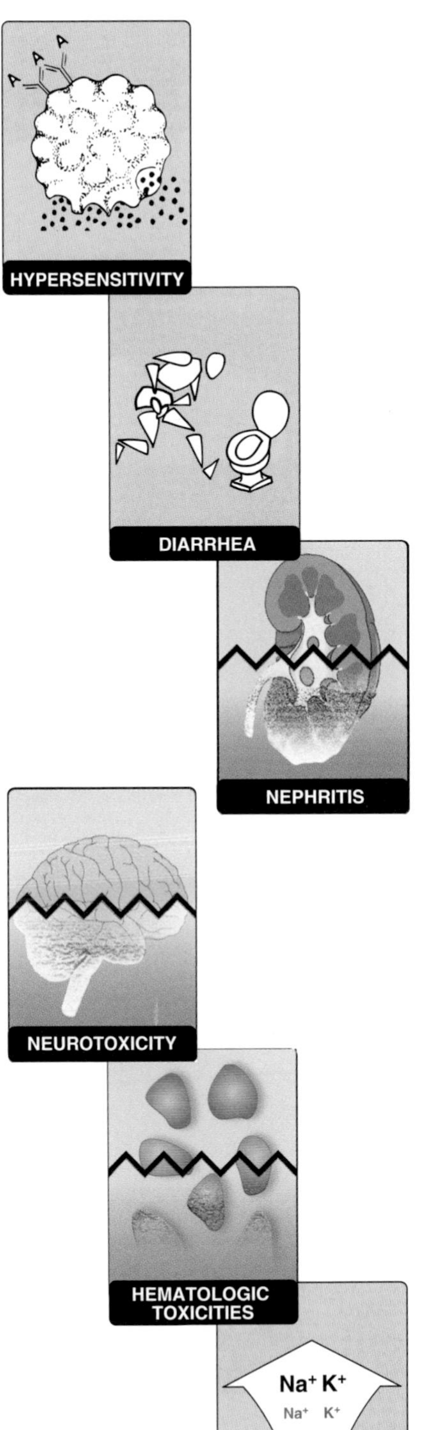

Figure 31.9
Summary of the adverse effects of *penicillin*.

III. CEPHALOSPORINS

The cephalosporins are β-lactam antibiotics that are closely related both structurally and functionally to the penicillins. Most cephalosporins are produced semisynthetically by the chemical attachment of side

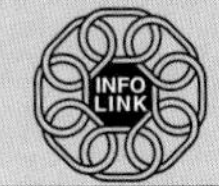

[2]See p. 217 in **Lippincott's Illustrated Reviews: Microbiology** for a discussion of pseudomembranous colitis.

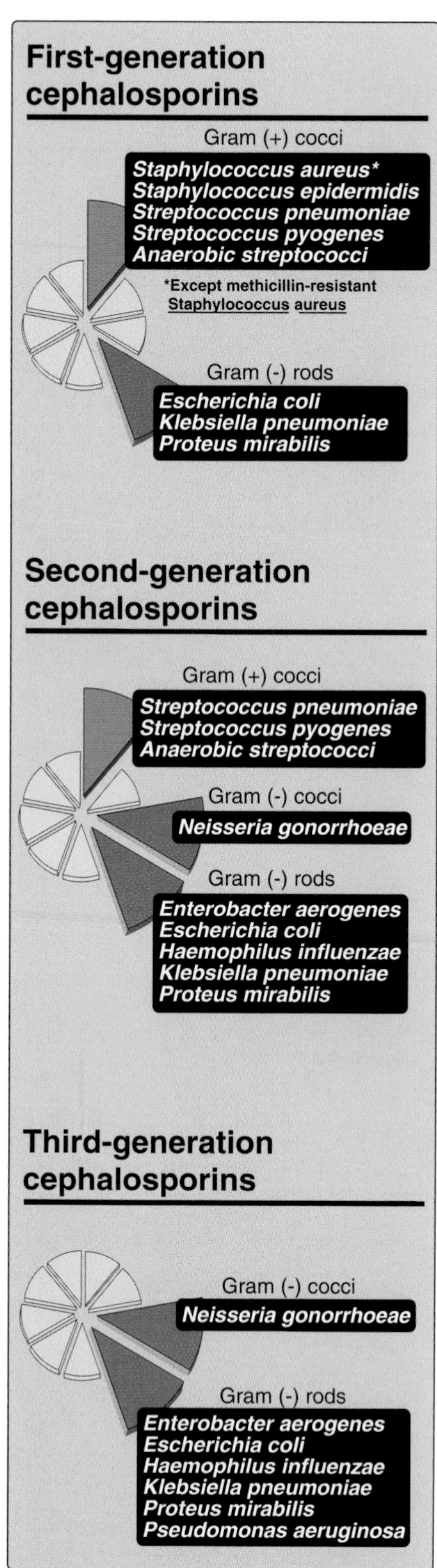

Figure 31.10
Summary of therapeutic applications of cephalosporins.

chains to 7-aminocephalosporanic acid. Cephalosporins have the same mode of action as penicillins, and they are affected by the same resistance mechanisms. However, they tend to be more resistant than the penicillins to β-lactamases.

A. Antibacterial spectrum

Cephalosporins have been classified as first, second, third, or fourth generation, based largely on their bacterial susceptibility patterns and resistance to β-lactamases (Figure 31.10). [Note: Cephalosporins are ineffective against MRSA, L. monocytogenes, Clostridium difficile, and the enterococci.]

1. **First generation:** Cephalosporins designated as "first generation" act as *penicillin G* substitutes. They are resistant to the staphylococcal penicillinase, and also have activity against Proteus mirabilis, E. coli, and Klebsiella pneumoniae (the acronym PEcK has been suggested).

2. **Second generation:** The second-generation cephalosporins display greater activity against three additional gram-negative organisms: H. influenzae, Enterobacter aerogenes, and some Neisseria species, whereas activity against gram-positive organisms is weaker. [Note: The exceptions to this generalization are the structurally related cephamycins, *cefoxitin* [sef OX i tin] and *cefotetan* [sef oh TEE tan], which have little activity against H. influenzae. They are, however, effective against Bacteroides fragilis, with *cefoxitin* being the most potent.]

3. **Third generation:** These cephalosporins have assumed an important role in the treatment of infectious disease. Although inferior to first-generation cephalosporins in regard to their activity against gram-positive cocci, the third-generation cephalosporins have enhanced activity against gram-negative bacilli, including those mentioned above, as well as most other enteric organisms plus Serratia marcescens. *Ceftriaxone* [sef tree AKS own] or *cefotaxime* [sef oh TAKS eem] have become agents of choice in the treatment of meningitis. *Ceftazidime* [sef TA zi deem] has activity against Pseudomonas aeruginosa.

4. **Fourth generation:** *Cefepime* [SEF eh peem] is classified as a fourth-generation cephalosporin, and must be administered parenterally. *Cefepime* has a wide antibacterial spectrum, being active against streptococci and staphylococci (but only those that are *methicillin*-susceptible). *Cefipime* is also effective against aerobic gram-negative organisms, such as enterobacter, E. coli, K. pneumoniae, P. mirabilis, and P. aeruginosa.

B. Resistance

Mechanisms of bacterial resistance to the cephalosporins are essentially the same as those described for the penicillins. [Note: Although they are not susceptible to hydrolysis by the staphylococcal penicillinase, cephalosporins may be susceptible to extended-spectrum β-lactamases.]

C. Pharmacokinetics

1. **Administration:** All of the cephalosporins must be administered IV or IM (Figure 31.11) because of their poor oral absorption, with the exceptions being those noted in Figure 31.12.

2. **Distribution:** All cephalosporins distribute very well into body fluids. However, adequate therapeutic levels in the CSF, regardless of inflammation, are achieved only with the third-generation cephalosporins. For example, *ceftriaxone* or *cefotaxime* are effective in the treatment of neonatal and childhood meningitis caused by H. influenzae). *Cefazolin* [se FA zo lin] finds application in prophylaxis prior to surgery because of its half-life and its activity against penicillinase-producing S. aureus. Its ability to penetrate bone is especially useful in orthopedic surgery. All cephalosporins cross the placenta.

3. **Fate:** Biotransformation of cephalosporins by the host is not clinically important. Elimination occurs through tubular secretion and/or glomerular filtration (see Figure 31.11). Therefore doses must be adjusted in cases of severe renal failure to guard against accumulation and toxicity. *Cefoperazone* [sef oh PER a zone] and *ceftriaxone* are excreted through the bile into the feces and, therefore, are frequently employed in patients with renal insufficiency.

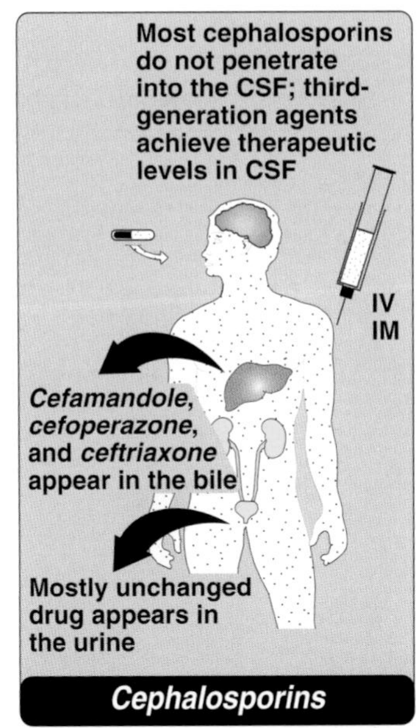

Most cephalosporins do not penetrate into the CSF; third-generation agents achieve therapeutic levels in CSF
IV
IM
Cefamandole, *cefoperazone*, and *ceftriaxone* appear in the bile
Mostly unchanged drug appears in the urine
Cephalosporins

Figure 31.11
Administration and fate of the cephalosporins.

D. Adverse effects

The cephalosporins produce a number of adverse affects, some of which are unique to particular members of the group.

1. **Allergic manifestations:** Patients who have had an anaphylactic response to penicillins should not receive cephalosporins. The cephalosporins should be avoided or used with caution in individuals who are allergic to penicillins (about five to fifteen percent show cross-sensitivity). In contrast, the incidence of allergic reactions to cephalosporins is one to two percent in patients without a history of allergy to penicillins.

2. **A disulfiram-like effect:** When *cefamandole* [sef a MAN dole], *cefotetan*, or *cefoperazone* is ingested with alcohol or alcohol-containing medications, a *disulfiram*-like effect is seen (see p. 112). This happens because these cephalosporins block the second step in alcohol oxidation, which results in the accumulation of acetaldehyde.[3] The toxicity is due to the presence of the methylthiotetrazole (MTT) group.

3. **Bleeding:** Bleeding is also associated with agents that contain the MTT group because of anti-vitamin K effects (see Figure 31.12). Administration of the vitamin corrects the problem.

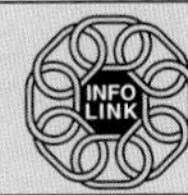

[3]See p. 315 in ***Lippincott's Illustrated Reviews: Biochemistry*** (3rd ed.) for a discussion of alcohol metabolism.

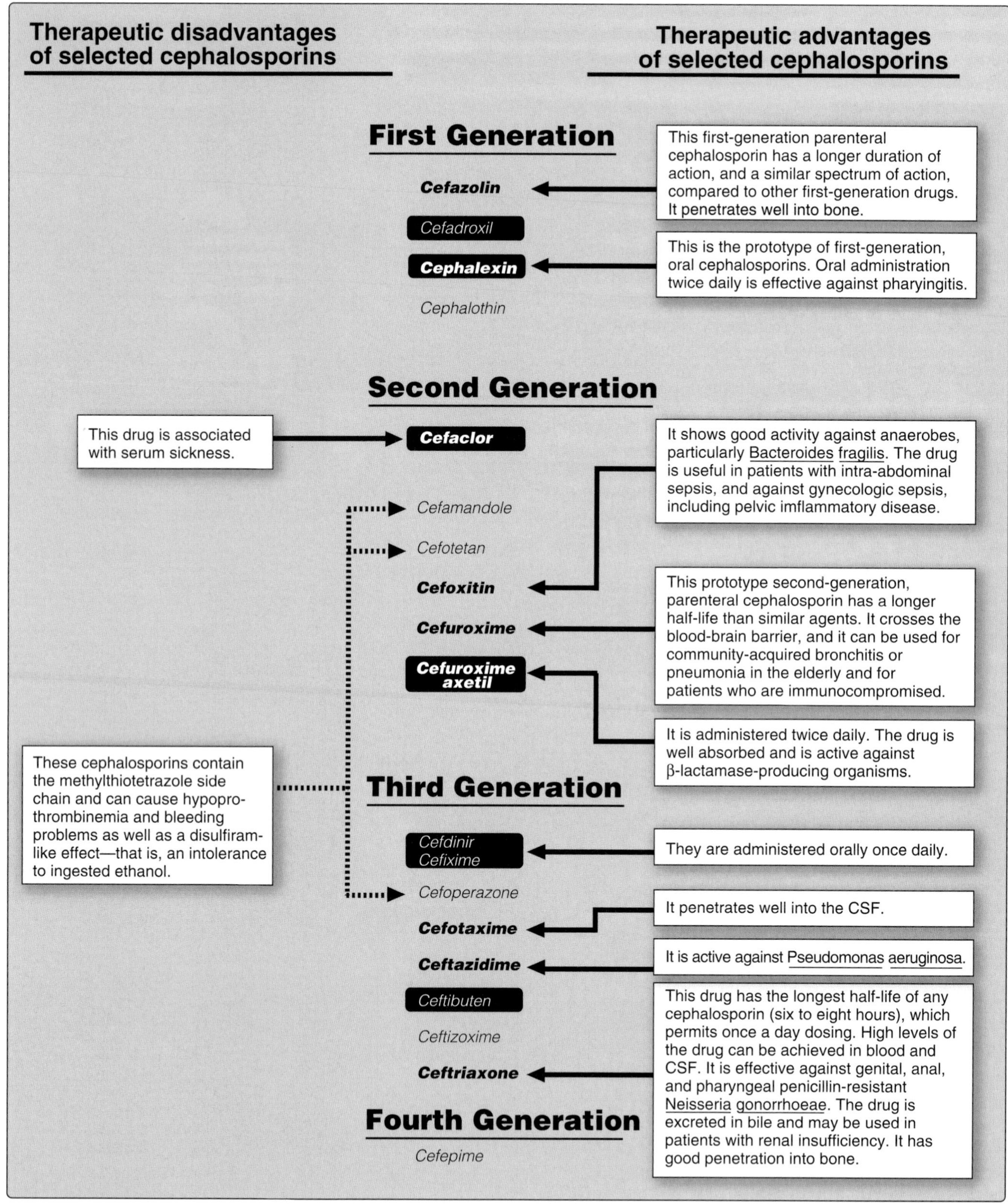

Figure 31.12
Characteristic of some clinically useful cephalosporins. [Note: Drugs that can be administered orally are shown in reverse type. More useful drugs shown in **bold**.] CSF = cerebrospinal fluid.

IV. OTHER β-LACTAM ANTIBIOTICS

A. Carbapenems

Carbapenems are synthetic β-lactam antibiotics that differ from the penicillins in that the sulfur atom of the thiazolidine ring (see Figure 31.2) has been externalized and replaced by a carbon atom (Figure 31.13). *Imipenem* [i mi PEN em] and *meropenem* [mer oh PEN em] are the only drugs of this group currently available. *Imipenem* is compounded with *cilastatin* to protect it from metabolism by renal dehydropeptidase.

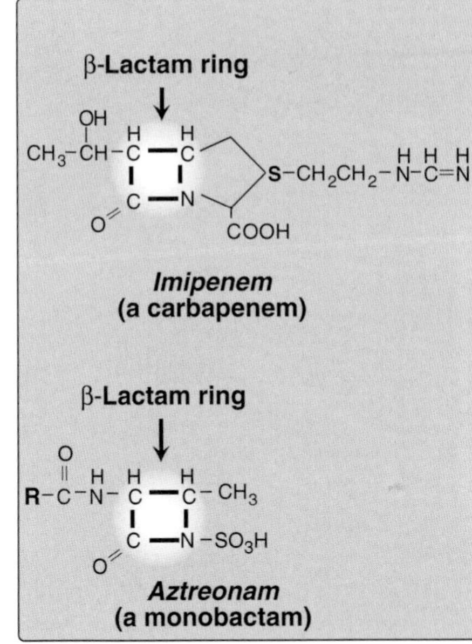

Figure 31.13
Structural features of *imipenem* and *aztreonam*.

1. **Antibacterial spectrum:** *Imipenem/cilastatin* and *meropenem* are the broadest-spectrum β-lactam antibiotic preparations currently available (Figure 31.14). *Imipenem* resists hydrolysis by most β-lactamases, but not the metallo-β-lactamases. The drug plays a role in empiric therapy, because it is active against penicillinase-producing gram-positive and gram-negative organisms, anaerobes, and Pseudomonas aeruginosa (although other pseudomonas strains are resistant, and resistant strains of P. aeruginosa have been reported to arise during therapy). *Meropenem* has antibacterial activity similar to that of *imipenem*.

2. **Pharmacokinetics:** *Imipenem* and *meropenem* are administered IV, and penetrate well into body tissues and fluids, including the CSF when the meninges are inflamed. They are excreted by glomerular filtration. *Imipenem* undergoes cleavage by a dehydropeptidase found in the brush border of the proximal renal tubule. This enzyme forms an inactive metabolite that is potentially nephrotoxic. Compounding the *imipenem* with *cilastatin* protects the parent drug and, thus, prevents the formation of the toxic metabolite. This allows the drug to be used in the treatment of urinary tract infections. *Meropenem* does not undergo metabolism. [Note: Doses of these agents must be adjusted in patients with renal insufficiency.]

3. **Adverse effects:** *Imipenem/cilastatin* can cause nausea, vomiting, and diarrhea. Eosinophilia and neutropenia are less common than with other β-lactams. High levels of *imipenem* may provoke seizures, but *meropenem* is less likely to do so.

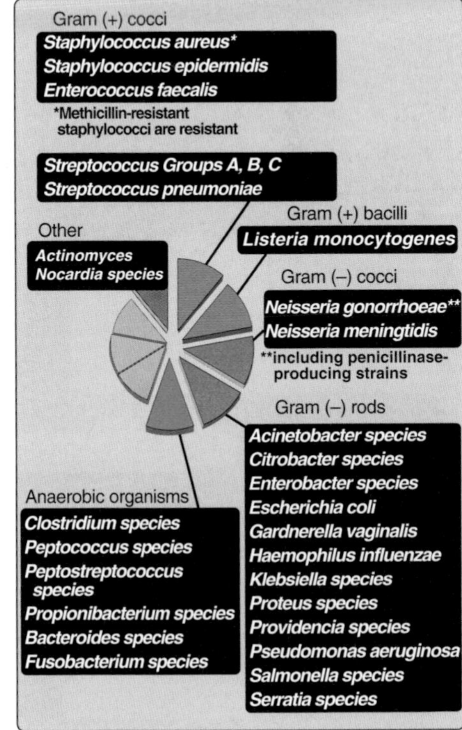

Figure 31.14
Antimicrobial spectrum of *imipenem*.

B. Monobactams

The monobactams, which also disrupt bacterial cell wall synthesis, are unique, because the β-lactam ring is not fused to another ring (see Figure 31.13). *Aztreonam* [az TREE oh nam], which is the only commercially available monobactam, has antimicrobial activity directed primarily against the Enterobacteriaceae, but it also acts against aerobic gram-negative rods, including P. aeruginosa. It lacks activity against gram-positive organisms and anaerobes. This narrow antimicrobial spectrum precludes its use alone in empiric therapy (see p. 342). *Aztreonam* is resistant to the action of β-lactamases. It is administered either IV or IM, and is excreted in the urine. It can accumulate in patients with renal failure. *Aztreonam* is

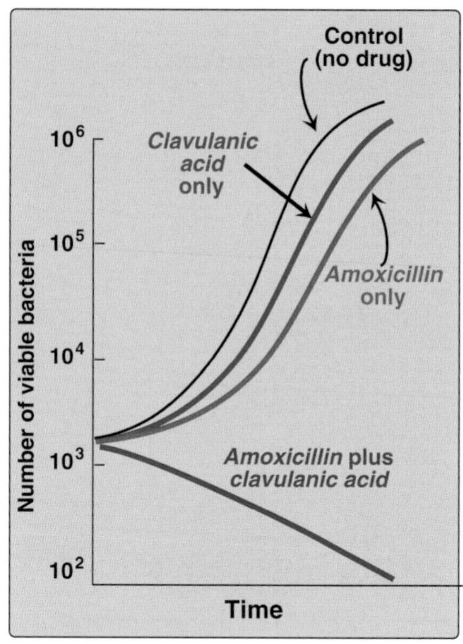

Figure 31.15
The in vitro growth of Escherichia coli in the presence of *amoxicillin*, with and without *clavulanic acid*.

relatively nontoxic, but it may cause phlebitis, skin rash, and occasionally, abnormal liver function tests. This drug has a low immunogenic potential, and it shows little cross-reactivity with antibodies induced by other β-lactams. Thus, this drug may offer a safe alternative for treating patients who are allergic to penicillins and/or cephalosporins.

V. β-LACTAMASE INHIBITORS

Hydrolysis of the β-lactam ring, either by enzymatic cleavage with a β-lactamase or by acid, destroys the antimicrobial activity of a β-lactam antibiotic. β-Lactamase inhibitors, such as *clavulanic acid* [cla vue LAN ick], *sulbactam* [sul BACK tam], and *tazobactam* [ta zoh BACK tam], contain a β-lactam ring but, by themselves, do not have significant antibacterial activity. Instead, they bind to and inactivate β-lactamases, thereby protecting the antibiotics that are normally substrates for these enzymes. The β-lactamase inhibitors are therefore formulated with β-lactamase-sensitive antibiotics. For example, Figure 31.15 shows the effect of *clavulanic acid* and *amoxicillin* on the growth of β-lactamase-producing E. coli. [Note: *Clavulanic acid* alone is nearly devoid of antibacterial activity.] Not all β-lactamases are inhibited. For example, *tazobactam*, which is compounded with *piperacillin*, does not affect P. aeruginosa β-lactamase. Therefore, this organism remains refractory to *piperacillin*.

VI. OTHER AGENTS AFFECTING THE CELL WALL

Vancomycin [van koe MYE sin] is a tricyclic glycopeptide that has become increasingly important because of its effectiveness against multiple drug-resistant organisms, such as MRSA and enterococci. The medical community is presently concerned with emergence of *vancomycin* resistance in these organisms. [Note: *Bacitracin* [bass i TRAY sin] is a mixture of polypeptides that also inhibits bacterial cell wall synthesis. It is active against a wide variety of gram-positive organisms. Its use is restricted to topical application because of its potential for nephrotoxicity.]

A. Mode of action

Vancomycin inhibits synthesis of bacterial cell wall phospholipids as well as peptidoglycan polymerization by binding to the D-Ala-D-Ala side chain of the precursor pentapeptide. This prevents the transglycosylation step in peptidoglycan polymerization, thus weakening the cell wall and damaging the underlying cell membrane.

B. Antibacterial spectrum

Vancomycin is effective primarily against gram-positive organisms (Figure 31.16). It has been lifesaving in the treatment of MRSA and *methicillin*-resistant Staphylococcus epidermidis (MRSE) infections, as well as enterococcal infections. With the emergence of resistant strains, it is important to curtail the increase in *vancomycin*-resistant bacteria (for example, Enterococcus faecium and Enterococcus fae-

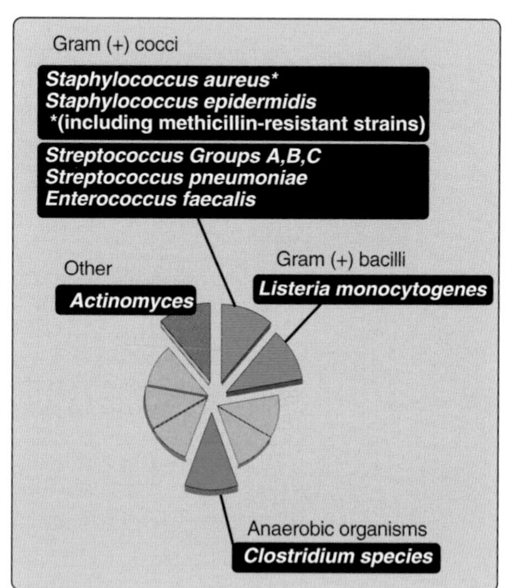

Figure 31.16
Antimicrobial spectrum of *vancomycin*.

calis) by restricting the use of *vancomycin* to the treatment of serious infections caused by β-lactam-resistant, gram-positive microorganisms, or for patients with gram-positive infections who have a serious allergy to the β-lactams. Oral *vancomycin* is limited to treatment for potentially life-threatening antibiotic-associated colitis due to C. difficile or staphylococci. *Vancomycin* is used in individuals with prosthetic heart valves and in patients undergoing implantation with prosthetic devices. [Note: The latter is of particular concern in those hospitals where there is a problem with MRSA or MRSE. Two new protein synthesis inhibitors—*quinopristin/dalfopristin* and *linezolid*—are currently available for the treatment of *vancomycin*-resistant organisms.] *Vancomycin* acts synergistically with the aminoglycosides, and this combination can be used in the treatment of enterococcal endocarditis.

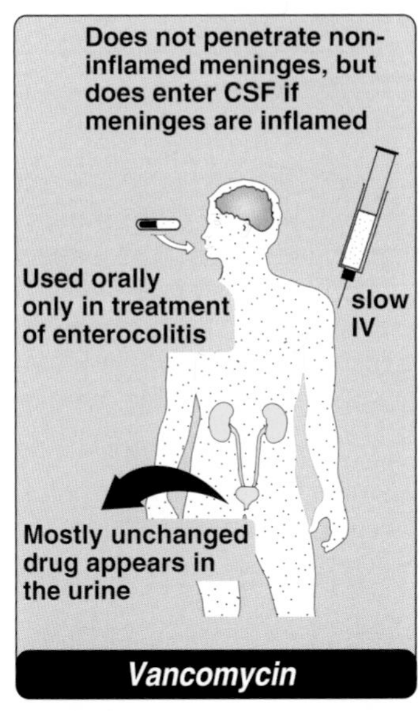

Figure 31.17
Administration and fate of *vancomycin*.

C. Resistance

Vancomycin resistance can be caused by plasmid-mediated changes in permeability to the drug or by decreased binding of *vancomycin* to receptor molecules. [Note: An example of the latter is caused by the replacement of a D-Ala by D-lactate in resistant organisms.]

D. Pharmacokinetics

Slow IV infusion is employed for treatment of systemic infections or for prophylaxis. Because *vancomycin* is not absorbed after oral administration, this route is only employed for the treatment of antibiotic-induced colitis due to C. difficile when *metronidazole* has proven ineffective. Inflammation allows penetration into the meninges. However, it is often necessary to combine *vancomycin* with other antibiotics, such as *ceftriaxone*. Metabolism of the drug is minimal, and 90 to 100 percent is excreted by glomerular filtration (Figure 31.17). [Note: Dosage must be adjusted in renal failure, because the drug will accumulate. The normal half-life of *vancomycin* is six to ten hours, compared to over 200 hours in end-stage renal disease.]

E. Adverse effects

Side effects are a serious problem with *vancomycin*, and include fever, chills, and/or phlebitis at the infusion site. Flushing ("red man syndrome") and shock result due to histamine release caused by rapid infusion (Figure 31.18). Dose-related hearing loss has occurred in patients with renal failure who accumulate the drug. Ototoxicity and nephrotoxicity are more common when *vancomycin* is administered with another drug (for example, an aminoglycoside) that can also produce these effects.

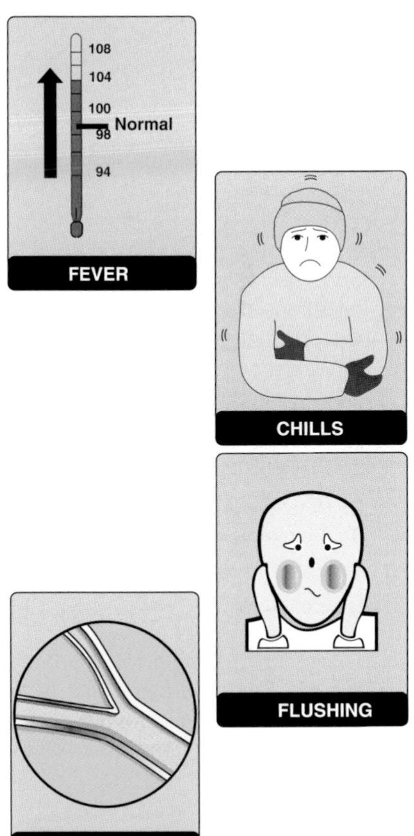

Figure 31.18
Some adverse effects of *vancomycin*.

Study Questions

Choose the ONE best answer

31.1 An elderly diabetic patient is admitted to the hospital with pneumonia. The sputum culture stains for a gram-negative rod. The patient is started on intravenous ampicillin. Two days later, the patient is not improving, and the microbiology laboratory reports the organism to be a β-lactamase-producing H. influenzae. What course of treatment is indicated?

A. Continue with the intravenous ampicillin
B. Switch to intravenous cefotaxime
C. Switch to oral vancomycin
D. Add gentamicin to the ampicillin therapy

Correct answer = B. Cefotaxime, a third-generation cephalosporin, is not susceptible to hydrolysis by β-lactamase, is bactericidal, and has few adverse effects. To continue the ampicillin is not appropriate, because the organism is resistant to it. Vancomycin is used in the treatment of serious infections caused by β-lactamase-resistant, gram-positive microorganisms (H. influenzae is gram-negative). Although gentamicin has some activity against H. influenzae, it also causes adverse effects, such as nephrotoxicity, which may harm the patient.

31.2 A seventy-year-old alcoholic male with poor dental hygiene is to have his remaining teeth extracted for subsequent dentures. He has mitral valve stenosis with mild cardiac insufficiency and is being treated with captopril, digoxin, and furosemide. The dentist decides that his medical history warrants prophylactic antibiotic therapy prior to the procedure and prescribes which of the following drugs?

A. Vancomycin
B. Amoxicillin
C. Tetracycline
D. Cotrimoxazole
E. Imipenem

Correct answer = B. Multiple tooth extractions can lead to bacteremia, and the mitral valve stenosis and cardiac insufficiency place him at risk for developing endocarditis. The present American Heart Association guidelines indicate amoxicillin (3 g, 1 hour prior to procedure, and 1.5 g, 6 hours after the original dose). Vancomycin would be appropriate only if the patient was allergic to penicillins. Tetracycline and cotrimoxazole are bacteriostatic and are not effective against the viridans group of streptococci, the usual causative organism. Imipenem is also inappropriate, because its spectrum is too broad.

31.3 A patient with degenerative joint disease is to undergo insertion of a hip prosthesis. To avoid complications due to postoperative infection, the surgeon will pretreat this patient with an antibiotic. This hospital has a significant problem with methicillin-resistant Staphylococcus aureus. Which of the following antibiotics should the surgeon select?

A. Ampicillin
B. Imipenem/cilastatin
C. Gentamicin/piperacillin
D. Vancomycin
E. Cefazolin

Correct answer = D. The only antibiotic on the list that is effective against methicillin-resistant Staphylococcus aureus is vancomycin.

31.4 A 25-year-old male returns home from a holiday in the Far East and complains of three days of dysuria and a purulent urethral discharge. You diagnose this to be a case of gonorrhea. Which of the following is appropriate treatment?

A. Ceftriaxone IM
B. Penicillin G IM
C. Gentamicin IM
D. Piperacillin/tazobactam IV
E. Vancomycin IV

Correct answer = A. Most gonoccocal infections are now resistant to penicillin, the previous drug of choice. The other antibiotics are inappropriate.

Protein Synthesis Inhibitors

32

I. OVERVIEW

A number of antibiotics exert their antimicrobial effects by targeting the bacterial ribosome, which has components that differ structurally from those of the mammalian cytoplasmic ribosome. In general, the bacterial ribosome is smaller (70S) than the mammalian ribosome (80S), and is composed of 50S and 30S subunits (as compared to 60S and 40S subunits).[1] The mammalian mitochondrial ribosome, however, more closely resembles the bacterial ribosome. Thus, although drugs that interact with the bacterial target usually spare the host cells, high levels of drugs such as *chloramphenicol* or the tetracyclines may cause toxic effects as a result of interaction with the mitochondrial ribosomes. Figure 32.1 lists the drugs discussed in this chapter.

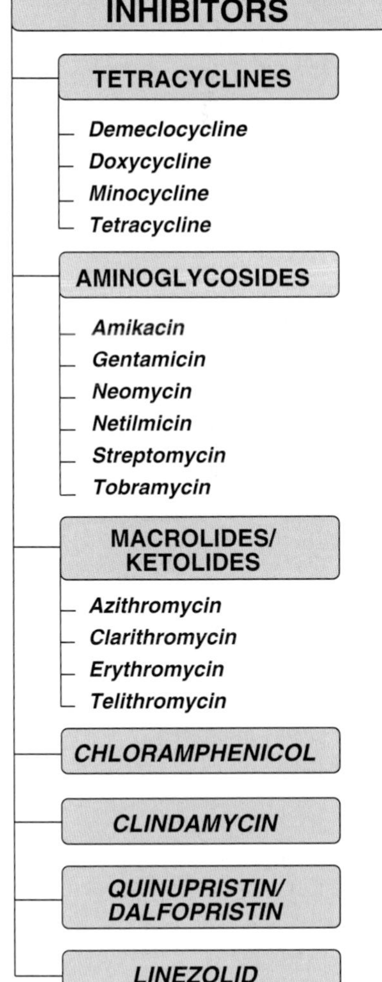

Figure 32.1
Summary of protein synthesis inhibitors.

II. TETRACYCLINES

The tetracyclines [tet ra SYE kleen] are a group of closely related compounds that, as the name implies, consist of four fused rings with a system of conjugated double bonds. Substitutions on these rings are responsible for a variation in the drugs' individual pharmacokinetics, which cause small differences in their clinical efficacy.

A. Mechanism of action

Entry of these agents into susceptible organisms is mediated both by passive diffusion and by an energy-dependent transport protein mechanism unique to the bacterial inner cytoplasmic membrane. Nonresistant strains concentrate the tetracyclines intracellularly. The drug binds reversibly to the 30S subunit of the bacterial ribosome, thereby blocking access of the amino acyl-tRNA to the mRNA-ribosome complex at the acceptor site. By this mechanism, bacterial protein synthesis is inhibited (Figure 32.2).

B. Antibacterial spectrum

As broad-spectrum, bacteriostatic antibiotics, the tetracyclines are effective against gram-positive and gram-negative bacteria as well as against organisms other than bacteria. Tetracyclines are the drugs of choice for infections such as those shown in Figure 32.3.

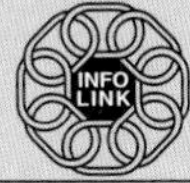

[1]See p. 433 in ***Lippincott's Illustrated Reviews: Biochemistry*** (3rd ed.) for a discussion of ribosomal structure and function.

Lippincott's Illustrated Reviews: Pharmacology, Third Edition,
by Richard D. Howland and Mary J. Mycek.

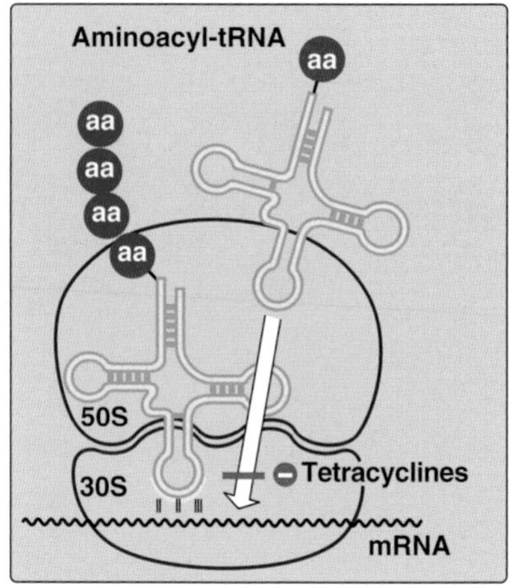

Figure 32.2
Tetracyclines binds to the 30S ribosomal subunit, thus preventing the binding of aminoacyl-tRNA to the ribosome. aa = amino acid.

C. Resistance

Widespread resistance to the tetracyclines limits their clinical use. The most commonly encountered, naturally occurring resistance ("R") factor[2] confers an inability of the organism to accumulate the drug, thus producing resistance. This is accomplished by Mg^{2+}-dependent, active efflux of the drug, mediated by the plasmid-encoded resistance protein, TetA. Other less important mechanisms of bacterial resistance to tetracyclines include enzymatic inactivation of the drug, and production of bacterial proteins that prevent tetracyclines from binding to the ribosome. Any organism resistant to one tetracycline is resistant to all. The majority of penicillinase-producing staphylococci are now insensitive to tetracyclines.

D. Pharmacokinetics

1. **Absorption:** All tetracyclines are adequately but incompletely absorbed after oral ingestion (Figure 32.4). However, taking these drugs concomitantly with dairy foods in the diet decreases absorption due to the formation of nonabsorbable chelates of the tetracyclines with calcium ions. Nonabsorbable chelates are also formed

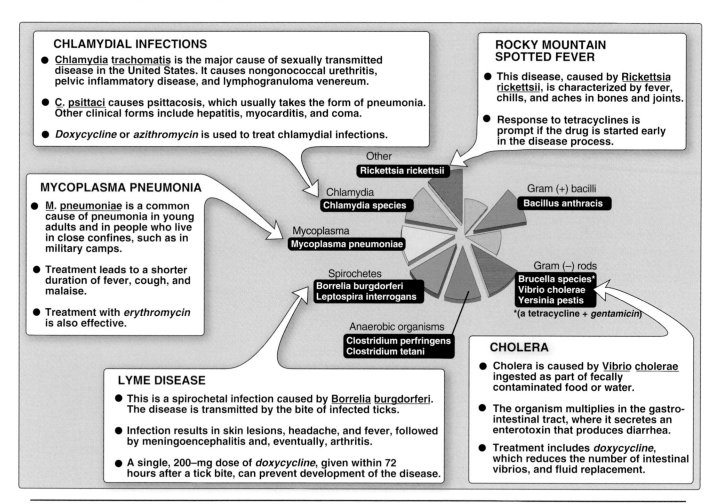

CHLAMYDIAL INFECTIONS

- Chlamydia trachomatis is the major cause of sexually transmitted disease in the United States. It causes nongonococcal urethritis, pelvic inflammatory disease, and lymphogranuloma venereum.
- C. psittaci causes psittacosis, which usually takes the form of pneumonia. Other clinical forms include hepatitis, myocarditis, and coma.
- *Doxycycline* or *azithromycin* is used to treat chlamydial infections.

ROCKY MOUNTAIN SPOTTED FEVER

- This disease, caused by Rickettsia rickettsii, is characterized by fever, chills, and aches in bones and joints.
- Response to tetracyclines is prompt if the drug is started early in the disease process.

MYCOPLASMA PNEUMONIA

- M. pneumoniae is a common cause of pneumonia in young adults and in people who live in close confines, such as in military camps.
- Treatment leads to a shorter duration of fever, cough, and malaise.
- Treatment with *erythromycin* is also effective.

Other
Rickettsia rickettsii

Chlamydia
Chlamydia species

Mycoplasma
Mycoplasma pneumoniae

Spirochetes
Borrelia burgdorferi
Leptospira interrogans

Anaerobic organisms
Clostridium perfringens
Clostridium tetani

Gram (+) bacilli
Bacillus anthracis

Gram (–) rods
Brucella species*
Vibrio cholerae
Yersinia pestis
*(a tetracycline + *gentamicin*)

LYME DISEASE

- This is a spirochetal infection caused by Borrelia burgdorferi. The disease is transmitted by the bite of infected ticks.
- Infection results in skin lesions, headache, and fever, followed by meningoencephalitis and, eventually, arthritis.
- A single, 200–mg dose of *doxycycline*, given within 72 hours after a tick bite, can prevent development of the disease.

CHOLERA

- Cholera is caused by Vibrio cholerae ingested as part of fecally contaminated food or water.
- The organism multiplies in the gastrointestinal tract, where it secretes an enterotoxin that produces diarrhea.
- Treatment includes *doxycycline*, which reduces the number of intestinal vibrios, and fluid replacement.

Figure 32.3
Typical therapeutic applications of tetracyclines.

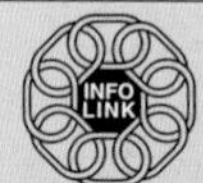

[2]See p. 133 in ***Lippincott's Illustrated Reviews: Microbiology*** for a discussion of bacterial resistance genes.

with other divalent and trivalent cations (for example, those found in magnesium and aluminum antacids and in iron preparations). [Note: This presents a problem if a patient self-treats the epigastric upsets caused by tetracycline ingestion with antacids (Figure 32.5).] *Doxycycline* [dox i SYE kleen] and *minocycline* [mine oh SYE kleen] are almost totally absorbed on oral administration. *Doxycycline* is preferred for parenteral administration.

2. **Distribution:** The tetracyclines concentrate in the liver, kidney, spleen, and skin, and they bind to tissues undergoing calcification (for example, teeth and bones) or to tumors that have a high calcium content (for example, gastric carcinoma). Penetration into most body fluids is adequate. Although all tetracyclines enter the cerebrospinal fluid (CSF), levels are insufficient for therapeutic efficacy, except for *minocycline*. *Minocycline* enters the brain in the absence of inflammation and also appears in tears and saliva. Although useful in eradicating the meningococcal carrier state, *minocycline* is not effective for central nervous system infections. All tetracyclines cross the placental barrier, and concentrate in fetal bones and dentition.

3. **Fate:** All the tetracyclines concentrate in the liver, where they are, in part, metabolized and conjugated to form soluble glucuronides. The parent drug and/or its metabolites are secreted into the bile. Most tetracyclines are reabsorbed in the intestine via the enterohepatic circulation and enter the urine by glomerular filtration. Obstruction of the bile duct and hepatic or renal dysfunction can increase their half-lives. Unlike other tetracyclines, *doxycycline* can be employed for treating infections in renally compromised patients, because it is preferentially excreted via the bile into the feces. [Note: Tetracyclines are also excreted in breast milk.]

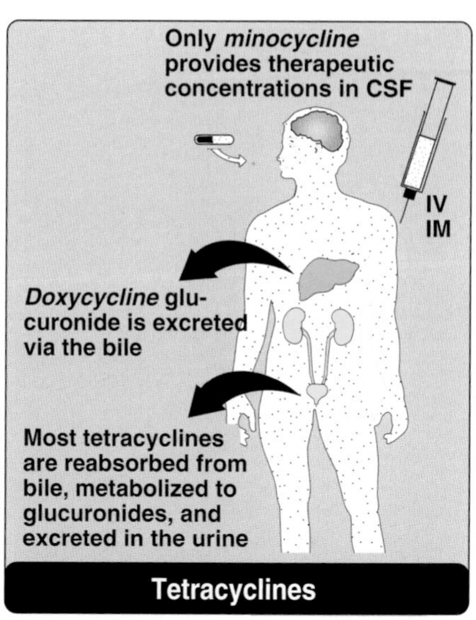

Figure 32.4
Administration and fate of tetracyclines.

E. Adverse effects

1. **Gastric discomfort:** Epigastric distress commonly results from irritation of the gastric mucosa (Figure 32.6), and is often responsible for noncompliance in patients treated with these drugs. The discomfort can be controlled if the drug is taken with foods other than dairy products.

2. **Effects on calcified tissues:** Deposition in the bone and primary dentition occurs during calcification in growing children. This causes discoloration and hypoplasia of the teeth and a temporary stunting of growth.

3. **Fatal hepatotoxicity:** This side effect has been known to occur in pregnant women who received high doses of tetracyclines, especially if they were experiencing pyelonephritis.

4. **Phototoxicity:** Phototoxicity, such as severe sunburn, occurs when a patient receiving a tetracycline is exposed to sun or ultraviolet rays. This toxicity is encountered most frequently with *tetracycline*, *doxycycline*, and *demeclocycline* [dem e kloe SYE kleen].

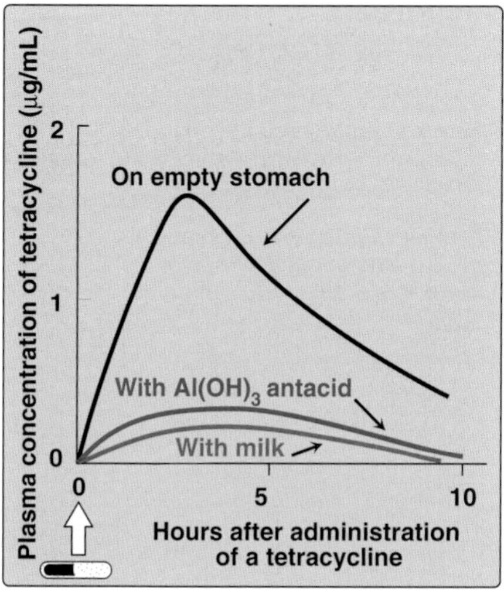

Figure 32.5
Effect of antacids and milk on the absorption of tetracyclines.

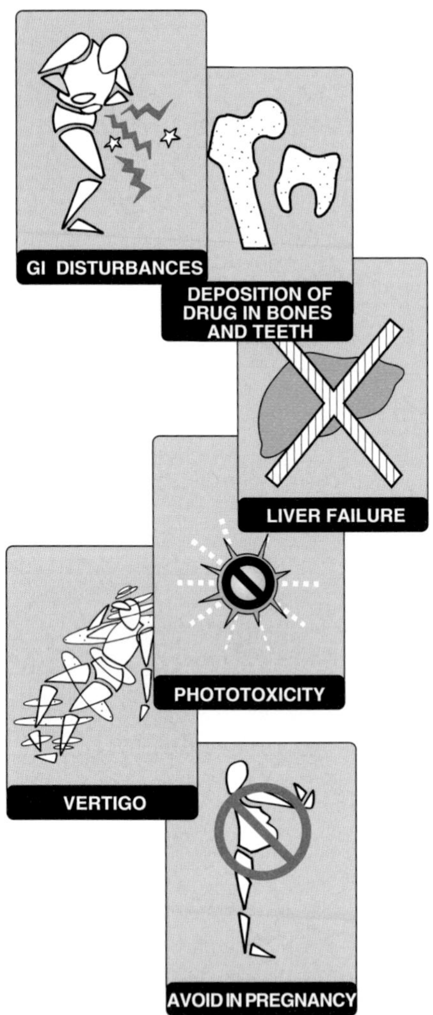

Figure 32.6
Some adverse effects of *tetracycline*.

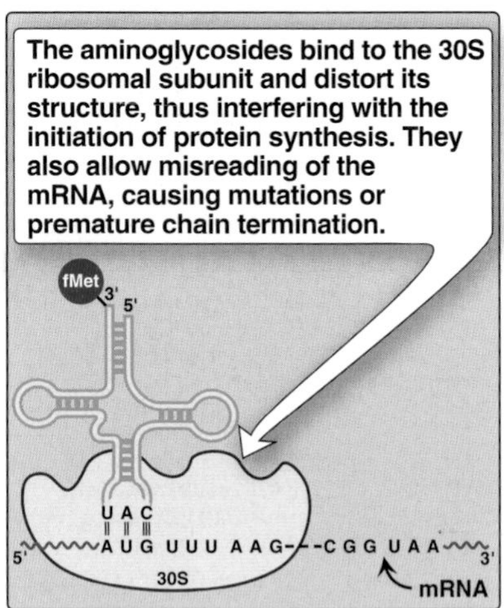

Figure 32.7
Mechanism of action of the aminoglycosides.

5. **Vestibular problems:** These side effects (for example, dizziness, nausea, and vomiting) occur particularly with *minocycline*, which concentrates in the endolymph of the ear and affects function. *Doxycycline* may also cause vestibular effects.

6. **Pseudotumor cerebri:** Benign, intracranial hypertension characterized by headache and blurred vision may occur rarely in adults. Although discontinuation of the drug reverses this condition, it is not clear whether permanent sequelae may occur.

7. **Superinfections:** Overgrowths of Candida (for example, in the vagina) or of resistant staphylococci (in the intestine) may occur. Pseudomembranous colitis due to an overgrowth of Clostridium difficile has also been reported.

8. **Contraindications:** Renally impaired patients should not be treated with any of the tetracyclines except *doxycycline*. Accumulation of tetracyclines may aggravate preexisting azotemia by interfering with protein synthesis, thus promoting amino acid degradation. The tetracyclines should not be employed in pregnant or breast-feeding women or in children under eight years of age.

III. AMINOGLYCOSIDES

Aminoglycoside antibiotics had been the mainstays for treatment of serious infections due to aerobic gram-negative bacilli. However, because their use is associated with serious toxicities, they have been replaced to some extent by safer antibiotics, such as the third-generation cephalosporins, the fluoroquinolones, and *imipenem/cilastatin*. Aminoglycosides that are derived from Streptomyces have -mycin suffixes, whereas those derived from Micromonospora end in -micin. The terms "aminoglycoside" and "aminocyclitol" stem from their structure—two amino sugars joined by a glycosidic linkage to a central hexose (aminocyclitol) nucleus. Their polycationic nature precludes their easy passage across tissue membranes. All members of this family are believed to inhibit bacterial protein synthesis by the mechanism determined for *streptomycin* [strep toe MYE sin] as described below.

A. Mechanism of action

Susceptible gram-negative organisms allow aminoglycosides to diffuse through porin channels in their outer membranes. These organisms also have an oxygen-dependent system that transports the drug across the cell membrane. The antibiotic then binds to the 30S ribosomal subunit prior to ribosome formation (Figure 32.7). There, it interferes with assembly of the functional ribosomal apparatus, and/or can cause the 30S subunit of the completed ribosome to misread the genetic code. Polysomes[3] become depleted, because the aminoglycosides interrupt the process of polysome disaggregation and assembly. [Note: The aminoglycosides synergize with β-lactam antibiotics, because of the latters' action on cell wall synthesis, which enhances diffusion of the aminoglycosides into the bacterium.]

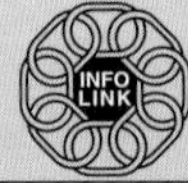

[3]See p. 440 in ***Lippincott's Illustrated Reviews: Biochemistry*** (3rd ed.) for a discussion of polysomes.

B. Antibacterial spectrum

The aminoglycosides are effective in the empirical treatment of infections suspected of being due to aerobic gram-negative bacilli, including Pseudomonas aeruginosa. To achieve an additive or synergistic effect, aminoglycosides are often combined with a β-lactam antibiotic, or *vancomycin*, or a drug active against anaerobic bacteria. All aminoglycosides are bactericidal. The exact mechanism of their lethality is unknown, because other antibiotics that affect protein synthesis are generally bacteriostatic. [Note: The aminoglycosides are only effective against aerobic organisms, because strict anaerobes lack the oxygen-requiring transport system.] Some therapeutic applications of four commonly used aminoglycosides—*amikacin* [am i KAY sin], *gentamicin* [jen ta MYE sin], *tobramycin* [toe bra MYE sin], and *streptomycin*—are shown in Figure 32.8.

C. Resistance

Resistance can be caused by 1) decreased uptake of drug when the oxygen-dependent transport system for aminoglycosides or porin channels are absent, 2) an altered 30S ribosomal subunit aminoglycoside-binding site that has a decreased affinity for the drugs, or 3) plasmid-associated synthesis of enzymes (for example, acetyl transferases, nucleotidyltransferases, and phosphotransferases) that modify and inactivate aminoglycoside antibiotics. Each of these enzymes has its own aminoglycoside specificity; therefore, cross-resistance is not an invariable rule. [Note: *Netilmicin* [ne TIL mye sin] and *amikacin* are less vulnerable to these enzymes than are the other antibiotics of this group.]

D. Pharmacokinetics

1. **Administration:** The highly polar, polycationic structure of the aminoglycosides prevents adequate absorption after oral administration (Figure 32.9). Therefore, all aminoglycosides (except *neomycin* [nee oh MYE sin]) must be given parenterally to achieve adequate serum levels. [Note: The severe nephrotoxicity associated with *neomycin* precludes parenteral administration, and its current use is limited to topical application for skin infections or oral administration to prepare the bowel prior to surgery.] The bactericidal effect is concentration and time dependent; that is, the greater the concentration of drug, the greater the rate at which the organisms die. They also have a postantibiotic effect. Because of these properties, once-daily dosing with the aminoglycosides can be employed. This results in fewer toxicities and is cheaper to administer. The exceptions are pregnancy, neonatal infections, and bacterial endocarditis, in which these agents are administered in divided doses every eight hours. [Note: The dose that is administered is calculated based on lean body mass, because these drugs do not distribute into fat.]

2. **Distribution:** All the aminoglycosides have similar pharmacokinetic properties. Levels achieved in most tissues are low, and penetration into most body fluids is variable. Concentrations in CSF are inadequate, even when the meninges are inflamed.

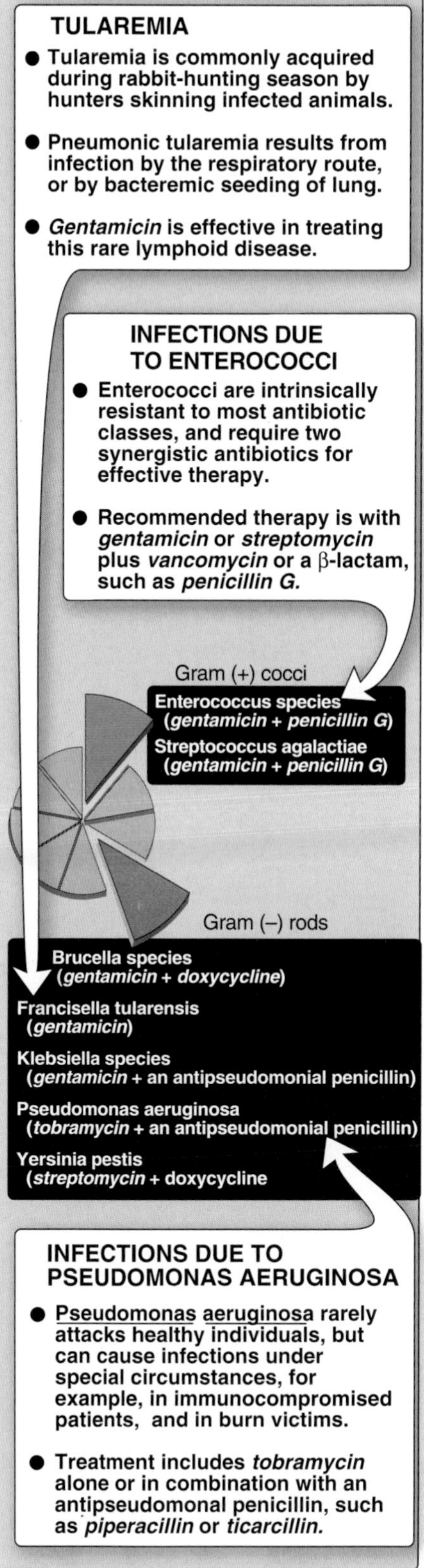

TULAREMIA
Tularemia is commonly acquired during rabbit-hunting season by hunters skinning infected animals.
Pneumonic tularemia results from infection by the respiratory route, or by bacteremic seeding of lung.
Gentamicin is effective in treating this rare lymphoid disease.
INFECTIONS DUE TO ENTEROCOCCI
Enterococci are intrinsically resistant to most antibiotic classes, and require two synergistic antibiotics for effective therapy.
Recommended therapy is with gentamicin or streptomycin plus vancomycin or a β-lactam, such as penicillin G.
Gram (+) cocci
Enterococcus species (gentamicin + penicillin G)
Streptococcus agalactiae (gentamicin + penicillin G)
Gram (–) rods
Brucella species (gentamicin + doxycycline)
Francisella tularensis (gentamicin)
Klebsiella species (gentamicin + an antipseudomonial penicillin)
Pseudomonas aeruginosa (tobramycin + an antipseudomonial penicillin)
Yersinia pestis (streptomycin + doxycycline
INFECTIONS DUE TO PSEUDOMONAS AERUGINOSA
Pseudomonas aeruginosa rarely attacks healthy individuals, but can cause infections under special circumstances, for example, in immunocompromised patients, and in burn victims.
Treatment includes tobramycin alone or in combination with an antipseudomonal penicillin, such as piperacillin or ticarcillin.

Figure 32.8
Typical therapeutic applications of aminoglycosides.

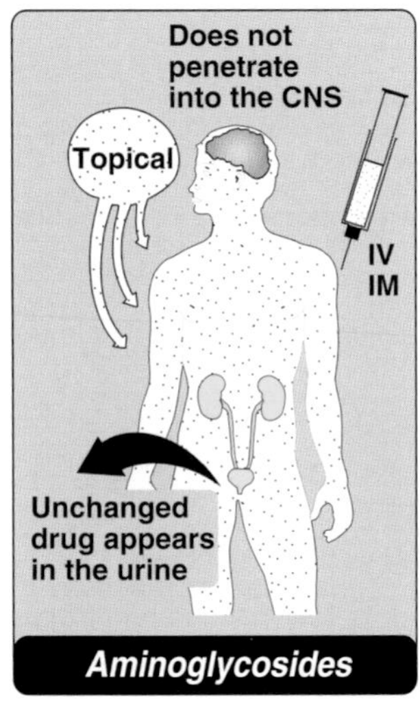

Figure 32.9
Administration and fate of aminoglycosides.

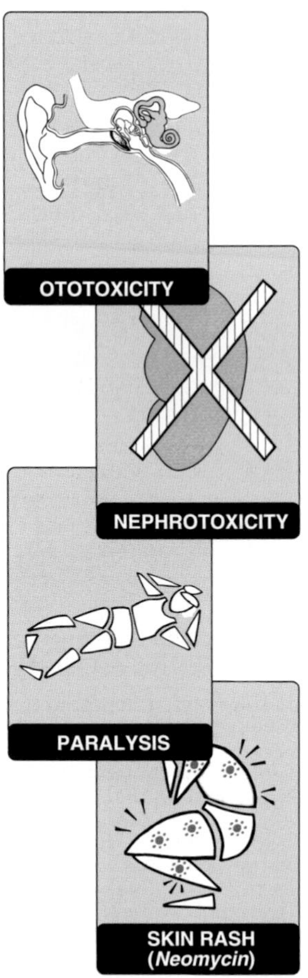

Figure 32.10
Some adverse effects of aminoglycosides.

Except for *neomycin*, the aminoglycosides may be administered intrathecally or intraventricularly. High concentrations accumulate in the renal cortex and in the endolymph and perilymph of the inner ear, which may account for their nephrotoxic and ototoxic potential. All aminoglycosides cross the placental barrier and may accumulate in fetal plasma and amniotic fluid.

3. **Fate:** Metabolism of the aminoglycosides does not occur in the host. All are rapidly excreted into the urine, predominantly by glomerular filtration (see Figure 32.9). Accumulation occurs in patients with renal failure and requires dose modification.

E. Adverse effects

It is important to monitor plasma levels of *gentamicin*, *tobramycin*, *netilmicin*, and *amikacin* to avoid concentrations that cause dose-related toxicities (Figure 32.10). [Note: When the drugs are administered two to three times daily, both peak and trough levels are measured. Peak levels are defined as those obtained thirty minutes to one hour after infusion. Trough levels are obtained immediately before the next dose. When once-daily dosing is employed, only the trough concentrations are monitored.] Patient factors, such as old age, previous exposure to aminoglycosides, gender, and liver disease, tend to predispose patients to adverse reactions. The elderly are particularly susceptible to nephrotoxicity and ototoxicity.

1. **Ototoxicity:** Ototoxicity (vestibular and cochlear) is directly related to high peak plasma levels and the duration of treatment. The antibiotic accumulates in the endolymph and perilymph of the inner ear, and toxicity correlates with the number of destroyed hair cells in the organ of Corti. Deafness may be irreversible and has been known to affect fetuses in utero. Patients simultaneously receiving another ototoxic drug, such as the loop diuretics *furosemide*, *bumetanide*, or *ethacrynic acid* or *cisplatin*, are particularly at risk. Vertigo and loss of balance (especially in patients receiving *streptomycin*) may also occur, because these drugs affect the vestibular apparatus.

2. **Nephrotoxicity:** Retention of the aminoglycosides by the proximal tubular cells disrupts calcium-mediated transport processes, and this results in kidney damage ranging from mild, reversible renal impairment to severe, acute tubular necrosis, which can be irreversible. However, the exact biochemical processes that lead to the toxicity remain to be elucidated.

3. **Neuromuscular paralysis:** This side effect most often occurs after direct intraperitoneal or intrapleural application of large doses of aminoglycosides. The mechanism responsible is a decrease in both the release of acetylcholine from prejunctional nerve endings and the sensitivity of the postsynaptic site. Patients with myasthenia gravis are particularly at risk. Prompt administration of *calcium gluconate* or *neostigmine* can reverse the block.

4. **Allergic reactions:** Contact dermatitis is a common reaction to topically applied *neomycin*.

IV. MACROLIDES

The macrolides are a group of antibiotics with a macrocyclic lactone structure to which one or more deoxy sugars are attached. *Erythromycin* [er ith roe MYE sin] was the first of these drugs to find clinical application, both as a drug of first choice, and as an alternative to *penicillin* in individuals who are allergic to β-lactam antibiotics. The newer members of this family, *clarithromycin* [kla rith roe MYE sin] (a methylated form of *erythromycin*) and *azithromycin* [az ith roe MYE sin] (having a larger lactone ring), have some features in common with, and others that improve on, *erythromycin*. *Telithromycin* [tel ith roe MYE sin]—an *erythromycin* derivative (a ketolide)—has recently been approved.

A. Mechanism of action

The macrolides bind irreversibly to a site on the 50S subunit of the bacterial ribosome, thus inhibiting the translocation steps of protein synthesis[4] (Figure 32.11). They may also interfere at other steps, such as transpeptidation. Generally considered to be bacteriostatic, they may be cidal at higher doses. Their binding site is either identical or in close proximity to that for *clindamycin* and *chloramphenicol*.

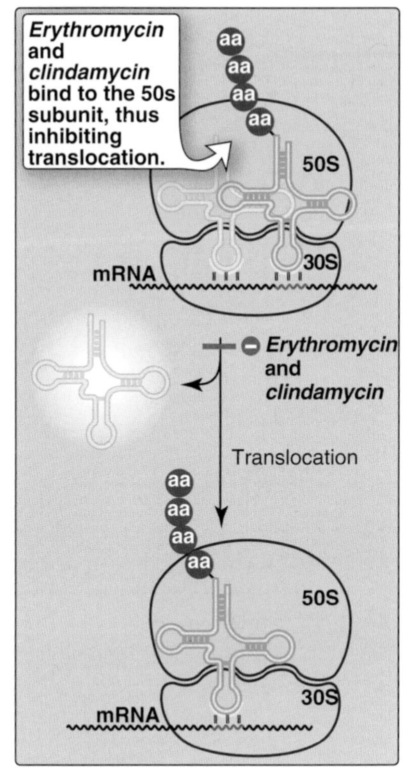

Figure 32.11
Mechanism of action of *erythromycin* and *clindamycin*.

B. Antibacterial spectrum

1. **Erythromycin:** This drug is effective against many of the same organisms as *penicillin G* (Figure 32.12); therefore, it is used in patients allergic to the penicillins.

2. **Clarithromycin:** This antibiotic has a spectrum of antibacterial activity similar to that of *erythromycin*, but it is also effective

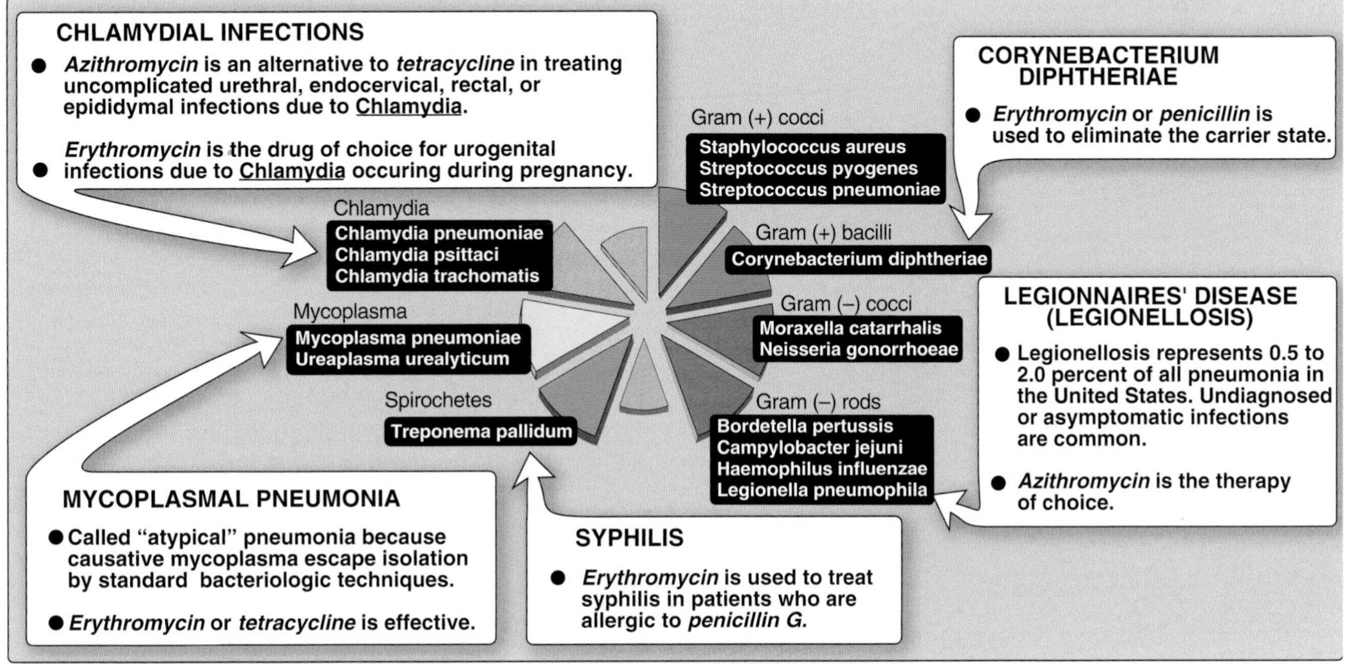

Figure 32.12
Typical therapeutic applications of macrolides.

[4]See p. 438 in ***Lippincott's Illustrated Reviews: Biochemistry*** (3rd ed.) for a discussion of protein synthesis.

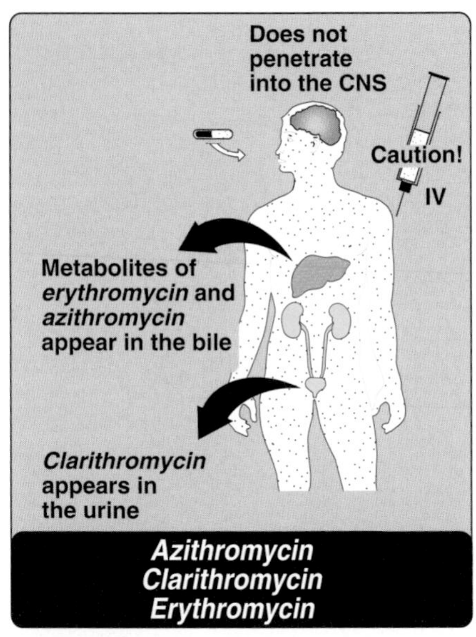

Figure 32.13
Administration and fate of the macrolide antibiotics.

against Haemophilus influenzae. Its activity against intracellular pathogens, such as Chlamydia, Legionella, Moraxella, and Ureaplasma species, and Helicobacter pylori, is higher than that of *erythromycin*.

3. **Azithromycin:** Although less active against streptococci and staphylococci than *erythromycin*, *azithromycin* is far more active against respiratory infections due to H. influenzae and Moraxella catarrhalis. Except for its cost, *azithromycin* is now the preferred therapy for urethritis caused by Chlamydia trachomatis. It also has activity against Mycobacterium avium-intracellulare complex in AIDS patients with disseminated infections.

4. **Telithromycin:** This drug has an antibacterial spectrum similar to that of *azithromycin*.

C. Resistance

Resistance to *erythromycin* is becoming a serious clinical problem. For example, most strains of staphylococci in hospital isolates are resistant to this drug. Several mechanisms have been identified: 1) the inability of the organism to take up the antibiotic or the presence of an efflux pump, both of which limit the amount of intracellular drug; 2) a decreased affinity of the 50S ribosomal subunit for the antibiotic, resulting from the methylation of an adenine in the 23S bacterial ribosomal RNA; and 3) the presence of a plasmid-associated *erythromycin* esterase. Both *clarithromycin* and *azithromycin* show cross-resistance with *erythromycin*, but *telithromycin* can be effective against macrolide-resistant organisms.

D. Pharmacokinetics

1. **Administration:** The *erythromycin* base is destroyed by gastric acid. Thus, either enteric-coated tablets or esterified forms of the antibiotic are administered. All are adequately absorbed on oral administration (Figure 32.13). *Clarithromycin, azithromycin*, and *telithromycin* are stable to stomach acid and are readily absorbed. Food interferes with the absorption of *erythromycin* and *azithromycin* but can increase that of *clarithromycin*. *Azithromycin* is available for intravenous (IV) infusion, but IV administration of *erythromycin* is associated with a high incidence of thrombophlebitis.

2. **Distribution:** *Erythromycin* distributes well to all body fluids except the CSF. It is one of the few antibiotics that diffuses into prostatic fluid, and it has the unique characteristic of accumulating in macrophages. All four drugs concentrate in the liver. Inflammation allows for greater tissue penetration. Similarly, *clarithromycin, azithromycin*, and *telithromycin* are widely distributed in the tissues. Serum levels of *azithromycin* are low; the drug is concentrated in neutrophils, macrophages, and fibroblasts. *Azithromycin* has the longest half-life and largest volume of distribution of the four drugs (see Figure 32.14).

	Erythromycin	*Clarithromycin*	*Azithromycin*	*Telithromycin*
Oral absorption	Yes	Yes	Yes	Yes
Half-life (hours)	2	3.5	>40	10
Conversion to an active metabolite	No	Yes	Yes	Yes
Percent excretion in urine	15	50	12	13

Figure 32.14
Some properties of the macrolide antibiotics.

3. **Fate:** *Erythromycin* and *telithromycin* are extensively metabolized, and are known to inhibit the oxidation of a number of drugs through their interaction with the cytochrome P450 system (see p.

14). Interference with the metabolism of drugs such as *theophylline* and *carbamazepine* has been reported for *clarithromycin* (see below). *Clarithromycin* is oxidized to the 14-hydroxy derivative, which retains antibiotic activity.

4. **Excretion:** *Erythromycin* and *azithromycin* are primarily concentrated and excreted in an active form in the bile (see Figure 32.13). Partial reabsorption occurs through the enterohepatic circulation. Inactive metabolites are excreted into the urine. In contrast, *clarithromycin* and its metabolites are eliminated by the kidney as well as the liver, and it is recommended that dosage of this drug be adjusted in patients with compromised renal function.

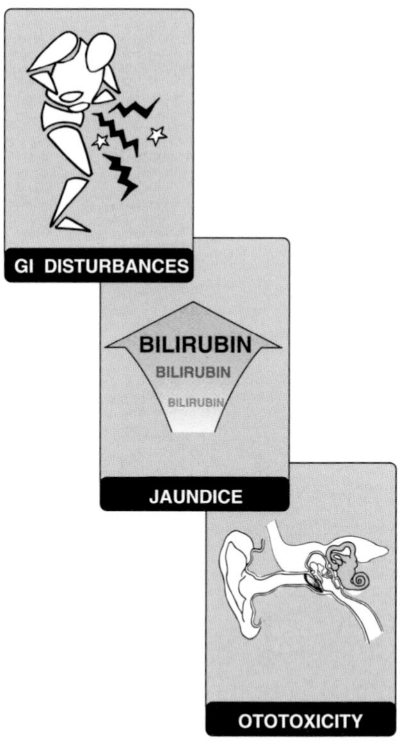

Figure 32.15
Some adverse effects of macrolide antibiotics.

E. Adverse effects

1. **Epigastric distress:** This side effect is common and can lead to poor patient compliance for *erythromycin*. *Clarithromycin* and *azithromycin* seem to be better tolerated by the patient, but gastrointestinal problems are their most common side effects (Figure 32.15).

2. **Cholestatic jaundice:** This side effect occurs especially with the estolate form of *erythromycin*, presumably as the result of a hypersensitivity reaction to the estolate form (the lauryl salt of the propionyl ester of *erythromycin*). It has also been reported for other forms of the drug.

3. **Ototoxicity:** Transient deafness has been associated with *erythromycin*, especially at high dosages.

4. **Contraindications:** Patients with hepatic dysfunction should be treated with caution—if at all—with *erythromycin*, *telithromycin*, or *azithromycin*, because these drugs accumulate in the liver. Similarly, patients who are renally compromised should be given *telithromycin* with caution. *Telithromycin* may worsen myasthenia gravis.

5. **Interactions:** *Erythromycin*, *telithromycin*, and *clarithromycin* inhibit the hepatic metabolism of a number of drugs, which can lead to toxic accumulations of these compounds (Figure 32.16). An interaction with *digoxin* may occur in some patients. In this case, the antibiotic eliminates a species of intestinal flora that ordinarily inactivates *digoxin*, thus leading to greater reabsorption of the drug from the enterohepatic circulation. No interactions have been reported for *azithromycin*.

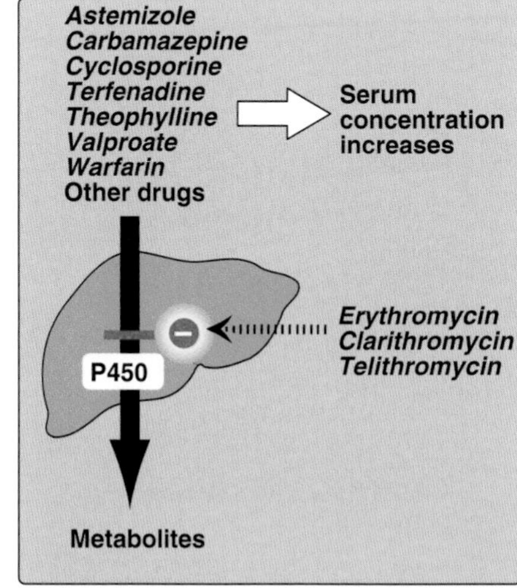

Figure 32.16
Inhibition of the cytochrome P450 system by *erythromycin,clarithromycin* and *telithromycin*.

V. CHLORAMPHENICOL

Chloramphenicol [klor am FEN i kole] is active against a wide range of gram-positive and gram-negative organisms. However, because of its toxicity, its use is restricted to life-threatening infections for which no alternatives exist.

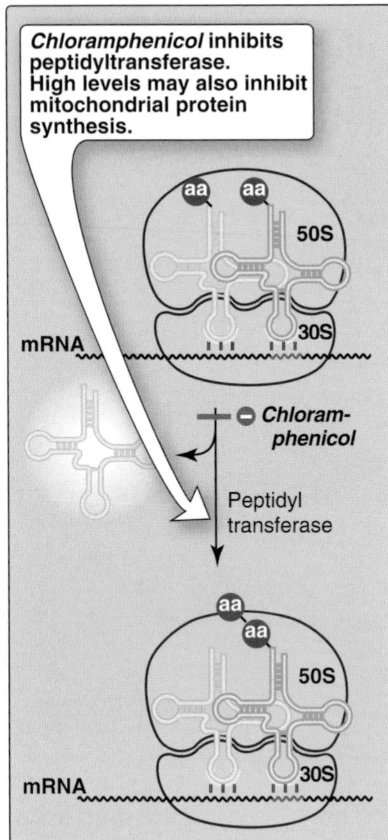

Figure 32.17
Mechanism of action of *chloramphenicol*.

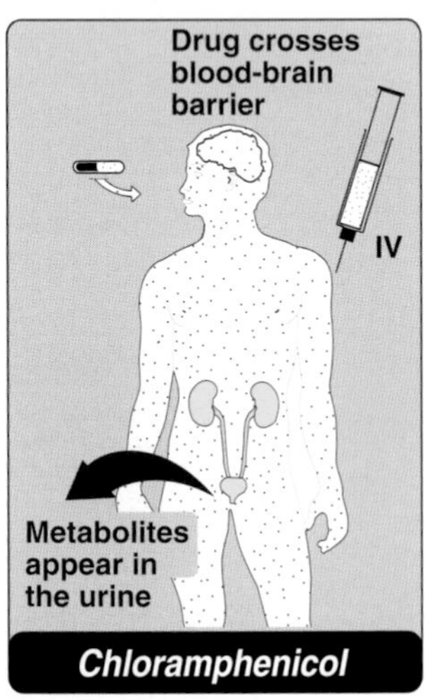

Figure 32.18
Administration and fate of *chloramphenicol*.

A. Mechanism of action

The drug binds to the bacterial 50S ribosomal subunit and inhibits protein synthesis at the peptidyl transferase reaction (Figure 32.17). Because of the similarity of mammalian mitochondrial ribosomes to those of bacteria, protein synthesis in these organelles may be inhibited at high circulating *chloramphenicol* levels, producing bone marrow toxicity.

B. Antimicrobial spectrum

Chloramphenicol, a broad-spectrum antibiotic, is active not only against bacteria but also against other microorganisms, such as rickettsiae. Pseudomonas aeruginosa is not affected, nor are the chlamydiae. *Chloramphenicol* has excellent activity against anaerobes. The drug is either bactericidal or (more commonly) bacteriostatic, depending on the organism.

C. Resistance

Resistance is conferred by the presence of an R factor that codes for an acetyl coenzyme A transferase. This enzyme inactivates *chloramphenicol*. Another mechanism for resistance is associated with an inability of the antibiotic to penetrate the organism. This change in permeability may be the basis of multidrug resistance.

D. Pharmacokinetics

Chloramphenicol may be administered either intravenously or orally (Figure 32.18). It is completely absorbed via the oral route because of its lipophilic nature, and is widely distributed throughout the body. It readily enters the normal CSF. The drug inhibits the hepatic mixed-function oxidases. Excretion of the drug depends on its conversion in the liver to a glucuronide, which is then secreted by the renal tubule. Only about ten percent of the parent compound is excreted by glomerular filtration. *Chloramphenicol* is also secreted into breast milk.

E. Adverse effects

The clinical use of *chloramphenicol* is limited to life-threatening infections because of the serious adverse effects associated with its administration. In addition to gastrointestinal upsets, overgrowth of Candida albicans may appear on mucuous membranes.

1. **Anemias:** Hemolytic anemia occurs in patients with low levels of glucose 6-phosphate dehydrogenase[5]. Other types of anemia occurring as a side effect of *chloramphenicol* include reversible anemia, which is apparently dose-related and occurs concomitantly with therapy, and aplastic anemia, which although rare is idiosyncratic and usually fatal. [Note: Aplastic anemia is independent of dose and may occur after therapy has ceased.]

2. **Gray baby syndrome:** This adverse effect occurs in neonates if the dosage regimen of *chloramphenicol* is not properly adjusted. Neonates have a low capacity to glucuronylate the antibiotic, and they have underdeveloped renal function. Ttherefore, neonates have a decreased ability to excrete the drug, which accumulates

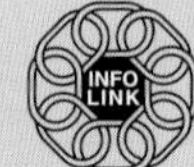

[5]See p. 149 in ***Lippincott's Illustrated Reviews: Biochemistry*** (3rd ed.) for a discussion of glucose 6-phosphate dehydrogenase deficiency.

to levels that interfere with the function of mitochondrial ribosomes. This leads to poor feeding, depressed breathing, cardiovascular collapse, cyanosis (hence the term "gray baby"), and death. Adults who have received very high doses of the drug can also exhibit this toxicity.

3. **Interactions:** *Chloramphenicol* is able to inhibit some of the hepatic mixed-function oxidases and, thus, blocks the metabolism of such drugs as *warfarin*, *phenytoin*, *tolbutamide* and *chlorpropamide*, thereby elevating their concentrations and potentiating their effects (Figure 32.19).

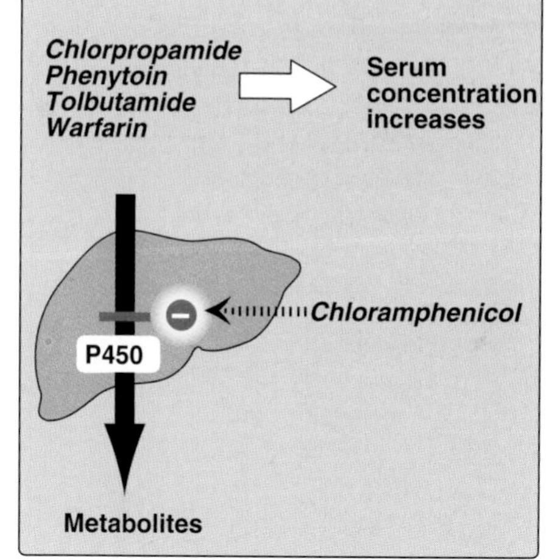

Figure 32.19
Inhibition of the cytochrome P450 system by *chloramphenicol*.

VI. CLINDAMYCIN

Clindamycin [klin da MYE sin] has a mechanism of action that is the same as that of *erythromycin*. *Clindamycin* is employed primarily in the treatment of infections caused by anaerobic bacteria, such as Bacteroides fragilis, which often causes abdominal infections associated with trauma. However, it is also significantly active against non-enterococcal, gram-positive cocci. Resistance mechanisms are the same as those for *erythromycin*, but cross-resistance is not a problem. [Note: Clostridium difficile is always resistant to *clindamycin*.] *Clindamycin* is well absorbed by the oral route. It distributes well into all body fluids except the CSF. Adequate levels of *clindamycin* are not achieved in the brain, even when meninges are inflamed. Penetration into bone occurs even in the absence of inflammation. *Clindamycin* undergoes extensive oxidative metabolism to inactive products. The drug is excreted into the bile or urine by glomerular filtration, but therapeutically effective levels of the parent drug are not achieved in the urine (Figure 32.20). Accumulation has been reported in patients with either severely compromised renal function or hepatic failure. In addition to skin rashes, the most serious adverse effect is potentially fatal pseudomembranous colitis caused by overgrowth of C. difficile, which elaborates necrotizing toxins.[6] Oral administration of either *metronidazole* or *vancomycin* is usually effective in controlling this serious problem. [Note: *Vancomycin* should be reserved for a condition that does not respond to *metronidazole*.] Impaired liver function has also been reported.

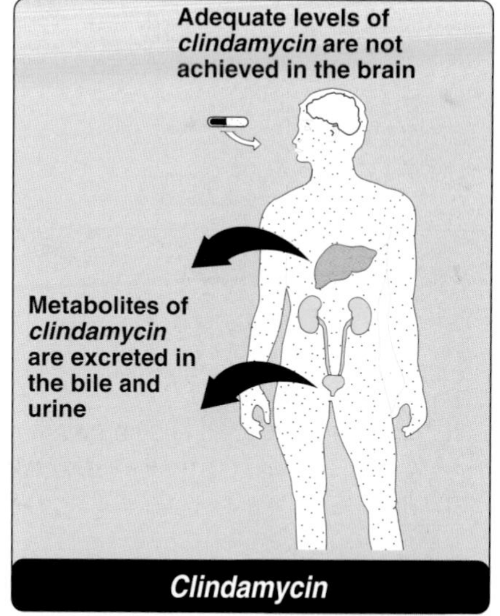

Figure 32.20
Administration and fate of *clindamycin*.

VII. QUINUPRISTIN/DALFOPRISTIN

Quinupristin/dalfopristin [KWIN oo pris tin, DAL foh pris tin] is a mixture of two streptogramins in a ratio of thirty to seventy, respectively. They are derived from a streptomycete and then chemically modified. The drug is reserved for the treatment of *vancomycin*-resistant Enterococcus faecium (VRE).

A. Mechanism of action

Each component of this combination drug binds to a separate site on the 50S bacterial ribosome, forming a stable ternary complex. Thus, they synergistically interrupt protein synthesis. The combination drug is bactericidal and has a long postantibiotic effect.

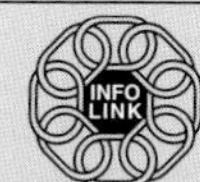

[6]See p. 217 in ***Lippincott's Illustrated Reviews: Microbiology*** for a discussion of Clostridium difficile toxins.

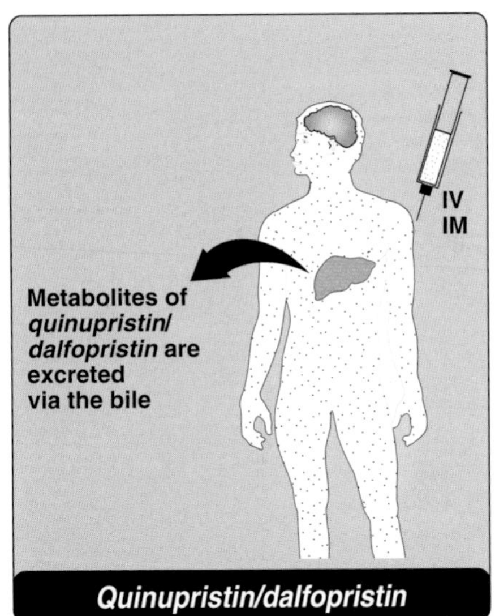

Figure 32.21
Administration and fate of *quinupristin/dalfopristin.*

B. Resistance

Enzymatic processes commonly account for resistance to these agents. For example, the presence of a ribosomal enzyme that methylates the target bacterial 23S ribosomal RNA site can interfere in *quinupristin* binding. In some cases, the enzymatic modification can change the action from bactericidal to bacteriostatic. Plasmid-associated acetyl transferase inactivates *dalfopristin.* An active efflux pump can also decrease levels of the antibiotics in bacteria.

C. Antibacterial spectrum

The combination drug is active primarily against gram-positive cocci, including those resistant to other antibiotics (for example, *methicillin*-resistant staphylococci). Its primary use is in the treatment of Enterococcus faecium infections, including VRE strains. [Note: In the latter case, the effect is bacteriostatic rather than cidal.] The drug is not effective against Enterococcus faecalis.

D. Pharmacokinetics

Quinupristin/dalfopristin are injected intravenously in a five percent dextrose solution (the drug is incompatible with a saline medium). The combination drug penetrates macrophages and polymorphonucleocytes, a property that is important, because VRE are intracellular. Levels in the CSF are low. In animal models, the lung, gallbladder, and bile levels of the drug exceed those in the blood. Both compounds undergo metabolism. The products are less active than the parent in the case of *quinupristin* and are equally active in the case of *dalfopristin.* Most of the parent drugs and metabolites are cleared through the liver and eliminated via the bile into the feces (Figure 32.21). Urinary excretion is secondary.

E. Adverse effects

1. **Venous irritation:** This commonly occurs when *quinupristin/dalfopristin* are administered through a peripheral rather than a central line.

2. **Arthralgia and myalgia:** These have been reported when higher levels of the drugs are employed.

3. **Hyperbilirubinemia:** Total bilirubin is elevated in about 25 percent of patients, resulting from a competition with the antibiotic for excretion.

4. **Interactions:** Because of the ability of *quinupristin/dalfopristin* to inhibit the cytochrome P450 (CYP3A4) isozyme, concomitant administration with drugs that are metabolized by this pathway may lead to toxicities (Figure 32.22). A drug interaction with *digoxin* appears to occur by the same mechanism as that caused by *erythromycin.*

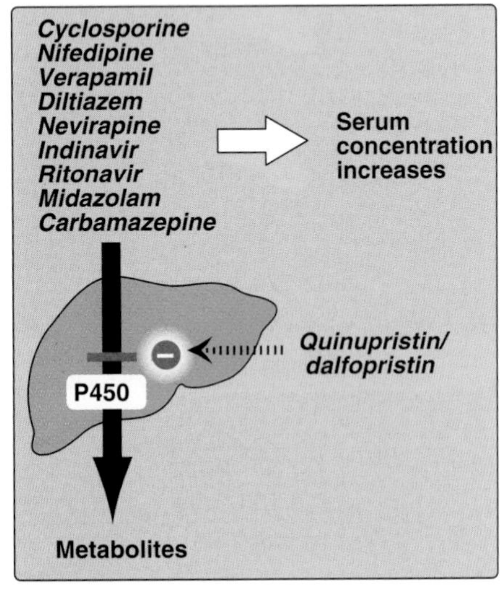

Figure 32.22
Inhibition of cytochrome P450 system by*quinupristin/dalfopristin.*

VIII. LINEZOLID

Linezolid was introduced recently to combat resistant gram-positive organisms, such as *methicillin*- and *vancomycin*-resistant Staphylococcus aureus, *vancomycin*-resistant Enterococcus faecium and Enterococcus faecalis, and *penicillin*-resistant streptococci. *Linezolid* is a totally synthetic oxazolidinone.

A. Mechanism of action

The drug inhibits bacterial protein synthesis by inhibiting the formation of the 70S initiation complex. *Linezolid* binds to a site on the 50S subunit near the interface with the 30S subunit (Figure 32.23).

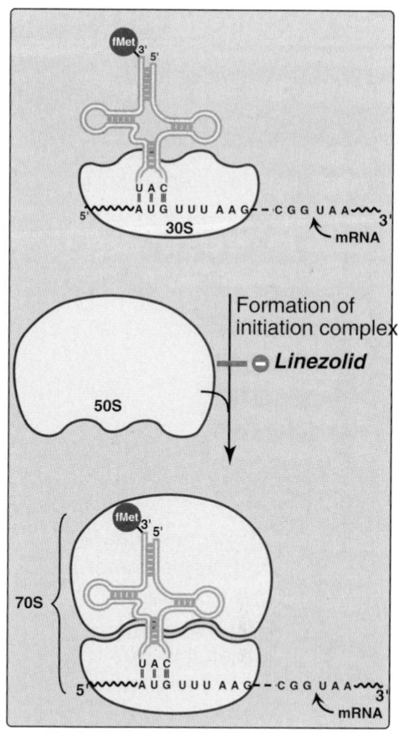

Figure 32.23
Mechanism of action of *linezolid*.

B. Resistance

Decreased binding to the target site confers resistance on the organism. Cross-resistance with other antibiotics does not occur.

C. Antibacterial spectrum

The antibacterial action of *linezolid* is directed primarily against gram-positive organisms, such as staphylococci, streptococci, and enterococci, as well as Corynebacterium species and Listeria monocytogenes (Figure 32.24). It is also moderately active against Mycobacterium tuberculosis. However, its main clinical use is against the resistant organisms mentioned above. Like other agents that interfere with bacterial protein synthesis, *linezolid* is bacteriostatic. However, it is cidal against the streptococci and Clostridium perfringens.

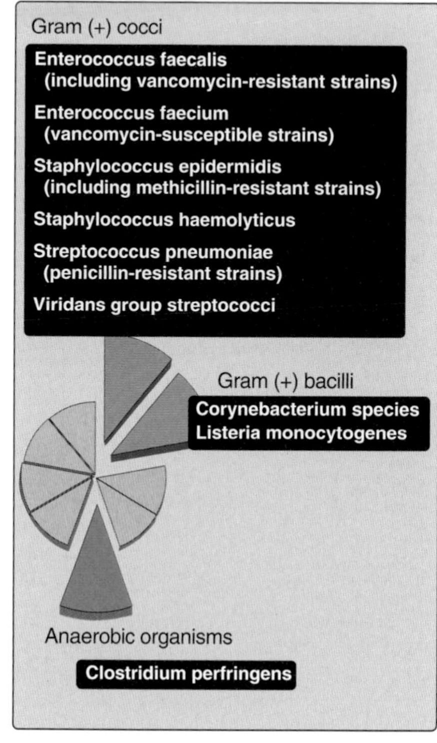

Figure 32.24
Antimicrobial spectrum of *linezolid*.

D. Pharmacokinetics

Linezolid is completely absorbed on oral administration. An intravenous preparation is also available. The drug is widely distributed throughout the body, having a volume of distribution of forty to fifty liters. Two metabolites that are oxidation products have been identified, one of which has antimicrobial activity. However, cytochrome P450 enzymes are not involved in their formation. The drug is excreted both by renal and nonrenal routes. The metabolites rely on the kidney for elimination

E. Adverse effects

Linezolid is well-tolerated, with some reports of gastrointestinal upset, nausea, and diarrhea, as well as headaches and rash. Thrombocytopenia was found to occur in about two percent of patients who were on the drug for longer than two weeks. The condition was reversible when the drug was suspended. Although no reports have appeared that *linezolid* inhibits monoamine oxidase activity, patients are cautioned not to consume large quantities of tyramine-containing foods. Early oxazolidinones had been shown to inhibit monoamine oxidase activity. Reversible enhancement of the pressor effects of *pseudoephedrine* or *phenylpropanolamine* was shown to occur. Further studies are required to establish whether interactions with dopaminergic or serotonergic agents occur.

Study Questions

Choose the ONE best answer.

32.1 A patient with a gunshot wound to the abdomen, which has resulted in spillage of intestinal contents, is brought to the emergency room. Which antibiotic would you select to effectively treat an infection due to Bacteroides fragilis?

A. Aztreonam
B. Clindamycin
C. Gentamicin
D. Azithromycin
E. Doxycycline

Correct answer = B. B. fragilis is an anaerobic organism. The only drug on the list that is effective against it is clindamycin.

32.2 A pregnant woman was hospitalized and catheterized with a Foley catheter. She developed a urinary tract infection caused by Pseudomonas aeruginosa, and was treated with gentamicin. Which of the following adverse effects was a risk to the fetus when the woman was on gentamicin?

A. Skeletal deformity
B. Hearing loss
C. Teratogenesis
D. Blindness
E. Mental retardation

Correct answer = B. Gentamicin can cross the placental barrier and cause hearing loss in the newborns of mothers who have received it.

32.3 Children younger than eight years of age should not receive tetracyclines, because these agents:

A. cause rupture of tendons.
B. do not cross into the cerebrospinal fluid.
C. are not bactericidal.
D. deposit in tissues undergoing calcification.
E. can cause aplastic anemia.

Correct answer = D. It is true that tetracyclines are not bactericidal, but the reason they are contraindicated in this age group is that they are deposited in tissues undergoing calcification, such as teeth and bone, and therefore can stunt growth. Ciprofloxacin can interfere in cartilage formation and cause rupture of tendons, and it is also contraindicated in children. Tetracyclines can cross into the CSF but do not cause aplastic anemia—a property usually associated with chloramphenicol.

32.4 A 46-year-old woman is in the intensive care unit for treatment of a vancomycin-resistant strain of Enterococcus faecium-caused bacteremia. You want to limit the risk of drug interactions in this woman who is receiving five other medications. Which one of the following antibiotics would you choose?

A. Azithromycin
B. Clindamycin
C. Doxycycline
D. Linezolid
E. Quinupristin/dalfopristin

Correct answer = D. Azithromycin, clindamycin and doxycycline do not have significant activity against this organism. Both linezolid and quinupristin/dalfopristin have activity against vancomycin-resistant Enterococcus faecium, but the latter antibiotic is a potent inhibitor of CYP3A4 isozymes. Linezolid is not an inhibitor of cytochrome P450 isozymes. Therefore it would be less likely to have interactions with other drugs.

Quinolones, Folic Acid Antagonists, and Urinary Tract Antiseptics

33

I. FLUOROQUINOLONES

Introduction of the first fluorinated quinolone, *norfloxacin*, was rapidly followed by development of other members of this group, such as *ciprofloxacin*, which has had wide clinical application. Newer fluorinated quinolones offer greater potency, a broader spectrum of antimicrobial activity, greater in vitro efficacy against resistant organisms, and in some cases, a better safety profile than older quinolones and other antibiotics. Compared to *ciprofloxacin*, the new compounds are more highly active against gram-positive organisms, yet retain favorable activity against gram-negative microorganisms. It seems likely that the number of drugs in this class of antibiotics will increase due to its wide antibacterial spectrum, favorable pharmacokinetic properties, and relative lack of adverse reactions. Unfortunately, their overuse has already led to the emergence of resistant strains, resulting in limitations to their clinical usefulness. The fluoroquinolones and other antibiotics discussed in this chapter are listed in Figure 33.1.

A. Mechanism of action

The fluoroquinolones enter the bacterium by passive diffusion through water-filled protein channels (porins) in the outer membrane. Once inside the cell, they inhibit the replication of bacterial DNA by interfering with the action of DNA gyrase (topoisomerase II) and topoisomerase IV during bacterial growth and reproduction. [Note: Topoisomerases are enzymes that change the configuration or topology of DNA by a nicking, pass-through, and re-sealing mechanism. They do not change the DNA's primary sequence[1] (Figure 33.2).] Binding of the quinolone to both the enzyme and the DNA forms a ternary complex that inhibits the resealing step, and

QUINOLONES, FOLATE ANTAGONISTS, AND URINARY TRACT ANTISEPTICS

FLUOROQUINOLONES

FIRST GENERATION
- ***Nalidixic acid***

SECOND GENERATION
- ***Ciprofloxacin***
- ***Norfloxacin***
- ***Ofloxacin***

THIRD GENERATION
- ***Gatifloxacin***
- ***Levofloxacin***
- ***Moxifloxacin***
- ***Sparfloxacin***

FOURTH GENERATION
- ***Trovafloxacin***

INHIBITORS OF FOLATE SYNTHESIS
- ***Mafenide***
- ***Silver sulfadiazine***
- ***Succinylsulfathiazole***
- ***Sulfacetamide***
- ***Sulfadiazine***
- ***Sulfamethoxazole***
- ***Sulfasalazine***
- ***Sulfisoxazole***

Figure 33.1
Summary of drugs described in this chapter. (The figure continues on the next page.)

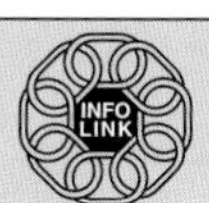

[1]See p. 398 in ***Lippincott's Illustrated Reviews: Biochemistry*** (3rd ed.) for a discussion of topoisomerase activity.

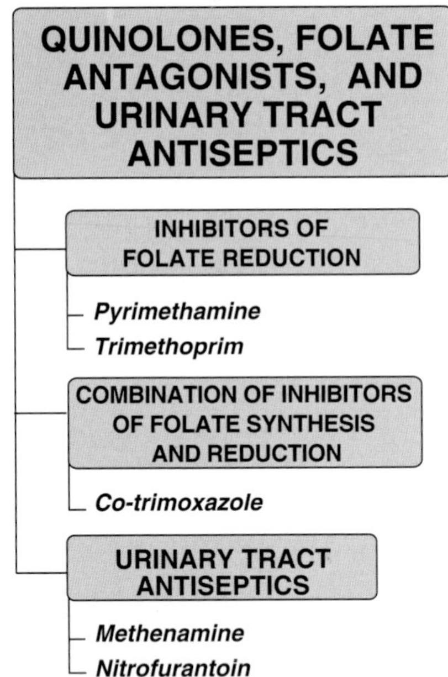

Figure 33.1 (continued)
Summary of drugs described in this chapter.

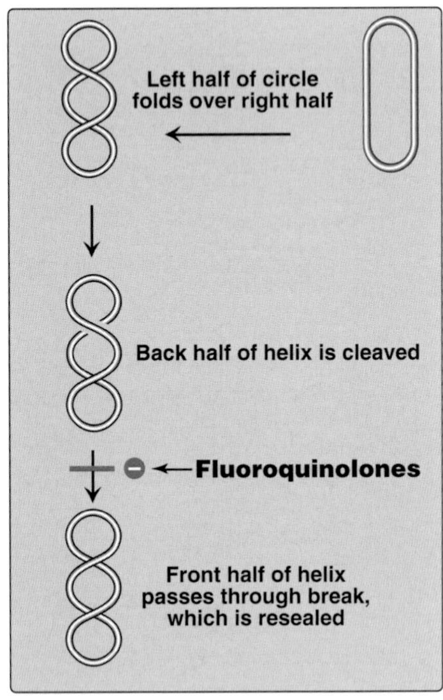

Figure 33.2
Action of type II DNA topoisomerase.

can cause cell death by inducing cleavage of the DNA. Because DNA gyrase is a bacteriospecific target for antimicrobial therapy, cross-resistance with other, more commonly used antimicrobial drugs is rare, but this is increasing in the case of multidrug-resistant organisms. The second site blocked by the fluoroquinolones—topoisomerase IV—is required by bacteria for cell division. It has been implicated in the process of segregating newly replicated DNA. In gram-negative organisms (for example, Escherichia coli), the inhibition of DNA gyrase is more significant than that of topoisomerase IV, whereas in gram-positive organisms (for example, the staphylococci), the opposite is true.

B. Antimicrobial spectrum

All the fluoroquinolones are bactericidal. Like aminoglycosides, the quinolones exhibit concentration-dependent bacterial killing. Bactericidal activity becomes more pronounced as the serum drug concentration increases to approximately thirty-fold the minimim inhibitory concentration. In general, they are effective against gram-negative organisms such as the Enterobacteriacea, Pseudomonas species, Haemophilus influenzae, Moraxella catarrhalis, Legionellaceae, chlamydia, and mycobacteria (except for Mycobacterium avium intracellulare complex). They are effective in the treatment of gonorrhea but not syphilis. The newer agents (for example, *levofloxacin*, *gatifloxacin*, *sparfloxacin*, *clinafloxacin*, and *moxifloxacin*) also have good activity against some gram-positive organisms, such as Streptococcus pneumoniae. Those with activity against some anaerobes are *sparfloxacin*, *gatifloxacin*, and *moxifloxacin*. If used prophylactically before transurethral surgery, they lower the incidence of postsurgical urinary tract infections (UTIs). It has become common practice to classify the fluoroquinolones into "generations," based on their antimicrobial targets (Figure 33.3). The nonfluorinated quinolone *nalidixic acid* is considered to be first generation, with a narrow spectrum of susceptible organisms usually confined to the urinary tract. *Ciprofloxacin*, *levofloxacin*, and *norfloxacin* are assigned to the second generation because of their activity against systemic aerobic gram-negative infections. In addition, these fluoroquinolones exhibit significant intracellular penetration, allowing therapy for infections in which a bacterium spends part or all of its life cycle inside a host cell (for example, chlamydia, mycoplasma, and legionella). *Sparfloxacin* and *gatifloxacin* are classified as third generation, because of their increased activity against gram-positive bacteria and atypical pathogens. Lastly, the fourth generation currently includes only *trovafloxacin*, which is active against many anaerobic as well as gram-positive organisms. The new fluoroquinolones are rarely appropriate as first-line drugs and should be used judiciously.

C. Examples of clinically useful fluoroquinolones

1. **Ciprofloxacin:** This is the most frequently used fluoroquinolone in the United States (Figure 33.4). The serum levels of *ciprofloxacin* [sip row FLOX a sin] that are achieved are effective against many systemic infections, with the exception of serious infections caused by *methicillin*-resistant Staphylococcus aureus (MRSA), the ente-

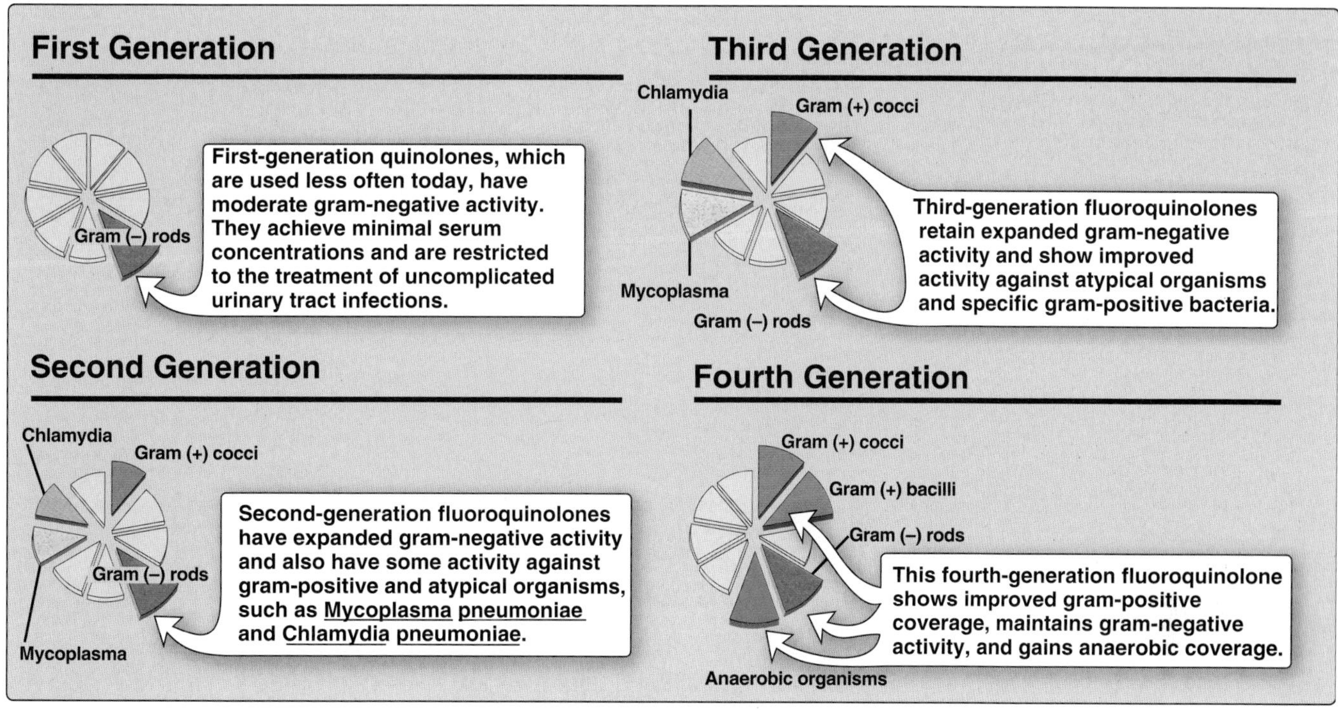

First Generation
First-generation quinolones, which are used less often today, have moderate gram-negative activity. They achieve minimal serum concentrations and are restricted to the treatment of uncomplicated urinary tract infections.
Gram (–) rods
Third Generation
Chlamydia
Gram (+) cocci
Third-generation fluoroquinolones retain expanded gram-negative activity and show improved activity against atypical organisms and specific gram-positive bacteria.
Mycoplasma
Gram (–) rods
Second Generation
Chlamydia
Gram (+) cocci
Second-generation fluoroquinolones have expanded gram-negative activity and also have some activity against gram-positive and atypical organisms, such as Mycoplasma pneumoniae and Chlamydia pneumoniae.
Gram (–) rods
Mycoplasma
Fourth Generation
Gram (+) cocci
Gram (+) bacilli
Gram (–) rods
This fourth-generation fluoroquinolone shows improved gram-positive coverage, maintains gram-negative activity, and gains anaerobic coverage.
Anaerobic organisms

Figure 33.3
Summary of antimicrobial spectrum of quinolones. [Note: The antimicrobial spectrum of specific agents may differ from the generalizations shown in this figure.]

rococci, and pneumococci. *Ciprofloxacin* is also particularly useful in treating infections caused by many Enterobacteriaceae and other gram-negative bacilli. For example, traveler's diarrhea caused by E. coli can be effectively treated. *Ciprofloxacin* is also the drug of choice for prophylaxis and treatment of anthrax. It is the most potent of the fluoroquinolones for Pseudomonas aeruginosa infections and, therefore, is used in the treatment of pseudomonal infections associated with cystic fibrosis. The drug is also used as an alternative to more toxic drugs, such as the aminoglycosides. It may act synergistically with β-lactams, and is also of benefit in treating resistant tuberculosis.

2. **Norfloxacin:** *Norfloxacin* (nor FLOX a sin] is effective against both gram-negative (including P. aeruginosa) and gram-positive organisms in treating complicated and uncomplicated UTIs and prostatitis. It is not effective in systemic infections.

3. **Levofloxacin:** *Levofloxacin* [leave oh FLOX a sin] is an isomer of *ofloxacin* [oh FLOX a sin], and has largely replaced it clinically. It is primarily used in the treatment of prostatitis due to E. coli and of sexually transmitted diseases, with the exception of syphilis. It may be used as alternative therapy in patients with gonorrhea. It has some benefit in the treatment of skin and lower respiratory tract infections. *Levofloxacin* has excellent activity against respiratory infections due to S. pneumoniae.

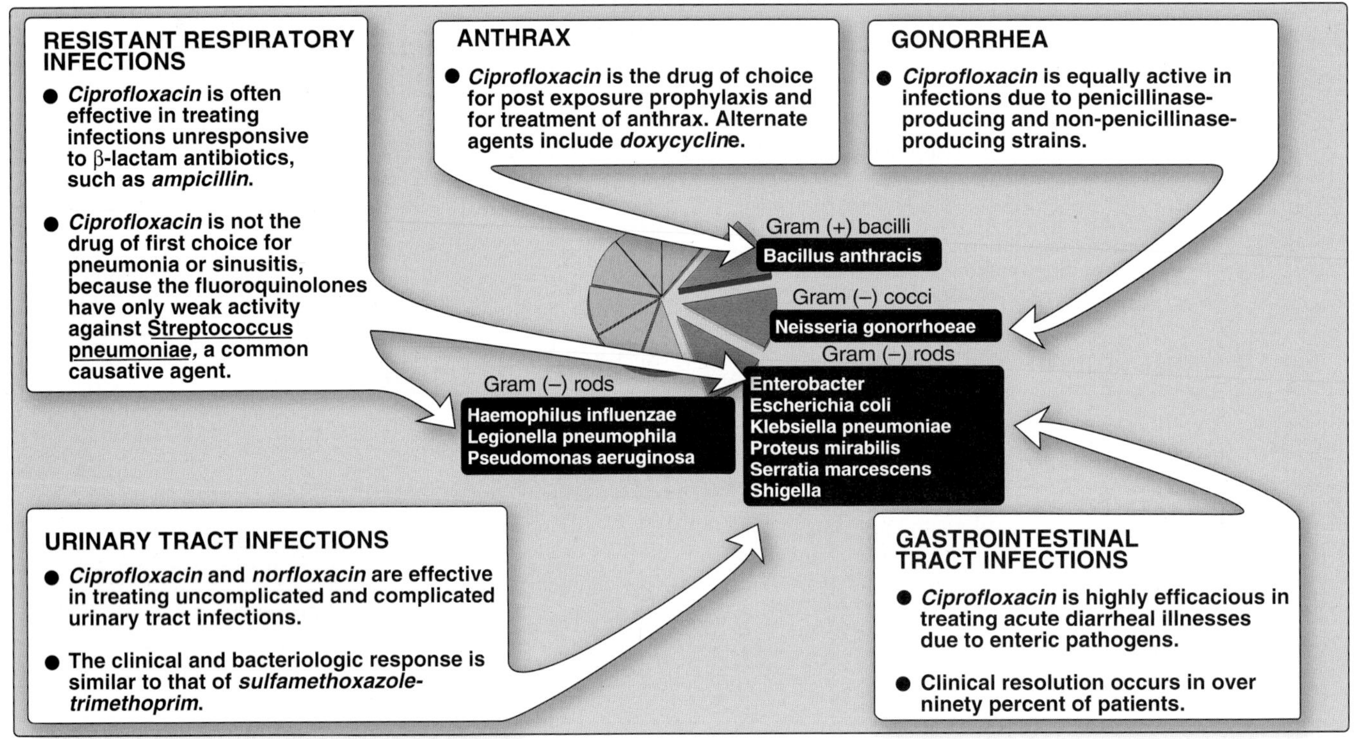

RESISTANT RESPIRATORY INFECTIONS
● *Ciprofloxacin* is often effective in treating infections unresponsive to β-lactam antibiotics, such as *ampicillin*.
● *Ciprofloxacin* is not the drug of first choice for pneumonia or sinusitis, because the fluoroquinolones have only weak activity against Streptococcus pneumoniae, a common causative agent.
ANTHRAX
● *Ciprofloxacin* is the drug of choice for post exposure prophylaxis and for treatment of anthrax. Alternate agents include *doxycycline*.
GONORRHEA
● *Ciprofloxacin* is equally active in infections due to penicillinase-producing and non-penicillinase-producing strains.
Gram (+) bacilli
Bacillus anthracis
Gram (–) cocci
Neisseria gonorrhoeae
Gram (–) rods
Enterobacter
Escherichia coli
Klebsiella pneumoniae
Proteus mirabilis
Serratia marcescens
Shigella
Gram (–) rods
Haemophilus influenzae
Legionella pneumophila
Pseudomonas aeruginosa
URINARY TRACT INFECTIONS
● *Ciprofloxacin* and *norfloxacin* are effective in treating uncomplicated and complicated urinary tract infections.
● The clinical and bacteriologic response is similar to that of *sulfamethoxazole-trimethoprim*.
GASTROINTESTINAL TRACT INFECTIONS
● *Ciprofloxacin* is highly efficacious in treating acute diarrheal illnesses due to enteric pathogens.
● Clinical resolution occurs in over ninety percent of patients.

Figure 33.4
Typical therapeutic applications of *ciprofloxacin*.

4. **Trovafloxacin and moxifloxacin:** These drugs not only have enhanced activity against gram-positive organisms (for example, S. pneumoniae) but also have excellent activity against anerobes (for example, Bacteroides fragilis). Although P. aeruginosa is susceptible to *trovafloxacin* [TRO vah flox a sin], the antibiotic is usually combined with aminoglycosides to treat this organism. *Moxifloxacin* [moxie FLOX a sin] has very poor activity against P. aeruginosa.

5. **Gatifloxacin:** *Gatifloxacin* [gat ee FLOX a sin] has excellent activity against respiratory infections due to S. pneumoniae.

D. Resistance

When the fluoroquinolones were first introduced, there was optimism that resistance would not develop. Although no plasmid-mediated resistance has been reported, resistant MRSA, pseudomonas, coagulase-negative staphylococci, and enterococci have unfortunately emerged due to chromosomal mutations. Cross-resistance exists among the quinolones. The mechanisms responsible for this resistance include the following.

1. **Altered target:** Mutations in the bacterial DNA gyrase have been associated with a decreased affinity for fluoroquinolones. Topoisomerase IV also undergoes mutations. Resistance is frequently associated with mutations in both gyrase and topoisomerase IV.

2. **Decreased accumulation:** Reduced intracellular concentration of the drugs in the bacterial cell is linked to two mechanisms. One involves a decreased number of porin proteins in the outer membrane of the resistant cell, thereby impairing access of the drugs to the intracellular topoisomerases. The other mechanism is associated with an energy-dependent efflux system in the cell membrane.

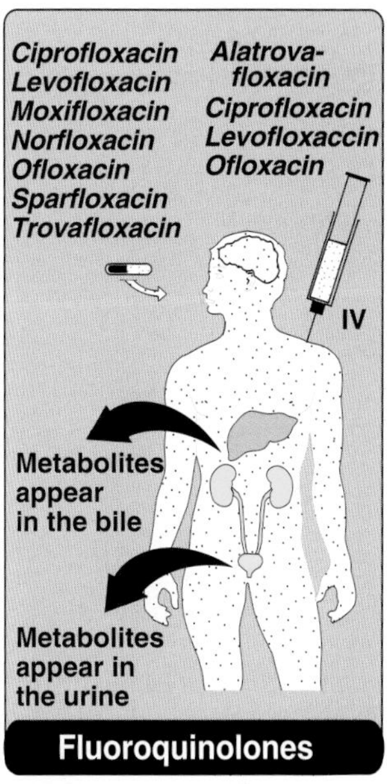

Figure 33.5
Administration and fate of the fluoroquinolones.

E. Pharmacokinetics

1. **Absorption:** Only 35 to 70 percent of orally administered *norfloxacin* is absorbed, compared with 85 to 95 percent of the other fluoroquinolones (Figure 33.5). Intravenous (IV) preparations of *ciprofloxacin*, *levofloxacin*, *gatifloxacin*, and *ofloxacin* are available. [Note: *Trovafloxacin* is available only as an IV preparation.] Ingestion of the fluoroquinolones with *sucralfate*, antacids containing aluminum or magnesium, or dietary supplements containing iron or zinc can interfere with the absorption of these antibacterial drugs. Calcium and other divalent cations have also been shown to interfere with the absorption of these agents (Figure 33.6). The fluoroquinolones with the longest half-lives (that is, *levofloxacin*, *moxifloxacin*, *sparfloxacin*, and *trovafloxacin*) permit once-daily dosing.

2. **Fate:** Binding to plasma proteins ranges from ten to forty percent. [Note: Achieved plasma levels of free *norfloxacin* are insufficient for treatment of systemic infections.] All the fluoroquinolones distribute well into all tissues and body fluids. Levels are high in bone, urine, kidney, and prostatic tissue (but not prostatic fluid), and concentrations in the lung exceed those in serum. Penetration into cerebrospinal fluid is low except for *ofloxacin*, for which concentrations can be as high as ninety percent of those in the serum. The fluoroquinolones also accumulate in macrophages and polymorphonuclear leukocytes, thus being effective against intracellular organisms such as Legionella pneumophila. They are excreted by the renal route.

F. Adverse reactions

In general, these agents are very well tolerated. Toxicities similar to those for *nalidixic acid* have been reported for the fluoroquinolones (Figure 33.7).

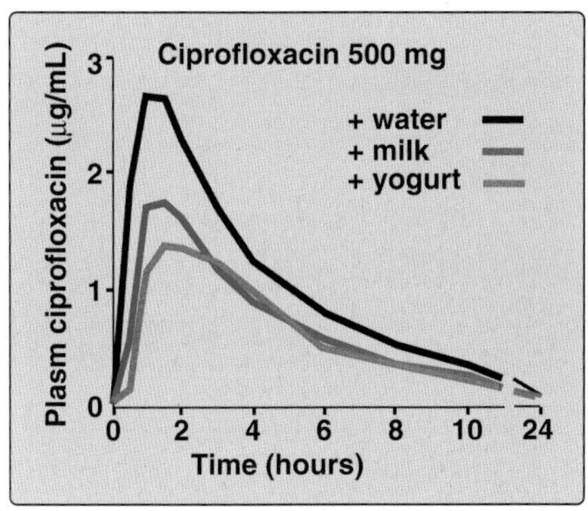

Figure 33.6
Effect of dietary calcium on the absorption of *ciprofloxaxin*.

1. **Gastrointestinal:** The most common adverse effects of the fluoroquinolones are nausea, vomiting, and diarrhea, which occur in three to six percent of patients.

2. **Central nervous system problems:** The most prominent central nervous system (CNS) effects of fluoroquinolone treatment are headache and dizziness or light-headedness. Thus, patients with CNS disorders, such as epilepsy, should be treated cautiously with these drugs. [Note: *Ciprofloxacin* interferes in the metabolism of *theophylline* and may evoke seizures.]

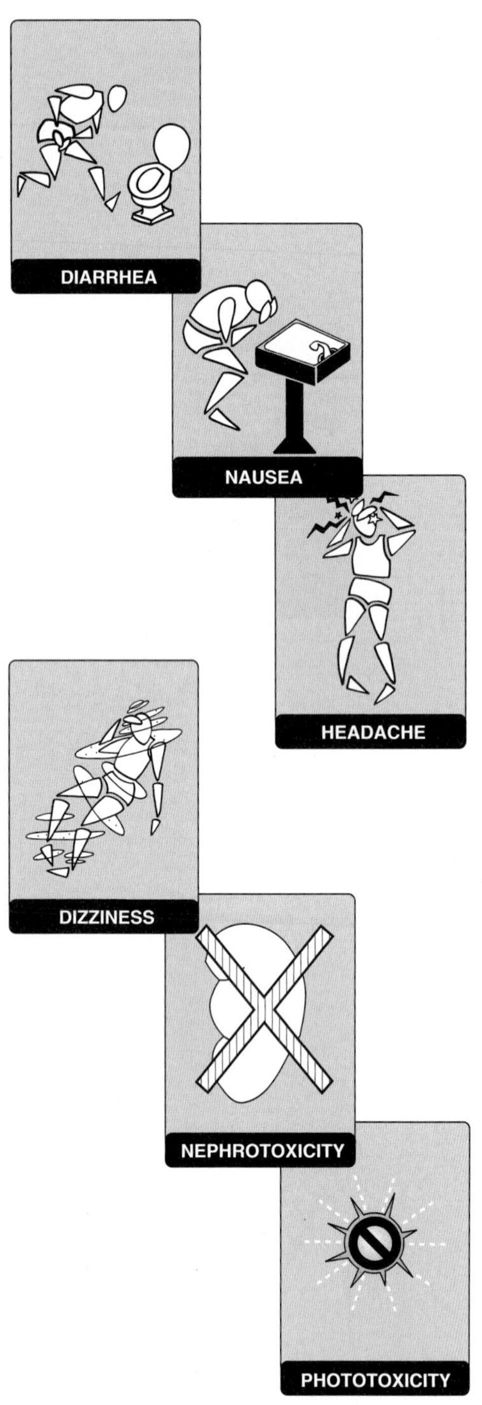

Figure 33.7
Some adverse reactions to fluoroquinolones.

3. **Phototoxicity:** Patients taking fluoroquinolones are advised to avoid excessive sunlight and to apply sunscreens. However, the latter may not protect completely. Thus, it is advisable that the drug should be discontinued at the first sign of phototoxicity.

4. **Liver toxicity:** *Trovafloxacin* is associated with serious liver injury, and therefore use of the drug is restricted to infections that are life-threatening (for example, pneumonia, intra-abdominal infections, or gynecologic and pelvic infections that do not respond to other antibiotics). Therapy with *trovafloxacin* should not continue for longer than fourteen days, and should only be used in hospitals and long-term nursing care facilities.

5. **Connective tissue problems:** Fluoroquinolones should be avoided in pregnancy, in nursing mothers, and in children under eighteen years of age, because articular cartilage erosion (arthropathy) occurs in immature experimental animals. [Note: Children with cystic fibrosis who receive *ciprofloxacin* have had few problems, but careful monitoring is indicated.] In adults, fluoroquinolones can infrequently cause ruptured tendons.

6. **Contraindications:** *Sparfloxacin* and *moxifloxacin* prolong the QT interval and, thus, should not be used in patients who are predisposed to arrhythmias or are taking antiarrhythmic medications.

7. **Drug interactions:** The effect of antacids and cations on the absorption of these agents was considered above. *Ciprofloxacin* and *ofloxacin* can increase the serum levels of *theophylline* by inhibiting its metabolism (Figure 33.8). This is not the case with the third- and fourth-generation fluoroquinolones, which may raise the serum levels of *warfarin*, *caffeine*, and *cyclosporine*. *Cimetidine* interferes with elimination of the fluoroquinolones.

II. OVERVIEW OF THE FOLIC ACID ANTAGONISTS

Coenzymes containing folic acid are required for the synthesis of purines and pyrimidines[2] (precursors of RNA and DNA) and other compounds necessary for cellular growth and replication. Therefore, in the absence of folic acid, cells cannot grow or divide. Humans cannot synthesize folic acid and, thus, must obtain preformed folate as a vitamin from the diet. In contrast, many bacteria are impermeable to folic acid, and therefore must rely on their ability to synthesize folate de novo. The sulfonamides (sulfa drugs) are a family of antibiotics that inhibit the synthesis of folic acid. A second type of folic acid antagonist—*trimethoprim*—prevents the conversion of folic acid to its active, coenzyme form (tetrahydrofolic acid). Thus, both compounds interfere with the ability of an infecting bacterium to divide. Compounding the sulfonamide *sulfamethoxazole* with *trimethoprim* (the generic name for the combination is *co-trimoxazole*) provides a synergistic combination that is used as effective treatment of a variety of bacterial infections.

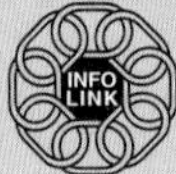

[2]See p. 299 in ***Lippincott's Illustrated Reviews: Biochemistry*** (3rd ed.) for a discussion of pyrimidine synthesis.

III. SULFONAMIDES

The sulfa drugs are seldom used when prescribed alone except in developing countries, where they are still employed because of their low cost and their efficacy in certain bacterial infections, such as trachoma and those of the urinary tract. However, when *co-trimoxazole* was introduced in the mid-1970s, there was a renewed interest in the sulfonamides. Sulfa drugs differ from each other not only in their chemical and physical properties but also in their pharmacokinetics.

A. Mechanism of action

Folic acid is synthesized from *p*-aminobenzoic acid (PABA), pteridine, and glutamate (Figure 33.9). All the sulfonamides currently in clinical use are synthetic analogs of PABA.[3] Because of their structural similarity to PABA, the sulfonamides compete with this substrate for the bacterial enzyme, dihydropteroate synthetase. They thus inhibit the synthesis of bacterial folic acid and, thereby, the formation of its essential cofactor forms.[4] The sulfa drugs, including *co-trimoxazole*, are bacteriostatic.

B. Antibacterial spectrum

Sulfa drugs are active against selected enterobacteria in the urinary tract and nocardia. In addition, *sulfadiazine* [sul fa DYE a zeen], in combination with the dihydrofolate reductase inhibitor *pyrimethamine* [py ri METH a meen], is the preferred form of treatment for toxoplasmosis and chloroquine-resistant malaria.

C. Resistance

Only organisms that synthesize their own folic acid are sensitive to the sulfonamides. Thus, humans are not affected, and bacteria that

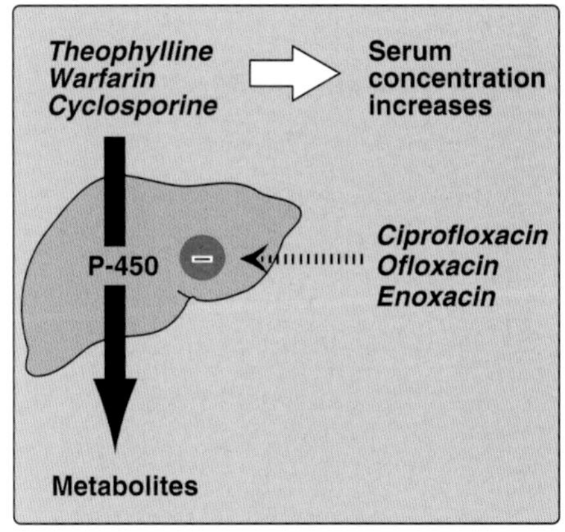

Figure 33.8
Drug interactions with fluoroquinolones.

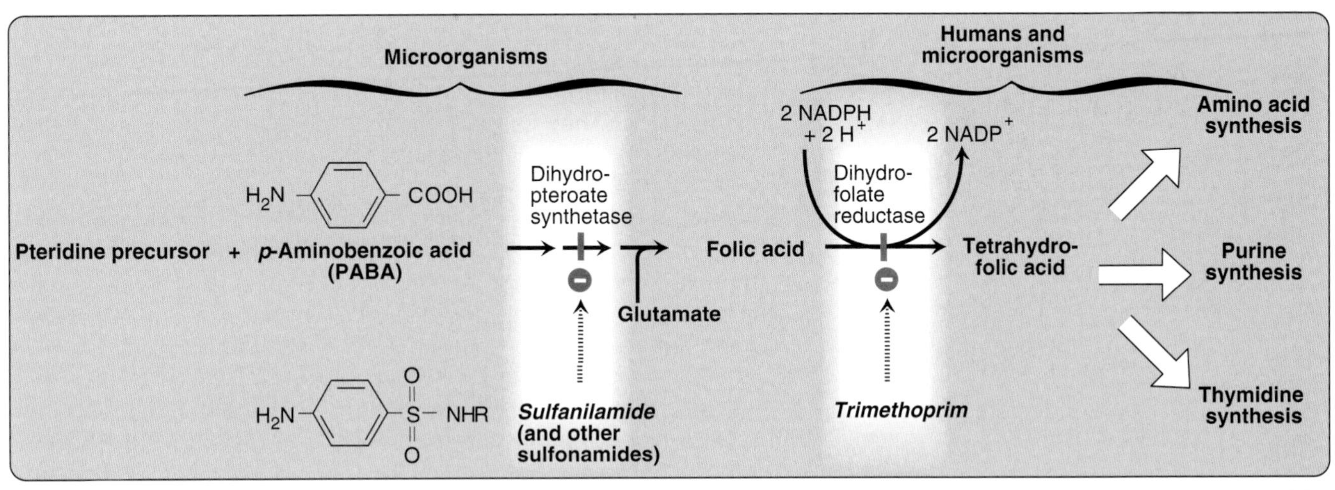

Figure 33.9
Inhibition of tetrahydrofolate synthesis by sulfonamides and *trimethoprim*.

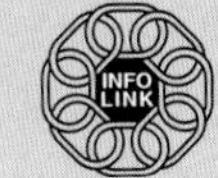

[3,4]See p. 272 in ***Lippincott's Illustrated Reviews: Biochemistry*** (3rd ed.) for a discussion of the synthesis and cofactor forms of folic acid.

do not synthesize folic acid are naturally resistant to these drugs. Acquired bacterial resistance to the sulfa drugs can arise from plasmid transfers or random mutations. [Note: Organisms resistant to one member of this drug family are resistant to all.] Resistance is generally irreversible and may be due to 1) an altered dihydropteroate synthetase, 2) decreased cellular permeability to sulfa drugs, or 3) enhanced production of the natural substrate, PABA.

D. Pharmacokinetics

1. **Administration:** After oral administration, most sulfa drugs are well absorbed via the small intestine (Figure 33.10). An exception is *sulfasalazine* [sul fa SAL a zeen]. It is not absorbed when administered orally or as a suppository and, therefore, is reserved for treatment of chronic inflammatory bowel disease (for example, Crohn disease or ulcerative colitis). [Note: Local intestinal flora split *sulfasalazine* into sulfapyridine and 5-aminosalicylate, with the latter exerting the anti-inflammatory effect. Absorption of the sulfapyridine can lead to toxicity in patients who are slow acetylators (see below).] Intravenous sulfonamides are generally reserved for patients who are unable to take oral preparations. Because of the risk of sensitization, sulfas are not usually applied topically. However, in burn units, creams of *silver sulfadiazine* or *mafenide* [mah FEN ide] *acetate* (*α-amino-p-toluene-sulfonamide*) have been effective in reducing burn-associated sepsis, because they prevent colonization of bacteria. Superinfections with resistant bacteria or fungi may still occur. [Note: *Silver sulfadiazine* is preferred, because *mafenide* produces pain on application. Furthermore, *mafenide* can be absorbed in burn patients, causing an increased risk of acid-base imbalance.]

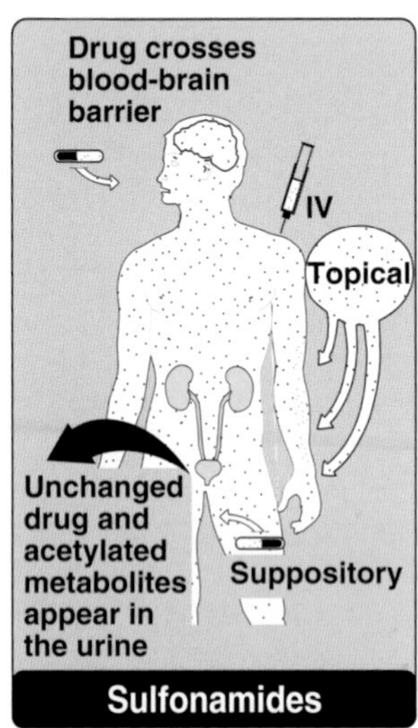

Figure 33.10
Administration and fate of the sulfonamides.

2. **Distribution:** Sulfa drugs are bound to serum albumin in the circulation, where the extent of binding depends on the particular agent's pK_a. In general, the lower the pK_a, the greater the binding.[5] Sulfa drugs distribute throughout the body's water and penetrate well into cerebrospinal fluid—even in the absence of inflammation. They can also pass the placental barrier and enter fetal tissues.

3. **Metabolism:** The sulfa drugs are acetylated, primarily in the liver. The product is devoid of antimicrobial activity but retains the toxic potential to precipitate at neutral or acidic pH. This causes crystalluria ("stone formation", see below) and, therefore, potential damage to the kidney.

4. **Excretion:** Sulfa drugs are eliminated by glomerular filtration. Therefore, depressed kidney function causes accumulation of both the parent compounds and their metabolites. The sulfonamides may also be eliminated in breast milk.

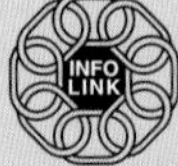

[5] See p. 6 in ***Lippincott's Illustrated Reviews: Biochemistry*** (3rd ed.) for a discussion of pK_a.

E. Adverse effects

1. **Crystalluria:** Nephrotoxicity develops as a result of crystalluria (Figure 33.11). Adequate hydration and alkalinization of urine prevent the problem by reducing the concentration of drug and promoting its ionization. Newer agents, such as *sulfisoxazole* [sul fi SOX a zole] and *sulfamethoxazole* [sul fa meth OX a zole] are more soluble at urinary pH than are the older sulfonamides (for example, *sulfadiazine*), and are less liable to cause crystalluria .

2. **Hypersensitivity:** Hypersensitivity reactions, such as rashes, angioedema, and Stevens-Johnson syndrome, are fairly common. The latter occurs more frequently with the longer-acting agents.

3. **Hemopoietic disturbances:** Hemolytic anemia is encountered in patients with glucose 6-phosphate dehydrogenase deficiency.[6] Granulocytopenia and thrombocytopenia can also occur.

4. **Kernicterus:** This disorder may occur in newborns because sulfa drugs displace bilirubin from binding sites on serum albumin. The bilirubin is then free to pass into the CNS, because the baby's blood-brain barrier is not fully developed (see below).

5. **Drug potentiation:** Transient potentiation of the hypoglycemic effect of *tolbutamide* or the anticoagulant effect of *warfarin* or *bishydroxycoumarin* results from their displacement from binding sites on serum albumin. Free *methotrexate* levels may also rise through displacement.

6. **Contraindications:** Due to the danger of kernicterus, sulfa drugs should be avoided in newborns and infants less than two months of age, as well as for pregnant women at term. Because sulfonamides condense with formaldehyde, they should not be given to patients receiving *methenamine* for UTIs (Figure 33.12).

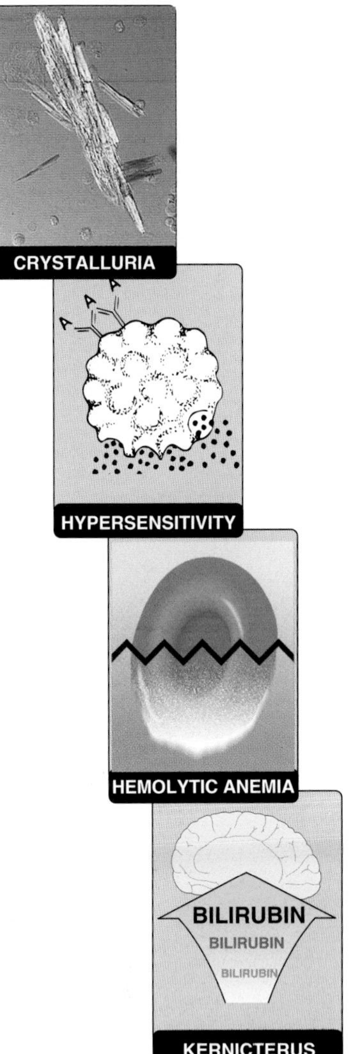

Figure 33.11
Some adverse reactions to sulfonamides.

IV. TRIMETHOPRIM

Trimethoprim [trye METH oh prim], a potent inhibitor of bacterial dihydrofolate reductase, exhibits an antibacterial spectrum similar to that of the sulfonamides. *Trimethoprim* is most often compounded with *sulfamethoxazole*, producing the combination called *co-trimoxazole*.

A. Mechanism of action

The active form of folate is the tetrahydro-derivative that is formed through reduction of dihydrofolate by dihydrofolate reductase.[7] This enzymatic reaction (see Figure 33.9) is inhibited by *trimethoprim*, leading to a decreased availability of the tetrahydrofolate coenzymes required for purine, pyrimidine, and amino acid synthesis.

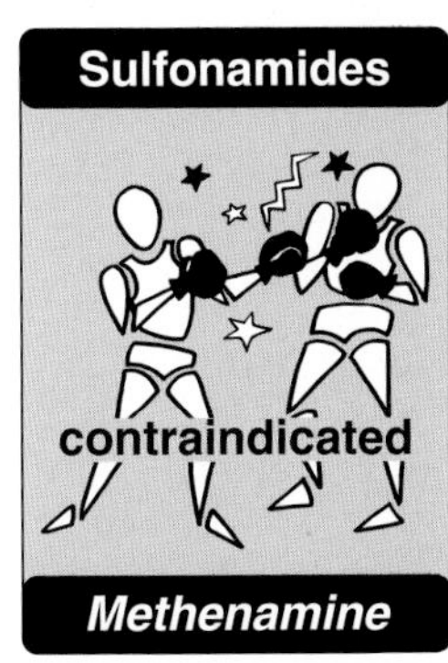

Figure 33.12
Contraindication for sulfonamide treatment.

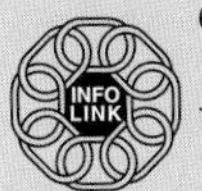

[6]See p. 149 in **Lippincott's Illustrated Reviews: Biochemistry** (3rd ed.) for a discussion of glucose 6-phosphate dehydrogenase deficiency.
[7]See p. 372 in **Lippincott's Illustrated Reviews: Biochemistry** (3rd ed.) for a discussion of the reaction catalyzed by dihydrofolate reductase.

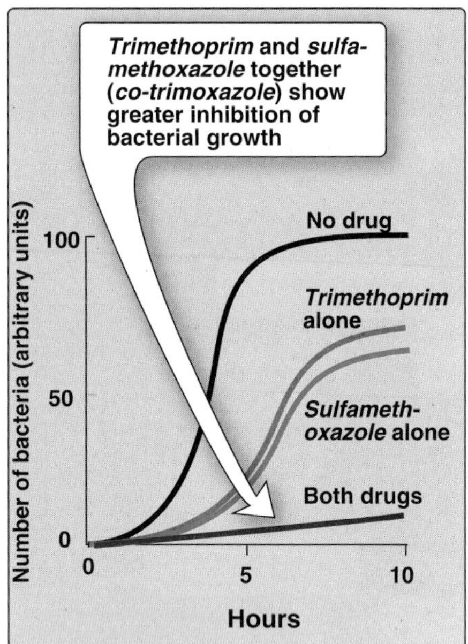

Figure 33.13
Synergism between *trimethoprim* and *sulfamethoxazole* on the inhibition of growth of Escherichia coli.

The bacterial reductase has a much stronger affinity for *trimethoprim* than does the mammalian enzyme, which accounts for the drug's selective toxicity. [Note: Examples of other drugs that function as folate reductase inhibitors include *pyrimethamine*, which is used with sulfonamides in treating parasitic infections, and *methotrexate*, which is used in cancer chemotherapy.]

B. Antibacterial spectrum

The antibacterial spectrum of *trimethoprim* is similar to that of *sulfamethoxazole*. However, *trimethoprim* is twenty- to fifty-fold more potent than the sulfonamide. *Trimethoprim* may be used alone in the treatment of acute UTIs, and in the treatment of bacterial prostatitis (although fluoroquinolones are preferred) and vaginitis (Figure 33.13).

C. Resistance

Resistance in gram-negative bacteria is due to the presence of an altered dihydrofolate reductase that has a lower affinity for *trimethoprim*. Overproduction of the enzyme may also lead to resistance, as this can decrease drug permeability.

D. Pharmacokinetics

The half-life of *trimethoprim* is similar to that of *sulfamethoxazole*. However, because the drug is a weak base, higher concentrations of *trimethoprim* are achieved in the relatively acidic prostatic and vaginal fluids. The drug also penetrates the cerebrospinal fluid. *Trimethoprim* undergoes some O-demethylation, but most of it is excreted unchanged through the kidney.

E. Adverse effects

Trimethoprim can produce the effects of folic acid deficiency.[8] These effects include megaloblastic anemia, leukopenia, and granulocytopenia, especially in pregnant patients and those having very poor diets. These blood disorders can be reversed by the simultaneous administration of *folinic acid*, which does not enter bacteria.

V. CO-TRIMOXAZOLE

The combination of *trimethoprim* with *sulfamethoxazole*, called *co-trimoxazole* [co try MOX a zole], shows greater antimicrobial activity than equivalent quantities of either drug used alone (see Figure 33.13). The combination was selected because of the similarity in the half-lives of the two drugs.

A. Mechanism of action

The synergistic antimicrobial activity of *co-trimoxazole* results from its inhibition of two sequential steps in the synthesis of tetrahydrofolic acid: *sulfamethoxazole* inhibits the incorporation of PABA into folic acid, and *trimethoprim* prevents reduction of dihydrofolate to tetrahydrofolate (see Figure 33.9).

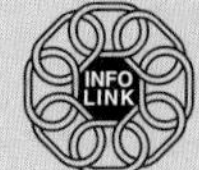

[8]See p. 372 in ***Lippincott's Illustrated Reviews: Biochemistry*** (3rd ed.) for a discussion of folic acid deficiency.

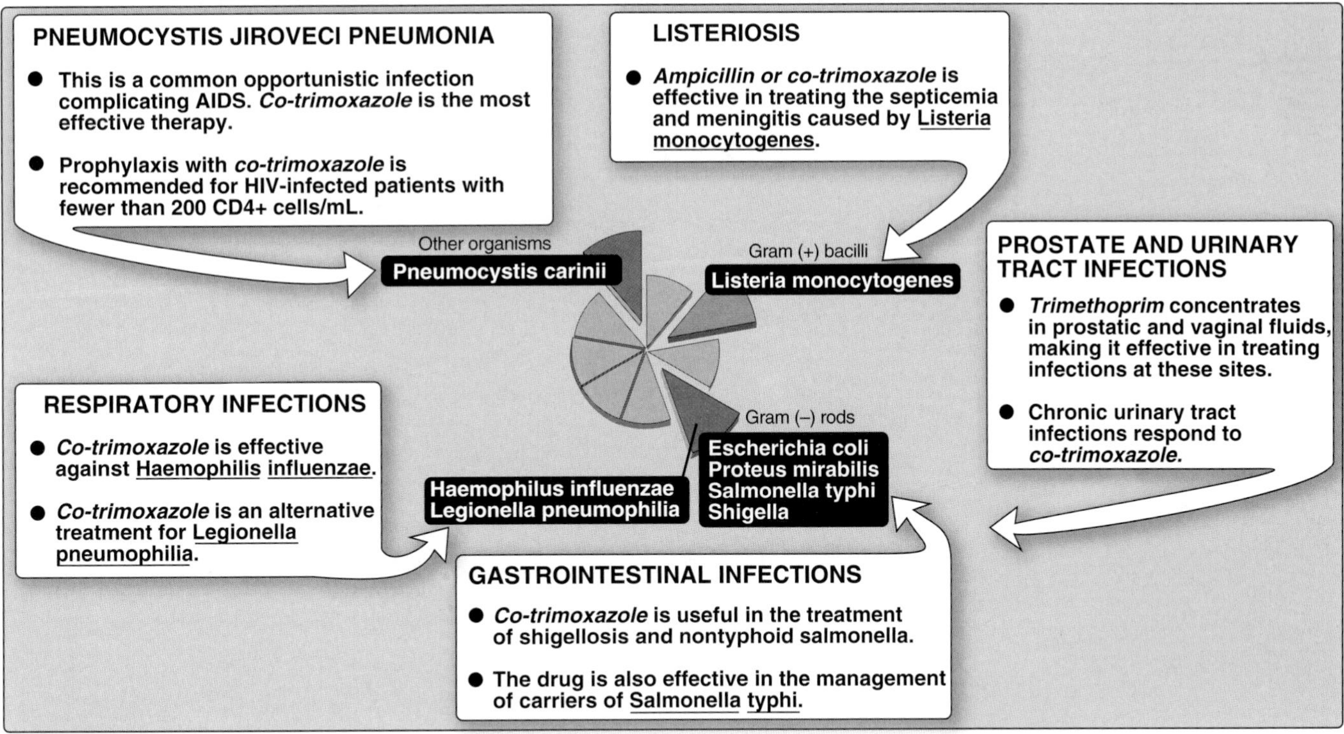

PNEUMOCYSTIS JIROVECI PNEUMONIA
This is a common opportunistic infection complicating AIDS. Co-trimoxazole is the most effective therapy.
Prophylaxis with co-trimoxazole is recommended for HIV-infected patients with fewer than 200 CD4+ cells/mL.
LISTERIOSIS
Ampicillin or co-trimoxazole is effective in treating the septicemia and meningitis caused by Listeria monocytogenes.
Other organisms
Pneumocystis carinii
Gram (+) bacilli
Listeria monocytogenes
PROSTATE AND URINARY TRACT INFECTIONS
Trimethoprim concentrates in prostatic and vaginal fluids, making it effective in treating infections at these sites.
Chronic urinary tract infections respond to co-trimoxazole.
RESPIRATORY INFECTIONS
Co-trimoxazole is effective against Haemophilis influenzae.
Co-trimoxazole is an alternative treatment for Legionella pneumophilia.
Gram (–) rods
Escherichia coli
Proteus mirabilis
Salmonella typhi
Shigella
Haemophilus influenzae
Legionella pneumophilia
GASTROINTESTINAL INFECTIONS
Co-trimoxazole is useful in the treatment of shigellosis and nontyphoid salmonella.
The drug is also effective in the management of carriers of Salmonella typhi.

Figure 33.14
Typical therapeutic applications of *co-trimoxazole* (*sulfamethoxazole* plus *trimethoprim*).

B. Antibacterial spectrum

Co-trimoxazole has a broader spectrum of antibacterial action than the sulfa drugs (Figure 33.14). It is effective in treating UTIs and respiratory tract infections, as well as Pneumocystis jeroveci pneumonia and *ampicillin*- or *chloramphenicol*-resistant systemic salmonella infections.

C. Resistance

Resistance to the *trimethoprim-sulfamethoxazole* combination is less frequently encountered than resistance to either of the drugs alone, because it would require that the bacterium have simultaneous resistance to both drugs.

D. Pharmacokinetics

Trimethoprim is more lipid soluble than *sulfamethoxazole* and has a greater volume of distribution. Administration of one part *trimethoprim* to five parts of the sulfa drug produces a ratio of the drugs in the plasma of twenty parts *sulfamethoxazole* to one part *trimethoprim*. This ratio is optimal for the antibiotic effect. *Co-trimoxazole* is generally administered orally (Figure 33.15). An exception involves intravenous administration to patients with severe pneumonia caused by P. jeroveci or to patients who cannot take the drug by mouth. Both agents distribute throughout the body. *Trimethoprim* concentrates in the relatively acidic milieu of prostatic and vaginal fluids, and accounts for the use of the *trimethoprim-sulfamethoxa-*

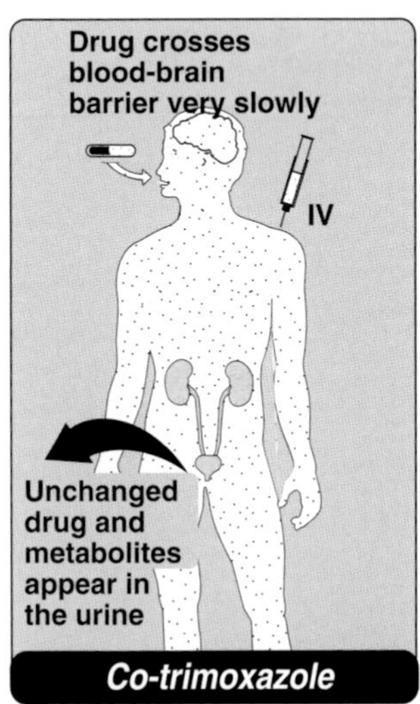

Figure 33.15
Administration and fate of the *co-trimoxazole*.

zole combination in infections at these sites. Both parent drugs and their metabolites are excreted in the urine.

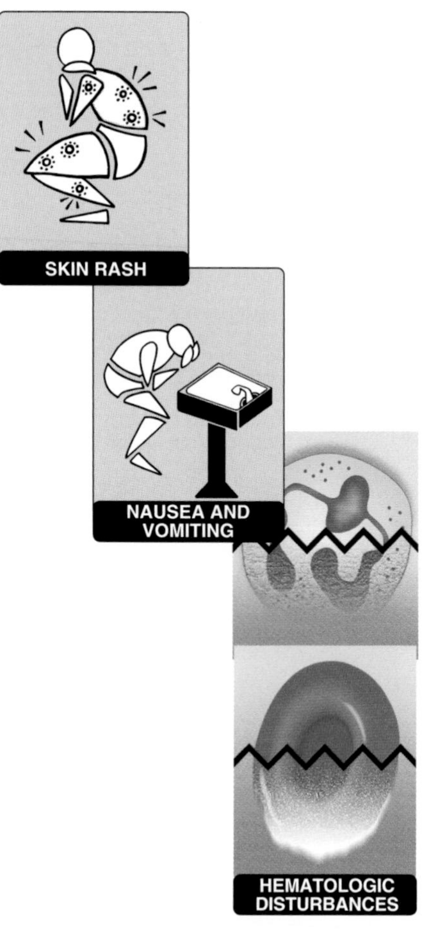

Figure 33.16
Some adverse reactions to *co-trimoxazole*.

E. Adverse effects

1. **Dermatologic:** Reactions involving the skin are very common and may be severe in the elderly (Figure 33.16).

2. **Gastrointestinal:** Nausea, vomiting, as well as glossitis and stomatitis are not unusual.

3. **Hematologic:** Megaloblastic anemia, leukopenia, and thrombocytopenia may occur. All these effects may be reversed by the concurrent administration of *folinic acid*, which protects the patient and does not enter the microorganism. Hemolytic anemia may occur in patients with glucose 6-phosphate dehydrogenase deficiency due to the *sulfamethoxazole*.

4. **HIV patients:** Immunocompromised patients with P. jeroveci pneumonia frequently show drug-induced fever, rashes, diarrhea, and/or pancytopenia.

5. **Drug Interactions:** Prolonged prothrombin times in patients receiving both *trimethoprim* and *warfarin* have been reported. The plasma half-life of *phenytoin* may be increased due to an inhibition of its metabolism. *Methotrexate* levels may rise due to displacement from albumin binding sites by *sulfamethoxazole*.

VI. URINARY TRACT ANTISEPTICS

Urinary tract infections (most commonly uncomplicated acute cystitis and pyleonephritis) in women of child bearing age and in the elderly are one of the most common problems seen by primary care physicians. Escherichia coli is the most common pathogen, causing about eighty percent of uncomplicated upper and lower UTIs. Staphylococcus saprophyticus is the second most common bacterial pathogen causing UTIs, with other common causes including Klebsiella pneumoniae and Proteus mirabilis. These infections may be treated with any one of a group of agents called urinary tract antiseptics, including *methenamine*, *nitrofurantoin*, and the quinolone *naladixic acid*. These drugs do not achieve antibacterial levels in the circulation, but because they are concentrated in the urine, microorganisms at that site can be effectively eradicated.

A. Methenamine

1. **Mechanism of action:** To act, *methenamine* [meth EN a meen] must decompose at an acidic pH of 5.5 or less in the urine, thus producing formaldehyde, which is toxic to most bacteria (Figure 33.17). The reaction is slow, requiring three hours to reach ninety percent decomposition. *Methenamine* should not be used in patients with indwelling catheters. Bacteria do not develop resistance to formaldehyde. [Note: *Methenamine* is frequently formulated with a weak acid, such as mandelic acid, which lowers the pH of the urine, thus aiding decomposition of the drug.]

2. **Antibacterial spectrum:** *Methenamine* is primarily used for chronic suppressive therapy. Urea-splitting bacteria that alkalinize the urine, such as *Proteus* species, are usually resistant to the action of *methenamine*. *Methenamine* is used to treat lower UTIs but is not effective in upper UTIs.

3. **Pharmacokinetics:** *Methenamine* is administered orally. In addition to formaldehyde, ammonium ion is produced in the bladder. Because the liver rapidly metabolizes ammonia to form urea, *methenamine* is contraindicated in patients with hepatic insufficiency, in which elevated levels of circulating ammonium ions would be toxic to the CNS. *Methenamine* is distributed throughout the body fluids, but no decomposition of the drug occurs at pH 7.4. Thus, systemic toxicity does not occur. The drug is eliminated in the urine.

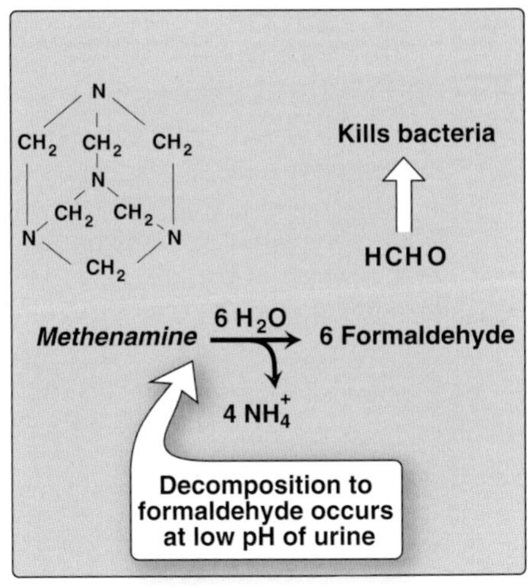

Figure 33.17
Formation of formaldehyde from *methenamine* at acid pH.

4. **Adverse effects:** The major side effect of *methenamine* treatment is gastrointestinal distress, although at higher doses, albuminuria, hematuria, and rashes may develop. *Methenamine mandelate* is contraindicated in patients with renal insufficiency, because mandelic acid may precipitate. [Note: Sulfonamides react with formaldehyde, and must not be used concomitantly with *methenamine* (Figure 33.18).]

B. Nitrofurantoin

Nitrofurantoin [nye troe FYOOR an toyn] is less commonly employed for treating UTIs because of its narrow antimicrobial spectrum and its toxicity. Sensitive bacteria reduce the drug to an active agent that inhibits various enzymes and damages DNA. Antibiotic activity is greater in acidic urine. The drug is bacteriostatic. It is useful against E. coli, but other common urinary tract gram-negative bacteria may be resistant. Gram-positive cocci are susceptible. Adverse effects include gastrointestinal disturbances, acute pneumonitis, and neurologic problems.

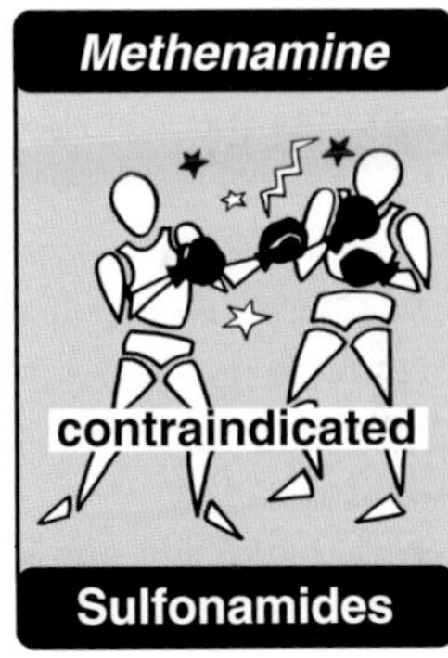

Figure 33 .18
Contraindication for *methenamine* treatment.

Study Questions

Choose the ONE best answer.

33.1 A 30 year old male is diagnosed to be HIV positive. His CD4+ count is 200 cells/cm and his viral load is 10,000 copies/mL. In addition to receiving antiviral therapy, which of the following is indicated to protect him against pneumonia due to Pneumocystis jiroveci?

A. Trimethoprim
B. Ciprofloxacin
C. Co-trimoxazole
D. Clindamycin

Correct answer = C. Prophylaxis with co-trimoxazole is the standard treatment for HIV patients with CD4+ counts at 200 cells/cm or lower. Clindamycin is effective in pneumonia, which has already developed due to this organism, but is not employed for prophylaxis because of its adverse effect on the gastrointestinal tract. Ciprofloxacin lacks activity versus this organism.

33.2 A 26-year-old young man presents with the symptoms of gonorrhea. Because this condition is often associated with an infection due to Chlamydia trachomatis, which of the following quinolones would be the best choice for treating him?

A. Ciprofloxacin
B. Nalidixic acid
C. Norfloxacin
D. Levofloxacin

Correct answer = D. Levofloxacin has the best activity of all the quinolones against both gonorrheal and chlamydial infections. Nalidixic acid is without activity in these conditions.

33.3 In which one of the following infections is ciprofloxacin ineffective?

A. Urinary tract infections due to a β-lactamase-producing strain of klebsiella
B. Pneumonia due to Streptococcus pneumoniae
C. Exacerbation of chronic bronchitis due to Moraxella catarrhalis
D. Urinary tract infection due to Escherichia coli
E. Urinary tract infections due to Pseudomonas aeruginosa

Correct answer = B. Ciprofloxacin does not have sufficient activity against S. pneumoniae to be effective. Because it is not a β-lactam, ciprofloxacin is effective in treating urinary tract infections caused by β-lactamase-producing organisms. Ciprofloxacin is indicated for treatment of the other infections listed.

33.4 Sulfonamides increase the risk of neonatal kernicterus because they

A. diminish the production of plasma albumin.
B. increase the turnover of red blood cells.
C. inhibit the metabolism of bilirubin.
D. compete for bilirubin binding sites on plasma albumin.
E. depress the bone marrow.

Correct answer = D. Increased release of albumin-bound bilirubin increases the plasma concentration of free bilirubin, which can penetrate the central nervous system.

Antimycobacterial Drugs

34

I. OVERVIEW

Mycobacteria are slender, rod-shaped bacteria with lipid-rich cell walls that stain poorly with the Gram stain, but once stained, the walls cannot be easily decolorized by treatment with acidified organic solvents. Hence, they are termed "acid-fast." The most widely encountered mycobacterial infections is tuberculosis—the leading cause worldwide of death from infection. Members of the genus Mycobacterium also cause leprosy as well as several tuberculosis-like human infections. Mycobacterial infections are intracellular and, generally, result in the formation of slow-growing granulomatous lesions that are responsible for major tissue destruction.[1] Five first-line antimicrobial agents are currently recommended for antituberculosis therapy (Figure 34.1). Second-line medications are either less effective, more toxic, or have not been studied as extensively. They are useful in patients who cannot tolerate the first-line drugs or who are infected with myobacteria that are resistant to the first-line agents.

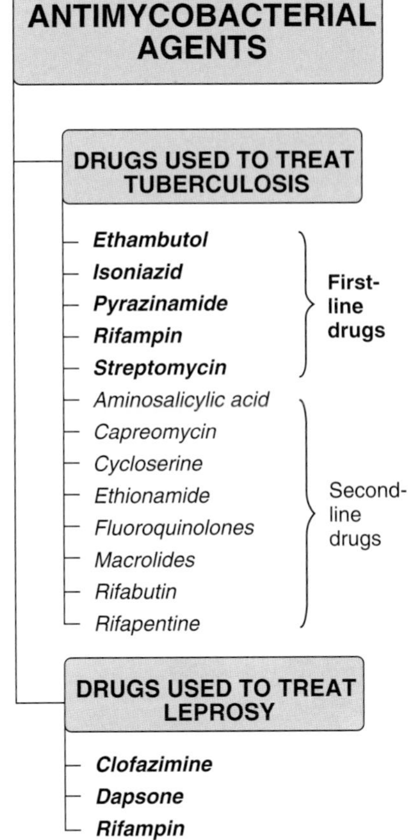

Figure 34.1
Summary of drugs used to treat mycobacterial infections.

II. CHEMOTHERAPY FOR TUBERCULOSIS

Mycobacterium tuberculosis, one of a number of mycobacteria, can lead to serious infections of the lungs, genitourinary tract, skeleton, and meninges. Treating tuberculosis as well as other mycobacterial infections presents therapeutic problems. The organism grows slowly; thus, the disease may have to be treated for six months to two years. Resistant organisms readily emerge, particularly in patients who have had prior therapy or who fail to adhere to the treatment protocol. It is currently estimated that about one-third of the world's population is infected with M. tuberculosis, with thirty million people having active disease. Worldwide, eight million new cases occur, and two million people die of the disease each year.

A. Strategies for addressing drug resistance

Strains of M. tuberculosis that are resistant to a particular agent emerge during treatment with a single drug. For example, Figure 34.2 shows that resistance rapidly develops in patients given only *streptomycin.* Therefore, multidrug therapy is employed when treating tuberculosis in an effort to delay or prevent the emergence of resistant

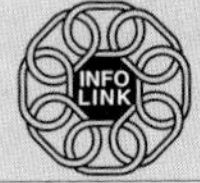

[1]See p. 245 in ***Lippincott's Illustrated Reviews: Microbiology*** for a discussion of mycobacterial infections.

Lippincott's Illustrated Reviews: Pharmacology, Third Edition,
by Richard D. Howland and Mary J. Mycek.

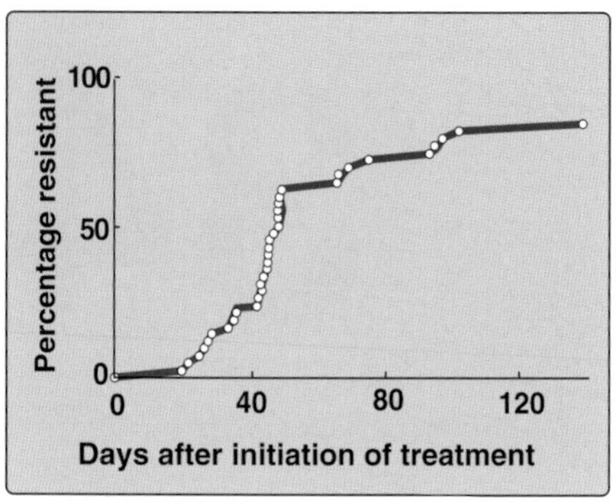

Figure 34.2
Cumulative percentage of strains of Mycobacterium tuberculosis showing resistance to *streptomycin*.

strains. *Isoniazid*, *rifampin*, *ethambutol*, *streptomycin*, and *pyrazinamide* are the principal or so-called "first-line" drugs because of their efficacy and acceptable degree of toxicity. However today, because of poor patient compliance and other factors, the number of multidrug-resistant organisms has risen. Some bacteria have been identified that are resistant to as many as seven antitubercular agents. Therefore, although treatment regimens vary in duration and in the agents employed, they always include a minimum of two drugs, preferably with both being bactericidal (see p. 342). The combination of drugs should prevent the emergence of resistant strains. The multidrug regimen is continued well beyond the disappearance of clinical disease to eradicate any persistent organisms. For example, the short-course chemotherapy for tuberculosis includes *isoniazid*, *rifampin*, and *pyrazinamide* for two months and then *isoniazid* and *rifampin* for the next four months (the "continuation phase," Figure 34.3). *Ethambutol* or *streptomycin* may also be added to this regimen. Patient compliance is often low when multidrug schedules last for six months or longer. One successful strategy for achieving better treatment completion rates is "directly observed therapy," in which patients take their medication while being supervised and observed.

B. Isoniazid

Isoniazid [eye soe NYE a zid], the hydrazide of isonicotinic acid, is a synthetic analog of pyridoxine. It is the most potent of the antitubercular drugs, but is never given as a single agent in the treatment of active tuberculosis. Its introduction revolutionized the treatment of tuberculosis.

1. **Mechanism of action:** *Isoniazid*, often referred to as *INH*, is a prodrug that is activated by a mycobacterial catalase-peroxidase (KatG). Genetic and biochemical evidence has implicated at least two different target enzymes for *isoniazid* within the unique Type II fatty acid synthase system involved in the production of mycolic acids. [Note: Mycolic acid is a unique class of very-long-chain, β-hydroxylated fatty acid found in mycobacterial cell walls. Decreased mycolic acid synthesis corresponds with the loss of acid-fastness after exposure to *isoniazid*.] The targeted enzymes are enoyl acyl carrier protein reductase (InhA) and a β-ketoacyl-ACP synthase (KasA). The activated drug covalently binds to and inhibits these enzymes, which are essential for the synthesis of mycolic acid.

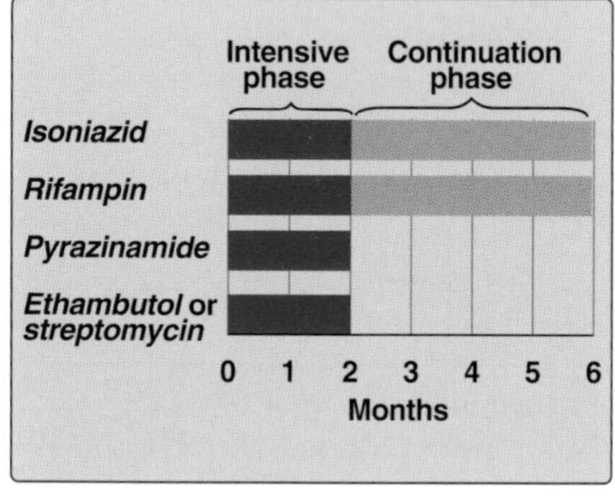

Figure 34.3
One of several recommended multidrug schedules for the treatment of tuberculosis.

2. **Antibacterial spectrum:** For bacilli in the stationary phase, *isoniazid* is bacteriostatic, but for rapidly dividing organisms, it is bactericidal. It is effective against intracellular bacteria. *Isoniazid* is specific for treatment of M. tuberculosis, although Mycobacterium kansasii (an organism that causes three percent of the clinical illness known as tuberculosis) may be susceptible at higher drug levels. When it is used alone, resistant organisms rapidly emerge.

3. **Resistance:** This is associated with several different chromosomal mutations, each of which results in one of the following: mutation or deletion of KatG (producing mutants incapable of prodrug activation), varying mutations of the acyl carrier proteins, or overexpression of InhA. Cross-resistance does not occur between *isoniazid* and other antitubercular drugs.

4. **Pharmacokinetics:** Orally administered *isoniazid* is readily absorbed. Absorption is impaired if *isoniazid* is taken with food, particularly carbohydrates, or with aluminum-containing antacids. The drug diffuses into all body fluids, cells, and caseous material (necrotic tissue resembling cheese that is produced in tubercles). Drug levels in the cerebrospinal fluid (CSF) are about the same as those in the serum. The drug readily penetrates host cells and is effective against bacilli growing intracellularly. Infected tissue tends to retain the drug longer. *Isoniazid* undergoes N-acetylation and hydrolysis, resulting in inactive products. [Note: Acetylation is genetically regulated, with the fast acetylator trait being autosomally dominant. A bimodal distribution of fast and slow acetylators exists (Figure 34.4).] Chronic liver disease decreases metabolism, and doses must be reduced. Excretion is through glomerular filtration, predominantly as metabolites (Figure 34.5). Slow acetylators excrete more of the parent compound. Severely depressed renal function results in accumulation of the drug, primarily in slow acetylators.

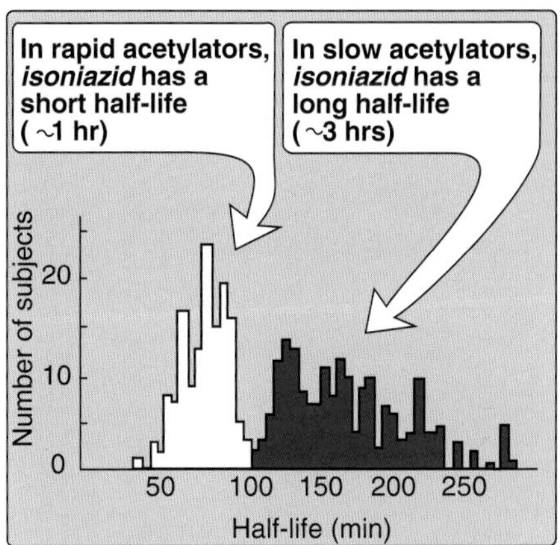

Figure 34 .4
Bimodal distribution of *isoniazid* half-lives caused by rapid and slow acetylation of the drug.

5. **Adverse effects:** The incidence of adverse effects is fairly low. Except for hypersensitivity, adverse effects are related to the dosage and duration of administration.

   a. **Peripheral neuritis:** Peripheral neuritis (manifest as paresthesia), which is the most common adverse effect, appears to be due to a relative pyridoxine deficiency. Most of the toxic reactions are corrected by pyridoxine (vitamin B_6) supplementation. [Note: *Isoniazid* can achieve levels in breast milk that are high enough to cause a pyridoxine deficiency in the infant unless the mother is supplemented with the vitamin.[2]]

   b. **Hepatitis and idiosyncratic hepatotoxicity:** Potentially fatal hepatitis is the most severe side effect associated with *isoniazid*. It has been suggested that this is caused by a toxic metabolite of monoacetylhydrazine, formed during the metabolism of *isoniazid*. Its incidence increases among patients with increasing age, among patients who also take *rifampin*, or among those who drink alcohol daily.

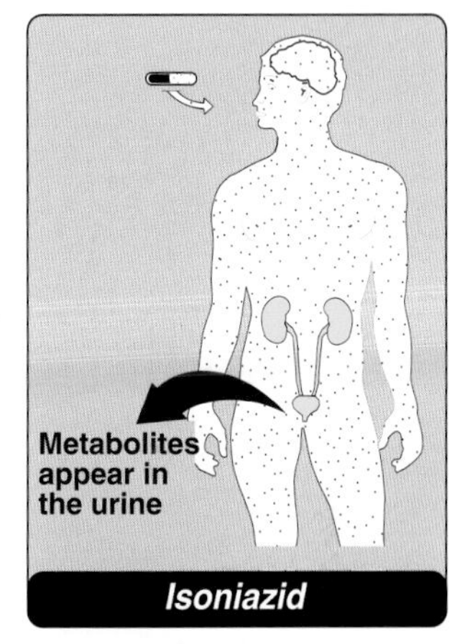

Figure 34.5
Administration and fate of *isoniazid*.

   c. **Drug interactions:** Because *isoniazid* inhibits metabolism of *phenytoin* (Figure 34.6), *isoniazid* can potentiate the adverse effects of that drug (for example, nystagmus and ataxia). Slow acetylators are particularly at risk .

   d. **Other adverse effects:** Mental abnormalities, convulsions in patients prone to seizures, and optic neuritis have been observed. Hypersensitivity reactions include rashes and fever.

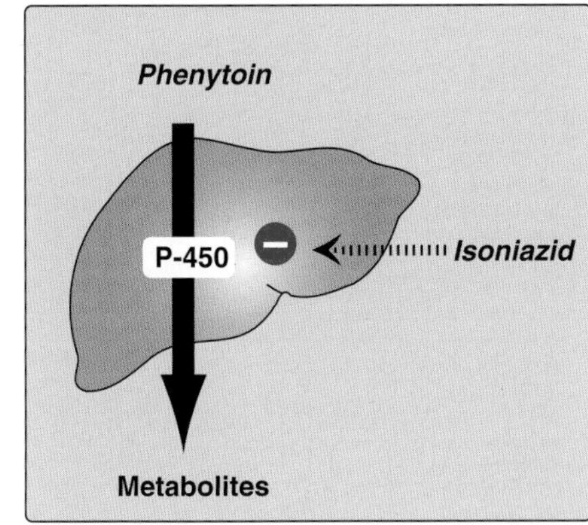

Figure 34.6
Isoniazid potentiates the adverse effects of *phenytoin*.

C. Rifampin

Rifampin [rif AM pin], which is derived from the soil mold Streptomyces, has a broader antimicrobial activity than *isoniazid,* and has found application in the treatment of a number of different bacterial infections. Because resistant strains rapidly emerge during therapy, it is never given as a single agent in the treatment of active tuberculosis.

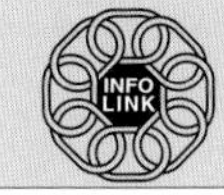

[2]See p. 376 in ***Lippincott's Illustrated Reviews: Biochemistry*** (3rd ed.) for a discussion of pyridoxine.

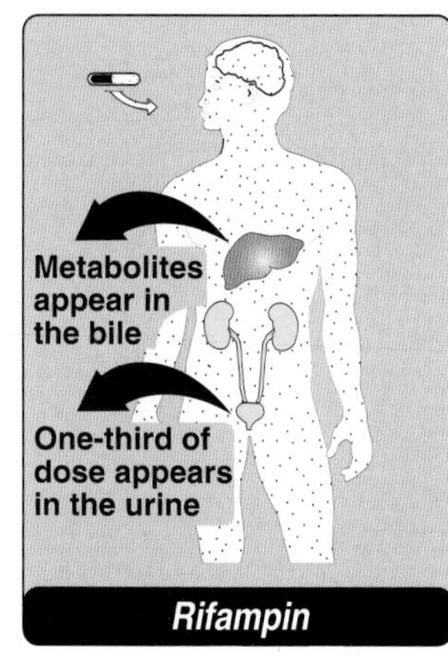

Figure 34.7
Administration and fate of *rifampin*. [Note: Patient should be warned that urine and tears may be orange-red in color.]

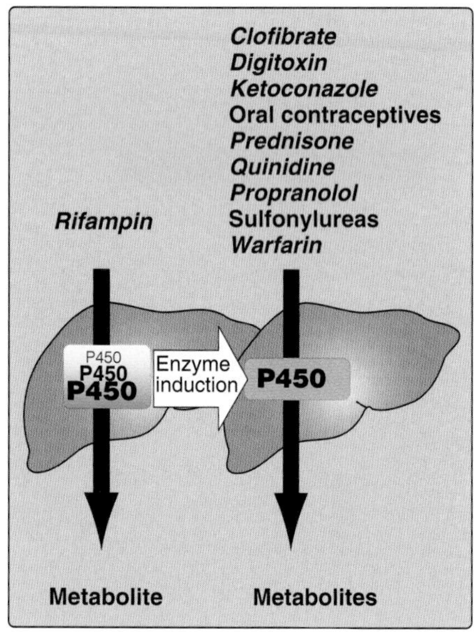

Figure 34.8
Rifampin induces cytochrome P450, which can decrease the half-lives of coadministered drugs that are metabolized by this system.

1. **Mechanism of action:** *Rifampin* blocks transcription by interacting with the β subunit of bacterial but not human DNA-dependent RNA polymerase.[3] [Note: The drug is thus specific for prokaryotes.] *Rifampin* inhibits RNA synthesis by suppressing the initiation step.

2. **Antimicrobial spectrum:** *Rifampin* is bactericidal for both intracellular and extracellular mycobacteria, including M. tuberculosis, and atypical mycobacteria, such as M. kansasii. It is effective against many gram-positive and gram-negative organisms, and is frequently used prophylactically for individuals exposed to meningitis caused by meningococci or Haemophilus influenzae. *Rifampin* is the most active antileprosy drug at present, but to delay the emergence of resistant strains, it is usually given in combination with other drugs. *Rifabutin*, an analog of *rifampin*, has some activity against Mycobacterium avium-intracellulare complex but is less active against tuberculosis.

3. **Resistance:** Resistance to *rifampin* can be caused by a mutation in the affinity of the bacterial DNA-dependent RNA polymerase for the drug or by decreased permeability.

4. **Pharmacokinetics:** Absorption is adequate after oral administration. Distribution of *rifampin* occurs to all body fluids and organs. Adequate levels are attained in the CSF even in the absence of inflammation. The drug is taken up by the liver and undergoes enterohepatic cycling. *Rifampin* itself can induce the hepatic mixed-function oxidases (see p. 14), leading to a shortened half-life. Elimination of metabolites and the parent drug is via the bile into the feces or via the urine (Figure 34.7). [Note: Urine and feces as well as other secretions have an orange-red color; patients should be forewarned. Tears may permanently stain soft contact lenses orange-red.]

5. **Adverse effects:** These are a minor problem with *rifampin* but can include nausea and vomiting, rash, and fever. The drug should be used judiciously in patients with hepatic failure because of the jaundice that occurs in patients with chronic liver disease, alcoholics, and the elderly.

6. **Drug interactions:** Because *rifampin* can induce a number of cytochrome P450 enzymes (see p. 14), it can decrease the half-lives of other drugs that are coadministered and metabolized by this system (Figure 34.8). This may lead to higher dosage requirements for these agents. [Note: Substitution of *rifabutin* for *rifampin* should be considered for HIV-infected individuals being treated with protease inhibitors or non-nucleoside reverse transcriptase inhibitors, because *rifabutin* does not increase the metabolism of these drugs.]

D. Pyrazinamide

Pyrazinamide [peer a ZIN a mide] is a synthetic, orally effective, bactericidal, antitubercular agent used in combination with *isoniazid* and *rifampin*. It is bactericidal to actively dividing organisms, but the mech-

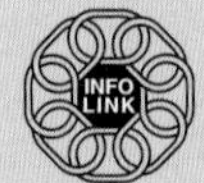

[3]See p. 414 in ***Lippincott's Illustrated Reviews: Biochemistry*** (3rd ed.) for a discussion of the role of DNA-dependent RNA polymerase.

anism of its action is unknown. *Pyrazinamide* must be enzymatically hydrolyzed to pyrazinoic acid, which is the active form of the drug. Some resistant strains lack the pyrazinamidase. *Pyrazinamide* is active against tubercle bacilli in the acidic environment of lysosomes as well as in macrophages. *Pyrazinamide* distributes throughout the body, penetrating the CSF. It undergoes extensive metabolism. About one to five percent of patients taking *isoniazid*, *rifampin*, and *pyrazinamide* may experience liver dysfunction. Urate retention can also occur and may precipitate a gouty attack[4] (Figure 34.9).

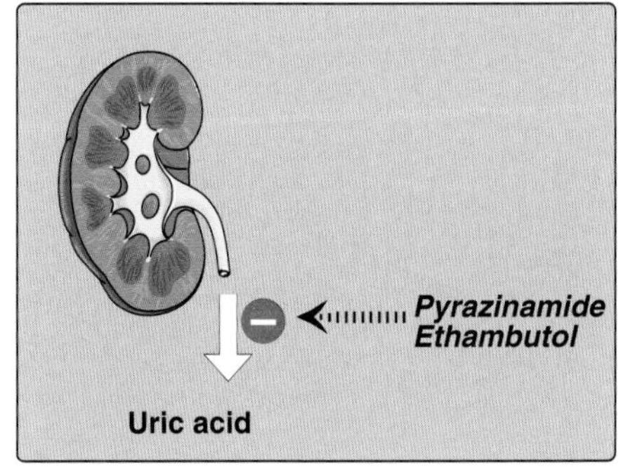

Figure 34.9
Pyrazinamide and *ethambutol* may cause urate retention and gouty attacks.

E. Ethambutol

Ethambutol [e THAM byoo tole] is bacteriostatic and specific for most strains of M. tuberculosis and M. kansasii. *Ethambutol* inhibits arabinosyl transferase—an enzyme that is important for the synthesis of the mycobacterial arabinogalactan cell wall. Resistance is not a serious problem if the drug is employed with other antitubercular agents. *Ethambutol* can be used in combination with *pyrazinamide*, *isoniazid*, and *rifampin* to treat tuberculosis. Absorbed on oral administration, *ethambutol* is well distributed throughout the body. Penetration into the central nervous system (CNS) is therapeutically adequate in tuberculous meningitis. Both parent drug and metabolites are excreted by glomerular filtration and tubular secretion. The most important adverse effect is optic neuritis, which results in diminished visual acuity and loss of ability to discriminate between red and green. Visual acuity should be periodically examined. Discontinuation of the drug results in reversal of the toxic symptoms. In addition, urate excretion is decreased by the drug; thus, gout may be exacerbated (see Figure 34.9). Figure 34.10 summarizes some of the characteristics of first-line drugs. [Note: As with any drug, antitubercular drugs have a therapeutic margin—that is, the difference between the minimum drug concentration required to inhibit the growth of M. tuberculosis and the maximum concentration that can be given without provoking drug toxicity. Figure 34.11 shows hows this therapeutic margin varies for the different first-line drugs.]

DRUG	ADVERSE EFFECTS	COMMENTS
Ethambutol	Optic neuritis with blurred vision, red-green color blindness	Establish baseline visual acuity and color vision; test monthly.
Isoniazid	Hepatic enzyme elevation, hepatitis, peripheral neuropathy	Take baseline hepatic enzyme measurements; repeat if abnormal or patient is at risk or symptomatic. Clinically significant interation with *phenytoin* and antifugal agents (azols).
Pyrazinamide	Nausea, hepatitis, hyperuricemia, rash, joint ache, gout (rare)	Take baseline hepatic enzymes and uric acid measurements; repeat if abnormal or patient is at risk or symptomatic.
Rifampin	Hepatitis, GI upset, rash, flu-like syndrome, significant interaction with several drugs	Take baseline hepatic enzyme measurements and CBC count; repeat if abnormal or patient is at risk or symptomatic. Warn patient that urine and tears may turn red-orange in color.
Streptomycin	Ototoxicity, nephrotoxiciity	Do baseline audiography and renal function tests; avoid or reduce doses in patients older than sixty years.

Figure 34.10
Some characteristics of first-line drugs used in treating tuberculosis. CBC = complete blood count.

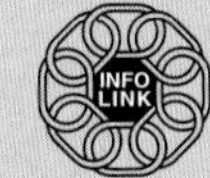

[4]See p. 296 in ***Lippincott's Illustrated Reviews: Biochemistry*** (3rd ed.) for a discussion of uric acid and gout.

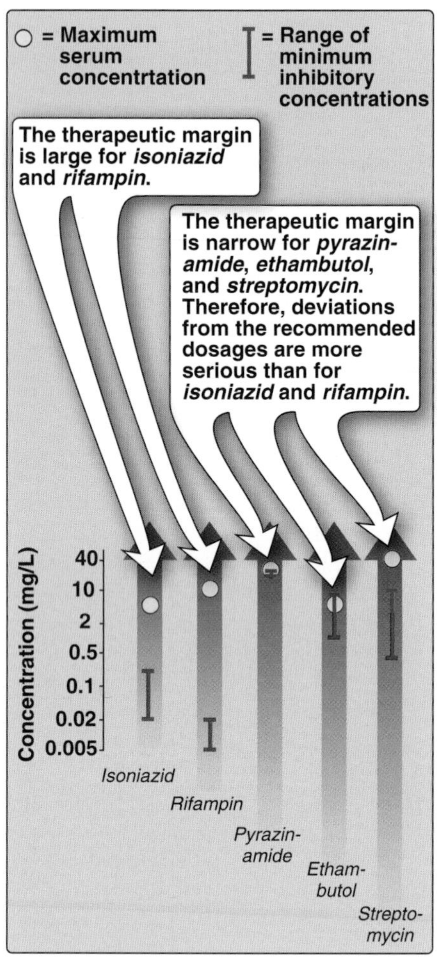

Figure 34.11
The therapeutic margins for different antitubercular drugs.

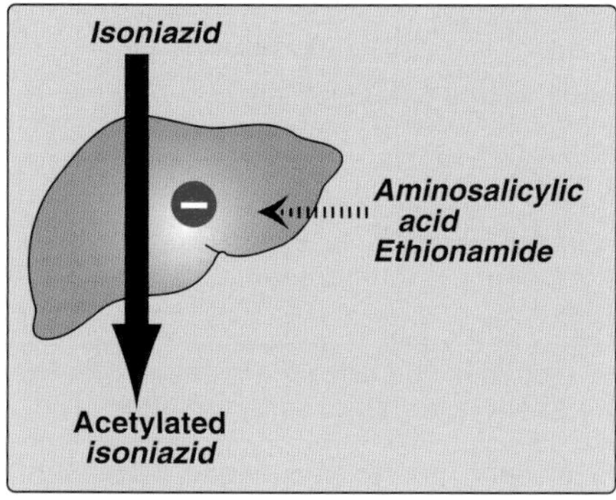

Figure 34.12
Aminosalicylic acid and *ethionamide* can inhibit the acetylation of *isoniazid*.

F. Alternate second-line drugs

A number of drugs—*aminosalicylic acid* [a mee noe sal i SIL ik], *ethionamide* [e thye ON am ide], *cycloserine* [sye kloe SER een], *capreomycin* [kap ree oh MYE sin], fluoroquinolones, and macrolides—are considered to be second-line drugs, either because they are no more effective than the first-line agents and their toxicities are often more serious, or because they are particularly active against atypical strains of mycobacteria. *Streptomycin*, the first antibiotic effective in the treatment of tuberculosis, is discussed with the aminoglycosides (see p. 370). Its action is directed against extracellular organisms. Infections due to *streptomycin*-resistant organisms may be treated with *amikacin*, to which these bacilli remain sensitive.

1. **Aminosalicylic acid** is used infrequently today, because it is poorly tolerated. It is a bacteriostatic agent that acts as a competitive inhibitor for *p*-aminobenzoic acid (PABA) in folate biosynthesis.[5]

2. **Capreomycin** is a peptide that inhibits protein synthesis. It is administered parenterally. *Capreomycin* is primarily reserved for the treatment of multidrug-resistant tuberculosis. Careful monitoring of the patient is necessary to prevent its nephrotoxicity and ototoxicity.

3. **Cycloserine** is an orally effective, tuberculostatic agent that appears to antagonize the steps in bacterial cell wall synthesis involving D-alanine.[6] It distributes well throughout body fluids, including the CSF. Cycloserine is metabolized, and both parent and metabolite are excreted in urine. Accumulation occurs with renal insufficiency. Adverse effects involve CNS disturbances, and epileptic seizure activity may be exacerbated. Peripheral neuropathies are also a problem, but they respond to pyridoxine.

4. **Ethionamide** is a structural analog of *isoniazid*, but it is not believed to act by the same mechanism. *Ethionamide* can inhibit acetylation of *isoniazid* (Figure 34.12). It is effective after oral administration and is widely distributed throughout the body, including the CSF. Metabolism is extensive, and the urine is the main route of excretion. Adverse effects that limit its use include gastric irritation, hepatotoxicity, peripheral neuropathies, and optic neuritis. Supplementation with vitamin B_6 (pyridoxine) may lessen the severity of the neurologic side effects.

5. **Fluoroquinolones** such as *ciprofloxacin* and *levofloxacin,* have an important place in the treatment of multidrug-resistant tuberculosis. Some atypical strains of mycobacteria are also susceptible. These drugs are discussed in detail in Chapter 33 (see p. 381).

6. **Macrolides** such as *azithromycin* and *clarithromycin*, are part of the regimen that includes *ethambutol* and *rifabutin* used for the treatment of infections by M. avium-intracellulare complex. *Azithromycin* is preferred for HIV-infected patients, because it is least likely to interfere with the metabolism of antiretroviral drugs. Details about the pharmacology of macrolides are found in Chapter 32 (see p. 373).

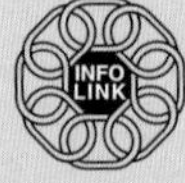

[5]See p. 372 in ***Lippincott's Illustrated Reviews: Biochemistry*** (3rd ed.) for a discussion of the role of *p*-aminobenzoic acid in folate biosynthesis.
[6] See p. 113 in ***Lippincott's Illustrated Reviews: Microbiology***) for a discussion of the role of D-alanine in bacterial cell wall synthesis.

III. CHEMOTHERAPY FOR LEPROSY

Leprosy (or, as it is specified by the United States Public Health Service, Hansen disease), is rare in the United States, but a small number of cases, both imported and domestically acquired, are reported each year. Worldwide, it is a much larger problem (Figure 34.13). Approximately seventy percent of all cases in the world are located in India. Bacilli from skin lesions or nasal discharges of infected patients enter susceptible individuals via abraded skin or the respiratory tract. The World Health Organization recommends the triple-drug regimen of *dapsone*, *clofazimine*, and *rifampin* for 6 to 24 months. Figure 34.14 shows the effects of multidrug therapy.

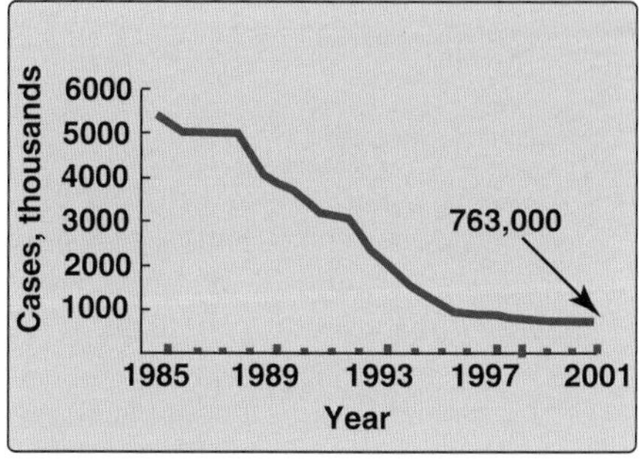

Figure 34.13
Reported prevalence of leprosy worldwide.

A. Dapsone

Dapsone [DAP sone] is structurally related to the sulfonamides. It is bacteriostatic for Mycobacterium leprae, but resistant strains are encountered. *Dapsone* is also employed in the treatment of pneumonia caused by Pneumocystis jiroveci in patients infected with the human immunodeficiency virus. *Dapsone* acts as a PABA antagonist to inhibit folate biosynthesis. The drug is well absorbed from the gastrointestinal tract and is distributed throughout the body, with high levels concentrated in the skin. The parent drug enters the enterohepatic circulation and undergoes hepatic acetylation. Both parent drug and metabolites are eliminated through the urine. Adverse reactions include hemolysis, especially in patients with glucose 6-phosphate dehydrogenase deficiency,[7] as well as methemoglobinemia, peripheral neuropathy, and the possibility of developing erythema nodosum leprosum (a serious and severe skin complication of leprosy). [Note: The latter is treated with corticosteroids or *thalidomide*.]

B. Clofazimine

Clofazimine [kloe FA zi meen] is a phenazine dye that binds to DNA, and prevents it from serving as a template for future DNA replication. Its redox properties may lead to the generation of cytotoxic oxygen radicals that are also toxic to the bacteria. *Clofazimine* is bactericidal to M. leprae and has some activity against M. avium-intracellulare complex. Following oral absorption, the drug accumulates in tissues, allowing for intermittent therapy, but it does not enter the CNS. Patients may develop a red-brown discoloration of the skin. Eosinophilic enteritis has been reported as an adverse effect. The drug also has some antiinflammatory activity; thus, erythema nodosum leprosum does not develop.

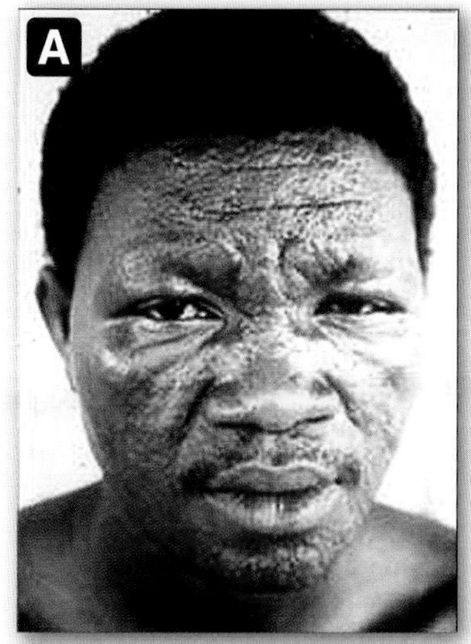

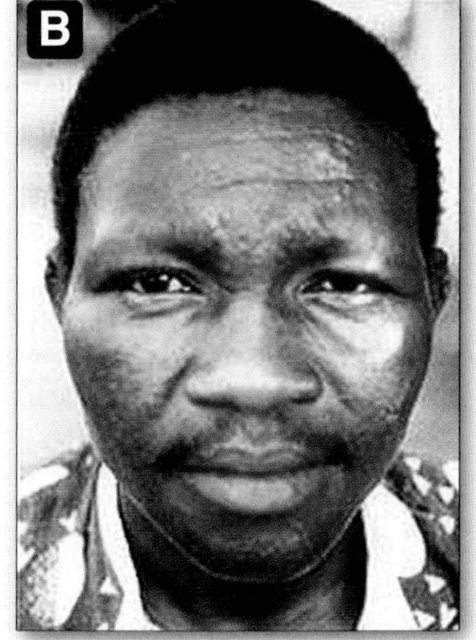

Figure 34.14
Leprosy patient. A. Before therapy. B. After six months of multidrug therapy.

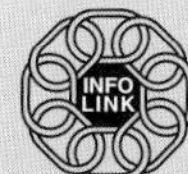

[7]See p. xxx in ***Lippincott's Illustrated Reviews: Biochemistry*** (3rd ed.) for a discussion of glucose-6-phosphate dehydrogenase deficiency.

Study Questions

Choose the ONE best answer.

34.1 A 31-year-old white intravenous drug user was admitted to the hospital with a four-week history of cough and fever. A chest radiograph showed left upper lobe cavitary infiltrate. Cultures of sputum yielded M. tuberculosis susceptible to all antimycobacterial drugs. The patient received isoniazid, rifampin, and pyrazinamide. The patient's sputum remained culture-positive for the subsequent four months. Which one of the following is the most likely cause of treatment failure?

A. False-positive cultures
B. Maladsorption of the medications
C. Concomitant infection with HIV
D. Noncompliance by the patient
E. Drug resistance

Correct answer = D. Although malabsorption of the drugs and the emergence of drug resistance are possibilities, the most common cause of treatment failure is nonadherence to the treatment protocol. Better treatment completion rates occur with "directly observed therapy." False-positive cultures is a possible but an unlikely explanation.

34.2 A forty-year-old man has been on primary therapy for active pulmonary tuberculosis for the past two months. At his regular clinic visit, he complains of a "pins and needles" sensation in his feet. You suspect that he might be deficient in which one of the following vitamins?

A. Ascorbic acid
B. Niacin
C. Pyridoxine
D. Calcitriol
E. Folic acid

Correct answer = C. Primary therapy for active pulmonary tuberculosis includes isoniazid. Isoniazid causes peripheral neuropathies with symptoms including paresthesias such as "pins and needles" and numbness. This relative deficiency of pyridoxine appears to be due to the interference of isoniazid with its activation, and by enhancing the excretion of pyridoxine. Concurrent administration of 10 mg of pyridoxine prevents the neuropathic actions of isoniazid.

34.3 A thirty-five-year-old male, formerly a heroin abuser, has been on methadone maintenance for the last thirteen months. Two weeks ago, he had a positive PPD test, and a chest radiograph showed evidence of right upper lobe infection. He was started on standard antimycobacterial therapy. He has come to the emergency department complaining of "withdrawal symptoms." Which of the following antimycobacterial drugs is likely to have caused this patient's acute withdrawal reaction?

A. Ethambutol
B. Isoniazid
C. Pyrazinamide
D. Rifampin
E. Streptomycin

Correct answer = D. Rifampin is a potent inducer of cytochrome P450-dependent drug metabolizing enzymes. The duration of action of methadone is dependent upon hepatic clearance, so enhanced drug metabolism will shorten the duration and increase the risk of withdrawal symptoms in individuals on methadone maintenance.

Antifungal Drugs

35

I. OVERVIEW

Infectious diseases caused by fungi are called mycoses, and are often chronic in nature.[1] Many common mycotic infections are superficial and only involve the skin (cutaneous mycoses), but fungi may also penetrate the skin, causing subcutaneous infections. The fungal infections that are most difficult to treat are the systemic mycoses, which are often life-threatening. Unlike bacteria, fungi are eukaryotic. They have rigid cell walls composed largely of chitin—a polymer of N-acetylglucosamine—rather than peptidoglycan (a characteristic component of most bacterial cell walls). The fungal cell membrane contains ergosterol rather than the cholesterol found in mammalian membranes. These chemical characteristics are useful in targeting chemotherapeutic agents against fungal infections. Fungal infections are generally resistant to antibiotics used in the treatment of bacterial infections, and conversely, bacteria are resistant to the antifungal agents. The last two decades have seen a rise in the incidence of fungal infections, so that candidemia is the fourth most common cause of septicemia. This increased incidence of fungal infections is associated with greater numbers of individuals who are on chronic immune suppression following organ transplant, undergoing chemotherapy for myelogenous and solid tumors, or infected with the human immunodeficiency virus (HIV). During this same period, there have been significant changes in the therapeutic options available to the clinician. For example, the ongoing development of new azole antifungal drugs offers effective therapy for all but the most serious mycotic infections. Clinically useful antifungal agents are listed in Figure 35.1.

ANTIFUNGAL DRUGS

DRUGS FOR SUBCUTANEOUS AND SYSTEMIC MYCOSES

- ***Amphotericin B***
- ***Caspofungin***
- ***Fluconazole***
- ***Flucytosine***
- ***Itraconazole***
- ***Ketoconazole***
- ***Voriconazole***

DRUGS FOR CUTANEOUS MYCOSES

- ***Butoconazole***
- ***Clotrimazole***
- ***Econazole***
- ***Griseofulvin***
- ***Miconazole***
- ***Nystatin***
- ***Terbinafine***
- ***Terconazole***

Figure 35.1
Summary of antifungal drugs.

II. DRUGS FOR SUBCUTANEOUS AND SYSTEMIC MYCOTIC INFECTIONS

The drugs used in the treatment of subcutaneous and systemic mycoses are listed in Figure 35.1. [Note: Additional azole drugs are effective in the topical treatment of candidiasis or dermatophytic infections.] The echinocandins are a new class of antifungal agents that exert their fungicidal activity by inhibiting 1,3-β-glucan synthesis for the fungal cell wall.

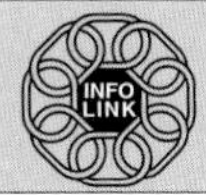

[1]See Chapter 23 in ***Lippincott's Illustrated Reviews: Microbiology*** for a discussion of fungal infections.

Lippincott's Illustrated Reviews: Pharmacology, Third Edition,
by Richard D. Howland and Mary J. Mycek.
Lippincott Williams & Wilkins, Baltimore, MD © 2006.

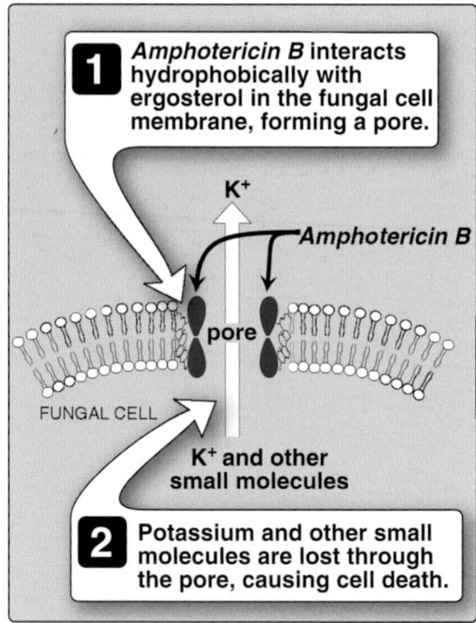

Figure 35.2
Model of a pore formed by *amphotericin B* in the lipid bilayer membrane.

A. Amphotericin B

Amphotericin B [am foe TER i sin] is a naturally occurring, polyene macrolide antibiotic produced by Streptomyces nodosus. In spite of its toxic potential, *amphotericin B* is the drug of choice for the treatment of life-threatening, systemic mycoses. [Note: *Amphotericin B* has undergone several formulation improvements that reduce the incidence of side effects, particularly nephrotoxicity.] The drug is also sometimes used in combination with *flucytosine* so that lower (less toxic) levels of *amphotericin B* are possible.

1. **Mechanism of action:** Several *amphotericin B* molecules bind to ergosterol in the plasma membranes of sensitive fungal cells. There, they form pores (channels) that require hydrophobic interactions between the lipophilic segment of the polyene antibiotic and the sterol (Figure 35.2). The pores disrupt membrane function, allowing electrolytes (particularly potassium) and small molecules to leak from the cell, resulting in cell death. [Note: Because the polyene antibiotics bind preferentially to ergosterol rather than to cholesterol—the sterol found in mammalian membranes—a relative (but not absolute) specificity is conferred.]

2. **Antifungal spectrum:** *Amphotericin B* is either fungicidal or **fungistatic**, depending on the organism and the concentration of the drug. It is effective against a wide range of fungi, including Candida albicans, Histoplasma capsulatum, Cryptococcus neoformans, Coccidioides immitis, Blastomyces dermatitidis, and many strains of aspergillus. [Note: *Amphotericin B* is also used in the treatment of the protozoal infection, leishmaniasis.]

3. **Resistance:** Fungal resistance, although infrequent, is associated with decreased ergosterol content of the fungal membrane.

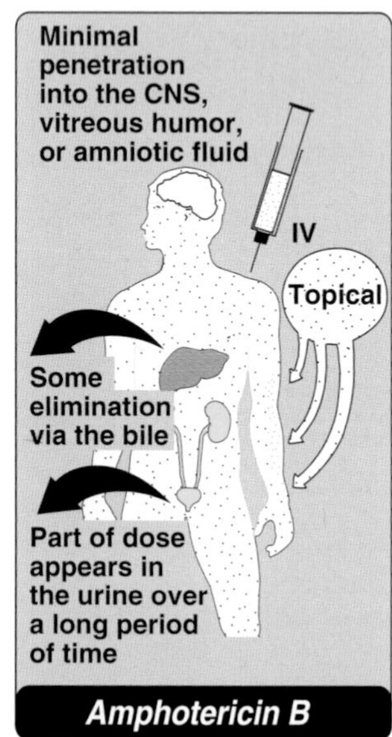

Figure 35.3
Administration and fate of *amphotericin B*.

4. **Pharmacokinetics:** *Amphotericin B* is administered by slow, intravenous infusion (Figure 35.3). *Amphotericin B* is insoluble in water, and injectable preparations require the addition of sodium deoxycholate, which produces a soluble colloidal dispersion. The more dangerous intrathecal route is sometimes chosen for the treatment of meningitis caused by fungi that are sensitive to the drug. *Amphotericin B* has also been formulated with a variety of artificial lipids that form liposomes. For example, the simplest and smallest of the liposome prepartions is produced by the incorporation of *amphotericin B* into a single liposomal bilayer composed of phopholipids and cholesterol (Figure 35.4) These liposomal preparations have the primary advantage of reduced renal and infusion toxicity. However, because of their high cost, they are reserved mainly as salvage therapy for those individuals who cannot tolerate conventional *amphotericin B*. *Amphotericin B* is extensively bound to plasma proteins and is distributed throughout the body, becoming highly tissue-bound. Inflammation favors penetration into various body fluids, but little of the drug is found in the cerebrospinal fluid (CSF), vitreous humor, or amniotic fluid. However, *amphotericin B* does cross the placenta. Low levels of the drug and its metabolites appear in the urine over a long period of time; some

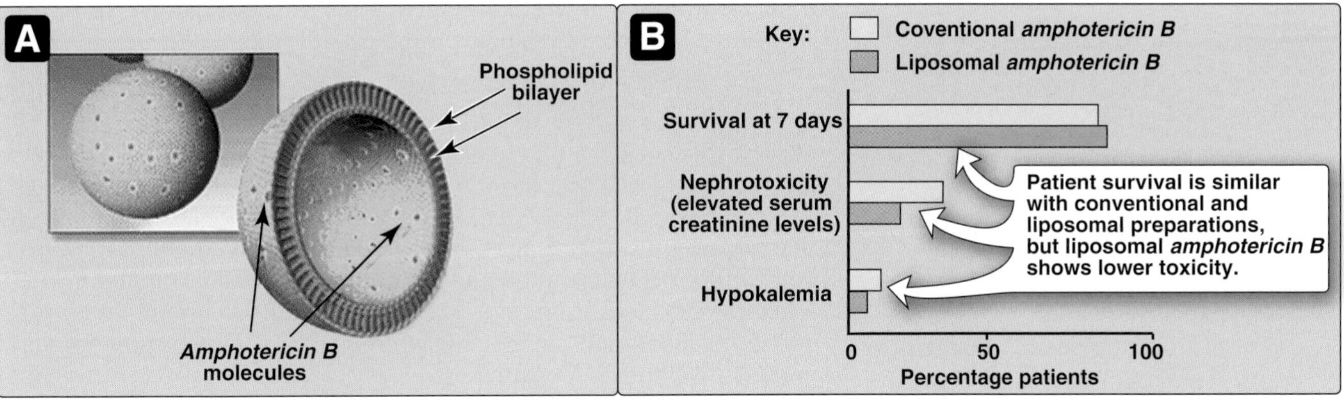

Figure 35.4
A. *Amphotericin B* intercalated between the phospholipids of a spherical liposome (AmBisome™). B. Outcomes of antifungal therapy in febrile, neutropenic cancer patients treated with conventional *amphotericin B* and liposomal *amphotericin B*.

are also eliminated via the bile. Dosage adjustment is not required in patients with compromised renal or hepatic function.

5. **Adverse effects:** *Amphotericin B* has a low therapeutic index. A total daily dose should not exceed 1.5 mg/kg. Small test doses are usually administered to assess the degree of a patient's negative responses, such as anaphylaxis or convulsions. Other toxic manifestations include the following (Figure 35.5).

   a. **Fever and chills:** These occur with intravenous administration, but they usually subside with repeated administration of the drug. Premedication with a corticosteroid or an antipyretic helps to prevent this problem.

   b. **Renal impairment:** Despite the low levels of the drug excreted in the urine, patients may exhibit a decrease in glomerular filtration rate and renal tubular function. Creatinine clearance can drop, and potassium and magnesium are lost. [Note: Nephrotoxicity may be potentiated by sodium depletion.] Normal renal function usually returns on suspension of the drug, but residual damage is likely at high doses. Azotemia (elevated blood urea) is exacerbated by other nephrotoxic drugs, such as aminoglycosides, *cyclosporine*, or *pentamidine*, although adequate hydration can decrease its severity.

   c. **Hypotension:** A shock-like fall in blood pressure accompanied by hypokalemia may occur, requiring potassium supplementation. Care must be exercised in patients taking *digitalis*.

   d. **Anemia:** Normochromic, normocytic anemia caused by a reversible suppression of erythrocyte production may occur. This may be exacerbated in patients infected with (HIV) who are taking *zidovudine*.

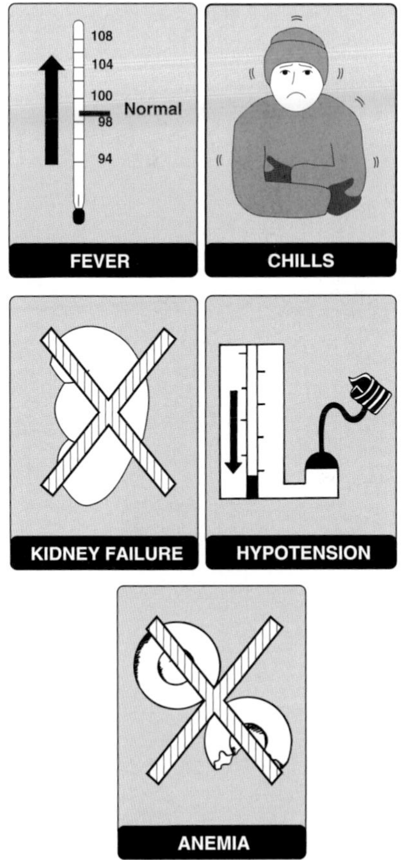

Figure 35.5
Adverse effects of *amphotericin B*.

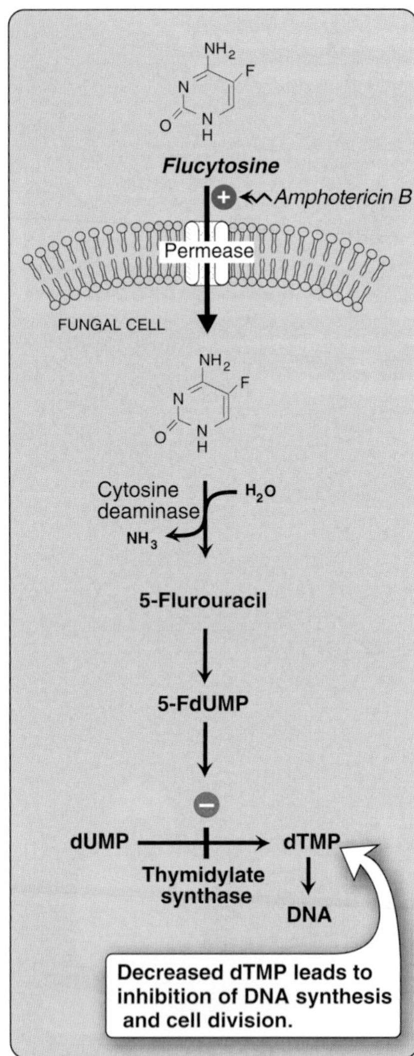

Figure 35.6
Mode of action of *flucytosine*. 5-FdUMP = 5-fluorodeoxyuridine 5'-monophosphate.

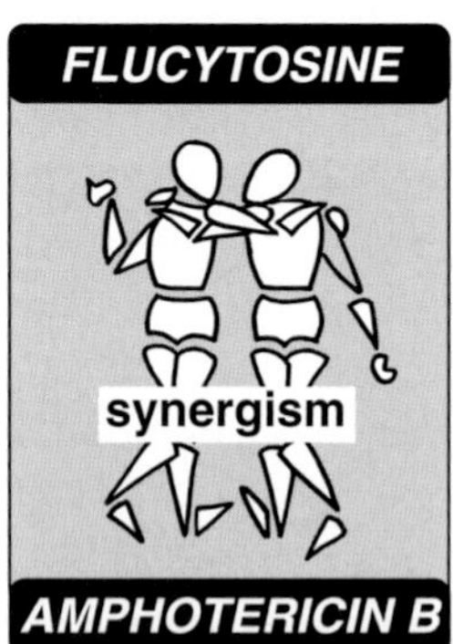

Figure 35.7
Synergism between *flucytosine* and *amphotericin B*.

e. **Neurologic effects:** Intrathecal administration can cause a variety of seriousneurologic problems.

f. **Thrombophlebitis:** Adding *heparin* to the infusion can alleviate this problem.

B. Flucytosine

Flucytosine [floo SYE toe seen] (*5-FC*) is a synthetic pyrimidine antimetabolite that is often used in combination with *amphotericin B*. This combination of drugs is administered for the treatment of systemic mycoses and for meningitis caused by Cryptococcus neoformans and Candida albicans.

1. **Mechanism of action:** *5-FC* enters fungal cells via a cytosine-specific permease—an enzyme not found in mammalian cells. *5-FC* is then converted by a series of steps to 5-fluorodeoxyuridine 5'-monophosphate (5-FdUMP). This false nucleotide inhibits thymidylate synthase, thus depriving the organism of thymidylic acid—an essential DNA component (Figure 35.6). The unnatural mononucleotide is further metabolized to a trinucleotide (5-fluorodeoxyuridine 5'-triphosphate), and is incorporated into fungal RNA, thus disrupting nucleic acid and protein synthesis. [Note: *Amphotericin B* increases cell permeability, allowing more *5-FC* to penetrate the cell. Thus, *5-FC* and *amphotericin B* are synergistic (Figure 35.7).]

2. **Antifungal spectrum:** *5-FC* is fungistatic. It is effective in combination with *itraconazole* for treating chromoblastomycosis and in combination with *amphotericin B* for treating candidiasis or cryptococcosis .

3. **Resistance:** Resistance due to decreased levels of any of the enzymes in the conversion of *5-FC* to *5-fluorouracil* (*5-FU*) and beyond, or increased synthesis of cytosine, can develop during therapy. This is the primary reason that *5-FC* is not used as a single antimycotic drug. The rate of emergence of resistant fungal cells is lower with a combination of *5-FC* plus a second antifungal agent than it is with *5-FC* alone.

4. **Pharmacokinetics:** *5-FC* is well absorbed by the oral route. It distributes throughout the body water and penetrates well into CSF. *5-FU* is detectable in patients and is probably the result of metabolism of *5-FC* by intestinal bacteria. Excretion of both the parent drug and its metabolites is by glomerular filtration, and the dose must be adjusted in patients with compromised renal function.

5. **Adverse effects:** *5-FC* causes reversible neutropenia, thrombocytopenia, and occasional bone marrow depression. Caution must be exercised in patients undergoing radiation or chemotherapy with drugs that depress bone marrow. Reversible hepatic dysfunction with elevation of serum transaminases and alkaline phosphatase may occur. Gastrointestinal disturbances, such as nausea, vomiting, and diarrhea, are common, and severe enterocolitis may occur. [Note: Some of these adverse effects may be related to *5-FU* formed by intestinal organisms from *5-FC*.]

C. Ketoconazole

Ketoconazole [kee toe KON a zole] was the first orally active azole available for the treatment of systemic mycoses.

1. **Mechanism of action:** Azoles are predominantly fungistatic. They inhibit C-14 α-demethylase (a cytochrome P450 enzyme), thus blocking the demethylation of lanosterol to ergosterol—the principal sterol of fungal membranes (Figure 35.8). This inhibition disrupts membrane structure and function and, thereby, inhibits fungal cell growth. [Note: Unfortunately, as is often the case for the initial member of a class of drugs, the selectivity of *ketoconazole* toward its target is not as precise as those of later azoles. For example, in addition to blocking fungal ergosterol synthesis, the drug also inhibits human gonadal and adrenal steroid synthesis, leading to decreased testosterone and cortisol production. In addition, *ketoconazole* inhibits cytochrome P450-dependent hepatic drug-metabolizing enzymes.]

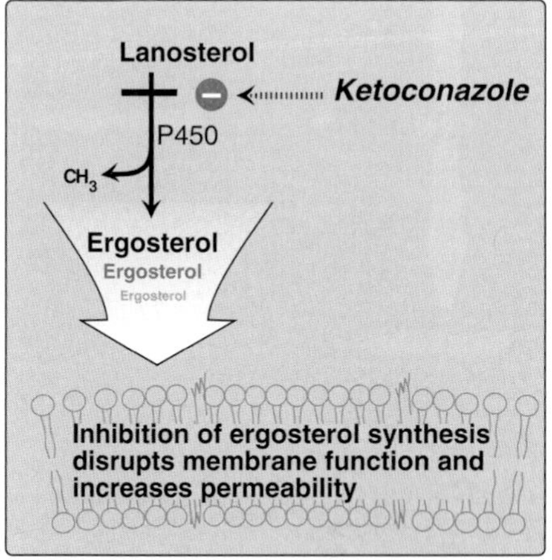

Figure 35.8
Mode of action of *ketoconazole*.

2. **Antifungal spectrum:** *Ketoconazole* is active against many fungi, including histoplasma, blastomyces, candida, and coccidioides, but not aspergillus species. Although *itraconazole* has largely replaced *ketoconazole* in the treatment of most mycoses because of its broader spectrum, greater potency, and fewer adverse effects, *ketoconazole*, as a second-line drug, is a less expensive alternative for the treatment of mucocutaneous candidiasis. Strains of several fungus species that are resistant to *ketoconazole* have been identified.

3. **Resistance:** This is becoming a significant clinical problem, particularly in the protracted therapy required for those with advanced HIV infection. Identified mechanisms of resistance include mutations in the C-14 α-demethylase gene, which cause decreased azole binding. Additionally, some strains of fungi have developed the ability to pump the azole out of the cell.

4. **Pharmacokinetics:** *Ketoconazole* is only administered orally (Figure 35.9). It requires gastric acid for dissolution and is absorbed through the gastric mucosa. Drugs that raise gastric pH, such as antacids, or that interfere with gastric acid secretion, such as H_2-histamine receptor blockers and proton-pump inhibitors, impair absorption. Administering acidifying agents, such as cola drinks, before taking the drug can improve absorption in patients with achlorhydria. *Ketoconazole* is extensively bound to plasma proteins. Although penetration into tissues is limited, it is effective in the treatment of histoplasmosis in lung, bone, skin, and soft tissues. The drug does not enter the CSF. Extensive metabolism occurs in the liver, and excretion is primarily through the bile. Levels of parent drug in the urine are too low to be effective against mycotic infections of the urinary tract.

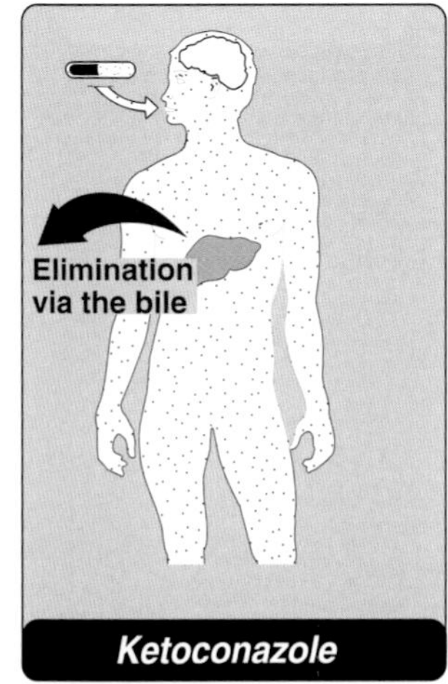

Figure 35.9
Administration and fate of *ketoconazole*.

5. **Adverse effects:** In addition to allergies, dose-dependent gastrointestinal disturbances, including nausea, anorexia, and vomiting, are the most common adverse effects of *ketoconazole* treatment. Endocrine effects, such as gynecomastia, decreased libido, impo-

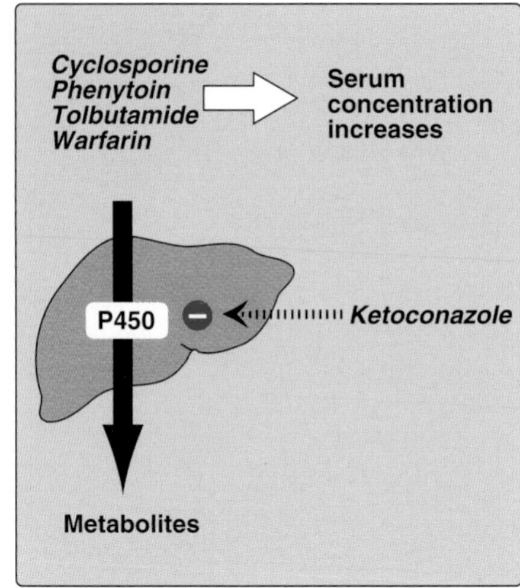

Figure 35.10
By inhibiting cytochrome P450, *ketoconazole* can potentiate the toxicities of other drugs.

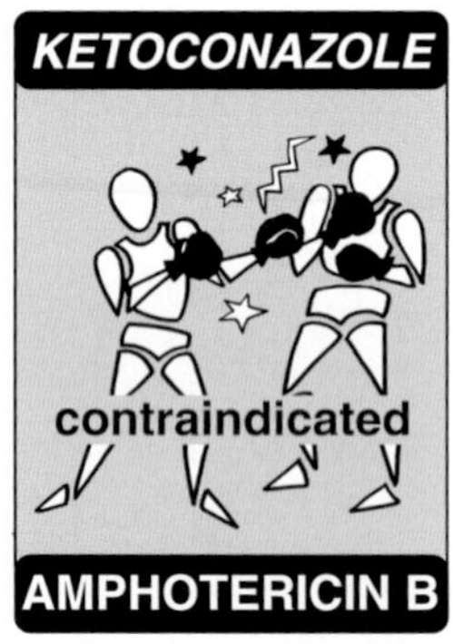

Figure 35.11
Ketoconazole and *amphotericin B* should not be used together.

tence, and menstrual irregularities, result from the blocking of androgen and adrenal steroid synthesis by *ketoconazole*. Transient increases in serum transaminases are found in from two to ten percent of patients. Frank hepatitis occurs rarely but requires immediate cessation of treatment. [Note: *Ketoconazole* may accumulate in patients with hepatic dysfunction. Plasma concentrations of the drug should be monitored in these individuals.]

6. **Drug interactions and contraindications:** By inhibiting cytochrome P450, *ketoconazole* can potentiate the toxicities of drugs such as *cyclosporine*, *phenytoin*, *tolbutamide*, and *warfarin*, among others (Figure 35.10). *Rifampin*, an inducer of the cytochrome P450 system, can shorten the duration of action of *ketoconazole* and the other azoles. Drugs that decrease gastric acidity, such as H_2-receptor blockers, antacids, and proton-pump inhibitors, as well as *sucralfate*, can decrease absorption of *ketoconazole*. *Ketoconazole* and *amphotericin B* should not be used together, because the decrease in ergosterol in the fungal membrane reduces the fungicidal action of *amphotericin B* (Figure 35.11). Finally, *ketoconazole* is teratogenic in animals, and should not be given during pregnancy.

D. Fluconazole

Fluconazole [floo KON a zole] is clinically important because of its lack of the endocrine side effects of *ketoconazole*, and its excellent penetrability into the CSF of both normal and inflamed meninges. *Fluconazole* is employed prophylactically, with some success, for reducing fungal infections in recipients of bone marrow transplants. It inhibits the synthesis of fungal membrane ergosterol in the same manner as *ketoconazole*, and is the drug of choice for Cryptococcus neoformans, for candidemia, and for coccidioidomycosis. *Fluconazole* is effective against all forms of mucocutaneous candidiasis. [Note: Treatment failures due to resistance have been reported in some HIV-infected patients.] *Fluconazole* is administered orally or intravenously. Its absorption is excellent and, unlike *ketoconazole*, is not dependent on gastric acidity. Binding to plasma proteins is minimal. Unlike *ketoconazole*, *fluconazole* is poorly metabolized. The drug is excreted via the kidney, and doses must be reduced in patients with compromised renal function. The adverse effects caused by *fluconazole* treatment are less of a problem than with *ketoconazole*. *Fluconazole* has no endocrinologic effects, because it does not inhibit the cytochrome P450 system responsible for the synthesis of androgens. However, it can inhibit the P450 cytochromes that metabolize other drugs listed in Figure 35.10. Nausea, vomiting, and rashes are a problem. Hepatitis is rare. *Fluconazole* is teratogenic, as are other azoles, and should not be used in pregnancy.

E. Itraconazole

Itraconazole [it ra KON a zole] is a recent addition to the azole family of antifungal agents, with a broad antifungal spectrum. Like *fluconazole*, it is a synthetic triazole and also lacks the endocrinologic side effects of *ketoconazole*. Its mechanism of action is the same as that of the other azoles. *Itraconazole* is now the drug of choice for the treatment of blastomycosis, aspergillosis, sporotrichosis, paracoccidioidomycosis, and histoplasmosis. Unlike *ketoconazole*, it is effective in AIDS-associated histoplasmosis. *Itraconazole* is well-absorbed orally, but it requires acid for dissolution. Food increases the bioavailability of some preparations. The drug is extensively bound to plasma proteins and distributes well throughout most tissues, including bone and adipose tissues. However, therapeutic concentrations are not attained in the CSF. Like *ketoconazole*, it is extensively metabolized by the liver but does not inhibit androgen synthesis. Its major metabolite, hydroxyitraconazole, is biologically active, with a similar antifungal spectrum. Little of the parent drug appears in the urine; thus, doses do not have to be reduced in renal failure. Adverse effects include nausea and vomiting, rash (especially in immunocompromised patients), hypokalemia, hypertension, edema, and headache. *Itraconazole* should be avoided in pregnancy. *Itraconazole* inhibits the metabolism of many drugs, including oral anticoagulants, statins, and *quinidine*. Inducers of the cytochrome P450 system increase the metabolism of *itraconazole*.

F. Newer azoles

Voriconazole [vor i KON a zole] has the advantage of being a broad-spectrum antifungal agent. *Voriconazole* is approved for the treatment of invasive aspergillosis and serious infections caused by Scedosporium apiospermum and fusarium species. *Voriconazole* is orally active and penetrates tissues well, including the CNS. Elimination is primarily by metabolism. Side effects are similar to those of the other azoles. One unique problem is a transient visual disturbance that occurs shortly after a dose of the drug. Figure 35.12 summarizes the azole antifungal agents.

G. Caspofungin

Caspofungin [kas poh FUN jin] is the first approved member of the echinocandins class of antifungal drugs. Echinocandins interfere with the synthesis of the fungal cell wall by inhibiting the synthesis of β(1,3)-D-glucan, leading to lysis and cell death. This drug's spectrum is limited to aspergillus and candida species. *Caspofungin* is

	KETOCONAZOLE	*FLUCONAZOLE*	*ITRACONAZOLE*
SPECTRUM	Narrow	Expanded	Expanded
ROUTE(S) OF ADMINISTRATION	Oral	Oral, IV	Oral
$t_{1/2}$ (HOURS)	6–9	30	30–40
CSF PENETRATION	No	Yes	No
RENAL EXCRETION	No	Yes	No
INTERACTION WITH OTHER DRUGS	Frequent	Occasional	Occasional
INHIBITION OF MAMMALIAN STEROL SYNTHESIS	Dose-dependent inhibitory effect	No inhibition	No inhibition

Figure 35.12
Summary of some azole fungistatic drugs.

not active by the oral route. The drug is highly bound to serum proteins and has a half-life of nine to eleven hours. It is slowly metabolized by hydrolysis and N-acetylation. Elimination is approximately equal between the urinary and fecal routes. Adverse effects include fever, rash, nausea, and phlebitis. Flushing occurs—probably due to the release of histamine from mast cells. *Caspofungin* should not be coadministered with *cyclosporine*. *Caspofungin* is a second-line antifungal for those who have failed or cannot tolerate *amphotericin B* or *itraconazole*. It is very expensive.

III. DRUGS FOR CUTANEOUS MYCOTIC INFECTIONS

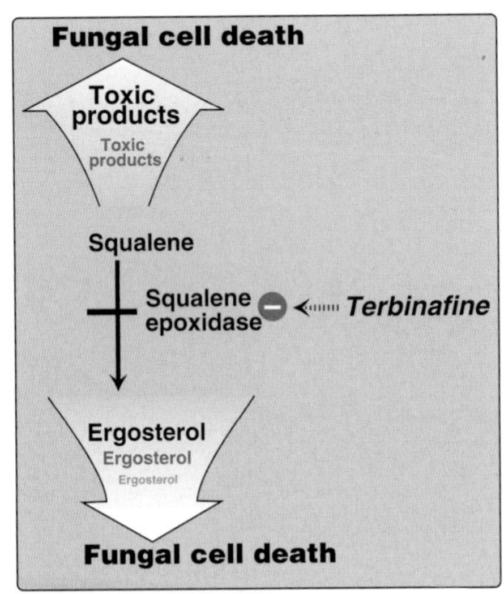

Figure 35.13
Mode of action of *terbinafine*.

Fungi that cause superficial skin infections are called dermatophytes. Common dermatomycoses, such as tinea infections, are often referred to as "ringworm." This is a misnomer, because fungi rather than worms cause the disease.

A. Terbinafine

Terbinafine [TER bin a feen] is the drug of choice for treating dermatophytoses and, especially, onychomycoses (fungal infections of nails). It is better tolerated, requires shorter duration of therapy, and is more effective than either *itraconazole* or *griseofulvin*.

1. **Mechanism of action:** *Terbinafine* inhibits fungal squalene epoxidase, thereby decreasing the synthesis of ergosterol (Figure 35.13). This plus the accumulation of toxic amounts of squalene result in the death of the fungal cell. [Note: Significantly higher concentrations of *terbinafine* are needed to inhibit human squalene epoxidase, an enzyme required for the cholesterol synthetic pathway.]

2. **Antifungal spectrum:** The drug is primarily fungicidal. Antifungal activity is limited to dermatophytes and Candida albicans. Therapy is prolonged—usually about three months—but considerably shorter than that with *griseofulvin*.

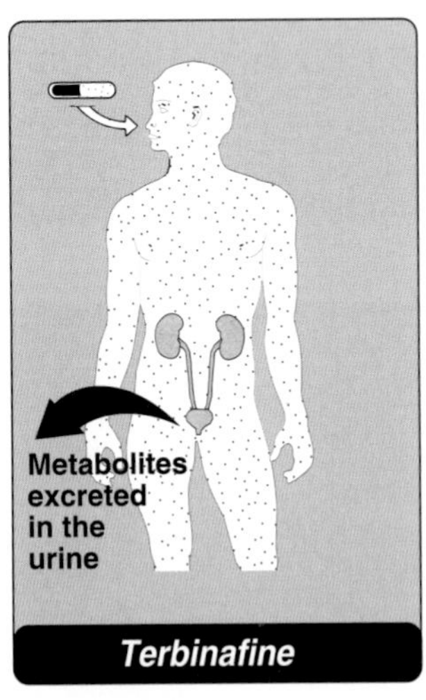

Figure 35.14
Administration and fate of *terbinafine*.

3. **Pharmacokinetics:** *Terbinafine* is orally active, although its bioavailability is only forty percent due to first-pass metabolism. Absorption is not significantly enhanced by food. *Terbinafine* is greater than 99 percent bound to plasma proteins. It is deposited in the skin, nails, and fat. *Terbinafine* accumulates in breast milk and, therefore, should not be given to nursing mothers. A prolonged terminal half-life of 200 to 400 hours may reflect the slow release from these tissues. *Terbinafine* is extensively metabolized prior to urinary excretion (Figure 35.14). Patients with either moderate renal impairment or hepatic cirrhosis have reduced clearance.

4. **Adverse effects:** The most common adverse effects due to *terbinafine* are gastrointestinal disturbances (diarrhea, dyspepsia, and nausea), headache, and rash. Taste and visual disturbances have been reported as well as transient elevations in serum liver

enzyme levels. All adverse effects resolve upon drug discontinuation. Rarely, *terbinafine* may cause hepatotoxicity and neutropenia. Although *terbinafine* is extensively metabolized, there does not seem to be a significant risk of reduced clearance of other drugs. *Rifampin* decreases blood levels of *terbinafine*, whereas *cimetidine* increases blood levels of *terbinafine*.

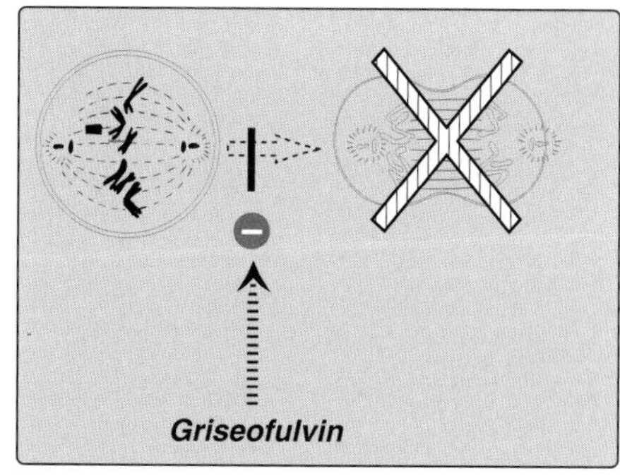

Figure 35.15
Inhibition of mitosis by *griseofulvin*.

B. Griseofulvin

Griseofulvin [gri see oh FUL vin] has been largely replaced by *terbinafine* for the treatment of dermatophytic infections of the nails. *Griseofulvin* requires treatment of six to twelve months in duration. It is only fungistatic, and it causes a number of significant drug interactions. *Griseofulvin* accumulates in newly synthesized, keratin-containing tissue, where it causes disruption of the mitotic spindle and inhibition of fungal mitosis (Figure 35.15). Duration of therapy is dependent on the rate of replacement of healthy skin or nails. Ultrafine crystalline preparations are absorbed adequately from the gastrointestinal tract; absorption is enhanced by high-fat meals. *Griseofulvin* induces hepatic cytochrome P450 activity (Figure 35.16). It also increases the rate of metabolism of a number of drugs, including anticoagulants. It may exacerbate intermittent porphyria. Patients should not drink alcoholic beverages during therapy, because griseofulvin potentiates the intoxicating effects of alcohol.

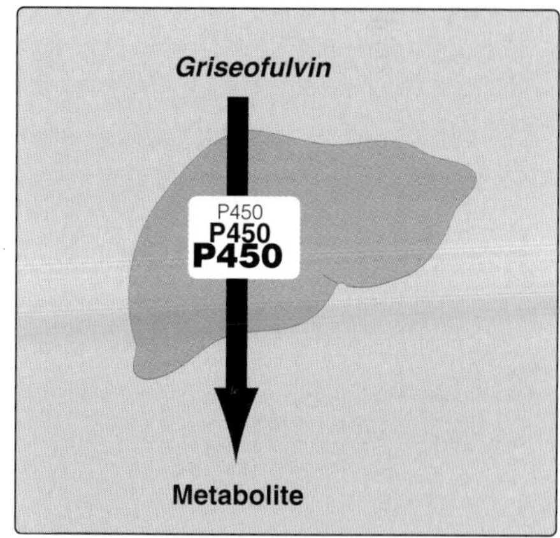

Figure 35.16
Induction of hepatic cytochrome P450 activity by *griseofulvin*.

C. Nystatin

Nystatin [nye STAT in] is a polyene antibiotic, and its structure, chemistry, mechanism of action, and resistance resemble those of *amphotericin B*. Its use is restricted to topical treatment of candida infections because of its systemic toxicity. The drug is negligibly absorbed from the gastrointestinal tract, and it is never used parenterally. It is administered as an oral agent ("swish and swallow") for the treatment of oral candidiasis. Excretion in the feces is nearly quantitative. Adverse effects are rare because of its lack of absorption, but nausea and vomiting occasionally occur.

D. Miconazole and other topical agents

Miconazole [my KON a zole], *clotrimazole* [kloe TRIM a zole], *butoconazole* [byoo toe KON a zole], and *terconazole* [ter KON a zole] are topically active drugs that are only rarely administered parenterally because of their severe toxicity. Their mechanism of action and antifungal spectrum are the same as *ketoconazole*. Topical use is associated with contact dermatitis, vulvar irritation, and edema. *Miconazole* is a potent inhibitor of warfarin metabolism, and has resulted in bleeding in warfarin-treated patients even when *miconazole* is applied topically. No significant difference in clinical outcomes is associated with any azole or *nystatin* in the treatment of vulvar candidiasis.

Study questions

Choose the ONE best answer.

35.1 A 25 year-old male AIDS patient has a fever of 102°F and complains of severe headaches during the past week. Staining of his CSF with India ink reveals Cryptococcus neoformans. The patient is admitted to the hospital and is treated with:

A. intravenous amphotericin B plus flucytosine.
B. oral ketoconazole.
C. intrathecal amphotericin B.
D. oral fluconazole.
E. intravenous amphotericin B plus ketoconazole.

Correct answer = C. Intrathecal administration of amphotericin B is indicated as the most effective way to treat cryptococcal meningitis. Although intravenous amphotericin B may be useful, the addition of flucytosine with its potential for bone marrow toxicity would not be appropriate therapy. Oral ketoconazole is also wrong because of its inability to cross into the CSF. Although fluconazole is very effective against Cryptococcus neoformans and does enter the CSF, the oral route is only used for chronic suppressive therapy and not as treatment for meningitis. The combination of amphotericin B and ketoconazole is a poor one, because ketoconazole disrupts fungal membrane function and, thus, interferes with the action of amphotericin B.

35.2 A 30-year-old male has had a heart transplant and is being maintained on the immunosuppressant, cyclosporine. He develops a Candida infection and is treated with ketoconazole. Why is this poor therapy?

A. Ketoconazole is not effective against Candida.
B. Ketoconazole reacts with cyclosporine to inactivate it.
C. Ketoconazole has a potential for cardiotoxicity.
D. Ketoconazole inhibits cytochrome P450 enzymes that inactivate cyclosporine.
E. Ketoconazole causes gynecomastia and decreased libido in the male.

Correct answer = D. Ketoconazole is effective against Candida, but it does not react with cyclosporine, and is not cardiotoxic. Ketoconazole inhibits the hepatic cytochrome P450 enzymes that inactivate cyclosporine. Thus, in this instance, the patient would be in danger of increased cyclosporine toxicity. Although ketoconazole does cause gynecomastia and decreased libido, this would not be of primary concern.

35.3 A 22-year-old male has been treating his "athlete's foot" with an over-the-counter drug without much success. Upon examination, it is found the nail bed of both great toes is infected. Which one of the following antifungal agents would be most appropriate for this patient?

A. Caspofungin
B. Fluconazole
C. Griseofulvin
D. Nystatin
E. Terbinafine

Correct answer = E. Terbinafine is the drug of choice for the treatment of dermatophytic infections. Because it is fungicidal, it requires a shorter course of therapy than griseofulvin. Drug interactions are also not a problem with terbinafine. Dermatophytes may respond to fluconazole, but this drug is reserved for more serious systemic infections. Nystatin and caspofungin are not useful in the treatment of dermatophytic infections.

Antiprotozoal Drugs

36

I. OVERVIEW

Protozoal infections are common among people in underdeveloped tropical and subtropical countries, where sanitary conditions, hygienic practices, and control of the vectors of transmission are inadequate. However, with increased world travel, protozoal diseases, such as malaria, amebiasis, leishmaniasis, trypanosomiasis, trichomoniasis, and giardiasis, are no longer confined to specific geographic locales. Because they are eukaryotes, the unicellular protozoal cells have metabolic processes closer to those of the human host than to prokaryotic bacterial pathogens. Protozoal diseases are thus less easily treated than bacterial infections, and many of the antiprotozoal drugs cause serious toxic effects in the host, particularly on cells showing high metabolic activity, such as neuronal, renal tubular, intestinal, and bone marrow stem cells. Most antiprotozoal agents have not proved to be safe for pregnant patients. Drugs used to treat protozoan infections are summarized in Figure 36.1.

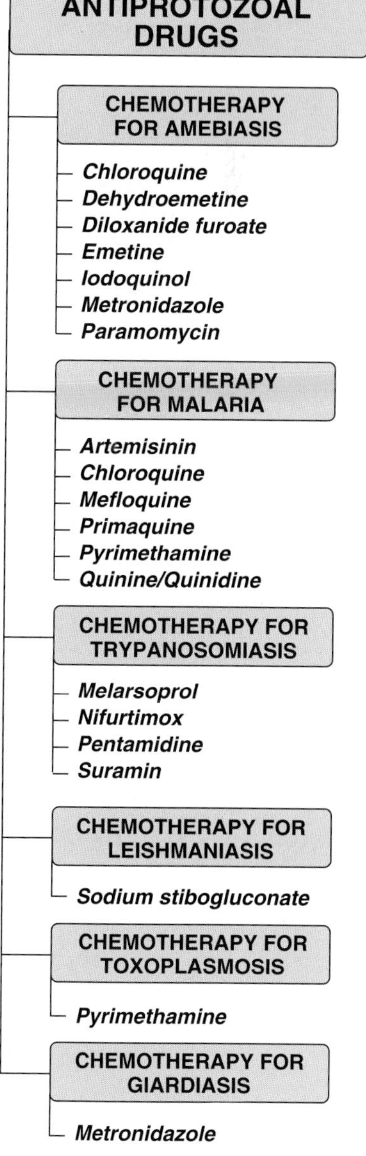

Figure 36.1
Summary of antiprotozoal agents.

II. CHEMOTHERAPY FOR AMEBIASIS

Amebiasis (also called amebic dysentery) is an infection of the intestinal tract caused by Entamoeba histolytica. The disease can be acute or chronic, with patients showing varying degrees of illness, from no symptoms to mild diarrhea to fulminating dysentery. The diagnosis is established by isolating E. histolytica from fresh feces. Therapy is aimed not only at the acutely ill patient but also at those who are asymptomatic carriers, because dormant E. histolytica may cause future infections in the carrier and be a potential source of infection for others.

A. Life cycle of E. histolytica

Entamoeba histolytica exists in two forms: cysts that can survive outside the body, and labile but invasive trophozoites that do not persist outside the body. Cysts, ingested through feces-contaminated food or water, pass into the lumen of the intestine, where the trophozoites are liberated. The trophozoites multiply, and they either invade and ulcerate the mucosa of the large intestine or simply feed on intestinal bacteria. [Note: One strategy for treating luminal amebiasis is to add antibiotics, such as *tetracycline*, to the treatment regimen, resulting in a reduction in intestinal flora—the ameba's

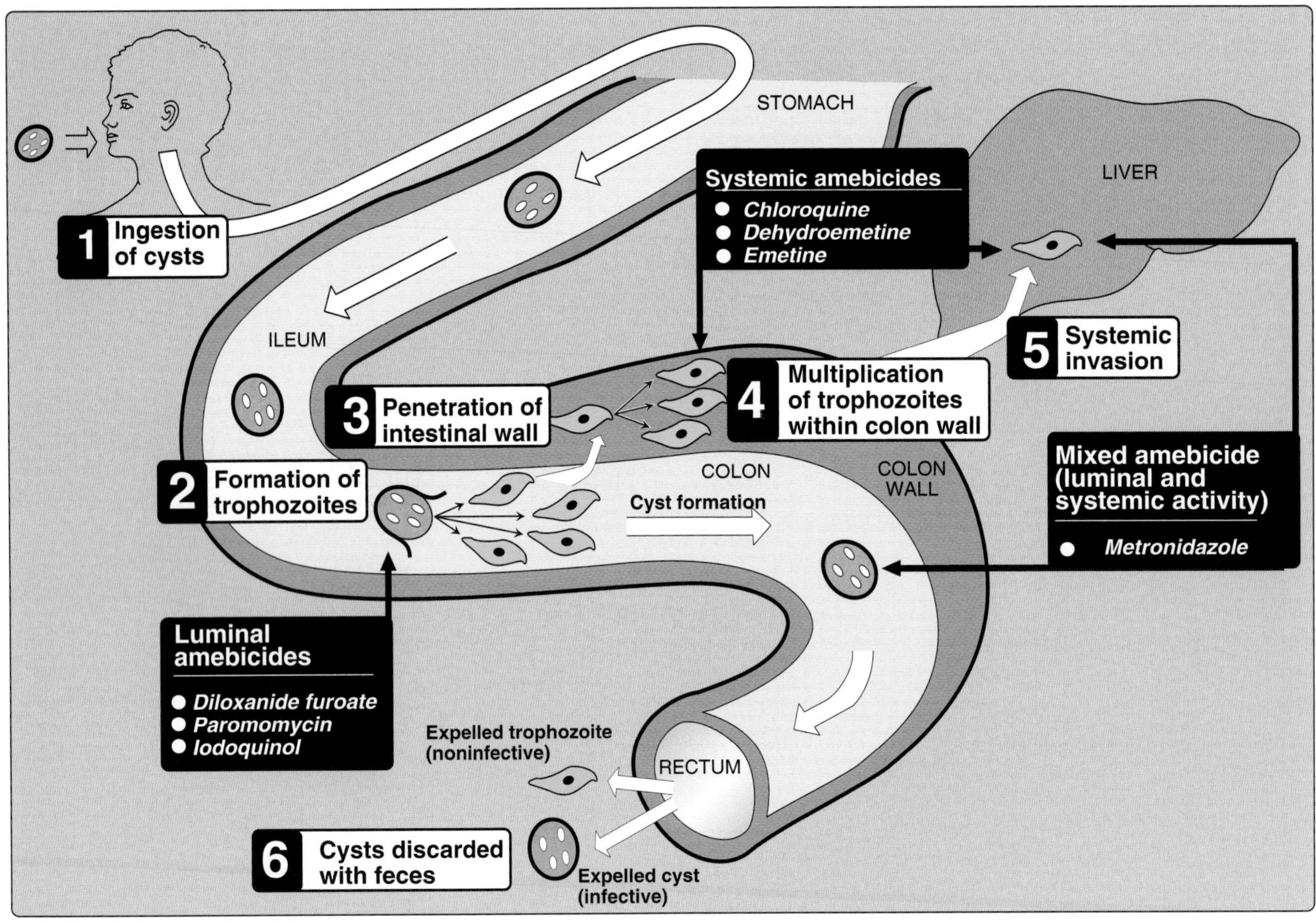

Figure 36.2
Life cycle of Entamoeba histolytica showing the sites of action of amebicidic drugs.

major food source.] The trophozoites within the intestine are slowly carried toward the rectum, where they return to the cyst form and are excreted in feces. Large numbers of trophozoites within the colon wall can also lead to systemic invasion. A summary of the life cycle of E. histolytica is presented in Figure 36.2.

B. Classification of amebicidal drugs

Therapeutic agents are classified as luminal, systemic, or mixed (luminal and systemic) amebicides according to the site where the drug is effective (see Figure 36.2). For example, luminal amebicides act on the parasite in the lumen of the bowel, whereas systemic amebicides are effective against amebas in the intestinal wall and liver. Mixed amebicides are effective against both the luminal and systemic forms of the disease, although luminal concentrations are too low for single-drug treatment.

C. Mixed amebicide

Metronidazole [me troe NYE da zole] is the mixed amebicide of choice for treating amebic infections; it kills the E. histolytica trophozoites. [Note: *Metronidazole* also finds extensive use in the treatment of infections caused by Giardia lamblia, Trichomonas vaginalis, anaerobic cocci, and anaerobic gram-negative bacilli (for example, Bacteroides species). *Metronidazole* is the drug of choice for the treatment of pseudomembranous colitis caused by the anaerobic, gram-positive bacillus Clostridium difficile, and is also effective in the treatment of brain abscesses caused by these organisms.]

1. **Mechanism of action:** Some anaerobic protozoan parasites (including amebas) possess ferrodoxin-like, low-redox-potential, electron-transport proteins that participate in metabolic electron removal reactions. The nitro group of *metronidazole* is able to serve as an electron acceptor, forming reduced cytotoxic compounds that bind to proteins and DNA, resulting in cell death.

2. **Pharmacokinetics:** *Metronidazole* is completely and rapidly absorbed after oral administration (Figure 36.3). [Note: For the treatment of amebiasis, it is usually administered with a luminal amebicide, such as *diloxanide furoate, iodoquinol*, or *paromomycin*. This combination provides cure rates of greater than ninety percent.] *Metronidazole* distributes well throughout body tissues and fluids. Therapeutic levels can be found in vaginal and seminal fluids, saliva, breast milk, and cerebrospinal fluid (CSF). Metabolism of the drug depends on hepatic oxidation of the *metronidazole* sidechain by mixed-function oxidase, followed by glucuronylation. Therefore, concomitant treatment with inducers of this enzymatic system, such as *phenobarbital*, enhances the rate of metabolism. Conversely, those drugs that inhibit this system, such as *cimetidine*), prolong the plasma half-life of *metronidazole*. The drug accumulates in patients with severe hepatic disease. The parent drug and its metabolites are excreted in the urine.

3. **Adverse effects:** The most common adverse effects are those associated with the gastrointestinal tract, including nausea, vomiting, epigastric distress, and abdominal cramps (Figure 36.4). An unpleasant, metallic taste is often experienced. Other effects include oral moniliasis (yeast infection of the mouth) and, rarely, neurotoxicologic problems, such as dizziness, vertigo, and numbness or paresthesias in the peripheral nervous system. [Note: The latter are reasons for discontinuing the drug.] If taken with alcohol, a *disulfiram*-like effect occurs (see p. 112).

4. **Resistance:** Resistance to *metronidazole* is not a therapeutic problem, although strains of trichomonads resistant to the drug have been reported.

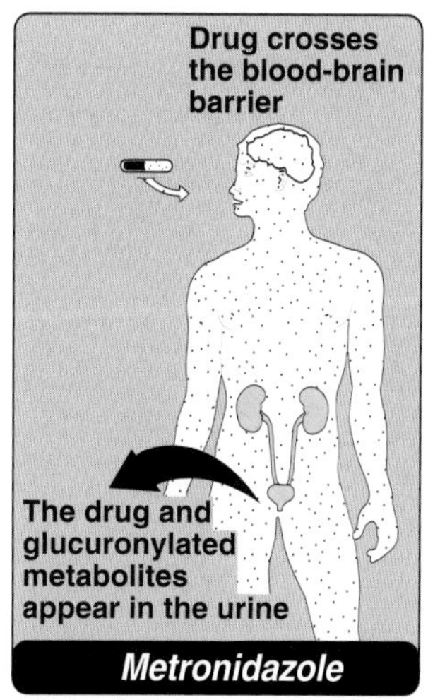

Figure 36.3
Administration and fate of *metronidazole*.

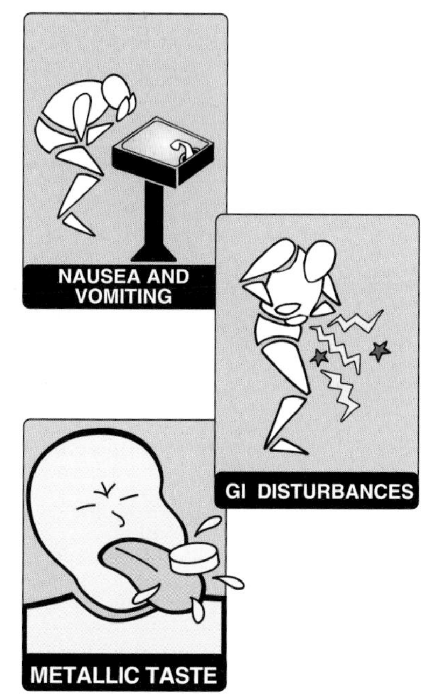

Figure 36.4
Adverse efffects of *metronidazole*.

D. Luminal amebicides

After treatment of invasive intestinal or extraintestinal amebic disease is complete, a luminal agent, such as *iodoquinol, diloxanide furoate*, or *paromomycin*, should be administered for treatment of asymptomatic colonization state.

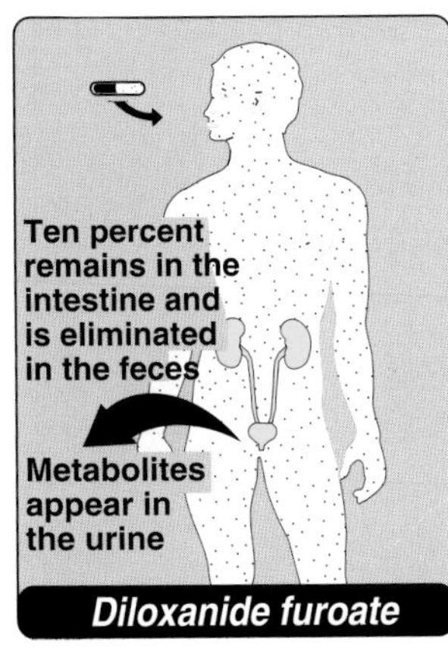

Figure 36.5
Administration and fate of *diloxanide furoate.*

1. ***Iodoquinol*** [eye oh doe QUIN ole], a halogenated 8-hydroxyquinolone, is amebicidal against E. histolytica, and is effective against the luminal trophozoite and cyst forms. Side effects from *iodoquinol* include rash, diarrhea, and dose-related peripheral neuropathy, including a rare optic neuritis. Long term use of this drug should be avoided.

2. ***Diloxanide furoate*** [dye LOKS a nide] is useful in the treatment of asymptomatic shedders of cysts. Its only indication is in the treatment of intestinal amebiasis. After oral administration, *diloxanide furoate* is hydrolyzed in the intestinal mucosa; the resulting free *diloxanide* is about ninety percent absorbed and is excreted via the urine (Figure 36.5). However, the unabsorbed drug is the active amebicide. Adverse effects are mild, and include flatulence, dryness of the mouth, pruritus, and urticaria. The drug is contraindicated in pregnant women and children under two years of age.

3. ***Paromomycin*** [par oh moe MYE sin], an aminoglycoside antibiotic, is only effective against the intestinal (luminal) forms of E. histolytica and tapeworm, because it is not significantly absorbed from the gastrointestinal tract. It is an alternative agent for cryptosporidiosis. Although directly amebicidal, *paromomycin* also exerts its antiamebic actions by reducing the population of intestinal flora. Its direct amebicidal action is probably due to the effects it has on cell membranes, causing leakage. Very little of the drug is absorbed on oral ingestion, but that which is absorbed is excreted in the urine. Gastrointestinal distress and diarrhea are the principal adverse effects.

E. Systemic amebicides

These drugs are useful for treating liver absesses or intestinal wall infections caused by amebas.

1. ***Chloroquine*** [KLOR oh kwin] is used in combination with *metronidazole* and *diloxanide furoate* to treat and prevent amebic liver abscesses. It eliminates trophozoites in liver abscesses, but it is not useful in treating luminal amebiasis. *Chloroquine* is also effective in the treatment of malaria.

2. ***Emetine*** [EM e teen] and ***dehydroemetine*** [de hye dro EM e teen] are alternative agents for the treatment of amebiasis. They inhibit protein synthesis by blocking chain elongation.[1] Intramuscular injection is the preferred route. *Emetine* is concentrated in the liver, where it persists for a month after a single dose. It is slowly metabolized and excreted, and it can accumulate. Its halflife in plasma is five days. The use of these ipecac alkaloids is limited by their toxicities (*dehydroemetine* is less toxic than *emetine*), and close clinical observation is necessary when these drugs are administered. They should not be taken for more than ten days. Among the untoward effects are pain at the site of injection, transient nausea, cardiotoxicity (for example, arrhythmias or congestive heart failure), neuromuscular weakness, dizziness, and rashes. A summary of the treatment of amebiasis is shown in Figure 36.6.

CLINICAL SYNDROME	DRUG
Asymptomatic cyst carriers	*Iodoquinol* or *Paromycin* or *Diloxanide furoate*
Diarrhea/dysentery Extraintestinal	*Metronidazole* plus *Iodoquinol* or *Paromycin* or *Diloxanide furoate*
Amebic liver absess	*Chloroquine* plus *Metronidazole* or *Emetine*

Figure 36.6
Some commonly used therapeutic options for the treatment of amebiasis.

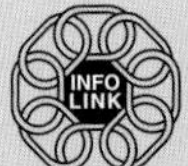

[1]See p. 429 in ***Lippincott's Illustrated Reviews: Biochemistry*** (3rd ed.) for a more detailed discussion of protein synthesis.

III. CHEMOTHERAPY FOR MALARIA

Malaria is an acute infectious disease caused by four species of the protozoal genus Plasmodium. The parasite is transmitted to humans through the bite of a female anopheles mosquito, which thrives in humid, swampy areas. Plasmodium falciparum is the most dangerous species, causing an acute, rapidly fulminating disease that is characterized by persistent high fever, orthostatic hypotension, and massive erythrocytosis (an abnormal elevation in the number of red blood cells accompanied by swollen and reddish condition of the limbs). P. falciparum infection can lead to capillary obstruction and death if treatment is not instituted promptly. Plasmodium vivax causes a milder form of the disease. Plasmodium malariae is common to many tropical regions, but Plasmodium ovale is rarely encountered. Resistance acquired by the mosquito to insecticides, and by the parasite to drugs, has led to new therapeutic challenges, particularly in the treatment of P. falciparum.

A. Life cycle of the malaria parasite

When an infected mosquito bites, it injects Plasmodium sporozoites into the bloodstream (Figure 36.7). The sporozoites migrate through

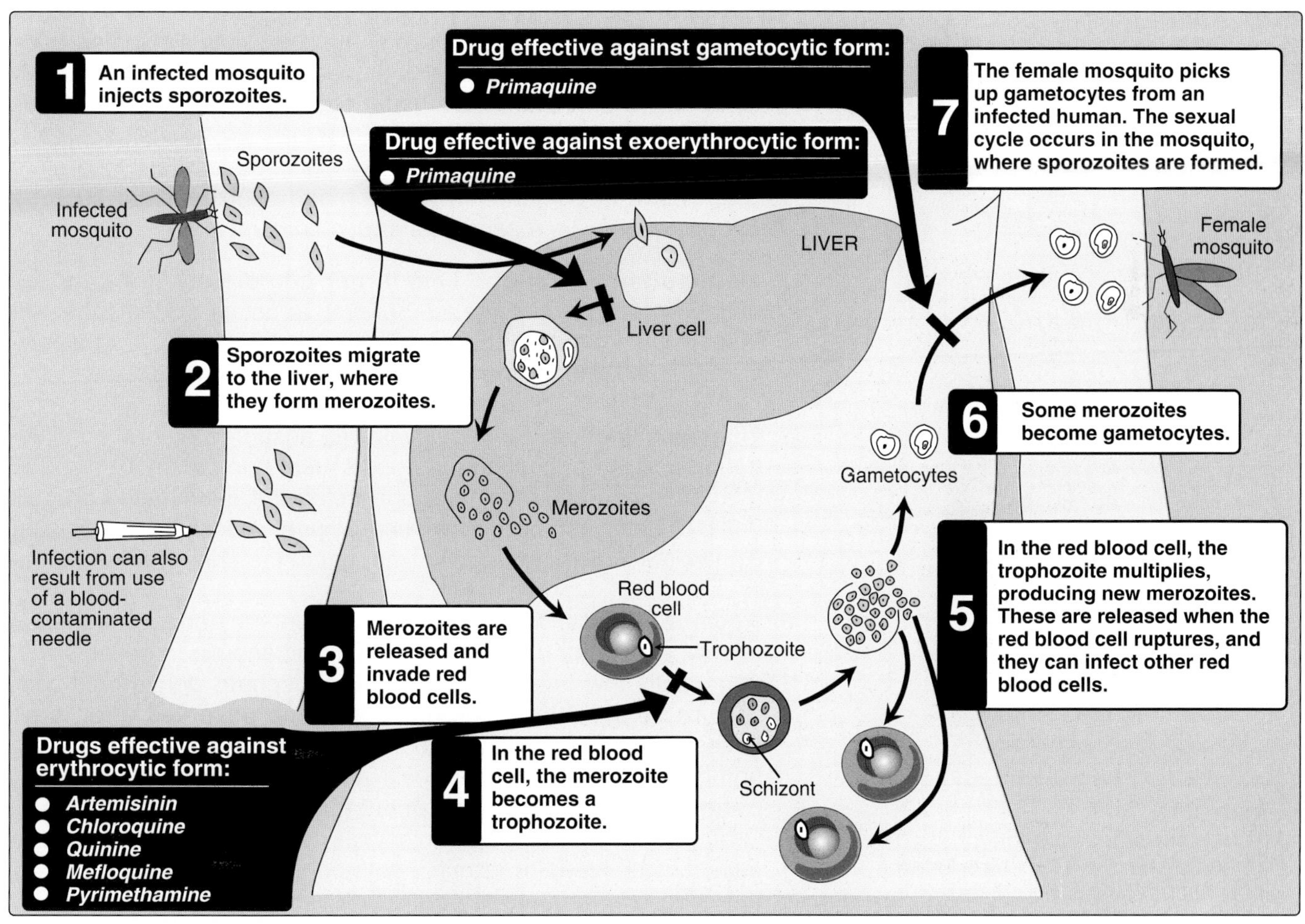

Figure 36.7
Life cycle of the malarial parasite, Plasmodium falciparum, showing the sites of action of antimalarial drugs.

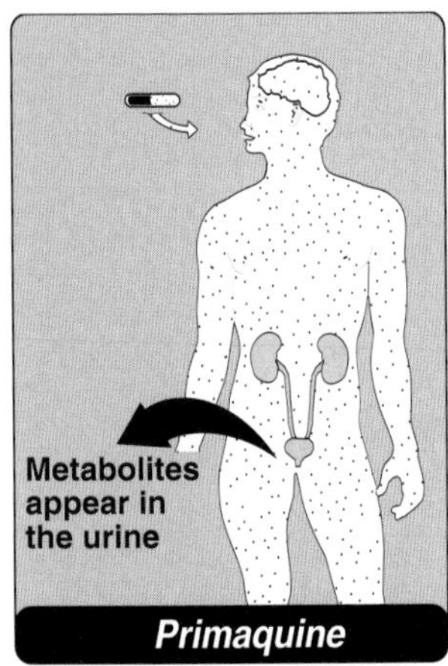
Metabolites appear in the urine
Primaquine

Figure 36.8
Administration and fate of *primaquine.*

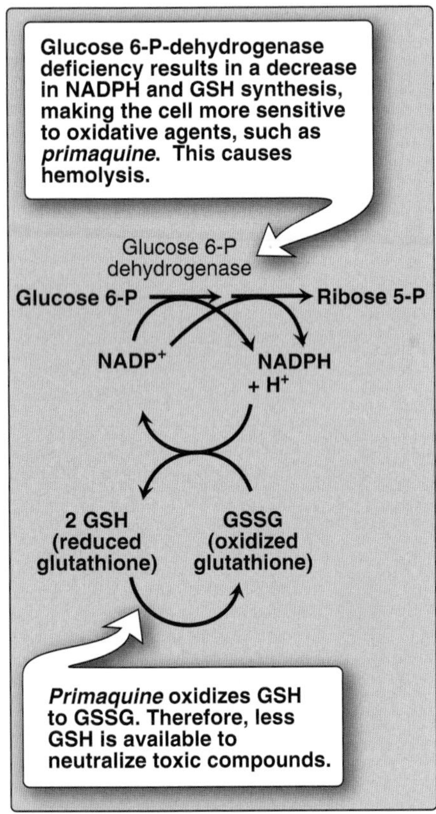
Glucose 6-P-dehydrogenase deficiency results in a decrease in NADPH and GSH synthesis, making the cell more sensitive to oxidative agents, such as *primaquine*. This causes hemolysis.
Glucose 6-P dehydrogenase
Glucose 6-P
Ribose 5-P
NADP+
NADPH + H+
2 GSH (reduced glutathione)
GSSG (oxidized glutathione)
Primaquine oxidizes GSH to GSSG. Therefore, less GSH is available to neutralize toxic compounds.

Figure 36.9
Mechanism of *primaquine*-induced hemolytic anemia. GSH = reduced glutathione; GSSG = oxidized glutathione; NADPH = reduced nicotinamide adenine dinucleotide phosphate.

the blood to the liver, where they form cyst-like structures containing thousands of merozoites. [Note: Diagnosis depends on laboratory identification of the parasites in red blood cells of peripheral blood smears.] Upon release, each merozoite invades a red blood cell, becoming a trophozoite and using hemoglobin as a nutrient. The trophozoites multiply and become merozoites. Eventually, the infected cell ruptures, releasing heme and merozoites that can enter other erythrocytes. [Note: Alternatively, released merozoites can become gametocytes, which are picked up by mosquitoes from the blood they ingest. The cycle thus begins again, with the gametocytes becoming sporozoites in the insect.] The effectiveness of a drug treatment is related to the particular species of infecting plasmodium and the stage of its life cycle that is targeted. A summary of the life cycle of the parasite and the sites of therapeutic interventions are presented in Figure 36.7.

B. Tissue schizonticide: Primaquine

Primaquine [PRIM a kwin] is an 8-aminoquinoline that eradicates primary exoerythrocytic forms of P. falciparum and P. vivax, and the secondary exoerythrocytic forms of recurring malarias (P. vivax and P. ovale). [Note: *Primaquine* is the only agent that can lead to radical cures of the P. vivax and P. ovale malarias, which may remain in the liver after the erythrocytic form of the disease is eliminated.] The sexual (gametocytic) forms of all four plasmodia are destroyed in the plasma or are prevented from maturing later in the mosquito, thus interrupting the transmission of the disease. [Note: *Primaquine* is not effective against the erythrocytic stage of malaria and, therefore is often used in conjunction with a blood schizonticide, such as *chloroquine*, *quinine*, *mefloquine*, or *pyrimethamine*.]

1. **Mechanism of action:** This is not completely understood. Metabolites of *primaquine* are believed to act as oxidants that are responsible for the schizonticidal action as well as for the hemolysis and methemoglobinemia encountered as toxicities.

2. **Pharmacokinetics:** *Primaquine* is well absorbed on oral administration and is not concentrated in tissues. It is rapidly oxidized to many compounds, the major one being the deaminated drug. It has not been established which compound possesses the schizontocidal activity. Metabolites appear in the urine (Figure 36.8).

3. **Adverse effects:** *Primaquine* has a low incidence of adverse effects, except for drug-induced hemolytic anemia in patients with genetically low levels of glucose-6-phosphate dehydrogenase[2] (Figure 36.9). Other toxic manifestations observed after large doses of the drug include abdominal discomfort, especially when administered in combination with *chloroquine* (which may affect patient compliance), and occasional methemoglobinemia. Granulocytopenia and agranulocytosis are rarely seen, except in patients with lupus or arthritis; both conditions are aggravated by the drug. *Primaquine* is contraindicated during pregnancy. All Plasmodium species may develop resistance to *primaquine*.

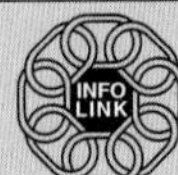
INFO LINK

[2]See p. 149 in ***Lippincott's Illustrated Reviews: Biochemistry*** (3rd ed.) for a discussion of glucose-6-phosphate dehydrogenase deficiency.

C. Blood schizontocide: Chloroquine

Chloroquine [KLOR oh kwin] is a synthetic 4-aminoquinoline that has been the mainstay of antimalarial therapy, and it is the drug of choice in the treatment of erythrocytic P. falciparum malaria, except in resistant strains. *Chloroquine* is less effective against P. vivax malaria. It is highly specific for the asexual form of plasmodia. *Chloroquine* is also effective in the treatment of extraintestinal amebiasis. [Note: The anti-inflammatory action of *chloroquine* explains its occasional use in rheumatoid arthritis and discoid lupus erythematosus.]

1. **Mechanism of action:** Although a detailed explanation of the mechanisms by which *chloroquine* kills plasmodial parasites is still incomplete, the following processes are essential for the drug's lethal action (Figure 36.10). After traversing the erythrocytic and plasmodial membranes, *chloroquine* (a diprotic weak base) is concentrated in the organism's acidic food vacuole, primarily by ion trapping. It is in the food vacuole that the parasite digests the host cell's hemoglobin to obtain essential amino acids. However, this process also releases large amounts of soluble heme (ferriprotoporphyrin IX), which is toxic to the parasite. To protect itself, the parasite ordinarily polymerizes the heme to hemozoin (a pigment), which is sequestered in the parasite's food vacuole. *Chloroquine* specifically binds to heme, preventing its polymerization to hemozoin. The increased pH and the accumulation of heme result in oxidative damage to the membranes, leading to lysis of both the parasite and the red blood cell. The binding to heme and prevention of its polymerization appear to be a crucial step in the drug's antiplasmodial activity, and may represent a unifying mechanism for such diverse compounds as *chloroquine*, *quinidine*, and *mefloquine*.

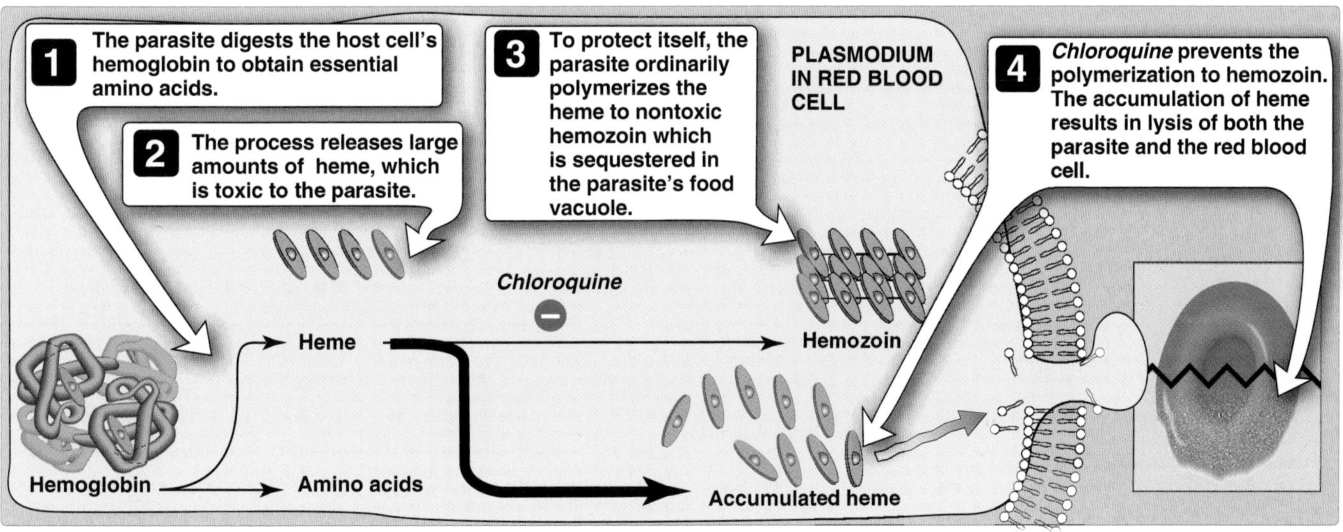

Figure 36.10
Action of *chloroquine* on the formation of hemozoin by Plasmodium species.

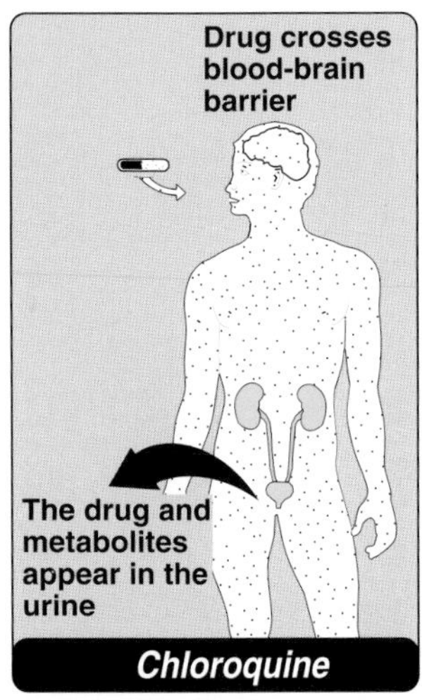

Figure 36.11
Administration and fate of *chloroquine*.

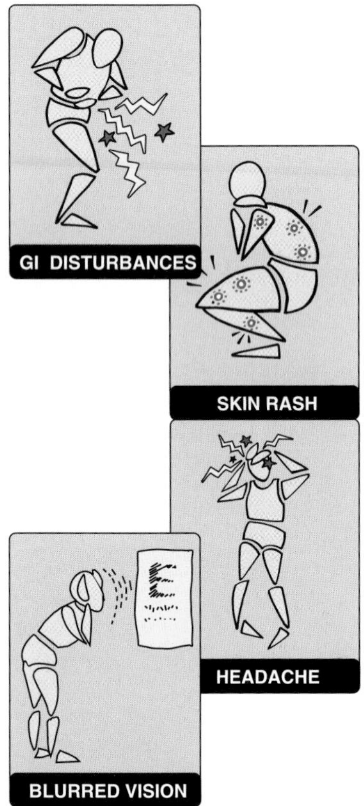

Figure 36. 12
Some adverse effects commonly associated with *chloroquine*.

2. **Pharmacokinetics:** *Chloroquine* is rapidly and completely absorbed following oral administration. Usually, four days of therapy suffice to cure the disease. The drug concentrates in erythrocytes, liver, spleen, kidney, lung, melanin-containing tissues, and leukocytes. Thus, it has a very large volume of distribution. It persists in erythrocytes (see "Mechanism of action" above). The drug also penetrates into the central nervous system (CNS) and traverses the placenta. *Chloroquine* is dealkylated by the hepatic mixed-function oxidase system, but some metabolic products retain antimalarial activity. Both parent drug and metabolites are excreted predominantly in the urine (Figure 36.11). The excretion rate is enhanced as urine is acidified.

3. **Adverse effects:** Side effects are minimal at the low doses used in the chemosuppression of malaria. At higher doses, many more toxic effects occur, such as gastrointestinal upset, pruritus, headaches, and blurring of vision (Figure 36.12). [Note: An ophthalmologic examination should be routinely performed.] Discoloration of the nail beds and mucous membranes may be seen on chronic administration. *Chloroquine* should be used cautiously in patients with hepatic dysfunction or severe gastrointestinal problems or in patients with neurologic or blood disorders. *Chloroquine* can cause electrocardiographic changes, because it has a quinidine-like effect. It may also exacerbate dermatitis produced by *gold* or *phenylbutazone* therapy. [Note: Patients with psoriasis or porphyria should not be treated with *chloroquine*, because an acute attack may be provoked.]

4. **Resistance:** Resistance of plasmodia to available drugs has become a serious medical problem throughout Africa, Asia, and most areas of Central and South America. *Chloroquine*-resistant P. falciparum exhibit multigenic alterations that confer a high level of resistance. [Note: When a *chloroquine*-resistant organism is encountered, therapy usually consists of an orally administered combination of *quinine*, *pyrimethamine*, and a sulfonamide, such as *sulfonadoxine*.]

D. Blood schizonticide: Mefloquine

Mefloquine [MEF lo kween] appears to be promising as an effective single agent for suppressing and curing infections caused by multidrug-resistant forms of P. falciparum. Its exact mechanism of action remains to be determined, but like *quinine*, it can apparently damage the parasite's membrane. Resistant strains have been identified. *Mefloquine* is absorbed well after oral administration and concentrates in the liver and lung. It has a long half-life (seventeen days) because of its concentration in various tissues and its continuous circulation through the enterohepatic and enterogastric systems. The drug undergoes extensive metabolism. Its major excretory route is the feces. Adverse reactions at high doses range from nausea, vomiting, and dizziness, to disorientation, hallucinations, and depression. Electrocardiographic abnormalities and cardiac arrest are possible if *mefloquine* is taken concurrently with *quinine* or *quinidine*.

E. Blood schizonticides: Quinine and quinidine

Quinine [KWYE nine] and its stereoisomer, quinidine [KWIH ni deen], interfere with heme polymerization, resulting in the death of the erythrocytic form of the plasmodial parasite. These drugs are reserved for severe infestations and for malarial strains that are resistant to other agents, such as *chloroquine*. Taken orally, *quinine* is well distributed throughout the body and can reach the fetus. Alkalinization of the urine decreases its excretion. The major adverse effect of *quinine* is cinchonism—a syndrome causing nausea, vomiting, tinnitus, and vertigo. These effects are reversible and are not considered to be reasons for suspending therapy. However, *quinine* treatment should be suspended if a positive Coombs test for hemolytic anemia occurs. Drug interactions include potentiation of neuromuscular-blocking agents and elevation of *digoxin* levels if taken concurrently with *quinine*. *Quinine* absorption is retarded when the drug is taken with aluminum-containing antacids. *Quinine* is fetotoxic.

F. Blood schizonticide: Artemisinin

Artemisinin [ar te MIS in in] is derived from the qinghaosu plant, which has been used in Chinese medicine for more than two millennia in the treatment of fevers and malaria. *Artemisinin* (or one of its derivatives) is available for the treatment of severe, multidrug-resistant P. falciparum malaria. Its antimalarial action involves the production of free radicals within the plasmodium food vacuole, following cleavage of the drug's endoperoxide bridge by heme iron in parasitized erythrocytes. It is also believed to covalently bind to and damage specific malarial proteins. Oral, rectal, and intravenous preparations are available, but the short half-lives preclude their use in chemoprophylaxis. They are metabolized in the liver and are excreted primarily in the bile. Adverse effects include nausea, vomiting, and diarrhea, but overall, *artemisinin is* remarkably safe. Extremely high doses may cause neurotoxicity and prolongation of the QT interval.

G. Blood schizonticide and sporontocide: Pyrimethamine

The antifolate agent *pyrimethamine* [peer i METH a meen] is frequently employed to effect a radical cure as a blood schizonticide. It also acts as a strong sporonticide in the mosquito's gut when the mosquito ingests it with the blood of the human host. *Pyrimethamine* inhibits plasmodial dihydrofolate reductase[3] at much lower concentrations than those needed to inhibit the mammalian enzyme. The inhibition deprives the protozoan of tetrahydrofolate—a cofactor required in the de novo biosynthesis of purines and pyrimidines and in the interconversions of certain amino acids. *Pyrimethamine* alone is effective against P. falciparum. In combination with a sulfonamide, it is also used against P. malariae and Toxoplasma gondii. If megaloblastic anemia occurs with *pyrimethamine* treatment, it may be reversed with *leucovorin*. Figure 36.13 shows some therapeutic options in the treatment of malaria.

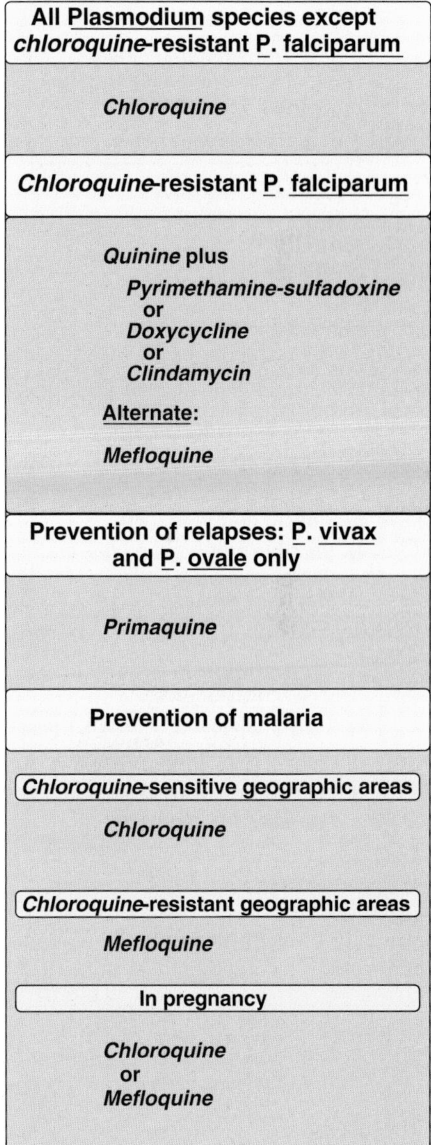

All Plasmodium species except chloroquine-resistant P. falciparum
Chloroquine
Chloroquine-resistant P. falciparum
Quinine plus
Pyrimethamine-sulfadoxine
or
Doxycycline
or
Clindamycin
Alternate:
Mefloquine
Prevention of relapses: P. vivax and P. ovale only
Primaquine
Prevention of malaria
Chloroquine-sensitive geographic areas
Chloroquine
Chloroquine-resistant geographic areas
Mefloquine
In pregnancy
Chloroquine
or
Mefloquine

Figure 36.13
Some commonly used therapeutic options for the treatment and prevention of malaria.

[3]See p. 293 in ***Lippincott's Illustrated Reviews: Biochemistry*** (3rd ed.) for a discussion of dihydrofolate reductase.

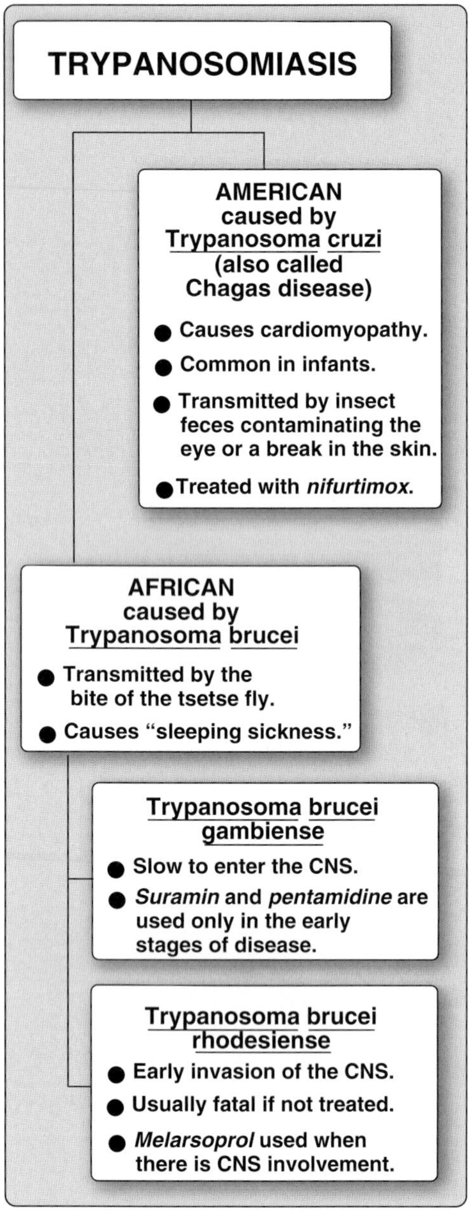

IV. CHEMOTHERAPY FOR TRYPANOSOMIASIS

Trypanosomiasis refers to two chronic and, eventually, fatal diseases caused by species of Trypanosoma: African sleeping sickness, and American sleeping sickness (Figure 36.14). In African sleeping sickness, the causative organisms, Trypanosoma brucei gambiense and Trypanosoma brucei rhodiense, initially live and grow in the blood. The parasite invades the CNS, causing an inflammation of the brain and spinal cord that produces the characteristic lethargy and, eventually, continuous sleep. Chagas' disease (American sleeping sickness) is caused by Trypanosoma cruzi and occurs in South America.

TRYPANOSOMIASIS

AMERICAN caused by Trypanosoma cruzi (also called Chagas disease)
- Causes cardiomyopathy.
- Common in infants.
- Transmitted by insect feces contaminating the eye or a break in the skin.
- Treated with *nifurtimox*.

AFRICAN caused by Trypanosoma brucei
- Transmitted by the bite of the tsetse fly.
- Causes "sleeping sickness."

Trypanosoma brucei gambiense
- Slow to enter the CNS.
- *Suramin* and *pentamidine* are used only in the early stages of disease.

Trypanosoma brucei rhodesiense
- Early invasion of the CNS.
- Usually fatal if not treated.
- *Melarsoprol* used when there is CNS involvement.

Figure 36.14
Summary of trypanosomiasis.

A. Melarsoprol

Melarsoprol [mel AR so prol] is a derivative of mersalyl oxide, a trivalent arsenical. Its use is limited to the treatment of trypanosomal infections—usually in the late stage with CNS involvement—and it is lethal for these parasites.

1. **Mechanism of action:** The drug reacts with sulfhydryl groups of various substances, including enzymes in both the organism and host. The parasite's enzymes may be more sensitive than those of the host. There is evidence that mammalian cells may be less permeable to the drug and, thus, are protected from its toxic effects. Trypanosomal resistance may also be due to decreased permeability of the drug.

2. **Pharmacokinetics:** *Melarsoprol* usually is slowly administered intravenously through a fine needle, even though it is absorbed from the gastrointestinal tract. Because it is very irritating, care should be taken not to infiltrate surrounding tissue. Adequate trypanocidal concentrations appear in the CSF, in contrast to nonpenetration of the CSF by *pentamidine*. *Melarsoprol* is therefore the agent of choice in the treatment of T. brucei rhodesiense, which rapidly invades the CNS, as well as for meningoencephalitis caused by T. brucei gambiense. The host readily oxidizes *melarsoprol* to a relatively nontoxic pentavalent arsenic compound. The drug has a very short half-life and is rapidly excreted into the urine (Figure 36.15).

3. **Adverse effects:** CNS toxicities are the most serious side effects of *melarsoprol* treatment. Encephalopathy may appear soon after the first course of treatment but usually subsides. It may, however, be fatal. Hypersensitivity reactions may also occur, and fever may follow injection. Gastrointestinal disturbances, such as severe vomiting and abdominal pain, can be minimized if the patient is in the fasting state during drug administration and for several hours thereafter. *Melarsoprol* is contraindicated in patients with influenza. Hemolytic anemia has been seen in patients with glucose 6-phosphate dehydrogenase deficiency.

B. Pentamidine isethionate

Pentamidine [pen TAM i deen] is active against a variety of protozoal infections, including many trypanosomes, such as T. brucei gambiense, for which *pentamidine* is used to treat and prevent the organism's hematologic stage. However, some trypanosomes, including T. cruzi, are resistant. *Pentamidine* is also effective in the treatment of systemic blastomycosis (caused by the fungus Blastomyces dermatitidis) and in treating infections caused by Pneumocystis jiroveci (formerly called P. carinii—a name now used to refer to the organism in animals). [Note: It is now considered to be a fungus, but it is not susceptible to antifungal drugs. *Trimethoprim–sulfamethoxazole* is preferred in the treatment of P. jiroveci infections. However, *pentamidine* is the drug of choice in treating patients with pneumonia caused by P. jiroveci who have failed to respond to *trimethoprim-sulfamethoxazole*. The drug is also used in treating P. jiroveci-infected individuals who are allergic to sulfonamides. Because of the increased incidence of pneumonia caused by this organism in immunocompromised patients, such as those infected with human immunodeficiency virus, *pentamidine* has assumed an important place in chemotherapy.] *Pentamidine* is also an alternative drug to *stibogluconate* in the treatment of leishmaniasis.

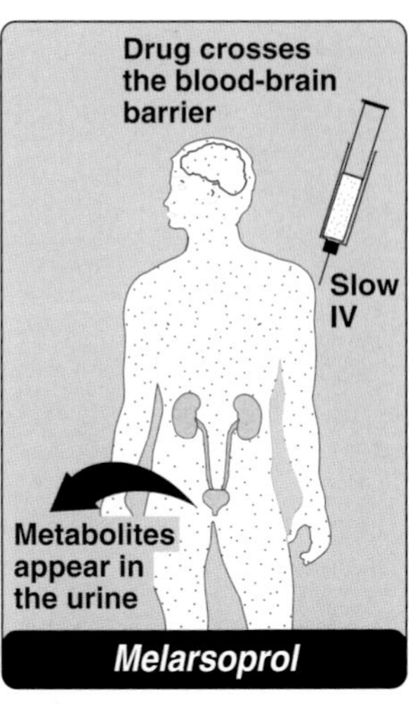

Figure 36.15
Administration and fate of *melarsoprol*.

1. **Mechanism of action:** T. brucei concentrates the *pentamidine* by an energy-dependent, high-affinity uptake system. [Note: Resistance is associated with an inability of the trypanosome to concentrate the drug.] Although its mechanism of action has not been defined, evidence exists that the drug binds to the parasite's DNA and interferes with the synthesis of RNA, DNA, phospholipid, and protein by the parasite.

2. **Pharmacokinetics:** Fresh solutions of *pentamidine* are administered intramuscularly or as an aerosol (Figure 36.16). [Note: The intravenous route is avoided because of severe adverse reactions, such as a sharp fall in blood pressure, and tachycardia.] The drug is concentrated and stored in the liver and kidney for a long period of time. Because it does not enter the CSF, it is ineffective against the meningoencephalitic stage of trypanosomiasis. The drug is not metabolized, and it is excreted very slowly into the urine. Its halflife in the plasma is about five days.

3. **Adverse effects:** Serious renal dysfunction may occur, which reverses on discontinuation of the drug. Other adverse reactions are hypotension, dizziness, rash, and toxicity to β cells of the pancreas.

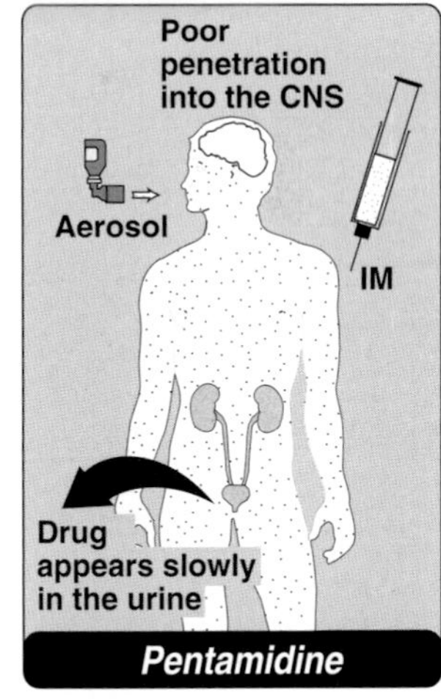

Figure 36.16
Administration and fate of *pentamidine*.

C. Nifurtimox

Nifurtimox [nye FER tim oks] has found use only in the treatment of acute T. cruzi infections (Chagas disease), although treatment of the chronic stage of such infections has led to variable results. [Note: *Nifurtimox* is suppressive, not curative.] Being a nitroaromatic compound, *nifurtimox* undergoes reduction and, eventually, generates intracellular oxygen radicals, such as superoxide radicals and hydrogen peroxide[4] (Figure 36.17). These highly reactive radicals are toxic to T. cruzi, which lacks catalase.[5] [Note: Mammalian cells are partially protected from such substances by the presence of enzymes such as catalase, glutathione peroxidase, and superoxide

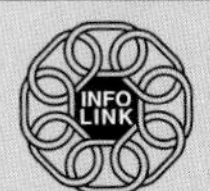

[4]See p. 145 in ***Lippincott's Illustrated Reviews: Biochemistry*** (3rd ed.) for a discussion of reactive oxygen intermediates.
[5]See p. 146 in ***Lippincott's Illustrated Reviews: Biochemistry*** (3rd ed.) for a discussion of catalase.

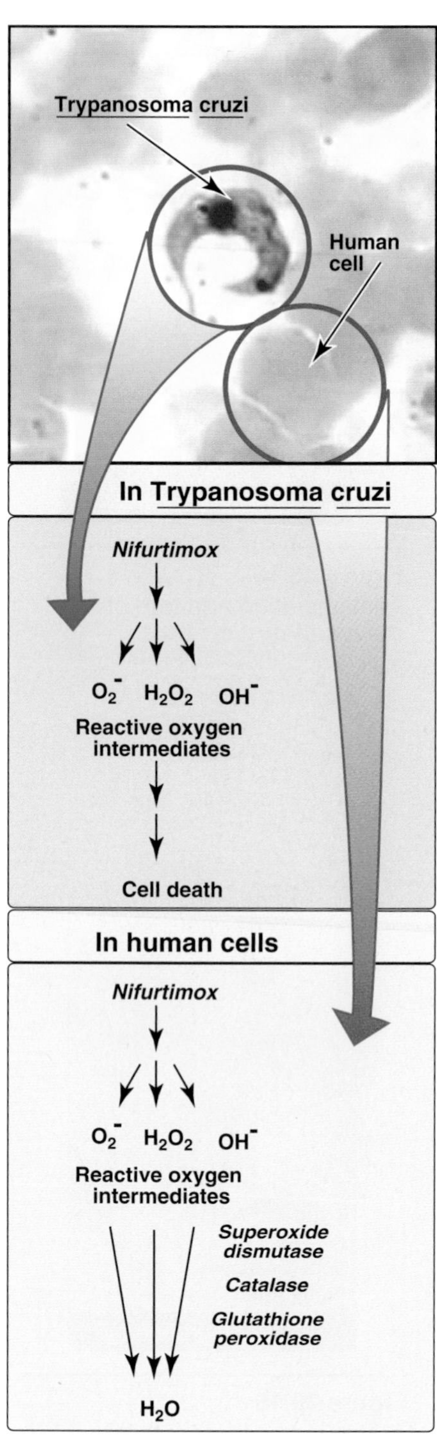

Figure 36.17
Generation of toxic intermediates by *nifurtimox*.

dismutase.] *Nifurtimox* is administered orally, and it is rapidly absorbed and metabolized to unidentified products that are excreted in the urine. Adverse effects are common following chronic administration, particularly among the elderly. Major toxicities include immediate hypersensitivity reactions such as anaphylaxis, delayed hypersensitivity reactions such as dermatitis and icterus, and gastrointestinal problems that may be so severe that they cause weight loss. Peripheral neuropathy is relatively common, and disturbances in the CNS may also occur. In addition, cell-mediated immune reactions may be suppressed.

D. Suramin

Suramin [SOO ra min] is used primarily in the early treatment and, especially, in the prophylaxis of African trypanosomiasis. It is very reactive and inhibits many enzymes, among them those involved in energy metabolism (for example, glycerol phosphate dehydrogenase[6]), which appears to be the mechanism most closely correlated with trypanocidal activity. The drug must be injected intravenously. It binds to plasma proteins and remains in the plasma for a long time, accumulating in the liver and in the proximal tubular cells of the kidney. The severity of the adverse reactions demands that the patient be carefully followed, especially if he or she is debilitated. Although infrequent, adverse reactions include nausea and vomiting (which cause further debilitation of the patient), shock and loss of consciousness, acute urticaria, and neurologic problems, including paresthesia, photophobia, palpebral edema (edema of the eyelids), and hyperesthesia of the hands and feet. Albuminuria tends to be common, but when cylindruria (the presence of renal casts in the urine) and hematuria occur, treatment should cease.

V. CHEMOTHERAPY FOR LEISHMANIASIS

There are three types of leishmaniasis: cutaneous, mucocutaneous, and visceral. [Note: In the visceral type (liver and spleen), the parasite is in the bloodstream and can cause very serious problems.] Leishmaniasis is transmitted from animals to humans (and between humans) by the bite of infected sandflies. The diagnosis is established by demonstrating the parasite in biopsy material and skin lesions. The treatments of leishmaniasis and trypanosomiasis are difficult, because the effective drugs are limited by their toxicities and failure rates. Pentavalent antimonials, such as *sodium stibogluconate*, are the conventional therapy used in the treatment of leishmaniasis, with *pentamidine* and *amphotericin B* as backup agents. *Allopurinol* has also been reported to be effective (it is converted to a toxic metabolite by the amastigote form[7] of the organism).

A. Life cycle of the causative organism: Leishmania

The sandfly transfers the flagellated promastigote form of the protozoa, which is rapidly phagocytized by macrophages. In the macrophage, the promastigotes rapidly change to nonflagellated

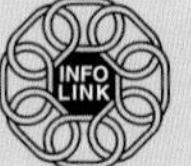

[6]See p. 186in ***Lippincott's Illustrated Reviews: Biochemistry*** (3rd ed.) for a discussion of glycerol phosphate dehydrogenase.
[7]See p. 286 in ***Lippincott's Illustrated Reviews: Microbiology*** for a discussion of leishmaniasis.

amastigotes and multiply, killing the cell. The newly released amastigotes are again phagocytized, and the cycle continues.

B. Sodium stibogluconate

Stibogluconate [stib o GLOO koe nate] is not effective in vitro. Therefore, it has been proposed that reduction to the trivalent antimony compound is essential for activity. The exact mechanism of action has not been determined. Evidence for inhibition of glycolysis in the parasite at the phosphofructokinase reaction[8] has been found. Because it is not absorbed on oral administration, *sodium stibogluconate* must be administered parenterally, and it is distributed in the extravascular compartment. Metabolism is minimal, and the drug is excreted in the urine (Figure 36.18). Adverse effects include pain at the injection site, gastrointestinal upsets, and cardiac arrhythmias. Renal and hepatic function should be monitored periodically.

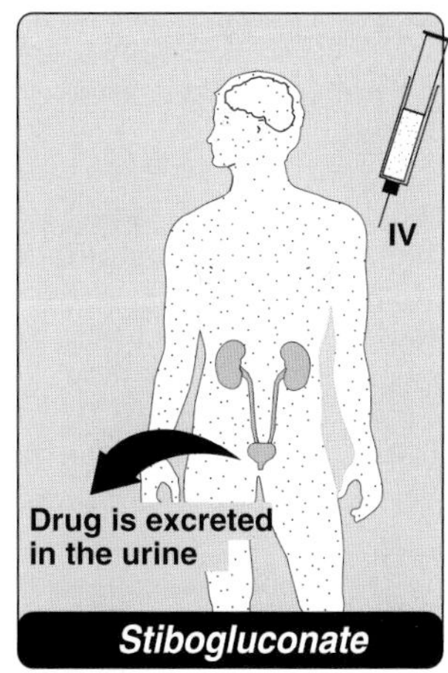

Figure 36.18
Administration and fate of *stibogluconate*.

VI. CHEMOTHERAPY FOR TOXOPLASMOSIS

One of the most common infections in humans is caused by the protozoan Toxoplasma gondii, which is transmitted to humans when they consume raw or inadequately cooked, infected meat.[9] An infected pregnant woman can transmit the organism to her fetus. Cats are the only animals that shed oocysts, which can infect other animals as well as humans. The treatment of choice for this condition is the antifolate drug *pyrimethamine*. A combination of *sulfadiazine* and *pyrimethamine* is also efficacious. *Leucovorin* is often administered to protect against folate deficiency. Other inhibitors of folate biosynthesis, such as *trimethoprim* and *sulfamethoxazole*, are without therapeutic efficacy in toxoplasmosis. [Note: At the first appearance of a rash, *pyrimethamine* should be discontinued, because hypersensitivity to this drug can be severe.]

VII. CHEMOTHERAPY FOR GIARDIASIS

Giardia lamblia is the most commonly diagnosed intestinal parasite in the United States.[10] It has only two life-cycle stages: the binucleate trophozoite with four flagellae, and the drug-resistant, four-nucleate cyst (Figure 36.19). Ingestion, usually from contaminated drinking water, leads to infection. The trophozoites exist in the small intestine and divide by binary fission. Occasionally, cysts are formed that pass out in the stool. Although some infections are asymptomatic, severe diarrhea can occur, which can be very serious in immune-suppressed patients. The treatment of choice is *metronidazole*.

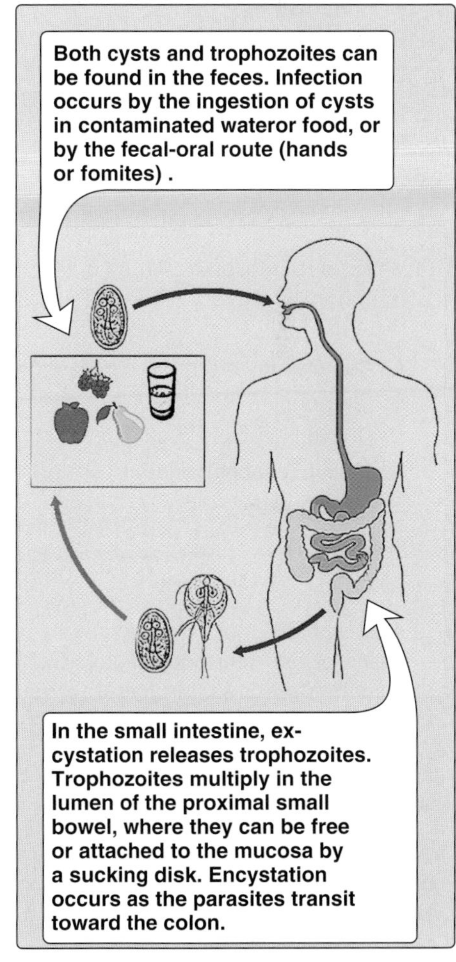

Both cysts and trophozoites can be found in the feces. Infection occurs by the ingestion of cysts in contaminated wateror food, or by the fecal-oral route (hands or fomites) .
In the small intestine, excystation releases trophozoites. Trophozoites multiply in the lumen of the proximal small bowel, where they can be free or attached to the mucosa by a sucking disk. Encystation occurs as the parasites transit toward the colon.

Figure 36.19
Life cycle of Giardia lamblia.

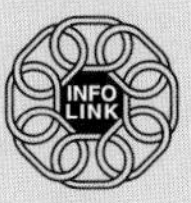

[8]See p. 97 in ***Lippincott's Illustrated Reviews: Biochemistry*** (3rd ed.) for a discussion of phosphofructokinase reaction.
[9]See p. 285 in ***Lippincott's Illustrated Reviews: Microbiology*** for a discussion of toxoplasmosis.
[10]See p. 281 in ***Lippincott's Illustrated Reviews: Microbiology*** for a discussion of giardiasis.

Study Questions

Choose the ONE best answer.

36.1 A 36-year-old male of Lebanese ancestry is being treated for vivax malaria. He experiences severe fatigue, back pain, and darkened urine. Which one of the following antimalarial drugs is most likely to have caused his symptoms?

A. Pyrimethamine
B. Artemisinin
C. Chloroquine
D. Quinine
E. Primaquine

Correct answer = E. The symptoms presented by the patient are consistent with hemolytic anemia. The patient is male and from the Mediterranean basin, both of which are factors associated with glucose 6-phosphate dehydrogenase deficiency. Primaquine is most likely to cause hemolytic anemia in such individuals.

36.2 Tinnitus, dizziness, blurred vision, and headache are indicative of toxicity to which one of the following antimalarial drugs?

A. Primaquine
B. Quinine
C. Pyrimethamine
D. Chloroquine
E. Sulfadoxine

Correct answer = B. The symptoms are characteristic of cinchonism, which is characteristic of quinine or quinidine.

37.4 Which of the following drugs is recommended for the treatment of severe, multidrug-resistant falciparum malaria?

A. Artemisinin
B. Chloroquine
C. Quinine
D. Sodium stibogluconate
E. Primaquine

Correct answer = A. Artemisinin is the antimalarial drug recommended for life-threatening, multidrug-resistant falciparum malaria. The parasite is resistant to chloroquine and quinine and would not be affected by primaquine or stibogluconate.

37.3 A 22-year-old man, who frequently back-packs, complains of diarrhea and fatigue. Examination of stool specimens shows binucleate organisms with four flagellae. Which one of the following drugs would be effective in treating this patient's infestation?

A. Metronidazole
B. Quinidine
C. Pentamidine
D. Sulfadoxine
E. Stibogluconate

Correct answer = A. The patient has giardiasis, and metronidazole is the drug of choice for this intestinal protozoal infection. He probably was infected by drinking contaminated water from a stream. The other drugs are not effective against giardia.

Anthelmintic Drugs

37

I. OVERVIEW

Three major groups of helminths (worms)—the nematodes, trematodes and cestodes—infect humans. As in all antibiotic regimens, the anthelminthic drugs (Figure 37.1) are aimed at metabolic targets that are present in the parasite, but are either absent from or have different characteristics than those of the host. Figure 37.2 illustrates the high incidence of helminthic infections.

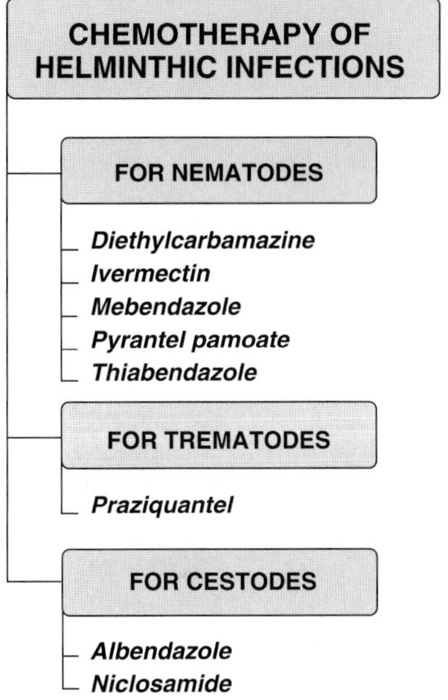

CHEMOTHERAPY OF HELMINTHIC INFECTIONS
FOR NEMATODES
Diethylcarbamazine
Ivermectin
Mebendazole
Pyrantel pamoate
Thiabendazole
FOR TREMATODES
Praziquantel
FOR CESTODES
Albendazole
Niclosamide

Figure 37.1
Summary of anthelmintic agents.

II. DRUGS FOR THE TREATMENT OF NEMATODES

Nematodes are elongated roundworms that possess a complete digestive system, including both a mouth and an anus. They cause infections of the intestine as well as the blood and tissues.

A. Mebendazole

Mebendazole [me BEN da zole], a synthetic benzimidazole compound, is effective against a wide spectrum of nematodes. It is a drug of choice in the treatment of infections by whipworm (Trichuris trichiura), pinworm (Enterobius vermicularis), hookworms (Necator americanus and Ancylostoma duodenale), and roundworm (Ascariasis lumbricoides). *Mebendazole* acts by binding to and interfering with the assembly of the parasites' microtubules and also by decreasing glucose uptake. Affected parasites are expelled with the feces. *Mebendazole* is nearly insoluble in aqueous solution. Little of an oral dose (that is chewed) is absorbed by the body, unless it is taken with a high-fat meal. It undergoes first pass metabolism to inactive compounds. *Mebendazole* is relatively free of toxic effects, although patients may complain of abdominal pain and diarrhea. It is, however, contraindicated in pregnant women (Figure 37.3), because it has been shown to be embryotoxic and teratogenic in experimental animals.

B. Pyrantel pamoate

Pyrantel pamoate [pi RAN tel], along with *mebendazole*, is effective in the treatment of infections caused by roundworms, pinworms, and hookworms (Figure 37.4). *Pyrantel pamoate* is poorly absorbed orally and exerts its effects in the intestinal tract. It acts as a depolarizing, neuromuscular-blocking agent, causing persistent activation of the parasite's nicotinic receptors. The paralyzed worm is then expelled from the host's intestinal tract. Adverse effects are mild and include nausea, vomiting, and diarrhea.

Lippincott's Illustrated Reviews: Pharmacology, Third Edition,
by Richard D. Howland and Mary J. Mycek.
Lippincott Williams & Wilkins, Baltimore, MD © 2006.

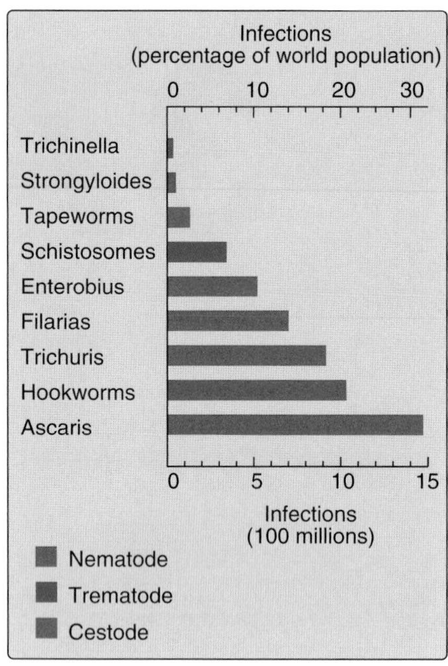

Figure 37.2
Relative incidence of helminth infections worldwide.

C. Thiabendazole

Thiabendazole [thye a BEN da zole], another synthetic benzimidazole, is effective against strongyloidiasis caused by Strongyloides stercoralis (threadworm), cutaneous larva migrans, and early stages of trichinosis (caused by Trichinella spiralis, see Figure 37.4). *Thiabendazole*, like the other benzimidazoles, affects microtubular aggregation. Although nearly insoluble in water, the drug is readily absorbed on oral administration. It is hydroxylated in the liver and excreted in the urine. The adverse effects most often encountered are dizziness, anorexia, nausea, and vomiting. There have been reports of central nervous system (CNS) symptomatology. Among the cases of erythema multiforme and Stevens-Johnson syndrome reportedly caused by *thiabendazole*, there have been a number of fatalities. Its use is contraindicated during pregnancy.

D. Ivermectin

Ivermectin [eye ver MEK tin] is the drug of choice for the treatment of onchocerciasis (river blindness) caused by Onchocerca volvulus, and is a drug of first choice for cutaneous larva migrans and strongyloides. *Ivermectin* targets the parasite's glutamate-gated Cl^- channel receptors. Chloride influx is enhanced, and hyperpolarization occurs, resulting in paralysis of the worm. The drug is given orally. It does not cross the blood-brain barrier and, thus, it has no pharmacologic effects in the CNS. However, it is contraindicated in patients with meningitis, because their blood-brain barrier is more permeable, and CNS effects might be expected. *Ivermectin* is also contraindicated in pregnancy (see Figure 37.3). The killing of the microfilaria can result in a Mazotti-like reaction (fever, headache, dizziness, somnolence, and hypotension).

E. Diethylcarbamazine

Diethylcarbamazine [dye eth il kar BAM a zeen] is used in the treatment of filariasis because of its ability to immobilize microfilariae, and render them susceptible to host defense mechanisms. Combined with *albendazole*, *diethylcarbamazine* is effective in the treatment of Wucheria bancrofti and Brugia malayi infections. It is rapidly absorbed following oral administration with meals and is excreted primarily in the urine. Urinary alkalosis or renal impairment may require dosage reduction. Adverse effects are primarily caused by host reactions to the killed organisms. The severity of symptoms is related to the parasite load, and include fever, malaise, rash, myalgias, arthralgias, and headache. Most patients have leukocytosis. Antihistamines or steroids may be given to ameliorate many of the symptoms. Figure 37.4 summarizes the major infections caused by nematodes, and the common therapies used for them.

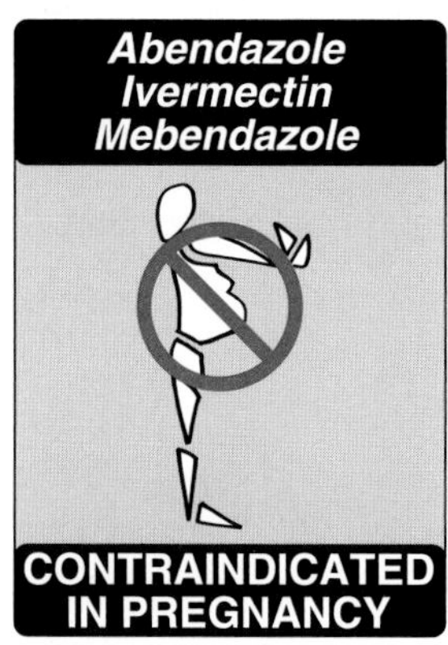

Figure 37.3
Albendazole, *ivermectin*, and *mebendazole* are contraindicated in pregnancy.

III. DRUGS FOR THE TREATMENT OF TREMATODES

The trematodes (flukes) are leaf-shaped flatworms that are generally characterized by the tissues they infect. For example, they may be categorized as liver, lung, intestinal, or blood flukes (Figure 37.5).

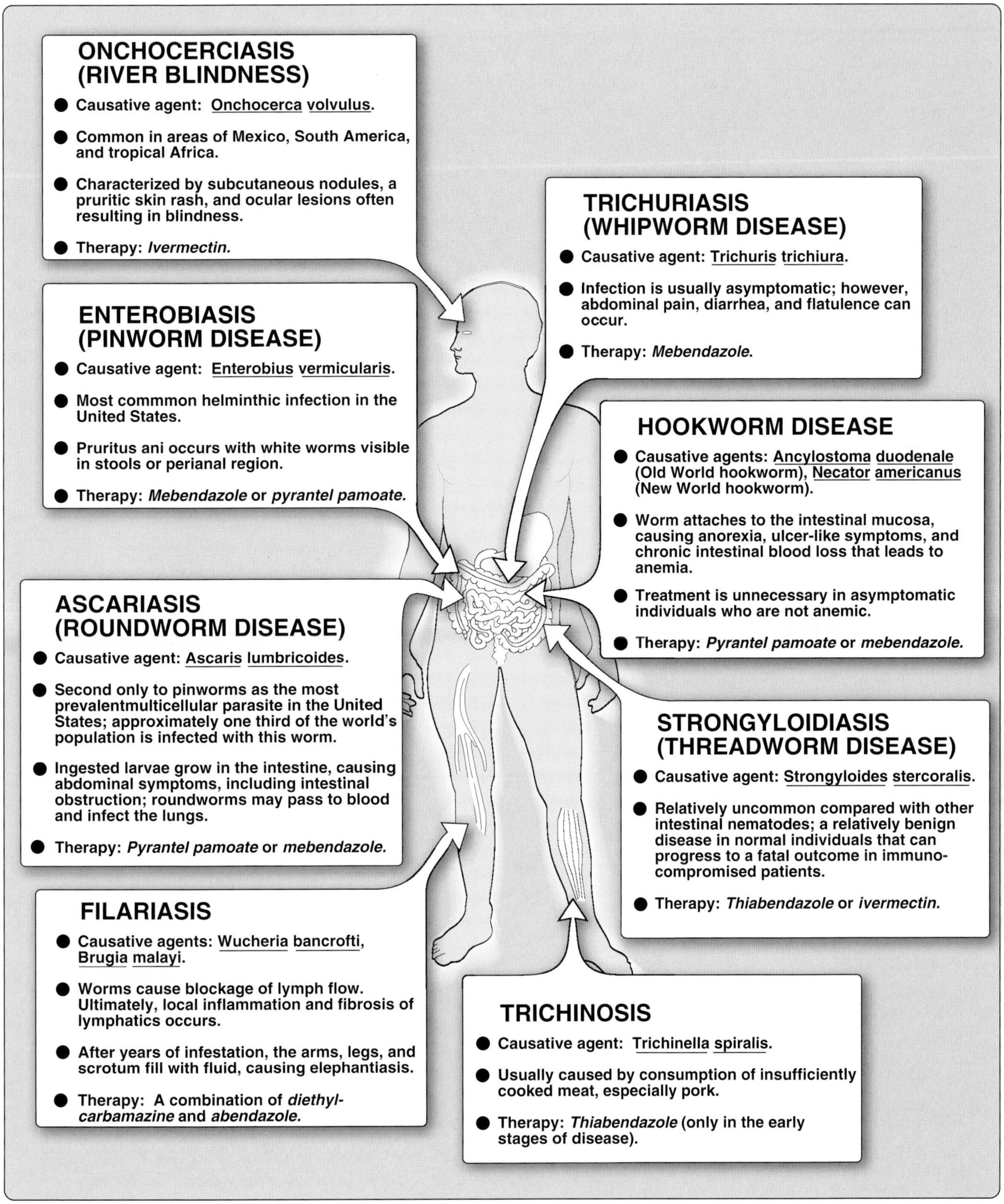

ONCHOCERCIASIS (RIVER BLINDNESS)

- Causative agent: Onchocerca volvulus.
- Common in areas of Mexico, South America, and tropical Africa.
- Characterized by subcutaneous nodules, a pruritic skin rash, and ocular lesions often resulting in blindness.
- Therapy: *Ivermectin.*

TRICHURIASIS (WHIPWORM DISEASE)

- Causative agent: Trichuris trichiura.
- Infection is usually asymptomatic; however, abdominal pain, diarrhea, and flatulence can occur.
- Therapy: *Mebendazole.*

ENTEROBIASIS (PINWORM DISEASE)

- Causative agent: Enterobius vermicularis.
- Most commmon helminthic infection in the United States.
- Pruritus ani occurs with white worms visible in stools or perianal region.
- Therapy: *Mebendazole* or *pyrantel pamoate.*

HOOKWORM DISEASE

- Causative agents: Ancylostoma duodenale (Old World hookworm), Necator americanus (New World hookworm).
- Worm attaches to the intestinal mucosa, causing anorexia, ulcer-like symptoms, and chronic intestinal blood loss that leads to anemia.
- Treatment is unnecessary in asymptomatic individuals who are not anemic.
- Therapy: *Pyrantel pamoate* or *mebendazole.*

ASCARIASIS (ROUNDWORM DISEASE)

- Causative agent: Ascaris lumbricoides.
- Second only to pinworms as the most prevalentmulticellular parasite in the United States; approximately one third of the world's population is infected with this worm.
- Ingested larvae grow in the intestine, causing abdominal symptoms, including intestinal obstruction; roundworms may pass to blood and infect the lungs.
- Therapy: *Pyrantel pamoate* or *mebendazole.*

STRONGYLOIDIASIS (THREADWORM DISEASE)

- Causative agent: Strongyloides stercoralis.
- Relatively uncommon compared with other intestinal nematodes; a relatively benign disease in normal individuals that can progress to a fatal outcome in immuno-compromised patients.
- Therapy: *Thiabendazole* or *ivermectin.*

FILARIASIS

- Causative agents: Wucheria bancrofti, Brugia malayi.
- Worms cause blockage of lymph flow. Ultimately, local inflammation and fibrosis of lymphatics occurs.
- After years of infestation, the arms, legs, and scrotum fill with fluid, causing elephantiasis.
- Therapy: A combination of *diethyl-carbamazine* and *abendazole.*

TRICHINOSIS

- Causative agent: Trichinella spiralis.
- Usually caused by consumption of insufficiently cooked meat, especially pork.
- Therapy: *Thiabendazole* (only in the early stages of disease).

Figure 37.4
Characteristics of and therapy for commonly encountered nematode infections.

A. Praziquantel

Trematode infections are generally treated with *praziquantel* [pray zi KWON tel]. This drug is an agent of choice for the treatment of all forms of schistosomiasis and other trematode infections and for cestode infections like cysticercosis. Permeability of the cell membrane to calcium is increased, causing contracture and paralysis of the parasite. *Praziquantel* is rapidly absorbed after oral administration and distributes into the cerebrospinal fluid. High levels occur in the bile. The drug is extensively metabolized oxidatively, resulting in a short half-life. The metabolites are inactive and are excreted through the urine and bile. Common adverse effects include drowsiness, dizziness, malaise, and anorexia, as well as gastrointestinal upsets. The drug is not recommended for pregnant women or nursing mothers. Drug interactions due to increased metabolism have been reported with *dexamethasone*, *phenytoin*, and *carbamazepine*. *Cimetidine*, which inhibits cytochrome P450 isozymes, causes increased *praziquantel* levels. *Praziquantel* is contraindicated for the treatment of ocular cysticercosis, because destruction of the organism in the eye may damage the organ.

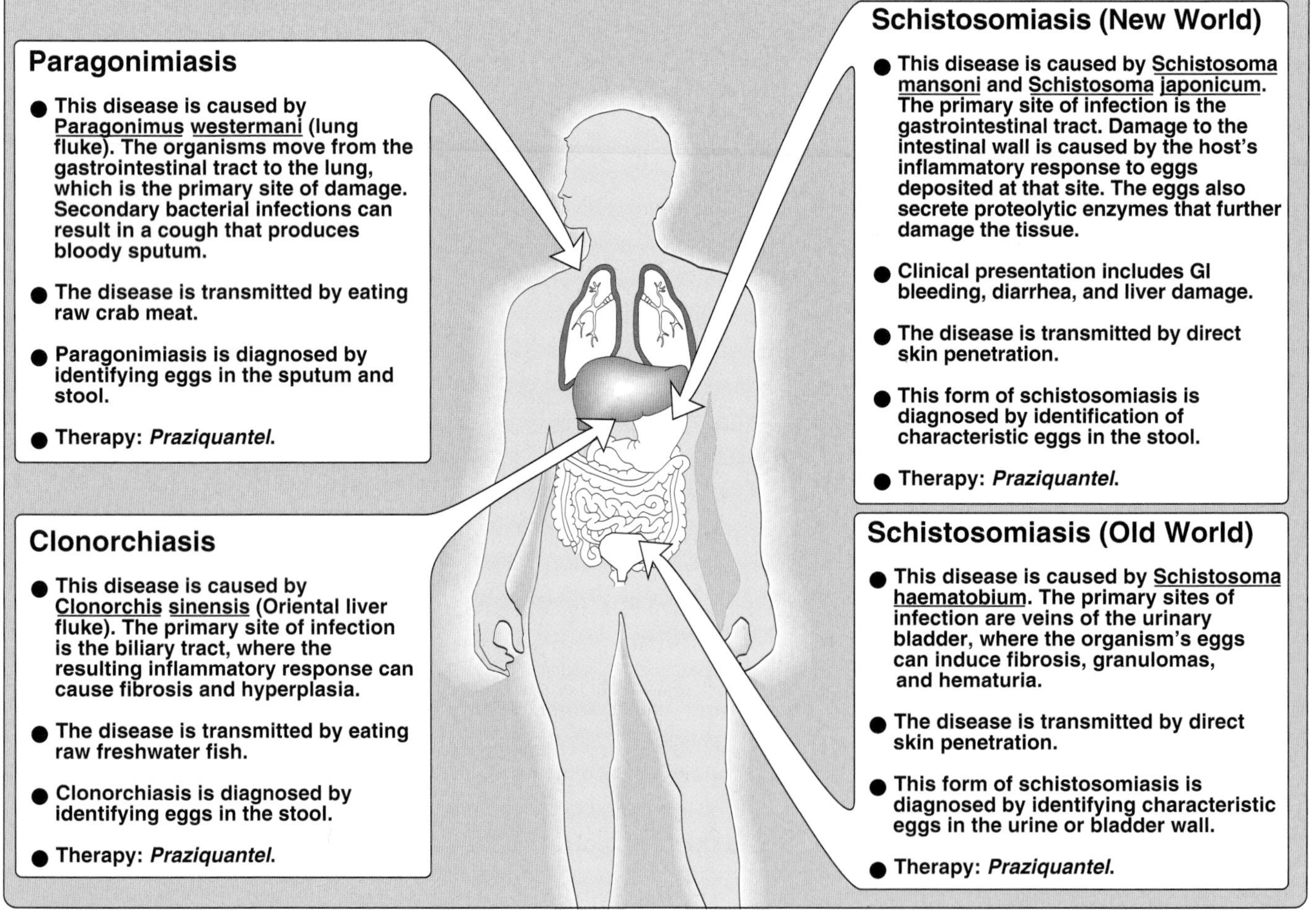

Figure 37.5
Characteristics of and therapy for commonly encountered trematode infections.

IV. DRUGS FOR THE TREATMENT OF CESTODES

The cestodes, or "true tapeworms," typically have a flat, segmented body and attach to the host's intestine (Figure 37.6). Like the trematodes, the tapeworms lack a mouth and a digestive tract throughout their life cycle.

A. Niclosamide

Niclosamide [ni KLOE sa mide] is the drug of choice for most cestode (tapeworm) infections. Its action has been ascribed to inhibition of the parasite's mitochondrial anaerobic phosphorylation of ADP, which produces usable energy in the form of ATP. The drug is lethal for the cestode's scolex and segments of cestodes, but not for the ova. A laxative is administered prior to oral administration of *niclosamide*. This is done to purge the bowel of all dead segments and so preclude digestion and liberation of the ova, which may lead to cysticercosis. Alcohol should be avoided within one day of *niclosamide*.

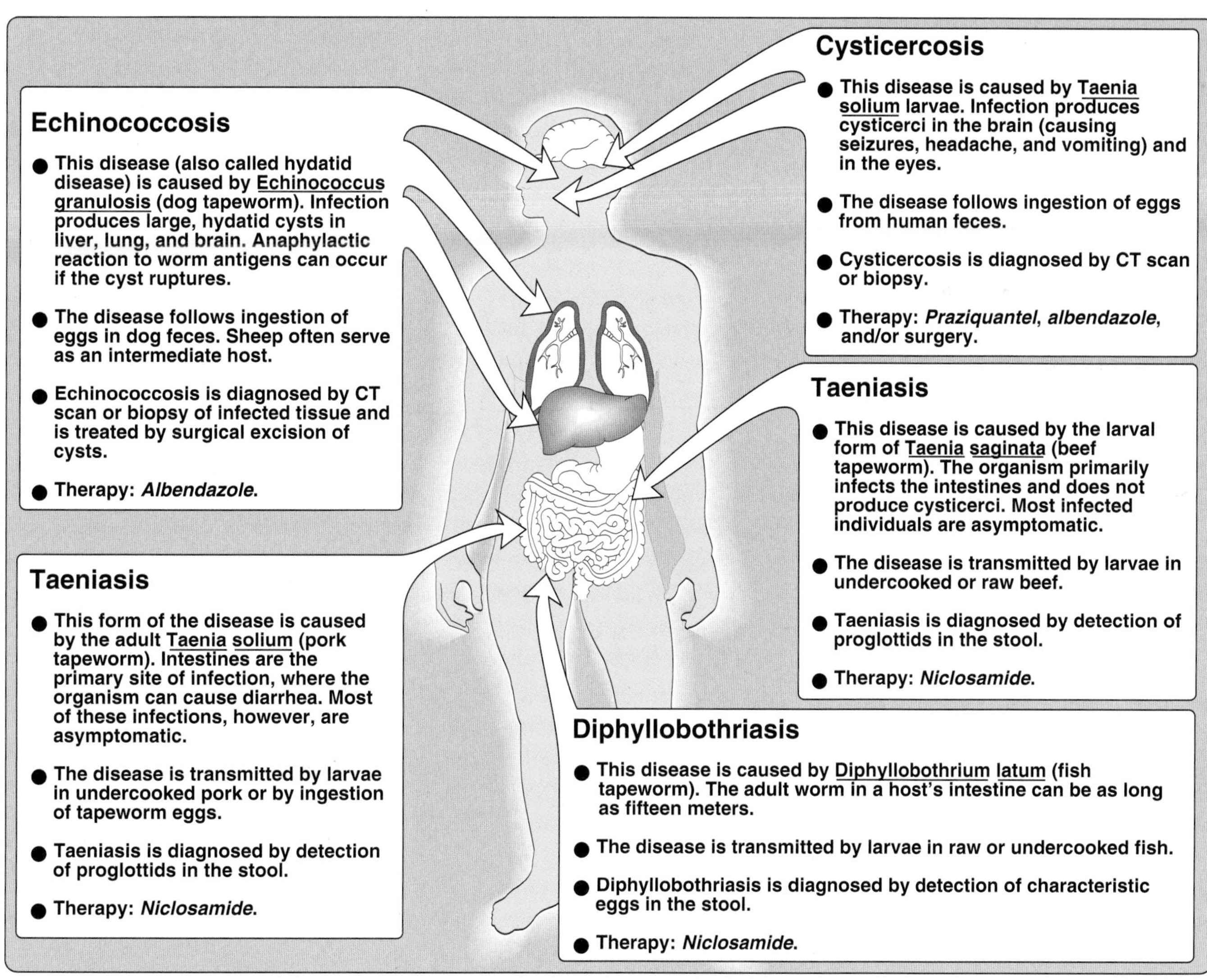

Echinococcosis
This disease (also called hydatid disease) is caused by Echinococcus granulosis (dog tapeworm). Infection produces large, hydatid cysts in liver, lung, and brain. Anaphylactic reaction to worm antigens can occur if the cyst ruptures.
The disease follows ingestion of eggs in dog feces. Sheep often serve as an intermediate host.
Echinococcosis is diagnosed by CT scan or biopsy of infected tissue and is treated by surgical excision of cysts.
Therapy: Albendazole.
Taeniasis
This form of the disease is caused by the adult Taenia solium (pork tapeworm). Intestines are the primary site of infection, where the organism can cause diarrhea. Most of these infections, however, are asymptomatic.
The disease is transmitted by larvae in undercooked pork or by ingestion of tapeworm eggs.
Taeniasis is diagnosed by detection of proglottids in the stool.
Therapy: Niclosamide.
Cysticercosis
This disease is caused by Taenia solium larvae. Infection produces cysticerci in the brain (causing seizures, headache, and vomiting) and in the eyes.
The disease follows ingestion of eggs from human feces.
Cysticercosis is diagnosed by CT scan or biopsy.
Therapy: Praziquantel, albendazole, and/or surgery.
Taeniasis
This disease is caused by the larval form of Taenia saginata (beef tapeworm). The organism primarily infects the intestines and does not produce cysticerci. Most infected individuals are asymptomatic.
The disease is transmitted by larvae in undercooked or raw beef.
Taeniasis is diagnosed by detection of proglottids in the stool.
Therapy: Niclosamide.
Diphyllobothriasis
This disease is caused by Diphyllobothrium latum (fish tapeworm). The adult worm in a host's intestine can be as long as fifteen meters.
The disease is transmitted by larvae in raw or undercooked fish.
Diphyllobothriasis is diagnosed by detection of characteristic eggs in the stool.
Therapy: Niclosamide.

Figure 37.6
Characteristics of and therapy for commonly encountered cestode infections.

B. Albendazole

Albendazole [al BEN da zole] is a benzimidazole that, like the others, inhibits microtubule synthesis and glucose uptake in nematodes. Its primary therapeutic application, however, is in the treatment of cestodal infestations, such as cysticercosis (caused by Taenia solium larvae) and hydatid disease (caused by Echinococcus granulosis). *Albendazole* is erratically absorbed after oral administration, but absorption is enhanced by a high-fat meal. It undergoes extensive first-pass metabolism, including formation of the sulfoxide, which is also active. *Albendazole* and its metabolites are primarily excreted in the urine. When used in short-course therapy (one to three days) for nematodal infestations, adverse effects are mild and transient, and include headache and nausea. Treatment of hydatid disease (three months) has risk of hepatotoxicity and, rarely, agranulocytosis or pancytopenia. Medical treatment of neurocysticercosis is associated with inflammatory responses to dying parasites in the CNS, including headache, vomiting, hyperthermia, convulsions, and mental changes. The drug should not be given during pregnancy (see Figure 37.3) or to children under two years of age.

Study Question

Choose the ONE best answer.

37.1 A 48-year-old immigrant from Mexico presents with seizures and other neurologic symptoms. Eggs of Taenia solium are found upon examination of a stool specimen. A magnetic resonance image of the brain shows many cysts, some of which are calcified. Which one of the following drugs would be of benefit to this individual?

A. Ivermectin
B. Pyrantel pamoate
C. Albendazole
D. Diethylcarbamazine
E. Niclosamide

Correct answer = C. The symptoms and other findings for this patient are consistent with neurocysticercosis. Albendazole is the drug of choice for the treatment of this infestation. The other drugs are not effective against the larval forms of tapeworms.

37.2 A 56-year-old man from South America is found to be parasitized by both schistosomes and Taenia solium—the pork tapeworm. Which of the following antihelmintic drugs would be effective for both infestations?

A. Albendazole
B. Ivermectin
C. Mebendazole
D. Niclosamide
E. Praziquantel

Correct answer = E. Praziquantel is a primary drug for the treatment of trematode and cestode infestations. Although albendazole is effective in cysticercosis, it is not active against flukes, and this patient has no evidence of cysticercosis. Niclosamide is also active against tape worms but has no activity against blood flukes.

Antiviral Drugs

38

I. OVERVIEW

Viruses are obligate intracellular parasites. They lack both a cell wall and a cell membrane, and they do not carry out metabolic processes. Viral reproduction uses much of the host's metabolic machinery, and few drugs are selective enough to prevent viral replication without injury to the host. Therapy for viral diseases is further complicated by the fact that the clinical symptoms appear late in the course of the disease, at a time when most of the virus particles have replicated. [Note: This contrasts with bacterial diseases, in which the clinical symptoms are usually coincident with bacterial proliferation.] At this late, symptomatic stage of the viral infection, administration of drugs that block viral replication has limited effectiveness. However, some antiviral agents are useful as prophylactic agents. Only a few virus groups, including those that cause the viral infections discussed in this chapter, respond to available anitviral drugs. To assist in the review of these drugs, they are grouped according to the organisms that are affected (Figure 38.1).

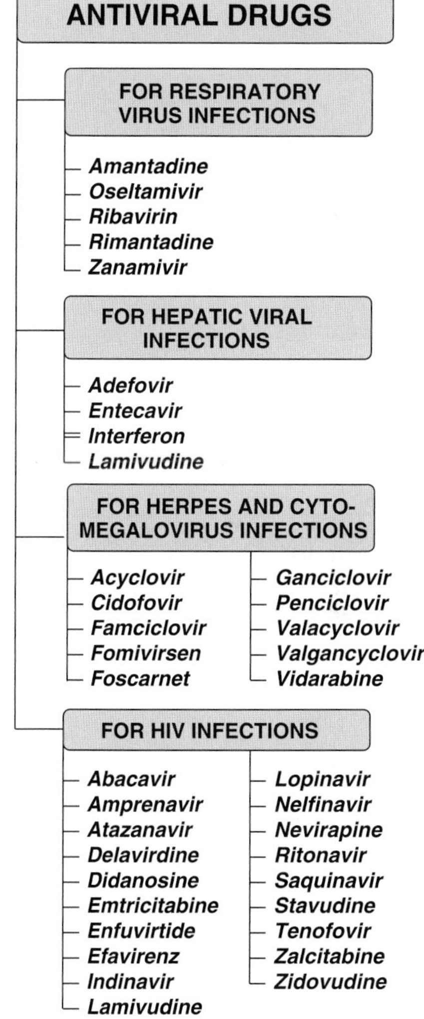

Figure 38.1
Summary of antiviral drugs. HIV = human immunodeficiency virus.

II. TREATMENT OF RESPIRATORY VIRUS INFECTIONS

Viral respiratory tract infections for which treatments exist include those of influenza types A and B and respiratory syncytial virus (RSV). [Note: Immunization against influenza A is the preferred approach. However, antiviral agents are employed when patients are allergic to the vaccine, or when the outbreak is due to an immunologic variant of the virus not covered by vaccines, or when outbreaks occur among unvaccinated individuals at risk who are in closed settings (for example, in nursing homes).]

A. Neuraminidase inhibitors

Orthomyxoviruses that cause influenza contain the enzyme neuraminidase, which is essential to the life cycle of the virus. Viral neuraminidase can be selectively inhibited by the sialic acid analogs, *oseltamivir* [os el TAM i veer] and *zanamivir* [za NA mi veer]. These drugs prevent the release of new virions, and their spread from cell to cell. Unlike the *adamantine* analogs discussed below, *oseltamivir* and *zanamivir* are effective against both type A and type B influenza viruses. They do not interfere with the immune response to influenza A vaccine. Administered prior to exposure, neuraminidase inhibitors prevent infection, and when administered within the first 24 to 48 hours of the onset of infection, they have a modest effect on the intensity and duration of symptoms.

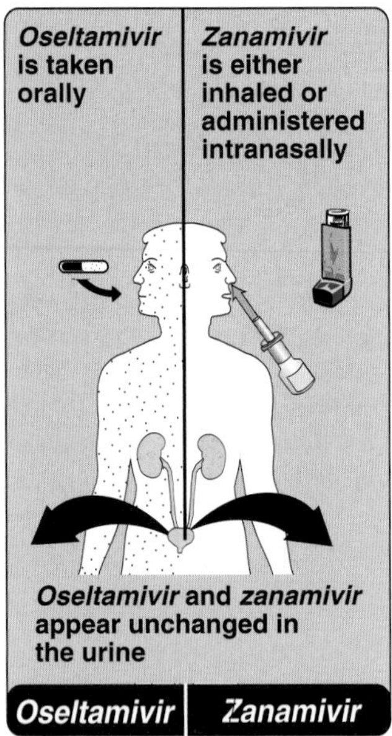

Figure 38.2
Administration and metabolism of *oseltamivir* and *zanamivir.*

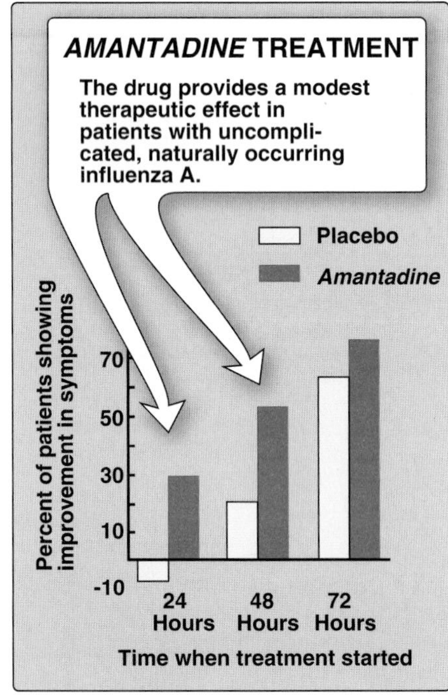

Figure 38.3
Improvement in symptoms of individuals with naturally occurring influenza infections treated with *amantadine.*

1. **Mode of action:** Influenza viruses employ a specific neuraminidase that is inserted into the host cell membrane for the purpose of releasing newly formed virions. *Oseltamivir* and *zanamivir* are transition-state analogs of the sialic acid substrate, and serve as inhibitors of the enzyme activity. Virions accumulate at the internal infected cell surface.

2. **Pharmacokinetics:** *Oseltamivir* is an orally active prodrug that is rapidly hydrolyzed by the liver to its active form. *Zanamivir,* on the other hand, is not active orally, and is either inhaled or administered intranasally. Both drugs are eliminated unchanged in the urine (Figure 38.2).

3. **Adverse effects:** The most common side effects of *oseltamivir* are gastrointestinal discomfort and nausea, which can be alleviated by taking the drug with food. *Zanamivir* is not associated with gastrointestinal disturbance, because it is administered directly to the airways. Irritation of the respiratory tract does occur, however. *Zanamivir* should be avoided in individuals with severe reactive asthma or chronic obstructive respiratory disease, because bronchospasm may occur with the risk of fatality. Neither drug has been reported to have clinically significant drug interactions.

4. **Resistance:** Mutations of the neuraminidase have been identified in adults treated with either of the neuraminidase inhibitors. These mutants, however, are often less infective and virulent than the wild type.

B. Inhibitors of viral uncoating

The therapeutic spectrum of the *adamantine* derivatives, *amantadine* [a MAN ta deen] and *rimantadine* [ri MAN ta deen], is limited to influenza A infections, for which the drugs have been shown to be equally effective in both treatment and prevention. For example, these drugs are seventy to ninety percent effective in preventing infection if treatment is begun at the time of—or prior to—exposure to the virus. Also, both drugs reduce the duration and severity of systemic symptoms if started within the first 48 hours after exposure to the virus (Figure 38.3). Neither impairs the immune response to influenza A vaccine, and either can be administered as a supplement to vaccination, thus providing protection until antibody response occurs (usually two weeks in healthy adults). Treatment is particularly useful in high-risk patients who have not been vaccinated and during epidemics. [Note: *Amantadine* is also effective in the treatment of some cases of Parkinson disease (see p. 100).]

1. **Mode of action:** The primary antiviral mechanism of *amantadine* and *rimantadine* is to block the viral membrane matrix protein, M2, which functions as an ion channel. This channel is required for the fusion of the viral membrane with the cell membrane that ultimately forms the endosome (created when the virus is internalized by endocytosis). [Note: The acid environment of the endosome is required for viral uncoating.] These drugs may also interfere with the release of new virions.

2. **Pharmacokinetics:** Both drugs are well absorbed orally. *Amantadine* distributes throughout the body and readily penetrates into the central nervous system (CNS), whereas *rimantadine* does not cross the blood-brain barrier to the same extent. *Amantadine* is not extensively metabolized. It is excreted into the urine and may accumulate to toxic levels in patients with renal failure. On the other hand, *rimantadine* is extensively metabolized by the liver, and both the metabolites and the parent drug are eliminated by the kidney (Figure 38.4).

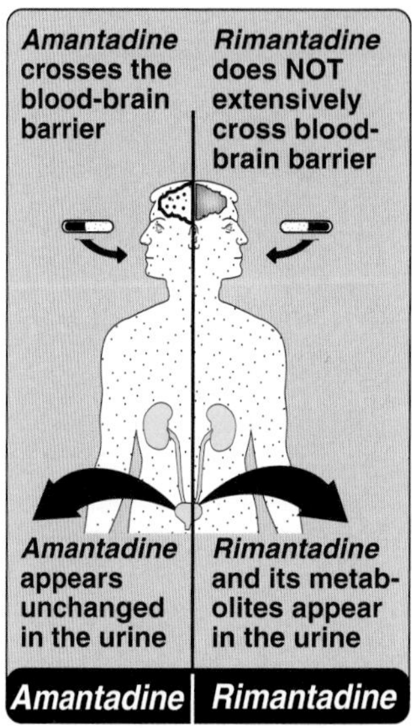

Figure 38.4
Administration and metabolism of *amantadine* and *rimantadine.*

3. **Adverse effects:** The side effects of *amantadine* are mainly associated with the CNS. Minor neurologic symptoms include insomnia, dizziness, and ataxia. More serious side effects have been reported (for example, hallucinations and seizures). The drug should be employed cautiously in patients with psychiatric problems, cerebral atherosclerosis, renal impairment, or epilepsy. *Rimantadine* causes fewer CNS reactions, because it does not efficiently cross the blood-brain barrier. Both drugs cause gastrointestinal intolerance. *Amantadine* and *rimantadine* should be used with caution in pregnant and nursing mothers, because they have been found to be embryotoxic and teratogenic in rats.

4. **Resistance:** Resistance can develop rapidly in up to fifty percent of treated individuals, and resistant strains can be readily transmitted to close contacts. Resistance has been shown to result from a change in one amino acid of the M2 matrix protein. Cross-resistance occurs between the two drugs.

C. Ribavirin

Ribavirin [rye ba VYE rin] is a synthetic guanosine analog. It is effective against a broad spectrum of RNA and DNA viruses. For example, *ribavirin* is used in treating infants and young children infected with severe RSV infections. [Note: It is not indicated for use in adults.] *Ribavirin* is also effective in chronic hepatitis C infections when used in combination with *interferon-α-2b*. *Ribavirin* may reduce the mortality and viremia of Lassa fever.

1. **Mode of action:** The mode of action of *ribavirin* has been studied only for the influenza viruses. The drug is first converted to the 5'-phosphate derivatives, the major product being the compound *ribavirin*-triphosphate, which exerts its antiviral action by inhibiting GTP formation, preventing viral mRNA capping,[1] and blocking RNA-dependent RNA polymerase. [Note: Rhinoviruses and enteroviruses, which contain preformed mRNA and do not need to synthesize mRNA in the host cell to initiate an infection, are relatively resistant to the action of *ribavirin*.]

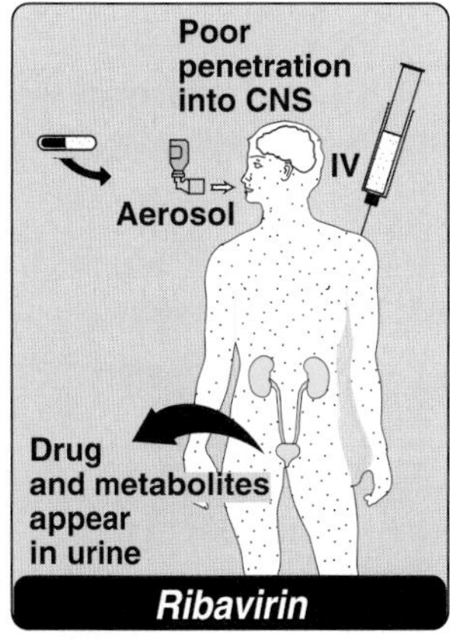

Figure 38.5
Administration and metabolism of *ribavirin*.

2. **Pharmacokinetics:** *Ribavirin* is effective orally and intravenously. Absorption is increased if the drug is taken with a fatty meal. An aerosol is used in certain respiratory viral conditions, such as the treatment of RSV infection. Studies of drug distribution in primates showed retention in all tissues, except brain. The drug and its metabolites are eliminated in the urine (Figure 38.5).

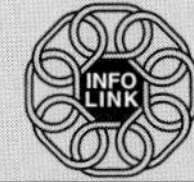

[1]See p. 423 in ***Lippincott's Illustrated Reviews: Biochemistry*** (3rd ed.) for a discussion of mRNA capping.

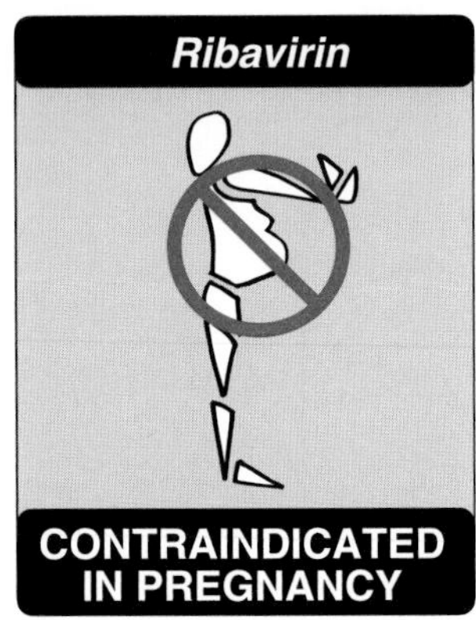

Figure 38.6
Ribavirin causes teratogenic effects.

3. **Adverse effects:** Side effects reported for oral or parenteral use of *ribavirin* have included dose-dependent transient anemia. Elevated bilirubin has been reported. The aerosol may be safer, although respiratory function in infants can deteriorate quickly after initiation of aerosol treatment. Therefore, monitoring is essential. Because of teratogenic effects in experimental animals, *ribavirin* is contraindicated in pregnancy (Figure 38.6).

III. TREATMENT OF HEPATIC VIRAL INFECTIONS

The hepatitis viruses thus far identified—A, B, C, D, and E—each have a pathogenesis specifically involving replication in and destruction of hepatocytes. Of this group, hepatitis B and hepatitis C are the most common causes of chronic hepatitis, cirrhosis, and hepatocellular carcinoma (Figure 38.7), and the are the only hepatic viral infections for which therapy is currently available. [Note: Hepatitis A is a commmonly encountered infection, but it is not a chronic disease.] Chronic hepatitis B is treated with *interferon-α* or *lamivudine*. Combination therapy of *interferon* plus *lamivudine* is no more effective than monotherapy with *lamivudine*. Chronic hepatitis C responds to the combination of *interferon-α* plus *ribavirin*.

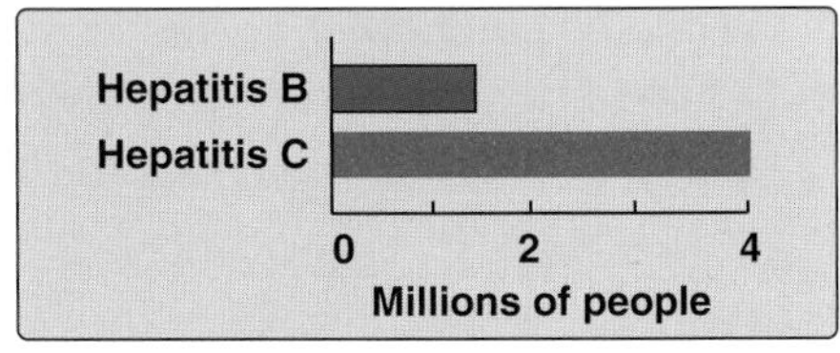

Figure 38.7
The prevalence of chronic hepatitis B and C in the United States.

A. Interferon

Interferon [in ter FEER on] is a family of naturally occurring, inducible glycoproteins that interfere with the ability of viruses to infect cells. Although *interferon* inhibits the growth of many viruses in vitro, its activity in vivo against viruses has been disappointing. The interferons are synthesized by recombinant DNA technology. At least three types of *interferon* exist, α, β, and γ (Figure 38.8). One of the fifteen *interferon-α*—*interferon-α-2b*—has been approved for treatment of hepatitis B and C, condylomata acuminata, and cancers such as hairy-cell leukemia and Kaposi sarcoma. *Interferon-β* has some effectiveness in the treatment of multiple sclerosis.

Interferon-α	*Interferon-β*	*Interferon-γ*
Chronic hepatitis B and C	Relapsing-remitting multiple sclerosis	Chronic granulomatous disease
Genital warts caused by papillomavirus		
Leukemia, hairy-cell Leukemia, chronic myelogenous		
Kaposi's sarcoma		

Figure 38.8
Some approved indications for *interferons*.

1. **Mode of action:** The antiviral mechanism is incompletely understood. It appears to involve the induction of host cell enzymes that inhibit viral RNA translation, ultimately leading to the degradation of viral mRNA and tRNA.

2. **Pharmacokinetics:** *Interferon* is not active orally, but it may be administered intralesionally, subcutaneously, or intravenously. Very little active compound is found in the plasma, and its presence is not correlated with clinical responses. Cellular uptake and metabolism by the liver and kidney account for the disappearance of interferons from the plasma. Negligible renal elimination occurs. Attachment to large polyethylene glycol molecules prolongs the half-life of *interferon*, so once-a-week dosing can be employed.

3. **Adverse effects:** Adverse effects include flu-like symptoms on injection, such as fever, chills, myalgias, arthralgias, and gastrointestinal disturbances. These symptoms subside with subsequent administrations. The principal dose-limiting toxicities are bone marrow suppression including granulocytopenia, neurotoxicity characterized by somnolence and behavioral disturbances, severe fatigue

and weight loss, autoimmune disorders such as thyroiditis, and rarely, cardiovascular problems such as congestive heart failure. Acute hypersensitivity reactions and hepatic failure are rare.

4. Drug interactions: Interferons interfere with hepatic drug metabolism, and toxic accumulations of *theophylline* have been reported. Interferons may also potentiate the myelosuppression caused by other bonemarrow-depressing agents, such as *zidovudine.*

B. Lamivudine

This cytosine analog is an inhibitor of both hepatitis B virus (HBV) DNA polymerase and human immunodeficiency virus (HIV) reverse transcriptase. *Lamivudine* [la MI vyoo deen] must be phosphorylated by host cellular enzymes to the triphosphate (active) form. This compound competitively inhibits HBV DNA polymerase at concentrations that have negligible effects on host DNA polymerase. As with many nucleotide analogs, the intracellular half-life of the triphosphate is many hours longer than its plasma half-life, which permits infrequent dosing. Chronic treatment is associated with decreased plasma HBV DNA levels, improved biochemical markers, and reduced hepatic inflammation. *Lamivudine* is well absorbed orally and is widely distributed. Its plasma half-life is about nine hours. Seventy percent is excreted unchanged in the urine. Dose reductions are necessary when there is moderate renal insufficiency (creatinine clearance less than fifty mL/min). *Lamivudine* is very well tolerated, with rare occurrences of headache and dizziness.

C. Adefovir

Adefovir dipivoxil [ah DEH for veer die pih VOCKS ill] is a nucleotide analog that is phosphorylated to adefovir diphosphate, which is then incorporated into viral DNA. This leads to termination of further DNA synthesis and prevents viral replication. *Adefovir* is administered once a day and is excreted in the urine—45 percent as the active compound. Clearance is influenced by renal function. Both decreased viral load and improved liver function occurred in patients treated with *adefovir.* As with other agents, discontinuation of *adefovir* results in severe hepatitis exacerbation in about 25 percent of patients. *Adefovir* does not seem to have significant drug interactions. The drug should be used cautiously in patients with existing renal dysfunction.

D. Entecavir

Entecavir [en TECK ah veer] is a guanosine analog approved for the treatment of HBV infections. Following intracellular phosphorylation to the triphosphate it competes with the natural substrate, deoxyguanosine triphosphate, for viral reverse transcriptase. *Entecavir* has been shown to be effective against *lamivudine*-resistant strains of HBV. Liver inflammation and scarring are improved. *Entecavir* need only be given once a day. *Entecavir* undergoes both glomerular filtration and tubular secretion. Very little, if any, drug is metabolized. Renal function must be assessed periodically and drugs that have renal toxicity should be avoided. Patients should be monitored closely for several months after discontinuation of therapy because of the possibility of severe hepatitis.

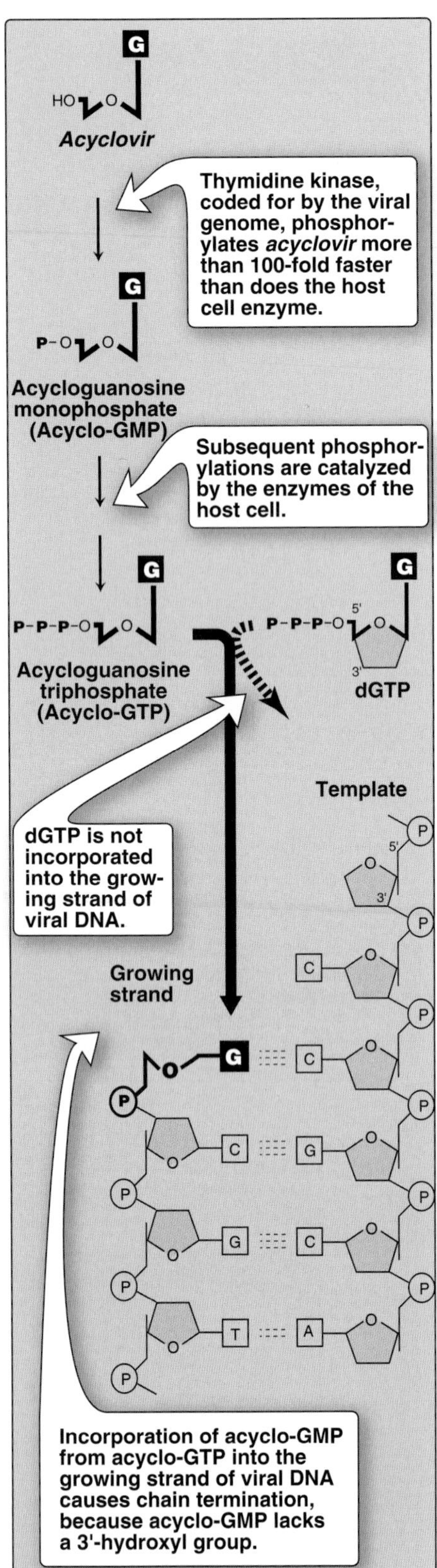

Figure 38.9
Incorporation of *acyclovir* into replicating viral DNA, causing chain termination. dGTP = deoxyguanosine triphosphate

IV. TREATMENT OF HERPESVIRUS INFECTIONS

Herpesviruses are associated with a broad spectrum of diseases—for example, cold sores, viral encephalitis, and genital infections (the latter being a hazard to the newborn during parturition). The drugs that are effective against these viruses exert their actions during the acute phase of viral infections and are without effect during the latent phase. Except for *foscarnet* and *fomivirsen*, all are purine or pyrimidine analogs that inhibit viral DNA synthesis.

A. Acyclovir

Acyclovir [ay SYE kloe ver] (acycloguanosine) is the prototypic antiherpetic therapeutic agent. It has a greater specificity than *vidarabine* against herpesviruses. Herpes simplex virus types 1 and 2 (HSV-1 and HSV-2), varicella-zoster virus (VZV), and some Epstein-Barr virus-mediated infections are sensitive to *acyclovir*. It is the treatment of choice in HSV encephalitis, and is more efficacious than *vidarabine* at increasing the rate of survival. The most common use of *acyclovir* is in therapy for genital herpes infections. It is also given prophylactically to seropositive patients before bone marrow and after heart transplants to protect such individuals during post-transplant immunosuppressive treatments.

1. **Mode of action:** *Acyclovir*, a guanosine analog that lacks a true sugar moiety, is monophosphorylated in the cell by the herpes virus-encoded enzyme, thymidine kinase (Figure 38.9). Therefore, virus-infected cells are most susceptible. The monophosphate analog is converted to the di- and triphosphate forms by the host cells. *Acyclovir* triphosphate competes with deoxyguanosine triphosphate as a substrate for viral DNA polymerase, and is itself incorporated into the viral DNA causing premature DNA-chain termination (see Figure 38.9). Irreversible binding of the *acyclovir*-containing template primer to viral DNA polymerase inactivates the enzyme. The drug is less effective against the host enzyme.

2. **Pharmacokinetics:** Administration of *acyclovir* can be by an intravenous, oral, or topical route. [Note: The efficacy of topical applications is doubtful.] The drug distributes well throughout the body, including the cerebrospinal fluid (CSF). *Acyclovir* is partially metabolized to an inactive product. Excretion into the urine occurs both by glomerular filtration and by tubular secretion (Figure 38.10). *Acyclovir* accumulates in patients with renal failure. The valyl ester, *valacyclovir* [val ay SYE kloe veer], has greater oral bioavailability than *acyclovir*. This ester is rapidly hydrolyzed to *acyclovir* and achieves levels of the latter comparable to those from intravenous *acyclovir* administration.

3. **Adverse effects:** Side effects of *acyclovir* treatment depend on the route of administration. For example, local irritation may occur from topical application; headache, diarrhea, nausea, and vomiting may result after oral administration. Transient renal dysfunction may occur at high doses or in a dehydrated patient receiving the drug intravenously. High-dose *valacyclovir* can cause gastrointestinal problems and thrombotic thrombocytopenia purpura in AIDs patients.

4. **Resistance:** Altered or deficient thymidine kinase and DNA polymerases have been found in some resistant viral strains and are most commonly isolated from immunocompromised patients. Cross-resistance to the other cyclovirs occurs. [Note: Cytomegalovirus (CMV) is resistant, because it lacks a specific viral thymidine kinase.]

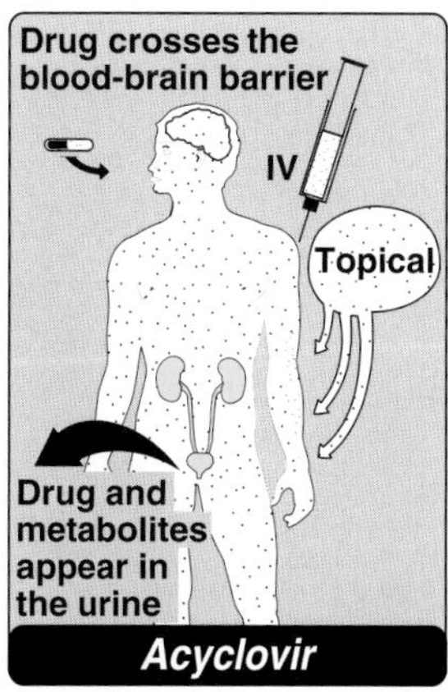

Figure 38.10
Administration and metabolism of *acyclovir.*

B. Cidofovir

Cidofovir [si DOE foe veer] is approved for treatment of CMV-induced retinitis in patients with AIDS. *Cidofovir* is a nucleotide analog of cytosine, the phosphorylation of which is not dependent on viral enzymes. It inhibits viral DNA synthesis. Slow elimination of the active intracellular metabolite permits prolonged dosage intervals and eliminates the permanent venous access used for *ganciclovir* therapy. *Cidofovir* is available for intravenous, intravitreal (injection into the eye's vitreous humor between the lens and the retina), and topical administration. *Cidofovir* produces significant toxicity to the kidney (Figure 38.11), and is contraindicated in patients with preexisting renal impairment, or in those who are taking concurrent nephrotoxic drugs including nonteroidal anti-inflammatory drugs. Neutropenia, metabolic acidosis, and ocular hypotony also occur. *Probenecid* is coadministered with *cidofovir* to reduce the risk of nephrotoxicity, but *probenecid* itself causes rash, headache, fever, and nausea. Since the introduction of HAART (highly active antiretroviral therapy), the prevalence of CMV infections in immunocompromised hosts has markedly declined, and the importance of *cidofovir* in the treatment of these patients has also diminished.

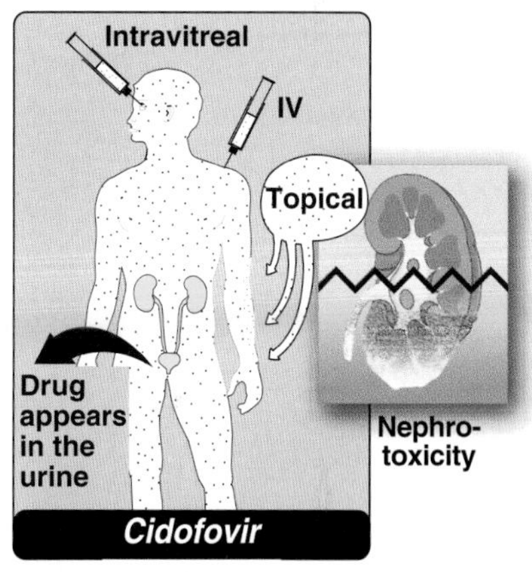

Figure 38.11
Administration, metabolism, and

C. Fomivirsen

Fomivirsen [foe MI veer sen] is an antisense oligonucleotide directed against CMV mRNA. Its use is limited to those who cannot tolerate—or have failed—other therapies for CMV retinitis. A two- to four-week hiatus after discontinuing *cidofovir* is desirable to reduce toxicity. The drug is administered intravitreally. The common adverse effects include iritis, vitritis, and changes in vision.

D. Foscarnet

Unlike most of the antiviral agents, *foscarnet* [fos KAR net] is not a purine or pyrimidine analog. Instead, it is phosphonoformate—a pyrophosphate derivative. *Foscarnet* has broad in vitro antiviral activity. It is apporoved for CMV retinitis in immunocompromised hosts and for *acyclovir*-resistant HSV and herpes zoster infections. *Foscarnet* works by reversibly inhibiting viral DNA and RNA polymerases, thereby terminating chain elongation. Mutation of the polymerase structure is responsible for resistant viruses. [Note: Cross-resistance between *foscarnet* and *ganciclovir* or *acyclovir* is uncommon.] *Foscarnet* is poorly absorbed orally and must be injected intravenously. It must also be given frequently to avoid relapse when plasma levels fall. It is dispersed throughout the body, and greater than ten percent enters the bone matrix, from which it slowly leaves. The parent drug is eliminated by glomerular filtration and tubular secretion into the urine (Figure 38.12). Adverse effects include nephrotoxicity, anemia, nausea, and fever. Due to chelation with divalent cations, hypocalcemia, and hypomagnesemia are also seen. In addition, hypokalemia, hypo- and hyperphosphatemia, seizures, and arrhythmias have been reported.

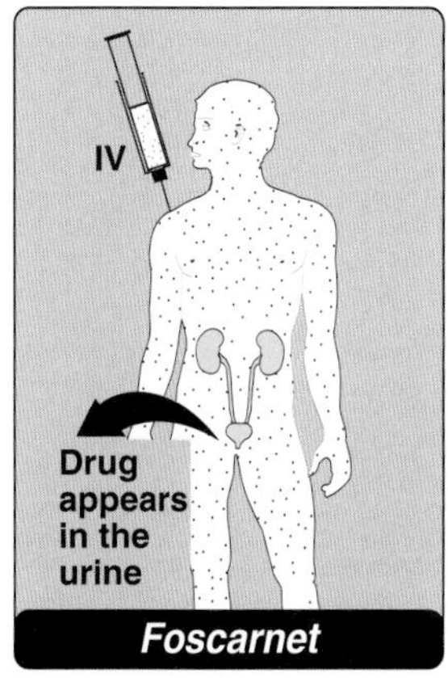

Figure 38.12
Administration and metabolism of *foscarnet.*

E. Ganciclovir

Ganciclovir [gan SYE kloe veer] is an analog of *acyclovir* that has eight- to twenty-times greater activity against CMV—the only viral infection for which it is approved. It is currently available for treatment of CMV retinitis in immunocompromised patients and for CMV prophylaxis in transplant patients.

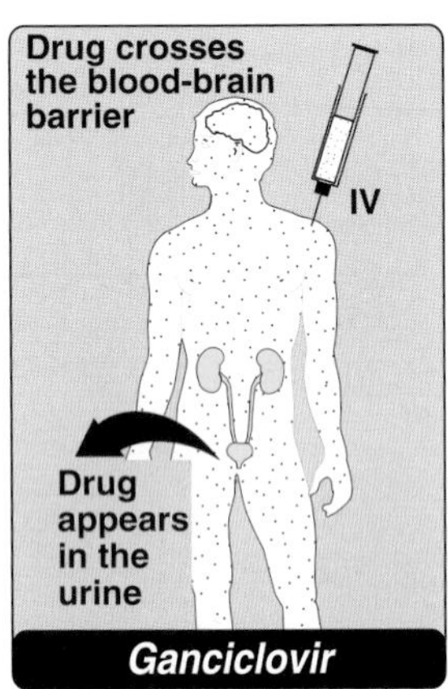

Figure 38.13
Administration and metabolism of *ganciclovir.*

1. **Mode of action:** Like *acyclovir*, *ganciclovir* is activated through conversion to the nucleoside triphosphate by viral and cellular enzymes, the actual pathway depending on the virus. CMV is deficient in thymidine kinase and, therefore, forms the triphosphate by another route. The nucleotide competitively inhibits viral DNA polymerase and can be incorporated into the DNA, thereby decreasing the rate of chain elongation.

2. **Pharmacokinetics:** *Ganciclovir* is administered intravenously, and distributes throughout the body, including the CSF. Excretion into the urine occurs through glomerular filtration and tubular secretion (Figure 38.13). Like *acyclovir*, *ganciclovir* accumulates in patients with renal failure. *Valganciclovir* [val gan SYE kloe veer] is the valyl ester of *ganciclovir*. Like *valacyclovir*, *valganciclovir* has high oral bioavailability, because rapid hydrolysis in the intestine and liver after oral administration leads to high levels of *ganciclovir*.

3. **Adverse effects:** Adverse effects include severe, dose-dependent neutropenia. [Note: Combined treatment with *zidovudine*, *azathioprine*, or *mycophenolate mofetil* can result in additive neutropenia.] *Ganciclovir* is carcinogenic as well as embryotoxic and teratogenic in experimental animals.

4. **Resistance:** Resistant CMV strains have been detected that have lower levels of *ganciclovir* triphosphate.

F. Penciclovir and famciclovir

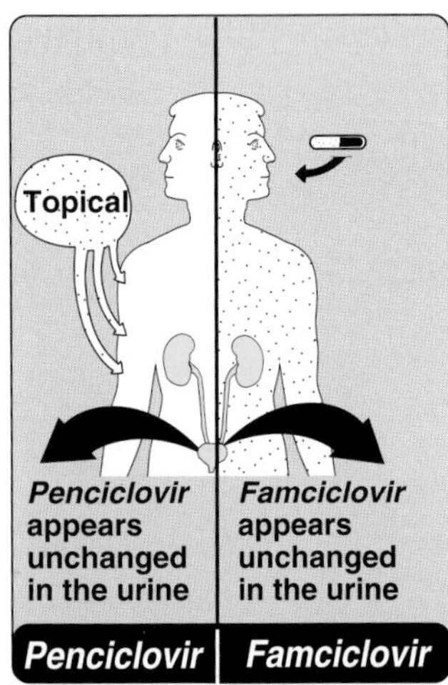

Figure 38.14
Administration and metabolism of *penciclovir* and *famciclovir*.

Penciclovir [pen SYE kloe veer] is an acyclic guanosine nucleoside derivative that is active against HSV-I, HSV-2, and VZV. *Penciclovir* is only administered topically (Figure 38.14). It is monophosphorylated by viral thymidine kinase, and cellular enzymes form the nucleoside triphosphate, which inhibits HSV DNA polymerase. *Penciclovir* triphosphate has an intracellular half-life twenty- to thirty-fold longer than does *acyclovir* triphosphate. *Penciclovir* is negligibly absorbed from topical application and is well tolerated. Both pain and healing are shortened approximately one-half day in duration compared to placebo-treated subjects. *Famciclovir* [fam SYE kloe veer], another acyclic analog of 2'-deoxyguanosine, is a prodrug that is metabolized to the active *penciclovir*. The antiviral spectrum is similar to that of *ganciclovir*, but it is presently approved only for treatment of acute herpes zoster. The drug is effective orally (see Figure 38.14). Adverse effects include headaches and nausea. Studies in experimental animals have shown an increased incidence of mammary adenocarcinomas and testicular toxicity.

G. Vidarabine (ara-A)

Vidarabine [vye DARE a been] (*arabinofuranosyl adenine*, *ara-A*, *adenine arabinoside*) is one of the most effective of the nucleoside analogs. However, it has been supplanted clinically by *acyclovir*, which is more efficacious and safe. Although *vidarabine* is active against HSV-1, HSV-2, and VZV, its use is limited to treatment of immunocompromised patients with herpetic and vaccinial keratitis, and in HSV keratoconjunctivitis. [Note: *Vidarabine* is only available as an opthalmic ointment.] *Vidarabine*, an adenosine analog, is converted in the cell to its 5'-triphosphate analog (*ara*-ATP), which is postulated to inhibit viral DNA synthesis. Some resistant HSV mutants have been detected that have altered DNA polymerase. Figure 38.15 summarizes selected antiviral agents.

Antiviral drug	Mechanism of action	Viruses or diseases affected
Acyclovir	Metabolized to acyclovir triphosphate, which inhibits viral DNA polymerase	Herpes simplex, varicella-zoster, cytomegalovirus
Amantadine	Blockage of the M2 protein ion channel and its ability to modulate intracellular pH	Influenza A
Cidofovir	Inhibition of viral DNA polymerase	Cytomegalovirus; indicated only for virus-induced retinitis
Famciclovir	Same as penciclovir	Herpes simplex, varicella-zoster
Foscarnet	Inhibition of viral DNA polymerase and reverse transcriptase at the pyrophosphate-binding site	Cytomegalovirus, acyclovir-resistant herpes simplex, acyclovir-resistant varicella-zoster
Ganciclovir	Metabolized to ganciclovir triphosphate,	Cytomegalovirus
Interferon-α	Induction of cellular enzymes that interfere with viral protein synthesis	Hepatitis B and C, human herpesvirus 8, papilloma virus, Kaposi's sarcoma, hairy-cell leukemia, chronic myelogenous leukemia
Lamivudine	Inhibition of viral DNA polymerase and reverse transcriptase	Hepatitis B (chronic cases), human immunodeficiency virus type 1
Oseltamivir	Inhibition of viral neuramidase	Influenza A
Penciclovir	Metabolized to penciclovir triphosphate, which inhibits viral DNA polymerase	Herpes simplex
Ribavirin	Interference with viral messenger RNA	Lassa fever, hantavirus (hemorrhagic fever renal syndrome) hepatitis C (in chronic cases in combination with interferon-α RSV in children and infants
Rimantadine	Blockage of the M2 protein ion channel and its ability to modulate intracellular pH	Influenza A
Valacyclovir	Same as acyclovir	Herpes simplex, varicella-zoster, cytomegalovirus
Vidarabine	inhibits viral DNA synthesis	HSV-1, HSV-2, and VZV, its use is limited to treatment of immunocompromised patients with HSV keratitis
Zanamivir	Inhibition of viral neuramidase	Influenza A

Figure 38.15
Summary of selected antiviral agents.

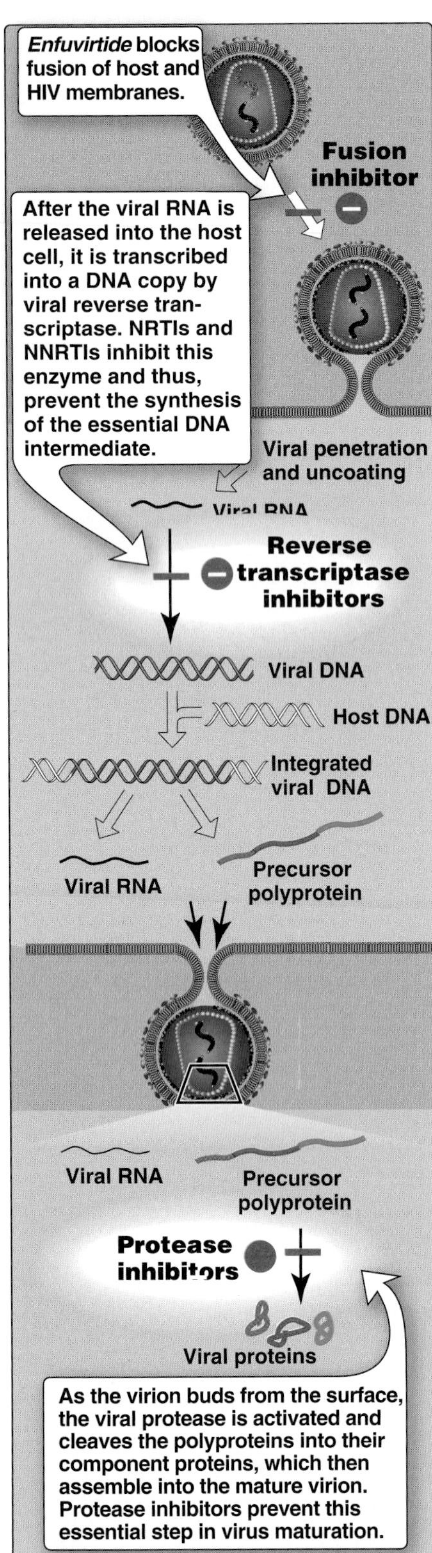

Figure 38.16
Drugs used to prevent HIV from replicating. [NRTI = nucleoside and nucleotide reverse transcriptase inhibitor, NNRTI = nonnucleoside reverse transcriptase inhibitor.

V. OVERVIEW OF THE TREATMENT FOR AIDS

Prior to approval of *zidovudine* in 1987, treatment of human immunodeficiency virus (HIV) infections focused on decreasing the occurrence of opportunistic infections that caused a high degree of morbidity and mortality in AIDS patients rather than on inhibiting HIV itself. Today, the viral life cycle is understood (Figure 38.16), and a highly active regimen is employed that uses combinations of drugs to suppress replication of HIV and restore a degree of immunocompetency to the host. This multidrug regimen is commonly referred to as "highly active antiretroviral therapy," or HAART (Figure 38.17). There are three classes of antiretroviral drugs, each of which targets one of two viral processes. These classes of drugs are nucleoside and nucleotide reverse transcriptase inhibitors (NRTIs), non-nucleoside reverse transcriptase inhibitors (NNRTIs), and protease inhibitors (PIs). The current recommendation for primary therapy is to administer two NRTIs with either a PI or a NNRTI. Selection of the appropriate combination is based on genotypic and phenotypic characteristics of the virus, viral load, patient factors such as disease symptoms and concurrent illnesses, impact of drug interactions, and ease of adherence to a frequently complex administration regimen. The principles that govern the use of multidrug therapy are 1) maximize the inhibition of viral replication and 2) minimize drug toxicities.

VI. NRTIs USED TO TREAT AIDS

Nucleoside and nucleotide reverse transcriptase inhibitors (NRTIs) are analogs of native ribosides (nucleosides or nucleotides containing ribose), which all lack a 3'-hydroxyl group. Once they enter cells, they are phosphorylated by a variety of cellular enzymes to the corresponding triphosphate analog, which is preferentially incorporated into the viral DNA by virus reverse transcriptase.[2] Because the 3'-hydroxyl group is not present, a 3'-5'-phosphodiester bond between an incoming nucleoside triphosphate and the growing DNA chain cannot be formed, and DNA chain elongation is terminated. Affinities of the drugs for many host cell DNA polymerases are lower than they are for HIV reverse transcriptase, although mitochondrial DNA polymerase γ appears to be susceptible at therapeutic concentrations. Many of the toxicities of the NRTIs are believed to be due to inhibition of the mitochondrial DNA polymerase in certain tissues. When more than one NRTI is given, care is taken not to have overlapping toxicities. Except for *lamivudine* and *abacavir*, all the NRTIs have been associated with a potentially fatal liver toxicity characterized by lactic acidosis and hepatomegaly with steatosis.

A. Zidovudine (AZT)

One of the mainstays for treatment of HIV infection and AIDS is the pyrimidine analog, *3'-azido-3'-deoxythymidine* (*AZT*). *AZT* has the generic name of *zidovudine* [zye DOE vyoo deen]. *AZT* is approved for use in children and adults and to prevent prenatal infection in pregnancy. It is also recommended for prophylaxis in individuals exposed to HIV infection. When used in HAART, *AZT* decreases the viral load and increases the number of CD4+ cells.[3] Presently, the only clinical use for *AZT* is in the treatment of patients infected with HIV.

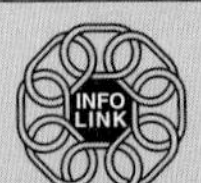

[2]See p. 303 in ***Lippincott's Illustrated Reviews: Microbiology*** for a discussion of viral reverse transcriptase.
[3]See p. 367 in ***Lippincott's Illustrated Reviews: Microbiology*** for a discussion of the decline in CD4+ cells in AIDS.

1. **Mode of action:** *AZT* must be converted to the corresponding nucleoside triphosphate by mammalian thymidine kinase for it to exert its antiviral activity. The relative lack of discrimination of the viral reverse transcriptase is believed to favor the introduction of *AZT* into virus-catalyzed DNA synthesis—the cellular DNA polymerase is more selective. In addition, the phosphorylation of deoxythymidylic acid (dTMP) to the corresponding diphosphate (dTDP) is inhibited by the azido-deoxythymidine monophosphate (*AZT*-MP).

2. **Pharmacokinetics:** The drug is well absorbed after oral administration. If taken with food, peak levels may be lower, but the total amount of drug absorbed is not affected. Penetration across the blood-brain barrier is excellent, and the drug has a half-life of one hour. The intracellular half-life, however, is approximately three hours. Most of the *AZT* is glucuronylated by the liver and then excreted in the urine (Figure 38.18).

3. **Adverse effects:** In spite of its seeming specificity, *AZT* is toxic to bone marrow. For example, severe anemia and leukopenia occur in patients receiving high doses. Headaches are also common. Seizures have been reported in patients with advanced AIDS. The toxicity of *AZT* is potentiated if glucuronylation is decreased by co-administration of drugs like *probenecid*, *acetaminophen*, *lorazepam*, *indomethacin*, and *cimetidine*. [Note: These drugs are themselves glucuronylated and, thus, can interfere with the glucuronylation of *AZT*. They should be avoided or used with caution in patients receiving *AZT*.] Both *stavudine* and *ribavirin* are activated by the same intracellular pathways, and should not be given with *AZT*.

4. **Resistance:** Resistance develops slowly over time, with approximately one-third of patients harboring resistant strains after one year of monotherapy. Resistance is associated with mutations at several codons. Cross-resistance to other nucleoside analogs also occurs.

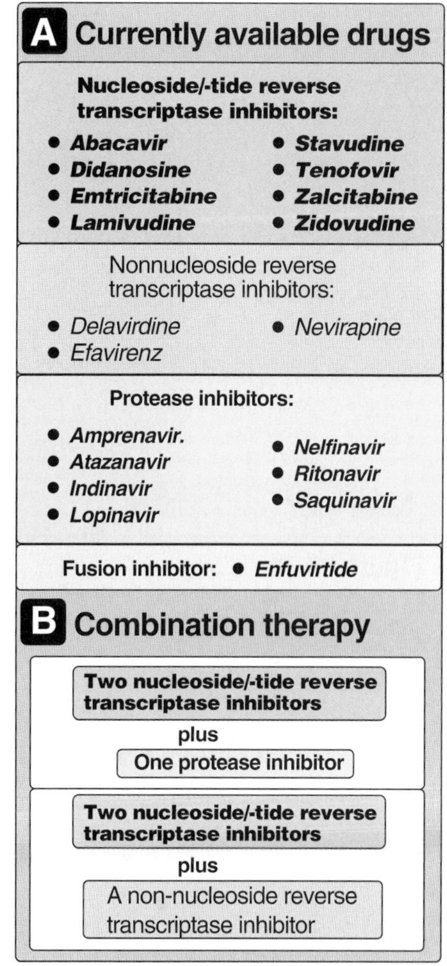

A Currently available drugs
Nucleoside/-tide reverse transcriptase inhibitors:
• Abacavir
• Didanosine
• Emtricitabine
• Lamivudine
• Stavudine
• Tenofovir
• Zalcitabine
• Zidovudine
Nonnucleoside reverse transcriptase inhibitors:
• Delavirdine
• Efavirenz
• Nevirapine
Protease inhibitors:
• Amprenavir.
• Atazanavir
• Indinavir
• Lopinavir
• Nelfinavir
• Ritonavir
• Saquinavir
Fusion inhibitor: • Enfuvirtide
B Combination therapy
Two nucleoside/-tide reverse transcriptase inhibitors
plus
One protease inhibitor
Two nucleoside/-tide reverse transcriptase inhibitors
plus
A non-nucleoside reverse transcriptase inhibitor

Figure 38.17
Highly active antiretroviral therapy (HAART).

B. Didanosine (ddI)

The second drug approved to treat HIV-1 infection was *didanosine* [dye DAN oh seen] (*dideoxyinosine*, *ddI*), which is missing both the 2'- and 3'-hydroxyl groups. Like *AZT*, *ddI* is administered along with other antiretroviral drugs and has demonstrated effectiveness in adults and children. Its activity is confined to HIV-1.

1. **Mechanism of action:** Upon entry into the host cell, *ddI* is biotransformed into dideoxyadenosine triphosphate (ddATP) through a series of reactions that involve phosphorylation of the *ddI*, amination to dideoxyadenosine monophosphate, and further phosphorylation. Like AZT, the resulting ddATP is incorporated into the DNA chain, causing termination of chain elongation.

2. **Pharmacokinetics:** Due to its acid lability, *ddI* is administered as either chewable, buffered tablets or in a buffered solution. Absorption is good if taken in the fasting state, but food causes decreased absorption. The drug penetrates into the CSF, but to a lesser extent than does *AZT*. About 55 percent of the parent drug

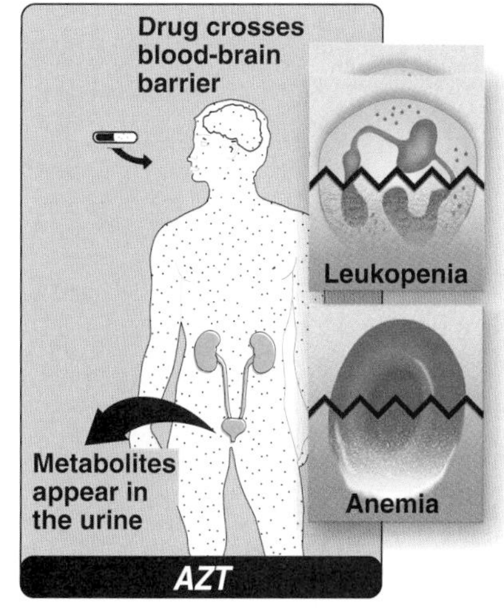

Figure 38.18
Administration, metabolism, and toxicity of *zidovudine (AZT)*.

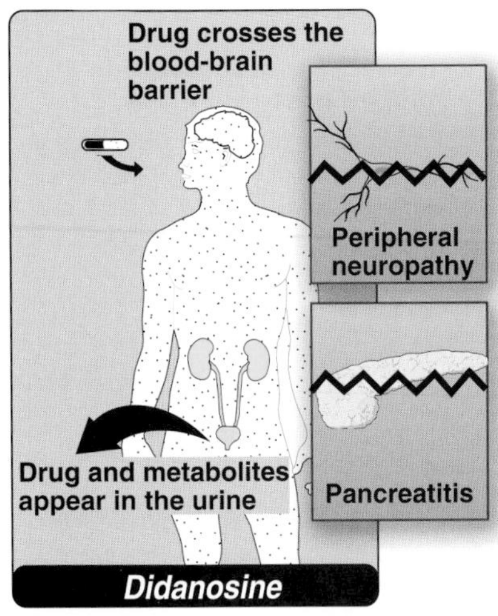

Figure 38.19
Administration, metabolism, and toxicity of *didanosine*.

appears in the urine (Figure 38.19). The present formulation contains considerable quantities of both phenylalanine and sodium, and it should be avoided in patients with phenylketonuria or sodium-restricted diets.

4. **Adverse effects:** Pancreatitis, which may be fatal, is a major toxicity of *ddI* treatment and requires monitoring of serum amylase. The dose-limiting toxicity of *ddI* is peripheral neuropathy. [Note: The buffering of stomach contents may interfere in the absorption of other drugs that require an acidic milieu for absorption, such as *ketoconazole*.] Because of its similar adverse effect profile, the concurrent use of *zalcitabine* is contraindicated.

5. **Resistance:** Viral isolates from patients who have undergone prolonged therapy with *ddI* contain reverse transcriptase with amino acid substitutions. Cross-resistance with other nucleoside agents has been reported.

C. Zalcitabine (ddC)

An analog of deoxycytidine, *zalcitabine* [zal SITE a been] (*dideoxycytidine*, *ddC*) is used with *AZT*. Like other drugs in this group, it is converted to the active triphosphate (ddCTP), which terminates chain elongation when incorporated into viral DNA and also inhibits viral reverse transcriptase. Point mutations in the reverse transcriptase lead to resistance. *ddC* is very well absorbed orally, but food or magnesium/aluminum-containing antacids reduces absorption. The drug is distributed throughout the body, but penetration into the CSF is lower than that obtained with *AZT*. Some of the drug is metabolized to the inactive dideoxyuridine (ddU). The urine is the main route of excretion of *ddC*, although fecal elimination of the drug, along with its metabolite, ddU, occurs (Figure 38.20). Rash and stomatitis are common but resolve on continued treatment. Peripheral neuropathy is the major toxicity and is probably a consequence of inhibition of the mammalian mitochondrial DNA polymerase γ. Pancreatitis resulting in death has occurred, especially if *ddC* is given with *pentamidine*. Concomitant use of *lamivudine* is not recommended.

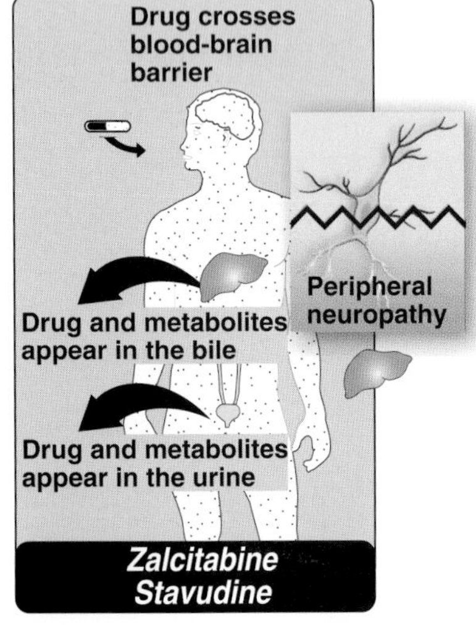

Figure 38.20
Administration, metabolism, and toxicity of *zalcitabine* and *stavudine*.

D. Stavudine (d4T)

Stavudine [STAV yoo deen] (*d4T*) is an analog of thymidine, in which a double bond joins the 2' and 3' carbons of the sugar. Like the others in this group of drugs, *d4T* must be converted by cellular kinases to the triphosphate (d4TTP), which inhibits the reverse transcriptase, causing DNA chain termination. In addition, it inhibits cellular enzymes such as the β and γ DNA polymerases, thus reducing mitochondrial DNA synthesis. The drug is almost completely absorbed on oral ingestion and is not affected by food. *d4T* penetrates the blood-brain barrier. About half of the parent drug can be accounted for in the urine (see Figure 38.20). Renal impairment interferes with clearance. The major and most common clinical toxicity is peripheral neuropathy.

E. Lamivudine (3TC)

Lamivudine [la MI vyoo deen] (*2'-deoxy-3'-thiacytidine, 3TC*) is approved for treatment of HIV in combination with *AZT*, but should not be used with ddC. This dideoxynucleoside terminates the synthesis of the proviral DNA chain, and also inhibits the reverse transcriptase of both HIV and HBV. However, it does not affect mitochondrial DNA synthesis or bone marrow precursor cells. A mutation at viral codon 184 confers a high degree of resistance to *3TC* but, more importantly, restores sensitivity to *AZT*. *3TC* has good bioavailability on oral administration and depends on the kidney for excretion. *3TC* is well tolerated.

F. Abacavir

Abacavir [a ba KA veer] is a guanosine analog available for children and adults with AIDS who cannot tolerate, or who are failing, current regimens. There may be some cross-resistance with strains resistant to *AZT* and *3TC*. *Abacavir* is well absorbed orally. Most of the drug is metabolized by non-cytochrome P450-dependent reactions. A carboxylic acid derivative and a glucuronylated form have been identified. Common side effects include gastrointestinal disturbances, headache, and dizziness. Approximately three percent of patients exhibit drug fever, gastrointestinal symptoms, malaise, and sometimes a rash. Sensitized individuals are never rechallenged, because of rapidly-appearing, severe reactions that lead to death.

G. Tenofovir

Tenofovir [te NOE fo veer] is the first approved drug that is a nucleotide analog—namely, an acyclic nucleoside phosphonate analog of adenosine-5'-monophosphate. It is converted by cellular enzymes to the diphosphate, which is the inhibitor of HIV reverse transcriptase. Cross-resistance with other NRTIs may occur, but some *AZT*-resistant strains retain susceptibility to *tenofovir*. *Tenofovir* should be taken with a meal to increase bioavailability. Most of the drug is recovered unchanged in the urine, and elimination is by filtration and active secretion. Gastrointestinal complaints are frequent and include nausea, diarrhea, and vomiting (Figure 38.21).

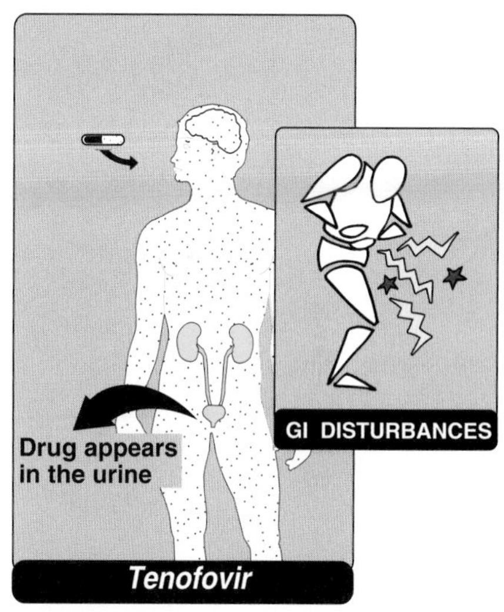

Figure 38.21
Administration, metabolism, and toxicity of *tenofovir*.

H. Emtricitabine

Emtricitabine [em tri SIGH ta been], a fluoro-derivative of *lamivudine*, inhibits both HIV and HBV reverse transcriptase. In a small clinical trial it was shown to be at least as effective as *lamivudine* in the treatment of HIV-infected individuals. *Emtricitabine* is orally active, with a mean bioavailability of 93 percent. Plasma half-life is about 10 hours, whereas it has a long intracellular half-life of 39 hours. Once-a-day dosing makes this unlike most other anti-HIV drugs. *Emtricitabine* is eliminated essentially unchanged in the urine. It does not affect CYP450 isozymes, and has no significant interactions with other drugs. Headache, diarrhea, nausea, and rash are its most common adverse effects. *Emtricitabine* causes hyperpigmentation of the soles and palms, and has been associated with lactic acidosis, fatty liver, and hepatomegaly. Withdrawal of *emtricitabine* in HBV-infected patients may result in worsening of the hepatitis.

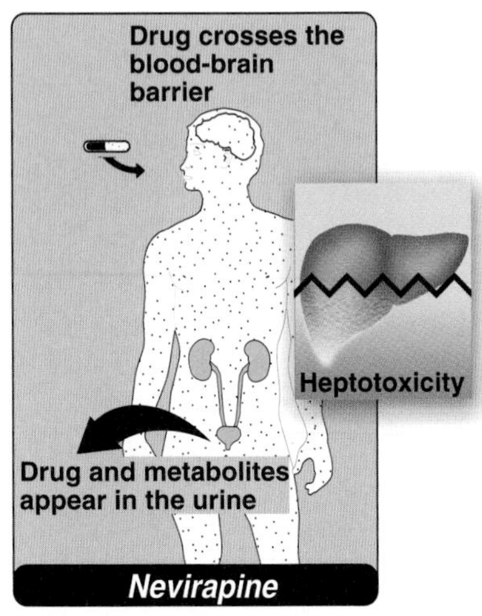

Figure 38.22
Administration, metabolism, and toxicity of *nevirapine*.

VII. NNRTIS USED TO TREAT AIDS

Non-nucleoside reverse transcriptase inhibitors (NNRTIs) are highly selective, noncompetitive inhibitors of HIV-1 reverse transcriptase. They bind to HIV reverse transcriptase at a site adjacent to the active site, inducing a conformational change that results in enzyme inhibition. They do not require activation by cellular enzymes. Their major advantage is their lack of effect on the host blood-forming elements, and lack of cross-resistance with NRTIs. These drugs, however, do have common characteristics that include cross-resistance, drug interactions, and a high incidence of hypersensitivity reactions, including rash.

A. Nevirapine

Nevirapine [ne VYE ra peen] is used in combination with other antiretroviral drugs for the treatment of HIV-1 infections in adults and children. It has recently been shown to be effective in reducing vertical transmission during pregnancy and may be used as a substitute for *AZT* for this purpose.

1. **Pharmacokinetics:** *Nevirapine* is well absorbed orally, and its absorption is not affected by food and antacids. The lipophilic nature of *nevirapine* accounts for its entrance into the fetus and mother's milk and for its wide tissue distribution, including the CNS. *Nevirapine* is dependent upon metabolism for elimination; most of the drug is excreted in the urine as the glucuronides of hydroxylated metabolites (Figure 38.22).

2. **Adverse effects:** The most frequently observed side effects are rash, fever, headache, and elevated serum transaminases. Severe dermatologic effects have been encountered, including Stevens-Johnson syndrome and toxic epidermal necrolysis. A fourteen-day titration period at one-half the dose is mandatory to reduce the risk of serious epidermal reactions. Fatal hepatotoxicity has occurred, and serum transaminase activity should be monitored closely during the first six months of therapy. *Nevirapine* is an inducer of the CYP3A4 family of cytochrome P450 drug-metabolizing enzymes. No dosage adjustments are necessary when *nevirapine* is given concomitantly with NRTIs, such as *ddI* or *AZT*. *Nevirapine* does increase the metabolism of protease inhibitors, but most combinations do not require dosage adjustment. *Nevirapine* should not be used with *saquinavir* because of the latter's low bioavailability. *Nevirapine* increases the metabolism of a number of drugs, such as oral contraceptives, *ketoconazole*, *methadone*, *metronidazole*, *quinidine*, *theophylline*, and *warfarin*.

B. Delavirdine

Delavirdine [de la VIR deen] has not undergone clinical trials as extensive as those of *nevirapine*, but in one study, *delavirdine* added to *AZT* and *ddI* was more effective than the NRTIs alone. As with other members of the class, resistance develops rapidly with monotherapy.

1. **Pharmacokinetics:** *Delavirdine* is rapidly absorbed after oral administration and is unaffected by the presence of food. It is extensively bound to plasma albumin (98 percent). *Delavirdine* is extensively metabolized, and very little is excreted as the parent compound. Fecal and urinary excretion each account for approximately one-half the elimination (Figure 38.23).

2. **Adverse effects:** Rash is the most common side effect of *delavirdine*. Nausea, dizziness, and headache have also been reported. *Delavirdine* is an inhibitor of cytochrome P450-mediated drug metabolism, including that of protease inhibitors. Although *ritonavir* levels are not altered significantly by the presence of *delavirdine*, the levels of *saquinavir* and *indinavir* are significantly increased. *Fluoxetine* and *ketoconazole* increase plasma levels of *delavirdine*, whereas *phenytoin*, *phenobarbital*, and *carbamazepine* result in substantial decreases in plasma levels of *delavirdine*.

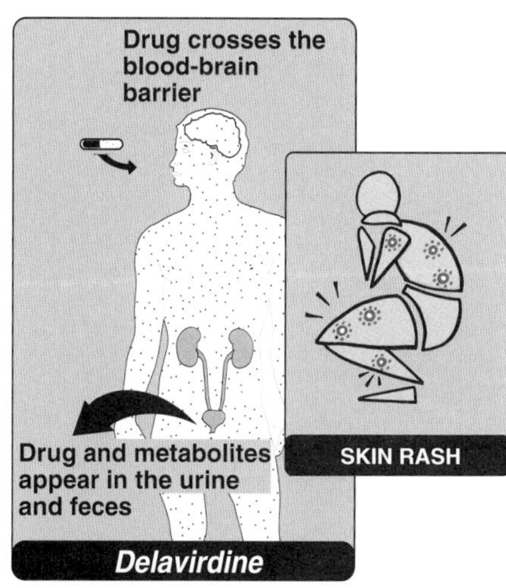

Figure 38.23
Administration, metabolism, and toxicity of *delavirdine*.

C. Efavirenz

Efavirenz [e fa VEER enz] treatment results in increases in CD4+ cell counts, and a decrease in viral load, comparable to that achieved by protease inhibitors when used in combination with NRTIs.

1. **Pharmacokinetics:** Following oral administration, *efavirenz* is well distributed, including to the CNS. Bioavailability is enhanced when taken with a high fat meal. Most of the drug is bound to plasma albumin (99 percent) at therapeutic doses. A half-life of more than forty hours accounts for its recommended once-a-day dosing. *Efavirenz* is extensively metabolized to inactive products.

2. **Adverse effects:** Most adverse effects are tolerable and are associated with the CNS, including dizziness, headache, vivid dreams, and loss of concentration. Nearly half of the patients experience these complaints, which usually resolve within a few weeks. Rash is the other most common side effect, with an incidence of approximately 25 percent. Severe, life-threatening reactions are rare. Pregnancy should be avoided in women who are taking *efavirenz*. *Efavirenz* is a modest inducer of cytochrome P450; therefore, the dose of *indinavir* may need to be increased when given with *efavirenz*.

VIII. HIV PROTEASE INHIBITORS

Inhibitors of HIV protease have significantly altered the course of this devastating viral disease. Within a year of their introduction in 1995, the number of deaths in the United States due to AIDS declined, although the trend appears to be leveling off (Figure 38.24).

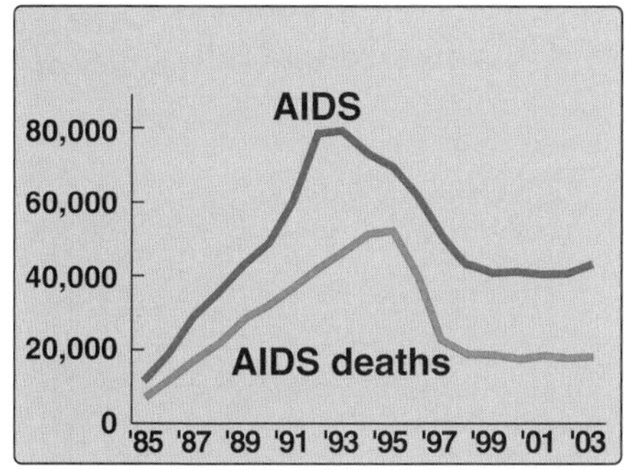

Figure 38.24
Estimated number of AIDS cases and deaths due to AIDS in the Unite States. Data on deaths were unreliable until 1987.

A. Overview

These potent agents have several common features that characterize their pharmacology.

1. **Mechanism of action:** All the drugs in this group are reversible inhibitors of the HIV aspartyl protease—the viral enzyme responsible for cleavage of the viral polyprotein into a number of essential enzymes (reverse transcriptase, protease, and integrase) and several structural proteins. The protease inhibitors exhibit at least a thousand-fold greater affinity for HIV-1 and HIV-2 enzymes than they have for comparable human proteases, such as renin and cathepsin D/E. This accounts for their selective toxicity. The inhibition prevents maturation of the viral particles and results in the production of non-infectious virions. Except for the hard-gelatin capsule of *saquinavir* (which has poor bioavailability), treatment of antiretrovirally naïve patients (that is, patients who have never had HIV therapy) with a protease inhibitor and two NRTIs results in a decrease in the plasma viral load to undetectable levels in 60 to 95 percent of patients. Treatment failures under these conditions are most likely due to a lack of patient adherence.

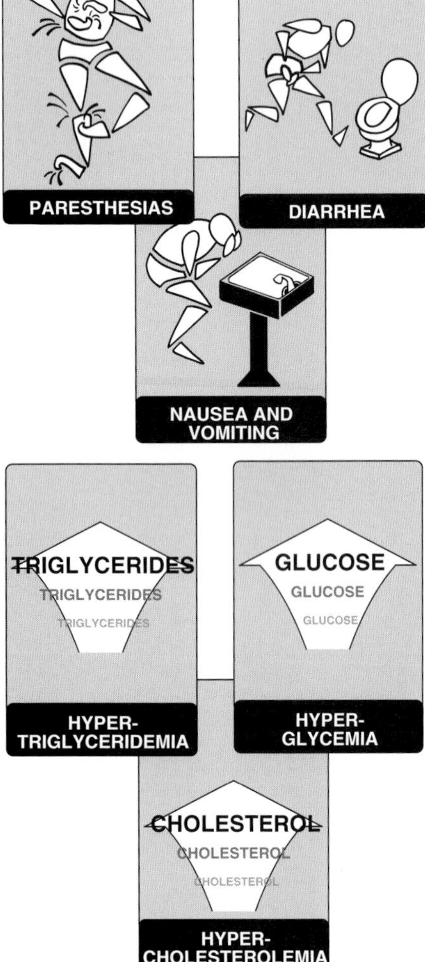

Figure 38.25
Some adverse effects of the HIV protease inhibitors.

2. **Pharmacokinetics:** Most protease inhibitors have poor oral bioavailability. High-fat meals substantially increase the bioavailability of some, such as *nelfinavir* and *saquinavir*, whereas the bioavailability of *indinavir* is decreased, and others are essentially unaffected. All are substrates for the CYP3A4 isozyme of cytochrome P450, and individual protease inhibitors are also metabolized by other P450 isozymes. Metabolism is extensive, and very little of the protease inhibitors are excreted unchanged in the urine. Dosage adjustments are unnecessary in renal impairment. Distribution into some tissues may be affected by the fact that the protease inhibitors are substrates for the P-glycoprotein multidrug efflux pump. Presence of this pump in endothelial cells of capillaries in the brain may limit protease inhibitor access to the CNS. The HIV protease inhibitors are all substantially bound to plasma proteins, specifically α_1-acid glycoprotein. This may be clinically important, because the concentration of α_1-acid glycoprotein increases in response to trauma and surgery.

3. **Adverse effects:** Protease inhibitors commonly cause paresthesias, nausea, vomiting, and diarrhea (Figure 38.25). Disturbances in glucose and lipid metabolism also occur, including diabetes, hypertriacylglycerolemia, and hypercholesterolemia. Chronic administration results in fat redistribution, including loss of fat from the extremities and its accumulation in the abdomen and the base of the neck ("buffalo hump", Figure 38.26), and breast enlargement. These physical changes may indicate to others that an individual is HIV positive.

4. **Resistance:** Resistance occurs as an accumulation of stepwise mutations of the protease gene. Initial mutations result in decreased ability of the virus to replicate, but as the mutations accumulate, virions with high levels of resistance to the protease emerge. Suboptimal concentrations result in the more rapid appearance of resistant strains.

5. **Drug Interactions:** Drug interactions are a common problem for all protease inhibitors, because they are not only substrates but also

potent inhibitors of CYP isozymes. The inhibitory potency of the compounds lies between that of *ritonavir,* the most potent, and that of *saquinavir*, the least potent inhibitor of CYP isozymes. Drug interactions are therefore quite common. Drugs that rely on metabolism for their termination of action may accumulate to toxic levels. Examples of potentially dangerous interactions include excessive sedation from *midazolam* or *triazolam*, bleeding from *warfarin*, and respiratory depression from *fentanyl* (Figure 38.27). In addition, inducers of CYP isozymes may result in the lowering of protease plasma concentrations to suboptimal levels, contributing to treatment failures. Thus, drugs such as *rifampin*, barbiturates, and *carbamazepine* should be avoided. Meticulous attention must be paid to all these detrimental interactions.

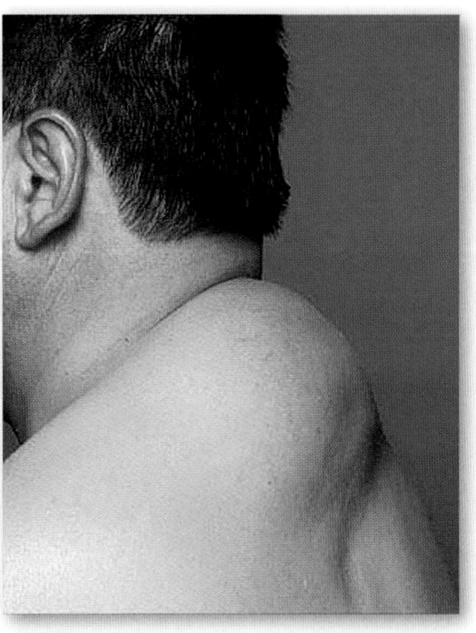

Figure 38.26
Accumulation of fat at base of the neck in a patient receiving a protease inhibitor.

B. Saquinavir

The soft-gel capsule formulation of *saquinavir* [sa KWIN a veer] improves its bioavailability, although the amount absorbed remains the lowest of all the protease inhibitors, at approximately twelve percent of the oral dose. To maximize bioavailability, *saquinavir* is given along with a low dose of *ritonavir*. High-fat meals also enhance absorption. Distribution into tissues is good, as evidenced by a large volume of distribution. Elimination of *saquinavir* is primarily by metabolism, followed by biliary excretion. Its half-life is seven to twelve hours, requiring multiple daily doses. Plasma levels can be significantly increased when *saquinavir* is combined with other antiretroviral agents that inhibit its metabolism, such as *delavirdine*. On the other hand, drugs that enhance the metabolism of *saquinavir*, such as *rifampin*, *rifabutin*, *nevirapine*, *efavirenz*, and other enzyme inducers, should be avoided if possible. The most common adverse effects of *saquinavir* treatment (five to ten percent of patients) include headache, fatigue, diarrhea, nausea, and other gastrointestinal disturbances. Increased levels of hepatic aminotransferases have been noted, particularly in patients with concurrent viral hepatitis B or C infections.

DRUG CLASS	EXAMPLE
ANTIARRHYTHMICS	*Quinidine*
ERGOT DERIVATIVES	*Ergotamine*
ANTIMYCOBACTERIAL DRUGS	*RIfampin*
BENZODIAZEPINES	*Midazolam*
BARBITURATES	Phenobarbital
ANTICOAGULANTS	Warfarin
HERBAL SUPPLEMENTS	St. John's wart

contraindicated

PROTEASE INHIBITORS

Figure 38.27
Drugs that should not be coadministered with any protease inhibitor.

C. Ritonavir

Ritonavir [ri TOE na veer] favorably alters the surrogate markers for HIV infection in both antiretroviral naïve and experienced patients (that is, those who have had previous HIV therapy). Bioavailability following oral administration is at least sixty percent, and is unaffected by food. However, *ritonavir* is unpalatable, and is taken with chocolate milk or nutritional supplements to improve palatability. Metabolism and biliary excretion are the primary methods of elimination. *Ritonavir* has a half-life of three to five hours. It is primarily an inhibitor of cytochrome P450 isozymes, resulting in numerous drug interactions. Because of this property, *ritonavir* has been increasingly employed as a "pharmacokinetic enhancer" of other protease inhibitors. Not only does concomitant *ritonavir* administration (at low doses) increase the bioavailability of the second protease inhibitor, it also diminishes the impact of meals. *Ritonavir* is a self-inducer of its own metabolism. Nausea, vomiting, diarrhea, and asthenia are among the more common adverse effects. Titration to the standard dose is effective in diminishing the gastrointestinal side effects. [Note: This maneuver is not effective with other protease inhibitors.] Circumoral paresthesia and headache frequently occur.

D. Indinavir

Clinical trials of *indinavir* [in DIN a veer] have demonstrated the efficacy of this drug in both antiretrovirally naïve and experienced patients. When used in combination with reverse transcriptase inhibitors, sustained effects have been demonstrated for as long as 100 weeks. *Indinavir* is well absorbed orally and, of all the protease inhibitors, is the least protein-bound, at sixty percent. [Note: Whether this accounts for its ability to reduce HIV RNA in tissue and fluids, such as lymph nodes, vaginal secretions, or semen, is unknown.] Acidic gastric conditions are necessary for absorption. Absorption is decreased when administered with meals, although a light, low-fat snack is permissible. *Ritonavir* overcomes this problem, and may also permit twice-a-day dosing. Metabolism and hepatic clearance account for elimination of *indinavir*. The dosage should therefore be reduced in the presence of hepatic insufficiency. *Indinavir* has the shortest half-life of the protease inhibitors, at 1.8 hours. It is well tolerated, with the usual gastrointestinal symptoms and headache predominating. *Indinavir* characteristically causes nephrolithiasis and hyperbilirubinemia. Adequate hydration is important to reduce the incidence of kidney stone formation, and patients should drink at least 1.5 L of water per day. Fat redistribution is particularly troublesome with this drug.

E. Nelfinavir

Nelfinavir [nel FIN a veer] is a nonpeptide protease inhibitor. It is well absorbed and does not require strict food or fluid conditions; however, it is usually given with food. *Nelfinavir* undergoes metabolism by several CYP isozymes. The major metabolite of *nelfinavir* produced by isozyme CYP2C19 has an antiviral activity equal to that of the parent compound, but it achieves plasma concentrations only forty percent of those of the parent compound. The half-life of *nelfinavir* is five hours. Diarrhea is the most common side effect and can be controlled by *loperamide*. Like other members of the class, *nelfinavir* can inhibit the metabolism of other drugs, resulting in required alterations of drug dosage or the prohibition of combined use.

F. Amprenavir

Like other protease inhibitors, *amprenavir* [am PREN a veer] is used in combination with at least two NRTIs. Its long plasma half-life permits twice-a-day dosing, but the large size and number of capsules per day (sixteen) may reduce patient compliance. Coadministration of *ritonavir* increases the plasma levels of *amprenavir* and lowers the total daily dose, thereby decreasing the complexity of the regimen. Nausea, vomiting, diarrhea, fatigue, paresthesias, and headache are common adverse effects.

G. Lopinavir

Lopinavir [loe PIN a veer] is the newest peptidomimetic protease inhibitor. It appears to have some benefit in patients who are not responding to other protease inhibitors. *Lopinavir* has very poor intrinsic bioavailability, which is substantially enhanced by including a low dose of *ritonavir* in the formulation. [Note: Only the coformulation known as *lopinavirR* is available in the United States.] *Lopinavir* is well tolerated, with gastrointestinal adverse effects being the most common. Enzyme inducers as well as St. John's wort should be avoided, because they lower the plasma concentrations of *lopinavir*. The oral solution contains alcohol and, thus, *disulfiram* or *metronidazole* administration can cause unpleasant reactions.

H. Atazanavir

Atazanavir [ah ta ZA na veer] inhibits HIV protease and is structurally unrelated to other HIV protease inhibitors. *Atazanavir* is well absorbed orally. Food increases absorption and bioavailability. The drug is highly protein bound (86 percent), undergoes extensive CYP3A4-catalyzed biotransformation. It is excreted primarily in the bile. Its half-life is about seven hours, but it only needs to be administered once a day. *Atazanavir* is a competitive inhibitor of glucuronyl transferase, and jaundice is a known side-effect. In the heart, atazanavir prolongs the PR interval and slows the heart rate. Early reports indicate a decreased risk of hyperlipidemia but it is not known if *atazanavir* is less likely to cause insulin resistance and lipodystrophy as seen with other protease inhibitors. Like the other protease inhibitors, *atazanavir* is a potent inhibitor of CYP3A4, and has the potential for many drug interactions.

A summary of protease inhibitors is presented in Figure 38.28.

DRUGS	MAJOR TOXICITIES AND CONCERNS
Amprenavir	Nausea, diarrhea, vomiting, oral and perioral paresthesia, and rash
Atazanavir	Nausea, abdominal discomfort, headache, skin rash
Indinavir	Benign hyperbilirubinemia, nephrolithiasis; Take one hour before or two hours after food; may take with skim milk or a low-fat meal; drink >1.5 L of liquid daily
Lopinavir	Gastrointestinal adverse effects are the most common
Nelfinavir	Diarrhea, nausea, flatulence, rash
Ritonavir	Diarrhea, nausea, taste perversion, vomiting, anemia, increased hepatic enzymes, increased triglycerides Requires refrigeration; take with meals; chocolate milk improves the taste
Saquinavir	Diarrhea, nausea, abdominal discomfort, elevated transaminase levels Take with high-fat meal or within 2 hours of a full meal

Figure 38.28
Summary of protease inhibitors. [Note: *Lopinavir* is co-formulated with *ritonavir*; *ritonavir* inhibits the metabolism of *lopinavir*, thereby increasing its level in the plasma.]

IX. VIRAL FUSION INHIBITOR

Enfuvirtide [en fu VEER tide] is the first of new class of antiretroviral drugs known as fusion inhibitors. In order for HIV to gain entry into the host cell, it must fuse its membrane with that of the host cell. This is accomplished by changes in the conformation of the viral transmembrane glycoprotein gp41, which occurs when HIV binds to the host cell surface. *Enfuvirtide* is a 36 amino acid peptide that binds to gp41, preventing the conformational change. *Enfuvirtide*, in combination with other antiretrovirals, is approved for therapy of treatment-experienced patients with evidence of viral replication despite ongoing antiretroviral drug therapy. As a peptide, it must be given subcutaneously. Most of the adverse effects are related to the injection, including pain, erythema, induration, and nodules, which occur in almost all patients. However, only three percent discontinue treatment because of them. *Enfuvirtide* must be reconstituted prior to administration. It is an expensive medication.

Study questions

Choose the ONE best answer.

38.1 A 30-year-old male patient with an HIV infection is being treated with a HAART regimen. Four weeks after initiating therapy, he comes to the emergency department complaining of severe flank pain, nausea, and frequent urination. Which one of the following drugs is most likely the cause of his symptoms?

A. Zidovudine
B. Nelfinavir
C. Indinavir
D. Efavirenz
E. Nevirapine

Correct answer = C. The protease inhibitor, indinavir, causes nephrolithiasis, which produces symptoms of pain, frequent urination, and nausea. The other drugs, although part of a HAART regimen, do not cause adverse effects with this cluster of symptoms. Zidovudine causes anemia. Nelfinavir causes nausea and diarrhea. Efavirenz and nevirapine cause rashes.

38.2 Chills, fever, and muscle aches are common reactions to which one of the following antiviral drugs?

A. Acyclovir
B. Ganciclovir
C. Oseltamivir
D. Interferon
E. Ribavirin

Correct answer = D. Interferon causes flu-like symptoms, including chills, fever, and myalgias, upon injection. Pretreatment with acetaminophen decreases the reaction. The other drugs do not cause this particular adverse effect.

38.3 An HIV-positive woman is diagnosed with CMV retinitis. She has been on a HAART regimen containing zidovudine. Which of the following anti-CMV drugs is likely to cause additive myelosuppression with zidovudine?

A. Acyclovir
B. Ganciclovir
C. Amantadine
D. Foscarnet
E. Ribavirin

Correct answer = B. Ganciclovir is myelosuppresive in and of itself and will add to the myelosuppression caused by zidovudine. The combination has an increased risk of neutropenia and anemia. Foscarnet has anti-CMV activity, but it does not cause myelosuppression. The other drugs are not effective against CMV.

38.4 A 25-year-old man is diagnosed with HIV, and therapy is initiated. After the first week of therapy, the patient complains of headaches, irritability, and nightmares. Which one of the following antiretroviral drugs is most likely to be causing these symptoms?

A. Efavirenz
B. Indinavir
C. Lamivudine
D. Nevirapine
E. Stavudine

Correct answer = A. CNS symptoms are characteristic of efavirenz, especially at the beginning of therapy, and occur in nearly fifty percent of patients. These adverse effects abate with continued administration of efavirenz. The other drugs are unlikely to cause CNS side effects.

Anticancer Drugs

39

I. OVERVIEW

It is estimated that 25 percent of the population of the United States will face a diagnosis of cancer during their lifetime, with one million new cancer patients diagnosed each year. Less than a quarter of these patients will be cured solely by surgery and/or local radiation. Most of the remainder will receive systemic chemotherapy at some time during their illness. In a small fraction (approximately ten percent) of patients with cancer representing selected neoplasms, the chemotherapy will result in a cure or a prolonged remission. However, in most cases, the drug therapy will produce only a regression of the disease, and complications and/or relapse may eventually lead to death. Thus, the overall five-year survival rate for cancer patients is about forty percent, ranking cancer second only to cardiovascular disease as a cause of mortality. (See Figure 39.1 for a list of the anticancer agents discussed in this chapter.)

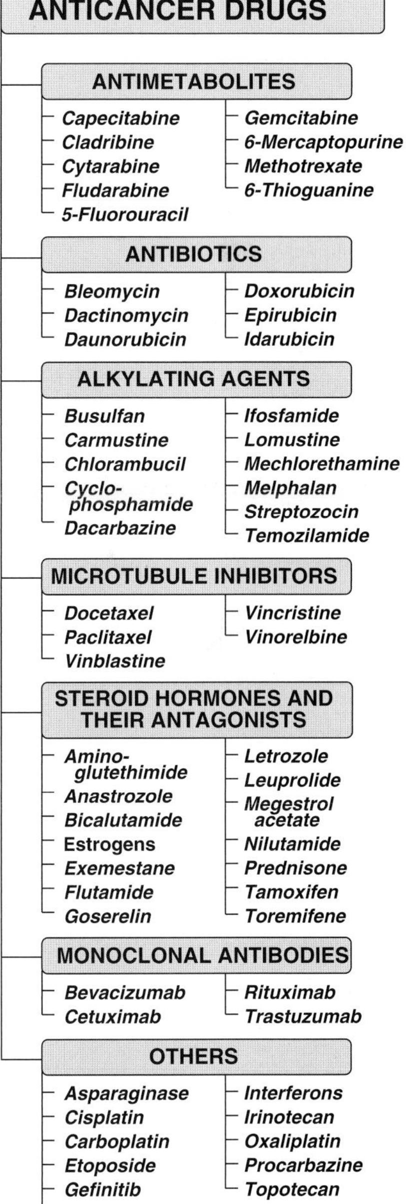

ANTICANCER DRUGS
ANTIMETABOLITES
Capecitabine
Cladribine
Cytarabine
Fludarabine
5-Fluorouracil
Gemcitabine
6-Mercaptopurine
Methotrexate
6-Thioguanine
ANTIBIOTICS
Bleomycin
Dactinomycin
Daunorubicin
Doxorubicin
Epirubicin
Idarubicin
ALKYLATING AGENTS
Busulfan
Carmustine
Chlorambucil
Cyclo-phosphamide
Dacarbazine
Ifosfamide
Lomustine
Mechlorethamine
Melphalan
Streptozocin
Temozilamide
MICROTUBULE INHIBITORS
Docetaxel
Paclitaxel
Vinblastine
Vincristine
Vinorelbine
STEROID HORMONES AND THEIR ANTAGONISTS
Amino-glutethimide
Anastrozole
Bicalutamide
Estrogens
Exemestane
Flutamide
Goserelin
Letrozole
Leuprolide
Megestrol acetate
Nilutamide
Prednisone
Tamoxifen
Toremifene
MONOCLONAL ANTIBODIES
Bevacizumab
Cetuximab
Rituximab
Trastuzumab
OTHERS
Asparaginase
Cisplatin
Carboplatin
Etoposide
Gefinitib
Imanitib
Interferons
Irinotecan
Oxaliplatin
Procarbazine
Topotecan

Figure 39.1
Summary of chemotherapeutic agents.

II. PRINCIPLES OF CANCER CHEMOTHERAPY

Cancer chemotherapy strives to cause a lethal cytotoxic event in the cancer cell that can arrest a tumor's progression. The attack is generally directed against metabolic sites essential to cell replication—for example, the availability of purines and pyrimidines that are the building blocks for DNA or RNA synthesis (Figure 39.2). Ideally, these anticancer drugs should interfere only with cellular processes that are unique to malignant cells. Unfortunately, most currently available anticancer drugs do not specifically recognize neoplastic cells but, rather, affect all proliferating cells—both normal and abnormal. Therefore, almost all antitumor agents have a steep dose-response curve for both toxic and therapeutic effects.

A. Treatment strategies

1. **Goal of treatment:** The ultimate goal of chemotherapy is a cure (that is, long-term, disease-free survival). A true cure requires the eradication of every neoplastic cell. If a cure is not attainable, then the goal becomes palliation (that is, alleviation of symptoms and avoidance of life-threatening toxicity). This allows the individual to maintain a "normal" existence, with the cancer thus being treated as a chronic disease. In either case, the neoplastic cell burden is

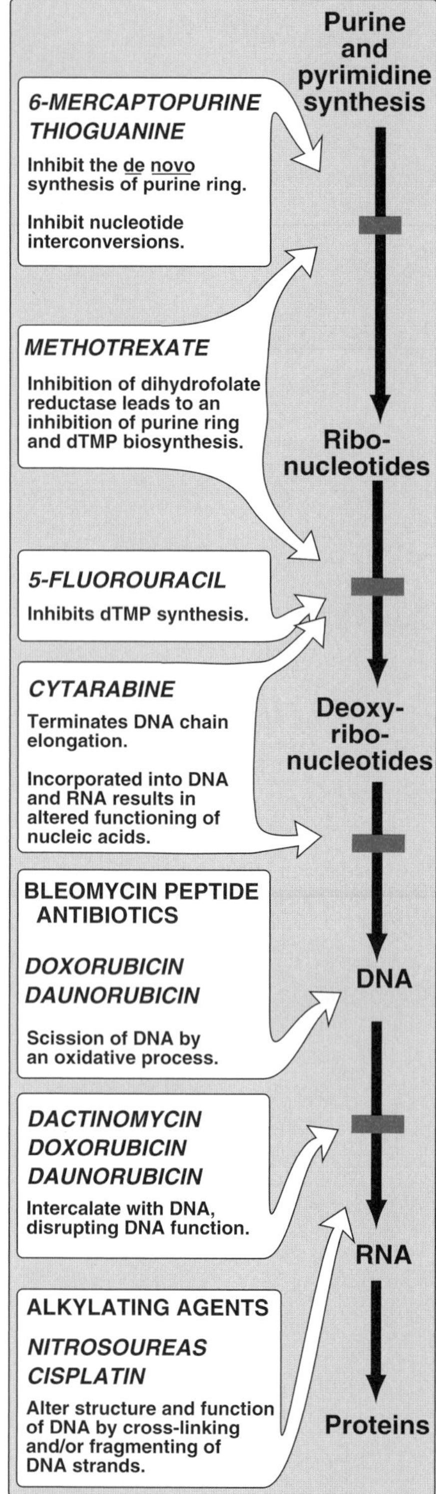

Figure 39.2
Examples of chemotherapeutic agents affecting the availability of RNA and DNA precursors. dTMP = deoxythymidine monophosphate.

initially reduced (debulked), either by surgery and/or radiation, followed by chemotherapy, immunotherapy, or a combination of these treatment modalities (Figure 39.3).

2. **Indications for treatment:** Chemotherapy is indicated when neoplasms are disseminated and are not amenable to surgery. Chemotherapy is also used as a supplemental treatment to attack micrometastases following surgery and radiation treatment.

3. **Tumor susceptibility and the growth cycle:** The fraction of tumor cells that are in the replicative cycle ("growth fraction") influences their susceptibility to most cancer chemotherapeutic agents. Rapidly dividing cells are generally more sensitive to anticancer drugs, whereas nonproliferating cells (those in the G_0 phase; Figure 39.4) usually survive the toxic effects of many of these agents.

   a. **Cell-cycle specificity of drugs:** Both normal cells and tumor cells go through growth cycles (Figure 39.4). However, normal and neoplastic tissues may differ in the number of cells that are in the various stages of the cycle. Chemotherapeutic agents that are effective only against replicating cells—that is those cells that are cycling—are said to be cell-cycle specific (see Figure 39.4), whereas other agents are said to be cell-cycle nonspecific. The nonspecific drugs, although having generally more toxicity in cycling cells, are also useful against tumors that have a low percentage of replicating cells.

   b. **Tumor growth rate:** The growth rate of most solid tumors in vivo is initially rapid, but growth rate decreases as the tumor size increases (see Figure 39.3). This is due to the unavailability of nutrients and oxygen caused by inadequate vascularization. Reducing the tumor burden through surgery or radiation promotes the recruitment of the remaining cells into active proliferation and increases their susceptibility to chemotherapeutic agents.

B. Treatment regimens and scheduling

Drugs are usually administered on the basis of body surface area, with an effort being made to tailor the medications to each patient.

1. **Log kill:** Destruction of cancer cells by chemotherapeutic agents follows first-order kinetics; that is, a given dose of drug destroys a constant fraction of cells. The term "log kill" is used to describe this phenomenon. For example, a diagnosis of leukemia is generally made when there are about 10^9 (total) leukemic cells. Consequently, if treatment leads to a 99.999-percent kill, then 0.001 percent of 10^9 cells (or 10^4 cells) would remain. This is defined as a five-log kill. At this point, the patient appears asymptomatic; that is, the patient is in remission (see Figure 39.3). For most bacterial infections, a five-log (100,000-fold) reduction in the number of microorganisms results in a cure, because the immune system can destroy the remaining bacterial cells. However, tumor cells are not as readily eliminated, and additional treatment is required to totally eradicate the leukemic cell population.

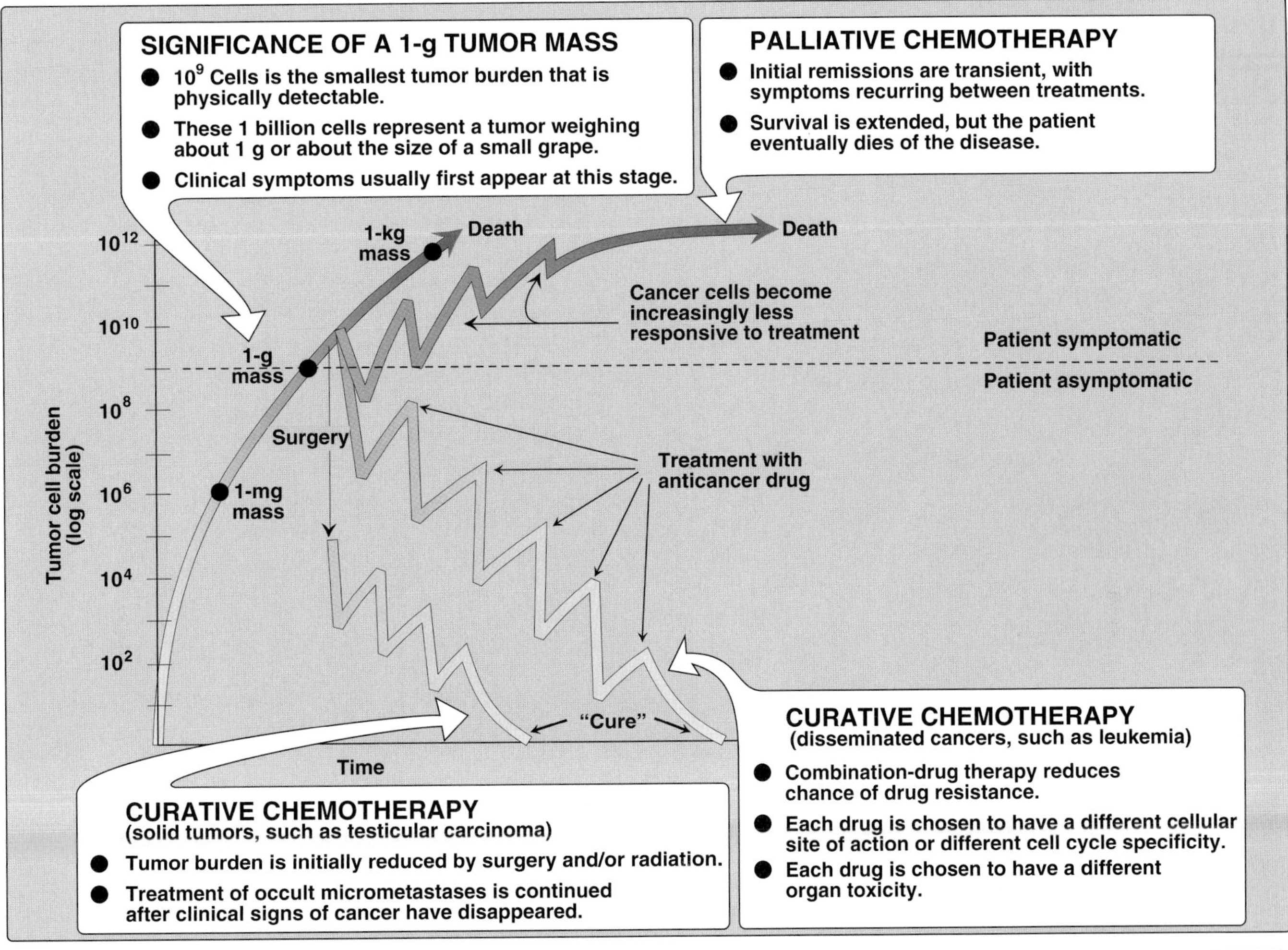

Figure 39.3
Effects of various treatments on the cancer cell burden in a hypothetical patient.

2. **Pharmacologic sanctuaries:** Leukemic or other tumor cells find sanctuary in tissues such as the central nervous system (CNS), where transport constraints prevent certain chemotherapeutic agents from entering. Therefore, a patient may require irradiation of the craniospinal axis or intrathecal administration of drugs to eliminate the leukemic cells at that site. Similarly, drugs may be unable to penetrate certain areas of solid tumors.

3. **Treatment protocols:** Combination-drug chemotherapy is more successful than single-drug treatment in most of the cancers for which chemotherapy is effective.

   a. **Combinations of drugs:** Cytotoxic agents with qualitatively different toxicities, and with different molecular sites and mechanisms of action, are usually combined at full doses. This results in higher response rates, due to additive and/or potentiated cytotoxic effects, and nonoverlapping host toxicities. In contrast, agents with similar dose-limiting toxicities, such as myelosuppression, can be combined safely only by reducing the doses of each.

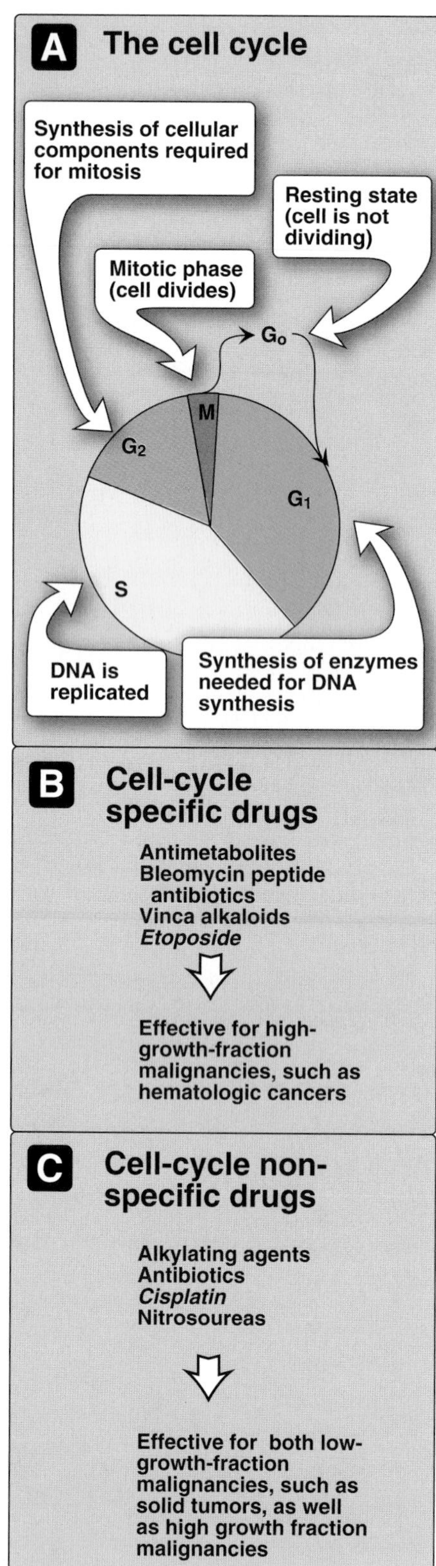

Figure 39.4
Effects of chemotherapeutic agents on the growth cycle of mammalian cells.

b. **Advantages of drug combinations**: The advantages of such combinations are that they 1) provide maximal cell killing within the range of tolerated toxicity, 2) are effective against a broader range of cell lines in the heterogeneous tumor population, and 3) may delay or prevent the development of resistant cell lines.

c. **Treatment protocols:** Many cancer treatment protocols have been developed, and each one is applicable to a particular neoplastic state. They are usually identified by an acronym, for example, a common regimen called POMP—used for the treatment of acute lymphocytic leukemia—consists of ***p**rednisone*, ***o**ncovin* (*vincristine*), ***m**ethotrexate*, and ***p**urinethol* (*mercaptopurine*). Therapy is scheduled intermittently to allow recovery of normal tissue, such as the patient's immune system, which is also affected by the drugs, thus reducing the risk of serious infection.

C. Problems associated with chemotherapy

Cancer drugs are toxins that present a lethal threat to the cell. It is therefore not surprising that cells have evolved elaborate defense mechanisms to protect themselves from chemical toxins, including chemotherapeutic agents.

1. **Resistance:** Some neoplastic cells (for example, melanoma) are inherently resistant to most anticancer drugs. Other tumor types may be selected for or acquire resistance to the cytotoxic effects of a medication by mutating, particularly after prolonged administration of low drug doses. The development of drug resistance is minimized by short-term, intensive, intermittent therapy with combinations of drugs. Drug combinations are also effective against a broader range of resistant cell lines in the tumor population. A variety of mechanisms are responsible for drug resistance, each of which is considered separately in the discussion of a particular drug.

2. **Multidrug resistance:** Stepwise selection of an amplified gene that codes for a transmembrane protein (P-glycoprotein for "permeability" glycoprotein; Figure 39.5) is responsible for multidrug resistance. This resistance is due to ATP-dependent pumping of drugs out of the cell in the presence of P-glycoprotein. Cross-resistance among structurally unrelated agents occurs. For example, cells that are resistant to the cytotoxic effects of the vinca alkaloids are also resistant to *dactinomycin*, the anthracycline antibiotics, as well as to *colchicine*, and vice versa. These drugs are all naturally occurring substances, each of which has a hydrophobic aromatic ring and a positive charge at neutral pH. [Note: P-glycoprotein is normally expressed at low levels in most cell types, but higher levels are found in the kidney, liver, pancreas, small intestine, colon, and adrenal gland. It has been suggested that the presence of P-glycoprotein may account for the intrinsic resistance to chemotherapy observed in adenocarcinomas in these tissues.] Certain drugs at high concentrations (for example, *verapamil*) can inhibit the pump and, thus, interfere with the efflux of the anticancer agent. However, these drugs are

undesirable because of adverse pharmacologic actions of their own. Pharmacologically inert pump blockers are being sought.

3. **Toxicity:** Therapy aimed at killing rapidly dividing cells also affects normal cells undergoing rapid proliferation (for example, cells of the buccal mucosa, bone marrow, gastrointestinal mucosa, and hair), contributing to the toxic manifestations of chemotherapy.

   a. **Common adverse effects:** Most chemotherapeutic agents have a narrow therapeutic index. Severe vomiting, stomatitis, and alopecia occur to a lesser or greater extent during therapy with all antineoplastic agents. Vomiting is often controlled by administration of antiemetic drugs. Some toxicities, such as myelosuppression that predisposes to infection, are common to many chemotherapeutic agents (Figure 39.6), whereas other adverse reactions are confined to specific agents, for example, cardiotoxicity with doxorubicin and pulmonary fibrosis with bleomycin. The duration of the side effects varies widely. For example, alopecia is transient, but the cardiac, pulmonary, and bladder toxicities are irreversible.

   b. **Minimizing adverse effects:** Some toxic reactions may be ameliorated by interventions, such as perfusing the tumor locally (for example, a sarcoma of the arm), removing some of the patient's marrow prior to intensive treatment and then reimplanting it, or promoting intensive diuresis to prevent bladder toxicities. The megaloblastic anemia that occurs with *methotrexate* can be effectively counteracted by administering *folinic acid* (*leucovorin, 5-formyltetrahydrofolic acid*; see below). With the availability of human granulocyte colony-stimulating factor (*filgrastim*), the neutropenia associated with treatment of cancer by many drugs can be partially reversed.

4. **Treatment-induced tumors:** Because most antineoplastic agents are mutagens, neoplasms (for example, acute nonlymphocytic leukemia) may arise ten or more years after the original cancer was cured. [Note: Treatment-induced neoplasms are especially a problem after therapy with alkylating agents.]

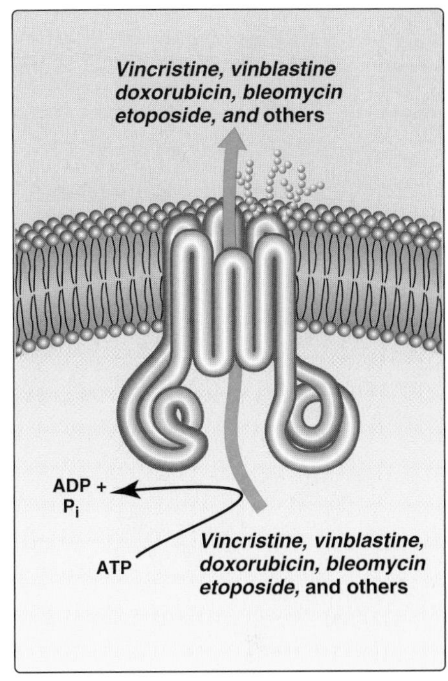

Figure 39.5
The six membrane-spanning loops of the P-glycoprotein form a central channel for the ATP-dependent pumping of drugs from the cell.

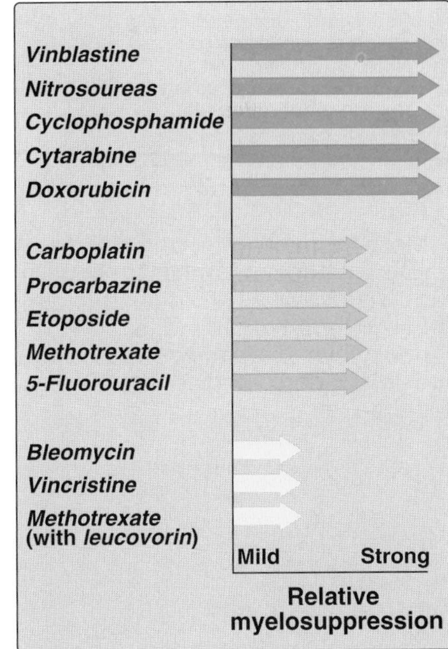

Figure 39.6
Comparison of myelosuppressive potential of chemotherapeutic drugs.

III. ANTIMETABOLITES

Antimetabolites are structurally related to normal compounds within the cell. They generally interfere with the availability of normal purine or pyrimidine nucleotide precursors either by inhibiting their synthesis, or by competing with them in DNA or RNA synthesis. Their maximal cytotoxic effects are S-phase (and, therefore, cell-cycle) specific.

A. Methotrexate

The vitamin folic acid plays a central role in a variety of metabolic reactions involving the transfer of one-carbon units[1] and is essential for cell replication. *Methotrexate* [meth oh TREK sate] (*MTX*) is struc-

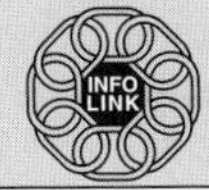

[1]See p. 265 in Lippincott's Illustrated Reviews: Biochemistry (3rd ed.) for a discussion of the one-carbon pool.

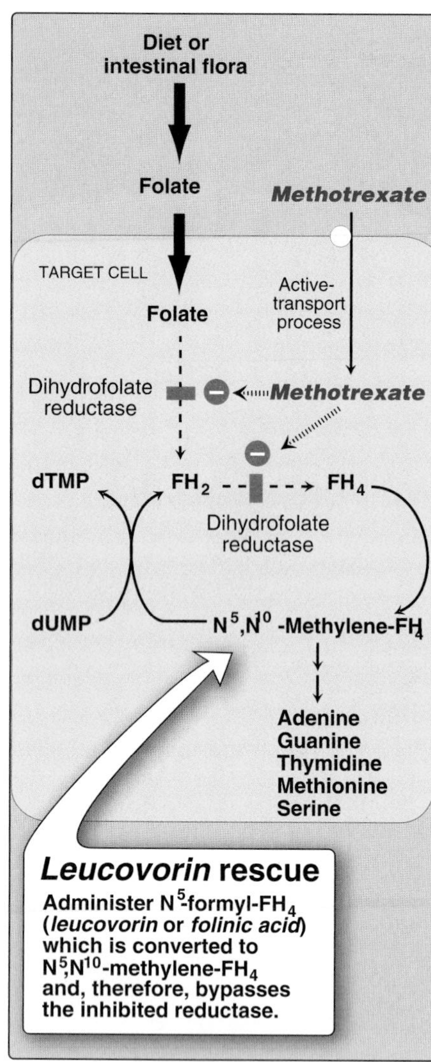

Figure 39.7
Mechanism of action of *methotrexate* and the effect of administration of *leucovorin.* FH_2 = dihydrofolate; FH_4 = tetrahydrofolate; dTMP = deoxythymidine monophosphate; dUMP = deoxyuridine mono phosphate.

turally related to folic acid, and acts as an antagonist of that vitamin by inhibiting dihydrofolate reductase[2]—the enzyme that converts folic acid to its active, coenzyme form, tetrahydrofolic acid (FH_4).

1. **Mechanism of action:** Folic acid is obtained from dietary sources or from that produced by intestinal flora. It undergoes reduction to the tetrahydrofolate form (FH_4) via a reaction catalyzed by intracellular nicotinamide adenine dinucleotide phosphate-dependent dihydrofolate reductase (DHFR; Figure 39.7). *MTX* enters the cell by active-transport processes that normally mediate the entry of N^5-methyl FH_4. At high concentrations, the drug can also diffuse into the cell. *MTX* has an unusually strong affinity for DHFR and effectively inhibits the enzyme. Like tetrahydrofolate itself, *MTX* becomes polyglutamated within the cell—a process that favors intracellular retention of the compound due to increased negative charge. *MTX*-polyglutamates also potently inhibit DHFR. This inhibition deprives the cell of folate coenzymes and leads to decreased production of compounds that depend on these coenzymes for their biosynthesis. These compounds include the nucleotides adenine, guanine, and thymidine and the amino acids methionine and serine. This leads to depressed DNA, RNA, and protein synthesis and ultimately to cell death (see Figure 39.7). The inhibition of DHFR can only be reversed by a thousand-fold excess of the natural substrate, dihydrofolate (FH_2; see Figure 39.7), or by administration of *leucovorin*, which bypasses the blocked enzyme and replenishes the folate pool. [Note: *Leucovorin*, or *folinic acid*, is the N^5-formyl group–carrying form of FH_4.].

2. **Resistance:** Nonproliferating cells are resistant to *MTX*, probably because of a relative lack of DHFR, thymidylate synthase, and/or the glutamylating enzyme. Resistance in neoplastic cells can be due to amplification (production of additional copies) of the gene that codes for DHFR, resulting in increased levels of this enzyme. The enzyme affinity for *MTX* may also be diminished. Resistance can also occur from a reduced influx of *MTX*, apparently caused by a change in the carrier-mediated transport responsible for pumping the drug into the cell. Decreased levels of the *MTX* polyglutamate have been reported in resistant cells, and may be due to its decreased formation or increased breakdown.

3. **Therapeutic uses:** *MTX*, usually in combination with other drugs, is effective against acute lymphocytic leukemia, choriocarcinoma, Burkitt lymphoma in children, breast cancer, and head and neck carcinomas. In addition, low-dose MTX is effective as a single agent against certain inflammatory diseases, such as severe psoriasis and rheumatoid arthritis, as well as Crohn disease. All patients receiving *methotrexate* require close monitoring for possible toxic sequelae.

4. **Pharmacokinetics:**

   a. **Administration and distribution:** *Methotrexate* is variably absorbed at low doses from the GI tract, but it can also be administered by intramuscular (IM), intravenous (IV), and

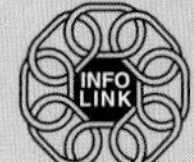

[2]See p. 265 in Lippincott's Illustrated Reviews: Biochemistry (3rd ed.) for a discussion of dihydrofolate reductase.

intrathecal routes (Figure 39.8). [Note: Because *MTX* does not penetrate the blood-brain barrier, it is administered intrathecally to destroy neoplastic cells in the central sanctuary sites.] High concentrations of the drug are found in the intestinal epithelium, liver, and kidney as well as in ascites and pleural effusions. *MTX* is also distributed to the skin.

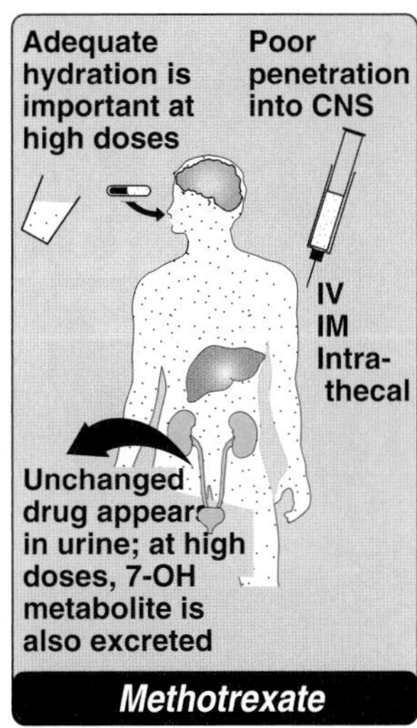

Figure 39.8
Administration and fate of *methotrexate*.

b. Fate: As previously mentioned, *MTX* is metabolized to polyglutamate derivatives. This property is important, because the polyglutamates, which also inhibit DHFR, remain within the cell even in the absence of extracellular drug. This is in contrast to *MTX* per se, which rapidly leaves the cell as the extracellular drug levels fall. High doses of *MTX* undergo hydroxylation at the 7-position. This derivative is much less active as an antimetabolite. It is less water soluble than *MTX* and may lead to crystalluria. Therefore, it is important to keep the urine alkaline and the patient well hydrated to avoid renal toxicity. Excretion of the parent drug and the 7-OH metabolite occurs primarily via the urine, although some of the drug and its metabolite appear in the feces due to enterohepatic excretion.

5. Adverse effects:

a. Commonly observed toxicities: In addition to nausea, vomiting and diarrhea, the most frequent toxicities occur in tissues that are constantly renewing. Thus, *MTX* causes stomatitis, myelosuppression, erythema, rash, urticaria, and alopecia. Some of these adverse effects can be prevented or reversed by administering *leucovorin* (see Figure 39.7), which is taken up more readily by normal cells than by tumor cells. Doses of *leucovorin* must be kept minimal to avoid interference with the antitumor action of *MTX*.

b. Renal damage: Although uncommon during conventional therapy, renal damage is a complication of high-dose *MTX* and its 7-OH metabolite, which can precipitate in the tubules. Alkalinization of the urine and hydration help to prevent this problem.

c. Hepatic function: Hepatic function should be monitored. Long-term use of *MTX* may lead to fibrosis or cirrhosis.

d. Pulmonary toxicity: This is a rare complication. Children who are being maintained on *MTX* may develop cough, dyspnea, fever, and cyanosis. Infiltrates are seen on radiographs. This toxicity is reversible on suspension of the drug.

e. Neurologic toxicities: These are associated with intrathecal administration of *MTX* and include subacute meningeal irritation, stiff neck, headache, and fever. Rarely, seizures, encephalopathy, or paraplegia occur. Long-lasting effects, such as learning disabilities, have been seen in children who received the drug by this route.

f. Contraindications: Because *MTX* is teratogenic in experimental animals and is an abortifacient, it should be avoided in

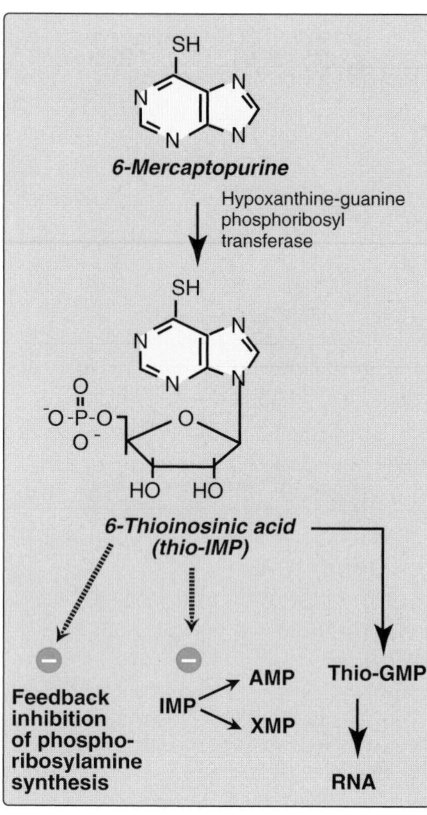

Figure 39.9
Actions of *6-mercaptopurine.*

pregnancy. [Note: *MTX* is used with *misoprostol* to induce abortion.]

B. 6-Mercaptopurine

The drug *6-mercaptopurine* [mer kap toe PYOOR een] (*6-MP*) is the thiol analog of hypoxanthine. *6-MP* and *6-thioguanine* (*6-TG*) were the first purine analogs to prove beneficial for treating neoplastic disease. [Note: *Azathioprine*, an immunosuppressant, exerts its effects after conversion to *6-MP*.] *6-MP* is used principally in the maintenance of remission in acute lymphoblastic leukemia. *6-MP* and its analog, *azathioprine*, are beneficial in the treatment of Crohn disease.

1. Mechanism of action:

a. **Nucleotide formation:** To exert its antileukemic effect, *6-MP* must penetrate target cells and be converted to the nucleotide analog, *6-mercaptopurine*-ribose-phosphate (better known as 6-thioinosinic acid, or TIMP; Figure 39.9). The addition of the ribose-phosphate is catalyzed by the salvage pathway enzyme, hypoxanthine-guanine phosphoribosyl transferase (HGPRT).[3]

b. **Inhibition of purine synthesis**: A number of metabolic processes involving purine biosynthesis and interconversions are affected by the nucleotide analog, TIMP. Like adenosine monophosphate (AMP), guanosine monophosphate (GMP), and inosine monophosphate (IMP), TIMP can inhibit the first step of de novo purine-ring biosynthesis (catalyzed by glutamine:phosphoribosyl pyrophosphate amidotransferase). TIMP also blocks the formation of AMP and xanthinylic acid from inosinic acid.[4]

c. **Incorporation into nucleic acids:** TIMP is converted to TGMP, which after phosphorylation to di- and triphosphates can be incorporated into RNA. The deoxyribonucleotide analogs that are also formed are incorporated into DNA. This results in nonfunctional RNA and DNA.

2. **Resistance:** Resistance is associated with 1) an inability to biotransform *6-MP* to the corresponding nucleotide because of decreased levels of HGPRT (for example, in Lesch-Nyhan syndrome, in which patients lack this enzyme), 2) an increased dephosphorylation, or 3) increased metabolism of the drug to thiouric acid or other metabolites.

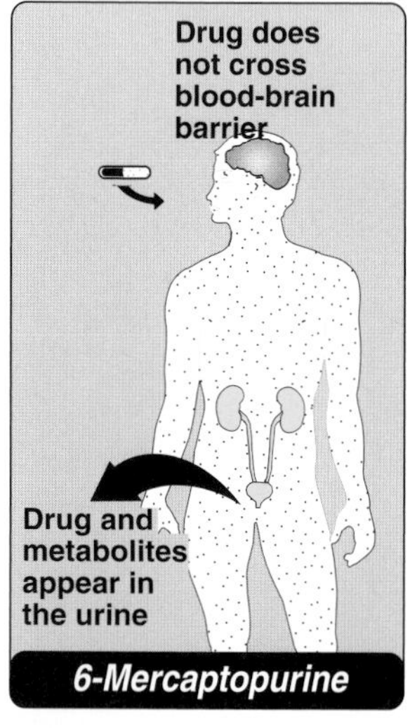

Figure 39.10
Administration and fate of *6-mercaptopurine.*

3. **Pharmacokinetics:** Absorption by the oral route is erratic. The drug is widely distributed throughout the body, except for the cerebrospinal fluid (CSF; Figure 39.10). *6-MP* undergoes metabolism in the liver to the 6-methylmercaptopurine derivative or to thiouric acid (an inactive metabolite). [Note: The latter reaction is catalyzed by xanthine oxidase.[5]] Because the xanthine oxidase inhibitor, *allopurinol*, is frequently used to reduce hyperuricemia in cancer patients receiving chemotherapy, it is important to

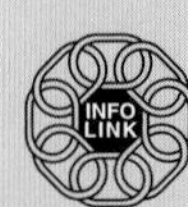

[3]See p. 294 in ***Lippincott's Illustrated Reviews: Biochemistry*** (3rd ed.) for a discussion of hypoxanthine-guanine phosphoribosyl transferase.
[4]See p. 293 in ***Lippincott's Illustrated Reviews: Biochemistry*** (3rd ed.) for a discussion of the conversion of IMP to other purine nucleotides.
[5]See p. 297 in ***Lippincott's Illustrated Reviews: Biochemistry*** (3rd ed.) for a discussion of xanthine oxidase.

decrease the dose of *6-MP* in these individuals to avoid accumulation of the drug and exacerbation of toxicities (Figure 39.11). The parent drug and its metabolites are excreted by the kidney.

4. **Adverse effects:** Bone marrow depression is the chief toxicity. Side effects also include nausea, vomiting, and diarrhea. Hepatotoxicity has been reported.

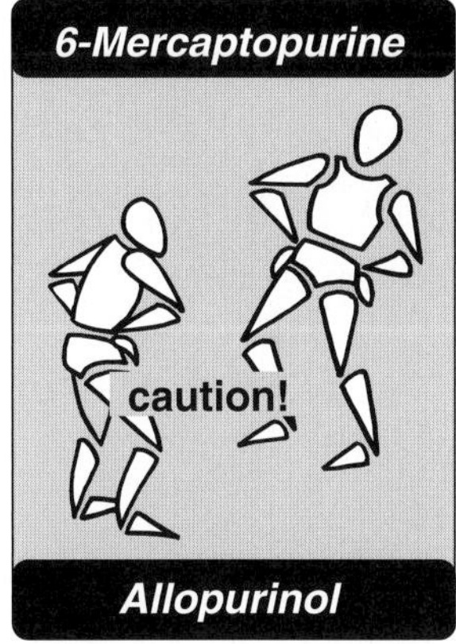

Figure 39.11
Potential drug interaction between *allopurinol* and *6-mercaptopurine*.

C. 6-Thioguanine

6-Thioguanine [thye oh GWAH neen] (*6-TG*), a purine analog, is primarily used in the treatment of acute nonlymphocytic leukemia in combination with *daunorubicin* and *cytarabine*. Like *6-MP*, *6-TG* must first be converted to the nucleotide form, which then inhibits the biosynthesis of the purine ring and the phosphorylation of GMP to guanosine diphosphate. The nucleotide form of *6-TG* can also be incorporated into RNA and DNA. Cross-resistance occurs between *6-MP* and *6-TG*. Toxicities are the same as those with *6-MP*.

D. Fludarabine

Fludarabine [floo DARE a been] is the 5'-phosphate of 2-fluoro-adenine arabinoside—a purine nucleotide analog. It is useful in the treatment of chronic lymphocytic leukemia and may replace *chlorambucil*, the present drug of choice. *Fludarabine* is also effective against hairy-cell leukemia and indolent non-Hodgkin lymphoma. *Fludarabine* is a prodrug, the phosphate being removed in the plasma to form 2-F-araA, which is taken up into cells and again phosphorylated (initially by deoxycytidine kinase). Although the exact cytotoxic lesion is uncertain, the triphosphate is incorporated into both DNA and RNA. This decreases their synthesis in the S-phase and affects their function. Resistance is associated with reduced uptake into cells, lack of deoxycytidine kinase, decreased affinity of DNA polymerase for the nucleotide analog, plus other mechanisms. *Fludarabine* is administered IV rather than orally, because intestinal bacteria split off the sugar to yield the very toxic metabolite, fluoroadenine. Urinary excretion accounts for partial elimination. In addition to nausea, vomiting, and diarrhea, myelosuppression is the dose-limiting toxicity. Fever, edema, and severe neurologic toxicity also occur. At high doses, progressive encephalopathy, blindness, and death have been reported.

E. Cladribine

Another purine analog, *2-chlorodeoxy adenosine*, or *cladribine* [KLA dri been], undergoes reactions similar to those of *fludarabine*; that is, it must be converted to a nucleotide to be cytotoxic. It becomes incorporated at the 3'-terminus of DNA and, thus, hinders elongation. It also affects DNA repair, and is a potent inhibitor of ribonucleotide reductase.[6] Resistance may be due to mechanisms analogous to those that affect *fludarabine*, although cross-resistance is not a problem. *Cladribine* is effective against chronic lymphocytic leukemia, non-Hodgkin lymphoma, and hairy-cell leukemia. It also has some activity versus multiple sclerosis. The drug is given as a single, continuous infusion. *Cladribine* distributes throughout

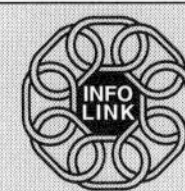

[6]See p. 295 in ***Lippincott's Illustrated Reviews: Biochemistry*** (3rd ed.) for a discussion of ribonucleotide reductase.

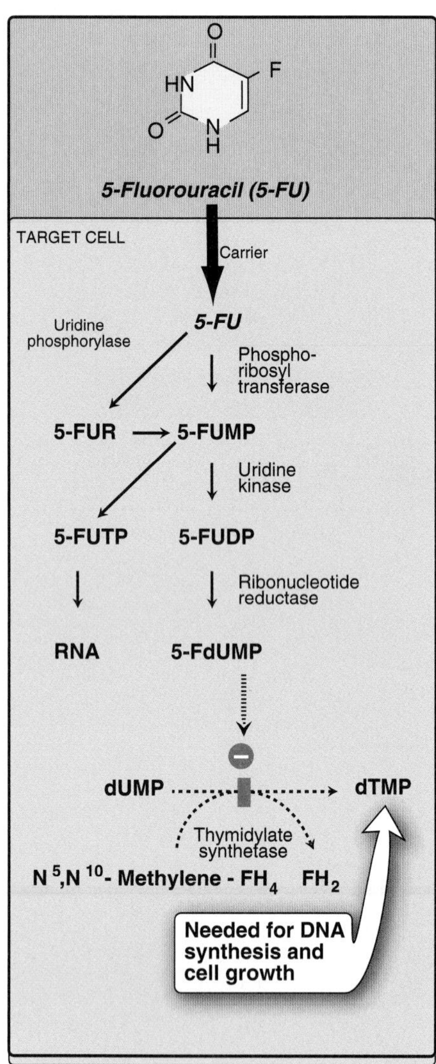

Figure 39.12
Mechanism of the cytotoxic action of *5-FU. 5-FU* is converted to 5-FdUMP, which competes with deoxyuridine monophosphate (dUMP) for the enzyme thymidylate synthetase. 5-FU = 5-fluorouracil; 5-FUR = 5-fluorouridine; 5-FUMP = 5-fluorouridine monophosphate; 5-FUDP = 5-fluorouridine diphosphate; 5-FUTP = 5-fluorouridine triphosphate; dUMP = deoxyuridine monophosphate; dTMP = deoxythymidine monophosphate. 5-FdUMP = 5-fluorodeoxyuridine monophosphate.

the body, including into the CSF. Severe bone marrow suppression is a common adverse effect, as is fever. Peripheral neuropathy has also been reported. The drug is teratogenic.

F. 5-Fluorouracil

5-Fluorouracil [flure oh YOOR ah sil] (*5-FU*), a pyrimidine analog, has a stable fluorine atom in place of a hydrogen atom at position 5 of the uracil ring. The fluorine interferes with the conversion of deoxyuridylic acid to thymidylic acid, thus depriving the cell of one of the essential precursors for DNA synthesis. *5-FU* is employed primarily in the treatment of slowly growing solid tumors (for example, colorectal, breast, ovarian, pancreatic, and gastric carcinomas). Adjuvant therapy with *levamisole*—a veterinary anthelmintic agent—improves the survival of some patients with colon cancer. When applied topically, *5-FU* is also effective for the treatment of superficial basal cell carcinomas.

1. **Mechanism of action:** *5-FU* per se is devoid of antineoplastic activity. It enters the cell through a carrier-mediated transport system and is converted to the corresponding deoxynucleotide (5-FdUMP, Figure 39.12), which competes with deoxyuridine monophosphate for thymidylate synthase.[7] 5-FdUMP acts as a pseudosubstrate and is trapped with the enzyme and its N^5,N^{10}-methylene tetrahydrofolic acid (*leucovorin*) coenzyme in a ternary complex that cannot proceed to products. DNA synthesis decreases due to lack of thymidine, leading to imbalanced cell growth and cell death. [Note: *Leucovorin* is administered with *5-FU* because the reduced folate coenzyme is required in the thymidylate synthase reaction. Lack of sufficient coenzyme reduces the effectiveness of the antipyrimidine. For example, the standard regimen for advanced colorectal cancer today is *irinotecan + 5-FU/leucovorin*.] *5-FU* is also incorporated into RNA, and low levels have been detected in DNA. In the latter case, a glycosylase excises the *5-FU* damaging the DNA.

2. **Resistance:** Resistant cells are encountered that have lost the ability to convert *5-FU* into its active form, that have altered or increased thymidylate synthase, or that have an increased rate of *5-FU* catabolism. Elevated levels of dihydropyrimidine dehydrogenase can decrease the availability of *5-FU*.

3. **Pharmacokinetics:** Because of its severe toxicity to the GI tract, *5-FU* is given IV or, in the case of skin cancer, topically (Figure 39.13). The drug penetrates well into all tissues, including the CNS. *5-FU* is rapidly metabolized in the liver, lung, and kidney. It is eventually converted to fluoro-β-alanine, which is removed in the urine, and to CO_2, which is exhaled. The dose of *5-FU* must be adjusted in the case of impaired hepatic function.

4. **Adverse effects:** In addition to nausea, vomiting, diarrhea, and alopecia, severe ulceration of the oral and GI mucosa, bone marrow depression (with bolus injection), and anorexia are frequently

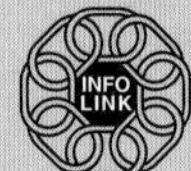

[7]See p. 300 in ***Lippincott's Illustrated Reviews: Biochemistry*** (3rd ed.) for a discussion of thymidylate synthase.

encountered. An *allopurinol* mouthwash has been shown to reduce oral toxicity. A dermopathy (erythematous desquamation of the palms and soles) called the "hand-foot syndrome" is seen after extended infusions.

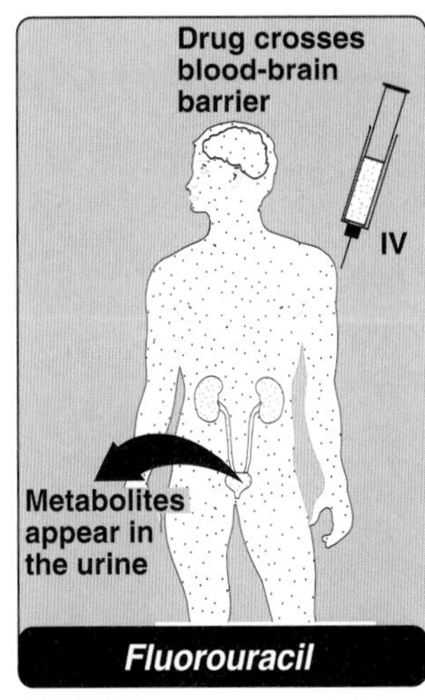

Figure 39.13
Administration and fate of *fluorouracil.*

G. Capecitabine

Capecitabine [cape SITE a been] is a novel, oral fluoropyrimidine carbamate. It is approved for the treatment of metastatic breast cancer that is resistant to first-line drugs (for example, *paclitaxel* and anthracyclines) and is currently also used for treatment of colorectal cancer.

1. **Mechanism of action:** After being absorbed, *capecitabine* (which is itself nontoxic) undergoes a series of enzymic reactions, the last of which is hydrolysis to *5-FU.* This step is catalyzed by thymidine phosphorylase—an enzyme that is concentrated primarily in tumors (Figure 39.14). Thus, the cytotoxic activity of *capecitabine* is the same as that of *5-FU,* and is tumor-specific. The most important reaction inhibited by *5-FU* (and, thus, *capecitabine*) is thymidylate synthase.

2. **Pharmacokinetics:** *Capecitabine* has the advantage of being well absorbed following oral administration. It is extensively metabolized to *5-FU* (as described above) and is eventually biotransformed into fluoro-β-alanine and CO_2. Metabolites are primarily eliminated in the urine or, in the case of CO_2, expired.

3. **Adverse effects:** These are similar to those with *5-FU,* with the toxicity occurring primarily in the GI tract. *Capecitabine* should be used cautiously in patients with hepatic or renal impairment. The drug is contraindicated in individuals who are hypersensitive to *5-FU,* are pregnant, or are lactating. Patients taking *coumarin* anticoagulants or *phenytoin* should be monitored for coagulation parameters and drug levels, respectively.

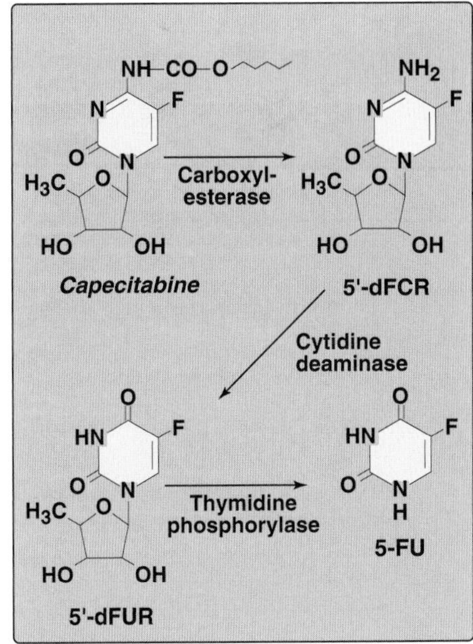

Figure 39.14
Metabolic pathway of *capecitabine* to 5-fluorouracil (5-FU). 5'-dFCR = 5'-deoxy-5-fluorocytidine; 5'-dFUR = 5'-deoxy-5-fluorouridine

H. Cytarabine

Cytarabine [sye TARE ah been] (*cytosine arabinoside,* or *ara-C*) is an analog of 2'-deoxycytidine in which the natural ribose residue is replaced by D-arabinose. *Ara-C* acts as a pyrimidine antagonist. The major clinical use of *ara-C* is in acute nonlymphocytic (myelogenous) leukemia in combination with *6-TG* and *daunorubicin.*

1. **Mechanism of action:** *Ara-C* enters the cell by a carrier-mediated process and, like the other purine and pyrimidine antagonists, must be sequentially phosphorylated to the nucleotide form (*cytosine arabinoside* triphosphate, or *ara*-CTP) in order to be cytotoxic. The nucleotide is incorporated into nuclear DNA and can retard chain elongation. It is therefore S-phase (and, hence, cell-cycle) specific.

2. **Resistance:** Resistance to *ara-C* may result from a defect in the transport process, a change in phosphorylating enzymes (especially deoxycytidine kinase), or an increased pool of the natural

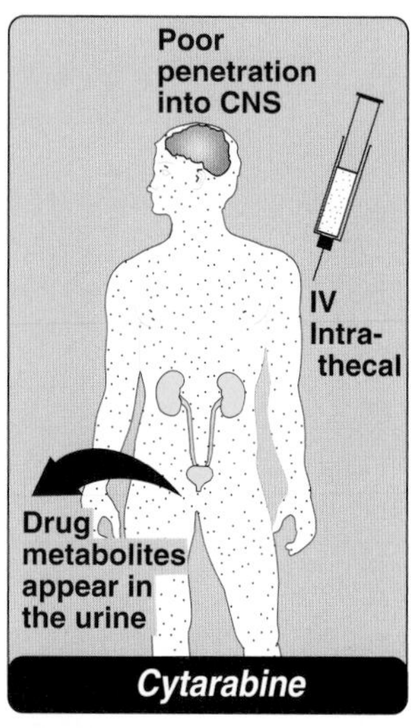

Figure 39.15
Administration and fate of *cytarabine*.

dCTP nucleotide. Increased deamination of the drug to ara-U can also cause resistance.

3. **Pharmacokinetics:** *Ara-C* is not effective when given orally, because of its deamination to the noncytotoxic uracil arabinoside (ara-U) by cytidine deaminase in the intestinal mucosa and liver. Given IV, it distributes throughout the body but does not penetrate the CNS in sufficient amounts to be effective against meningeal leukemia (Figure 39.15). However, it may be injected intrathecally. A new preparation that provides slow release into the CSF is also available. *Ara-C* undergoes extensive oxidative deamination in the body to ara-U—a pharmacologically inactive metabolite. Both *ara-C* and ara-U are excreted in the urine.

4. **Adverse effects:** Nausea, vomiting, diarrhea, and severe myelosuppression (primarily granulocytopenia) are the major toxicities associated with *ara-C*. Hepatic dysfunction is also occasionally encountered. At high doses or with intrathecal injection, *ara-C* may cause seizures or altered mental states.

I. Gemcitabine

Gemcitabine [jem SITe ah been] is an analog of the nucleoside deoxycytidine. It is used for the first-line treatment of locally advanced or metastatic adenocarcinoma of the pancreas. It also is effective against non–small cell lung cancer and several other tumors.

1. **Mechanism of action:** *Gemcitabine* is a substrate for dexoxycytidine kinase, which phosphorylates the drug to 2',2'-difluorodeoxycytidine triphosphate (Figure 39.16). The latter compound inhibits DNA synthesis by being incorporated into sites in the growing strand that ordinarily would contain cytosine. Evidence suggests that DNA repair does not readily occur. Levels of the natural nucleotide, dCTP, are lowered, because *gemcitabine* competes with the normal nucleoside substrate for deoxycytidine kinase. *Gemcitabine* may also inhibit ribonucleotide reductase.

2. **Resistance:** Resistance to the drug is probably due to its inability to be converted to a nucleotide, caused by an alteration in deoxycytidine kinase. In addition, the tumor cell can produce increased levels of endogenous deoxycytidine that compete for the kinase, thus bypassing the inhibition.

3. **Pharmacokinetics:** *Gemcitabine* is infused IV. It is deaminated to difluorodeoxyuridine, which is not cytotoxic, and is excreted in the urine.

4. **Adverse effects:** Myelosuppression is the dose-limiting toxicity of *gemcitabine*. Other toxicities include nausea, vomiting, alopecia, rash, and a flu-like syndrome. Transient elevations of serum transaminases, proteinuria, and hematuria are common.

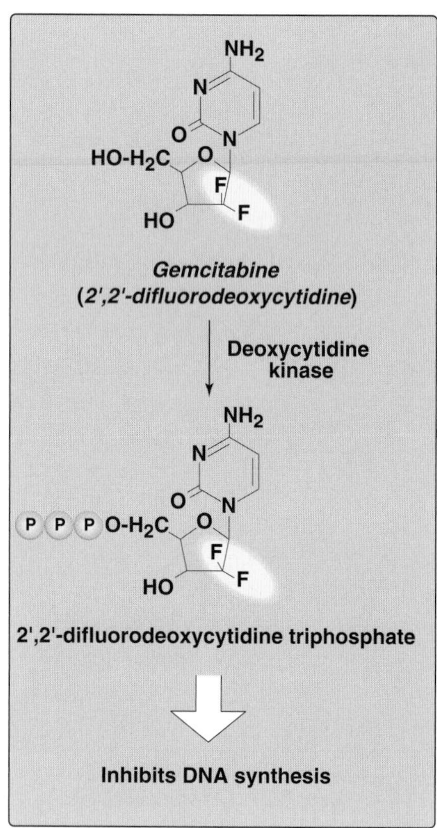

Figure 39.16
Mechanism of action of *gemcitabine*.

IV. ANTIBIOTICS

The antibiotics owe their cytotoxic action to their interactions with DNA, leading to disruption of DNA function. They are cell-cycle specific.

A. Dactinomycin

Dactinomycin [dak ti noe MYE sin], known to biochemists as *actinomycin D*, was the first antibiotic to find therapeutic application in tumor chemotherapy. *Dactinomycin* is used in combination with surgery and *vincristine* for the treatment of Wilms tumor. With *MTX*, *dactinomycin* is effective in the treatment of gestational choriocarcinoma. Some soft-tissue sarcomas also respond.

1. **Mechanism of action:** The drug intercalates into the minor groove of the double helix between guanine-cytosine base pairs of DNA,[8] forming a stable *dactinomycin*-DNA complex. The complex interferes primarily with DNA-dependent RNA polymerase, although at high doses, *dactinomycin* also hinders DNA synthesis. The drug also causes single-strand breaks, possibly due to action on topoisomerase II or by generation of free radicals.

2. **Resistance:** Resistance is due to an increased efflux of the antibiotic from the cell via P-glycoprotein. DNA repair may also play a role.

3. **Pharmacokinetics:** The drug, administered IV, distributes to many tissues but does not enter the cerebrospinal fluid (Figure 39.17). The drug is minimally metabolized. Most of the parent drug and its metabolites are excreted via the bile, and the remainder are excreted via the urine.

4. **Adverse effects:** The major dose-limiting toxicity is bone marrow depression. The drug is immunosuppressive. Other adverse reactions include nausea, vomiting, diarrhea, stomatitis, and alopecia. Extravasation during injection produces serious problems. *Dactinomycin* sensitizes to radiation, and inflammation at sites of prior radiation therapy may occur.

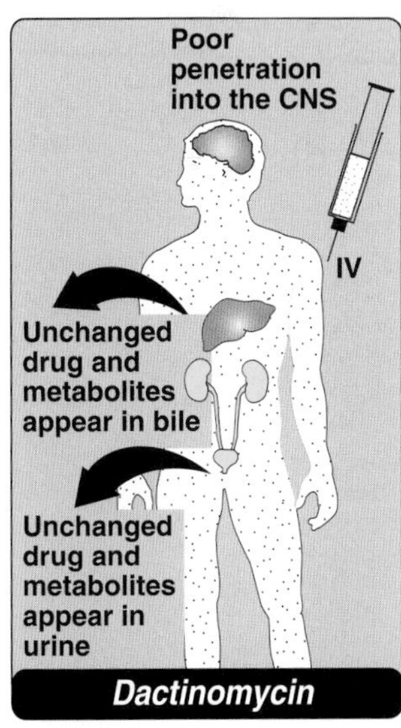

Figure 39.17
Administration and fate of *dactinomycin*.

B. Doxorubicin and daunorubicin

Doxorubicin [dox oh ROO bi sin] and *daunorubicin* [daw noe ROO bi sin] are classified as anthracycline antibiotics. *Doxorubicin* is the hydroxylated analog of *daunorubicin*. *Idarubicin* [eye da RUE bi sin], the 4-demethoxy analog of *daunorubicin*, and *epirubicin* [eh pee ROO bih sin] are also available. Applications for these agents differ despite their structural similarity and their apparently similar mechanisms of action. *Doxorubicin* is one of the most important and widely used anticancer drugs. It is used in combination with other agents for treatment of sarcomas and a variety of carcinomas, including breast and lung, as well as for treatment of acute lymphocytic leukemia and lymphomas. *Daunorubicin* and *idarubicin* are used in the treatment of acute leukemias.

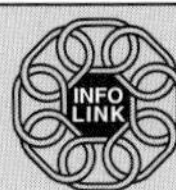

[8]See p. 395 in ***Lippincott's Illustrated Reviews: Biochemistry*** (3rd ed.) for a discussion of DNA structure.

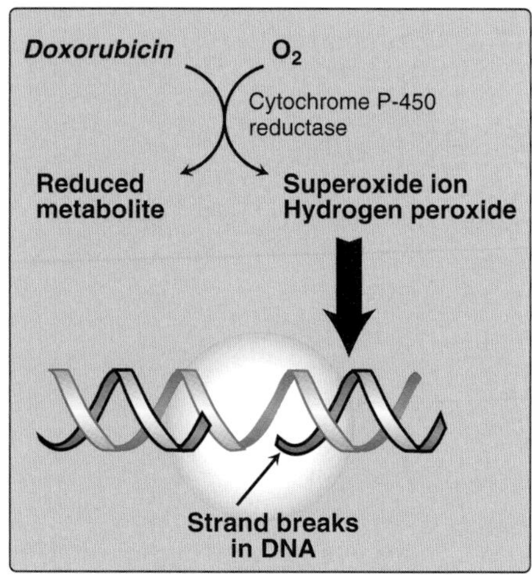

Figure 39.18
Doxorubicin interacts with molecular oxygen, producing superoxide ions and hydrogen peroxide, which cause single-strand breaks in DNA.

1. **Mechanism of action:** The anthracyclines have three major activities that may vary with the type of cell. All three are maximal in the S and G_2 phases.

   a. **Intercalation in the DNA:** The drugs insert nonspecifically between adjacent base pairs and bind to the sugar-phosphate backbone of DNA. This causes local uncoiling and, thus, blocks DNA and RNA synthesis. Intercalation can interfere with the topoisomerase II–catalyzed breakage/reunion reaction of DNA strands, causing irreparable breaks.

   b. **Binding to cell membranes:** This action alters the function of transport processes coupled to phosphatidylinositol activation.[9]

   c. **Generation of oxygen radicals:** Cytochrome P450 reductase (present in cell nuclear membranes) catalyzes reduction of the anthracyclines to semiquinone free radicals. These in turn reduce molecular O_2, producing superoxide ions and hydrogen peroxide, which mediate single-strand scission of DNA (Figure 39.18). Tissues with ample superoxide dismutase (SOD) or glutathione peroxidase activity are protected.[10] Tumors and heart tissue are generally low in SOD. In addition, cardiac tissue lacks catalase and, thus, cannot dispose of hydrogen peroxide. Lipid peroxidation therefore may explain the cardiotoxicity of anthracyclines.

2. **Pharmacokinetics:** All these drugs must be administered IV because they are inactivated in the GI tract. Extravasation is a serious problem that can lead to tissue necrosis. The anthracycline antibiotics bind to plasma proteins as well as to tissues, where they are widely distributed. They do not penetrate the blood-brain barrier or the testes. All these drugs undergo extensive hepatic metabolism. The bile is the major route of excretion, and the drug dose must be modified in patients with impaired hepatic function (Figure 39.19). Some renal excretion also occurs, but the dose generally need not be adjusted in patients with renal failure. The drugs impart a red color to the urine.

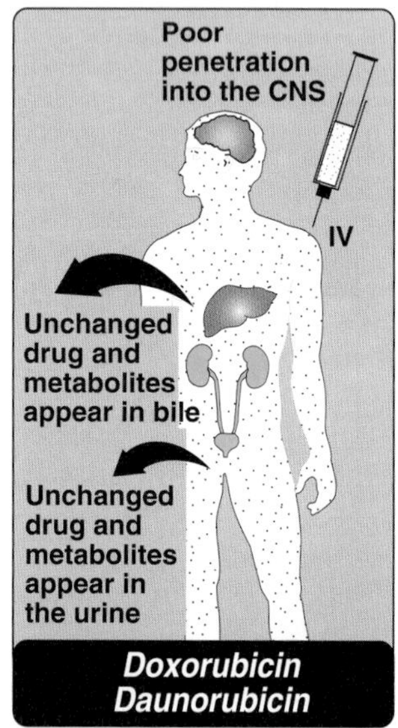

Figure 39.19
Administration and fate of *doxorubicin* and *daunorubicin*.

3. **Adverse effects:** Irreversible, dose-dependent cardiotoxicity, apparently a result of the generation of free radicals and lipid peroxidation, is the most serious adverse reaction and is more common with *daunorubicin* and *doxorubicin* than with *idarubicin* or *epirubicin*. Irradiation of the thorax increases the risk of cardiotoxicity. Addition of *trastuzumab* to protocols with *doxorubicin* or *epirubicin* increases congestive heart failure. There has been some success with the iron-chelator *dexrazone* in protecting against the cardiotoxicity of *doxorubicin*. [Note: A new liposomal-encapsulated *doxorubicin* has been reported to be less cardiotoxic than the usual formulation.] As with *dactinomycin*, both *doxorubicin* and *daunorubicin* also cause transient bone marrow suppression, stomatitis, and GI tract disturbances. Increased skin pigmentation is also seen. Alopecia is usually severe.

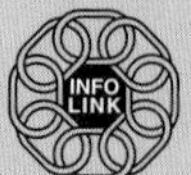

[9]See p. 203 in ***Lippincott's Illustrated Reviews: Biochemistry*** (3rd ed.) for a discussion of phosphatidylinositol activation.
[10]See p. 146 in ***Lippincott's Illustrated Reviews: Biochemistry*** (3rd ed.) for a discussion of super oxide dismutase and glutathione.

C. Bleomycin

Bleomycin [blee oh MYE sin] is a mixture of different copper-chelating glycopeptides that, like the anthracycline antibiotics, cause scission of DNA by an oxidative process. *Bleomycin* is cell-cycle specific and causes cells to accumulate in the G_2 phase. It is primarily employed in the treatment of testicular tumors in combination with *vinblastine* or *etoposide*. Response rates are close to 100 percent if *cisplatin* is added to the regimen. *Bleomycin* is also effective, although not curative, for squamous cell carcinomas and lymphomas.

1. **Mechanism of action**: A DNA-bleomycin-Fe^{2+} complex appears to undergo oxidation to bleomycin-Fe^{3+}. The liberated electrons react with oxygen to form superoxide or hydroxide radicals, which in turn attack the phosphodiester bonds of DNA, resulting in strand breakage and chromosomal aberrations (Figure 39.20).

2. **Resistance:** Although the mechanisms of resistance have not been elucidated, experimental systems have implicated increased levels of *bleomycin* hydrolase (or deamidase), glutathione-S-transferase, and possibly, increased efflux of the drug. DNA repair also may contribute.

3. **Pharmacokinetics:** *Bleomycin* is administered by a number of routes, including subcutaneous, intramuscular, IV, and intracavitary. The *bleomycin*-inactivating enzyme (a hydrolase) is high in a number of tissues (for example, liver and spleen) but is low in lung and is absent in skin (accounting for the drug's toxicity in those tissues). Most of the parent drug is excreted unchanged into the urine by glomerular filtration, necessitating dose adjustment in patients with renal failure.

4. **Adverse effects:** Pulmonary toxicity is the most serious adverse effect, progressing from rales, cough, and infiltrate to potentially fatal fibrosis. Mucocutaneous reactions and alopecia are common. Hypertrophic skin changes and hyperpigmentation of the hands are prevalent. There is a high incidence of fever and chills and a low incidence of serious anaphylactoid reactions. *Bleomycin* is unusual in that myelosuppression is rare.

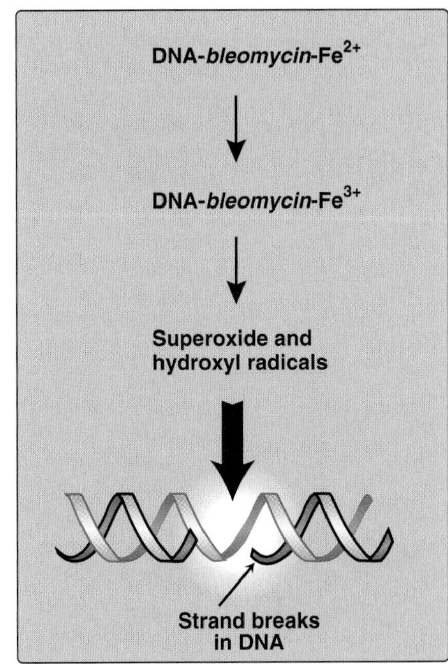

Figure 39.20
Bleomycin causes breaks in DNA by an oxidative process.

V. ALKYLATING AGENTS

Alkylating agents exert their cytotoxic effects by covalently binding to nucleophilic groups on various cell constituents. Alkylation of DNA is probably the crucial cytotoxic reaction that is lethal to the tumor cell. Alkylating agents do not discriminate between cycling and resting cells, but they are most toxic for rapidly dividing cells. They are used in combination with other agents to treat a wide variety of lymphatic and solid cancers. In addition to being cytotoxic, all are mutagenic and carcinogenic and can lead to a second malignancy, such as acute leukemia.

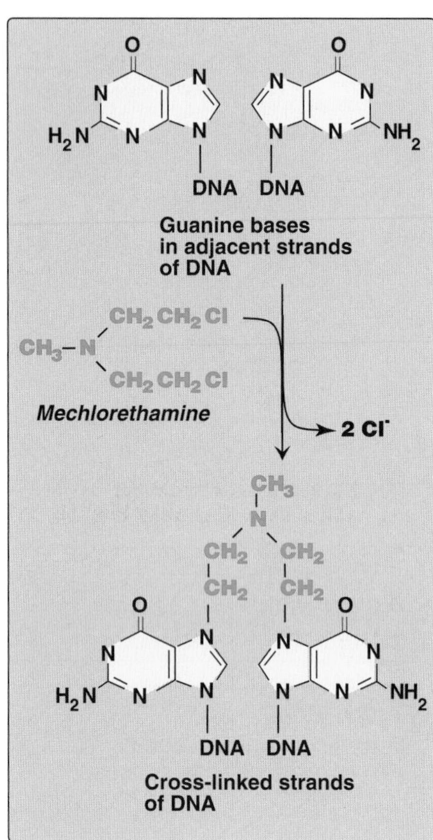

Figure 39.21
Alkylation of guanine bases in DNA is responsible for the cytotoxic effect of *mechlorethamine.*

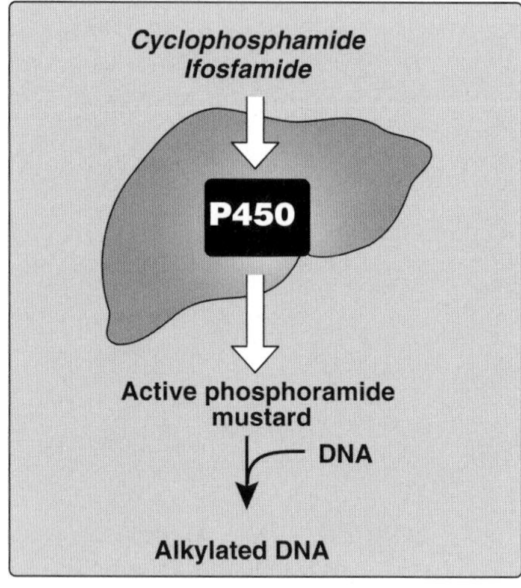

Figure 39.22
Activation of *cyclophosphamide* and *ifosfamide* by hepatic cytochrome P450.

A. Mechlorethamine

Mechlorethamine [mek lor ETH ah meen] was developed as a vesicant (nitrogen mustard) during World War I. Its ability to cause lymphocytopenia led to its use in lymphatic cancers. Because it can bind and react at two separate sites, it is called a "bifunctional agent." *Mechlorethamine* was used primarily in the treatment of Hodgkin disease and may find use in the treatment of some solid tumors.

1. **Mechanism of action:** *Mechlorethamine* is transported into the cell where the drug forms a reactive intermediate that alkylates the N7 nitrogen of a guanine residue in one or both strands of a DNA molecule (Figure 39.21). This alkylation leads to cross-linkages between guanine residues in the DNA chains and/or depurination, thus facilitating DNA strand breakage. Alkylation can also cause miscoding mutations. Although alkylation can occur in both cycling and resting cells (and, therefore, is cell-cycle nonspecific), proliferating cells are more sensitive to the drug, especially those in G_1 and S phases.

2. **Resistance:** Resistance has been ascribed to decreased permeability of the drug, increased conjugation with thiols such as glutathione, and possibly, increased DNA repair.

3. **Pharmacokinetics:** *Mechlorethamine* is very unstable, and solutions must be made up just prior to administration. *Mechlorethamine* is also a powerful vesicant (blistering agent), and is only administered IV. Because of its reactivity, scarcely any drug is excreted.

4. **Adverse effects:** The adverse effects caused by *mechlorethamine* include severe nausea and vomiting (centrally mediated). [Note: These effects can be diminished by pretreatment with *palonosetron* and *dexamethasone.*] Severe bone marrow depression limits extensive use. Latent viral infections (for example, herpes zoster) may appear because of immunosuppression. Extravasation is a serious problem. If it occurs, the area should be infiltrated with isotonic sodium thiosulfite to inactivate the drug.

B. Cyclophosphamide and ifosfamide

These drugs are very closely related mustard agents that share most of the same toxicities. They are unique in that they can be taken orally, and are cytotoxic only after generation of their alkylating species, which are produced through hydroxylation by cytochrome P450. These agents have a broad clinical spectrum, being used either singly or as part of a regimen in the treatment of a wide variety of neoplastic diseases, such as Burkitt lymphoma and breast cancer. Non-neoplastic disease entities, such as nephrotic syndrome and intractable rheumatoid arthritis, are also effectively treated with *cyclophosphamide.*

1. **Mechanism of action:** *Cyclophosphamide* [sye kloe FOSS fah mide] is the most commonly used alkylating agent. Both *cyclophosphamide* and *ifosfamide* [eye FOSS fah mide] are first

biotransformed to hydroxylated intermediates by the cytochrome P450 system (Figure 39.22). The hydroxylated intermediates then undergo breakdown to form the active compounds, phosphoramide mustard and acrolein. Reaction of the phosphoramide mustard with DNA is considered to be the cytotoxic step.

2. **Resistance:** Resistance results from increased DNA repair, decreased drug permeability, and reaction of the drug with thiols (for example, glutathione). Cross-resistance does not always occur.

3. **Pharmacokinetics:** Unlike most of the alkylating agents, *cyclophosphamide* and *ifosfamide* are preferentially administered by the oral route (Figure 39.23). Minimal amounts of the parent drug are excreted into the feces (after biliary transport), or into the urine by glomerular filtration.

4. **Adverse effects:** The most prominent toxicities of both drugs (after alopecia, nausea, vomiting, and diarrhea) are bone marrow depression, especially leukocytosis, and hemorrhagic cystitis, which can lead to fibrosis of the bladder. The latter toxicity has been attributed to acrolein in the urine in the case of *cyclophosphamide* and to toxic metabolites of *ifosfamide*. [Note: Adequate hydration as well as IV injection of MESNA (sodium 2-mercaptoethane sulfonate), which inactivates the toxic compounds, minimizes this problem.] Other toxicities include effects on the germ cells, resulting in amenorrhea, testicular atrophy, and sterility. Veno-occlusive disease of the liver is seen in about 25 percent of the patients. A fairly high incidence of neurotoxicity has been reported in patients on high-dose *ifosfamide*, probably due to the metabolite, chloroacetaldehyde. Secondary malignancies may appear years after therapy.

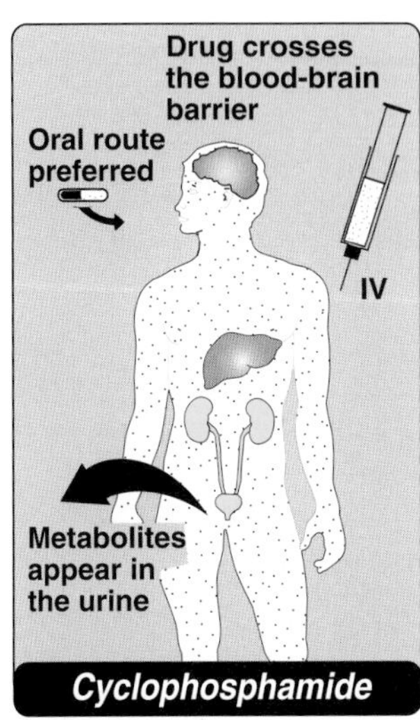

Figure 39.23
Administration and fate of *cyclophosphamide*.

C. Nitrosoureas

Carmustine [kar MUS teen] and *lomustine* [loe MUS teen] are closely related nitrosoureas. Because of their ability to penetrate into the CNS, the nitrosoureas are primarily employed in the treatment of brain tumors. They find limited use in the treatment of other cancers. [Note: *Streptozocin* [strep toe ZOE sin] is another nitrosourea that is specifically toxic to the β-cells of the islets of Langerhans, hence its use in the treatment of insulinomas.]

1. **Mechanism of action:** The nitrosoureas exert cytotoxic effects by an alkylation that cross-links strands of DNA to inhibit its replication and, eventually, RNA and protein synthesis. Although they alkylate DNA in resting cells, cytotoxicity is expressed only on cell division. Therefore, nondividing cells can escape death if DNA repair occurs.

2. **Resistance:** Although the true nature of resistance to nitrosoureas is unknown, it probably results from DNA repair and reaction of the drugs with thiols.

3. **Pharmacokinetics:** In spite of the similarities in their structures, *carmustine* is administered IV, whereas *lomustine* is given orally.

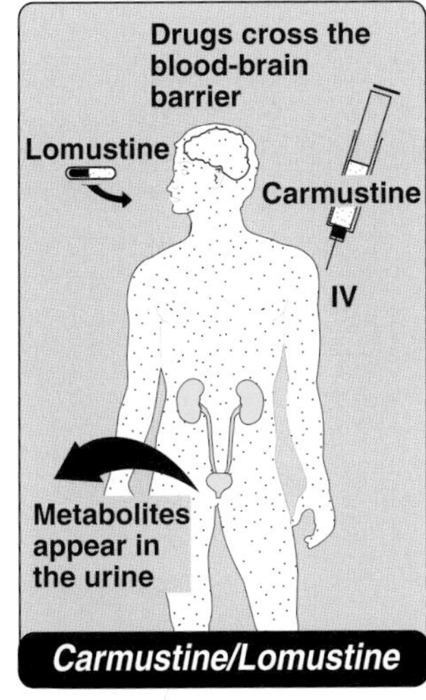

Figure 39.24
Administration and fate of *carmustine/lomustine*.

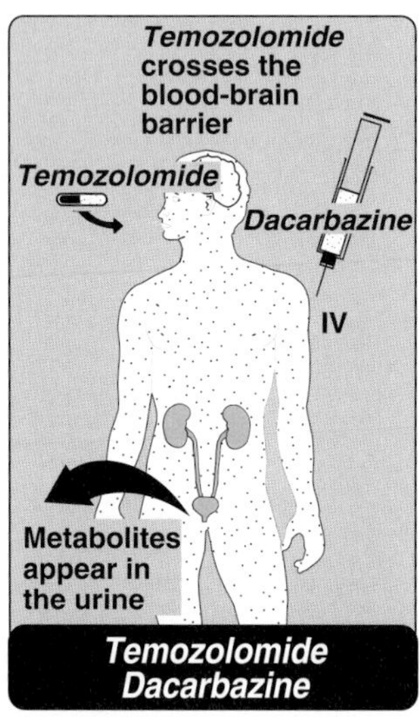

Figure 39.25
Administration and fate of *temozolomide/dacarbazine.*

Because of their lipophilicity, they distribute to many tissues, but their most striking property is their ability to readily penetrate into the CNS. The drugs undergo extensive metabolism. *Lomustine* is metabolized to active products. The kidney is the major excretory route for the nitrosoureas (Figure 39.24).

4. **Adverse effects:** These include delayed hematopoietic depression, which may be due to metabolic products. An aplastic marrow may develop on prolonged use. Renal toxicity and pulmonary fibrosis related to duration of therapy is also encountered. [Note: *Streptozotocin* is also diabetogenic.]

D. Temozolamide and dacarbazine

The treatment of tumors in the brain is particularly difficult. Recently, *temozolomide* [te moe ZOE loe mide], a triazene agent, has been approved for use against treatment-resistant gliomas and anaplastic astrocytomas. *Temozolomide* is related to *dacarbazine* [dah KAR bah zeen]—an agent that has found some use in the treatment of melanoma. Both must undergo biotransformation to an active metabolite, methylhydrazine, which is probably responsible for the drugs' activity. The cytotoxic action of these agents has been attributed to their ability to methylate DNA on the O6 position of guanine. *Temozolomide* also has the property of inhibiting the repair enzyme, O^6-guanine-DNA-alkyltransferase. A property that distinguishes *temozolomide* from *dacarbazine* is the former's ability to cross the blood-brain barrier. Whereas *dacarbazine* is administered IV, *temozolomide* is taken orally and has excellent oral bioavailability. The parent drugs and metabolites are excreted in the urine (Figure 39.25). *Temozolomide* is taken for five consecutive days and repeated every 28 days. Its major initial toxicities are nausea and vomiting. Myelosuppression (thrombocytopenia and neutropenia) occur later in the treatment cycle.

E. Other alkylating agents

Melphalan [MEL fah lan], a phenylalanine derivative of nitrogen mustard, and *chlorambucil* [clor AM byoo sil] are oral agents used in the treatment of multiple myeloma and chronic lymphocytic leukemia, respectively. They have moderate hematologic toxicities and upset the GI tract. *Busulfan* [byoo SUL fan] is another oral agent that is effective against chronic granulocytic leukemia. Myelosuppression is its major toxicity. It can also cause pulmonary fibrosis. Like other alkylating agents, all these agents are leukemogenic.

VI. MICROTUBULE INHIBITORS

The mitotic spindle is part of a larger, intracellular skeleton (cytoskeleton) that is essential for the movements of structures occurring in the cytoplasm of all eukaryotic cells. The mitotic spindle consists of chromatin plus a system of microtubules composed of the protein tubulin. The mitotic spindle is essential for the equal partitioning of DNA into the two daughter cells that are formed when a eukaryotic cell divides. Several plant-derived substances used as anticancer drugs disrupt this process by affecting the equilibrium between the polymerized and depolymerized forms of the microtubules, thereby causing cytotoxicity.

A. Vincristine and vinblastine

Vincristine [vin KRIS teen] (*VX*) and *vinblastine* [vin BLAS teen] (*VBL*) are structurally related compounds derived from the periwinkle plant, Vinca rosea. They are therefore referred to as the vinca alkaloids. A structurally related, new (and less toxic) agent is *vinorelbine* [vye NOR el been] (*VRB*). Although the vinca alkaloids are structurally very similar to each other, their therapeutic indications are different. They are generally administered in combination with other drugs. *VX* is used in the treatment of acute lymphoblastic leukemia in children, Wilms tumor, Ewing soft-tissue sarcoma, and Hodgkin and non-Hodgkin lymphomas, as well as some other rapidly proliferating neoplasms. [Note: *VX* (trade name is *oncovin*) is the "O" in the POMP regimen for leukemia and a number of other protocols.] *VBL* is administered with *bleomycin* and *cisplatin* for the treatment of metastatic testicular carcinoma. It is also used in the treatment of systemic Hodgkin and non-Hodgkin lymphomas. *VRB* is beneficial in the treatment of advanced non–small cell lung cancer, either as a single agent or with *cisplatin.*

1. **Mechanism of action:** *VX* and *VBL* are both **cell cycle-specific** and **phase-specific**, because they block mitosis in metaphase. Their binding to the microtubular protein, tubulin, is GTP–dependent and blocks the ability of tubulin to polymerize to form microtubules. Instead, paracrystalline aggregates consisting of tubulin dimers and the alkaloid drug are formed. The resulting dysfunctional spindle apparatus, frozen in metaphase, prevents chromosomal segregation and cell proliferation (Figure 39.26).

2. **Resistance:** Resistant cells have been shown to have an enhanced efflux of *VX*, *VBL,* and *VRB* via P-glycoprotein in the cell membrane. Alterations in tubulin structure may also affect binding of the vinca alkaloids.

3. **Pharmacokinetics:** Intravenous injection of these agents leads to rapid cytotoxic effects and cell destruction. This in turn can cause hyperuricemia due to the oxidation of purines to uric acid. The hyperuricemia is ameliorated by administration of the xanthine oxidase–inhibitor *allopurinol.* The vinca alkaloids are concentrated and metabolized in the liver by the cytochrome P450 pathway. They are excreted into bile and feces. Doses must be modified in patients with impaired hepatic function or biliary obstruction.

4. **Adverse effects:** Both *VX* and *VBL* have certain toxicities in common. These include phlebitis or cellulitis, if the drugs extravasate during injection, as well as nausea, vomiting, diarrhea, and alopecia. However, the adverse effects of *VX* and *VBL* are not identical. *VBL* is a more potent myelosuppressant than *VX*, whereas peripheral neuropathy (paresthesias, loss of reflexes, footdrop, and ataxia) is associated with *VX*. Constipation is more frequently encountered with *VX*, which can also cause inappropriate antidiuretic hormone secretion. The anticonvulsants *phenytoin*, *pheno-*

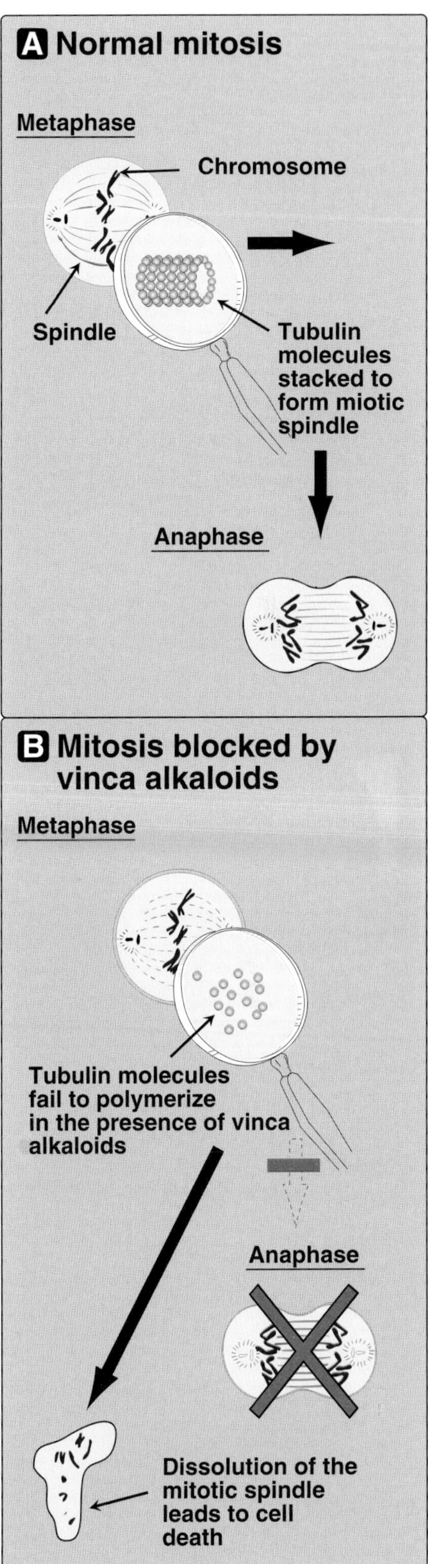

Figure 39.26
Mechanism of action of the microtubule inhibitors.

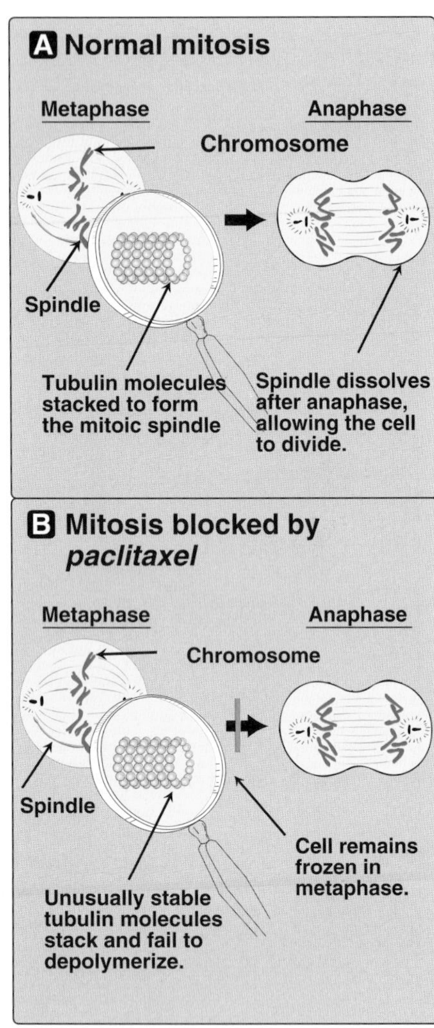
A Normal mitosis
Metaphase
Anaphase
Chromosome
Spindle
Tubulin molecules stacked to form the mitoic spindle
Spindle dissolves after anaphase, allowing the cell to divide.
B Mitosis blocked by paclitaxel
Metaphase
Anaphase
Chromosome
Spindle
Cell remains frozen in metaphase.
Unusually stable tubulin molecules stack and fail to depolymerize.

Figure 39.27
Paclitaxel stabilizes microtubules, rendering them nonfunctional.

barbital, and *carbamazepine* can accelerate the metabolism of *VX*, whereas the azole antifungal drugs can slow its metabolism. Granulocytopenia is dose-limiting for *VRB*.

G. Paclitaxel and docetaxel

Better known as *taxol*, *paclitaxel* [PAK li tax el] is the first member of the taxane family to be used in cancer chemotherapy. A semi-synthetic *paclitaxel* is now available through chemical modification of a precursor found in the needles of yew species. Substitution of a side chain has resulted in *docetaxel* [doe see TAX el], which is the more potent of the two drugs. *Paclitaxel* has shown good activity against advanced ovarian cancer and metastatic breast cancer. Favorable results have been obtained in non–small cell lung cancer when administered with *cisplatin*. *Docetaxel* is showing impressive benefits, with fewer side effects, in these conditions.

1. **Mechanism of action:** Both drugs are active in the G_2/M phase of the cell cycle. They bind reversibly to the β-tubulin subunit, but unlike the vinca alkaloids, they promote polymerization and stabilization of the polymer rather than disassembly (Figure 39.27). Thus, they shift the depolymerization-polymerization process to favor the formation of microtubules. The overly stable microtubules formed are nonfunctional, and chromosome desegregation does not occur. This results in death of the cell.

2. **Resistance:** Like the vinca alkaloids, resistance has been associated with the presence of amplified P-glycoprotein or a mutation in tubulin structure.

3. **Pharmacokinetics:** These agents are infused and have similar pharmacokinetics. Both have a large volume of distribution, but neither enters the brain. Hepatic metabolism by the cytochrome P450 system and biliary excretion are responsible for their elimination into the stool. Thus, dose modification is not required in patients with renal impairment, but doses should be reduced in patients with hepatic dysfunction.

4. **Adverse effects:** The dose-limiting toxicity of *paclitaxel* and *docetaxel* is neutropenia. [Note: Patients with fewer than 1500 neutrophils/mm^3 should not be given these agents.] Treatment with granulocyte colony-stimulating factor (*filgrastim*) can prevent the problems associated with this condition. Peripheral neuropathy can develop with either of these drugs. A transient, asymptomatic bradycardia is sometimes observed with *paclitaxel*, and fluid retention is seen with *docetaxel*. The latter drug is contraindicated in patients with cardiac disease. Alopecia occurs, but vomiting and diarrhea are uncommon. Because of serious hypersensitivity reactions (including dyspnea, urticaria, and hypotension), a patient who is to be treated with *paclitaxel* is premedicated with *dexamethasone* and *diphenhydramine* as well as with an H_2 blocker.

VII. STEROID HORMONES AND THEIR ANTAGONISTS

Tumors that are steroid hormone–sensitive may be either 1) hormone-responsive, in which the tumor regresses following treatment with a specific hormone; 2) hormone–dependent, in which removal of a hormonal stimulus causes tumor regression; or 3) both. Hormone treatment of responsive tumors usually is only palliative, except in the case of the cytotoxic effect of glucocorticoids (for example, *prednisone*) on lymphomas. Removal of hormonal stimuli from hormone-dependent tumors can be accomplished by surgery (for example, in the case of orchiectomy for patients with advanced prostate cancer) or by drugs (for example in breast cancer, for which treatment with the antiestrogen *tamoxifen* is used to prevent estrogen stimulation of breast cancer cells). For a steroid hormone to influence a cell, that cell must have cytosolic receptors that are specific for that hormone (Figure 39.28A).

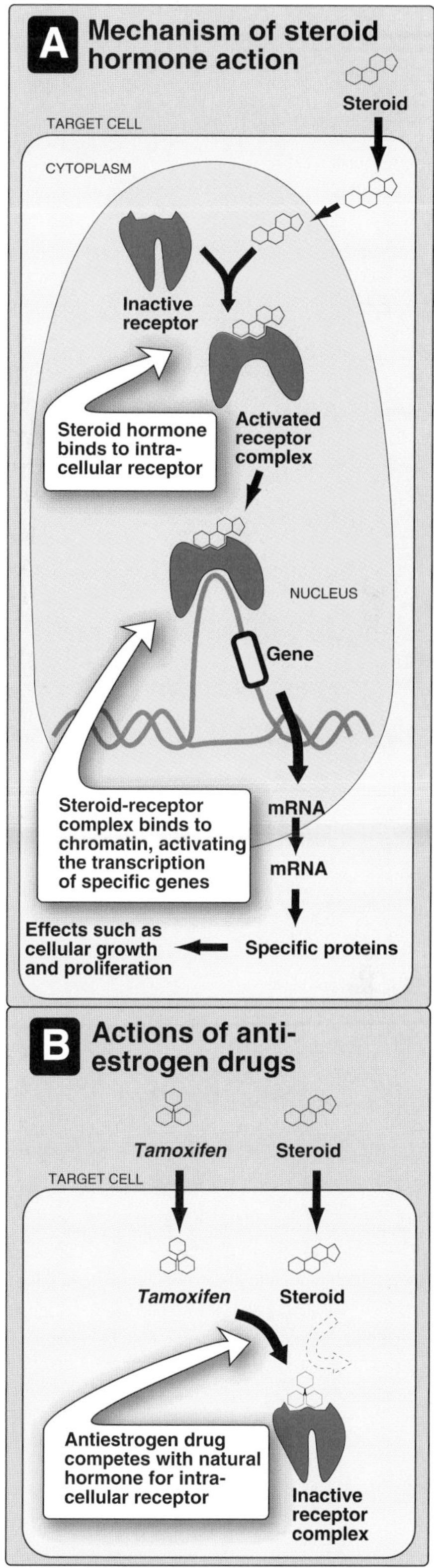

Figure 39.28
Action of steroid hormones and antiestrogen agents.

A. Prednisone

Prednisone [PRED ni sone] is a potent, synthetic, anti-inflammatory corticosteroid with less mineralocorticoid activity than *cortisol*. The use of this compound in the treatment of lymphomas arose when it was observed that patients with Cushing syndrome, which is associated with hypersecretion of cortisol, have lymphocytopenia and decreased lymphoid mass. [Note: At high doses, *cortisol* is also lymphocytolytic and leads to hyperuricemia due to the breakdown of lymphocytes.] *Prednisone* is primarily employed to induce remission in patients with acute lymphocytic leukemia and in the treatment of both Hodgkin and non-Hodgkin lymphomas.

1. **Mechanism of action:** *Prednisone* itself is inactive, and must first be reduced to prednisolone by 11-β-hydroxysteroid dehydrogenase.[11] This steroid then binds to a receptor that triggers the production of specific proteins (see Figure 39.28A).

2. **Resistance:** Resistance is associated with an absence of the receptor protein or a mutation that lowers receptor affinity for the hormone. However, in some resistant cells, a receptor-hormone complex is formed, although a stage of gene expression is apparently affected.

3. **Pharmacokinetics:** *Prednisone* is readily absorbed orally. Like other glucocorticoids it is bound to plasma albumin and transcortin. It undergoes 11-β-hydroxylation to prednisolone in the liver. Prednisolone is the active drug. The latter is glucuronidated and excreted into the urine along with the parent compound.

4. **Adverse effects:** *Prednisone* has many of the adverse effects associated with glucocorticoids. It can predispose to infection (due to its immunosuppressant action) and to ulcers and pancreatitis. Other effects include hyperglycemia, cataract formation, glaucoma, osteoporosis, and change in mood (euphoria or psychosis).

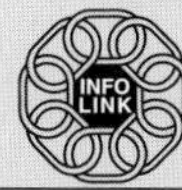

[11]See p. 236 in ***Lippincott's Illustrated Reviews: Biochemistry*** (3rd ed.) for the reaction catalyzed by 11-β-hydroxysteroid dehydrogenase.

B. Tamoxifen

Tamoxifen [tah MOX ih fen] is an estrogen antagonist. It is structurally related to the synthetic estrogen *diethylstilbestrol* and is used for first-line therapy in the treatment of estrogen receptor–positive breast cancer. *Tamoxifen* has weak estrogenic activity, and is classified as a selective estrogen-receptor modulator (SERM). Another SERM that has been approved for advanced breast cancer in postmenopausal women is *toremifene* [tore EM ih feen]. It also finds use prophylactically in reducing breast cancer in women who are at high risk. However, because of possible effects stimulating premalignant lesions due to its estrogenic properties, *tamoxifen* is presently approved only for five years of use.

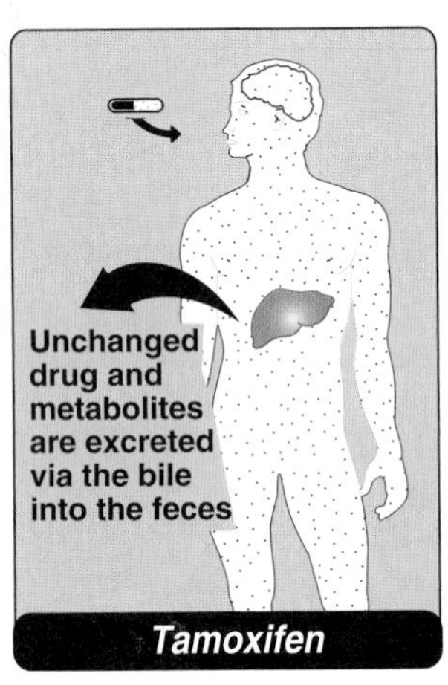
Unchanged drug and metabolites are excreted via the bile into the feces
Tamoxifen

Figure 39.29
Administration and fate of *tamoxifen*.

1. **Mechanism of action:** *Tamoxifen* binds to the estrogen receptor, but the complex is not productive. That is, the complex fails to induce estrogen-responsive genes, and RNA synthesis does not ensue (Figure 39.28B). The result is a depletion of estrogen receptors, and the growth-promoting effects of the natural hormone and other growth factors are suppressed. [Note: Estrogen competes with *tamoxifen*. Therefore, in premenopausal women, the drug is used with a gonadotropin-releasing analog such as *leuprolide*, which lowers estrogen levels.] The action of *tamoxifen* is not related to any specific phase of the cell cycle.

2. **Resistance:** Resistance is associated with a decreased affinity for the receptor, a decreased number of receptors, or the presence of a dysfunctional receptor.

3. **Pharmacokinetics:** *Tamoxifen* is effective on oral administration. It is partially metabolized by the liver. Some metabolites possess antagonist activity, whereas others have agonist activity. Unchanged drug and its metabolites are excreted predominantly through the bile into the feces (Figure 39.29).

4. **Adverse effects:** Side effects caused by *tamoxifen* are similar to the effects of natural estrogen, including hot flashes, nausea, vomiting, skin rash, vaginal bleeding, and discharge (due to some slight estrogenic activity of the drug and some of its metabolites). Hypercalcemia requiring cessation of the drug may occur. *Tamoxifen* can also lead to increased pain if the tumor has metastasized to bone. *Tamoxifen* has the potential to cause endometrial cancer. Other toxicities include thromboembolism and effects on vision. [Note: Because of a more favorable adverse effect profile, aromatase inhibitors are making an impact in the treatment of breast cancer.]

C. Aromatase inhibitors

The aromatase reaction is responsible for the extra-adrenal synthesis of estrogen from androstenedione, which takes place in liver, fat, muscle, skin, and breast tissue, including breast malignancies. Peripheral aromatization is an important source of estrogen in postmenopausal women. Aromatase inhibitors decrease the production of estrogen in these women .

1. **Aminoglutethimide:** *Aminoglutethimide* [ah mee noe glue TETH ih mide] was the first aromatase inhibitor to be identified for the treatment of metastatic breast cancer in postmenopausal women. *Aminoglutethimide* was shown to inhibit both the adrenal synthesis of pregnenolone (a precursor of estrogen) from cholesterol as well as the extra-adrenal synthesis. Because the drug also inhibits hydrocortisone synthesis, which evokes a compensatory rise in adrenocorticotropic hormone secretion sufficient to overwhelm the blockade of the adrenal, the drug is usually taken with *hydrocortisone*. Due to its nonselective properties and unfavorable side effects, as well as the need to concomittantly administer *hydrocortisone* (*cortisol*), newer aromatase inhibitors (described below) have been developed

2. **Anastrozole and letrozole:** The imidazole aromatase inhibitors, *anastrozole* [an AS troe zole] and *letrozole* [LE troe zole], are nonsteroidal. They have gained favor in the treatment of breast cancer because 1) they are more potent (they inhibit aromatization by greater than 96 percent, compared to less than ninety percent with *aminoglutethimide*), 2) they are more selective than *aminoglutethimide*, 3) they do not need to be supplemented with hydrocortisone, 4) they do not predispose to endometrial cancer, and 5) they are devoid of the androgenic side effects that occur with the steroidal aromatase inhibitors. Although *anastrozole* and *letrozole* are considered to be second-line therapy after *tamoxifen* for hormone-dependent breast cancer in the United States, they have become first-line drugs in other countries for the treatment of breast cancer in postmenopausal women They are orally active and cause almost a total suppression of estrogen synthesis. They are cleared primarily by liver metabolism.

3. **Exemestane:** A steroidal, irreversible inhibitor of aromatase, *exemestanei* [ex uh MES tane] is orally well-absorbed and widely distributed. Hepatic metabolism is by the CYP3A4 isozyme, but to date, no interactions have been reported. Because the metabolites are excreted into the urine, doses of the drug must be adjusted in patients with renal failure. Its major toxicities are nausea, fatigue, and hot flashes. Acne and hair changes also occur.

D. Progestins

Megestrol acetate [me JESS trole] was formerly the progestin used most widely in treating metastatic hormone-responsive breast and endometrial neoplasms. It is orally effective. Other agents are usually compared to it in clinical trials. However, the aromatase inhibitors are replacing it in therapy.

E. Leuprolide and goserelin

Gonadotropin-releasing hormone (GnRH) is normally secreted by the hypothalamus and stimulates the anterior pituitary to secrete the gonadotropic hormones, leuteinizing hormone (LH; the primary stimulus for the secretion of testosterone by the testes), and follicle-stimulating hormone (FSH; which stimulates the secretion of estrogen). The synthetic nonapeptides, *leuprolide* [loo PROE lide] and

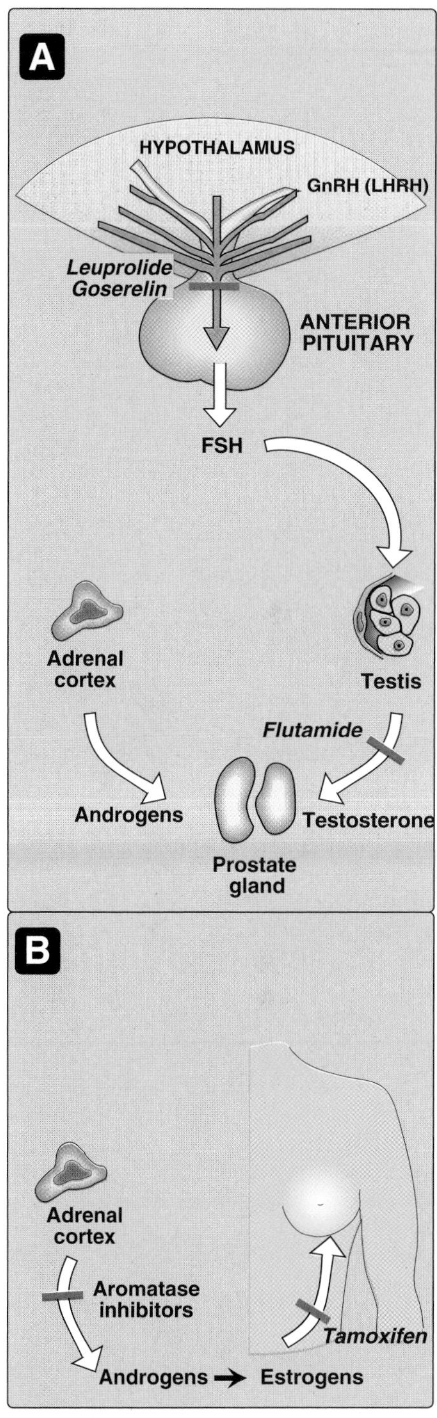

Figure 39.30
Effects of some anticancer drugs on the endocrine system. A. In therapy for prostatic cancer. B. In therapy of postmenopausal breast cancer. GnRH (LHRH) = gonadotropin-releasing hormone (leuteinizing hormone-releasing hormone).

goserelin [GOE se rel in], are analogs of GnRH. As GnRH agonists, they occupy the GnRH receptor in the pituitary, which leads to its desensitization and, consequently, inhibition of release of FSH and LH. Thus, both androgen and estrogen syntheses are reduced (Figure 39.30). Response to *leuprolide* in prostatic cancer is equivalent to that of orchiectomy (surgical removal of one or both testes), with regression of tumor and relief of bone pain. These drugs have some benefit in premenopausal women with advanced breast cancer and have largely replaced estrogens in therapy for prostate cancer. *Leuprolide* is available 1) as a sustained-release preparation, 2) subcutaneously, or 3) as a depot intramuscular injection, to treat metastatic carcinoma of the prostate. *Goserelin acetate* is implanted intramuscularly. Levels of androgen may initially rise but then fall to castration levels. The adverse effects of these drugs, including impotence, hot flashes, and tumor flare, are minimal compared to those experienced with estrogen treatment.

F. Estrogens

Estrogens, such as *ethinyl estradiol* or *diethylstilbestrol*, had been used in the treatment of prostatic cancer. However, they have been largely replaced by the GnRH analogs because of fewer adverse effects. Estrogens inhibit the growth of prostatic tissue by blocking the production of LH, thereby decreasing the synthesis of androgens in the testis. Thus, tumors that are dependent on androgens are affected. Estrogen treatment can cause serious complications, such as thromboemboli, myocardial infarction, strokes, and hypercalcemia. Men who are taking estrogens may experience gynecomastia and impotence.

G. Flutamide, nilutamide and bicalutamide

Flutamide [FLOO tah mide], *nilutamide* [nye LOO ta mide], and *bicalutamide* [bye ka LOO ta mide] are synthetic, nonsteroidal antiandrogens used in the treatment of prostate cancer. They compete with the natural hormone for binding to the androgen receptor and prevent its translocation into the nucleus (see Figure 39.30). *Flutamide* is metabolized to an active hydroxy derivative that binds to the androgen receptor. *Flutamide* blocks the inhibitory effects of testosterone on gonadotropin secretion, causing an increase in serum LH and testosterone levels. *Flutamide* is always administered in combination with *leuprolide* or *goserelin*. These antiandrogens are taken orally. [Note: *Flutamide* requires dosing three times a day and the others once a day.] These agents are cleared through the kidney. Side effects include gynecomastia and GI distressand, in the case of *flutamide*, liver failure. *Nilutamide* can cause visual problems.

VIII. MONOCLONAL ANTIBODIES

Monoclonal antibodies have become an active area of drug development for anticancer therapy and other non-neoplastic diseases, because they are directed at specific targets, and often have fewer adverse effects. They are created from B lymphocytes (from immunized mice or hamsters) fused with “immortal” B lymphocyte tumor cells. The resulting hybrid cells can be individually cloned, and each clone will produce antibodies directed against a single antigen type. Recombinant technology has led to the creation of "humanized" antibodies that overcome the immunologic problems previously observed following administration of mouse antibodies. Currently there are several monoclonal antibodies available in the United States for the treatment of cancer. *Trastuzumab*, *rituximab*, *bevacizumab* and *cetuximab* are described below. Others include: *gemtuzumab ozogamicin,* which is a monoclonal antibody conjugated with a plant toxin and binds to CD33—a cell-surface receptor that is present on the leukemia cells of eighty percent of patients with acute myelocytic leukemia; *alemtuzumab,* which is effective in treatment of B-cell chronic lymphocytic leukemia that no longer responds to other agents; and I^{131}-*tositumomab*, which is used in relapsed non-Hodgkin lymphoma.

A. Trastuzumab

In patients with metastatic breast cancer, overexpression of transmembrane human epidermal growth factor–receptor protein 2 (HER2) is seen in 25 to 30 percent of patients. *Trastuzumab* [tra STEW zoo mab], a recombinant DNA–produced, humanized monoclonal antibody, specifically targets the extracellular domain of the HER2 growth receptor that has intrinsic tyrosine kinase activity. The drug, usually administered with *paclitaxel*, can cause regression of breast cancer and metastases in a small percentage of these individuals. [Note: There are at least fifty tyrosine kinases that mediate cell growth or division by phosphorylating signaling proteins. They have been implicated in the development of many neoplasms by an unknown mechanism.] *Trastuzumab* binds to HER2 sites in breast cancer tissue and inhibits the proliferation of cells that overexpress the HER2 protein, thereby decreasing the number of cells in the S phase.

1. **Mechanism of action:** How the antibody causes its anticancer effect remains to be elucidated. Several mechanisms have been proposed—for example, down-regulation of HER2-receptor expresssion, an induction of antibody-dependent cytoxicity, or a decrease in angiogenesis due to an effect on vascular endothelial growth factor. Efforts are being directed toward identifying those patients with tumors that are sensitive to the drug.

2. **Pharmacokinetics:** *Trastuzumab* is administered IV. *Trastuzumab* does not penetrate the blood-brain barrier.

3. **Adverse effects:** The most serious toxicity associated with the use of *trastuzumab* is congestive heart failure. The toxicity is worsened if given in combination with *anthracycline*. Extreme caution should be exercised when giving the drugs to patients with preexisting cardiac dysfunction. Other adverse effects include infusion-related fever and chills, headache, dizziness, nausea, vomiting, abdominal pain, and back pain, but these effects are well-tolerated. Cautious use of the drug is recommended in patients who are hypersensitive to it, to Chinese hamster ovary cell proteins, or to benzyl alcohol (in which case sterile water can be used in place of the bacteriostic solution provided for preparation of the injection).

B. Rituximab

Rituximab (ri TUCX ih mab) was the first monoclonal antibody TO BE approved for the treatment of cancer. It is a genetically engineered, chimeric monoclonal antibody directed against the CD20 antigen on the surfaces of normal and malignant B lymphocytes. CD20 plays a role in the activation process for cell-cycle initiation and differentiation. The CD20 antigen is expressed on nearly all B-cell non-Hodgkin lymphomas, but not in other bone marrow cells. *Rituximab* has proven to be effective in the treatment of post-transplant lymphoma and in chronic lymphocytic leukemia.

1. **Mechanism of action:** The Fab domain of *rituximab* binds to the CD20 antigen on the B lymphocytes, and its Fc domain recruits immune effector functions, inducing complement and antibody-dependent, cell-mediated cytotoxicity of the B cells. The antibody is commonly used with other combinations of anticancer agents, such as *cyclophosphamide*, *doxorubicin*, *VX,* and *prednisone* (*CHOP*).

2. **Pharmacokinteics:** *Rituximab* is infused IV, and causes a rapid depletion of B cells (both normal and malignant). The fate of the antibody has not been described.

3. **Adverse effects:** Severe adverse reactions have been fatal. It is important to infuse *rituximab* slowly. Hypotension, bronchospasm, and angioedema may occur. Chills and fever frequently accompany the first infusion, especially in patients with high circulating levels of neoplastic cells, because of rapid activation of complement, which results in the release of tumor necrosis factor α and interleukins. Pretreatment with *diphenhydramine*, *acetaminophen*, and bronchodilators can ameliorate these problems. Cardiac arrhythmias can also occur. Tumor lysis syndrome has been reported within 24 hours of the first dose of *rituximab*. This syndrome consists of acute renal failure that may require dialysis, hyperkalemia, hypocalcemia, hyperuricemia, and hyperphosphatasemia (an abnormally high content of alkaline phosphatase in the blood). Leukopenia, thrombocytopenia, and neutropenia have been reported in less than ten percent of patients.

C. Bevacizumab

The monoclonal antibody, *bevacizumab* [be va SEE zoo mab] is the first in a new class of anticancer drugs called antiangiogenesis agents. *Bevacizumab* is approved for use as a first-line drug against metastatic colorectal cancer, and is given with 5-FU-based chemotherapy. *Bevacizumab* is infused intravenously. It attaches to and stops vascular endothelial growth factor from stimulating the formation of new blood vessels. Without new blood vessels, tumors do not receive oxygen and essential nutrients necessary for growth and proliferation. The most common adverse effects of this treatment are hypertension, stomatitis, and diarrhea. Less common are bleeding in the intestines, protein in the urine, and heart failure. Among the rare serious side effects are bowel perforation, opening of healed wounds, and stroke.

D. Cetuximab

Cetuximab [see TUX i mab] is another chimeric monoclonal antibody that has recently been approved to treat colorectal cancer. It is believed to exert its antineoplastic effect by targeting the epidermal growth factor receptor on the surface of cancer cells and interfering with their growth. It is usually used with *irinotecan*. Like other antibodies, it is administered intravenously. *Cetuximab* has caused difficulty breathing and low blood pressure during the first treatment, and interstitial lung disease has been reported. Other side effects include rash, fever, constipation, and abdominal pain.

IX. OTHER CHEMOTHERAPEUTIC AGENTS

A. Platinum coordination complexes

Cisplatin [SIS pla tin] was the first member of the platinum coordination complex class of anticancer drugs, but because of its severe toxicity, *carboplatin* [KAR boe pla tin] was developed. The mechanisms of action of the two drugs is similar, but their potency, pharmacokinetics, patterns of distribution, and dose-limiting toxicities differ. *Cisplatin* has synergistic cytotoxicity with radiation and other chemotherapeutic agents. *Oxaliplatin* [ox AL ih pla tin], a new member of this class of drugs, is a closely-related analog of *carboplatin*. *Cisplatin* has found wide application in the treatment of solid tumors, such as metastatic testicular carcinoma in combination with *VBL* and *bleomycin*, ovarian carcinoma in combination with *cyclophosphamide*, or alone for bladder carcinoma. *Carboplatin* is employed when patients cannot be vigorously hydrated, as is required for *cisplatin* treatment, or if they suffer from kidney dysfunction or are prone to neuro- or ototoxicity. *Oxaliplatin* is showing excellent activity against advanced colorectal cancer.

1. **Mechanism of action:** The mechanism of action for this class of drugs is similar to that of the alkylating agents. In the high-chloride milieu of the plasma, *cisplatin* persists as the neutral species, which enters the cell and loses its chlorides in the low-chloride milieu. It then binds to the N7 of guanine in DNA, forming inter- and intrastrand cross-links. The resulting cytotoxic lesion inhibits both DNA replication and RNA synthesis. Similarly, the chemical moieties that replace the chlorides in the *carboplatin* structure are removed hydrolytically to form the active drug. Cytotoxicity can occur at any stage of the cell cycle, but cells are most vulnerable to the actions of these drugs in the G_1 and S phases. Both drugs can also bind proteins and other compounds containing thiol (–SH) groups.

2. **Resistance:** Sensitivity to these agents is decreased if cells have elevated glutathione levels or increased DNA repair or if metallothionein (a protein rich in –SH groups) is induced. Decreased cellular uptake has also been implicated. Cross-resistance between *cisplatin* and *carboplatin* is not invariable. However, there is none with *oxaliplatin*.

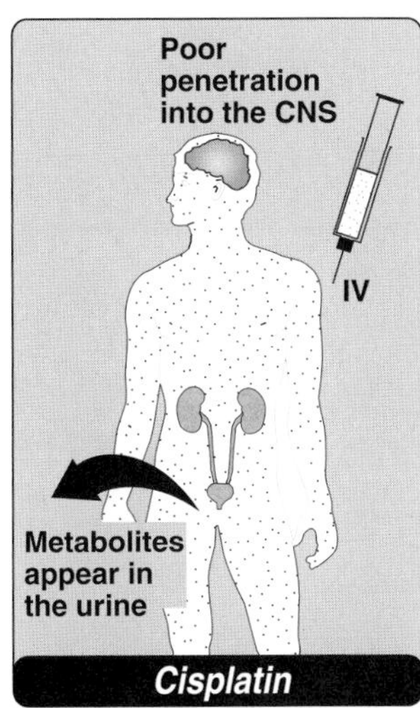

Figure 39.31
Administration and fate of *cisplatin*.

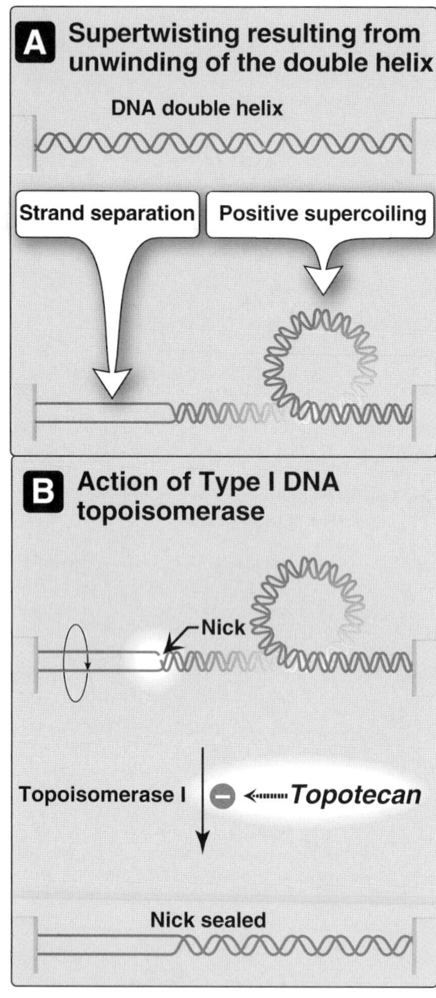

Figure 39.32
Action of Type I DNA topoisomerases.

3. **Pharmacokinetics:** These agents are administered IV in saline solution. They can also be given intraperitoneally for ovarian cancer and intra-arterially to perfuse other organs. More than ninety percent of *cisplatin* is covalently bound to plasma proteins, but the binding of *carboplatin* to plasma proteins is very low. The highest concentrations of the drugs are found in the liver, kidney, and intestinal, testicular, and ovarian cells, but little penetrates into the cerebral spinal fluid. The renal route is the main avenue for excretion (Figure 39.31).

4. **Adverse effects:** Severe, persistent vomiting occurs for at least one hour after administration of *cisplatin*, and may continue for as long as five days. Premedication with antiemetic agents is usually helpful. The major limiting toxicity is dose-related nephrotoxicity, involving the distal convoluted tubule and collecting ducts. This can be ameliorated by aggressive hydration and diuresis. Hypomagnesemia and hypocalcemia usually occur concurrently. [Note: It is important to correct calcium levels before correcting magnesium levels.] Other toxicities include ototoxicity with high-frequency hearing loss and tinnitus, mild bone marrow suppression, some neurotoxicity characterized by paresthesia and loss of proprioception, and hypersensitivity reactions ranging from skin rashes to anaphylaxis. Patients concomitantly receiving aminoglycosides are at greater risk for nephrotoxicity and ototoxicity. Unlike *cisplatin*, *carboplatin* causes only mild nausea and vomiting, and it is not nephro-, neuro-, or ototoxic. Its dose-limiting toxicity is myelosuppression.

B. Irinotecan and topotecan

Irinotecan [eye rin oh TEE kan] and *topotecan* [toe poe TEE kan]] are semisynthetic derivatives of an earlier, more toxic drug, *camptothecin* [camp toe THEE sin]. They have a complicated multi-ring structure containing a lactone ring that is essential for activity. *Topotecan* is employed in metastatic ovarian cancer when primary therapy has failed, and also in the treatment of small-cell lung cancer. *Irinotecan* is used as a first-line drug together with *5-FU* and *leucovorin* for the treatment of colon or rectal carcinoma.

1. **Mechanism of action:** These drugs are S-phase specific.They inhibit topoisomerase I, which is essential for the replication of DNA in human cells (Figure 39.32). Unlike *etoposide*, which inhibits the related enzyme topoisomerase II (see below), *topotecan* was the first clinically useful toposisomerase I inhibitor. The topoisomerases relieve torsional strain in DNA by causing reversible, single-strand breaks. By binding to the enzyme-DNA complex, these agents prevent reannealing of the single-strand breaks.

2. **Resistance:** Several mechanisms may explain resistance. Among them are the ability to transport the drugs out of the cell, decreased ability to convert *irinotecan* to the active SN40 metabolite, or a down-regulation or mutation in topoisomerase I.

3. **Pharmacokinetics:** *Topotecan* and *irinotecan* are infused IV. Hydrolysis of the lactone ring destroys the activity of these drugs. Both the drugs and their metabolites are eliminated in the urine. Therefore, the dose may have to be modified in patients with impaired kidney function.

4. **Adverse effects:** Bone marrow suppression—particularly neutropenia—is the dose-limiting toxicity for *topotecan*. Frequent peripheral blood counts should be performed on patients taking this drug. [Note: *Topotecan* should not be used in patients with a baseline neutrophil count of less than 1500 cells/mm^3. Doing so could result in infection and death.] Other hematologic complications, including thrombocytopenia and anemia, may also occur. Non-hematologic effects include diarrhea, nausea, vomiting, alopecia, and headache. Myelosuppression is also seen with *irinotecan*, and delayed diarrhea may be severe and require treatment with *loperamide*.

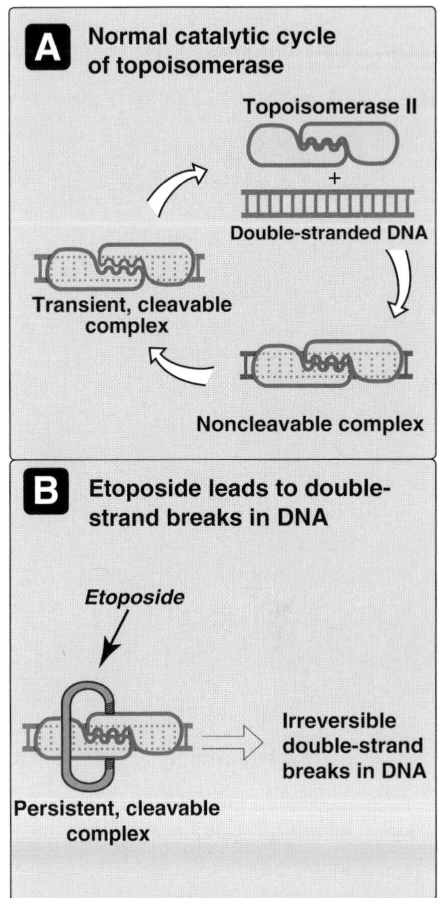

Figure 39.33
Mechanism of action of *etoposide*.

C. Etoposide (VP-16)

Etoposide [e toe POE side] and its analog, *teniposide* [ten i POE side] are semisynthetic derivatives of the plant alkaloid, podophyllotoxin. They block cells in the late S-G_2 phase of the cell cycle. Their major target is topoisomerase II. Binding of the drugs to the enzyme-DNA complex results in persistence of the transient, cleavable form of the complex and, thus, renders it susceptible to irreversible double-strand breaks (Figure 39.33). Resistance to topoisomerase inhibitors is conferred either by presence of the multi-drug resistant P-glycoprotein or by mutation of the enzyme. *Etoposide* finds its major clinical use in the treatment of oat-cell carcinoma of the lung and in combination with *bleomycin* and *cisplatin* for testicular carcinoma. *Teniposide* is used as a second-line agent in the treatment of acute lymphocytic leukemia. *Etoposide* may be administered either IV or orally, whereas *teniposide* is only administered IV. They are highly bound to plasma proteins and distribute throughout the body, but they enter the CSF poorly. Despite this, *teniposide* has shown effectiveness against gliomas and neuroblastomas. Metabolites are converted to glucuronide and sulfate conjugates and are excreted in the urine. Drugs that induce the cytochrome P450 system lead to an acceleration of *teniposide* metabolism. Dose-limiting myelosuppression (primarily leukopenia) is the major toxicity for both drugs. Leukemia may develop in patients who were treated with *etoposide*. Other toxicities are alopecia, anaphylactic reactions, nausea, and vomiting.

D. Imatinib

Imatinib mesylate [i MAT in tib] is used for the treatment of chronic myeloid leukemia in blast crisis, and gastrointestinal stromal tumor (GIST). It acts as a signal transduction inhibitor, used specifically to inhibit tumor tyrosine kinase activity. A deregulated kinase is associated with the BCR-ABL fusion protein that is present in the leukemia cells of almost every patient with chronic myeloid leukemia. In the case of GI stromal tumor, there is an unregulated expression of tyrosine kinase associated with a growth factor. The ability of *imatinib* to occupy the "kinase pocket" prevents the phosphorylation of tyrosine on the substrate molecule, and hence inhibits subsequent steps that lead to cell proliferation. *Imatinib* has the advantage over *interferon-α* in that it can be given orally. It also has a more rapid hematologic response than *interferon-α* plus *cytarabine*. Studies of cell lines indicate that resistance may occur by amplification of the BCR/ABL gene and/or by increased efflux due to increased multi-drug-resistance protein. The drug is very well absorbed orally. It undergoes metabolism by the cytochrome P450 system to several compounds, of which the N-demethyl derivative is active. Excretion is predominantly through the feces. Adverse effects include fluid retention and edema, hepatotoxicity, thrombocytopenia or neutropenia, as well as nausea and vomiting.

E. Gefinitib (Iressa)

Gefinitib [ge FIN ih tib] targets the epidermal growth factor receptor. It is approved for the treatment of non-small cell lung cancer that has failed to respond to other therapy, and is effective in ten to twenty percent of patients with this cancer. *Gefinitib* is usually used as a single agent. *Gefinitib* is absorbed after oral administration and undergoes extensive metabolism in the liver by the cytochrome P450 enzyme CYP3A4. At least five metabolites have been identified, only one of which has significant antitumor activity. The major route of excretion of the drug and its metabolites is the feces. The most common adverse effects are diarrhea, nausea, and acne-like skin rashes. A rare but potentially fatal adverse effect is interstitial lung disease, which presents as acute dyspnea with cough.

F. Procarbazine

Procarbazine [proe KAR ba zeen] is used in the treatment of Hodgkin disease and other cancers. *Procarbazine* rapidly equilibrates between the plasma and the CSF after oral or parenteral administration. It must undergo a series of oxidative reactions to exert its cytotoxic action that causes inhibition of DNA, RNA, and protein synthesis. Metabolites and the parent drug are excreted via the kidney. Bone marrow depression is the major toxicity, and nausea, vomiting, and diarrhea are common. The drug is also neurotoxic, causing symptoms ranging from drowsiness to hallucinations to paresthesias. Because it inhibits monoamine oxidase, patients should be warned against ingesting foods that contain tyramine (for example, aged cheeses, beer, and wine). Ingestion of alcohol leads to a disulfiram-type reaction). *Procarbazine* is both mutagenic and teratogenic. Nonlymphocytic leukemia has developed in patients treated with the drug.

G. L-Asparaginase

L-Asparaginase [ah SPAR a gi nase] catalyzes the deamination of asparagine to aspartic acid and ammonia. The form of the enzyme used chemotherapeutically is derived from bacteria. *L-Asparaginase* is used to treat childhood acute lymphocytic leukemia in combination with *VX* and *prednisone*. Its mechanism of action is based on the fact that some neoplastic cells require an external source of asparagine because of their limited capacity to synthesize sufficient amounts of that amino acid to support growth and function. *L-asparaginase* hydrolyzes blood asparagine and, thus, deprives the tumor cells of this nutrient, which is needed for protein synthesis (Figure 39.34). Resistance to the drug is due to increased capacity of tumor cells to synthesize asparagine. The enzyme must be administered either IV or intramuscularly because it is destroyed by gastric enzymes. Toxicities include a range of hypersensitivity reactions (because it is a foreign protein), a decrease in clotting factors, liver abnormalities, pancreatitis, seizures, and coma due to ammonia toxicity.

H. Interferons

Human interferons have been classified into three types—alpha, beta, and gamma (IFN-α, IFN-β, IFN-γ)—on the basis of their antigenicity. The alpha interferons are primarily leukocytic, whereas the beta and gamma interferons are produced by connective tissue fibroblasts and T lymphocytes, respectively. Recombinant DNA techniques in bacteria have made available large quantities of pure interferons, including two species designated *interferon alpha-2a* and *2b* that are employed in treating neoplastic diseases. *Interferon alpha-2a* is presently approved for the management of hairy-cell leukemia, chronic myeloid leukemia, and AIDS-related Kaposi sarcoma. *Interferon alpha-2b* is approved for the treatment of hairy-cell leukemia, melanoma, AIDS-related Kaposi sarcoma, and follicular lymphoma.

1. **Mechanism of action:** Interferons secreted from producing cells interact with surface receptors on other cells, at which site they exert their effects. Bound interferons are neither internalized nor degraded. The alpha and beta interferons compete with each other for binding and, therefore, presumably bind at the same receptor or in close proximity; gamma interferons bind at different receptors. As a consequence of the binding of interferon, a series of complex intracellular reactions take place. These include synthesis of enzymes, suppression of cell proliferation, activation of macrophages, and increased cytotoxicity of lymphocytes. However, the exact mechanism by which the interferons are cytotoxic is unknown

2. **Pharmacokinetics:** Interferons are well absorbed after intramuscular or subcutaneous injections. An intravenous form of *interferon alpha-2b* is also available. Interferons undergo glomerular filtration and are degraded during reabsorption, but liver metabolism is minimal.

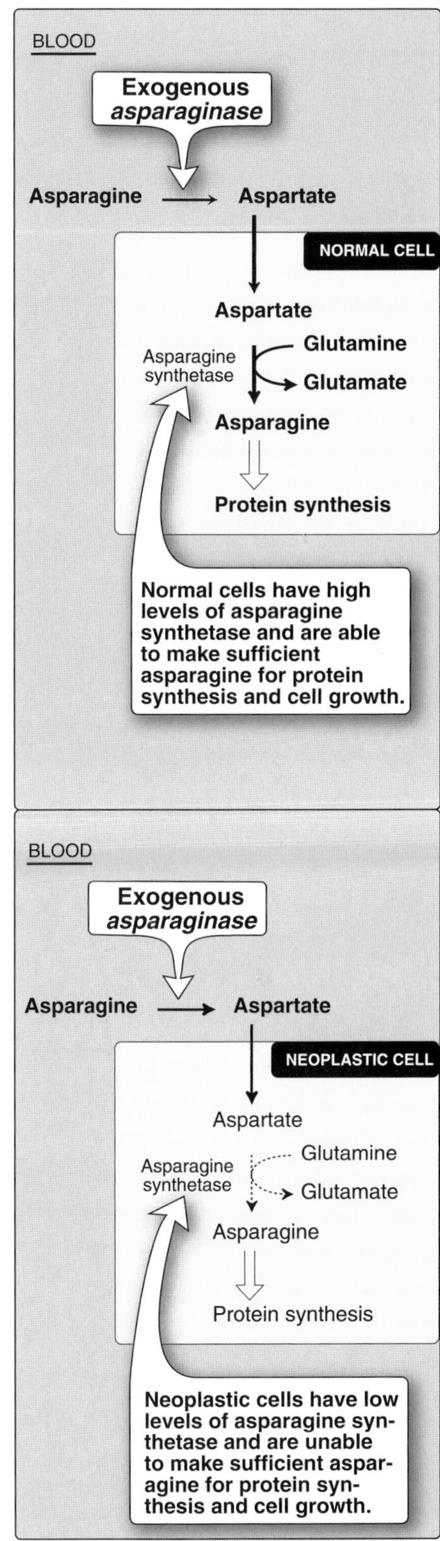

Figure 39.34
Activity of asparagine synthetase in normal and neoplastic cells.

3. Adverse effects: Depression is associated with the alpha interferons. Fever with chills occurs during the first few days of treatment. Dose-related toxicities includes leukopenia and, possibly, thrombocytopenia. Fatigue, malaise, anorexia, weight loss, alopecia, and transient elevation of liver enzymes have also been reported. Transient and reversible nephrotoxicity with proteinuria have been seen at high doses. Interferon α-2b should be used cautiously in patients with cardiovascular disease.

Study Questions

Choose the ONE best answer.

39.1 A patient with colonic cancer is being treated with 5-fluorouracil as well as leucovorin (N^5,N^{10}-methylene tetrahydrofolate). The rationale for administering the coenzyme depends on its being essential for:

A. conversion of 5-fluorouracil to fluorodeoxyuridylic acid (FdUMP).

B. protection against the anemia caused by 5-fluorouracil treatment.

C. the inhibition of thymidylate synthase by FdUMP.

D. prolongation of the antitumor effect of 5-fluorouracil.

Correct answer = C. Thymidylate synthase forms a ternary complex with thymidine and N^5,N^{10}-methylene tetrahydrofolic acid. Consequently, the coenzyme is required for 5-fluorouracil to be effective, albeit as the mononucleotide metabolite (FdUMP). It plays no role in the conversion of 5-FU to FdUMP. 5-FU does not cause megaloblastic anemia. The coenzyme does not affect the pharmacokinetics of 5-FU.

40.2 Neutropenia develops in a patient undergoing cancer chemotherapy. Administration of which one of the following agents would accelerate recovery of neutrophil counts?

A. Leucovorin

B. Filgrastim

C. Prednisone

D. Vitamin B_{12}

Correct answer = B. Filgrastim is a a human granulocyte colony-stimulating factor that can act on hematopoietic cells to stimulate proliferation. It regulates production of neutrophils in the bone marrow and, thus, is effective in reversing neutropenia in patients undergoing cancer chemotherapy. Leucovorin, the N^5,N^{10}-derivative of tetrahydrofolic acid, and vitamin B_{12}, although they would be effective in the treatment of anemias, do not increase neutrophil counts. The glucocorticoid, prednisone, is also ineffective.

40.3 Hydration and/or diuresis can prevent the renal toxicity associated with:

A. cisplatin.

B. chlorambucil.

C. tamoxifen.

D. gemcitabine.

E. methotrexate.

Correct answer = A. Only cisplatin in the list above causes renal toxicity.

40.4 A patient is being treated with allopurinol to control hyperuricemia resulting from chemotherapy. Which of the following would have to have its dose reduced to prevent toxicity?

A. 5-Fluorouracil

B. 6-Mercaptopurine

C. 6-Thioguanine

D. Fludarabine

E. Cytarabine

Correct answer = B. Mercaptopurine is metabolized to 6-thiouric acid by xanthine oxidase. Prevention of this reaction by allopurinol would divert more of the antimetabolite to cytotoxic pathways. 6-Thioguanine undergoes minimal metabolism by the xanthine oxidase pathway and thus is not affected by allopurinol. Nor is fludarabine metabolized by this pathway, because it does not undergo deamination by adenosine deaminase, which would be required to be metabolized by xanthine oxidase. The other two agents are pyrimidine compounds and, thus, are not biotransformed to uric acid.

Immunosuppressive Drugs

40

I. OVERVIEW

The importance of the immune system in protecting the body against harmful foreign molecules is well-recognized. However, in some instances, this protection can result in serious problems. For example, the introduction of an allograft (that is, the graft of an organ or tissue from one individual to another who is not genetically identical) can elicit a damaging immune response, causing rejection of the transplanted tissue. Transplantation of organs and tissues (for example, kidney, heart, or bone marrow) has become routine due to improved surgical techniques and better tissue typing. Also, drugs are now available that more selectively inhibit rejection of transplanted tissues while preventing the patient from becoming immunologically compromised (Figure 40.1). Earlier drugs were nonselective, and patients frequently succumbed to infection due to suppression of both the antibody-mediated (humoral) and cell-mediated arms of the immune system.[1] Today, theprincipal approach to immunosuppressive therapy is to alter lymphocyte function using drugs, or antibodies against immune proteins. Because of their severe toxicities when used as monotherapy, a combination of immunosuppressive agents, usually at lower doses, is generally employed. [Note: Immunosuppressive therapy is also used in the treatment of autoimmune diseases; for example, steroids can control acute glomerulonephritis.] Immunosuppressive drugs can be categorized according to their mechanisms of action: 1) some agents interfere with cytokine production or action, 2) others disrupt cell metabolism, preventing lymphocyte proliferation, and 3) mono- and polyclonal antibodies block T cell surface molecules.

IMMUNOSUPPRESSIVE DRUGS

- **SELECTIVE INHIBITORS OF CYTOKINE PRODUCTION AND FUNCTION**
  - ***Cyclosporine***
  - ***Sirolimus***
  - ***Tacrolimus (FK506)***
- **IMMUNOSUPPRESSIVE ANTIMETABOLITES**
  - ***Azathioprine***
  - ***Mycophenolate mofetil***
- **ANTIBODIES**
  - ***Antithymocyte globulins***
  - ***Basiliximab***
  - ***Daclizumab***
  - ***Muromonab-CD3 (OKT3)***
- **ADRENOCORTICOIDS**
  - ***Methylprednisolone***
  - ***Prednisolone***
  - ***Prednisone***

Figure 40.1
Immunosuppressant drugs.

II. SELECTIVE INHIBITORS OF CYTOKINE PRODUCTION AND FUNCTION

Cytokines are soluble, antigen-nonspecific, signaling proteins that bind to cell surface receptors on a variety of cells. The term cytokine includes the molecules known as interleukins (ILs), interferons (IFNs), tumor neucrosis factors (TNFs), transforming growth factors, and colony-stimulating factors. Of particular interest when discussing

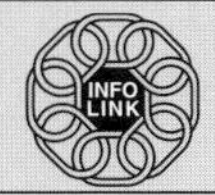

[1]See p. 59 in ***Lippincott's Illustrated Reviews: Microbiology*** for a discussion of humoral and cell-mediated immunity.

Lippincott's Illustrated Reviews: Pharmacology, Third Edition,
by Richard D. Howland and Mary J. Mycek.
Lippincott Williams & Wilkins, Baltimore, MD © 2006.

Cytokine	Actions
IL-1	• Enhances activity of NK cells • Attracts neutrophils and macrophages
IL-2	• Induces proliferation of antigen-primed T cells • Enhances activity of NK cells
IFN-γ	• Enhances activity of macrophages and NK cells • Increases expression of MHC molecules • Enhances production of IgG_{2a}
TNF-α	• Cytotoxic effect on tumor cells • Induces cytokine secretion in the inflammatory response

Figure 40.2
Summary of selected cytokines.

immunosuppresive drugs is IL-2—a compound that stimulates the proliferation of antigen-primed (helper) T cells, which subsequently produce more IL-2, IFN-γ, and TNF-β (Figure 40.2). These cytokines collectively activate natural killer cells, macrophages, and cytotoxic T lymphocytes. Clearly, drugs that interfere with the production or activity of IL-2, such as *cyclosporine*, will significantly dampen the immune response and, thereby, decrease graft rejection.

A. Cyclosporine

Cyclosporine [sye kloe SPOR een] (*CsA*) is a cyclic peptide composed of eleven amino acids (several are methylated on the peptidyl nitrogen). The drug is extracted from a soil fungus. *CsA* is used to prevent rejection of kidney, liver, and cardiac allogeneic transplants. Although *CsA* can be used alone, it is more effective when glucocorticoids are also administered, and this is the usual practice (Figure 40.3). *CsA* is an alternative to *methotrexate* for the treatment of severe, active rheumatoid arthritis. It can also be used for patients with recalcitrant psoriasis that does not respond to other therapies.

1. **Mechanism of action:** *Cyclosporine* preferentially suppresses cell-mediated immune reactions, whereas humoral immunity is affected to a far lesser extent. After diffusing into the T cell, *CsA* binds to a cyclophilin (more generally called an immunophilin) to form a complex that binds to calcineurin (Figure 40.4). The latter is responsible for dephosphorylating NFATc (**c**ytosolic **N**uclear **F**actor of **A**ctivated **T** cells). The *CsA*-calcineurin complex cannot perform this reaction; thus, NFATc cannot enter the nucleus to promote the reactions that are required for the synthesis of a number of cytokines, including IL-2. The end result is a decrease in IL-2—the primary chemical stimulus for increasing the number of T lymphocytes.

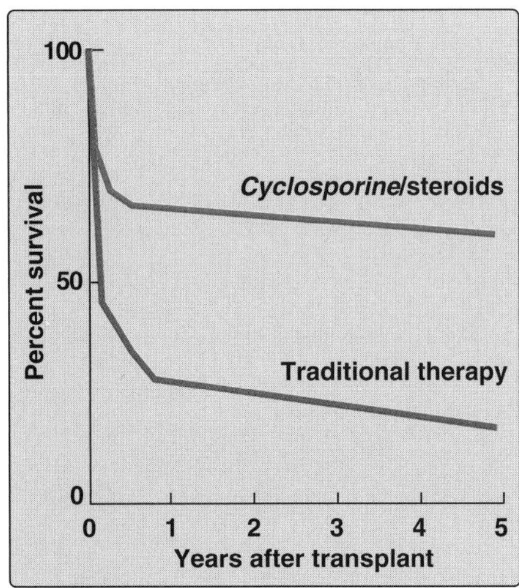

Figure 40.3
Effect of *cyclosporine* on liver transplant survival.

2. **Pharmacokinetics:** *Cyclosporine* may be given either orally or by intravenous infusion. Oral absorption is variable. Interpatient variability may be due to metabolism by a cytochrome P450 (CYP3A4) in the gastrointestinal tract, where the drug is metabolized. About fifty percent of the drug is associated with the blood fraction. Half of this is in the erythrocytes, and less than one-tenth is bound to the lymphocytes. *CsA* is extensively metabolized, primarily by hepatic CYP3A4. [Note: When other drug substrates for this enzyme are given concomittantly, many drug interactions have been reported.] It is not clear whether any of the 25 or more metabolites have any activity. Excretion of the metabolites is through the biliary route, with only a small fraction of the parent drug appearing in the urine.

3. **Adverse effects:** Many of the adverse effects caused by *CsA* are dose-dependent; therefore, it is important to monitor levels of the drug. Nephrotoxicity is the most common and important adverse effect of *CsA*. It is therefore critical to monitor kidney function. Reduction of the *CsA* dosage can result in reversal of nephrotoxicity. [Note: Coadministration of drugs that also can cause kidney dysfunction, for example, the aminoglycoside antibiotics; anti-inflammatories such as *diclofenac*, *naproxen*, or *sulindac*; and

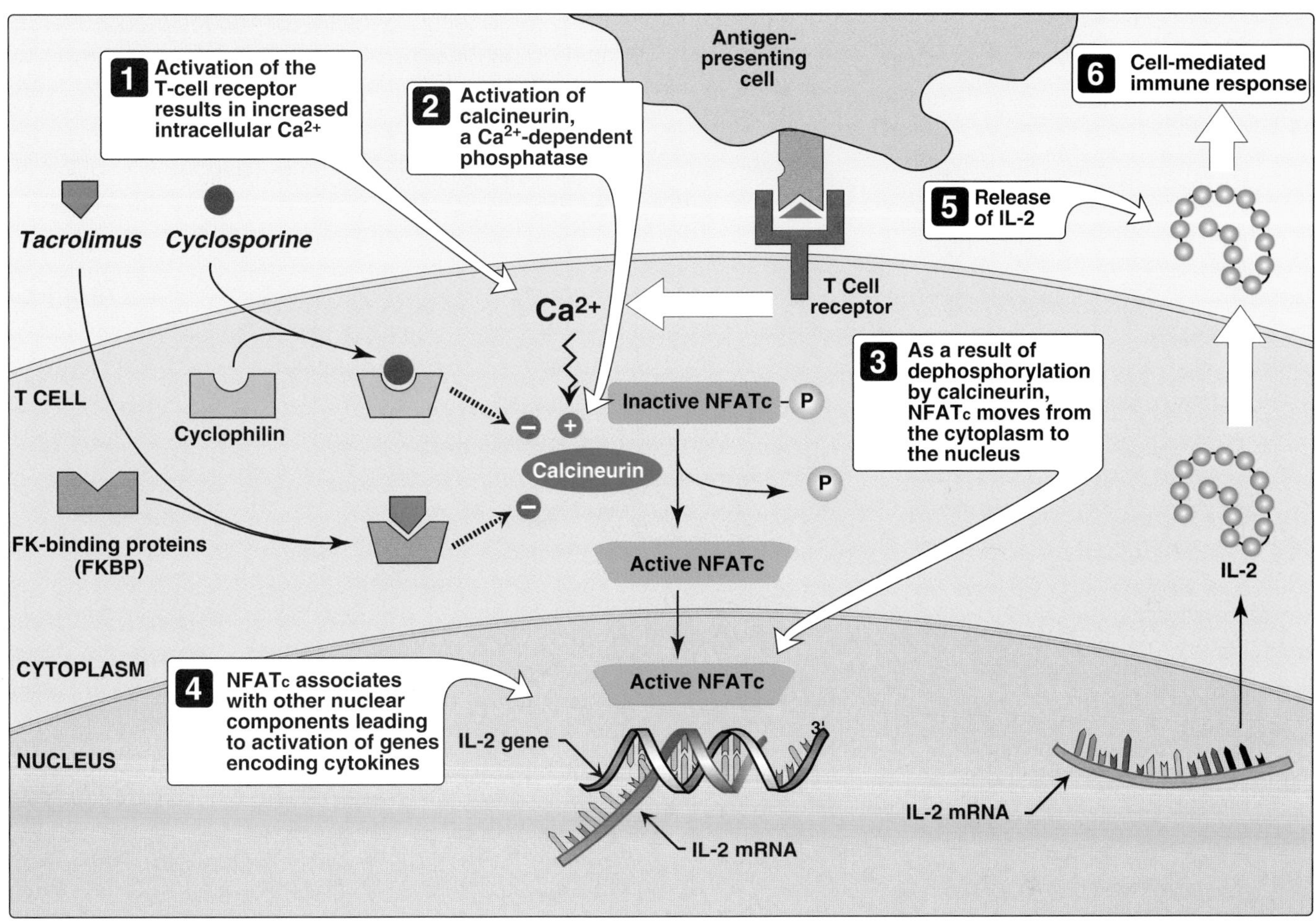

Figure 40.4
Mechanism of action of *cyclosporine* and *tacrolimus*. Il-2 = interleukin-2. NFATc = cytosolic nuclear factor of activated T cells.

proton-pump inhibitors like *cimetidine* or *ranitidine* can potentiate the nephrotoxicity of *CsA*.] Hepatotoxicity can also occur; therefore, liver function should be periodically assessed. Infections in patients taking *CsA* are common and may be life-threatening. Viral infections due to herpes group and cytomegalovirus are prevalent. Lymphoma may occur, presumably due to immunosuppression, although recent evidence has raised the question regarding whether *CsA* itself may promote lymphoma formation. Anaphylactic reactions can occur on parenteral administration. Other toxicities include hypertension, hyperkalemia (it is important not to use K^+-sparing diuretics in these patients), tremor, hirsutism, glucose intolerance, and gum hyperplasia.

B. Tacrolimus

Tacrolimus [ta CRAW lih mus] (*TAC*, originally called FK506) is a macrolide that is isolated from a soil fungus. *Tacrolimus* is approved for the prevention of rejection of liver and kidney transplants and is given with a glucocorticoid. This drug has found favor over *CsA*, not only because of its potency and decreased episodes of rejection (Figure 40.5) but also because lower doses of glucocorticoid can be

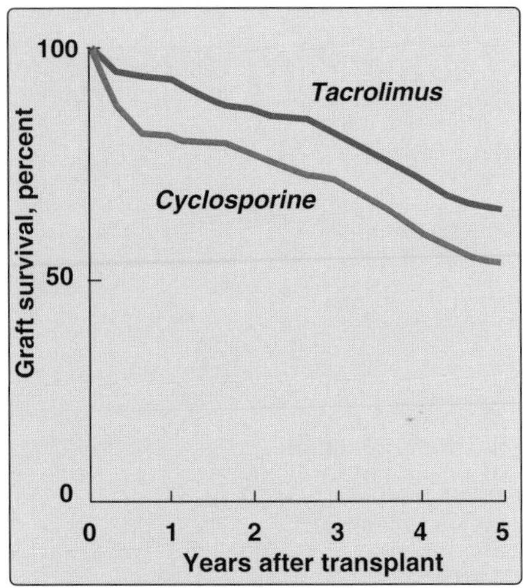

Figure 40.5
Five-year renal allograft survival in patients treated with *cyclosporine* or *tacrolimus*.

used, thus reducing the likelihood of steroid-associated adverse effects. An ointment preparation has been approved for moderate to severe atopic dermatitis that does not respond to conventional therapies.

1. **Mechanism of action:** *TAC* exerts its immunosuppressive effect in the same manner as *CsA*, except that it binds to a different immunophilin, FKBP-12 (FK-**b**inding **p**rotein; Figure 40.6).

2. **Pharmacokinetics:** *TAC* may be administered orally or intravenously. The oral route is preferable, but as with *CsA*, oral absorption of *TAC* is incomplete and variable, requiring tailoring of doses. Absorption is decreased if the drug is taken with high-fat or high-carbohydrate meals. *TAC* is from 10- to 100-fold more potent than *CsA*. It is highly bound to serum proteins and is also concentrated in erythrocytes. Like *CsA*, *TAC* undergoes hepatic metabolism by the CYP3A4 isozyme; thus, the same drug interactions occur. At least one metabolite of *TAC* has been shown to have immunosuppressive activity. Renal excretion is very low, and most of the drug and its metabolites are found in the feces.

3. **Adverse effects:** Nephrotoxicity and neurotoxicity (tremor, seizures, hallucinations) tend to be more severe in patients who are treated with *TAC* than in patients treated with *CsA*, but careful dose adjustment can minimize this problem. Development of post-transplant, insulin-dependent diabetes mellitus is a problem, especially in black and Hispanic patients. Other toxicities are the same as those for *CsA*, except that *TAC* does not cause hirsutism or gingival hyperplasia. Anaphylactoid reactions to the injection vehicle have been reported. The drug interactions are the same as those described above for *CsA*.

C. Sirolimus

Sirolimus [sih ROW lih mus] (*SRL*) is a recently approved macrolide obtained from fermentations of a soil mold. The earlier name—and one that is sometimes still used—is *rapamycin*. It is equipotent to *CsA*. *SRL* is approved for use in renal transplantation, to be used together with *CsA* and glucocorticoids, thereby allowing lower doses of those medications to be employed and, thus, lowering their toxic potential. The combination of *SRL* and *CsA* are apparently synergistic. The antiproliferative action of *SRL* has found use in cardiology. *SRL*-coated stents inserted into the cardiac vasculature inhibit restenosis of the blood vessels by reducing proliferation of the endothelial cells. In addition to its immunosuppressive effects, *SRL* also inhibits proliferation of cells in the graft intimal areas and, thus, is effective in halting graft vascular disease.

1. **Mechanism of action:** *SRL* and *TAC* bind to the same cytoplasmic FK-binding protein, but instead of forming a complex with calcineurin, *SRL* binds to mTOR (**m**ammalian **T**arget **O**f **R**apamycin). The latter is a serine-threonine kinase. [Note: TOR proteins are essential for many cellular functions, such as cell-cycle progression, DNA repair, and as regulators involved in protein translation.] Binding of *SRL* to mTOR blocks the progression of activated

T cells from the G_1 to the S phase of the cell cycle and, consequently, the proliferation of these cells (see Figure 40.6). Unlike *CsA* and *TAC*, *SRL* does not owe its effect to lowering IL-2 production but, rather, to inhibiting the cellular responses to IL-2.

2. **Pharmacokinetics:** The drug is available only as oral preparations. Although it is readily absorbed, high-fat meals can decrease the drug's absorption. *SRL* is extensively bound to plasma proteins, and its immunosuppressive actions persist for six months after suspension of therapy. Like both *CsA* and *TAC*, *SRL* is metabolized by the CYP3A4 isozyme and probably interacts with the same drugs as do *CsA* and *TAC*. The parent drug and its metabolites are predominantly eliminated in the feces.

3. **Adverse effects:** A frequent side effect of *SRL* is hyperlipidemia (elevated cholesterol and triacylglycerol), which can require treatment. The combination of *CsA* and *SRL* is more nephrotoxic than *CsA* alone; however, administration of *SRL* with *TAC* appears to be less toxic. Other untoward problems are headache, nausea and diarrhea, hypertension, leukopenia, and thrombocytopenia.

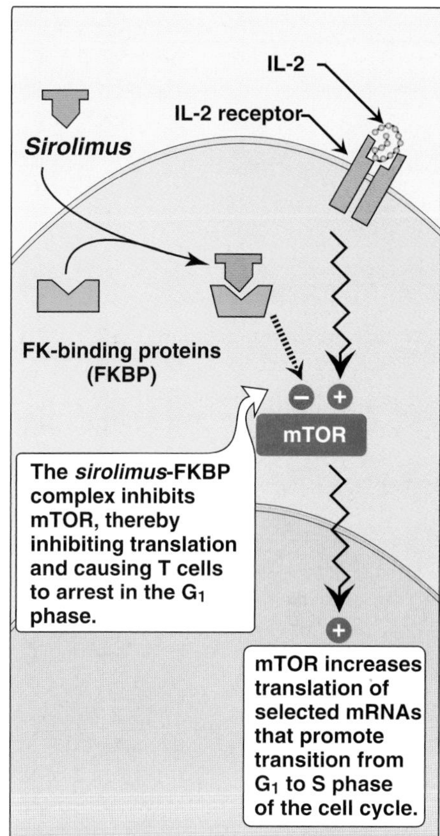
IL-2
IL-2 receptor
Sirolimus
FK-binding proteins (FKBP)
mTOR
The sirolimus-FKBP complex inhibits mTOR, thereby inhibiting translation and causing T cells to arrest in the G1 phase.
mTOR increases translation of selected mRNAs that promote transition from G1 to S phase of the cell cycle.

Figure 40.6
Mechanism of action of *sirolimus*. mTOR = molecular target of *rapamycin* (*sirolimus*).

III. IMMUNOSUPPRESSIVE ANTIMETABOLITES

These antimetabolite agents are generally used in combination with glucocorticoids, and the calcineurin inhibitors, *CsA* and *TAC*.

A. Azathioprine

Azathioprine [ay za TYE oh preen] has been the cornerstone of immunosuppressive therapy during the last several decades. It is a prodrug that is converted first to *6-mercaptopurine* (*6-MP*), and then to the corresponding nucleotide, thioinosinic acid. The immunosuppressive effects of *azathioprine* are due to this nucleotide analog. Because of their rapid proliferation in the immune response and their dependence on the de novo synthesis of purines required for cell division, lymphocytes are predominantly affected by the cytotoxic effects of *azathioprine*. [Note: The drug has little effect on suppressing a chronic immune response.] Its major nonimmune toxicity is bone marrow suppression. Concomittant use with angiotensin-converting enzyme inhibitors or *cotrimoxazole* in renal transplant patients can lead to an exaggerated leukopenic response. Nausea and vomiting are also encountered. (See p. 460 for a discussion of the mechanism of action, resistance, and pharmacokinetics of *6-MP*.)

B. Mycophenolate mofetil

Azathioprine is being replaced by *mycophenolate mofetil* [mye koe FEN oh late MAW feh til] because of the latter's safety and efficacy in prolonging graft survival. It has been successfully used in heart, kidney, and liver transplants. As an ester, it is rapidly hydrolyzed in the gastrointestinal tract to mycophenolic acid (MPA), which is a potent, reversible, uncompetitive inhibitor of inosine monophosphate dehydrogenase, blocking the de novo formation of guanosine phosphate. Thus, like *6-MP*, it deprives the rapidly proliferating T and B

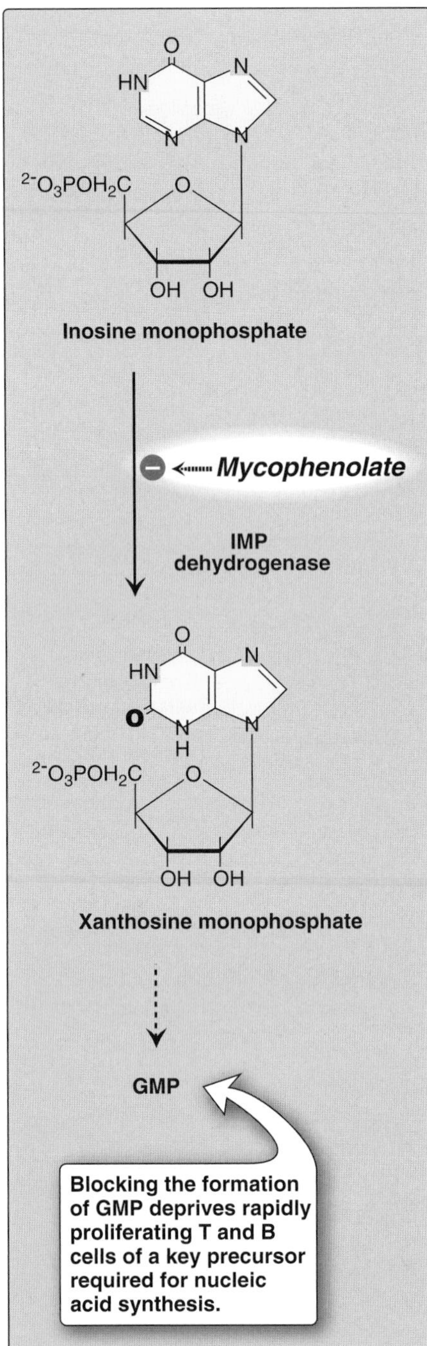

Figure 40.7
Mechanism of action of *mycophenolate.*

cells of a key component of nucleic acids (Figure 40.7). [Note: Lymphocytes lack the salvage pathway for purine synthesis and, therefore, are dependent on de novo purine production.] Mycophenolic acid is quickly and almost completely absorbed after oral administration. Both MPA and its glucuronidated metabolite are highly bound (greater than ninety percent) to plasma albumin, but no displacement-type interactions have been reported. The glucuronide is excreted predominantly in the urine. Adverse effects include pain, diarrhea, leukopenia, opportunistic infections, sepsis, and lymphoma. [Note: MPA is less mutagenic or carcinogenic than *azathioprine*.] Concomittant administration with antacids containing magnesium or aluminum, or with *cholestyramine*, can decrease absorption of the drug.

IV. ANTIBODIES

The use of antibodies plays a central role in prolonging allograft survival. They are prepared either by immunization of rabbits or horses with human lymphoid cells (producing a mixture of polyclonal antibodies directed against a number of lymphocyte antigens), or by hybridoma technology (producing antigen-specific, monoclonal antibodies). [Note: Hybridomas are produced by fusing mouse antibody-producing cells with immortal, malignant plasma cells (Figure 40.8). Hybrid cells are selected and cloned, and the antibody specificity of the clones is determined. Clones of interest can be cultured in large quantities to produce clinically useful amounts of the desired antibody. Recombinant DNA technology can also be used to replace part of the mouse gene sequence with human genetic material, thus "humanizing" the antibodies produced, making them less antigenic.] The names of monoclonal antibodies conventionally contain "muro" if they are from a murine (mouse) source, and "xi" or "iz" if they are humanized (see Figure 40.8). The suffix "mab" (monoclonal antibody) identifies the category of drug. The polyclonal antibodies, although relatively inexpensive to produce, are variable and less specific, which is in contrast to monoclonal antibodies, which are homogeneous and specific.

A. Antithymocyte globulins

Thymocytes are cells that develop in the thymus and serve as T-cell precursors. The antibodies developed against them are prepared by immunization of large rabbits or horses with human lymphoid cells and, thus, are polyclonal. They are primarily employed, together with other immunosuppressive agents, to treat the hyperacute phase of allograft rejection. The antibodies bind to the surface of circulating T lymphocytes, which then undergo various reactions, such as complement-mediated destruction, antibody-dependent cytotoxicity, apoptosis, and opsonization. The antibody-bound cells are phagocytosed in the liver and spleen, resulting in lymphopenia and impaired T-cell responses. The antibodies are administered intramuscularly or are slowly infused intravenously, and their half-life extends from three to nine days. Because the humoral (B cell–mediated) antibody mechanism remains active, antibodies can be formed against these foreign proteins. [Note: This is less of a problem with the humanized antibodies.] Other adverse effects include chills and fever, leukopenia and thrombocytopenia, infections due to cytomegalovirus (CMV) or other viruses, and skin rashes.

B. Muromonab-CD3 (OKT3)

Muromonab-CD3 [myoo roe MOE nab] is a murine monoclonal antibody that is synthesized by hybridoma technology and directed against the glycoprotein CD3 antigen of human T cells. *Muromonab-CD3* is used for treatment of acute rejection of renal allografts as well as for steroid-resistant acute allograft rejection in cardiac and hepatic transplant patients. It is also used to deplete T cells from donor bone marrow prior to transplantation.

1. **Mechanism of action:** Binding to the CD3 protein results in a disruption of T-lymphocyte function, because access of antigen to the recognition site is blocked. Circulating T cells are depleted; thus, their participation in the immune response is decreased. Because *muromonab-CD3* recognizes only one antigenic site, the immunosuppression is less broad than that seen with the polyclonal antibodies. T cells usually return to normal within 48 hours of discontinuation of therapy.

2. **Pharmacokinetics:** The antibody is administered intravenously. Initial binding of *muromonab-CD3* to the antigen transiently activates the T cell and results in cytokine release (cytokine storm). It is therefore customary to premedicate the patient with *methylprednisolone*, *diphenhydramine*, and *acetaminophen* to alleviate the cytokine release syndrome. The antibody is extensively metabolized and is eliminated predominantly in the bile.

3. **Adverse effects:** Anaphylactoid reactions may occur. Cytokine release syndrome may follow the first dose. The symptoms can range from a mild, flu-like illness to a life-threatening, shock-like reaction. High fever is common. Central nervous system effects, such as seizures, encephalopathy, cerebral edema, aseptic meningitis, and headache, may occur. Infections can increase, including some due to CMV. *Muromonab-CD3* is contraindicated in patients with a history of seizures, in those with uncompensated heart failure, in pregnant women, and in those who are breast-feeding. Because of these adverse effects and the availability of *basiliximab* and *daclizumab*, *muromonab-CD3* is being less widely used.

C. IL-2-receptor antagonists

The antigenicity and short serum half-life of the murine monoclonal antibody has been averted by replacing most of the murine amino acid sequences with human ones by genetic engineering. *Basiliximab* [bah si LIK si mab] is said to be "chimerized" because it consists of 25-percent murine and 75-percent human protein. *Daclizumab* [dah KLIZ yoo mab] is 90-percent human protein, and is designated "humanized." Both agents have been approved for prophylaxis of acute rejection in renal transplantation. They are used with *CsA* and corticosteroids.

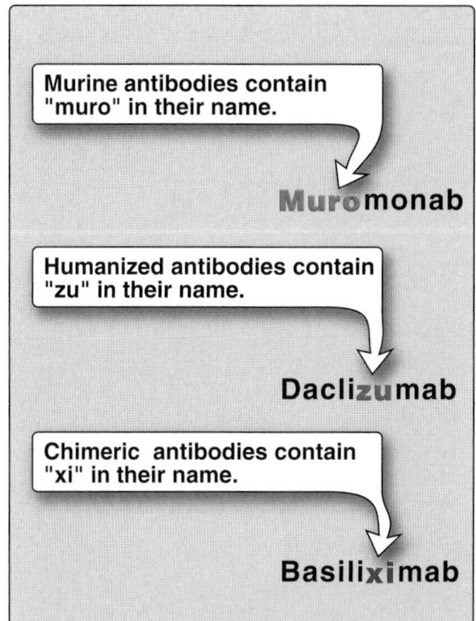

Figure 40.8
Conventions for naming monoclonal antibodies. [Note: *Muromonab* was named before the convention was adopted to make the last three letters in their names *mab*.]

1. **Mechanism of action:** Both compounds are anti-CD25 antibodies, and bind to the α-chain of the IL-2 receptor on activated T cells. They thus interfere with the proliferation of these cells. *Basiliximab* is about ten-fold more potent than *daclizumab* as a blocker of IL-2-stimulated T-cell replication. Blockade of this receptor foils the ability of any antigenic stimulus to activate the T cell-response system.

2. **Pharmacokinetics:** Both antibodies are given intravenously. The serum half-life of *daclizumab* is about 20 days, and the blockade of the receptor is 120 days. Five doses of *daclizumab* are usually administered—the first at 24 hours before transplantation, and the next four doses at fourteen-day intervals. The serum half-life of *basiliximab* is about seven days. Usually, two doses of this drug are administered—the first at two hours prior to transplantation, and the second at four days after the surgery (Figure 40.9).

3. **Adverse effects:** Both *daclizumab* and *basiliximab* are well-tolerated. Their major toxicity is gastrointestinal. No clinically relevant antibodies to the drugs have been detected, and malignancy does not appear to be a problem.

A summary of the major immunosuppressive drugs is presented in Figure 40.9

V. ADRENOCORTICOIDS

The glucocorticoids were the first pharmacologic agents to be used as immunosuppressives both in transplantation and in various autoimmune disorders. They are still one of the mainstays for attenuating rejection episodes. For transplantation, the most common agents are *prednisone* or *methylprednisolone*, whereas *prednisone* or *prednisolone* are employed for autoimmune conditions. [Note: In transplantation, they are used in combination with agents described previously in this chapter.] The steroids are used to suppress acute rejection of solid organ allografts and in chronic graft-versus-host disease. In addition, they are effective against a wide variety of autoimmune conditions, including refractory rheumatoid arthritis, systemic lupus erythematosus, temporal arthritis, and asthma. The exact mechanism responsible for the immunosuppressive action of the glucocorticoids is unclear. The T lymphocytes are affected most. The steroids are able to rapidly reduce lymphocyte populations by lysis or redistribution. On entering cells, they bind to the glucocorticoid receptor. The complex passes into the nucleus and regulates the translation of DNA. Among the genes affected are those involved in inflammatory responses. The use of these agents is associated with numerous adverse effects. For example, they are diabetogenic, and they can cause hypercholesterolemia, cataracts, osteoporosis, and hypertension on prolonged use. Consequently, efforts are being directed toward reducing or eliminating the use of steroids in the maintenance of allografts.

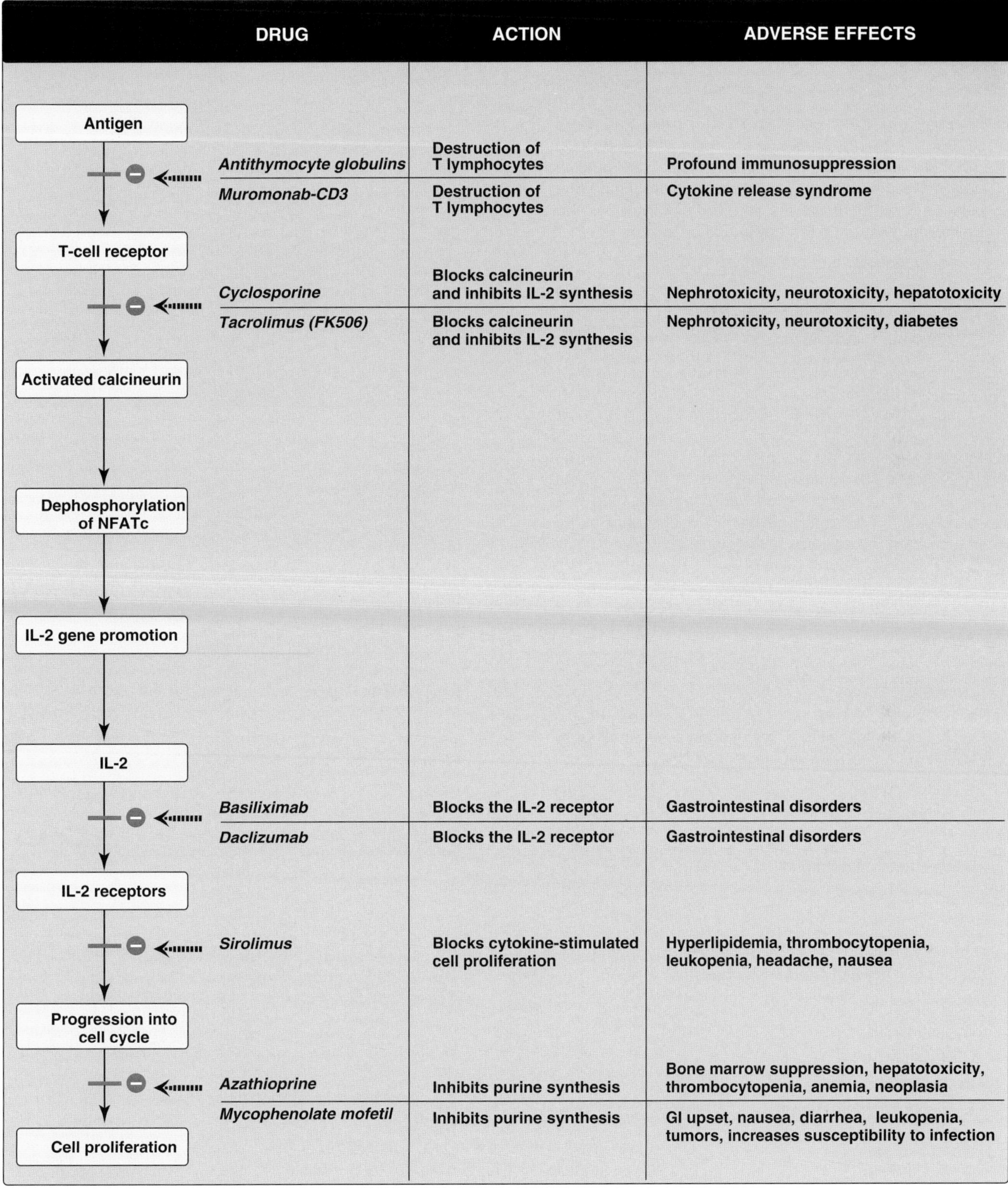

DRUG	ACTION	ADVERSE EFFECTS
Antithymocyte globulins	Destruction of T lymphocytes	Profound immunosuppression
Muromonab-CD3	Destruction of T lymphocytes	Cytokine release syndrome
Cyclosporine	Blocks calcineurin and inhibits IL-2 synthesis	Nephrotoxicity, neurotoxicity, hepatotoxicity
Tacrolimus (FK506)	Blocks calcineurin and inhibits IL-2 synthesis	Nephrotoxicity, neurotoxicity, diabetes
Basiliximab	Blocks the IL-2 receptor	Gastrointestinal disorders
Daclizumab	Blocks the IL-2 receptor	Gastrointestinal disorders
Sirolimus	Blocks cytokine-stimulated cell proliferation	Hyperlipidemia, thrombocytopenia, leukopenia, headache, nausea
Azathioprine	Inhibits purine synthesis	Bone marrow suppression, hepatotoxicity, thrombocytopenia, anemia, neoplasia
Mycophenolate mofetil	Inhibits purine synthesis	GI upset, nausea, diarrhea, leukopenia, tumors, increases susceptibility to infection

Figure 40.9
Sites of action of commonly used immunosuppressants. Il-2 = interleukin-2. NFATc = cytosolic nuclear factor of activated T cells.

Study Questions

Choose the ONE best answer.

40.1 A 45-year-old male who received a renal transplant three months previously and is being maintained on methylprednisolone, cyclosporine, and mycophenolate mofetil is found to have increased creatinine levels, indicating possible rejection. Which of the following courses of therapy would be appropriate?

A. Increased dose of methylprednisolone
B. Hemodialysis
C. Treatment with muromonab-CD3
D. Treatment with sirolimus
E. Treatment with azathioprine

Correct answer = C. This patient is apparently undergoing an acute rejection of the kidney. The most effective treatment would be administration of an antibody, and muromonab-CD3 is indicated for this condition. Increasing the dose of methylprednisolone may have some effect, but this exposes the patient to the adverse effects of glucocorticoids. Sirolimus is used prophylactically with cyclosporine to prevent renal rejection but is less effective when an episode is occurring. Furthermore, the combination of cyclosporine and sirolimus is more nephrotoxic than cyclosporine alone. Azathioprine has no benefit over mycophenolate.

40.2 A 23-year-old female suffering from grand mal epilepsy is being controlled with phenytoin. She is a candidate for a renal transplant. Which agent might exacerbate the seizures in this patient?

A. Mycophenolate mofetil
B. Sirolimus,
C. Cyclosporine
D. Tacrolimus

Correct answer = D. Central nervous system problems such as headache and tremor as well as seizures are among the adverse effects commonly associated with tacrolimus. Cyclosporine, sirolimus, and tacrolimus are metabolized by the CYP3A4 isozyme of the P450 oxidases. Phenytoin can induce this enzyme; thus, the doses of these agents must be carefully adjusted and their blood levels carefully monitored in this patient. Mycophenolate mofetil has predominantly gastrointestinal side effects.

40.3 Which of the following drugs used to prevent allograft rejection can cause hyperlipidemia?

A. Azathioprine
B. Basiliximab
C. Tacrolimus
D. Mycophenolate mofetil
E. Sirolimus

Correct answer = E. Patients who are receiving sirolimus can develop elevated cholesterol and triacylglycerol levels, which can be controlled by statin therapy. None of the other agents has this adverse effect.

40.4 Which of the following drugs specifically inhibit calcineurin in the activated T lymphocytes?

A. Daclizumab
B. Tacrolimus
C. Prednisone
D. Sirolimus
E. Mycophenolate mofetil

Correct answer = B. Tacrolimus binds to FKBP-12, which in turn inhibits calcineurin and interferes in the cascade of reactions that synthesize IL-2 and lead to T-lymphocyte proliferation. Although daclizumab also interferes with T-lymphocyte proliferation, it does so by binding to the CD25 site on the IL-2 receptor. Prednisone can affect not only T-cell proliferation but also that of B cells; therefore, it is not specific. Sirolimus, while also binding to FKBP-12, does not inhibit calcineurin. Mycophenolate mofetil exerts its immunosuppressive action by inhibiting inosine monophosphate dehydrogenase, thus depriving the cells of guanosine—a key component of nucleic acids.

UNIT VIII: Anti-inflammatory Drugs and Autacoids

Anti-inflammatory Drugs 41

I. OVERVIEW

Inflammation is a normal, protective response to tissue injury caused by physical trauma, noxious chemicals, or microbiologic agents. Inflammation is the body's effort to inactivate or destroy invading organisms, remove irritants, and set the stage for tissue repair. When healing is complete, the inflammatory process usually subsides. However, inflammation is sometimes inappropriately triggered by an innocuous agent, such as pollen, or by an autoimmune response, such as in asthma or rheumatoid arthritis. In such cases, the defense reactions themselves may cause progressive tissue injury, and anti-inflammatory or immunosuppressive drugs may be required to modulate the inflammatory process. Inflammation is triggered by the release of chemical mediators from injured tissues and migrating cells. The specific chemical mediators vary with the type of inflammatory process and include amines, such as histamine and 5-hydroxytryptamine; lipids, such as the prostaglandins; small peptides, such as bradykinin; and larger peptides, such as interleukin-1 (IL-1). Discovery of the wide variation among chemical mediators has clarified the apparent paradox in which an anti-inflammatory drug may interfere with the action of a particular mediator important in one type of inflammation but be without effect in inflammatory processes not involving the drug's target mediator. The drugs described in this chapter are summarized in Figure 41.1.

II. PROSTAGLANDINS

All of the nonsteroidal anti-inflammatory drugs (NSAIDs) act by inhibiting the synthesis of prostaglandins. Thus, an understanding of NSAIDs requires comprehension of the actions and biosynthesis of prostaglandins—unsaturated fatty acid derivatives containing twenty carbons that include a cyclic ring structure. [Note: These compounds are sometimes referred to as eicosanoids; "eicosa" refers to the twenty carbon atoms.]

ANTI-INFLAMMATORY DRUGS

- **NSAIDs**
  - ***Aspirin***
  - ***Diflunisal***
  - ***Diclofenac***
  - ***Etodolac***
  - **Fenamates**
  - ***Fenoprofen***
  - ***Flurbiprofen***
  - ***Ibuprofen***
  - ***Indomethacin***
  - ***Ketoprofen***
  - ***Meloxicam***
  - ***Methylsalicylate***
  - ***Nabumetone***
  - ***Naproxin***
  - ***Nimesulide***
  - ***Oxaprazin***
  - ***Piroxicam***
  - ***Sulindac***
  - ***Tolmetin***
- **COX-2 INHIBITORS**
  - ***Celecoxib***
- **OTHER ANALGESICS**
  - ***Acetaminophen***

Figure 41.1
Summary of anti-inflammatory drugs. NSAIDs = nonsteroidal anti-inflammatory drugs; COX = cyclooxygenase. (Continued on next page.)

Lippincott's Illustrated Reviews: Pharmacology, Third Edition,
by Richard D. Howland and Mary J. Mycek.

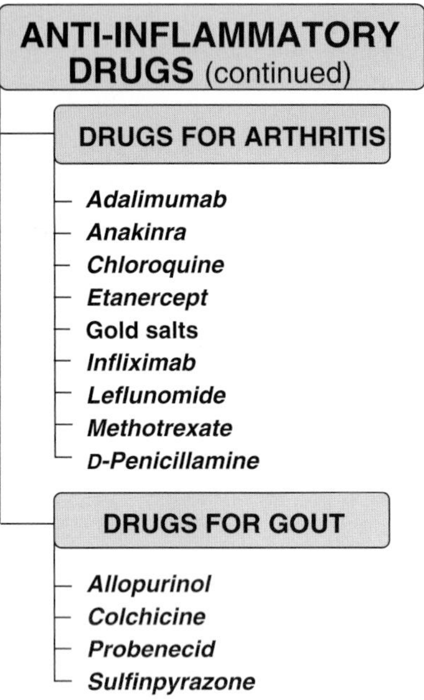

Figure 41.1 (continued)
Summary of anti-inflammatory drugs.

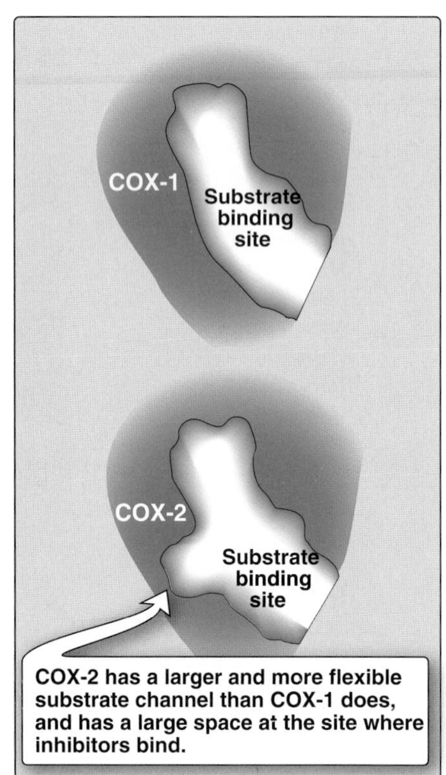

Figure 41.2
Structural differences in active sites of cyclooxygenase (COX)-1 and COX-2.

A. Role of prostaglandins as local mediators

Prostaglandins and related compounds are produced in minute quantities by virtually all tissues. They generally act locally on the tissues in which they are synthesized, and they are rapidly metabolized to inactive products at their sites of action. Therefore, the prostaglandins do not circulate in the blood in significant concentrations. Thromboxanes, leukotrienes, and the hydroperoxyeicosatetraenoic and hydroxyeicosatetraenoic acids (HPETEs and HETEs, respectively) are related lipids, synthesized from the same precursors as the prostaglandins are, and using interrelated pathways.

B. Synthesis of prostaglandins

Arachidonic acid, a twenty-carbon fatty acid, is the primary precursor of the prostaglandins and related compounds. Arachidonic acid is present as a component of the phospholipids of cell membranes—primarily phosphatidyl inositol and other complex lipids.[1] Free arachidonic acid is released from tissue phospholipids by the action of phospholipase A_2 and other acyl hydrolases via a process controlled by hormones and other stimuli. There are two major pathways in the synthesis of the eicosanoids from arachidonic acid.

1. **Cyclooxygenase pathway:** All eicosanoids with ring structures—that is, the prostaglandins, thromboxanes, and prostacyclins—are synthesized via the cyclooxygenase pathway. Two related isoforms of the cyclooxygenase enzymes have been described. Cyclooxygenase-1 (COX-1) is responsible for the physiologic production of prostanoids, whereas cyclooxygenase-2 (COX-2) causes the elevated production of prostanoids that occurs in sites of disease and inflammation. COX-1 is described as a "housekeeping enzyme" that regulates normal cellular processes, such as gastric cytoprotection, vascular homeostasis, platelet aggregation, and kidney function. COX-2 is constitutively expressed in some tissues, such as the brain, kidney, and bone. Its expression at other sites is increased during states of inflammation. The two enzymes share sixty-percent homology in amino acid sequence. However, the conformation for the substrate binding sites and catalytic regions are slightly different. For example, COX-2 has a larger and more flexible substrate channel than COX-1 has, and COX-2 has a large space at the site where inhibitors bind (Figure 41.2). [Note: The structural differences between COX-1 and COX-2 permitted the development of COX-2-selective inhibitors. Another distinguishing characteristic of COX-2 is that its expression is inhibited by glucocorticoids (Figure 41.3), which may contribute to the significant anti-inflammatory effects of these drugs.

2. **Lipoxygenase pathway:** Alternatively, several lipoxygenases can act on arachidonic acid to form 5-HPETE, 12-HPETE, and 15-HPETE, which are unstable peroxidated derivatives that are converted to the corresponding hydroxylated derivatives (the HETES) or to leukotrienes or lipoxins, depending on the tissue (see Figure 41.3).[2] Antileukotriene drugs, such as *zileuton, zafirlukast*, and *mon-*

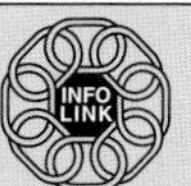

[1]See p. 180 in ***Lippincott's Illustrated Reviews: Biochemistry*** (3rd ed.) for a discussion of the chemistry of arachidonic acid.
[2]See p. 211 in ***Lippincott's Illustrated Reviews: Biochemistry*** (3rd ed.) for a discussion of prostaglandin synthesis.

telukast, are useful for the treatment of moderate to severe allergic asthma.

C. Actions of prostaglandins

Many of the actions of prostaglandins are mediated by their binding to a wide variety of distinct cell membrane receptors that operate via G proteins, which subsequently activate or inhibit adenylyl cyclase or stimulate phospholipase C.[3] This causes an enhanced formation of diacylglycerol and inositol 1,4,5-trisphosphate (IP_3). Prostaglandin $F_{2\alpha}$ ($PGF_{2\alpha}$), the leukotrienes, and thromboxane A_2 (TXA_2) mediate certain actions by activating phosphatidylinositol metabolism and causing an increase of intracellular Ca^{2+}.

D. Functions in the body

Prostaglandins and their metabolites produced endogenously in tissues act as local signals that fine-tune the response of a specific cell type. Their functions vary widely depending on the tissue. For example, the release of TXA_2 from platelets triggers the recruitment of new platelets for aggregation (the first step in clot formation). However, in other tissues, elevated levels of TXA_2 convey a different signal; for example, in certain smooth muscle, this compound induces contraction. Prostaglandins are also among the chemical mediators that are released in allergic and inflammatory processes.

III. NONSTEROIDAL ANTI-INFLAMMATORY DRUGS

The NSAIDs are a group of chemically dissimilar agents that differ in their antipyretic, analgesic, and anti-inflammatory activities. They act primarily by inhibiting the cyclooxygenase enzymes that catalyze the first step in prostanoid biosynthesis. This leads to decreased prostaglandin synthesis with both beneficial and unwanted effects. Long-term treatment with COX-2-specific inhibitors have been shown to increase the risks of myocardial infarctions and strokes, and several of these drugs have been withdrawn. Many experts believe that long-term therapy with older, nonspecific NSAIDs (not including *aspirin*) may also cause similar problems. Patients are now advised to take the lowest dose that is effective for as short a period as possible.

A. Aspirin and other salicylates

Aspirin [AS pir in] is the prototype of traditional NSAIDs. It is the most commonly used and is the drug to which all other anti-inflammatory agents are compared. However, about fifteen percent of patients show an intolerance to aspirin. Therefore, these individuals may benefit from other NSAIDs. In addition, some of the newer NSAIDs are superior to aspirin in certain patients, either because they have greater anti-inflammatory activity and/or cause less gastric irritation, or because they can be taken less frequently. However, the newer NSAIDs are considerably more expensive than aspirin, and some have proved to be more toxic in other ways.

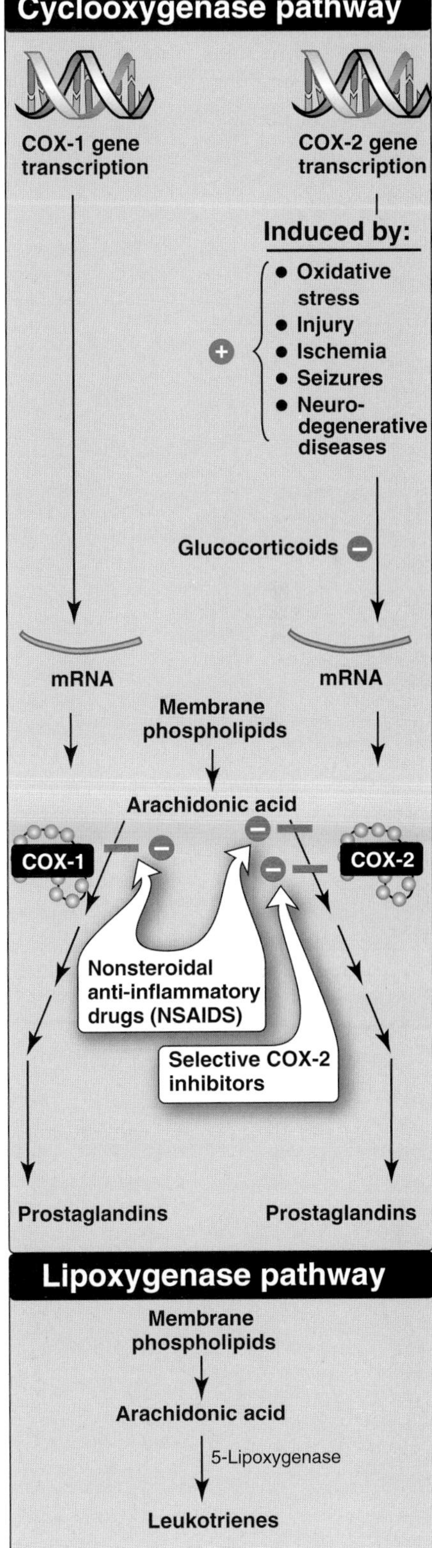

Figure 41.3
Synthesis of prostaglandins and leukotrienes. COX = cyclooxygenase.

[3]See p. 203 in ***Lippincott's Illustrated Reviews: Biochemistry*** (3rd ed.) for a discussion of the role of phospholipase C in signal transmission.

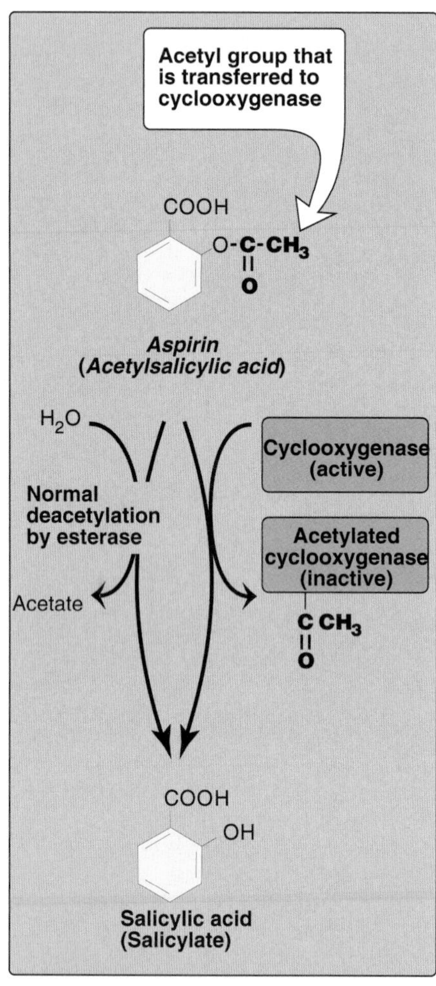

Figure 41.4
Metabolism of *aspirin* and acetylation of cyclooxygenase by *aspirin*.

1. **Mechanism of action:** Aspirin is a weak organic acid that is unique among the NSAIDs in that it irreversibly acetylates (and thus inactivates) cyclooxygenase (Figure 41.4). The other NSAIDs, including salicylate, are all reversible inhibitors of cyclooxygenase. Aspirin is rapidly deacetylated by esterases in the body, producing salicylate, which has anti-inflammatory, antipyretic, and analgesic effects. The antipyretic and anti-inflammatory effects of the salicylates are due primarily to the blockade of prostaglandin synthesis at the thermoregulatory centers in the hypothalamus and at peripheral target sites. Furthermore, by decreasing prostaglandin synthesis, the salicylates also prevent the sensitization of pain receptors to both mechanical and chemical stimuli. *Aspirin* may also depress pain stimuli at subcortical sites (that is, the thalamus and hypothalamus).

2. **Actions:** The NSAIDs, including *aspirin*, have three major therapeutic actions—namely, they reduce inflammation (anti-inflammation), pain (analgesia), and fever (antipyrexia; Figure 41.5). However, as described later in this section, not all NSAIDs are equally potent in each of these actions.

   a. **Anti-inflammatory actions:** Because *aspirin* inhibits cyclooxygenase activity, it diminishes the formation of prostaglandins and, thus, modulates those aspects of inflammation in which prostaglandins act as mediators. *Aspirin* inhibits inflammation in arthritis, but it neither arrests the progress of the disease nor induces remission. [Note: *Acetaminophen*, although a useful analgesic and antipyretic, has weak anti-inflammatory activity, and, therefore, is not useful in the treatment of inflammation, such as that seen with rheumatoid arthritis (see Figure 41.5). *Acetaminophen* is therefore discussed separately.]

   b. **Analgesic action:** Prostaglandin E_2 (PGE_2) is thought to sensitize nerve endings to the action of bradykinin, histamine, and other chemical mediators released locally by the inflammatory process. Thus, by decreasing PGE_2 synthesis, *aspirin* and other NSAIDs repress the sensation of pain. The salicylates are used mainly for the management of pain of low to moderate intensity arising from integumental structures rather than that arising from the viscera. NSAIDs are superior to opioids for the management of pain in which inflammation is involved. However, combinations of opioids and NSAIDs are effective in treating pain caused by a malignancy.

   c. **Antipyretic action:** Fever occurs when the set-point of the anterior hypothalamic thermoregulatory center is elevated. This can be caused by PGE_2 synthesis, stimulated when an endogenous fever-producing agent (pyrogen), such as a cytokine, is released from white cells that are activated by infection, hypersensitivity, malignancy, or inflammation. The salicylates lower body temperature in patients with fever by impeding PGE_2 synthesis and release. *Aspirin* resets the "thermostat" toward normal, and it rapidly lowers the body temperature of febrile patients by increasing heat dissipation as a result of peripheral vasodilation and sweating. *Aspirin* has no effect on normal body temperature.

d. **Respiratory actions:** At therapeutic doses, *aspirin* increases alveolar ventilation. [Note: Salicylates uncouple oxidative phosphorylation, which leads to elevated CO_2 and increased respiration.] Higher doses work directly on the respiratory center in the medulla, resulting in hyperventilation and respiratory alkalosis that is usually compensated for adequately by the kidney. At toxic levels, central respiratory paralysis occurs, and respiratory acidosis ensues due to continued production of CO_2.

e. **Gastrointestinal effects:** Normally, prostacyclin (PGI_2) inhibits gastric acid secretion, whereas PGE_2 and $PGF_{2\alpha}$ stimulate synthesis of protective mucus in both the stomach and small intestine. In the presence of *aspirin*, these prostanoids are not formed, resulting in increased gastric acid secretion and diminished mucus protection. This may cause epigastric distress, ulceration, and/or hemorrhage. At ordinary *aspirin* doses, as much as 3 to 8 ml of blood may be lost in the feces per day. [Note: Buffered and enteric-coated preparations are only marginally helpful in dealing with this problem. The PGE_1 derivative *misoprostol*, the proton pump inhibitor *omeprazol*, and H_2-antihistamines also reduce the risk of gastric ulcer, and are used in the treatment of gastric damage induced by NSAIDs.]

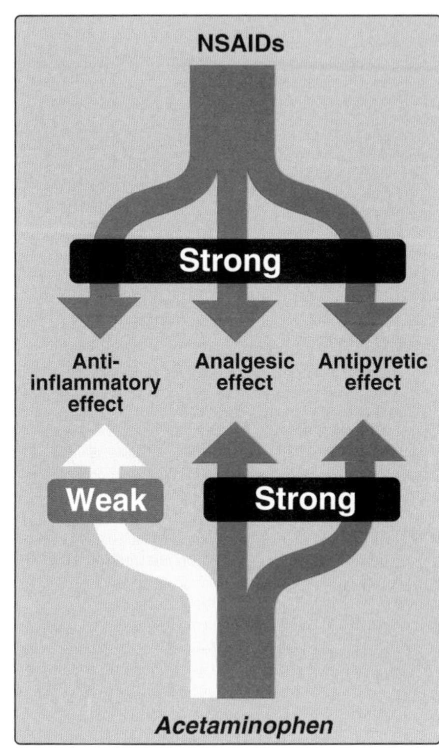

Figure 41.5
Actions of nonsteroidal anti-inflammatory drugs (NSAIDs) and *acetaminophen*.

f. **Effect on platelets:** TXA_2 enhances platelet aggregation, whereas PGI_2 decreases it. Low doses (60–80 mg daily) of *aspirin* can irreversibly inhibit thromboxane production in platelets without markedly affecting TXA_2 production in the endothelial cells of the blood vessel. [Note: The acetylation of cyclooxygenase is irreversible. Because platelets lack nuclei, they cannot synthesize new enzyme, and the lack of thromboxane persists for the lifetime of the platelet (three to seven days). This contrasts with the endothelial cells, which have nuclei and, therefore, can produce new cyclooxygenase.] As a result of the decrease in TXA_2, platelet aggregation (the first step in thrombus formation) is reduced, producing an anticoagulant effect with a prolonged bleeding time.

g. **Actions on the kidney:** Cyclooxygenase inhibitors prevent the synthesis of PGE_2 and PGI_2—prostaglandins that are responsible for maintaining renal blood flow, particularly in the presence of circulating vasoconstrictors (Figure 41.6). Decreased synthesis of prostaglandins can result in retention of sodium and water and may cause edema and hyperkalemia in some patients. Interstitial nephritis can also occur with all NSAIDs except *aspirin*.

3. **Therapeutic uses:**

a. **Antipyretics and analgesics:** *Sodium salicylate*, *choline salicylate* (in the liquid formulation), *choline magnesium salicylate*,

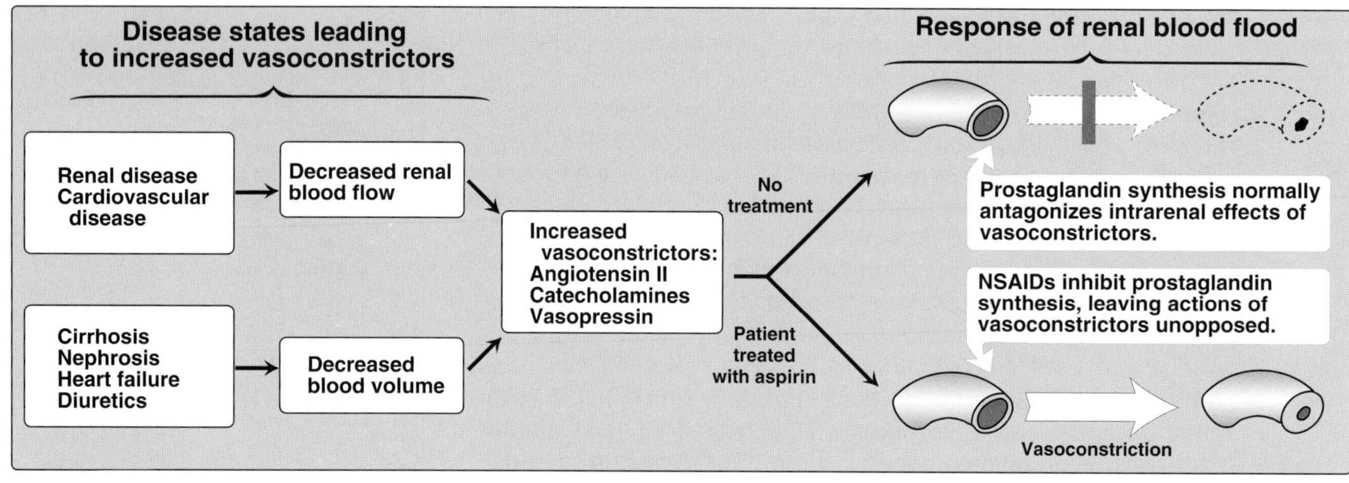

Figure 41.6
Renal effect of *aspirin* inhibition of prostaglandin synthesis. NSAIDS = nonsteroidal anti-inflammatory drugs.

and *aspirin* are used as antipyretics and analgesics in the treatment of gout, rheumatic fever, and rheumatoid arthritis. [Note: Salicylates are the drugs of choice in the treatment of rheumatoid arthritis.] Commonly treated conditions requiring analgesia include headache, arthralgia, and myalgia.

b. **External applications:** *Salicylic acid* is used topically to treat corns, calluses, and epidermophytosis (an eruption caused by fungi). *Methyl salicylate* ("oil of wintergreen") is used externally as a cutaneous counterirritant in liniments.

c. **Cardiovascular applications:** Salicylates are used to inhibit platelet aggregation (see above). Low doses of *aspirin* are used prophylactically to decrease the incidence of transient ischemic attack and unstable angina in men as well as that of coronary artery thrombosis. *Aspirin* also facilitates closure of the patent ductus arteriosus (PGE_2 is responsible for keeping the ductus arteriosus open).

d. **Colon cancer:** There is evidence that chronic use of *aspirin* reduces the incidence of colorectal cancer.

4. **Pharmacokinetics:**

a. **Administration and distribution:** Salicylates, especially *methyl salicylate*, are absorbed through intact skin. After oral administration, the un-ionized salicylates are passively absorbed from the stomach and the small intestine (dissolution of the tablets is favored at the higher pH of the gut). Rectal absorption of the salicylates is slow and unreliable, but it is a useful route for administration to vomiting children. Salicylates (except for *diflunisal*) cross both the blood-brain barrier and the placenta.

b. **Dosage:** The salicylates exhibit analgesic activity at low doses; only at higher doses do these drugs show anti-inflammatory activity (Figure 41.7). For example, two 325 mg *aspirin* tablets administered four times a day produce analgesia, whereas twelve to twenty tablets per day produce both analgesic and anti-inflammatory activity. Low dosages of *aspirin* (160 mg every other day) have been shown to reduce the incidence of recurrent myocardial infarction, and to reduce the mortality in post-myocardial infarction patients. Furthermore, *aspirin* in a dose of 160 to 325 mg/day appears to be beneficial in the prevention of a first myocardial infarction, at least in men over the age of fifty years. Thus, prophylactic *aspirin* therapy is advocated in patients with clinical manifestations of coronary disease if no specific contraindications are present.

c. **Fate:** At normal low dosages (650 mg/day), *aspirin* is hydrolyzed to salicylate and acetic acid by esterases in tissues and blood (see Figure 41.4). Salicylate is converted by the liver to water-soluble conjugates that are rapidly cleared by the kidney, resulting in elimination with first-order kinetics and a serum half-life of 3.5 hours. At anti-inflammatory dosages (>4 g/day), the hepatic metabolic pathway becomes saturated, and zero-order kinetics are observed, with the drug having a half-life of fifteen hours or more (Figure 41.8). Saturation of the hepatic enzymes requires treatment for several days to one week. Being an organic acid, salicylate is secreted into the urine and can affect uric acid excretion—namely, at low doses of *aspirin*, uric acid secretion is decreased, whereas at high doses, uric acid secretion is increased.

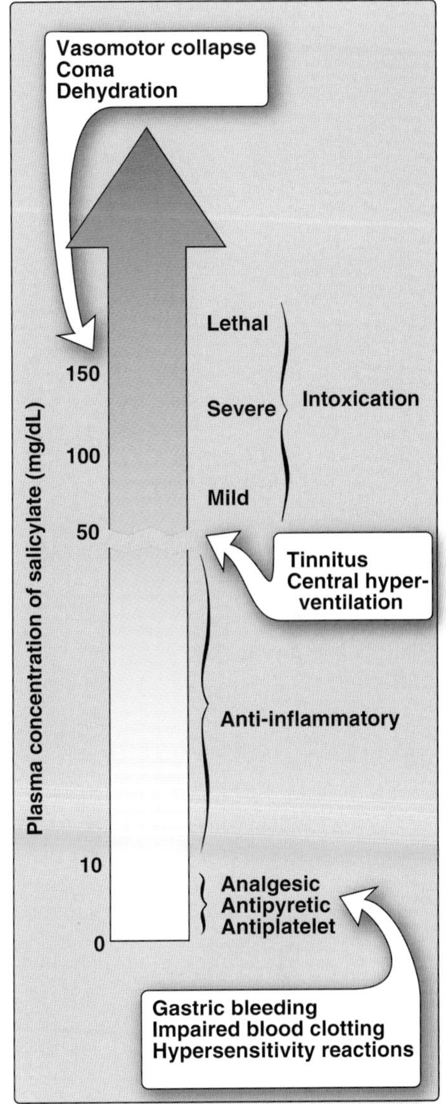

Figure 41.7
Dose-dependent effects of salicylate.

5. **Adverse effects:**

a. **Gastrointestinal:** The most common gastrointestinal (GI) effects of the salicylates are epigastric distress, nausea, and vomiting. Microscopic GI bleeding is almost universal in patients treated with salicylates. [Note: *Aspirin* is an acid. At stomach pH, *aspirin* is uncharged; consequently, it readily crosses into mucosal cells, where it ionizes (becomes negatively charged) and becomes trapped, thus potentially causing direct damage to the cells. *Aspirin* should be taken with food and large volumes of fluids to diminish GI disturbances. Alternatively, *misoprostol* may be taken concurrently.]

b. **Blood:** The irreversible acetylation of platelet cyclooxygenase reduces the level of platelet TXA_2, resulting in inhibition of platelet aggregation and a prolonged bleeding time. For this reason, *aspirin* should not be taken for at least one week prior to surgery. When salicylates are administered, anticoagulants may have to be given in reduced dosage.

c. **Respiration:** In toxic doses, salicylates cause respiratory depression and a combination of uncompensated respiratory and metabolic acidosis.

d. **Metabolic processes:** Large doses of salicylates uncouple oxidative phosphorylation.[4] The energy normally used for the production of ATP is dissipated as heat, which explains the hyperthermia caused by salicylates when taken in toxic quantities.

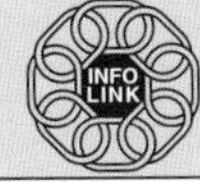

[4]See p. 78 in ***Lippincott's Illustrated Reviews: Biochemistry*** (3rd ed.) for a discussion of uncoupling of oxidative phosphorylation and heat production.

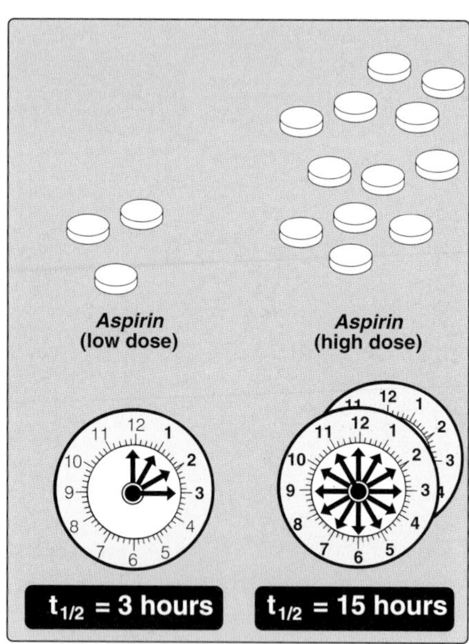

Figure 41.8
Effect of dose on the half-life of *aspirin*.

e. **Hypersensitivity:** Approximately fifteen percent of patients taking *aspirin* experience hypersensitivity reactions. Symptoms of true allergy include urticaria, bronchoconstriction, or angioneurotic edema. Fatal anaphylactic shock is rare.

f. **Reye syndrome:** *Aspirin* given during viral infections has been associated with an increased incidence of Reye syndrome, which is an often fatal, fulminating hepatitis with cerebral edema. This is especially encountered in children, who therefore should be given *acetaminophen* instead of *aspirin* when such medication is required to reduce fever.

g. **Drug interactions:** Concomitant administration of salicylates with many classes of drugs may produce undesirable side effects (Figure 41.9).

6. **Toxicity:** Salicylate intoxication may be mild or severe. The mild form is called salicylism, and is characterized by nausea, vomiting, marked hyperventilation, headache, mental confusion, dizziness, and tinnitus (ringing or roaring in the ears). When large doses of salicylate are administered, severe salicylate intoxication may result (see Figure 41.7). The symptoms listed above are followed by restlessness, delirium, hallucinations, convulsions, coma, respiratory and metabolic acidosis, and death from respiratory failure. Children are particularly prone to salicylate intoxication. Ingestion of as little as 10 g of *aspirin* (or 5 g of *methyl salicylate*, with the latter being used as a counterirritant in liniments) can cause death in children. Treatment of salicylism should include measurement of serum salicylate concentrations and of pH to determine the best form of therapy. In mild cases, symptomatic treatment is usually sufficient. Increasing the urinary pH enhances the elimination of salicylate. In serious cases, mandatory measures include the intravenous administration of fluid, dialysis (hemodialysis or peritoneal dialysis), and the frequent assessment and correction of acid-base and electrolyte balances. [Note: *Diflunisal* does not cause salicylism.]

B. Propionic acid derivatives

Ibuprofen [eye BYOO proe fen] was the first in this class of agents to become available in the United States. It has been joined by *naproxen* [nah PROX en], *fenoprofen* [fen oh PROE fen], *ketoprofen* [key toe PROE fen], *flurbiprofen* [flur bye PROE fen], and *oxaprozin* [ox ah PROE zin]. All these drugs possess anti-inflammatory, analgesic, and antipyretic activity. They have gained wide acceptance in the chronic treatment of rheumatoid arthritis and osteoarthritis, because their gastrointestinal effects are generally less intense than that of *aspirin*. These drugs are reversible inhibitors of the cyclooxygenases, and thus, like *aspirin*, inhibit the synthesis of prostaglandins but not that of leukotrienes. All are well absorbed on oral administration, and are almost totally bound to serum albumin. [Note: *Oxaprozin* has the longest half-life, and is administered once daily.] They undergo hepatic metabolism, and are excreted by the kidney. The most common adverse effects are GI, ranging from dyspepsia to bleeding. Side effects involving the central nervous system (CNS), such as headache, tinnitus, and dizziness, have also been reported.

C. Acetic acid derivatives

This group of drugs includes *indomethacin* [in doe METH a sin], *sulindac* [sul IN dak], and *etodolac* [eh TOE doh lak]. All have anti-inflammatory, analgesic, and antipyretic activity. They act by reversibly inhibiting cyclooxygenase. They are generally not used to lower fever. Despite its potency as an anti-inflammatory agent, the toxicity of *indomethacin* limits its use to the treatment of acute gouty arthritis, ankylosing spondylitis, and osteoarthritis of the hip. *Sulindac* is an inactive prodrug that is closely related to *indomethacin.* Although the drug is less potent than *indomethacin*, it is useful in the treatment of rheumatoid arthritis, ankylosing spondylitis, osteoarthritis, and acute gout. The adverse reactions caused by *sulindac* are similar to, but less severe than, those of the other NSAIDs, including *indomethacin. Etodolac* has effects similar to those of the other NSAIDs. GI problems may be less common.

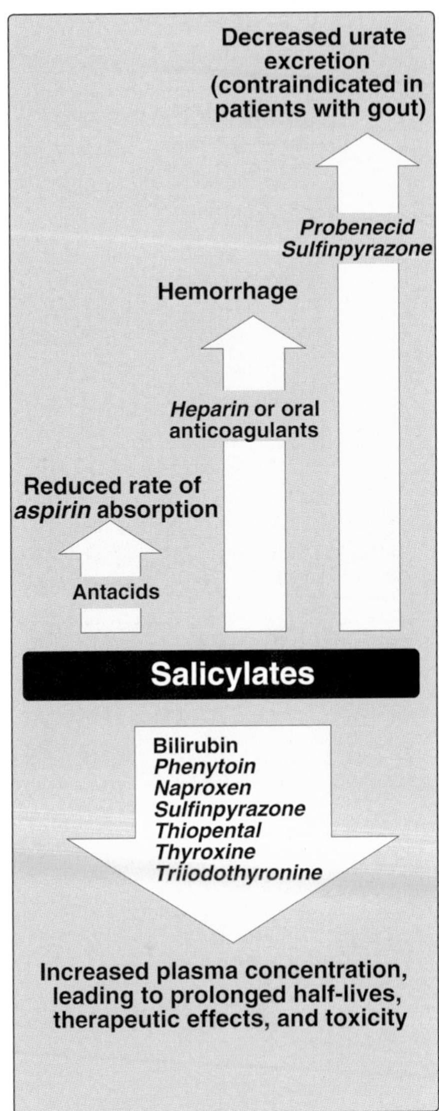

Figure 41.9
Drugs interacting with salicylates.

D. Oxicam derivatives

Piroxicam [peer OX i kam] and *meloxicam* [mel OX i kam] are used to treat rheumatoid arthritis, ankylosing spondylitis, and osteoarthritis. They have long half-lives, which permit administration once a day. GI disturbances are encountered in approximately twenty percent of patients treated with *piroxicam. Meloxicam* is relatively COX-2 selective (Figure 41.10) and at low to moderate doses shows less GI irritation than *piroxicam.* However, the ability of *meloxicam* at therapeutic dosage to spare COX-1 is dose-related. At high doses, *meloxicam* is a nonselective NSAID, inhibiting both COX-1 and COX-2. *Piroxicam* and its metabolites are excreted in the urine. *Meloxicam* excretion is predominantly in the form of metabolites and occurs to equal extents in the urine and feces.

E. Fenamates

Mefenamic acid [meh FEN a mick] and *meclofenamate* [meh KLO fen a mate] have no advantages over other NSAIDs as anti-inflammatory agents. Their side effects, such as diarrhea, can be severe, and are associated with inflammation of the bowel. Cases of hemolytic anemia have been reported.

F. Other agents

1. **Diclofenac:** A cyclooxygenase inhibitor, *diclofenac* [dye KLO fe nak] is approved for long-term use in the treatment of rheumatoid arthritis, osteoarthritis, and ankylosing spondylitis. It is more potent than *indomethacin* or *naproxen.* An ophthalmic preparation is also available. *Diclofenac* accumulates in synovial fluid. The urine is the primary route of excretion for the drug and its metabolites. Its toxicities are similar to those of the other NSAIDs.

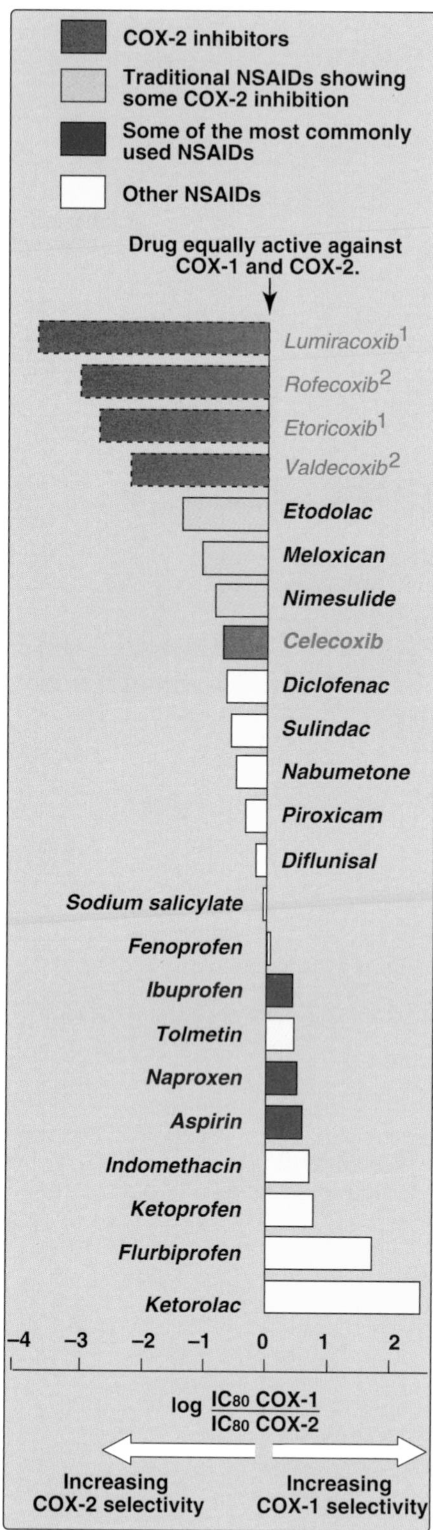

Figure 41.10
Relative selectivity of COX-1 and COX-2 inhibitors, shown as the logarithm of their ratio of IC_{80} (drug concentration to achieve eighty percent inhibition). [1]Not yet approved by the FDA. [2]Withdrawn from the market.

2. **Ketorolac:** This drug acts like the other NSAIDs. In addition to the oral route, *ketorolac* [key toe ROLE ak] can be administered intramuscularly in the treatment of postoperative pain and topically for allergic conjunctivitis. *Ketorolac* undergoes hepatic metabolism; the drug and its metabolites are eliminated via the urine. *Ketorolac* causes the same side effects as the other NSAIDs.

3. **Tolmetin and nabumetone:** *Tolmetin* [TOLL met in] and *nabumetone* [na BYOO me tone] are as potent as *aspirin* in treating adult or juvenile rheumatoid arthritis or osteoarthritis, but they may have fewer adverse effects.

4. **Diflunisal:** A diflurophenyl derivative of salicylic acid, *diflunisal* [dye FLOO ni sal] is not metabolized to salicylate and, therefore, cannot cause salicylate intoxication. *Diflunisal* is three- to four-fold more potent than *aspirin* as an analgesic and an anti-inflammatory agent, but it has no antipyretic properties. *Diflunisal* does not enter the CNS and, therefore, cannot relieve fever.

IV. COX-2-SELECTIVE NSAIDs

The substrate binding site of COX-1 differs from that of COX-2. COX-2 has a larger and more flexible substrate channel than that in COX-1 and a larger space at the site where inhibitors bind (see Figure 41.2). The structural difference between COX-1 and COX-2 has allowed the development of COX-2-selective agents, such as *celecoxib* and *valdecoxib*. These differ from most of the traditional NSAIDs, which inhibit both COX-1 and COX-2. However, some traditional NSAIDs, most notably *etodolac, meloxicam*, and *nimesulide*, display some level of COX-2 selectivity. For example, Figure 41.10 shows the relative inhibition selectivities of NSAIDs on COX-1 and COX-2. COX-2 inhibitors, as a group, have an advantage by showing a lower risk for the development of GI bleeding (Figure 41.11). These selective agents also have no significant effects on platelets. However, the COX-2 drugs (like the traditional NSAIDs) may cause renal insufficiency and increase the risk of hypertension. However, for patients who require chronic use of NSAIDs and are at high risk for NSAID-related gastroduodenal toxicity, primary therapy with a COX-2-selective inhibitor is a reasonable option.

A. Celecoxib

Celecoxib [sel eh COCKS ib] is significantly more selective for inhibition of COX-2 than of COX-1 (see Figure 41.10). In fact, at concentrations achieved in vivo, *celecoxib* does not block COX-1. Unlike the inhibition of COX-1 by *aspirin* (which is rapid and irreversible), the inhibition of COX-2 is time-dependent and reversible. *Celecoxib* was approved for treatment of osteoarthritis and rheumatoid arthritis. Unlike aspirin, *celecoxib* does not inhibit platelet aggregation and does not increase bleeding time.

1. **Pharmacokinetics:** *Celecoxib* is readily absorbed, reaching a peak concentration in about three hours. It is extensively metabolized in the liver by cytochrome P450 (CYP2C9) and is excreted in

the feces and urine. Its half-life is about eleven hours; thus, the drug is usually taken once a day.

2. **Adverse effects:** Abdominal pain, diarrhea, and dyspepsia are the most common adverse effects. The incidence of gastroduodenal ulcers in patients taking *celecoxib* was less that found in patients taking *naproxen*, *diclofenac*, or *ibuprofen* (see Figure 41.11). *Celecoxib* is contraindicated in patients who are allergic to sulfonamides. [Note: If there is a history of sulfonamide drug allergy, then use of a nonselective NSAID along with a proton-pump inhibitor is recommended.] As with other NSAIDs, kidney toxicity may occur. Selective COX-2 inhibitors should be avoided in patients with chronic renal insufficiency, severe heart disease, volume depletion, and/or hepatic failure. Patients who have had anaphylactoid reactions to *aspirin* or nonselective NSAIDs may be at risk for similar effects when challenged with COX-22selective agents. Inhibitors of CYP2C9, such as *fluconazole*, *fluvastatin*, and *zafirlukast*, may increase serum levels of *celecoxib*. *Celecoxib* has the ability to inhibit CYP2D6 and, thus, could lead to elevated levels of some β-blockers, antidepressants, and antipsychotic drugs.

Figure 41.12 summarizes some of the therapeutic advantages and disadvantages of members of the NSAID family.

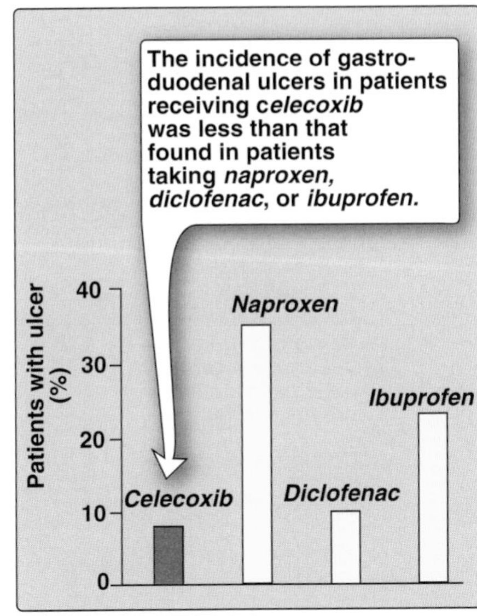

Figure 41.11
Cumulative incidence of of gastro-duodenal ulcers over twelve weeks in patients treated with NSAIDS.

V. OTHER ANALGESICS

Unlike the NSAIDs, analgesics such as *acetaminophen* have little or no anti-inflammatory activity. They have a therapeutic advantage over narcotic analgesics in that they do not cause physical dependence or tolerance.

A. Acetaminophen

Acetaminophen [a seat a MIN oh fen] inhibits prostaglandin synthesis in the CNS. This explains its antipyretic and analgesic properties. *Acetaminophen* has less effect on cyclooxygenase in peripheral tissues, which accounts for its weak anti-inflammatory activity. *Acetaminophen* does not affect platelet function or increase blood clotting time, but it does have many of the side effects of *aspirin*.

1. **Therapeutic uses:** *Acetaminophen* is a suitable substitute for the analgesic and antipyretic effects of *aspirin* for those patients with gastric complaints, for those for whom prolongation of bleeding time would be a disadvantage, or those who do not require the anti-inflammatory action of *aspirin*. *Acetaminophen* is the analgesic/antipyretic of choice for children with viral infections or chickenpox (recall that *aspirin* increases the risk of Reye syndrome). *Acetaminophen* does not antagonize the uricosuric agent *probenecid* and, therefore, may be used in patients with gout who are taking that drug.

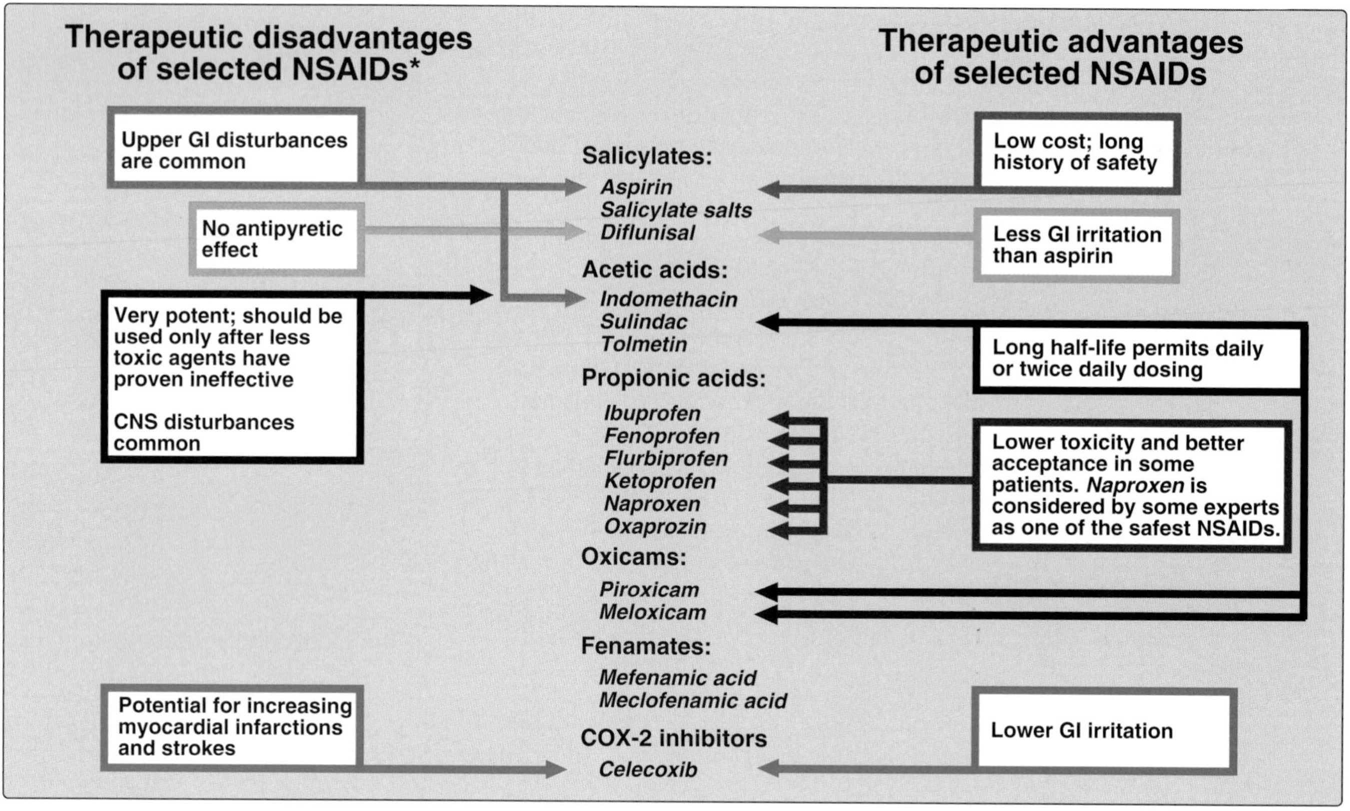

Figure 41.12
Summary of nonsteroidal anti-inflammatory agents (NSAIDs). *As a group, with the exception of *aspirin*, these drugs may have the potential to increase myocardial infarctions and strokes.

2. **Pharmacokinetics:** *Acetaminophen* is rapidly absorbed from the GI tract. A significant first-pass metabolism occurs in the luminal cells of the intestine and in the hepatocytes. Under normal circumstances, *acetaminophen* is conjugated in the liver to form inactive glucuronidated or sulfated metabolites. A portion of *acetaminophen* is hydroxylated to form N-acetylbenzoiminoquinone—a highly reactive and potentially dangerous metabolite that reacts with sulfhydryl groups. At normal doses of *acetaminophen*, the N-acetylbenzoiminoquinone reacts with the sulfhydryl group of glutathione, forming a nontoxic substance (Figure 41.13). *Acetaminophen* and its metabolites are excreted in the urine.

3. **Adverse effects:** With normal therapeutic doses, *acetaminophen* is virtually free of any significant adverse effects. Skin rash and minor allergic reactions occur infrequently. There may be minor alterations in the leukocyte count, but these are generally transient. Renal tubular necrosis and hypoglycemic coma are rare complications of prolonged, large-dose therapy. With large doses of *acetaminophen,* the available glutathione in the liver becomes depleted, and N-acetylbenzoiminoquinone reacts with the sulfhydryl groups of hepatic proteins, forming covalent bonds (see

Figure 41.13). Hepatic necrosis, a very serious and potentially life-threatening condition, can result. Renal tubular necrosis may also occur. [Note: Administration of N-acetylcysteine, which contains sulfhydryl groups to which the toxic metabolite can bind, can be lifesaving if administered within ten hours of the overdose.]

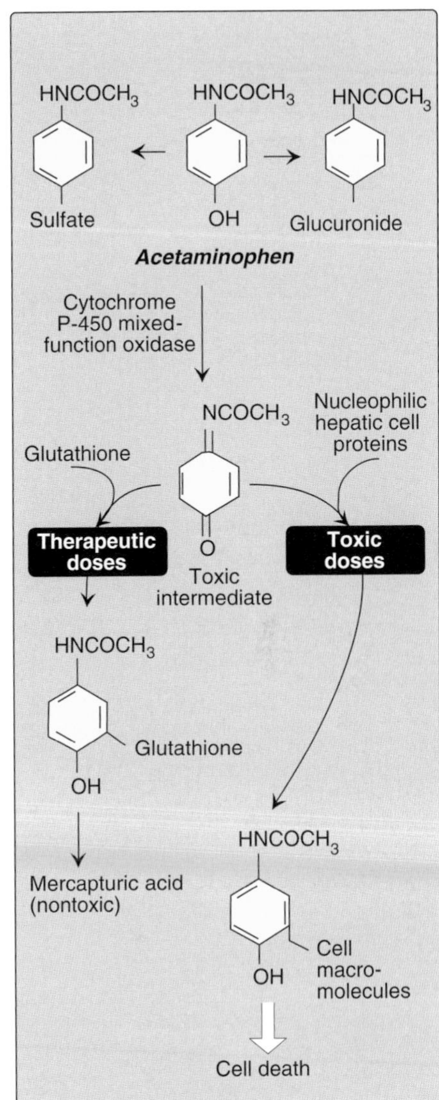

Figure 41.13
Metabolism of *acetaminophen*.

VI. DISEASE-MODIFYING ANTIRHEUMATIC AGENTS

A miscellaneous group of drugs termed disease-modifying antirheumatic drugs (DMARDs), or slow-acting anti-rheumatic drugs (SAARDs), have the potential to reduce or prevent joint damage. These drugs are used primarily for rheumatic disorders, especially cases in which the inflammatory disease does not respond to cyclooxygenase inhibitors. The DMARDs slow the course of the disease and can induce remission, preventing further destruction of the joints and involved tissues. They have a long onset of action, sometimes taking three to four months.

A. Choice of drug

No one DMARD is efficacious and safe in every patient, and trials of several different drugs may be necessary. Most experts begin DMARD therapy with one of the traditional small molecules, such as *methotrexate* or *hydroxychloroquine*. These agents are efficacious and are generally well tolerated, with well-known side-effect profiles. Inadequate response to the traditional agent may be followed by use newer DMARDs, such as *leflunomide*, *adalimumab*, *anakinra*, *etanercept*, and *infliximab*. Combination therapies are both safe and efficacious. In most cases, *methotrexate* is combined with one of the other DMARDs.

B. Methotrexate

Methotrexate [meth oh TREX ate], used alone or in combination therapy, has become the mainstay of treatment in patients with severe rheumatoid or psoriatic arthritis who have not responded adequately to NSAIDs. *Methotrexate* slows the appearance of new erosions within involved joints. Response to *methotrexate* occurs sooner than is usual for other slow-acting agents—often within three to six weeks of starting treatment. It is an immunosuppressant, and this may account for its effectiveness in arthritis, an autoimmune disease. Doses of *methotrexate* required for this treatment are much lower than those needed in cancer chemotherapy and are given once a week; therefore, the adverse effects are minimized. The most common side effects observed after *methotrexate* treatment of rheumatoid arthritis are mucosal ulceration and nausea. Cytopenias (particularly depression of the white-blood-cell count), cirrhosis of the liver, and an acute pneumonia-like syndrome may occur on chronic administration. [Note: Taking *leucovorin* a day after *methotrexate* reduces the severity of the adverse effects.] Contrary to early concerns, there have been minimal unexpected side effects after more than twenty years of surveillance.

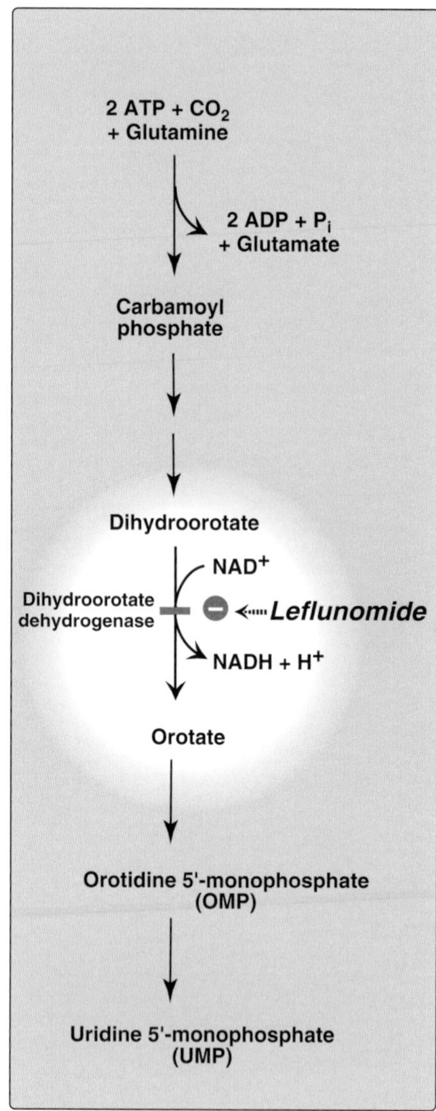

Figure 41.14
Site of action of *leflunomide*.

C. Leflunomide

Leflunomide (le FLOO na mide) is an immunomodulatory agent that preferentially causes cell arrest of the autoimmune lymphocytes through its action on dihydroorotate dehydrogenase (DHODH). Stimulation of a T cell by an antigen-presenting cell drives the lymphocyte into its replicative cycle. Many enzymes, including those required for de novo purine, pyrimidine, RNA, and membrane synthesis, are upregulated in the G_1 phase of the cycle. DHODH, which catalyzes the formation of orotate (a precursor of the pyrimidines from dihydroorotate in the mitochondria, is among these (Figure 41.14). [Note: Resting lymphocytes can meet their requirements for ribonucleotides through the salvage pathway, but cell division requires an 8- to 16-fold expansion of the ribonucleotide pool.] Inhibition of DHODH deprives the cell of the precursor for uridine monophosphate—a necessary component for RNA synthesis and a precursor of the thymidine-containing nucleotide required for DNA synthesis. After biotransformation, *leflunomide* is a reversible inhibitor of DHODH. *Leflunomide* has been approved for the treatment of rheumatoid arthritis. It not only reduces pain and inflammation associated with the disease but also appears to slow the progression of structural damage. *Leflunomide* can be used in monotherapy as an alternative to *methotrexate* or as an addition to *methotrexate* in combination therapy.

1. **Pharmacokinetics:** *Leflunomide* is well absorbed after oral administration. It is extensively bound to albumin (>90 percent) and has a half-life of fourteen to eighteen days. [Note: Because of its long half-life, loading doses are necessary.] *Leflunomide* is rapidly converted to the active metabolite. The metabolites are excreted in the urine and the feces. The active metabolite undergoes biliary recycling.

2. **Adverse effects:** The most common of these are headache, diarrhea, and nausea. Other untoward effects are weight loss, allergic reactions including a flu-like syndrome, skin rash, alopecia, and hypokalemia. *Leflunomide* is teratogenic in experimental animals and, therefore, is contraindicated in pregnancy and in women of child-bearing potential. It should be used with caution in patients with liver disease, because it is cleared by both biliary and renal excretion.

D. Chloroquine and hydroxychloroquine

The pharmacology of these drugs, which are also used in the treatment of malaria, is presented on p. 419. In treating inflammatory disorders, they are reserved for rheumatoid arthritis that has been unresponsive to NSAIDs or else are used in conjunction with an NSAID, which allows a lower dose of *chloroquine* or *hydroxychloroquine* to be administered. These drugs have been shown to slow progression of erosive bone lesions and may induce remission. They do cause serious adverse effects.

E. D-Penicillamine

D-Penicillamine [pen i SILL a meen], an analog of the amino acid cysteine, slows the progress of bone destruction and rheumatoid arthritis. Prolonged treatment with *penicillamine* has serious side effects, ranging from dermatologic problems to nephritis and aplastic anemia; therefore, it is used primarily in the treatment of rheumatoid arthritis after use of gold salts has failed but before use of corticosteroids has been attempted. [Note: *D-Penicillamine* is used as a chelating agent in the treatment of poisoning by heavy metals. It is also of benefit in treating cystinuria.]

F. Gold salts

Gold compounds, like the other drugs in this group, cannot repair existing damage. Rather, they can only prevent further injury. The currently available gold preparations are *gold sodium thiomalate* and *aurothioglucose*. It is believed that gold salts are taken up by macrophages and suppress phagocytosis and lysosomal enzyme activity. This mechanism retards the progression of bone and articular destruction. The gold compounds are being used less and less by rheumatologists, because of the need for meticulous monitoring for serious toxicity and the costs of administration and monitoring.

VII. ANTICYTOKINE THERAPIES IN RHEUMATOID ARTHRITIS

Interleukin-1b (IL-1b) and tumor necrosis factor-α (TNF-α) are proinflammatory cytokines involved in the pathogenesis of rheumatoid arthritis. When secreted by synovial macrophages, IL-1b and TNF-α stimulate synovial cells to proliferate and synthesize collagenase, thereby degrading cartilage, stimulating bone resorption, and inhibiting proteoglycan synthesis. Drug antagonists of these cytokines are proving to be effective in treating rheumatoid arthritis.

A. Etanercept

Tumor necrosis factor plays a key role in the host's immune system. The targeting of TNF-α rests on the observation that cytokines produced by macrophages (TNF-α, IL-1, IL-6, and IL-8) predominate in the rheumatoid synovium. *Etanercept*, *infliximab*, and *adalimumab* decrease the activity of TNF. *Etanercept* has been approved for the treatment of rheumatoid and psoriatic arthritis. [Note: Upon discontinuation of *etanercept*, the symptoms of arthritis generally return within a month.] The combination of *etanercept* and *methotrexate* was more effective than *methotrexate* or *etanercept* alone in retarding the disease process, achieving remission (Figure 41.15), and improving function. Many experts propose that an anti-TNF drug plus *methorexate* be considered as standard therapy for patients with rheumatoid and psoriatic arthritis.

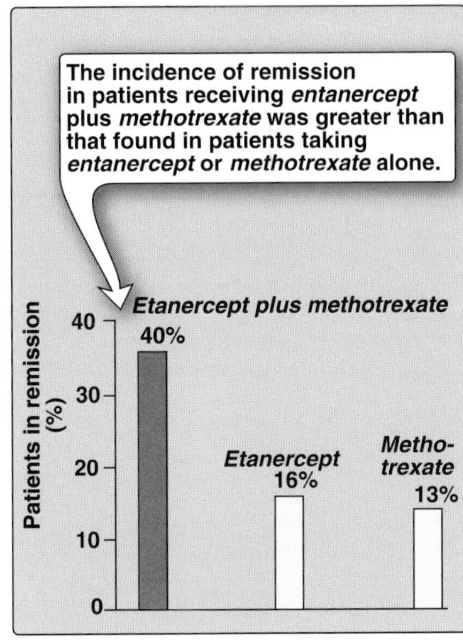

Figure 41.15
Incidence of remission from the symptoms of rheumatoid arthritis after one year of therapy.

1. **Mechanism of action:** *Etanercept* [ee tan ER sept] is a genetically engineered fusion protein composed of two identical chains of the recombinant human TNF-receptor p75 monomer fused with the Fc domain of human immunoglobin IgG_1. This soluble fusion protein binds two molecules of TNF and prevents them from binding to cellular receptors. The protein does not discriminate between TNF-α and TNF-β (lymphotoxin). [Note: Because TNF is important in modulating cellular immune responses to infection and tumors, some concern exists about the long-term use of *etanercept.*]

2. **Pharmacokinetics:** *Etanercept* is given subcutaneously twice a week. The time to maximum serum concentration after a single injection is about 72 hours. Its median half-life is 115 hours. Data on elimination are not available.

3. **Adverse effects:** *Etanercept* is well tolerated. No toxicities or antibodies have been reported. However, it can produce local inflammation at the site of injection. Patients with life-threatening infection, such as sepsis, should not receive therapy with *etanercept.*

B. Infliximab

Infliximab (in FLIX i mab) is a chimeric IgGκ monoclonal antibody composed of human and murine regions. The antibody binds specifically to human TNF-α, thereby neutralizing that cytokine. *Infliximab* has been approved for Crohn disease for both fistulizing and non-fistula disease. [Note: Increased levels of TNF-α are found in fecal samples of patients with Crohn disease.]. It is not approved for maintenance therapy beyond six weeks. *Infliximab* is approved for the treatment of rheumatoid arthritis. It inhibits the progression of structural damage and improves physical function in patients with moderate to severe disease. It is often used in combination with *methotrexate.*

1. **Pharmacokinetics:** *Infliximab* is infused intravenously over at least two hours. It distributes in the vascular compartment and has a half-life of 9.5 days. Its metabolism and elimination have not been described.

2. **Adverse effects:** Long-term use of *infliximab* is associated with development of anti-*infliximab* antibodies unless the drug is used in combination with *methotrexate*. Infusion reactions, such as fever, chill, pruritus, or urticaria, have occurred. Infections leading to pneumonia, cellulitis, and other conditions have also been reported. Leukopenia, neutropenia, thrombocytopenia, and pancytopenia have occurred. Whether treatment with *infliximab* predisposes to lymphoma, a condition that occurs with immunosuppressive or immune-altering drugs, remains to be established. [Note: *Infliximab* treatment does predispose to infections, which may be life-threatening.]

C. Adalimumab

Adalimumab [a dal AYE mu mab] is used in the treatment of active rheumatoid arthritis (moderate to severe) in patients with inadequate response to one or more DMARDs. *Adalimumab* is a recombinant monoclonal antibody that binds to human TNF-α receptor sites, thereby interfering with endogenous TNF-α activity. Elevated TNF levels in the synovial fluid are involved in the pathologic pain and joint destruction in rheumatoid arthritis. *Adalimumab* decreases signs and symptoms of rheumatoid arthritis and inhibits progression of structural damage. This medication may be administered by subcutaneous injection only. It may cause headache, nausea, rash, or reaction at the injection site. [Note: An increased predisposition to infections may reactivate pneumonia.]

D. Anakinra

Interleukin-1 is induced by inflammatory stimuli and mediates a variety of immunologic responses, including degradation of cartilage and stimulation of bone resorption.*Anakinra* [an a KIN ra] is an IL-1 receptor antagonist. (It binds to IL-1 receptor, thus preventing IL-1 actions.) *Anakinra* treatment leads to the reduction of signs and symptoms of moderately to severely active rheumatoid arthritis in adult patients who have failed one or more DMARDs. The drug may be used alone or in combination with DMARDs (other than TNF-blocking agents).

VIII. DRUGS EMPLOYED IN THE TREATMENT OF GOUT

Gout is a metabolic disorder characterized by high levels of uric acid in the blood. This hyperuricemia results in the deposition of sodium urate crystals in tissues, especially the kidney and joints. Hyperuricemia does not always lead to gout, but gout is always preceded by hyperuricemia. In humans, sodium urate is the end product of purine metabolism.[5] The deposition of urate crystals initiates an inflammatory process involving the infiltration of granulocytes that phagocytize the urate crystals (Figure 41.16). This process generates oxygen metabolites, which damage tissue, resulting in the release of lysosomal enzymes that evoke an inflammatory response. In addition, lactate production in the synovial tissues increases. The resulting local decrease in pH fosters further deposition of urate crystals. The cause of hyperuricemia is an overproduction of uric acid relative to the patient's ability to excrete it. Most therapeutic strategies for gout involve lowering the uric acid level below the saturation point, thus preventing the deposition of urate crystals. This can be accomplished by 1) interfering with uric acid synthesis with *allopurinol*, 2) increasing uric acid excretion with *probenecid* or *sulfinpyrazone*, 3) inhibiting leukocyte entry into the affected joint with *colchicine*, or 4) administration of NSAIDs.

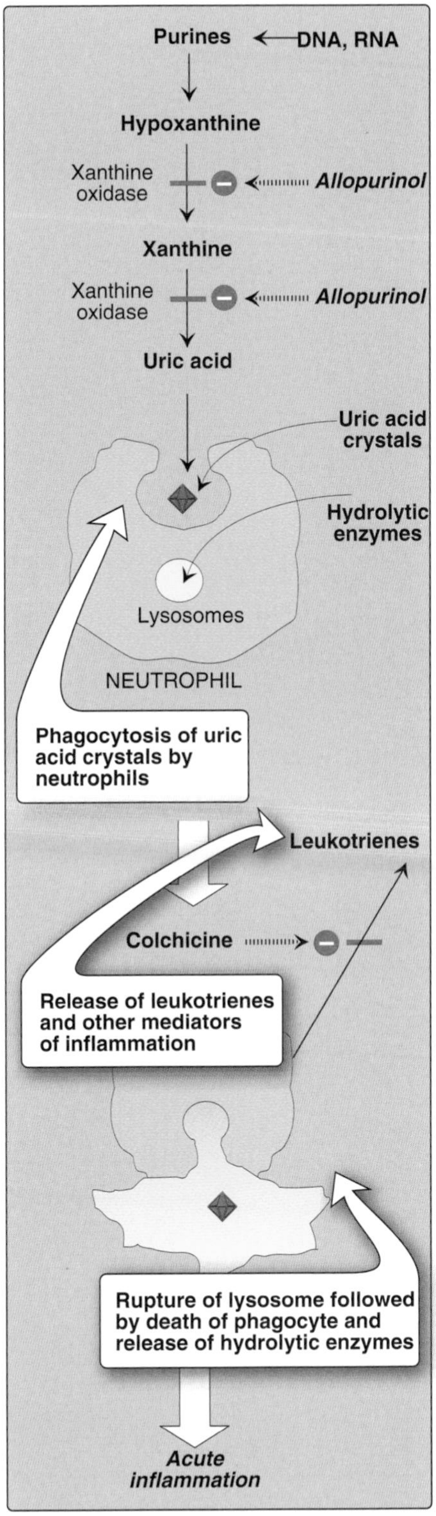

Figure 41.16
Role of uric acid in the inflammation of gout.

A. Treating acute gout

Acute gouty attacks can result from a number of conditions, including excessive alcohol consumption, a diet rich in purines, or kidney

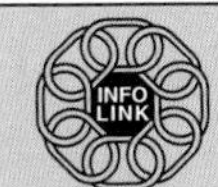

[5]See p. 299 in ***Lippincott's Illustrated Reviews: Biochemistry*** (3rd ed.) for a discussion of purine metabolism.

disease. Acute attacks are treated with *indomethacin* to decrease movement of granulocytes into the affected area and with NSAIDs to decrease pain and inflammation. [Note: *Aspirin* is contraindicated, because it competes with uric acid for the organic acid secretion mechanism in the proximal tubule of the kidney.]

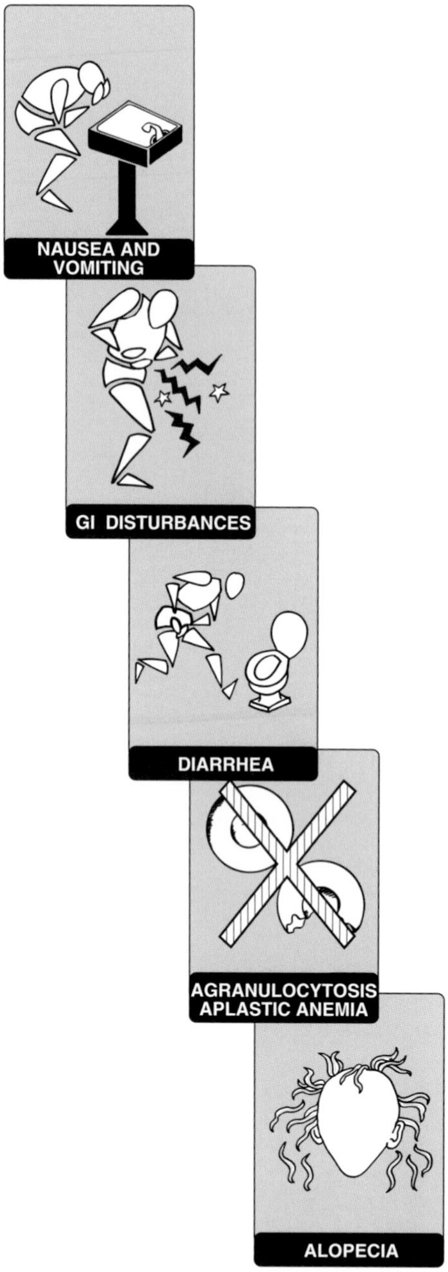

B. Treating chronic gout

Chronic gout can be caused by 1) a genetic defect, such as one resulting in an increase in the rate of purine synthesis; 2) renal deficiency; 3) Lesch-Nyhan syndrome;[6] or 4) excessive synthesis of uric acid associated with cancer chemotherapy. Treatment strategies for chronic gout include the use of uricosuric drugs that increase the excretion of uric acid, thereby reducing its concentration in plasma, and the use of *allopurinol*, which is a selective inhibitor of the terminal steps in the biosynthesis of uric acid. Uricosuric agents are first-line agents for patients with gout associated with normal urinary uric acid excretion. *Allopurinol* is preferred in patients with excessive uric acid excretion, with previous histories of uric acid stones, or with renal insufficiency.

C. Colchicine

Colchicine [KOL chi seen], a plant alkaloid, is reserved for the treatment of acute gouty attacks. It is neither a uricosuric nor an analgesic agent, although it relieves pain in acute attacks of gout. *Colchicine* does not prevent the progression of gout to acute gouty arthritis, but it does have a suppressive, prophylactic effect that reduces the frequency of acute attacks and relieves pain.

1. **Mechanism of action:** *Colchicine* binds to tubulin, a microtubular protein, causing its depolymerization. This disrupts cellular functions, such as the mobility of granulocytes, thus decreasing their migration into the affected area. Furthermore, *colchicine* blocks cell division by binding to mitotic spindles. *Colchicine* also inhibits the synthesis and release of the leukotrienes (see Figure 41.16).

2. **Therapeutic uses:** The anti-inflammatory activity of *colchicine* is specific for gout, usually alleviating the pain of acute gout within twelve hours. *Indomethacin* has largely replaced *colchicine* in the treatment of acute gouty attacks. *Colchicine* is currently used for prophylaxis of recurrent attacks. It is only rarely effective in other kinds of arthritis.

3. **Pharmacokinetics:** *Colchicine* is administered orally, followed by rapid absorption from the GI tract. It is also available combined with *probenecid* (see below). *Colchicine* is recycled in the bile and is excreted unchanged in the feces or urine.

4. **Adverse effects:** *Colchicine* treatment may cause nausea, vomiting, abdominal pain, and diarrhea (Figure 41.17). Chronic administration may lead to myopathy, agranulocytosis, aplastic anemia, and alopecia. The drug should not be used in pregnancy, and it should be used with caution in patients with hepatic, renal, or cardiovascular disease.

Figure 41.17
Some adverse effects of *colchicine*.

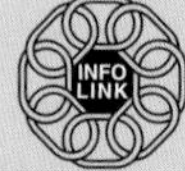

[6]See p. 296 in ***Lippincott's Illustrated Reviews: Biochemistry*** (3rd ed.) for a discussion of Lesch-Nyhan syndrome.

D. Allopurinol

Allopurinol [al oh PURE i nole] is a purine analog. It reduces the production of uric acid by competitively inhibiting the last two steps in uric acid biosynthesis that are catalyzed by xanthine oxidase (see Figure 41.16). [Note: Uric acid is less water soluble than its precursors. When xanthine oxidase is inhibited, the circulating purine derivatives (xanthine and hypoxanthine) are more soluble and, therefore, are less likely to precipitate.]

1. **Therapeutic uses:** *Allopurinol* is effective in the treatment of primary hyperuricemia of gout, and hyperuricemia secondary to other conditions, such as that associated with certain malignancies (those in which large amounts of purines are produced, particularly after treatment with chemotherapeutic agents.) or in renal disease.

2. **Pharmacokinetics:** *Allopurinol* is completely absorbed after oral administration. The primary metabolite is alloxanthine (oxypurinol), which is also a xanthine oxidase inhibitor. The pharmacologic effect of administered *allopurinol* results from the combined activity of these two compounds. The plasma half-life of *allopurinol* is short (two hours), whereas the half-life of oxypurinol is long (fifteen hours). Thus, effective inhibition of xanthine oxidase can be maintained with once-daily dosage. The drug and its metabolite are excreted in the feces and urine.

3. **Adverse effects:** *Allopurinol* is well tolerated by most patients. Hypersensitivity reactions, especially skin rashes, are the most common adverse reactions, occurring among approximately three percent of patients. The reactions may occur even after months or years of chronic administration. Acute attacks of gout may occur more frequently during the first several weeks of therapy; therefore *colchicine* and NSAIDs should be administered concurrently. GI side effects, such as nausea and diarrhea, are common. *Allopurinol* interferes with the metabolism of the anti-cancer agent *6-mercaptopurine* and the immunosuppressant *azathioprine*, requiring a reduction in dosage of these drugs.

E. Uricosuric agents: probenecid and sulfinpyrazone

The uricosuric drugs are weak organic acids that promote renal clearance of uric acid by inhibiting the urate-anion exchanger in the proximal tubule that mediates urate reabsorption. *Probenecid* [proe BEN e sid], a general inhibitor of the tubular secretion of organic acids, and *sulfinpyrazone* [sul fin PEER a zone], a derivative of *phenylbutazone*, are the two most commonly used uricosuric agents. At therapeutic doses, they block proximal tubular resorption of uric acid. [Note: At low dosage, these agents block proximal tubular secretion of uric acid.] These drugs have few adverse effects, although gastric distress may force discontinuance of *sulfinpyrazone*. *Probenecid* blocks the tubular secretion of *penicillin* and is sometimes used to increase levels of the antibiotic. It also inhibits excretion of *naproxen*, *ketoprofen,* and *indomethacin*.

Study Questions

Choose the ONE best answer.

41.1 In which one of the following conditions would aspirin be contraindicated?

A. Myalgia
B. Fever
C. Peptic ulcer
D. Rheumatoid arthritis
E. Unstable angina

Correct answer = C. Among the NSAIDs, aspirin is one of the worst for causing gastric irritation. Aspirin is an effective analgesic and is used to reduce muscle pain. It also has antipyretic actions so that it can be used to treat fever. Because of its anti-inflammatory properties, aspirin is used to treat pain related to the inflammatory process—for example, in the treatment of rheumatoid arthritis. Low doses of aspirin also decrease the incidence of transient ischemic attacks.

41.2 Which one of the following statements concerning COX-2 inhibitors is correct?

A. The COX-2 inhibitors show greater analgesic activity than traditional NSAIDs.
B. The COX-2 inhibitors decrease platelet function.
C. The COX-2 inhibitors do not affect the kidney.
D. The COX-2 inhibitors show anti-inflammatory activity similar to that of the traditional NSAIDs.
E. The COX-2 inhibitors are cardioprotective.

Correct answer = D. The COX-2 inhibitors show similar analgesic and anti-inflammatory activity compared to traditional NSAIDs. They do not affect platelets. Like NSAIDs, COX-2 inhibitors may cause the development of acute renal failure due to renal vasoconstriction. COX-2 inhibitors have the potential for increasing myocardial infarction.

41.3 An 8-year-old girl has a fever and muscle aches from a presumptive viral infection. Which one of the following drugs would be most appropriate to treat her symptoms?

A. Acetaminophen
B. Aspirin
C. Celecoxib
D. Codeine
E. Indomethacin

Correct answer = A. Aspirin should be avoided in children because of an association with Reye's syndrome. Indomethacin has antipyretic activity but is too toxic to use in these circumstances. Celecoxib is indicated for alleviation of pain and codeine has no antipyretic effects.

41.3 A 70-year-old man has a history of ulcer disease. He has recently experienced swelling and pain in the joints of his hands. His physician wants to begin therapy with a non-steroidal anti-inflammatory drug. Which one of the following drugs might also be prescribed along with the NSAID in order to reduce the risk of activating this patient's ulcer disease?

A. Allopurinol
B. Colchicine
C. Misoprostol
D. Probenecid
E. Sulindac

Correct answer = C. Misoprostol is a prostaglandin analog that can reduce gastric acid and pepsin secretion and promote the formation of mucus in the stomach. It is indicated for the purpose of decreasing the risk of ulcer activation in patient's taking NSAIDs. The other choices are not appropriate for alleviating the gastric irritation caused by NSAIDs.

Autacoids and Autacoid Antagonists

42

I. OVERVIEW

Prostaglandins, histamine, and serotonin belong to a group of compounds called autacoids. These heterogeneous substances have widely differing structures and pharmacologic activities. They all have the common feature of being formed by the tissues on which they act; thus, they function as local hormones. [Note: The word autacoid comes from the Greek: autos (self) and akos (medicinal agent, or remedy).] The autacoids also differ from circulating hormones in that they are produced by many tissues rather than in specific endocrine glands. The drugs described in this chapter (Figure 42.1) are either autacoids or autacoid antagonists (compounds that inhibit the synthesis of certain autacoids or interfere with their interactions with receptors).

II. PROSTAGLANDINS

Prostaglandins are unsaturated fatty acid derivatives that act on the tissues in which they are synthesized and are rapidly metabolized to inactive products at the site of action.[1]

A. Therapeutic uses of prostaglandins

Systemic administration of prostaglandins evokes a bewildering array of effects—a fact that limits the therapeutic usefulness of these agents.

1. **Abortion:** Several of the prostaglandins find use as abortifacients (agents causing abortions). The most effective option available involves oral administration *mifepristone* [mi FEP ri stone] (RU-486, a synthetic steroid with antiprogestational effects) followed at least 24 hours later by the the synthetic prostaglandin E_1 analog *misoprostol* [mye so PROST ole] administered vaginally (Figure 42.2). Women can self-administer this regimen with complete abortion rates exceeding 95 percent. The overall case-fatality rate

AUTACOIDS

PROSTAGLANDINS
- *Misoprostol*

H_1 ANTIHISTAMINES
- *Acrivastine*
- *Cetirizine*
- *Chlorpheniramine*
- *Cyclizine*
- *Desloratadine*
- *Diphenhydramine*
- *Dimenhydrinate*
- *Doxepin*
- *Doxylamine*
- *Fexofenadine*
- *Hydroxyzine*
- *Loratadine*
- *Meclizine*
- *Promethazine*

DRUGS USED TO TREAT MIGRAINE HEADACHE
- *Almotriptan*
- *Dihydroergotamine*
- *Eletriptan*
- *Naratriptan*
- *Rizatriptan*
- *Sumatriptan*
- *Zolmitriptan*

Figure 42.1
Summary of drugs affecting the autacoids.

INFO LINK

[1]See p. 211 in ***Lippincott's Illustrated Reviews: Biochemistry*** (3rd ed.) for a discussion of prostaglandin synthesis and actions.

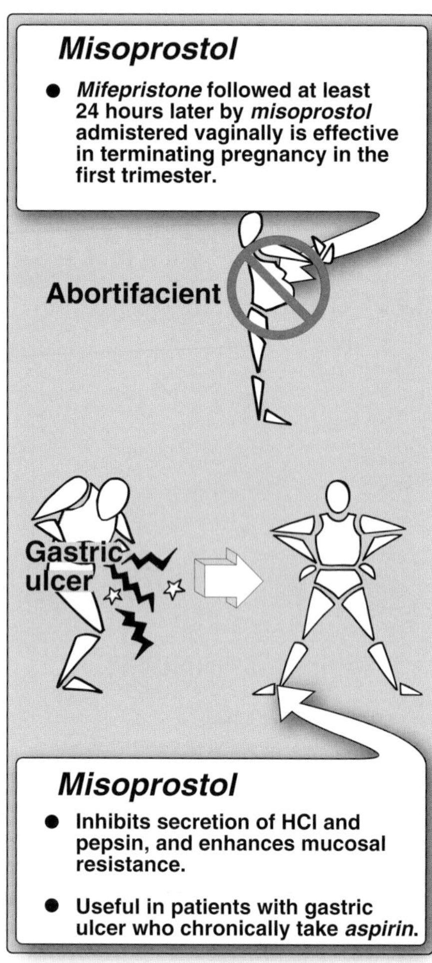

Figure 42.2
Therapeutic applications of *misoprostol*.

for abortion is less than one death per 100,000 procedures. Infection, hemorrhage, and retained tissue are among the more common complications.

2. **Peptic ulcers:** *Misoprostol* is sometimes used to inhibit the secretion of gastric acid and to enhance mucosal resistance to injury in patients with gastric ulcer who are chronically taking nonsteroidal anti-inflammatory agents. Proton-pump inhibitors, such as *omeprazol*, and H_2 antihistamines also reduce the risk of gastric ulcer, and are better tolerated than *misoprostol*, which induces intestinal disorders.

III. HISTAMINE

Histamine is a chemical messenger that mediates a wide range of cellular responses, including allergic and inflammatory reactions, gastric acid secretion, and neurotransmission in parts of the brain. Histamine has no clinical applications, but agents that interfere with the action of histamine (antihistamines) have important therapeutic applications.

A. Location, synthesis, and release

1. **Location:** Histamine occurs in practically all tissues, but it is unevenly distributed, with high amounts found in lung, skin, and the gastrointestinal tract (sites where the “inside” of the body meets the “outside”). It is found at high concentration in mast cells or basophils. Histamine also occurs as a component of venoms and in secretions from insect stings.

2. **Synthesis:** Histamine is an amine formed by the decarboxylation of the amino acid histidine by histidine decarboxylase[2], an enzyme that is expressed in cells throughout the body, including central nervous system neurons, gastric-mucosa parietal cells, mast cells, and basophils (Figure 42.3). In mast cells, histamine is stored in granules as an inactive complex composed of histamine and the polysulfated anion, heparin, along with an anionic protein. If histamine is not stored, it is rapidly inactivated by amine oxidase enzymes.

3. **Release of histamine:** The release of histamine may be the primary response to some stimuli, but most often, histamine is just one of several chemical mediators released. Stimuli causing the release of histamine from tissues include the destruction of cells as a result of cold, bacterial toxins, bee sting venoms, or trauma. Allergies and anaphylaxis can also trigger release of histamine.

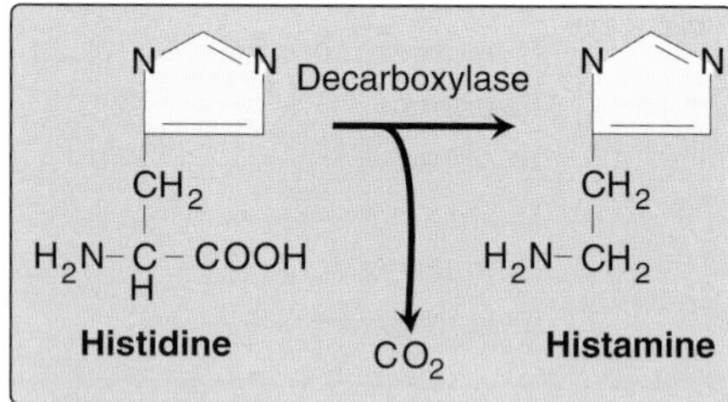

Figure 42.3
Biosynthesis of histamine.

B. Mechanism of action

Histamine released in response to various stimuli exerts its effects by binding to one or more of four types of histamine receptors—H_1, H_2, H_3, and H_4 receptors. H_1 and H_2 receptors are widely expressed and are the targets of clinically useful drugs. H_3 and H_4 receptors are expressed in only a few cell types, and their roles in drug action are unclear. All types of histamine receptors have seven transmem-

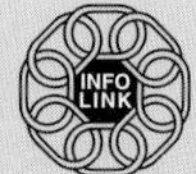

[2]See p. 285 in ***Lippincott's Illustrated Reviews: Biochemistry*** (3rd ed.) for a discussion of histamine.

brane helical domains and transduce extracellular signals by way of G protein–mediated second messenger systems. Some of histamine's wide range of pharmacologic effects are mediated by both H_1 and H_2 receptors, whereas others are mediated by only one class. For example, the H_1 receptors are important in producing smooth muscle contraction and increasing capillary permeability (Figure 42.4). Histamine promotes vasodilation by causing vascular endothelium to release nitric oxide.[3] This chemical signal diffuses to the vascular smooth muscle, where it stimulates cyclic guanosine monophosphate production, causing vasodilation. Histamine H_2 receptors mediate gastric acid secretion. The two most common histamine receptors exert their effects by different second messenger pathways. The actions of H_1 antihistamines occur through at least two mechanisms. Antiallergic activities of H_1 antihistamines, such as inhibition of the release of mediators from mast cells and basophils, involves stimulation of the intracellular activity of the polyphosphatidylinositol pathway.[4] Other actions of H_1 antihistamines involve the down-regulation of nuclear transcription factors that regulate the production of proinflammatory cytokines and adhesion proteins. In contrast, stimulation of H_2 receptors enhances the production of cyclic adenosine monophosphate (cAMP) by adenylyl cyclase.

C. Role in allergy and anaphylaxis

The symptoms resulting from intravenous injection of histamine are similar to those associated with anaphylactic shock and allergic reactions. These include contraction of smooth muscle, stimulation of secretions, dilation and increased permeability of the capillaries, and stimulation of sensory nerve endings.

1. **Role of mediators:** Symptoms associated with allergy and anaphylactic shock result from the release of certain mediators from their storage sites. Such mediators include histamine, serotonin, leukotrienes, and the eosinophil chemotactic factor of anaphylaxis. In some cases, these cause a localized allergic reaction, producing, for example, actions on the skin or respiratory tract. Under other conditions, these mediators may cause a full-blown anaphylactic response. It is thought that the difference between these two situations results from differences in the sites from which mediators are released and their rates of release. For example, if the release of histamine is slow enough to permit its inactivation before it enters the bloodstream, a local allergic reaction results. However, if histamine release is too fast for inactivation to be efficient, a full-blown anaphylactic reaction occurs.

IV. H_1 ANTIHISTAMINES

The term antihistamine, without a modifying adjective, refers to the classic H_1 receptor blockers. These compounds do not influence the formation or release of histamine; rather, they block the receptor-mediated response of a target tissue. [Note: This contrasts with the action of *cro-*

H_1 Receptors

EXOCRINE EXCRETION
Increased production of nasal and bronchial mucus, resulting in respiratory symptoms.

BRONCHIAL SMOOTH MUSCLE
Constriction of bronchioles results in symptoms of asthma and decreased lung capacity.

INTESTINAL SMOOTH MUSCLE
Constriction results in intestinal cramps and diarrhea.

SENSORY NERVE ENDINGS
Causes itching and pain.

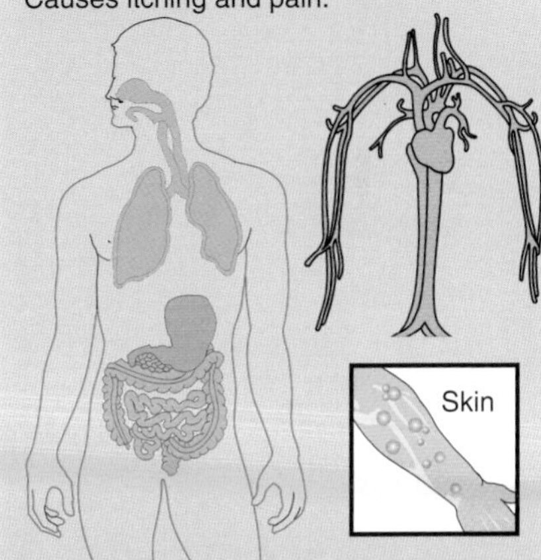

H_1 and H_2 Receptors

CARDIOVASCULAR SYSTEM
Lowers systemic blood pressure by reducing peripheral resistance. Causes positive chronotropism (mediated by H_2 receptors) and a positive inotropism (mediated by both H_1 and H_2 receptors).

SKIN
Dilation and increased permeability of the capillaries results in leakage of proteins and fluid into the tissues. In the skin, this results in the classic "triple response": wheal formation, reddening due to local vasodilation, and flare ("halo").

H_2 Receptors

Stomach
Stimulation of gastric hydrochloric acid secretion.

Figure 42.4
Actions of histamine.

INFO LINK

[3]See p. 148 in ***Lippincott's Illustrated Reviews: Biochemistry*** (3rd ed.) for a discussion of nitric oxide.
[4]See p. 203 in ***Lippincott's Illustrated Reviews: Biochemistry*** (3rd ed.) for a discussion of the polyphosphatidylinositol pathway.

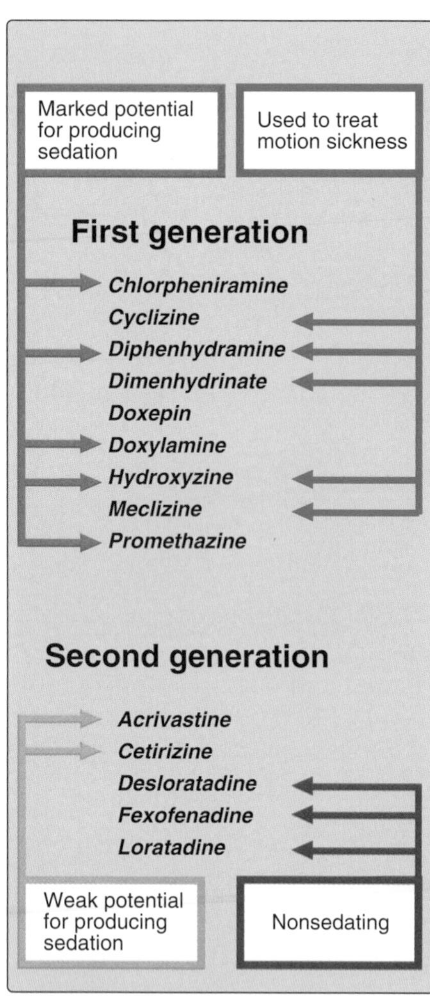

Figure 42.5
Summary of therapeutic advantages and disadvantages of some H_1 histamine–receptor blocking agents.

molyn, which inhibits the release of histamine from mast cells and is useful in the treatment of asthma.] The H_1 receptor blockers can be divided into first- and second-generation drugs (Figure 42.5). The older first-generation drugs are still widely used, because they are effective and inexpensive. However, most of these drugs penetrate the CNS and cause sedation. Furthermore, they tend to interact with other receptors, producing a variety of unwanted adverse effects. By contrast, the second-generation agents are specific for H_1 receptors, and because they do not penetrate the blood-brain barrier, they show less CNS toxicity than the first-generation drugs. Among these agents *desloratadine* [des lor AH tah deen], *fexofenadine* [fex oh FEN a deen], and *loratadine* [lor AT a deen] show the least sedation (Figure 42.6). [Note: The histamine receptors are distinct from those that bind serotonin, acetylcholine, and the catecholamines.]

A. Actions

The action of all the H_1 receptor blockers is qualitatively similar. However, most of these blockers have additional effects unrelated to their blocking of H_1 receptors; these effects probably reflect binding of the H_1 antagonists to cholinergic, adrenergic, or serotonin receptors (Figure 42.7).

B. Therapeutic uses

1. **Allergic and inflammatory conditions:** H_1 Receptor blockers are useful in treating allergies caused by antigens acting on immunoglobulin E (IgE) antibody-sensitized mast cells. For example, antihistamines are the drugs of choice in controlling the symptoms of allergic rhinitis and urticaria because histamine is the principal mediator. However, the H_1 receptor blockers are ineffective in treating bronchial asthma, because histamine is only one of several mediators of that condition. [Note: *Epinephrine* has actions on smooth muscle that are opposite to those of histamine, and it acts at different receptors. Therefore, *epinephrine* is the drug of choice in treating systemic anaphylaxis and other conditions that involve massive release of histamine.] Glucocorticoids show greater anti-inflammatory effects than the H_1 antihistamines.

2. **Motion sickness and nausea:** Along with the antimuscarinic agent *scopolamine*, certain H_1 receptor blockers, such as *diphenhydramine* [dye fen HYE dra meen], *dimenhydrinate* [dye men HYE dri nate], *cyclizine* [SYE kli zeen], *meclizine* [MEK li zeen], and hydroxyzine [hye DROX ee zeen] (see Figure 42.5), are the most effective agents for prevention of the symptoms of motion sickness. The antihistamines prevent or diminish vomiting and nausea mediated by both the chemoreceptor and vestibular pathways. The antiemetic action of these substances seems to be independent of their antihistaminic and other actions.

3. **Somnifacients:** Although they are not the medication of choice, many first-generation antihistamines, such as *diphenhydramine* and *doxylamine* [dox IL a meen], have strong sedative properties and are used in the treatment of insomnia (see Figure 42.5). The use of first-generation H_1 antihistamines is contraindicated in the treatment of individuals working in jobs where wakefulness is critical.

C. Pharmacokinetics

H_1 receptor blockers are well absorbed after oral administration, with maximum serum levels occurring at one to two hours. The average plasma half-life is four to six hours except for *meclizine*, which has a half-life of 12 to 24 hours. H_1 receptor blockers have high bioavailability and are distributed in all tissues, including the CNS. All first-generation H_1 antihistamines and some second-generation H_1 antihistamines, such as *desloratadine* and *loratadine*, are metabolized by the hepatic cytochrome P450 (CYP450) system. *Cetirizine* [seh TEER ih zeen] is excreted largely unchanged in the urine, and *fexofenadine* is excreted largely unchanged in the feces. After a single oral dose, the onset of action occurs within one to three hours. The duration of action for many oral H_1 antihistamines is at least 24 hours, facilitating once-daily dosing. They are most effective when used prophylactically before allergen exposure rather than as needed. Tolerance to the action of H_1 antihistamines has not been observed.

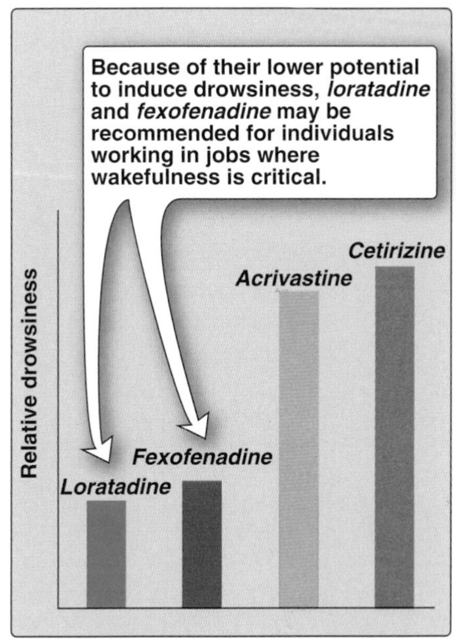

Figure 42.6
Relative potential for causing drowsiness in patients receiving second-generation H_1 antihistamines.

D. Adverse effects

First-generation H_1 receptor blockers have a low specificity; that is, they interact not only with histamine receptors but also with muscarinic cholinergic receptors, α-adrenergic receptors, and serotonin receptors (see Figure 42.7). The extent of interaction with these receptors and, as a result, the nature of the side effects vary with the structure of the drug. Some side effects may be undesirable, and others may have therapeutic value. Furthermore, the incidence and severity of adverse reactions for a given drug varies between individual subjects.

1. **Sedation:** First-generation H_1 antihistamines, such as *chlorpheniramine* [klor fen IR a meen], *diphenhydramine*, *hydroxyzine*, and *promethazine* [proe METH a zeen], bind to H_1 receptors and block the neurotransmitter effect of histamine in the CNS. The most fre-

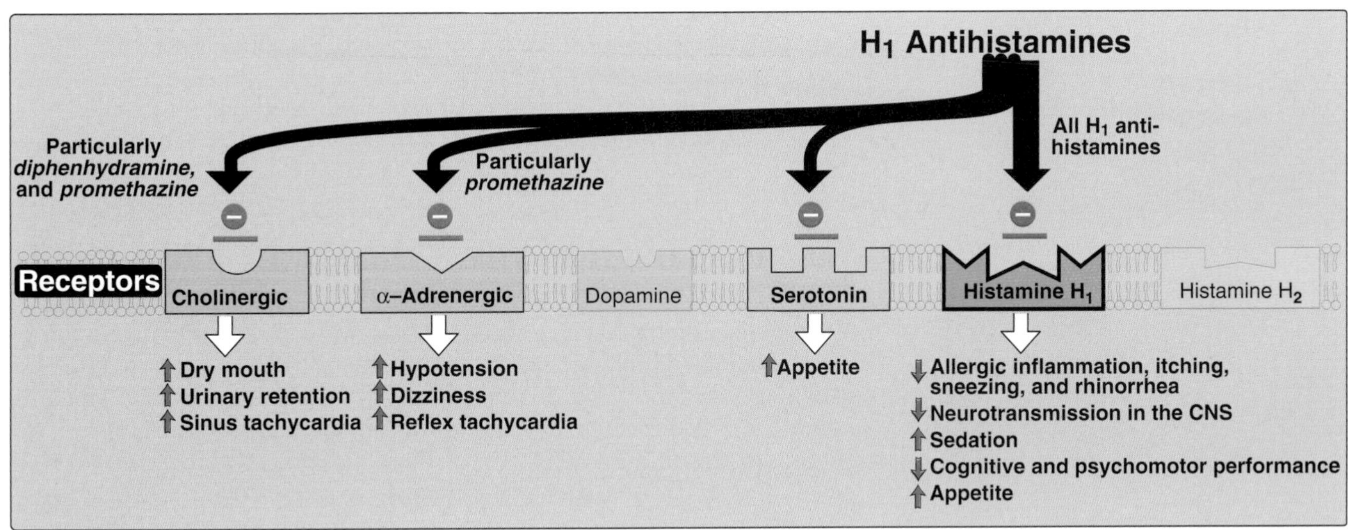

Figure 42.7
Effects of H_1 antihistamines at histamine, adrenergic, cholinergic, and serotonin-binding receptors. Many second generation antihistamines do not enter the brain and, therefore, show minimal CNS effects.

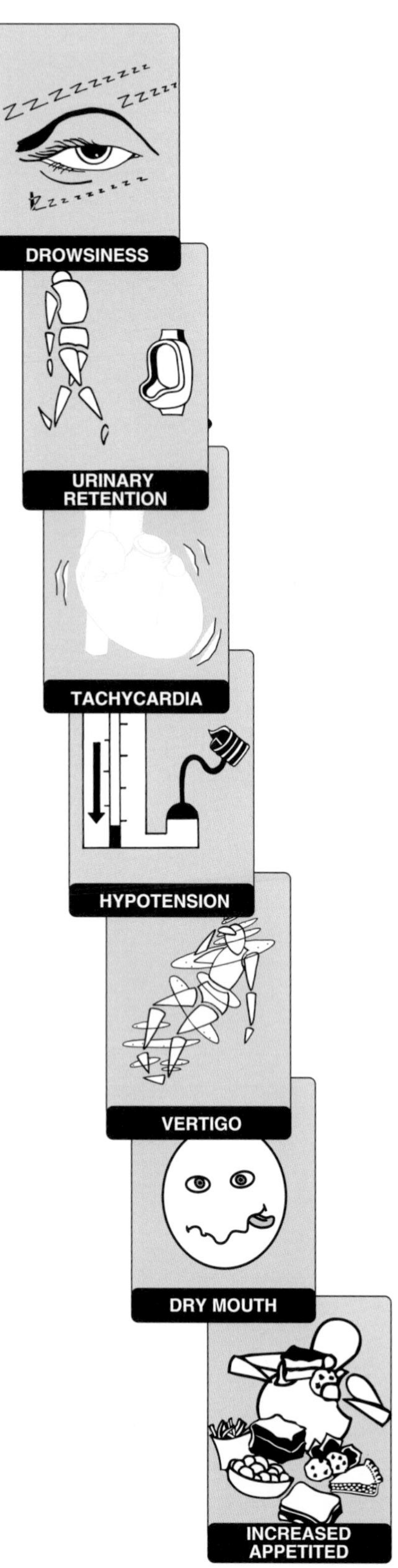

Figure 42.8
Some adverse effect observed with first-generation H_1 antihistamines.

quently observed adverse reaction is sedation (Figure 42.8). Other central actions include tinnitus, fatigue, dizziness, lassitude, incoordination, blurred vision, and tremors. Sedation is less common with the second-generation drugs, which do not readily enter the CNS. Second-generation H_1 antihistamines are specific for H_1 receptors and penetrate the CNS poorly. They show less sedation and other CNS effects.

2. **Dry mouth:** Oral antihistamines also exert weak anticholinergic effects, leading not only to a drying of the nasal passage but also to a tendency to dry the oral cavity. Blurred vision can occur as well with some drugs.

3. **Drug interactions:** Interaction of H_1 receptor blockers with other drugs can cause serious consequences, such as the potentiation of the effects of all other CNS depressants, including alcohol. Persons taking monoamine oxidase (MAO) inhibitors should not take antihistamines, because the MAO inhibitors can exacerbate the anticholinergic effects of the antihistamines.

4. **Overdoses:** Although the margin of safety of H_1 receptor blockers is relatively high and chronic toxicity is rare, acute poisoning is relatively common, especially in young children. The most common and dangerous effects of acute poisoning are those on the CNS, including hallucinations, excitement, ataxia, and convulsions. If untreated, the patient may experience a deepening coma and collapse of the cardiorespiratory system.

V. HISTAMINE H_2 RECEPTOR BLOCKERS

Histamine H_2 receptor blockers have little, if any, affinity for H_1 receptors. Although antagonists of the histamine H_2 receptor (H_2 antagonists) block the actions of histamine at all H_2 receptors, their chief clinical use is as inhibitors of gastric acid secretion in the treatment of ulcers. By competitively blocking the binding of histamine to H_2 receptors, these agents reduce intracellular concentrations of cAMP and, thereby, secretion of gastric acid. The four drugs used in the United States—*cimetidine*, *ranitidine*, *famotidine*, and *nizatidine*—are discussed in Chapter 28.

VI. DRUGS USED TO TREAT MIGRAINE HEADACHE

It has been estimated that eighteen million women and six million men in the United States suffer from severe migraine headaches. Migraine can usually be distinguished clinically from the two other common types of headaches—the cluster headache and tension-type headache—by its characteristics (Figure 42.9). For example, migraines present as a pulsatile, throbbing pain; cluster headaches as excruciating, sharp, steady pain; and tension-type headaches as dull pain, with a persistent tightening feeling in the head. Patients with severe migraine headaches report one to five attacks per month of moderate to severe pain, usually unilateral. The

	MIGRAINE	CLUSTER	TENSION TYPE
Family history	Yes	No	Yes
Sex	Females more often than males	Males more often than females	Females more often than males
Onset	Variable	During sleep	Under stress
Location	Usually unilateral	Behind or around one eye	Bilateral in band around head
Character and severity	Pulsating, throbbing	Excruciating, sharp, steady	Dull, persistent, tightening
Duration	2–72 hours per episode	15–90 minutes per episode	30 minutes to 7 days per episode
Associated symptoms	Visual auras, sensitivity to light and sound, pale facial appearance, nausea and vomiting	Unilateral or bilateral sweating, facial flushing, nasal congestion, lacrimation, pupillary changes	Mild intolerance to light and noise, anorexia

Figure 42.9
Characteristics of migraine, cluster, and tension-type headaches.

headaches affect patients for a major part of their lives and result in considerable health costs.

A. Types of migraine

There are two main types of migraine headaches. The first, migraine without aura (previously called common migraine), is a severe, unilateral, pulsating headache that typically lasts from 2 to 72 hours. These headaches are often aggravated by physical activity and are accompanied by nausea, vomiting, photophobia (hypersensitivity to light), and phonophobia (hypersensitivity to sound). Approximately 85 percent of patients with migraine do not have aura. In the second type, migraine with aura (previously called classic migraine), the headache is preceded by neurologic symptoms called auras, which can be visual, sensory, and/or cause speech or motor disturbances. Most commonly these prodromal symptoms are visual, occurring approximately 20 to 40 minutes before headache pain begins. In the fifteen percent of migraine patients whose headache is preceded by an aura, the aura itself allows diagnosis. The headache itself in migraines with or without auras is similar. For both types of migraines, women are three-fold more likely than men to experience either type of migraine.

B. Biologic basis of migraine headaches

The first manifestation of migraine with aura is a spreading depression of neuronal activity accompanied by reduced blood flow in the most posterior part of the cerebral hemisphere. This hypoperfusion gradually spreads forward over the surface of the cortex to other contiguous areas of the brain. The vascular alteration is accompanied by functional changes, for example, the hypoperfused regions show an abnormal response to changes in arterial partial pressure of CO_2. The hypoperfusion persists throughout the aura and well into the headache phase, after which hyperperfusion occurs. Patients who have migraine without aura do not show hypoperfusion. However, the pain of both types of migraine may be due to extracranial and intracranial arterial dilation. This stretching leads to release of neuroactive molecules, such as substance P.

C. Symptomatic treatment of acute migraine

Acute treatments can be classified as nonspecific (symptomatic) or migraine-specific. Nonspecific treatment incudes analgesics, such as nonsteroidal anti-inflammatory drugs, and antiemetics, such a *prochlorperazine*, to control vomiting. Opioids are reserved as rescue medication when other treatments of a severe migraine attack are not successful. Specific migraine therapy includes triptans and *dihydroergotamine*, both of which are 5-HT_{1D} receptor agonists. It has been proposed that activation of 5-HT_{1D} receptors by these agents leads either to vasoconstriction or to inhibition of the release of proinflammatory neuropeptides. Despite their high cost, most patients prefer triptans over ergot derivatives.

1. **Triptans:** This class of drugs includes *sumatriptan* [SOO ma trip tan], *naratriptan* [NAR a trip tan], *rizatriptan* [rye za TRIP tan], *eletriptan* [EH leh trip tan], *almotriptan* [AL moh trip tan], and *zolmitriptan* [zole ma TRIP tan]. These agents rapidly and effectively abort or markedly reduce the severity of migraine headaches in about seventy percent of patients. The triptans are serotonin agonists, acting at a subgroup of serotonin receptors found on small, peripheral nerves that innervate the intracranial vasculature. The nausea that occurs with *dihydroergotamine* and the vasoconstriction caused by *ergotamine* (see below) are much less pronounced with the triptans, particularly *rizatriptan* and *zolmitriptan*. *Sumatriptan* is given subcutaneously, intranasally, or orally. [Note: All other agents are taken orally.] The onset of the parenteral drug is about twenty minutes, compared with one to two hours when the drug is administered orally. The drug has a short duration of action, with an elimination half-life of two hours. Headache commonly recurs within 24 to 48 hours after a single dose of drug, but in most patients, a second dose is effective in aborting the headache. *Rizatriptan* and *eletriptan* are modestly more effective than *sumatriptan*, the prototype drug, whereas *naratriptan* and *almotriptan* are better tolerated. Individual responses to triptans vary, and more than one drug trial may be necessary before treatment is successful.

2. **Dihydroergotamine:** *Dihydroergotamine* [dye hye droe er GOT a meen], a derivative of *ergotamine*, is administered intravenously and has an efficacy similar to that of *sumatriptan*, but nausea is a common adverse effect.

D. Prophylaxis

Therapy to prevent migraine is indicated if the attacks occur two or more times a month and if the headaches are severe or complicated by serious neurologic signs. *Propranolol* is the drug of choice, but other β-blockers, particularly *nadolol*, have been shown to be effective. Other drugs that are effective for prevention of recurrent, refractory, severe migraine are shown in Figure 42.10.

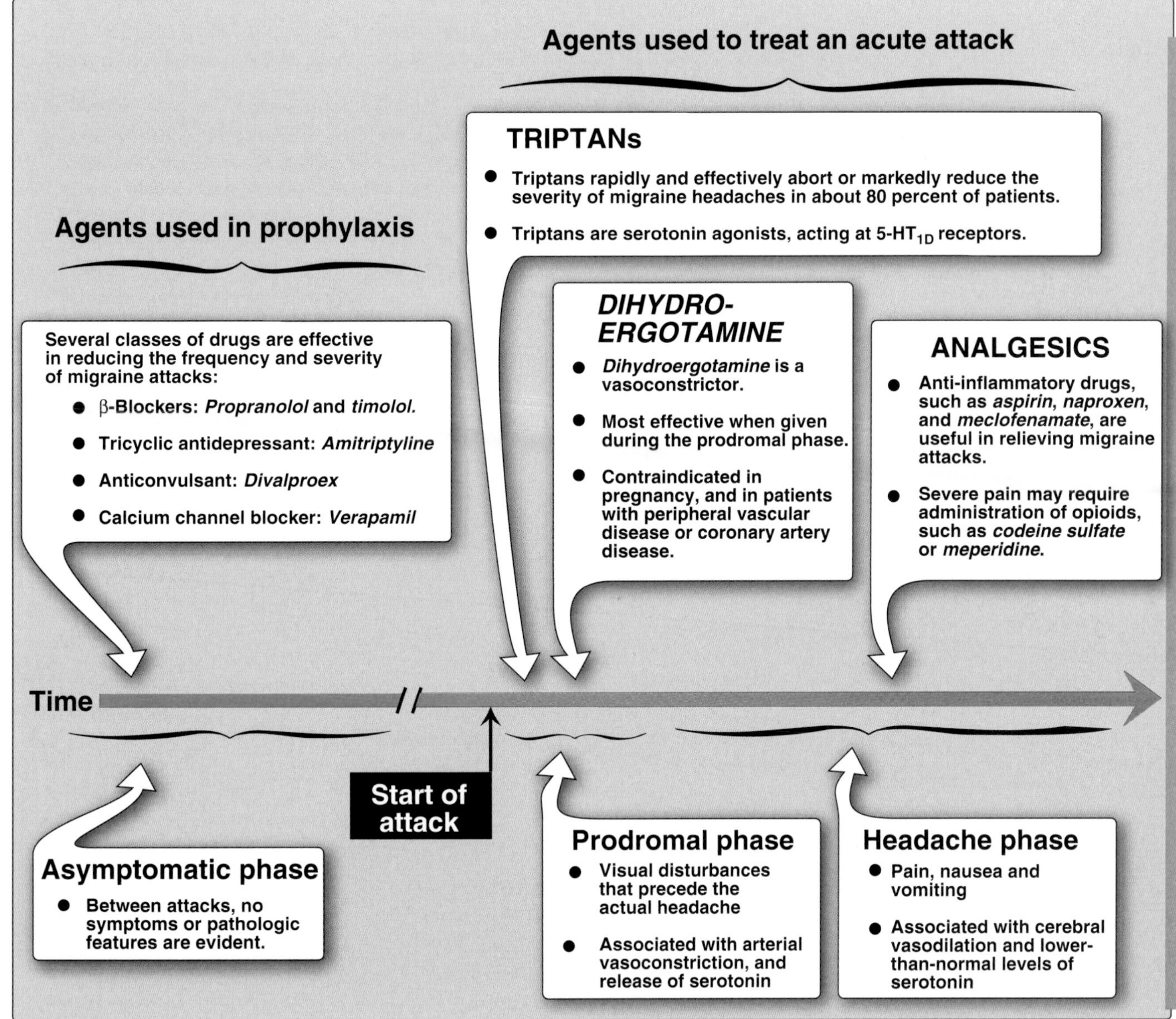

Agents used to treat an acute attack
TRIPTANs
Triptans rapidly and effectively abort or markedly reduce the severity of migraine headaches in about 80 percent of patients.
Triptans are serotonin agonists, acting at 5-HT1D receptors.
Agents used in prophylaxis
Several classes of drugs are effective in reducing the frequency and severity of migraine attacks:
β-Blockers: Propranolol and timolol.
Tricyclic antidepressant: Amitriptyline
Anticonvulsant: Divalproex
Calcium channel blocker: Verapamil
DIHYDRO-ERGOTAMINE
Dihydroergotamine is a vasoconstrictor.
Most effective when given during the prodromal phase.
Contraindicated in pregnancy, and in patients with peripheral vascular disease or coronary artery disease.
ANALGESICS
Anti-inflammatory drugs, such as aspirin, naproxen, and meclofenamate, are useful in relieving migraine attacks.
Severe pain may require administration of opioids, such as codeine sulfate or meperidine.
Time
Start of attack
Asymptomatic phase
Between attacks, no symptoms or pathologic features are evident.
Prodromal phase
Visual disturbances that precede the actual headache
Associated with arterial vasoconstriction, and release of serotonin
Headache phase
Pain, nausea and vomiting
Associated with cerebral vasodilation and lower-than-normal levels of serotonin

Figure 42.10
Drugs useful in the treatment and prophylaxis of migraine headaches.

Study Questions

Choose the ONE best answer.

42.1 Dihydroergotamine:

A. causes vasodilation.
B. exerts its actions by binding to specific ergotamine receptors.
C. is useful in treating acute migraine headaches.
D. is useful for maintaining uterine muscle tone during pregnancy.
E. has actions similar to those of nitroprusside.

Correct answer = C. Ergotamines act to counteract cerebral vasodilation that plays a role in migraine headaches. Vasoconstriction leading to tissue ischemia is one of the toxic complications associated with an overdose of these drugs. The ergot alkaloids interact with adrenergic, dopaminergic, and serotonin receptors. They are contraindicated in pregnancy because of their ability to cause uterine contraction and abortion. Nitroprusside is a powerful vasodilator used to treat the vasoconstriction that is characteristic of an overdose with ergot alkaloids.

43.2 A 43-year-old ship's captain complained of seasonal allergies. Which one of the following would be indicated?

A. Cyclizine
B. Doxepin
C. Doxylamine
D. Hydroxyzine
E. Fexofenadine

Correct answer = E. The use of first-generation H_1 antihistamines is contraindicated in the treatment of pilots and others who must remain alert. Because of its lower potential to induce drowsines, fexofenadine may be recommended for individuals working in jobs where wakefulness is critical.

43.3 Which one of the following statements concerning H_1 antihistamines is corrrect?

A. Second-generation H_1 antihistamines are relatively free of adverse effects.
B. Because of the established long-term safety of first-generation H_1 antihistamines, they are the first choice for initial therapy.
C. The motor coordination involved in driving an automobile is not affected by the use of first-generation H_1 anthistamines.
D. H_1 antihistamines can be used in the treatment of acute anaphylaxis.
E. Both first-generation and second-generation H_1 antihistamines readily penetrate the blood-brain barrier.

Correct answer = A. Second-generation H_1 antihistamines are preferred over first-generation agents because they are relatively free of adverse effects. Driving performance is adversely affected by first-generation H_1 antihistamines. Epinephrine, not antihistamine, is an acceptable treatment for acute anaphylaxis. Second-generation H_1 antihistamines penetrate the blood-brain barrier to a lesser degree than the first-generation drugs.

42.4 Which one of the following drugs could significantly impair the ability to drive an automobile?

A. Diphenhydramine
B. Ergotamine
C. Fexofenadine
D. Ranitidine
E. Sumatriptan

Correct answer = A. Diphenhydramine can impair operation of an automobile by causing drowsiness and by impairing accommodation. The other agents do not have this restriction.

Index

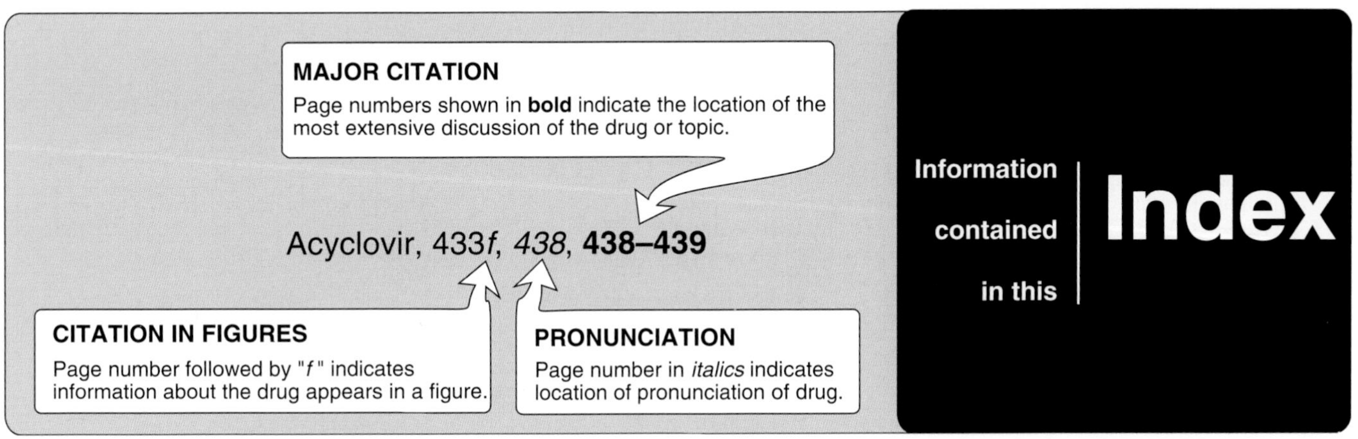
MAJOR CITATION
Page numbers shown in **bold** indicate the location of the most extensive discussion of the drug or topic.
Acyclovir, 433*f*, *438*, **438–439**
CITATION IN FIGURES
Page number followed by "*f*" indicates information about the drug appears in a figure.
PRONUNCIATION
Page number in *italics* indicates location of pronunciation of drug.
Information contained in this
Index

"*See*" cross-references direct the reader to the synonymous term. [Note: Positional and configurational designations in chemical names (for example, "3-", "α-", "N-", "D-") are ignored in alphabetizing.] Trade names of drugs are shown in CAPITAL LETTERS.

Figure Sources

Figure 1.23 modified from H. P. Range and M. M. Dale, Pharmacology, Churchill Livingstone (1987).

Figures 6.9, 6.11 and 6.11 modified from Allwood, Cobbold and Ginsburg, British Medical Bulletin 19:132 (1963).

Figure 8.14, modified from R. Young, American Family Physician, 59:2155 (1999).

Figure 9.5 modified from A. Kales, Excertpa Medical Congress Series 899:149 (1989).

Figure 9.6 from data of E. C. Dimitrion, A. J. Parashos, J. S. Giouzepas, Drug Invest. 4:316 (1992).

Figure 10.5 modified from N. L. Benowitz, Science 319:1318 (1988).

Figure 16.6 data from Results of the Cooperative North Scandinavian Enalapril Survival Study, N. Engl. J. Med. 316:80 (1988).

Figure 16.7 modified from the Effect of metoprolol CR/XL in chronic heart failure: Metoprolol CR/XL Randomised Intervention Trial in Congestive Heart Failure (MERIT-HF), Lancet 353:2001 (1999).

Figure 16.12 modified from M. Jessup, and S Brozena, N. Engl. J. Med. 348: 2007 (2003).

Figure 16.13 modified from T.B Young, M. Gheorghiade, and B. F. Uretsky, J. Am. Coll Cardiol. 32:686 (1998).

Figure 17.3 modified from J. A. Beven and J. H. Thompson, Essentials of Pharmacology, Harper and Row (1983).

Figure 17.9 modified from J. W. Mason, N. Engl. J. Med., 329:452 (1993).

Figure 19.5 modified from B. J. Materson, Drug Therapy, November p. 157 (1985).

Figure 20.8, modified from D. J. Schneider, P. B. Tracy, and B. E. Sobel, Hospital Practice, May 15, (1998), p. 107.

Figure 20.15, Effects of glycoprotein IIb/IIIa receptor antagonists on the incidence of death or nonfatal myocardial infarction followingpercutaneous transluminal coronary angioplasty. [Note: Data are from several studies; thus reported incidence of complicationswith standard therapy is not the same for each drug.] data from D.A. Vorchheimer, J. J. Badimon, and V. Fuster, Journal American Medical Association 281: 1407 (1999).

Figure 21.6. Modified from M. K. S. Leow, C. L. Addy, and C. S. Mantzoros. J. Clin. Endocrinol. Metab., 88:1961 (2003).

Figure 21.7, modified from Knopp, R. H., N. Engl. J. Med. 341:498 (1999).

Figures 21.10 modified from R. H. Knopp, Hospital Practice 23:22 (1988).

Figures 23.2 modified from B. G. Katzung, Basic and Clinical Pharmacology, Appleton and Lange (1987).

Figure 24.5 modified from M. C. Riddle, Postgraduate Med. 92:89 (1992).

Figure 24.7 modified from I. R. Hirsch, N. Engl. J. Med. 352:174 (2005).

Figure 24.9 modified from O. B Crofford, Ann. Rev. Medicine 46:267 (1995).

Figures 25.6 and 25.7 modified from D. R. Mishell, Jr., N. Engl. J. Med. 320:777 (1989).

Figure 25.8 modified from M. Polaneczky, G. S. Slap, C.F. Forke, A. R. Rappaport, and S. Sondheimer, N. Engl. J. Med 331:1201 (1994).

Figure 25.9 modified from A. S. Dobs, A. W. Meikle, S. Arver, S. W. Sanders, Ki. E. Caramelli and N. A. Mazer. J. Clin Endo & Met: 84:3469 (1999).

Figure 25.10 modified from J. D. McConnell, C. G. Roehrborn, O. M Bautista. N. Engl. J. Med. 349:2387 (2003).

Figure 28.2 modified from D. Cave, Hospital Practice, Sept 30, 1992.

Figure 28.6 modified from F. E. Silverstein, D. Y. Graham, J. R. Senior. Ann. Intern. Med 123:241 (1995).

Figure 28.7 modified from S. M. Grunberg and P. J. Hesketh, N. Engl. J. Med. 329: 1790 (1993).

Figures 28.9, 28.10 from data of S. Bilgrami and B. G. Fallon, Postgraduate Medicine, 94:55 (1993).

Figure 29.5 photo from Jordan, V. C., Scientific American, October, p. 60 (1998).

Figure 34.4 modified from data of D. A. Evans, K. A. Maley and V. A. McRusick, British Medical Journal 2:485 (1960).

Figure 34.5 modified from data of Neuvonen, P. J., Kivisto, K. T., and Lehto, P. Clin. Pharm Therap., 50: 499 (1991).

Figure 38.3 modified from R. Dolin, Science 227:1296 (1985).

Figure 38.15 modified from Balfour, H. H., N. Engl. J. Med. 340:1255 (1999).

Figure 39.5 modified from N. Kartner and V. Ling. Scientific American, March (1989).

Figure 42.9 modified from D. D. Dubose, A. C. Cutlip, and W. D. Cutlip. American Family Medicine 51:1498 (1995).